Leishmaniasis

The Current Status and
New Strategies for Control

NATO ASI Series

Advanced Science Institutes Series

A series presenting the results of activities sponsored by the NATO Science Committee, which aims at the dissemination of advanced scientific and technological knowledge, with a view to strengthening links between scientific communities.

The series is published by an international board of publishers in conjunction with the NATO Scientific Affairs Division

A	**Life Sciences**	Plenum Publishing Corporation
B	**Physics**	New York and London
C	**Mathematical and Physical Sciences**	Kluwer Academic Publishers Dordrecht, Boston, and London
D	**Behavioral and Social Sciences**	
E	**Applied Sciences**	
F	**Computer and Systems Sciences**	Springer-Verlag
G	**Ecological Sciences**	Berlin, Heidelberg, New York, London,
H	**Cell Biology**	Paris, and Tokyo

Recent Volumes in this Series

Volume 159—Biologically Based Methods for Cancer Risk Assessment
　　　edited by Curtis C. Travis

Volume 160—Early Influences Shaping the Individual
　　　edited by Spyros Doxiadis

Volume 161—Research in Congenital Hypothyroidism
　　　edited by F. Delange, D. A. Fisher, and D. Glinoer

Volume 162—Nematode Identification and Expert System Technology
　　　edited by Renaud Fortuner

Volume 163—Leishmaniasis: The Current Status and New Strategies for Control
　　　edited by D. T. Hart

Volume 164—Cochlear Mechanisms: Structure, Function, and Models
　　　edited by J. P. Wilson and D. T. Kemp

Volume 165—The Guanine-Nucleotide Binding Proteins: Common Structural and Functional Properties
　　　edited by L. Bosch, B. Kraal, and A. Parmeggiani

Series A: Life Sciences

Leishmaniasis

The Current Status and New Strategies for Control

Edited by

D. T. Hart

King's College London
London, United Kingdom

Springer Science+Business Media, LLC

Proceedings of a NATO Advanced Study Institute on
Leishmaniasis: The First Centenary (1885-1985)
New Strategies for Control,
held September 20-27, 1987,
on the Island of Zakinthos, Greece

Library of Congress Cataloging in Publication Data

NATO Advanced Study Institute on Leishmaniasis: the First Centenary (1885-
1985), New Strategies for Control (1987: Zakynthos, Greece)
   Leishmaniasis: the current status and new strategies for control / edited by D.
T. Hart.
      p.   cm.—(NATO ASI series. Series A, Life sciences; v. 163)
   "Proceedings of a NATO Advanced Study Institute on Leishmaniasis: the First
Centenary (1885-1985), New Strategies for Control, held September 20-27, 1987,
on the island of Zakynthos, Greece"—T.p. verso.
   "Published in cooperation with NATO Scientific Affairs Division."
   Includes bibliographical references and indexes.

   ISBN 978-1-4612-8862-6   ISBN 978-1-4613-1575-9 (eBook)
   DOI 10.1007/978-1-4613-1575-9

   1. Leishmaniasis—Congresses. I. Hart, D. T. (David Thomas) II. Series.
RC153.N38 1987   89-30745
616.9'364—dc19   CIP

© 1989 Springer Science+Business Media New York
Originally published by Plenum Press, New York in 1989.
Softcover reprint of the hardcover 1st edition 1989

All rights reserved

No part of this book may be reproduced, stored in a retrieval system, or transmitted
in any form or by any means, electronic, mechanical, photocopying, microfilming,
recording, or otherwise, without written permission from the Publisher

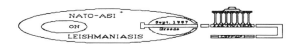

PREFACE

Leishmaniasis is at present the focus of considerable interest and attention. This is a most encouraging situation for both scientific and medical leishmaniacs! The recent celebration of the Centenary of the first description of the causative agents of the disease[1] was an occasion for leishmaniacs to reflect on the progress made towards our understanding and the control of this highly underrated tropical and subtropical disease.

It was during the Centenary celebrations that the need for an International meeting on Leishmaniasis was suggested. The support of a large number of people was then required to realize the NATO-Advanced Study Institute on Leishmaniasis. The remit of this ASI was to review the current status of our understanding of *Leishmania* and highlight new strategies for control.

Very special thanks are therefore due to Douglas Barker, David Bradley, David Evans, Len Goodwin, Bob Killick-Kendrick and Keith Vickerman in Great Britain, Craig Sinclair and Fred Opperdoes in Belgium, and Apolon Garifallow in Greece, for their invaluable support in the genesis and maturation of the ASI.

The ASI Secretariate was composed of Little Mac Plus and Big Mac II, Helen Lysandrides, Andrew Langridge, Nishi Mayer, Nancy Khammo and most importantly Barbara Hart. All of whom gave unquestioning and invaluable support in Bruxelles, London and finally on the Island of Zakinthos.

The Chairmen, Rapporteurs and Editors of the Lecture Sessions, New Strategies for Control Fora, Workshops and Field Trip are most warmly thanked for their considerable contribution to both the ASI and this monograph.

The ASI attracted participants from 22 countries and of the 257 applicants our finance supported 170 participants. However, due to the surprising large number of leishmaniacs who just happened to be in Zakinthos for their vacation (!), some 200 participants were regularly in attendance.

Indeed the final thanks must go to the participants who made the ASI the success it was attending the Lectures, Fora and Workshops with devotion and enthusiasm. It was a great privilege to organize such an event, the wonderful weather, good food and extremely good company made Zakinthos both a stimulating experience and very fond memory.

The very small word of thanks must surely go to the Daily Telegraph reporter Robert Bedlow who also attended the ASI and duly published the now famous headline "Sandfly brings killer disease to med beaches"[2]. Even with the great personal anguish which this highly contorted sensationalism and gross misquotation has evoked the resultant publicity has most fortunately heightened the publics awareness to Leishmaniasis - and this can only be constructive!

---

1   Leishmaniasis: The First Centenary 1885-1985, J. Royal Army Medical Corps 1986. 132, 127-152.

It is therefore hoped that this monograph will serve three function. Firstly, publication of the lecture sessions (Chapters 1,2,3,4 & 5) should act as a topical reference source to the most pertinent aspects of leishmanial research Secondly, the publication of the concise and succinct reflections of the experts in the field on "New Strategies for Control" (Chapters 6,7,8 & 9) should focus multidisciplinary interest in the most appropriate areas for fruitful future research. Finally, the Workshops (Chapters 10,11,12, & 13) deal with several controversial or equivocal topics in the field of leishmaniasis and give them new clarity.

This monograph should thus help focus the aforementioned renaissance in interest in Leishmaniasis. I hope it will encourage new and old leishmaniacs to strive, with focused enthusiasm, for a rational control and management mechanism for a disease which is still the cause of considerable morbidity and mortality more than a century after its discovery.

January 1988

David Thomas Hart

---

2   Daily Telegraph 22 September 1987. page 2

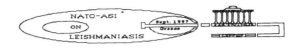

CONTENTS

CHAPTER 1	Page 1
AETIOLOGY & EPIDEMIOLOGY	

CHAPTER 2	173
ECOLOGY & ENTOMOLOGY	

CHAPTER 3	253
CELL BIOLOGY & IMMUNOLOGY	

CHAPTER 4	467
MOLECULAR BIOLOGY & BIOCHEMISTRY	

CHAPTER 5	691
CHEMOTHERAPY	

CHAPTER 6	819
NEW STRATEGIES FOR CONTROL	
I. VECTOR CONTROL	

CHAPTER 7	825
NEW STRATEGIES FOR CONTROL	
II. RESERVOIR CONTROL	

CHAPTER 8	833
NEW STRATEGIES FOR CONTROL	
III. VACCINATION	

CHAPTER 9	845
NEW STRATEGIES FOR CONTROL	
IV. CHEMOTHERAPY	

CHAPTER 10	895
WORKSHOP I	
CHARACTERIZATION & TAXONOMY	

CHAPTER 11	945
WORKSHOP II	
SANDFLY SYSTEMATICS & GENETICS	

CHAPTER 12	973
WORKSHOP III	
MOLECULAR GENETICS OF DEVELOPMENT	

CHAPTER 13	989
WORKSHOP IV	
CHEMOTHERAPY & IMMUNE RESPONSE	

CHAPTER 14	1001
FIELD TRIP	

CHAPTER 15	1017
NATO-ASI PHOTOGRAPHS	

CHAPTER 16	1023
LIST OF PARTICIPANTS	

CHAPTER 17	
AUTHOR INDEX	1037
SUBJECTS INDEX	1039

CHAPTER
1
AETIOLOGY & EPIDEMIOLOGY

AETIOLOGY AND EPIDEMIOLOGY: AN OVERVIEW
D.J.Bradley..................................3

THE GENUS *LEISHMANIA* IN THE MIDDLE EAST AND USSR
W.Peters.....................................9

EPIDEMIOLOGY OF MEDITERRANEAN LEISHMANIASIS BY *LEISHMANIA INFANTUM*: ISOENZYME AND kDNA ANALYSIS FOR THE IDENTIFICATION OF PARASITES FROM MAN, VECTORS AND RESERVOIRS
M. Gramiccia, L. Gradoni & M. Angelici....................................21

LEISHMANIASIS: STATUS IN TUNISIA (1986)
R. Ben Ismail, M. Ben Said & M.S. Ben Rachid...........................39

A REVIEW OF THE STATUS OF LEISHMANIASIS IN PAKISTAN FROM 1960-1986
M.A. Munir, M.A. Rab, J. Iqbal, A. Ghafoor, M.A. Khan & M.I.Burney.................47

ZOONOSES AND LEISHMANIASIS
R.S. Bray....................................57

RESERVOIRS OF VISCERAL LEISHMANIASIS
P.Abranches.................................61

EFFECTIVENESS OF CONTROL MEASURES AGAINST CANINE LEISHMANIASIS IN THE ISLE OF ELBA, ITALY
L. Gradoni, M. Gramiccia, F. Mancianti & S. Pieri...............................71

THE INCIDENCE OF CANINE LEISHMANIASIS IN NORTHERN GREECE (AN EPIZOOTIOLOGICAL STUDY OF THE DECADE 1977-1987)
V.I. Kontos & A.G. Spais...................77

STUDIES ON THE ROLE OF THE GROUND SQUIRREL (*CITELLUS CITELLUS*) IN THE EPIDEMIOLOGY OF LEISHMANIASIS
V.I. Kontos, G.S. Koptopoulos, S.Th. Haral-Abidis & A. G. Spais........................83

FIELD APPLICATION OF A DIRECT AGGLUTINATION TEST FOR VISCERAL LEISHMANIASIS
P.A. Kager, J. Leeuwenburg, R. Mugai, S. Kiugu, D.W. Iha, J.K. Mwaniki, D.K. Koech & A.E. Harith..................89

LEISHMANIASIS IN THE LOWLANDS OF BOLIVIA (LEISHBOL): PART I. AN OVERVIEW OF THE INTEGRATED PROJECT FOR THE CHARACTERIZATION, VIGILANCE AND CONTROL OF LEISHMANIASIS
M.Recacoechea, G.Villarroel, H. Bermundez R. Urjel, J.C.Dujardin & D.LE Ray.............95

LEISHMANIASIS IN THE LOWLANDS OF BOLIVIA (LEISHBOL): PART II. COMMUNITY HEALTH CARE FOR SPONTANEOUS SETTLERS IN ENDEMIC TROPICAL FOREST
G. Villarroel, M. Recacoechea & S. Balderrama..........................103

LEISHMANIASIS IN THE LOWLANDS OF BOLIVIA (LEISHBOL): PART III. STATUS OF THE DISEASE IN AN AREA OF SPONTANEOUS AGRICULTURAL COLONIZATION
M. Recacoechea, G. Villarroel, S. .Balderrama, R. Urjel, S. de Donker, D. Jacquet & D. LE Ray...............................109

LEISHMANIASIS IN THE LOWLANDS OF BOLIVIA (LEISHBOL): PART IV. FIELD IDENTIFICATION KEY FOR *LUTZOMYA* SPP. BASED ON THORACIC EXTERNAL CHARACTERS
H. Bermudez, A. Rivero, J.L. Claure, B. Montalvan & S. Rocha..................117

LEISHMANIASIS IN THE LOWLANDS OF BOLIVIA (LEISHBOL): PART V. MONTHLY DENSITY OF *LUTZOMYA YUCUMENSIS*, *LU.DAVISI* AND *LU.CARRERAI CARRERAI* IN THE RAIN FOREST OF YAPACANI, DEPARTMENT OF SANTA CRUZ
H. Bermudez, A. Rivero, B. Montalvan, J.L. Claure & S. Rocha.....................123

LEISHMANIASIS IN THE LOWLANDS OF BOLIVIA (LEISHBOL): PART VI. FLAGELLATE INFECTION IN SANDFLIES FROM THE RAIN FOREST OF YAPACANI
H. Bermudez, R. Urjel, A. Rivero, J.L. Claure & B. Montalban.................129

LEISHMANIASIS IN THE LOWLANDS OF BOLIVIA (LEISHBOL): PART VII. PRELIMINARY CHARACTERIZATION OF ELEVEN *LEISHMANIA* ISOLATES
R. Urjel, M. Recacoechea, Ph. Desjeux, H.Bermudez, G.Villarroel, S.Balderrama, J. Carrasco, O.Aguilar, J.Cl.Dujardin & D. LE Ray....................131

LEISHMANIASIS IN THE LOWLANDS OF BOLIVIA (LEISHBOL): PART VIII. CHARACTERIZATION AND IDENTIFICATION OF BOLIVIAN ISOLATES BY PFG KARYOTYPING
J.Cl. Dujardin, N. Gajendran, R. Hamers, G. Matthijsen, R. Urjel, M.Recacoechea, G. Villarroel, H. Bermudez, Ph.Desjeux, S. de Doncker & D. LE Ray....................137

THE DISTRIBUTION AND AETIOLOGY OF DIFFUSE CUTANEOUS LEISHMANIASIS IN THE NEW WORLD.
B.C. Walton & O. Velasco....................149

EPIDEMIOLOGICAL STUDIES ON CUTANEOUS LEISHMANIASIS IN THE STATE OF RIO DE JANEIRO, BRAZIL. DOMESTIC AND PERIDOMESTIC SANDFLY FAUNA
R.P. Brazil, B.G. Brazil, M.C. Gouvea, D.C. De Almeida, S.M.P. De Oliveira & J.A. De Memezes....................159

EVALUATION OF THE CANINE RESERVOIR OF VISCERAL LEISHMANIASIS: A METHODOLOGICAL REVIEW
R. Houin....................165

2
ECOLOGY & ENTOMOLOGY

THE ECOLOGY AND ENTOMOLOGY OF THE LEISHMANIASES
R. Killick-Kendrick....................175

SANDFLY BREEDING SITES
S. Bettini....................179

LEISHMANIASIS RESEARCH IN KENYA: PARASITE-VECTOR-HOST ASSOCIATION
P. Lawyer, J. Githure, Y. Mebrahtu, P. Perkins, R. Muigai & J. Leeuwenburg....................189

SANDFLIES AND DISEASE IN CYPRUS; 1944-1985
D.M. Minter & U. R. Eitrem....................207

THE EFFECT OF PERMETHRIN IMPREGNATED NETS ON *PHLEBOTOMUS* (DIPTERA:PSYCHODIDAE) IN CENTRAL ITALY
M. Maroli & R.P. Lane....................217

CUTICULAR HYDROCARBON ANALYSIS AS A TOOL IN SANDFLY IDENTIFICATION
A. Phillips, S. Kamhawi, P.J.M. Milligan & D.H. Molyneux....................225

BIOASSAYS AS AN INDICATOR OF PHEROMONE COMMUNICATION IN *LUTZOMYIA LONGIPALPIS* (DIPTERA: PSYCHODIDAE)
R.D. Ward, I. Morton, V. Lancaster, P. Smith & A. Swift....................235

WHY MEASURE THE VECTORIAL CAPACITY OF SANDFLIES?
C. Dye....................245

3
CELL BIOLOGY & IMMUNOLOGY

CELL BIOLOGY AND IMMUNOLOGY OF LEISHMANIASIS
F.E.G. Cox....................255

STUDIES OF IMMUNE MECHANISMS IN H-11-LINKED GENETIC SUSCEPTIBILITY TO MURINE VISCERAL LEISHMANIASIS
M. Roberts, P.M. Kaye, G. Milon & J.M. Blackwell....................259

CHARACTERIZATION OF *LEISHMANIA DONOVANI* INFECTIVE (METACYCLIC) PROMASTIGOTES FROM AXENIC CULTURES
M.K. Howard, G. Sayers & M.A. Miles....................267

DIFFERENT EPITOPES OF THE MACROPHAGE TYPE THREE COMPLEMENT RECEPTOR (CR3) ARE USED TO BIND *LEISHMANIA* PROMASTIGOTES HARVESTED AT DIFFERENT PHASES OF THEIR GROWTH CYCLE.
A. Cooper, A.O. Wozencraft, T.I.A. Roach & J.M. Blackwell....................271

IMMUNODOMINANT EPITOPES OF THE *LEISHMANIA* SURFACE MEMBRANE.
R.L.Anthony,J.B.Sacci&K.M.WilliamS..281

ANTIGENS RECOGNISED BY SERA FROM PATIENTS WITH VISCERAL LEISHMANIASIS
C.L. Jaffe, S. Argov, M. Zalis, N. Rachamim, M. Krup & Y. Shoenfeld....................295

INTERACTIONS BETWEEN LEISHMANIASIS AND MALARIA
F.E.G. Cox....................309

MODULATION OF CELL-MEDIATED IMMUNITY IN EXPERIMENTAL CUTANEOUS LEISHMANIASIS
F.Y. Liew....................315

THE LOCAL T-CELL RESPONSE IN EXPERIMENTAL LEISHMANIASIS
M.J. McElrath, H.W. Murray & Z.A. Cohn....................325

THE ROLE OF SPECIFIC T-CELL SUBSETS IN THE IMMUNOLOGICAL CONTROL OF EXPERIMENTAL CUTANEOUS LEISHMANIASIS
Th. Pedrazzini, V. Kindler, P. Vassalli, G. Marchal, G. Milon & J.A. Louis....................329

PARAMETERS OF T-CELL ACTIVATION IN MURINE LEISHMANIASIS
P.M. Kaye, A. Monroy-Ostria, T.I.A. Roach & J.M. Blackwell....................335

A POSSIBLE ROLE FOR PROSTAGLANDINS IN REGULATION OF DISEASE IN MURINE CUTANEOUS LEISHMANIASIS
J.P. Farrell, T.J. Nolan, W.L. Croop & C.E. Kirkpatrick....................345

USE OF A DOT-ELISA PROCEDURE FOR THE DETECTION OF SPECIFIC ANTIBODIES IN CUTANEOUS LEISHMANIASIS.
L.Guevara, L.Paz, E.Nieto & A.Llanos....................353

A NOVEL METHOD OF VACCINATION USING MEMBRANE ANTIGENS
J. Alexander & D.G. Russell....................359

LEISHMANIA MAJOR: IMMUNE RESPONSES ELICITED BY CARBOHYDRATE-LIPID CONTAINING FRACTIONS (C.L.F.)
M.V. Londner, G. Rosen, S. Frankenburg, D. Sevlever & C.L. Greenblatt..................367

PREMUNITION, A POSSIBLE LIMITATION IN THE PREVENTION OF THE LEISHMANIASES BY VACCINATION
L.F. Schnur...379

IMMUNOLOGICAL PROFILES IN INDIAN POST KALA-AZAR DERMAL LEISHMANIASIS
J.P. Haldar, K.C. Saha & A.C. Ghose........387

EVALUATION OF NON-SPECIFIC IMMUNITY IN CANINE LEISHMANIASIS.
O. Brandonisio, M. Altamura, L. Ceci, S. Antonaci, & E. Jirillo...........................395

ANTIGENIC VARIATION IN LEISHMANIA SPECIES EXPRESSED BY ANTIGENIC GLYCOCONJUGATES AND EXCRETED FACTOR
R.L. Jacobson, L.F. Schnur & C.L. Greenblatt..401

PRELIMINARY STUDIES ON THE DETECTION OF CIRCULATING ANTIGEN IN VISCERAL LEISHMANIASIS
M. Chance, S. Heath, J.M. Crampton & M. Hommel..409

THE 63KDA PROMASTIGOTE PROTEASE OF LEISHMANIA: ASSESSMENT OF HOST-PROTECTION IN BALB/C MICE USING LIPOSOMES AS ADJUVANT
L.P. Kahl, K-P. Chang & F.Y. Liew............417

STUDIES ON ANTIGENICITY OF AMPHIPHILIC AND HYDROPHILIC FORMS OF LEISHMANIA MAJOR PROMASTIGOTE SURFACE PROTEASE IN THE MOUSE
D. Rivier, S. Didisheim, R. Etges, C. Bordier & J. Mauel..............................423

HISTOPATHOGENIC MECHANISMS IN AMERICAN CUTANEOUS LEISHMANIASIS OF MICE
A. Monroy-Ostria, E. Velez-Castro & T. Monroy-Ostria..................................431

THE ROLE OF MEMBRANE-STABILIZING DRUGS ON UPTAKE OF LEISHMANIA PARASITES BY HUMAN MACROPHAGES.
A. Kharazmi, A.L. Sorensen & H. Nielsen...441

GENERATION OF MEGASOMES DURING THE PROMASTIGOTE - AMASTIGOTE TRANSFORMATION OF LEISHMANIA MEXICANA MEXICANA IN VITRO.
L. Tetley, C.A. Hunter, G.H. Coombs & K. Vickerman...449

TREATMENT OF EXPERIMENTAL CUTANEOUS AND VISCERAL MURINE LEISHMANIASIS WITH RECOMBINANT GAMMA-INTERFERON
A. Kiderlen & M-L. Lohmann-Matthes...457

4 MOLECULAR BIOLOGY & BIOCHEMISTRY

MOLECULAR BIOLOGY & BIOCHEMISTRY: AN OVERVIEW
G.H. Coombs...469

BIOCHEMICAL MECHANISMS OF PENTOSTAM
J.D. Berman & M. Grogl...........................473

EFFECTS OF SINEFUNGIN ON CELLULAR AND BIOCHEMICAL EVENTS IN PROMASTIGOTES OF LEISHMANIA D. DONOVANI
F. Lawrence & M. Robert-Gero.................479

METABOLISM AND FUNCTIONS OF TRYPANOTHIONE WITH SPECIAL REFERENCE TO LEISHMANIASIS
A.H. Fairlamb..487

THE STEROLS OF LEISHMANIA PROMASTIGOTES AND AMASTIGOTES: POSSIBLE IMPLICATIONS FOR CHEMOTHERAPY
L.J. Goad, J.S. Keithly, J.D. Berman, D.H. Beach & G.G. Holz.............................495

ASSESSMENT OF THE USE IN THE DIAGNOSIS OF LEISHMANIASIS OF BIOTINYLATED KINETOPLAST DERIVED DNA SEQUENCES
D.C. Barker...503

APPLICATION OF TOTAL AND RECOMBINANT DNA PROBES IN THE DIAGNOSIS OF LEISHMANIA INFECTIONS
G.J. Van Eys, G.J. Schoone, G.S. Ligthart, J.A. Schalken, & W.J. Terpstra................515

BIOTINYLATED KDNA FROM LEISHMANIA BRAZILIENSIS
M. Lopez, Y. Montoya, A. Llanos-Cuentas & J. Arevalo..525

KARYOTYPE ANALYSIS OF LEISHMANIA DONOVANI.
R.P. Bishop & M.A. Miles..........................533

ABNORMALLY MIGRATING CHROMOSOME IDENTIFIES LEISHMANIA DONOVANI POPULATIONS
N. Gajendran, J.Cl. Dujardin, D. LE Ray, G. Matthyssens, S. Muyldermans & R. Hamers..539

KINETOPLAST DNA PROBES FOR THE IDENTIFICATION OF THE OLD WORLD CUTANEOUS LEISHMANIASES
C.J. Chapman, W.P.K. Kennedy & D.A. Evans..549

SMALL NUCLEIC ACIDS IN LEISHMANIA
K. Stuart, P. Tarr, R. Aline, B. Smiley, J. Scholler & J. Keithly................................555

GENE EXPRESSION IN THE INFECTIVE PROMASTIGOTES OF LEISHMANIA MAJOR
D.F. Smith, P.D. Ready, R.M.R. Coulson, S. Searle & A.J.R. Campos......................563

IN VITRO AND IN VIVO DIFFERENTIATION OF L. MEXICANA-HSP70 GENE EXPRESSION
M. Shapira, J.G. McEwen & C.L. Jaffe.....575

THERMOREGULATED ANTIGEN EXPRESSION BY LEISHMANIA PROMASTIGOTES
T.E. Fehniger, G. Mengistu, A. Gessese, H. Mariam & Y. Negesse..........................581

A SIMPLE, HIGHLY REPETITIVE SEQUENCE IN THE LEISHMANIA GENOME
J. Ellis & J. Crampton.............................589

CLONING AND CHARACTERISATION OF *LEISHANIA DONOVANI* GENES CODING FOR IMMUNODOMINANT ANTIGENS
J.M. Kelly, M.L. Blaxter, E. Kellet & M.A. Miles.................597

SURFACE ANTIGENS OF *LEISHMANIA INFANTUM* IDENTIFIED BY MONOCLONAL ANTIBODIES: ISOLATION OF A MONOMERIC AND AN OLIGOMERIC FORM OF A MAJOR *L. INFANTUM* ANTIGEN
K.Ph. Soteriadou, A.K. Tzinia, M.G. Hadziantoniou & S.J. Tzartos....................603

SEQUENCE ANALYSIS OF THE MAJOR SURFACE GLYCOPROTEIN OF *LEISHMANIA MAJOR*.
L.L. Button, R.W. Olafson & W. McMaster..611

STRUCTURE FUNCTION STUDIES ON *LEISHMANIA* SURFACE MEMBRANE PROTEINS
R.W. Olafson, R.A. Dwek, T.W. Rademacher, K-P. Chang & M.A.J. Ferguson.............619

THE PROMASTIGOTE SURFACE PROTEASE OF *LEISHMANIA*: pH OPTIMUM AND EFFECTS OF PROTEASE INHIBITORS
R. Etges, J. Bouvier & C. Bordier..............627

PROTEOLYSIS IN *LEISHMANIA*: SPECIES DIFFERENCES AND DEVELOPMENTAL CHANGES IN PROTEINASE ACTIVITY
M.J. North, B.C. Lockwood, D.J. Mallinson & G.H. Coombs..........................635

THE *LEISHMANIA DONOVANI* LIPOPHOSPHOGLYCAN: STRUCTURE AND FUNCTION
S.J. Turco...................643

IMMUNOCHEMICAL CHARACTERIZATION OF THE *LEISHMANIA DONOVANI* 3'-NUCLEOTIDEASE
K.B. Pastakia & D.M. Dwyer....................651

INTERRELATIONS BETWEEN GLUCOSE AND ALANINE CATABOLISM, AMMONIA PRODUCTION, AND THE D-LACTATE PATHWAY IN *LEISHMANIA BRAZILIENSIS*.
J.J. Blum, D.G. Davis, T.N. Darling & R.E. London.............................659

LEISHMANIA AMASTIGOTES: ADAPTATIONS FOR GROWTH IN AN ACIDIC *IN VIVO* ENVIRONMENT
A.J. Mukkada, T.A. Glaser, S.A. Anderson & S.K. Wells................667

ABROGATION OF SKIN LESIONS IN CUTANEOUS LEISHMANIASIS BY ULTRAVIOLET B IRRADIATION
S.H. Giannini & E.C. De Fabo..................677

EVIDENCE FOR HYBRID FORMATION IN THE GENUS *LEISHMANIA*.
D.A. Evans, V. Smith, R. Killick-Kendrick, R.A. Neal & W. Peters................685

5
CHEMOTHERAPY

CHEMOTHERAPY: AN OVERVIEW
L.G. Goodwin.............................693

THE FUTURE FOR ANTILEISHMANIAL CHEMOTHERAPEUTIC AGENTS: A REVIEW
J.D. Berman..............................699

CHEMOTHERAPY OF MEDITERRANEAN VISCERAL LEISHMANIASIS WITH MEGLUMINE ANTIMONIATE
L. Tavares, C. Carvalho & E. Monteiro......705

THE *IN VITRO* SUSCEPTIBILITY OF MACROPHAGES INFECTED WITH AMASTIGOTES OF *LEISHMANIA* SPP. TO PENTAVALENT ANTIMONIAL DRUGS AND OTHER COMPOUNDS WITH SPECIAL RELEVANCE TO CUTANEOUS ISOLATES
S. Allen & R.A. Neal................711

RELAPSE IN KALA-AZAR: FAILURE OF SODIUM STIBOGLUCONATE TO CLEAR PARASITES FROM ORGANS OTHER THAN THE LIVER
K.C. Carter, J. Alexander, A.J. Baillie & T.F. Dolan............................721

FROM LYSOSOMES TO CELLS, FROM CELLS TO *LEISHMANIA*. AMINO ACID ESTERS, POTENTIAL CHEMOTHERAPEUTIC AGENTS?
M. Rabinovitch........................729

ANTILEISHMANIAL ACTIVITY OF L-LEUCINE METHYL ESTER AND L-TRYPTOPHANAMIDE
C.A. Hunter, L.M. Macpherson & G.H. Coombs..........................741

INHIBITION OF *LEISHMANIA* SPECIES BY DIFLUOROMETHYLORNITHINE
J.S. Keithly & A.H. Fairlamb..................749

ANTILEISHMANIAL EFFECT OF SINEFUNGIN AND ITS DERIVATIVES
M. Robert-Gero, F. Lawrence, P. Blanchard, N. Dodic, P. Paolantonacci, H. Malina & A. Mouna..............................757

EFFECTS OF LANOSTEROL-DEMETHYLATION INHIBITORS ON PROPAGATION AND STEROL BIOSYNTHESIS OF *LEISHMANIA* PROMASTIGOTES AND AMASTIGOTES
D.H. Beach, L.J. Goad, J.D. Berman & G.G. Holz...........................765

EFFECT OF RIBOSOME-INACTIVATING PROTEINS ON RIBOSOMES FROM *LEISHMANIA* AND THEIR POSSIBLE USES IN CHEMOTHERAPY
P. Cenini & F. Stirpe........................773

LEISHMANIASIS - AIDS: FAILURE TO RESPOND TO CHEMOTHERAPY
J. Alvar.......................781

LIPOSOMES AND OTHER DRUG DELIVERY SYSTEMS IN THE TREATMENT OF LEISHMANIASIS
S.L. Croft, R.A. Neal & L.S. Rao...............783

CARRIER-MEDIATED THERAPY OF MURINE VISCERAL LEISHMANIASIS
T.F. Dolan, C.A. Hunter, T. Laakso, G.H. Coombs, A.J. Baillie, P. Stjarnkvist & I. Sjoholm.............................793

SITE SPECIFIC ANTILEISHMANIAL DRUG DELIVERY
D.T Hart & M.J. Lawrence.......................807

6 NEW STRATEGIES FOR CONTROL
I: VECTOR CONTROL

NEW STRATEGIES FOR CONTROL FORUM: VECTOR CONTROL
R. Killick-Kendrick..................821

SQUASH BLOTTING *PHLEBOTOMUS PAPATASI* TO ESTIMATE RATES OF INFECTION BY *LEISHMANIA MAJOR*
P.D. Ready, D.F. Smith, R. Killick-Kendrick & R. Ben Ismail..................823

7 NEW STRATEGIES FOR CONTROL
II. RESERVOIR CONTROL

NEW STRATEGIES FOR CONTROL FORUM: RESERVOIR CONTROL
R.W. Ashford..................827

8 NEW STRATEGIES FOR CONTROL
III. VACCINATION

NEW STRATEGIES FOR CONTROL FORUM: VACCINATION
F.Y. Liew..................835

VACCINATION AND THE IMMUNOLOGICAL CONTROL OF LEISHMANIASIS.
J. Alexander..................839

9 NEW STRATEGIES FOR CONTROL
IV. CHEMOTHERAPY

NEW STRATEGIES FOR CONTROL FORUM: CHEMOTHRAPY
S.L. Croft & R.A. Neal..................847

STRATEGIES FOR THE DESIGN OF NEW ANTILEISHMANIAL DRUGS.
G.H. Coombs..................851

THE GLYCOSOME OF *LEISHMANIA* AS A POSSIBLE TARGET FOR CHEMOTHERAPEUTIC ATTACK
F.R. Opperdoes..................859

MOLECULAR STRATEGIES FOR ANTILEISHMANIAL DRUG DESIGN
D.T Hart, A. Langridge, D.J. Barlow & B.J. Sutton..................865

UNSTABLE AND STABLE GENE AMPLIFICATION IN METHOTREXATE-RESISTANT *L. MAJOR* AND NATURAL ISOLATES OF *L. TARENTOLAE*.
S.M. Beverley, T.E. Ellenberger & M. Petrillo-Peixoto..................873

POTENTIAL CLINICAL USE OF SINEFUNGIN: REDUCTION OF TOXICITY AND ENHANCEMENT OF ACTIVITY
M. Robert-Gero, F. Lawrence & E. Lederer..................879

EFFECTS OF A SQUALINE-2,3-EPOXIDASE INHIBITOR ON PROPAGATION AND STEROL BIOSYNTHESIS OF *LEISHMANIA* PROMASTIGOTES AND AMASTIGOTES
D.H. Beach, L.J. Goad, J.D. Berman, T.E. Ellenberger, S.M. Beverley & G.G. Holz..................885

RIBOSOME-INACTIVATING PROTEINS AND *LEISHMANIA*: NEW STRATEGIES FOR FUTURE RESEARCH
P. Cenini & F. Stirpe..................891

10 WORKSHOP I:
CHARACTERIZATION & TAXONOMY

WORKSHOP I: CHARACTERIZATION AND TAXONOMY OF *LEISHMANIA*
D.A. Evans..................897

CHARACTERISATION BY LIGHT MICROSCOPE *IN SITU'* HYBRIDISATION WITHIN 12 HOURS OF LIVE *LEISHMANIA* OBSERVATION
D.C. Barker..................901

ENZYME ELECTROPHORETIC EVIDENCE FOR THE IMPORTATION OF *L. INFANTUM* INTO THE NEW WORLD
H. Momen & G. Grimaldi Jr..................911

CHROMOSOME SIZE HOMOLOGIES IN *LEISHMANIA MAJOR* DETERMINED BY MOLECULAR KARYOTYPING
S.H. Giannini..................917

IDENTIFICATION OF *LEISHMANIA TROPICA* BY SPECIES SPECIFIC MONOCLONAL ANTIBODIES
R. Sarfstein & C.L. Jaffe..................925

FLOW CYTOMETRIC ANALYSIS OF *LEISHMANIA* SURFACE MEMBRANE ANTIGEN EXPRESSION
R.L. Anthony & J.B. Sacci..................931

ON THE CLINICAL MANIFESTATIONS AND PARASITES OF OLD WORLD LEISHMANIASIS AND *LEISHMANIA TROPICA* CAUSING VISCERAL LEISHMANIASIS
L.F. Schnur..................939

11 WORKSHOP II:
SANDFLY SYSTEMATICS & GENETICS

WORKSHOP II: SANDFLY SYSTEMATICS AND GENETICS
R.D. Ward..................947

SANDFLY SYSTEMATICS: EPIDEMIOLOGICAL REQUIREMENTS AND CURRENT DEVELOPMENTS
R.P. Lane..................951

DNA PROBES FOR VECTOR TAXONOMY
J. Crampton, T. Knapp & R. Ward..................957

DNA SEQUENCE POLYMORPHISMS AS GENOTYPIC MARKERS FOR PHLEBOTOMINE VECTORS OF *LEISHMANIA*
P.D. Ready & D.F. Smith..................965

12 WORKSHOP III:
MOLECULAR GENETICS & DEVELOPMENT

WORKSHOP III: MOLECULAR GENETICS OF *LEISHMANIA* DEVELOPMENT
D.F. Smith & P.D. Ready..................975

TRANSCRIPT ALTERATION IN *LEISHMANIA*
K. Stuart & J.E. Feagin..................977

CIRCULAR AND LINEAR FORMS OF SMALL NUCLEIC ACIDS IN *LEISHMANIA*
R. Hamers, N. Gajendran, J.C. Dujardin & K. Stuart 985

13
WORKSHOP IV:
CHEMOTHERAPY & IMMUNE RESPONSE

WORKSHOP IV: CHEMOTHERAPY AND THE IMMUNE RESPONSE
J. Alexander & S.L. Croft 991

CLEARANCE OF *L. DONOVANI* FROM THE LIVER OF BALB/c MICE RESULTS IN LOCAL RESISTANCE TO REINFECTION
K.C. Carter, A.J. Baillie, J. Alexander & T.F. Dolan 993

14
FIELD TRIP
ON THE ISLAND OF ZAKINTHOS

I - THE FIELD TRIP
FIELD TRIP ON THE ISLAND OF ZAKINTHOS: AN OVERVIEW
N. Leger 1003

II - FERAL RESERVOIRS OF LEISHMANIASIS ON THE ISLAND OF ZAKINTHOS
L.F. Schnur, C. Stamatopoulos, A. Garifallou, M. Patrikoussis & R.L. Jacobson 1007

III - EPIDEMIOLOGY OF HUMAN AND CANINE LEISHMANIASIS ON THE ISLAND OF ZAKINTHOS
A. Garifallou, M. Hadziandoniou, L.F. Schnur, B. Yuval, A. Warburg, R.L. Jacobson, E. Pateraki, M. Patrikoussis, Y. Schlein & C. Serie 1011

15
NATO-ASI PHOTOGRAPHS 1017

16
LIST OF PARTICIPANTS 1023

17
AUTHOR INDEX 1037
SUBJECT INDEX 1039

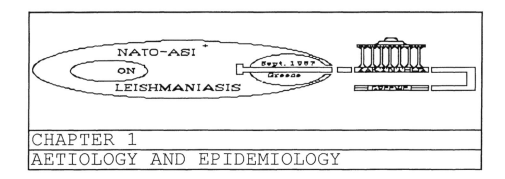

CHAPTER 1
AETIOLOGY AND EPIDEMIOLOGY

AETIOLOGY AND EPIDEMIOLOGY: OVERVIEW

David J Bradley

Department of Tropical Hygiene and Ross Institute
London School of Hygiene and Tropical Medicine
Keppel Street, London WC1E 7HT

The striking feature of the aetiology and epidemiology of the leishmaniases is qualitatitive complexity. In no other parasitic genus infecting man is there such a diversity of species and strains, variety of pathogenic manifestations, plethora of reservoir hosts and ecological richness of transmission patterns. Add to this the small size, species complexity and taxonomic horrors of the vector sandflies and it is remarkable that epidemiologists do not abandon the field to those rudely called by Lord Rutherford "stamp collectors" (whom he contrasted with physicists!) The task of an overview must therefore be to see how far we can progress to either finding order within this exuberant complexity, or if this is not yet possible, how far some order may be imposed, so that our understanding can be used to predict and thus to control human and animal leishmaniasis.

The papers in this section go far to set out both the current position and also aspects of progress for the future. Inevitably they cannot describe the global picture fully, and emphasis is naturally more on the Mediterranean situation, which so often gets neglected. There is relatively less on India and almost nothing on Africa. The Latin American data places more emphasis on the Andes and other less often described areas, rather than on the Amazon forests of Brazil which have been so carefully studied and usually tend to dominate the literature.

This overview will therefore tend towards over-sweeping generalizations, which may be corrected by reading the papers that follow, and which may be set against the general tendency of the field towards splitting and minute qualitative detail, which too often has either necessitated, or less laudably permitted, workers to avoid a more quantitative approach to their epidemiology. Recommendations and indications for future work will tend to arise from the broad issues discussed, rather than being listed as a formal series at the end. The overview will also incorporate many of the points raised in discussion after delivery of each of the papers.

The Leishmania Parasites

The decade has been dominated by the application of biochemical techniques to define similarities and differences between isolates of Leishmania from man and other mammals: a move in taxonomy from pathogenetic effects, culture characteristics, that Peters has conveniently called extrinsic characteristics toward the use, above all, of isoenzymes but more recently of other "intrinsic" characters which relate more closely and directly to the parasite genome. More recently still, methods involving the DNA itself such as restriction enzyme fragments (Gramiccia et al., this volume) have been used to complement the data from isozyme patterns. DNA hybridization is rapidly increasing in importance taxonomically, though it is probably true that this approach has so far been more used for identification and diagnosis rather than to develop taxonomic schemes, though this is only a matter of time.

The isoenzyme patterns have given an immense number of zymodemes, so that one approach to handling them is by numerical taxonomic methods to give some measure of taxonomic distance between strains, as was clearly shown in the paper by Rioux. Two other aspects have become clearer also.

The original leishmanial taxonomy had three species, each corresponding to a particular disease pattern in man: cutaneous, visceral or muco-cutaneous. Every year has seen more evidence that a precise correspondence between strains and disease is not the case. Initially the isozyme diversity of the aetiological agents of cutaneous lesions was apparent, with L. major and L. tropica not just different, but some way apart from each other. More recently in Europe the frequency of dermotropic strains of L. infantum has become clear (elegantly set out by Gramiccia et al.) and the general disparity in both Europe and the Americas between pathology and taxonomy clearly shown, There is, of course, a tendency to examine parasites from anomalous cases (a cutaneous lesion in a visceral leishmaniasis area, for example) by sophisticated means, so that in the literature such cases achieve disproportionate prominence. But the cumulative evidence now available shows that, in some areas at least, "atypical" pathology is common. Further progress will need a much greater understanding of pathogenesis in man and its determinants, a topic returned to later.

The second emerging feature from the taxonomic profusion is that in several areas, and areas of Mediterranean L. infantum are among them, there is great homogeneity of strains, as shown for dogs in N. Greece by Kostos et al. and in Italian foci. This has two research advantages: it simplifies one variable and it clears the way for the rigorous quantitative epidemiological analysis that is so intractable where several strains of parasite are circulating simultaneously.

Rioux's careful descriptive analysis of zymodemes points research in two ways. First, what is the meaning of small isozyme differences? Are they recurrently occurring neutral mutations that act as convenient labels for stocks of the parasites but have little or no biological significance beyond this, or are they adaptive in some way and biologically relevant in a deeper sense? The degree of sexual recombination that occurs in the life of Leishmania will be relevant to any answer to this question.

The versatility of biochemists and molecular biologists is such that soon we shall have, in addition to isoenzymes and restriction enzyme DNA fragments, DNA probes of all sorts, cytogenetic analysis and many other methods. The degree of diversity likely to be uncovered is likely to be enormous and very confusing. A few groups of taxa will be rapidly tidied up, but the residual chaos may be great. There is clearly a need to investigate the parasite genetic bases of pathogenicity for man and domestic animals and the determinants of visceralization, as well as variation that affects transmissibility by sandfly species. In other words, in the face of bewildering diversity, there will be a need to focus on relevant diversity, and we do not yet know in what this relevance consists, at the molecular level.

Most studies of diversity have been driven parasitologically: it is the parasite taxonomy that has tended to dominate our approach. But Bryce Walton's paper illustrates how productive another starting point can be. He starts from the rigorous clinical definition of diffuse cutaneous leishmaniasis and then seeks cases that fit it throughout the New World. Several conclusions are clear and striking. One is the diversity of Leishmania species (not just strains) which may cause it, so pushing the focus of relevant research towards the host features permitting this horrible condition to develop. Secondly, it becomes clear that diffuse leishmaniasis is not always a rare variant of the localized cutaneous disease: all the cutaneous leishmaniasis recorded from the Dominican Republic (all 23 cases!) is of the diffuse form, encouraging work in those situations on the parasite characters that predispose to the condition.

Epidemiology

The qualitative complexity of transmission and of epidemiological study has tended to attract the naturalist more than the quantitatively minded epidemiologist, so that with a few notable exceptions (for example the studies at Jacobina in Brazil) community-based epidemiological studies have been less frequent and less comprehensive than might have been expected, and the population biologists have tended to focus more on the sandfly dynamics than on other aspects of the transmission cycle. The sheer manpower demands of the ideal interdisciplinary study are too great and there are further problems of scale, of spatial heterogeneity and of diagnostic methodology related to "silent" cases of infection in man. Each of these aspects is considered below. With these limitations, can epidemiological thinking successfully guide control? The answer given at the meeting is that it can, as seen from the elegant work on Elba of Gradoni and his colleagues.

Endemic human leishmaniasis is in most circumstances a relatively rare infection. Cases of infantile Kala-azar in most Mediterranean countries are few in numbers, even where the dog infection rate may reach a prevalence exceeding 20%. Therefore if we are interested in human disease, large populations need to be studied. Yet work on dogs could utilize a much smaller population and it is frankly not feasible to carry out detailed sandfly studies over hundreds of square kilometres. Different sampling frames are needed for each component of the transmission cycle. But this may omit the crucial place and event responsible for the spillover of infection into man as a dead end host. One suspects that the way forward, already being followed in practice by some groups, is to combine a study of the dynamics of transmission between sandflies and dogs with another superimposed larger scale study of risk factors for human infection in the area.

The situation in some tropical areas, and especially during epidemic outbreaks, may give incidences much higher, to 50% in a few years for immigrant miners in Bolivia for example and above 20% for farming communities at the forest edge. Under these circumstances more conventional village-scale community based studies become both feasible and productive.

Another major problem for the epidemiologist is the great heterogeneity of sandfly distribution. Assumptions of even distribution of vectors over the study area, which are so convenient a simplifying assumption, are untrue for all vectors but more dramatically so in the case of sandflies. This creates great problems for sampling and design of field studies as well as for epidemiological modelling of results.

Work on visceral leishmaniasis in recent years, both due to _L. infantum_ and _L.donovani_, has demonstrated that subclinical infections in man are common and in many cases self-healing. There is some sort of threshold of development of a clinical case beyond which the disease becomes progressive and unlikely to show spontaneous recovery, but in many other people a transient period of seropositivity may be the only detectable sign of infection, and after it the patient may be resistant to re-infection. The full extent of such transient infections is not at all clear, and solution of the problem is exacerbated in the case of _L.infantum_ by the increase in innate resistance to infection with increasing age, and in some areas of _L.donovani_ (such as East Africa) by the concurrent circulation of other leishmanias not pathogenic for man but which may be responsible for transient responses or skin test conversion. These phenomena make it hard to measure the true rate of human infection. It may be considerably under-estimated by the approach based on clinical cases and in the extreme example, human inoculation with the parasites could be a much less rare event than usually accepted, and the focus of research should be more on the determinants of pathogenesis in those infected rather than the risk factors for inoculation of the parasite. These complexities may also apply to cutaneous infections, though with less force.

In the midst of these relatively intractable complexities, an effective way forward to understanding the dynamics of transmission may be to intervene in some clear and well-measured way in the cycle and determine the effects on the system. This approach was most elegantly shown in the paper by Gradoni and colleagues. Having determined on Elba that symptomatic dogs were the main source of sandfly infections, that serodiagnosis was effective and the limited transmission season gave an annual crop of new infections that could be efficiently detected, they operated a programme of treating preclinical infections and destroying dogs sick from leishmaniasis, and found a fall in incidence proportional to the reduction in infective dogs. They thus both tested their hypotheses and controlled the disease.

At the level of macro-epidemiology, the meeting showed that many countries had encountered similar experiences to that well documented for the USSR in the past. The leishmaniases, and particularly large outbreaks of the disease, are closely related to agricultural development and the related migrations of people. In South America forests are cut down and those who move in to farm, in such places as Bolivia are exposed to a high risk of infection. The ecotones of the forest edge, as in Brazil, provide a major health problem for the migrant-settler-farmer sequence of activities. The relation of leishmaniasis to agricultural development is also clearly shown in the papers from North Africa.

As epidemiology and pathogenesis are brought together, many unsolved problems remain, both of a practical applied type and also of a more general theoretical nature. The role of transient subclinical infections in changing the immune status of populations subject to _L. donovani_ and _L. infantum_ challenge in endemic areas is steadily becoming more thoroughly defined. The role of such sub-clinical infections in transmission is not known and may well be unimportant in man, but in reservoir host infections, of dogs particularly, is of interest and importance. The whole question of persistent infections, reservoir host pathology and transmission, and their inter-relations is still far from clear.

It is clear that many of the unsolved problems depend for their elucidation on epidemiological studies of defined populations in which sophisticated immunological studies are combined with the more usual types of observation, together with analysis of pathogenesis in the field in reservoir hosts. Leishmaniasis is not easy to study in this way because of the relatively low prevalence in most communities, the limited knowledge of reservoir host immunology, and the patchy distribution of sandflies. Nevertheless both the _Leishmania_ parasites and their epidemiology and immunology over the last two decades make such population-based multisciplinary studies a realistic challenge.

THE GENUS LEISHMANIA IN THE MIDDLE EAST AND USSR

Wallace Peters

Department of Medical Protozoology
London School of Hygiene and Tropical Medicine
London WC1E 7HT, England

INTRODUCTION

The subdivision of Old World leishmaniases into visceral infections, on the one hand, and cutaneous on the other, with the latter being subdivided into zoonotic rural and anthroponotic urban disease, must now be considered far too simplistic. So too must the concept that visceral disease (kala-azar, VL) is caused, in the areas under discussion, by Leishmania infantum, zoonotic cutaneous leishmaniasis (ZCL) by L.major and anthroponotic cutaneous leishmaniasis (ACL) by L.tropica. Advances in methods for the characterisation of the Kinetoplastida may truly be said to have revolutionised the picture of the genus Leishmania, not only here, but wherever in the world it occurs and, in parallel, understanding of the epidemiology of the infections and the aetiology of different clinical syndromes. Our ideas on the control of those members of the genus that are responsible for human disease must, therefore, now be revised.

This paper aims not to provide a comprehensive review of the leishmaniases in the Middle East and USSR but to examine the present state of knowledge of the different organisms in the context of their public health significance and the possible measures available for their control. The terminology used is that of Lainson and Shaw (1987).

MATERIALS AND METHODS

The principles of biochemical and immuno-taxonomy of the Leishmania were outlined at a Workshop held in 1980 (Chance and Walton 1982) and by Lainson and Shaw (1987). More details of the techniques for isoenzyme characterisation are given by Le Blancq et al. (1986). The writer and his colleagues, first in the Liverpool School of Tropical Medicine and, since 1979, in the London School of Hygiene and Tropical Medicine, have been privileged to study a large number of isolates of Leishmania from the majority of endemic countries, sent to the International Reference Centre established in the UK by the UNDP/World

Table 1. Species of _Leishmania_ and Disease Associations

Species	Disease
L.(L.)major (zymodemes LON-1, 2, 3, 4)	ZCL
L.(L.)tropica (various zymodemes)	ACL, "recidiva" CL, rarely VL
L.(L.)infantum (zymodemes LON-42, 43, 49)	VL, ? CL
L.(L.)gerbilli	non-pathogenic
L.(L.)arabica	non-pathogenic
_L.(L.)_ sp.USSR	?? VL

Bank/WHO Special Programme for Research and Training in Tropical Diseases. Liaison with other reference centres is maintained through the exchange of computerised data bases, as well as the free interchange of well characterised, reference isolates. Cryobanks are maintained in each reference centre for the conservation of isolates and reference material is supplied to any _bona fide_ research worker on request.

While isoenzyme characterisation provided the first baseline data on which most investigators still lean heavily, immunotaxonomic methods using monoclonal antibodies and DNA technology are coming into increasing use. DNA probes, for example, developed at a number of centres, are coming into prominence for the identification not only of _Leishmania_ in vertebrate and invertebrate hosts, but also for the identification of the sandfly vectors.

THE PARASITES AND VECTORS

Parasites (Table)

It is difficult to be sure, from a scrutiny of many early records, which species of _Leishmania_ are present in the different countries composing the Middle East and USSR, or which mammalian and insect vectors are infected, in the absence of a precise identification. The problem is especially serious in references to "Cutaneous leishmaniasis" (CL) or its various synonyms. However, from overall knowledge of the historical basis of their nomenclature, one can accept the old classification of "dry, urban" CL as being largely caused by _Leishmania (Leishmania) tropica_ and "wet, rural" CL as being caused by _L.(L.) major_. The terms "Anthroponotic cutaneous leishmaniasis" (ACL) and "Zoonotic cutaneous leishmaniasis" (ZCL) are also useful working terms for infection with _L.(L.) tropica_ and _L.(L.)major_ respectively. There is now, however, abundant evidence to indicate that CL, sometimes even with mucosal involvement, may be caused by infection with one or more variants of _L.(L.) infantum_.

Visceral infection. Visceral leishmaniasis (VL) is a condition that affects mostly infants and young children in the area under consideration. While there is general agreement that parasites of the _L.(L.) donovani_ - _L.(L.) infantum_ complex are responsible, other parasites may involve the viscera. A number of reports, the most recent among them that of Al-Hussayni _et al_. (1987), have implicated _L.(L.) tropica_ as an agent of VL on the basis of isoenzyme characterisation. The correct identification and, indeed, terminology of the visceralising parasites has been a moot point for some years. Isoenzyme studies have helped to resolve the question in some ways by illuminating the wide gap between typical L.(L.) donovani of the east of India and the rest but, at the same time, pointed to the heterogeneity that exists in parasites akin to L.(L.) infantum of which the type locality is Tunisia. Le Blancq and Peters (1986b) identified 12 enzyme profiles (zymodemes) among 67 stocks (including several from India). The greatest level of homogeneity existed between two isolates from the southwest of Saudia Arabia and a marker stock from Humera in Ethiopia. Further stocks identical to the first two, from infants with VL, have been isolated recently in the southwest of Saudi Arabia by Al-Zahrani (personal communication). It is interesting to note that Al-Hussayni et al. (1987) found a close homology between Iraqi isolates obtained from VL patients in central Iraq and the same Ethiopian marker, whereas a VL isolate from the Georgian SSR corresponded to the typical L.(L.) infantum marker from Tunisia (Le Blancq and Peters, 1986b). The latter authors reported that an Iraqi dog isolate and one from a patient with VL were identical to each other and differed in only a single enzyme (out of 13 examined) from the Ethiopian marker and Saudi isolates. On the contrary, another isolate from the viscera of an Iraqi dog was typed by Al-Hussayni et al. (1987) as L.(L.) tropica. We have recently examined several isolates obtained by Al-Zahrani from dogs in

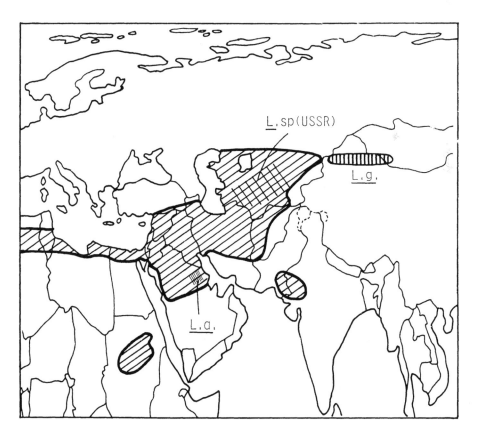

Figure. Distribution of L.(L.)major, tropica, gerbilli, arabica and L.(L.) sp.USSR.

11

the southwest of Saudi Arabia. While similar to the organism causing human VL, they differ in several enzymes but do not appear to correspond to L.(L.) tropica which is common in an area above the VL region, the Asir plateau. This situation is being further investigated. In summary, it would appear that VL in the USSR is caused by L.(L.) infantum of a variant similar to the type species. From Iraq, through Saudi Arabia and across the Red Sea to Ethiopia another variant is responsible, its full geographical distribution remaining undefined. [While one Sudanese isolate, reputedly from Khartoum, appears to be identical (Le Blancq and Peters, 1986b), others from that country and from Kenya belong to different zymodemes.]

Cutaneous infection. In spite of the difficulty of defining which is which, as noted above, there is no doubt that both L.(L.) tropica and L.(L.) major are, or in recent times were, widely distributed throughout the USSR and Middle East. However, in addition, two other Leishmania (Leishmania) species exist in the USSR and one in Saudi Arabia. L.(L.) gerbilli which was originally described as a parasite of the great gerbil (Rhombomys opimus) in southern Mongolia by Wang, Qu and Guan (1964), has recently been isolated from the same species of rodent in neighbouring areas of the USSR (Strelkova, personal communication). Another parasite, so far unnamed, has been identified in R.opimus in other parts of the USSR. This parasite has caused much confusion in the literature. Soviet scientists had long reported marked variability in the virulence of "L.major" isolated from this rodent when the parasites were inoculated into hamsters and noted that isolates from ZCL lesions in man appeared to be all of high virulence. Following the discovery by Le Blancq (1983) that a marked difference existed between the isoenzyme profiles of clones of high or low virulence, a preliminary note was published (Kellina et al., 1985) drawing attention to the need for caution in the interpretation of these data pending further field and clinical studies. The Soviet workers have since made many more isolates of the unnamed parasite which has proved, in some areas, to be far more common than L.(L.) major in R.opimus (Strelkova, personal communication). The questions of its infectivity to man and its vectors are still under investigation. It seems likely that different species of Phlebotomus are responsible for the transmission of L.(L.) major and L.(L.) spp. USSR.

A somewhat similar situation has been shown to exist in the Eastern Province of Saudi Arabia. The Al-Ahsa oasis is highly endemic for ZCL caused by L.(L.) major, the local zymodeme of which (LON 4) differs slightly from the classical marker of the USSR, as well as from isolates from Iran, parts of Iraq, Syria, Israel, the Sudan, Kenya and Senegal. LON 4 has also been identified in an isolate from Sinjar (Iraq) and two isolates from Kuwait (Le Blancq et al., 1986). [Since Sinjar is located in the northwestern corner of Iraq, near Mosul, it would be interesting to know if the individual from whom this isolate was made had been infected there or nearer Saudi Arabia.] The main reservoir of this parasite in Al-Ahsa is the fat-tailed sand rat, Psammomys obesus (Peters et al., 1985). The dominant phlebotomine species in the area is P.papatasi which was incriminated as the vector of L.(L.) major by Killick-Kendrick et al. (1985). A second parasite was isolated from P.obesus, quite distinctive from L.(L.) major. Named Leishmania (Leishmania) arabica by Peters, Elbihari and Evans

(1986), it has been shown by Killick-Kendrick (personal communication) to be capable of developing in P.papatasi, but proof of its development to the infective, metacyclic stage is not yet to hand. Like the new Russian parasite, L.arabica has never been isolated from CL lesions in man. Unlike the Russian parasite, however, it seems most likely that human beings are inoculated with L.arabica since P.papatasi is a common man-biter in Al-Ahsa, and almost the only fly in this genus present in the area, whereas the Russian parasite may be transmitted by a different species of Phlebotomus which is less anthropophilic. It will be interesting to learn whether L.arabica exists in rodents in other areas of Saudi Arabia or in other countries (eg, Israel) where P.obesus is common and, indeed, whether the unnamed Russian species infects R.opimus in other parts of its range (eg, in northern Iran) (see Figure).

The descriptions of CL in urban areas make it almost certain that the main pathogenic agent was L.(L.) tropica. From the isoenzyme studies of Lanotte et al. (1981) and Le Blancq and Peters (1986a) it has become clear that this is a very heterogeneous parasite. These investigations, supported recently by that of Al-Hussayni et al. (1987), have also pointed to the phyletic closeness of this species with the variants of L.(L.) infantum, compared with the distance of both from L.(L.) major. Le Blancq and Peters (1986a) defined 18 zymodemes among 27 stocks of L.(L.) tropica isolated from man in the USSR (Baku and Ashkabad), Afghanistan, India (Bikaner), Iran, Iraq, Israel and Saudi Arabia, as well as Greece. The isolate from Bikaner and one from Iraq were from animals, the former from a dog and the latter from Rattus rattus. Al-Hussayni et al. (1987) identified a visceral isolate from a dog near Baghdad as L.(L.) tropica. The role of dogs or other animals as reservoirs of different species of Leishmania is still open to discussion. While there is no question of the key role played by dogs and wild Canidae as reservoirs of classical L.(L.) infantum, their significance in relation to the species causing CL in man is uncertain. One confusing difficulty is that L.(L.) infantum produces both cutaneous and visceral disease in dogs. In 1910 Wenyon (1911) was unable to identify any Leishmania in the skin or viscera of 110 wild dogs in Baghdad which was a major centre of CL due, almost certainly, to L.(L.) tropica. As Pringle (1957) recalled, subsequent investigators did find cutaneous infections in dogs in several cities of Iraq where CL was common. Visceral infections were not identified. Adler and Theodor (1930) produced a typical "Oriental sore" in a human volunteer with a canine isolate from Baghdad. From Pringle's (1957) data it appeared that Phlebotomus sergenti was the vector in cities where CL was prevalent and this fly is now accepted as being the most important species to transmit this parasite in the USSR and Middle East. Recently Al-Zahrani (personal communication) has made numerous isolates of L.(L.) tropica from patients in the Asir plateau of Saudi Arabia (altitude circa 2,000 m), as well as from two P.sergenti. These isolates are still in the process of being fully characterised by isoenzyme and DNA techniques.

Dogs may also harbour other species of Leishmania. In the Al-Ahsa area of Saudi Arabia (Elbihari et al., 1984; Peters et al., 1985) and Alexandria, Egypt (Morsy et al., 1987) L.(L.) major has been isolated from dogs, but only on a few occasions, suggesting that the dog is a victim, rather than a reservoir of infection with this parasite. These observations do, however, stress the need for biochemical or other typing of isolates from canids before concluding which parasite is present, just as in man. [In the New World the dog is also infected with L.(V.) braziliensis and L.(V.) peruviana as well as the visceralising L.(L.) chagasi.]

Vectors

Numerous references have been made above to known or suspected vectors of the different species of Leishmania. In the Lebanon, Israel, Syria and Iran, P.major is believed to be the most important vector of L.(L.) infantum. According to Saf'janova (1985), a species of the P.caucasicus group is believed to transmit this parasite in Turkmenia, whereas the most likely vectors in Kazakhistan are P.smirnovi and P.longiductus. P.kandelakii is suspected in Azerbaidjan and possibly in Armenian SSR, with P.perfiliewi transcaucasicus and P.brevis acting as vectors in parts of the former area.

P.papatasi is undoubtedly the most important and widely distributed host of L.(L.) major, with other species coming into prominence in some regions. Very high infection rates have been reported in Israel (20 to 50% - Schlein et al., 1982) and Saudi Arabia (21% - Killick-Kendrick et al., 1985a). P.salehi has been found infected in the west of India, P.caucasicus, P.andrejevi and P.mongolensis in the USSR. P.alexandri, P.grimmi and P.sergenti have been suspected in other parts of the Middle East (Lewis and Ward, 1987). It must be borne in mind again, however, that in most cases no definitive, eg, biochemical, characterisation has been carried out on many isolates, leaving some question as to their true identity. This remark applies also to reports that P.papatasi transmits L.(L.) tropica.

The vectors in nature of the unnamed Russian Leishmania and L.(L.) arabica are still undetermined. It is possible that a member of the P.caucasicus complex plays this role in the USSR and most likely that P.papatasi transmits L.(L.) arabica in the Eastern Province of Saudi Arabia.

Animal reservoirs

There is, as stated above, no doubt that dogs, domestic or feral, are the most important reservoir hosts of classical L.(L.) infantum, with various species of wild Canidae such as foxes and jackals serving as secondary reservoirs where they occur. The role of the dog as the reservoir of VL in Saudia Arabia has still to be confirmed, although it seems to be the most likely candidate. Whether any animal reservoir of significance exists for L.(L.) tropica is open to question. While both dogs and Rattus rattus have been found to harbour this parasite, both animals may only be victims rather than reservoirs of what is probably an anthroponosis.

The situation with L.(L.) major is also fairly clear. A variety of rodents serve as reservoir hosts in different parts of its range. In the USSR, adjacent parts of Iran and Afghanistan Rhombomys obesus is the predominant reservoir. The most important host in much of Saudi Arabia and Israel, as well as parts of North Africa such as Libya is Psammomys obesus, while various species of Meriones act as secondary hosts in these and other Middle East countries. Rattus rattus appears to play a role in parts of Israel and Jordan, while a few non-rodents such as hedgehogs, hares and mustelids have been found infected in the USSR, whether as reservoirs or victims is uncertain. L.(L.) major causes enzootics in the main reservoirs, infection rates of P.obesus in Israel (Greenblatt et al., 1985) and Saudi Arabia (Elbihari et al., 1984) probably approaching 100% in some foci. The masterly review of Ashford and Bettini (1987) should be consulted for further information on the ecology and epidemiology of the leishmaniases in the USSR and Middle East.

POSSIBILITIES FOR CONTROL

General principles

Before control measures can be considered at the community level it is necessary to analyse the epidemiological situation in the area involved. For this purpose the mathematical models and guidelines set out by Lysenko and Beljaev (1987) are invaluable. WHO (1984) and Vioukov (1987) have reviewed available control methods, relating them to control of the vectors, the parasites and the reservoirs, while Greenblatt (1985) and Gunders (1987) have focussed on the role of and approaches to vaccination. The treatment of individual patients is not dealt with in this paper (but see Bryceson, 1987).

Anthroponotic cutaneous leishmaniasis. Of all the forms of leishmaniasis, ACL is probably the easiest to control in the community. It occurs mainly in larger towns or settled villages in which the vectors bite in or near the houses. Flies such as P.sergenti are readily controlled by the use of such residual insecticides as DDT in dwellings. Sayedi-Rashti and Nadim (1975) showed that ACL in Iran could be markedly reduced as a "spinoff" from the use of this insecticide to kill malaria-carrying mosquitoes as, indeed, was ZCL carried by P.papatasi. The problem of the control of ACL, therefore, is essentially one of finance and organisation. Once under control there is no animal reservoir from which L.tropica can reappear even if P.sergenti returns. The main source of residual foci appears to be the relatively small number of people who develop the chronic form of infection, "leishmaniasis recidivans". The identification and treatment of infected individuals and especially those with chronic infections therefore becomes an integral part of any campaign to control the transmission of ACL. Health education is an essential measure in such a programme

Zoonotic cutaneous leishmaniasis. Unlike ACL, ZCL is the most difficult type of leishmaniasis to control. The use of residual insecticides is only effective up to a point, and makes no lasting impact on transmission since the vectors, P.papatasi in particular, which breed and rest in the burrows of infected rodents, rapidly return to bite man once the effect of the insecticides has been lost (Seyedi-Rashti and Nadim, 1975). Other means of vector control such as the pumping of DDT into the burrows of R.opimus, has only had a short-term effect (Vioukov, 1987). Insecticide resistance does not, so far, appear to have been an important obstacle to control.

The control measures most likely to succeed in the long term are biological methods designed to destroy or distance the animal reservoirs. In the USSR the destruction of the colonial burrows of R.opimus by deep ploughing or crushing, followed in some communities by the construction of a surrounding moat to prevent recolonisation, resulted in a massive decline of sandflies and the transmission of L.(L.) major. In Libya some degree of control was achieved by bulldozing and flooding the burrows of P.obesus but the long-term effects of this have not been documented. This rodent is entirely dependent upon various xerophytic plants such as species of Chenopodium for its food. In the Al-Ahsa focus of ZCL in Saudi Arabia a pilot scheme is planned in which all food plants within 2 km of the periphery of infected villages will be removed mechanically, the re-invasion of the plants then being maintained by labourers employed by the villages. It is hoped that this measure will force P.obesus to emigrate beyond the flight range of P.papatasi, or even diminish in numbers so as to reduce the reservoir of L.(L.) major, of rodent-feeding sandflies and hence of transmission to the human population of the area.

Visceral leishmaniasis. In addition to the identification and treatment of cases in medical centres, the detection of cases by serological surveying of known endemic areas forms an important part of any control campaign. The elimination of canid reservoirs is, however, one of the main means of reducing transmission and one that is particularly applicable where feral dogs, often existing in large packs in the Middle East, are involved. The outstanding example of the success of this method is the People's Republic of China where it was, in fact, domestic rather than feral dogs that were concerned (Leng, 1982). This campaign has been followed by the establishment of a surveillance system since 1970 (Wang, 1985).

The role of vaccination

Once healed, CL confers lifelong immunity against serious reinfection with homologous organisms, although minor, self-healing lesions can develop (Killick-Kendrick et al., 1985b). The recognition of this principle has encouraged efforts to employ active vaccination as a method of limiting the effects of CL where other control methods have failed, or as an accessory tool. This approach has been employed mainly against CL due to L.(L.) major. [Unfortunately, many papers describing experimental studies on immunity and immunisation have failed to distinguish between this species and L.(L.) tropica.] Of the several directions that have been followed, including the use of living promastigotes, attenuated vaccines and killed vaccines, the first has, to date, met with most success. Traditionally, for example in Iraq, children were exposed to sandfly bite where a lesion will show least (eg, the buttocks) (Greenblatt, 1985) or deliberately inoculated on an inconspicuous site with material from an ulcer on another child (Gunders, 1987). Vaccination campaigns were carried out from 1937 onwards among settlers in highly endemic ZCL areas of the USSR where more than 20,000 people were inoculated with promastigotes of virulent strains of L.(L.) major. The same method was later employed among Israeli settlers and soldiers. As Gunders (1987) pointed out, vaccination with virulent L.(L.) major strains was followed not only by cell-mediated immunity as reflected by a positive leishmanin skin test, but also by a positive serological response. Over the past few years well over a million Iranian soldiers and villagers have been given live vaccination with an average 70% of leishmanin conversions. So far, under natural challenge, the incidence in those vaccinated was 2.5% as against 14% in the non-vaccinated population. It must be noted, however, that between 2 and 3% of those vaccinated developed chronic lesions requiring specific therapy (Peters and Killick-Kendrick, 1987).

Although no data have been published recently on the use of killed vaccines in the USSR or Middle East, reports from Brazil indicate that a "cocktail" of New World species of Leishmania (Viannia) and Leishmania (Leishmania) has given a significant level of protection against natural challenge with L.(V.) guyanensis (Antunes et al., 1987).

To date it would appear that attenuated strains of L.(L.) major) are of little value for vaccination. However, evidence from field observations in the Al-Ahsa area of Saudi Arabia suggests that inapparent (ie, sub-clinical) infection with L.(L.) arabica may give active protection against subsequent infection with virulent strains of L.(L.) major. Studies are currently under way in our laboratory to explore this hypothesis. It seems likely that similar observations have been made in the USSR where it is understood that the unnamed Russian parasite is being considered for a similar investigation. Clearly the deployment of a live vaccine, virulent or attenuated, poses many logistical problems and a killed vaccine would be preferable. While many studies are currently under way to develop vaccines against VL and CL based on defined antigens, the use of whole organisms would appear, at present, to be the most rational since immunity against CL (if not also VL) is primarily cell-mediated. Defined antigens are most effective in inducing humoral immunity which seems to be the least important way of affording protection against the leishmaniases.

CONCLUSIONS

The leishmaniases in the USSR and Middle East are caused by different variants (zymodemes) of L.(L.) major, tropica and infantum. Three other parasites, L.(L.) gerbilli, arabica and an unnamed Russian parasite infect rodents. While VL caused by L.(L.) infantum can be controlled, primarily by destroying the canid reservoir, and the transmission of ACL due to L.(L.) tropica can be interrupted by the use of insecticides, the control of ZCL poses a much greater problem. The value of measures aimed against the vectors, the rodent reservoirs and against the parasites themselves are discussed. Species of Leishmania such as L.(L.) arabica that are normally non-pathogenic for man may have some value as live vaccines against virulent L.(L.) major.

ACKNOWLEDGEMENTS

The writer wishes to thank Dr.David Hart and the organisers for supporting his participation in this NATO-ASI meeting. His original studies in Saudi Arabia were funded in part by the King Abdulaziz City for Science and Technology in the context of the National Leishmaniasis Research Programme centred on King Faisal University, Dammam, and in part by the Ministry of Health, Riyadh. The Leishmaniasis Reference Centre in London is funded in part by the UNDP/World Bank/WHO Special Programme for Research and Training in Tropical Diseases.

REFERENCES

Adler, S. and Theodor, O., 1930, The inoculation of canine leishmaniasis into man, Ann.Trop.Med.Parasitol., 24:197.

Al-Hussayni, N.K., Rassam, M.B., Jawdat, S.Z. and Wahid, F.N., 1987, Numerical taxonomy of some Old World Leishmania species, Trans.R.Soc.Trop.Med.Hyg., 81:581.

Antunes, C.M.F., Mayrink, W., Magalhaes, P.A., Costa, C.A., Melo, M.N., Dias, M., Michalick, M.S.M., Williams, P., Lima, A.O., Vieira, J.B.F. and Schettini, A.P.M., 1986, Controlled field trials of a vaccine against New World cutaneous leishmaniasis, Int.J.Epidemiol., 15:572.

Ashford, R.W. and Bettini, S., 1987, Ecology and epidemiology: Old World, in: "The leishmaniases in biology and medicine. Vol.1 Biology and epidemiology", W.Peters and R.Killick-Kendrick, eds., Academic Press, London.

Bryceson, A., 1987, Therapy in man, in: "The leishmaniases in biology and medicine. Vol.2 Clinical aspects and control", W.Peters and R.Killick-Kendrick, eds., Academic Press, London.

Chance, M.L. and Walton, B.C., eds., 1982, "Biochemical characterization of Leishmania", UNDP/World Bank/WHO Special Programme for Research and Training in Tropical Diseases, Geneva.

Elbihari, S., Kawasmeh, Z.A. and Al Naiem, A.H., 1984, Possible reservoir host(s) of zoonotic cutaneous leishmaniasis in Al-Hassa oasis, Saudi Arabia, Ann.Trop.Med.Parasitol., 78:543.

Greenblatt, C.L., 1985, Vaccination for leishmaniasis, in: "Leishmaniasis", K-P. Chang and R.S.Bray, eds., Elsevier, Amsterdam, New York, Oxford.

Greenblatt, C.L., Schlein, Y. and Schnur, L.F., 1985, Leishmaniasis in Israel and vicinity, in: "Leishmaniasis", K-P. Chang and R.S.Bray, eds., Elsevier, Amsterdam, New York, Oxford.

Gunders, A.E., 1987, Vaccination: past and future role in control, in: "The leishmaniases in biology and medicine. Vol.2 Clinical aspects and control", W.Peters and R. Killick-Kendrick, eds., Academic Press, London.

Kellina, O.I., Passova, O.M., Saf'janova, V.M., Le Blancq, S.M. and Peters, W., 1985, A new leishmanial parasite of the great gerbil (Rhombomys opimus) in the USSR, Trans.R. Soc.Trop.Med.Hyg., 79:872.

Killick-Kendrick, R., Leaney, A.J., Peters, W., Rioux, J-A. and Bray, R.S., 1985a, Zoonotic cutaneous leishmaniasis in Saudi Arabia: the incrimination of Phlebotomus papatasi as the vector in the Al-Hassa oasis, Trans.R.Soc.Trop.Med. Hyg., 79:252.

Killick-Kendrick, R., Bryceson, A.D.M., Peters, W., Evans, D.A., Leaney. A.J. and Rioux, J-A., 1985b, Zoonotic cutaneous leishmaniasis in Saudi Arabia: lesions healing naturally in man followed by a second infection with the same zymodeme of Leishmania major, Trans.R.Soc.Trop.Med. Hyg., 79:363.

Lanotte, G., Rioux, J-A., Maazoun, R., Pasteur, N., Pratlong, F. and Lepart, J., 1981, Application de la méthode numérique à la taxonomie du genre *Leishmania* Ross, 1903. A propos de 146 souches originaires de l'Ancien Monde. Utilisation des allozymes. Corollaires épidémiologiques et phylétiques, Ann. Parasitol. (Paris), 56:575.

Lainson R. and Shaw, J.J., 1987, Evolution, classification and distribution, in: "The leishmaniases in biology and medicine. Vol.1 Biology and epidemiology," W.Peters and R.Killick-Kendrick, eds., Academic Press, London.

Le Blancq, S.M., "An epidemiological and taxonomic study of Old World *Leishmania* using isoenzymes", PhD thesis, University of London.

Le Blancq, S.M., Schnur, L.F. and Peters, W., 1986a, *Leishmania* in the Old World: 1. The geographical and hostal distribution of *L.major* zymodemes, Trans.R.Soc.Trop.Med.Hyg., 80:99.

Le Blancq, S.M. and Peters, W., 1986a, *Leishmania* in the Old World: 2. Heterogeneity among *L.tropica* zymodemes, Trans.R.Soc.Trop.Med.Hyg., 80:113.

Le Blancq, S.M. and Peters, W., 1986b, *Leishmania* in the Old World: 4. The distribution of *L.donovani* sensu lato zymodemes, Trans.R.Soc.Trop.Med.Hyg., 80:367.

Leng, Y., 1982, A review of kala-azar in China from 1949 to 1959, Trans.R.Soc.Trop.Med.Hyg., 76:531.

Lysenko, A.J. and Beljaev, A.E., 1987, Quantitative approaches to epidemiology, in: "The leishmaniases in biology and medicine. Vol.1 Biology and epidemiology", W.Peters and R.Killick-Kendrick, eds., Academic Press, London.

Morsy, T.A., Schnur, L.F., Feinsod, F.M., Salem, A.M., Wahba, M.M. and El Said, S.M., 1987, Natural infections of *Leishmania major* in domestic dogs from Alexandria, Egypt, Am.J.Trop.Med.Hyg., 37:49.

Peters, W., Elbihari, S., Ching Liu, Le Blancq, S.M., Evans, D.A., Killick-Kendrick, R., Smith, V. and Baldwin, C.I., 1985, *Leishmania* infecting man and wild animals in Saudi Arabia 1. General survey, Trans.R.Soc.Trop.Med.Hyg., 79:831.

Peters, W., Elbihari, S. and Evans, D.A., 1986, *Leishmania* infecting man and wild animals in Saudi Arabia. 2. *Leishmania arabica* n.sp., Trans.R.Soc.Trop.Med.Hyg., 80:497.

Peters, W. and Killick-Kendrick, R., eds., 1987, "The leishmaniases in biology and medicine. Vol. 2 Clinical aspects and control", p.941, Academic Press, London.

Pringle, G., 1957, Oriental sore in Iraq: historical and epidemiological problems, Bull. Endemic Dis., 2:41.

Saf'janova, V.M., 1985, Leishmaniasis in the USSR, in: "Leishmaniasis", K-P. Chang and R.S.Bray, eds., Elsevier, Amsterdam, New York, Oxford.

Schlein, Y., Warburg, A., Schnur, L.F. and Gunders, A.E., 1982, Leishmaniasis in the Jordan Valley II. Sandflies and transmission in the central endemic area, Trans.R.Soc.Trop.Med.Hyg., 76:582.

Seyedi-Rashti, M.A. and Nadim, A., 1975, Re-establishment of cutaneous leishmaniasis after cessation of anti-malaria spraying, Trop.Geog.Med., 27:79.

Sukkar, F., 1985, Leishmaniasis in the Middle East, in: "Leishmaniasis", K-P. Chang and R.S.Bray, eds., Elsevier, Amsterdam, New York, Oxford.

Vioukov, V.N., 1987, Control of transmission, in: "The

leishmaniases in biology and medicine. Vol.2 Clinical aspects and control", W.Peters and R.Killick-Kendrick, eds., Academic Press, London.

Wang, C-T., 1985, Leishmaniasis in China: epidemiology and control program, in: "Leishmaniasis", K-P. Chang and R.S.Bray, eds., Elsevier, Amsterdam, New York, Oxford.

Wang, J., Qu, J-q. and Guan, Li-r., 1964, A study on the Leishmania parasite of the big gerbil in northeast China, Acta Parasitol. Sinica, 1:105.

Wenyon, C.M., 1911, Oriental sore in Bagdad, together with observations on a gregarine in Stegomyia fasciata, the haemogregarine of dogs and the flagellates of house flies. Parasitology, 4:273.

WHO, 1984, The leishmaniases, Techn. Rep. Ser. No.701, WHO, Geneva.

EPIDEMIOLOGY OF MEDITERRANEAN LEISHMANIASIS CAUSED BY LEISHMANIA INFANTUM: ISOENZYME AND kDNA ANALYSIS FOR THE IDENTIFICATION OF PARASITES FROM MAN, VECTORS AND RESERVOIRS

M. Gramiccia, L. Gradoni and M.C. Angelici

Istituto Superiore di Sanita
Department of Parasitology
Viale Regina Elena 299
00161 Rome
Italy

INTRODUCTION

Leishmania infantum Nicolle, 1908, has been considered in the past as the aethiological agent of human visceral leishmaniasis (VL) and canine leishmaniasis (CanL) in the Mediterranean basin. Biochemical techniques like isoenzyme electrophoresis, which were developed since the seventies for the identification of Leishmania isolates, have shown that L.infantum is also the cause of human cutaneous leishmaniasis in wide areas of the Mediterranean regions. Furthermore, new mammalian reservoirs of the parasite have been identified, and a number of Phlebotomus species (belonging to subgenus Laroussius) have been definitively incriminated as vectors, having previously been suspected on epidemiological grounds.

In the present note, the contributions of isoenzyme electrophoresis and kDNA analysis techniques to the study of the epidemiology of leishmaniasis by L.infantum in the Mediterranean areas are reviewed.

MATERIALS AND METHODS

Isolation

The techniques employed for the isolation and maintenance of parasites which have been subsequently typed as L.infantum *sensu lato* are as follows:

In vivo isolation. In vivo parasite isolation has been attempted through inoculation of infected material in outbred hamster (Bettini et al., 1980, 1986; Abranches et al., 1983; Rioux et al., 1985). Inbred LHC hamsters (Charles River, Massachussets), cortisone-treated, were used for the isolation of Italian dermotropic parasites which showed difficulty in growing in vitro (Pozio et al., 1985a). Balb/c mice were also used for the laboratory maintenance of strains isolated.

In vitro isolation. Different culture media were used for the primary culture of L.infantum: NNN (Nicolle, 1908) by Maazoun et al. (1981), Abranches et al. (1983) and Belazzoug et al. (1985); Tobie (Tobie et al., 1950) by Gramiccia et al. (1982) and Tzamouranis et al. (1984); EMTM (Evans, 1978) by Le Blancq and Peters (1986) and Gramiccia et al. (1984, 1987); BHI-CCS (Rioux et al., 1970) by Ben Ismail et al. (1986); Schneider (Hendricks et al., 1978) by Gramiccia et al. (1984, 1987). When strains showed difficulty in growing in vitro, two culture media, Schneider and EMTM, in sequence have been tried (Gramiccia et al., 1987); "sloppy Evans" (Evans et al., 1984) by Gramiccia (unpublished).

In vitro maintenance. Parasites and mass cultures were maintained in the aforementioned media, as well as in a number of liquid media, such as HO-MEM (Chance et al., 1977; Schnur et al., 1981), MEM (Le Blancq and Peters, 1986) and Grace (Gramiccia et al., 1985).

The selective property of some culture media (which are commonly employed in several laboratories) on different L.infantum stocks has been tested by us. Mixed parasite suspensions containing different ratios (9/1, 1/1, 1/9) of amastigotes or promastigotes of dermotropic and viscerotropic strains enzymatically characterized, were seeded into EMTM, BHI and Schneider's media. Different incubation periods and sub-inoculations were tested (Gramiccia, unpublished).

Parasite Characterization. The Leishmania characterization techniques which have been widely used in epidemiological investigations carried out in the Mediterranean basin and which allowed the identification of L. infantum from various hosts are isoenzyme electrophoresis and restriction enzyme kDNA analysis.

Isoenzyme electrophoresis. In Table 1 the technique employed for isoenzyme electrophoresis and the number of enzymes tested by different authors are reported. Twenty enzymes were examined: PGM, GPI, ASAT, G6PD, GPGD, ME, MDH, MPI, ICD, HK, FH, NH, ES, GD, GLUD, SOD, PEPD, PK, DIA. The WHO recommended reference strains (WHO, 1984) used were: MHOM/TN/80/IPT1 for L.infantum, MHOM/IN/80/DD8 for L.donovani, MHOM/SU/74/K27 and MHOM/SU/58/STRAIN-OD for L.tropica, MHOM/IL/67/JERICHO II, MHOM/SU/73/5ASKH and MRHO/SU/59/P-strain for L.major and MHOM/ET/72/L100 for L.aethiopica. Local reference strains were used for the analysis of particular enzymic variants: MHOM/FR/78/LEM75 and MCAN/TN/78/LEM78 for L.infantum infantum ZMON1=ZLON49, MHOM/FR/80/LEM189 for L.infantum ZMON11, MHOM/DZ/82/LIPA59 for L.infantum ZMON24.

Restriction enzymes kDNA analysis. This technique was employed by us for the identification of 29 stocks representing different L.infantum zymodemes. The technique for the kDNA extraction was that described by Morel and Simpson (1980). Eight restriction enzymes were employed:

AluI, BamHI, HindIII, HinfI, MspI, TaqI and HaeIII. All digests were performed under the conditions suggested by the manufacturer (Boehringer). Digestions were carried out overnight. 2% agarose plus 1 µg/ml ethidium bromide gels were run in Tris-borate/EDTA (TBE).

TABLE 1. ISOENZYME ANALYSIS OF LEISHMANIA INFANTUM

TECHNIQUE	NO. OF ENZYMES	REFERENCES
THIN-LAYER STARCH-GEL ELECTROPHORESIS	4-13	Chance et al., 1977; Schnur et al., 1981; Tzamouranis et al., 1984; Le Blancq & Peters, 1986
THICK-LAYER STARCH-GEL ELECTROPHORESIS	8-12	Maazoun et al., 1981; Gramiccia et al., 1984
POLYACRYLAMIDE GEL DISC ELECTROPHORESIS	1	Chance et al., 1977; Schnur et al 1981; Tzamouranis et al., 1984

RESULTS

Isolation

Some Leishmania stocks were obtained by isolation in outbred hamsters, such as those from black rats (Rattus rattus) and Ph. perniciosus in Italy (Bettini et al., 1980, 1986; Pozio et al., 1981). Primary isolation in LHC hamsters was the only method by which cultures of Italian dermotropic strains were established (Pozio et al., 1985a).

Most isolates were obtained in blood-agar media (Maazoun et al., 1981; Belazzoug, 1984; Gramiccia et al., 1982, 1984, 1987, unpublished data; Evans, D.A., personal communication; Le Blancq and Peters, 1986; Ben Ismail et al., 1986). These media were shown to be much more effective than liquid media for primary isolation of L.infantum. However, the inoculum of an infected LHC hamster spleen in Schneider's medium was essential in establishing cultures of dermotropic Italian strains, to be subsequently maintained in EMTM (Gramiccia et al., 1987).

The experiments on the selective property of culture media (Table 2) showed that blood-agar media selected viscerotropic strains, whereas Schneider's medium (liquid medium) selected dermotropic strains (unpublished data).

Parasite Characterization
Isoenzyme characterization. The results obtained by several authors in the isoenzyme characterization of L.infantum stocks from the Mediterranean basin are reported in Tables 3 and 4. Stocks were isolated from human visceral and cutaneous leishmaniasis cases, as well as from dog, fox (Vulpes vulpes), black rat (Rattus rattus) and three sandfly

species belonging to the subgenus Laroussius (Ph. ariasi, Ph. perniciosus, Ph.perfiliewi). Nine zymodemes were identified. One of them, corresponding to L.infantum.st. was classified both by the Reference Centre of Montpellier (ZMON1) and by the Reference Centre of London (ZLON49). The remaining 8 zymodemes were classified by the Montpellier Centre only. In Table 5 the enzymes discriminating between different zymodemes are reported.

Restriction enzyme kDNA analysis. Twenty-nine stocks, including the WHO reference strain for L.infantum, were examined through kDNA analysis with restriction enzymes (Table 6). The stocks were isolated from human VL (10) and CL (6) cases, 6 from dogs, 4 from black rats (R.rattus) and 3 from sandflies (Ph.perniciosus and Ph.perfiliewi). In Table 7 the results of schizodeme analysis compared with those of

TABLE 2. MIXED PARASITE POPULATION COMPOSED OF A VISCERTROPIC (ZMON1=ZLON49) AND A DERMOTROPIC (ZMON24) LEISHMAANIA INFANTUM STRAIN INOCULATED INTO THREE DIFFERENT CULTURE MEDIA. ZYMODEME ANALYSIS OF THE STRAINS OBTAINED

MEDIUM	ZMON1/ZMON24 RATIO IN THE INOCULUM.			INCUBATION PERIOD	ZYMODEME
BLOOD-AGAR (EMTM,BHI)	1/9	1/1	9/1	SHORT	ZMON1=ZLON49
				LONG	
LIQUID (Schneider's)	1/9	1/1	9/1	SHORT	ZMON24
				LONG	

zymodeme analysis are reported. In Table 8 the kDNA restriction enzymes by which each schizodeme was identified are shown. Eight schizodemes have been found, distinguished through 1-4 restriction enzymes. Most viscerotropic stocks, including the reference strain for L.infantum, were found to belong to one schizodeme (S1) (Angelica, unpublished).

TABLE 3. ISOENZYME CHARACTERIZATION OF LEISHMANIA INFANTUM STOCKS ISOLATED FROM MAN IN THE MEDITERRANEAN BASIN

PATHOLOGY	ZYMODEME	PLACE OF ORIGIN	REFERENCES
VISCERAL	ZMON1=ZLON49	ALGERIA	Belazzoug, 1982; 1984; 1986; Lanotte et al., 1981
		CYPRUS	Schnur et al., 1981
		EGYPT	Schnur, 1986
		FRANCE	Maazoun et al., 1981; Lanotte et al., 1981
		GREECE	Tzamouranis et al., 1984; Le Blancq and Peters, 1986
		ISRAEL	Schnur et al., 1981;
		ITALY	Gramiccia et al., 1982; 1984; Le Blancq and Peters, 1986
		MALTA	Schnur et al., 1981
		TUNISIA	Lanotte et al., 1981; Ben Ismail et al., 1986
	ZMON27	ITALY	Gramiccia et al., 1984
	ZMON72	ITALY	Gradoni et al., in press
	ZMON??	SPAIN	Gallego and Portus, 1984
	ZMON24	TUNISIA	Gramiccia, unpublished
CUTANEOUS	ZMON1=ZLON49	FRANCE	Rioux et al., 1980; 1986
		ITALY	Gramiccia et al., 1984; 1986
	ZMON11	FRANCE	Lanotte et al., 1981
	ZMON24	ALGERIA	Belazzoug et al., 1985b
		ITALY	Gramiccia et al., 1986; 1987
	ZMON24 MPI variant (to be named)	ITALY	Gramiccia, unpublished
	ZMON29	FRANCE	Rioux et al., 1986
		SPAIN	Gallego and Portus, 1984
	ZMON33	FRANCE	Moreno et al., 1984

TABLE 4. CHARACTERIZATION OF LEISHMANIA INFANTUM STOCKS ISOLATED FROM MAMMALS AND PHLEBOTOMINE VECTORS

HOST	ZYMODEME	PLACE OF ORIGIN	REFERENCES
DOG	ZMON1=ZLON49	ALGERIA	Belazzoug, 1984; 1986
		EGYPT	Azab et al., 1984
		FRANCE	Maazoun et al., 1981; Lanotte et al., 1981
		GREECE	Tzamouranis et al., 1984; Le Blancq and Peters, 1986
		ITALY	Gramiccia et al., 1982; 1984; Lanotte et al., 1981 Le Blancq and Peters, 1986
		MALTA	Gradoni, unpublished
		PORTUGAL	Lanotte et al., 1981; Abranches et al., 1984; Le Blancq and Peters, 1986
		SPAIN	Lanotte et al., 1981; Gallego and Portus, 1981
		TUNISIA	Maazoun et al., 1981; Ben Ismail et al., 1986
VULPES VULPES		PORTUGAL	Abranches et al., 1983; 1984
RATTUS RATTUS		ITALY	Gramiccia et al., 1982
		SPAIN	Gonzalez Castro et al., 1987
PHLEBOTOMUS ARIASI		FRANCE	Rioux et al., 1984
PH. PERNICIOSUS		ITALY	Bettini et al., 1986; Maroli et al., in preparation
PH. PERFILIEWI		ITALY	Maroli et al., 1987

TABLE 5. ENZYMES DISCRIMINATING BETWEEN LEISHMANIA INFANTUM ZYMODEMES

ZYMODEME	MARKER ENZYME
ZMON1=ZLON49	$G6PD_{100}$, PGM_{100}, MPI_{100}, NH_{100}
ZMON24	NH_{140}
ZMON27	NH_{130}
ZMON33	$G6PD_{105}$
ZMON72	PGM_{109}
ZMON11	$G6PD_{105}$, NH_{130}
ZMON24 MPI variant	$MPI_{100/117}$, NH_{140}
ZMON29	$G6PD_{105}$, NH_{140}
ZMON??	$G6PD_{102}$, NH_{140}

TABLE 6. ORIGIN OF 29 LEISHMANIA INFANTUM STOCKS EXAMINED FOR SCHIZODEME ANALYSIS

HOST	PATHOLOGY	LOCALITY
MAN	VL	ITALY
		TUNISIA
	CL	ITALY
		FRANCE
DOG	CANL	ITALY
		MALTA
RATTUS RATTUS	VL	ITALY
PHLEBOTOMUS PERNICIOSUS		ITALY
PH.PERFILIEWI		ITALY

TABLE 7. RESULTS OF SCHIZODEME ANALYSIS OF LEISHMANIA INFANTUM STOCKS COMPARES WITH ZYMODEME ANALYSIS

NO.OF STOCKS	TROPISM	SCHIZODEME	ZYMODEME
18	VISCEROTROPIC	S1	ZMON1=ZLON49
2		S2	ZMON1=ZLON49
1		S3	ZMON1=ZLON49
1		S4	ZMON27
1		S5	ZMON24
3	DERMOTROPIC	S	ZMON11; ZMON24
1		S	ZMON24
1		S	ZMON24
1		S	ZMON1=ZLON49

TABLE 8. kDNA RESTRICTION ENZYMES BY WHICH DIFFERENT SCHIZODEMES WERE IDENTIFIED

SCHIZODEME	MARKER kDNA RESTRICTION ENZYMES
S1	$AluI_a$, $BamHI_a$, $HaeIII_a$, $HinfI_a$, $MspI_a$, $TaqI_a$
S2	$HaeIII_b$
S3	$HinfI_b$
S4	$MspI_b$, $TaqI_b$
S5	$HaeIII_c$
S6	$TaqI_c$
S7	$AluI_b$, $BamHI_b$, $HaeIII_c$, $HinfI_c$
S8	$AluI_c$, $HaeIII_d$, $HinfI_d$

note: a, b, c and d represent different banding patterns.

TABLE 9. EPIDEMIOLOGICAL CHARACTERISTICS OF A VL FOCUS BY LEISHMANIA INFANTUM

PATHOLOGY	VL
CANINE LEISHMANIASIS	PRESENT, FREQUENTLY WITH HIGH PREVALENCES
WILD LEISHMANIASES	PRESENT
PROVEN VECTOR	PHLEBOTOMUS ARIASI
	PH.PERNICIOSUS
	PH.LONGICUSPIS
SUSPECTED VECTOR	PH.PERFILIEWI
	PH.MAJOR
	PH.TOBBI
PREVALENT ZYMODEME	ZMON1=ZLON49

DISCUSSION

The isolation and the biochemical characterization of L.infantum stocks have extended, and also even complicated, the epidemiological picture of leishmaniasis due to this species. L.infantum has been confirmed as being genetically different from L.donovani (Lanotte et al., 1981; Moreno et al., 1984), and it was found to cause both visceral and cutaneous leishmaniasis.

Visceral leishmaniasis

The distribution of VL in the Mediterranean basin should coincide with that of L.infantum. However, in Yugoslavia, Albania, Turkey, Lebanon and Libya the presence of L.infantum as the agent of VL is suspected on the basis of clinical and epidemiological findings only.

The zymodeme which shows the higher prevalence is ZMON1=ZLON49, which was isolated from man, dog, wild mammals and sandflies. Other viscerotropic zymodemes have been isolated from man only, in Italy (Gramiccia et al., 1984, 1985; Gradoni et al., in press), Spain (Gallego and Portus, 1984) and Tunisia (unpublished data). In Italy and Tunisia, these viscerotropic enzymatic variants represent about 18% of stocks examined.

Generally, the kDNA analysis seems to confirm the results of the symodeme analysis, though on some stocks it provides further information.

The dog was confirmed to be the domestic reservoir of visceral leishmaniasis, but the isolation of L.infantum from black rats and foxes supports the hypothesis of a sylvatic cycle of this parasite (Gradoni et al., 1983; Abranches et al., 1983). The proven vectors of VL in the Mediterranean area are Ph.ariasi, Ph.perniciosus, Ph.longicuspis, Ph.major syriacus and Ph.tobbi (Rioux et al., 1984; Adler and Theodor, 1935; Pozio et al., 1985b; Bettini et al., 1986; WHO, 1984; Maroli et al., in preparation). Suspected vectors are Ph.major neglectus and Ph.perfiliewi (WHO, 1984). A typical Mediterranean VL focus can be characterized as in Table 9.

Cutaneous leishmaniasis

The distribution of cutaneous leishmaniasis due to L.infantum in the Mediterranean basin is shown in Figure 1. Dermotropic L.infantum appears to be distributed in the Central-Western Mediterranean area. The isolation of L.infantum only from CL cases in the North-Western Mediterranean, supports the hypothesis of the absence of L.tropica and L.major in this area.

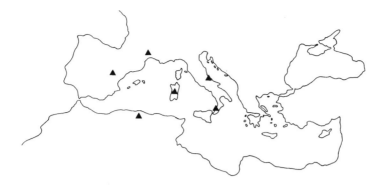

FIGURE 1   DISTRIBUTION OF DERMOTROPIC LEISHMANIA INFANTUM IN THE MEDITERRANEAN BASIN

The parasites isolated from CL cases belong to 6 different zymodemes: ZMON1=ZLON49, ZMON11, ZMON24, ZMON24 MPI variant (to be named), ZMON29 and ZMON33. One of them (ZMON1) is enzymatically identical to the agent of VL. In Italy, this zymodeme represents 21% of stocks isolated from CL cases. The other dermotropic zymodemes differ from ZMON1=ZLON49 for 1-3 enzymes (Table 5). The geographical distribution of each zymodeme appears to be a limited one, except for ZMON24 which was isolated both in Algeria and Italy. The recent identification of a stock from an infantile VL case in Tunisia as belonging to this zymodeme is of interest.

The cutaneous lesions retained as due to L.infantum are usually single ones, varying from inpetigous to ulcerative forms. The incubation period is very long, lasting from 1 to 3 years (Belazzoug et al., 1985; Rioux et al., 1985; unpublished observations of the authors). Considering that, for instance, the annual number of CL cases recorded in Italy (40-50) is about twice the number of VL cases (20-30), and assuming that all CL cases are due to L.infantum, this species cannot be considered any more an exclusively viscerotropic parasite.

Dermotropic parasites enzymatically different from ZMON1=ZLON49 have never been found in domestic or wild mammals, and in sandflies (Pozio et al., 1982; Rioux et al., 1985). Thus, the reservoir(s) and the vector(s) of these variant zymodemes are still unknown. L.infantum ZMON1=ZLON49 was isolated from Ph.perfiliewi in a typical CL focus at Abruzzi, Italy, where the disease was mainly due to variant zymodemes (Maroli et al., 1987). The sandfly species which have been suspected to transmit dermotropic L.infantum are Ph.ariasi in France (Rioux et al., 1985), Ph.perniciosus in Spain (Martinez-Ortega, 1984) and in Algeria (Belazzoug et al., 1985a) and Ph.longicuspis in Algeria (Belazzoug et al., 1985a).

Table 10 shows the association of intrinsic and extrinsic characters (Peters, 1980) of Italian viscerotropic and dermotropic *L.infantum* zymodemes. From this association, it appears that the dermotropic stocks enzymatically identical to ZMON1=ZLON49 show extrinsic characters different from those of viscerotropic zymodemes but similar to those of the other dermotropic zymodemes. Therefore, dermotropic ZMON1=ZLON49 could be genetically different from viscerotropic parasites belonging to the same zymodeme. It is also possible that this difference could not be revealed through electrophoresis of the enzymes so far examined. This hypothesis is supported also by preliminary data on kDNA analysis (Table 6).

The existence of mixed populations of different *L.infantum* zymodemes circulating through the same vector(s) and reservoir(s), as already shown by Kellina et al., (1985) in *L.major* cannot be excluded. This eventuality arises from the data on *L.infantum* recently reported by Rioux et al., (1986). If this is so, the use of highly selective culture media would eliminate some of the components of a mixed population.

The use of a technique which would reveal genetic differences in parasite populations directly from infected material, thus excluding a selective process due to culture, is therefore needed. A promising technology is that of recombinant DNA, by which rare or unique repetitive sequences are identified and used as probes (Barker and Butcher, 1983; Barker et al., 1985). Preliminary work with the objective of identifying specific probes from stocks representative of dermotropic *L.infantum* zymodemes, is being carried out in collaboration with Dr D. Smith and Dr P.D. Ready of Imperial College, London.

TABLE 10. EXTRINSIC CHARACTERS OF LEISHMANIA INFANTUM ZYMODEMES FOUND IN ITALY. VL: VISCERAL LEISHMANIA; CL: CUTANEOUS LEISHMANIASIS

ZYMODEME	HOST	CLINICAL OUTCOME	BEHAVIOUR IN VITRO	BEHAVIOUR IN VIVO
MON27	MAN	VL		
MON72	MAN	VL	EASILY ISOLATED IN BLOOD-AGAR MEDIA. SLOW GROWTH IN INSECT TISSUE CULTURE MEDIA.	EASILY ISOLATED IN OUTBRED SYRIAN HAMSTER. VISCERALIZATION OF PARASITES.
MON1	MAN, DOG, RATTUS RATTUS, PHLEBOTOMUS PERNICIOSUS PH. PERFILIEWI	VL		
	MAN	CL		
MON24	MAN	CL	EXTREMELY DIFFICULT TO ISOLATE IN BLOOD-AGAR MEDIA. FAST AND TRANSIENT GROWTH IN INSECT TISSUE CULTURE MEDIA.	ISOLATED ONLY IN CORTISONE-TREATED LHC INBRED HAMSTER. VISCERALIZATION OF PARASITES.
MON24 MPI VARIANT	MAN	CL		

REFERENCES

Abranches, P., Conceição Silva, F. M., and Silva Pereira, M. C. D., 1984, Le foyer de leishmaniose viscérale de la Région de Lisbonne. Application du typage enzymatique des souches y isolées à l'interpretation de sa structure. Proc.Int.Coll.Taxonom.Phylog.Leishmania, Montpellier, 1984.

Abranches, P., Conceição Silva, F. M., Ribeiro, M. M. S., Lopes, F. J., and Teixeira Gomes, L., 1983, Kala-azar in Portugal-IV. The wild reservoir: the isolation of a Leishmania from a fox, Trans.R.Soc.Trop.Med.Hyg., 77:420.

Adler, S., and Theodor, O., 1935, Investigation on Mediterranean kala-azar.IX. Feeding experiments with Phlebotomus perniciosus and other species on animals infected with Leishmania infantum, Proc.R.Soc., London(B), 116:516.

Azab, M. E., Rifaat, M. A., Schnur, L. F., Makhlouf, S. A., El Sherif, E., and Salem, A. M., 1984, Canine and rodent leishmanial isolates from Egypt, Trans.R.Soc.Trop.Med.Hyg., 78:263.

Barker, D. C., and Butcher, J., 1983, The use of DNA probes in the identification of leishmaniasis: discrimination between isolates of the Leishmania mexicana and L. braziliensis complexes, Trans.R.Soc.Trop.Med.Hyg., 77:285.

Barker, D. C., Butcher, J., Gibson, L. J., and Williams, R. H., 1985, Characterization of Leishmania sp. by DNA hybridization probes. A laboratory manual of simplified methods. UNDP/WORLD BANK/WHO/TDR.

Belazzoug, S., 1984, La leishmaniose en Algérie à travers l'identification des souches, Proc.Int.Coll.Taxonom.Phylog. Leishmania, Montpellier, 1984.

Belazzoug, S., 1986, Leishmania infantum, causative organism of visceral leishmaniasis at Biskra (Algeria), Trans.R.Soc.Trop. Med.Hyg., 80:1002.

Belazzoug, S., and Tabet-Derraz, O., 1982, La leishmaniose viscérale en Algérie. Récensement de cas diagnostiques entre 1975 et 1980, Bull.Soc.Path.Ex., 75:169.

Belazzoug, S., Ammar-Khodja, A., Belkaid, M., and Tabet-Derraz, O., 1985a, La leishmaniose cutanée du Nord de l'Algérie, Bull.Soc.Path.Ex., 78:615.

Belazzoug, S., Lanotte, G., Maazoun, R., Pratlong, F., and Rioux, J. A., 1985b, Un nouveau variant enzymatique de Leishmania infantum Nicolle, 1908, agent de la leishmaniose cutanée du Nord de l'Algérie. Ann.Parasitol.Hum.Comp., 60:1.

Ben Ismail, R., Gramiccia, M., Gradoni, L., Ben Saìd, M., and Ben Rachid, M. S., 1986, Identificazione biochimica di isolati di Leishmania dalla Tunisia, XIV Congr.Naz.Soc.It.Parassitologia, Pisa, 21-24 May, 1986, Parassitologia, in press.

Bettini, S., Pozio, E., and Gradoni, L., 1980, Leishmaniasis in Tuscany (Italy): (II) Leishmania from wild Rodentia and Carnivora in a human and canine leishmaniasis focus, Trans.R.Soc.Trop.Med.Hyg., 74:77.

Bettini, S., Gramiccia, M., Gradoni, L., and Atzeni, M.C., 1986, Leishmaniasis in Sardinia: II. Natural infection of Phlebotomus perniciosus Newstead 1911, by Leishmania infantum Nicolle, 1908, in the province of Cagliari, Trans.R.Soc.Trop.Med.Hyg., 80:458.

Chance, M. L., Gardener, P. J. and Peters, W., 1977, Biochemical taxonomy of Leishmania as an ecological tool. in: "Ecologie des Leishmanioses", Coll.Int.C.N.R.S., N.239.

Evans, D. A., 1978, Kinetoplastida, in: "Methods of cultivating parasites in vitro," A. E. R. Taylor, and J. R. Baker, eds., Academy Press, London.

Evans, D. A., Lanham, S. M., Baldwin, C. I., and Peters, W., 1984, The isolation and isoenzyme characterization of Leishmania braziliensis subsp. from patients with cutaneous leishmaniasis acquired in Belize, Trans.R.Soc.Trop.Med.Hyg., 78:35.

Gallego, J., and Portus, M., 1984, Etude preliminaire de la leishmaniose humaine et canine en Catalogne-Sud: à propos de l'étude enzymatique de quatre souches, Proc.Int.Coll.Taxonom. Phylog.Leishmania, Montpellier, 1984.

Gonzales Castro, J., Morillas Marquez, F., and Benavides Delgado, I., 1987, Leishmania infantum s.str., parasite du rat noir (Rattus rattus). A propos du typage enzymatique d'une souche isolée en Espagne, dans la province de Grenade, Ann.Parasitol.Hum.Comp., 62:101.

Gradoni, L., Gramiccia, M., Pettoello, M., Di Martino, L., and Nocerino, A., in press, A new Leishmania infantum enzymatic variant, agent of an urban visceral case unresponsive to drugs, Trans.R.Soc.Trop.Med.Hyg.

Gradoni, L., Pozio, E., Gramiccia, M., Maroli, M., and Bettini, S., 1983, Leishmaniasis in Tuscany (Italy). VII. Studies on the role of the black rat, Rattus rattus, in the epidemiology of visceral leishmaniasis. Trans.R.Soc.Trop.Med.Hyg., 77:427.

Gramiccia, M., Gradoni, L., and Bettini, S., 1986, Focolai di leishmaniosi cutanea da Leishmania infantum s.l. in Italia, XIV Congr.Naz.Soc.It. Parassitologia, Pisa, 21-24 May, 1986, Parassitologia, in press.

Gramiccia, M., Gradoni, L., and Pozio, E., 1984, Charactérisation enzymatique des leshmanies isolées en Italie. Proc.Int.Coll. Taxonom.Phylog.Leishmania, Montpellier, 1984.

Gramiccia, M., Gradoni, L., and Pozio, E., 1985, Il genere Leishmania in Italia, Parassitologia, 27:187.

Gramiccia, M., Gradoni, L., and Pozio, E., 1987, Leishmania infantum sensu lato as an agent of cutaneous leishmaniasis in Abruzzi region (Italy), Trans.R.Soc.Trop.Med.Hyg., 81:235.

Gramiccia, M., Maazoun, R., Lanotte, G., Rioux, J. A., Le Blancq, S., Evans, D. A., Peters, W., Bettini, S., Gradoni, L., and Pozio, E., 1982, Typage enzymatique de onze souche de Leishmania isolées, en Italie Continentale, à partir de formes viscérales murines, canines et vulpines. Mise en evidence d'un variant enzymatique chez le Renard (Vulpes vulpes) et le Chien, Ann.Parasitol.Hum.Comp., 57:527.

Hendricks, L. D., Wood, D. E., and Hajduk, M. E., 1978, Haemoflagellates: commercially available liquid media for rapid cultivation, Parasitology, 76: 309.

Kellina, O. I., Passova, O. M., Saf'yanova, V. M., Le Blancq, S., and Peters, W., 1985, A new leishmanial parasite of the great gerbil (Rhombomys opimus) in the USSR, Trans.R.Soc.Trop.Med. Hyg., 79:872.

Lanotte, G., Rioux, J. A., Maazoun, R., Pasteur, N., Pratlong, F., and Lepart, J., 1981, Application de la methode numérique à la taxonomie du genre Leishmania Ross, 1903. A propos de 146 souches de l'Ancien Monde. Utilisation des allozymes. Corollaires épidémiologiques et phylétiques. Ann.Parasitol.Hum. Comp., 56:575.

Le Blancq, S. M., and Peters, W., 1986, Leishmania in the Old World; 4. The distribution of L. donovani sensu lato zymodemes, Trans.R.Soc.Trop.Med.Hyg., 80:367.

Maazoun, R., Lanotte, G., Pasteur, N., Rioux, J. A., Kennou, M. F., and Pratlong,, F., 1981, Ecologie des leshimanioses dans le Sud de la France. 16. Contribution à l'analyse chimiotaxonomique des parasites de la leishmaniose viscérale méditerranéenne. A propos de 55 souches isolées en Cévennes, Côte d'Azur, Corse et Tunisie, Ann.Parasitol.Hum.Comp., 56:131

Maroli, M., Gramiccia, M., and Gradoni, L., 1987, Natural infection of Phlebotomus perfiliewi with Leishmania infantum in a cutaneous leishmaniasis focus of the Abruzzi region, Italy, Trans.R.Soc. Trop.Med.Hyg., 81: 596.

Maroli, M., Gramiccia, M., Gradoni, L., Ready, P.D., Smith, D. F., and Aquino, C., in preparation, A survey on natural infection of phlebotomine sandflies with Leishmania spp. in Central and South Italy.

Martinez-Ortega, E., 1984, Phlebotomus perniciosus, Newstead, 1911, posible vector le la leishmaniasis cutanea (Dipt.Psychod.), Rev.Iber.Parasitol., 44:59.

Morel, C., and Simpson, L., 1980, Characterization of pathogenic Trypanosomatidae by restriction endonuclease finger-printing of kinetoplast DNA minicircles, Am.J.Trop.Med.Hyg., 29 (Suppl.): 1070.

Moreno, G., Lanotte, G., Rioux, J. A., and Maazoun, R., 1984, Leishmania infantum Nicolle, 1908, complexe systematique ? Proc.Int.Coll.Taxonom.Phylog.Leishmania, Montpellier, 1984.

Nicolle, C., 1908, Culture du parasite du Bouton d'Orient, C.R.Acad. Sci.Paris, 146:842.

Peters, W., 1982, Introduction to the workshop, in: "Biochemical characterization of Leishmania", M. L. Chance, and B. C. Walton, eds., UNDP/WORLD BANK/WHO/TDR.

Pozio, E., Gramiccia, M., Gradoni, L., and Amerio, P., 1985a, Isolation of the agent causing cutaneous leishmaniasis in Italy and its visceralization in inbred hamsters, Trans.R.Soc.Trop. Med.Hyg., 79:260.

Pozio, E., Gradoni, L., Bettini, S., and Gramiccia, M., 1981, Leishmaniasis in Tuscany (Italy): V. Further isolation of Leishmania from Rattus rattus in the province of Grosseto, Ann.Trop.Med.Parasitol., 75:393.

Pozio, E., Maroli, M., Gradoni, L., and Gramiccia, M., 1985b, Laboratory transmission of Leishmania infantum to Rattus rattus by the bite of experimentally infected Phlebotomus perniciosus, Trans.R.Soc.Trop.Med.Hyg., 79:524.

Pozio, E., Gradoni, L., Gramiccia, M., Bettini, S., and Pampiglione, S., 1982, The "puzzle" of cutaneous leishmaniasis epidemiology in Italy, Acta Medit.Patol.Inf.Trop., 1:109.

Rioux, J. A., Lanotte, G., Dedet, J. P., and Martini-Dumas, A., 1970, Utilisation du milieu "coeur-cerveau-sang de mouton" pour la culture en masse de formes promastigotes des Leishmanies, Ann.Parasitol.Hum.Comp., 45:381.

Rioux, J. A., Jarry, D. M., Lanotte, G., Maazoun, R., and Killick-Kendrick, R., 1984, Ecologie des Leishmanioses dans le Sud de la France. 18. Identification enzymatique de Leishmania infantum Nicolle, 1908, isolé de Phlebotomus ariasi Tonnoir, 1921, spontanément infesté en Cevennes, Ann.Parasitol.Hum. Comp., 59:331.

Rioux, J. A., Lanotte, G., Maazoun, R., Perello, R., and Pratlong, F., 1980, Leishmania infantum Nicolle, 1908, agent du Bouton d'Orient autochtone. A propos de l'identification biochimique de deux souches isolées dans le Pyrénées-Orientales, C.R.Acad. Sci.Paris, 291:701.

Rioux, J. A., Moreno, G., Lanotte, G., Pratlong, F., Dereure, J., and Rispail, P., 1986, Two episodes of cutaneous leishmaniasis in man caused by different zymodemes of Leishmania infantum s.l., Trans.R.Soc.Trop.Med.Hyg., 80:1004.

Rioux, J. A., Lanotte, G., Pratlong, F., Dereure, J., Jarry, D., Moreno, G., Killick-Kendrick, R., Perieres, J., Guilvard, E., Belmonte, A., and Portus, M., 1985, La leishmaniose cutanée autochtone dans le Sud-Est de la France. Résultats d'une enquête éco-épidémiologique dans les Pyrénées-Orientales. Méd.Malad.Infect., 11:650.

Schnur, L. F., 1986, Kala-azar in Egypt and its cause. Trans.R.Soc.Trop.Med.Hyg., 80: 671.

Schnur, L. F., Chance, M. L., Ebert, F., Thomas, S. C., and Peters, W., 1981, The biochemical and serological taxonomy of visceralising Leishmania, Ann.Trop.Med.Parasitol., 75:3.

Tobie, E. J., Von Brand, T., and Nehlman, B., 1950, Cultural and physiological observations on Trypanosoma rhodesiense and Trypanosoma gambiense, J. Parasitol., 36:48.

Tzamouranis, N., Schnur, L. F., Garifallou, A., Pateraki, E., and Série, C., 1984, Leishmaniasis in Greece I. Isolation and identification of the parasite causing human and canine visceral leishmaniasis. Ann.Trop.Med.Parasitol., 78:363.

WHO, 1984, The leishmaniases, Techn.Rep.Series 701, WHO, Geneva.

LEISHMANIASIS : STATUS IN TUNISIA (1986)

R. Ben Ismail, M. Ben Said and M.S. Ben Rachid

Department de Parasitologie - Faculte de Medicine
Tunis, Tunisia

INTRODUCTION

Visceral (VL) and cutaneous (CL) leishmaniasis both occur in Tunisia. The first CL cases have been reported in Gafsa by Deperet and Boinet [1,2] in 1884 and the first infantile CL case was detected by Laveran [3] in 1903, in a suburb of Tunis. Since then, records on leishmaniasis were regularly reported by several workers [4-14]. The recent occurrence of severe outbreaks of zoonotic CL in the centre of the country [15] has modified the epidemiological picture and has made it necessary to give an up-to-date outline of the leishmaniasis situation in Tunisia.

MATERIALS AND METHODS

VL records, from the beginning of the century until 1981, were obtained from the literature [4-14]. From 1982 to 1986, data were collected from the paediatric services of the hospitals of Tunis, Sousse, Kairouan and Sfax and concerned parasitologically confirmed cases.

The data on CL were obtained by the analysis of 1566 observations of patients, from the whole territory. The following parameters: geographical distribution, epidemiological presentation (sporadic, endemic, epidemic), the number, site, suration and clinical appearance of lesions, the size of the amastigotes in subcutaneous smears and the behaviour of the parasite in culture, were studied.

RESULTS

Visceral Leishmaniasis

From 1903 to 1981, 470 VL cases were reported [4-14]. 278 new cases were recorded from 1982 to 1986. The analysis of the

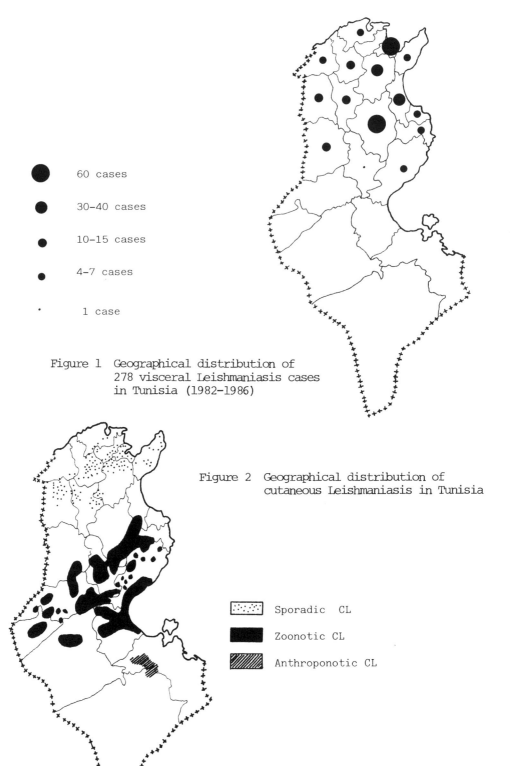

Figure 1 Geographical distribution of 278 visceral Leishmaniasis cases in Tunisia (1982-1986)

Figure 2 Geographical distribution of cutaneous Leishmaniasis in Tunisia

geographical distribution of the cases (Figure 1) shows that the foci are stable and almost all cases are from the sub-humid and semi-arid zones of the North. 77% of cases are less than 5 years old and of all the cases reported since the discovery of the disease in Tunisia, only 20 (2.8%) were in patients over 14 years of age. The disease appears to occur in sporadic form. Current annual incidence is about 50 reported cases. Patients are generally of modest and rural origins. Splenomegaly (99.2%), fever (93.2%), hepatomegaly (64%), weight loss (62.4%) and anaemia (98.2%) are the most frequent clincial signs. Mortality is 5-8%, in spite of the use of Glucantime R.

Cutaneous Leishmaniasis

Three noso-geographical forms of CL can be distinguished in Tunisia (Figure 2).

1. Sporadic CL of the North (SCL) : The analysis of 71 observations shows the following characteristics. The cases are sporadic and originate from northern areas which are known to be VL foci. Over 96% of cases have a single lesion of the face that may last up to 24 months without healing. Typically, the lesions consist of small crusty ulcers surrounded by a notable erythematous reaction. Presentation of cases reveals no particular transmission season. About 20 cases are observed each year. The amastigotes are 3 microns in diameter or less. Promastigotes are very difficult to maintain in culture and the strains are usually lost within the third passage.

2. Zoonotic CL (ZCL) : ZCL is epidemic in the centre and the south-west (semi-arid and arid zones). The analysis of 1412 observations shows that this form produces multiple lesions (more than 2 lesions in 66% of cases), localized most commonly on the limbs (67%). Self-healing usually occurs in 3 to 5 months in 82% of cases. Clinically, the lesions are mostly large and wet. Secondary infection is frequent. There is a seasonal occurrence of the outbreaks (aestivo-autumnal). Amastigotes are large (up to 6.5 microns in diameter) and it is easy to obtain promastigotes in culture.

3. Anthroponotic CL (ACL) : ACL is endemic and occurs in microfoci principally in the south-east of the country (presaharian zone, from Toujene to Tataouine). About 70% (50 out of 71) of cases have only one lesion. Over half the lesions are on the face. Unlike ZCL healing is delayed and exceptional cases have been seen of six years duration. The lesions are most often dry and vegetative. The amastigotes are 4 to 5 microns in diameter. The parasites are easy to obtain in culture.

DISCUSSION

It appears from this study that the geographical distribution of VL in man remains unchanged since the early records of the disease [4-14], the foci being confined to the sub-humid and semi-arid bioclimatic areas, in the north of the country. The pattern is of classical mediterranean infantile type and is sporadic. The causative agent is *Leishmania infantum* s.st. zymodeme LON.49 (= MON.1) [16]. Dogs are a proven reservoir host [13,16], while foxes and jackels are suspected of playing a role. It is notable that canine VL is more widely distributed than the disease in man [17] (unpublished data) especially in urban areas. Phlebotomus perniciosus is distributed in all the VL affected areas [18] and represents the most important potential vector, *P. perfiliewi* and *P. Longicuspis* are also suspected vectors.

The analysis of 1566 CL observations indicates tht 3 noso-geographical forms can be distinguished in Tunisia. The sporadic CL of the north is probably the same as that found in similar biotopes in neighbouring Algeria [19] where it is known to be caused by a variant of *L. infantum* [20]. In addition, the same species was identified in Italy from CL lesions [21,22], where the parasite was very difficult to maintain in culture. The vector and the reservoir(s) of SCL are unknown.

ZCL is known in Tunisia since 1884 [1,2]. A new outbreak arose in 1982 in the central area where the disease was previously unknown [7,15]. Since 1982, the epidemic has rapidly spread from the governate of Kairouan to cover parts of 8 other governorates (Sidi-Bouzid, Gafsa, Sfax, Mahdia, Tozeur, Kebili, Gabes and Kasserine). More than 20,000 cases were reported by the ministry of health (unpublished report) since the beginning of the epidemic. The causative agent was shown to be *L. major* zymodeme MON.25 [24]. *Phlebotomus papatasi* is a grade III [25] proven vector [26,27] of this form. *L.major* MON. 25 was also isolated from 3 rodent species : *Psammomys obesus*, *Meriones shawi* and *M. libycus*. However, further investigations are needed to confirm the incrimination of *M. Libycus* as reservoir host of ZCL in Tunisia [28].

Concerning ACL, the current prevalence is unknown due to the lack of active case detection in the affected areas, but it is clearly less than that of ZCL. The causative agent was identified, in the focus of Tataouine, as being *L. tropica* zymodeme MON.8 [29]. *Phlebotomus sergenti* is the suspected vector of ACL.

CONCLUSION

VL and CL both occur in Tunisia. Infantile VL is confined to the north of the country and is caused by *L. infantum* s.st. MON. 1. Dogs are a proven reservoir. Further investigations are needed to detect other possible reservoirs (wild canids, rodents) and to incriminate the vector(s).

Three CL forms, with particular clinical and epidemiological features can be distinguished in Tunisia. These forms affect separate areas of the country and are caused by three different species of *Leishmania*. Further studies are necessary to identify the SCL and ACL vectors and the SCL reservoir(s). Different control measures may be adapted for each of these particular forms.

REFERENCES

1. DEPERET C., BOINET, E. 1884. Du bouton de Gafsa au camp de Sathonay. Arch. Med. Pharm. Milit. 3, 296-302.

2. DEPERET, C., BOINET, E. 1884. Du bouton de Gafsa au camp de Sathonay.(suite). Arch. Med. Pharm. Milit. 3, 302-329.

3. LAVERAN A. 1904. Presentation de Parasite : (M. Cathoire), Piroplasma denovani. Bull. Acad. Med. 51, 247-248.

4. ANDERSON C. 1934. Chronique du kala-azar en Tunisie. Arch.Inst.Pasteur - Tunis. 23, 455-464.

5. ANDERSON C. 1938. Chronique du kala-azar. Arch. Inst. Pasteur - Tunis 27, 96-104.

6. BADER R. 1909. Contribution a l'etude de bouton d'Orient en Tunisie (Clou de Gafsa). These Medecine - Montpellier - 1909 - 73pp.

7. BEN RACHID M.S., HAMZA B., TABBANE C., GHARBI R., JEDDI H., BEN SAID M. 1983. Etat actuel des Leishmanioses en Tunisie. Ann. Soc.Belge Med.Trop. 63, 29-40.

8. CHATTON E. 1914. Le bouton d'Orient (Clou de Gafsa) dans le Djerid. Ses relations avec le facies rupestre du sol. Bull Soc. Path. Exot.,7, 30-35.

9. CHADLI A., BEN RACHID M.S., FHAIEL A. 1968. Chronique des Leishmanioses en Tunisie. Arch. Inst. Pasteur - Tunis. 45, 1-14.

10. LADJIMI R., LAKHOUA M. 1953. Premier cas de Bouton d'Orient dans la banlieue de Tunis. Arch. Inst. Pasteur - Tunis 1955, 32, 331-336.

11. NICOLLE C. 1912. Statistique des 30 premieres observations de kala-azar Arch. Inst. Pasteur. tunis 2, 65-67.

12. NICOLLE C., BLANC G. 1917. Extension de la region a bouton d'Orient tunisienne. Bull. Soc. Path. Excot. 10, 378-379.

13. NICOLLE C., COMTE C. 1908. Origine canine du kala-azar. Arch. Inst. Pasteur Tunis. 3, 99-103.

14. VERMEIL C. 1956. Chronique des Leishmanioses en Tunisie. Arch. Inst. Pasteur - TUNIS. 33, 195-201.

15. BEN-AMMAR R., BEN ISMAIL R., HELAL H., BACH-HAMBA D., CHAOUCH A., BOUDEN L., HANSACHI A., ZEMZARI A., BEN RACHID M.S. 1984. Un noveau foyer de Leishmaniose cutanee de type rural dans la region de Sidi-Saad (Tunisie). Bull. Soc. Franc. Parasitol., 2, 9-12

16. BEN ISMAIL R., GRAMICCIA M., GRADONI L., BED SAID M., BEN RACHID M.S. 1986 Identificazione biochemica di isolati di *Leishmania* della Tunisia. Parasitologia, 28, (in press).

17 DEDET J.P. 1971. Epidemiologie de la leishmaniose viscerale en Tunisie. Etude des reservoirs de virus. Incidence et reparation de la leishmaniose canine. These Sciences - Montpellier - 161 pp.

18 CROSET H., RIOUX J.A., MAISTRE M., N. BAYAR. 1978. Les phlebotomes de Tunisie. Mise au point systematique, chorologique et ethologique. Ann. Parasitol. (Paris) 53 711-749.

19 BELLAZOUG S., AMMAR-KHODJA A., BELKAID M. TABET-DERRAZ O. 1985 La Leishmaniose cutanee de nord de l'algerie. Bull. Soc. Ex. 78, 615-622.

20 BELLAZOUG S., LANOTTE G., MAAZOUN R., PRATLONG F., RIOUS J.A. 1985. Un nouveau variant enzymatique de *Leishmania infantum* Nicolle, 1908, agent de la leishmaniose cutanee du nord de l'Algerie. Ann. Parasit. Hum. Comp. 60, 1-3.

21 POZZIO E., GRAMICCIA M. GRADONI L. AMERO P. 1985 Isolation of the agent causing cutaneous leishmaniasis in Italy and visceralization in inbred hamsters. Trans. R. Soc. Trop. Med. Hyg. 79, 260-261

22 GRAMICCIA M., GRADONI L., POZIO E. 1987. *Leishmania infantum* sensu lato as an agent of cutaneous leishmaniasis in Abruzzi region (Italy). Trans. R. Soc. Trop. Med. Hyg. 81, 235-237.

23 POZIA E., GRADONI L. GRAMICCIA M., BETTINI S. PAMPIGLIONE S. 1982. The "puzzle" of cutaneous leishmaniasis epidemiology in Italy. Acta. Medit. Patol. Inf. Trop. 1 (S), 109-115.

24 BEN ISMAIL R., GRADONI L. GRAMICCIA M., BETTINI S., BEN RACHID M.S. 1986. Epidemic cutaneous leishmaniasis in Tunisia. Biochemical characterization of parasites. Trans. R. Soc. Trop. Med. Hyg. 80, 669-670.

25 KILLICK-KENDRICK R., WARD R.D. 1981. Ecology of *Leishmania*. Parasitology, 82, 143-152.

26 HELAL H., BEN-ISMAIL R., BACH-HAMBA D., SIDMON M., BETTINI S., BEN RACHID M.S. 1987. Enquete entomologique dans le foyer de leishmaniose cutanee zoonotique *(Leishmania major)* de Sidi Bouzid (Tunisie) en 1985. Bull. Soc. Path. Exot. 80, 349-356.

27 BEN-ISMAIL R., GRAMICCIA M., GRADONI L., HELAL H., BEN RACHID M.S. Isolation of *Leishmania major* (Yakimoff & Shokhor, 1914) from *Phlebotomus papatasi* (Scopili, 1786) in Tunisia. Trans. R. Soc. Trop. Med. Hyg. 81 (in press).

28 BEN-ISMAIL R., BEN RACHID M.S. GRADONI L., GRAMICIA M., HELAL H., BACH-HAMBA D. 1987. La leishmaniose cutanee zoonotique en Tunisie. I. Isolement de *Leishmania major* Yakimoff & Schokhor, 1914 chez *Psammomys obesus* Cretzchmar, 1828, *Meriones shawi* Duvernoy, 1842 et *Meriones libycus* Lichtenstein 1910 (Rongeurs, Gerbillises) dan le foyer de Douara. Ann. Soc. Belge Med. Trop. 67 (in press).

29 Rioux J.A., LANOTTE G., FOURATI K., KENNOU M.F., KILLICK-KENDRICK R., MAAZOUN R., PERRIERS J. 1980. Resurgence de la Leishmaniose cutanee dan le Sud Tunisien. Cambridge - Abstracts - 3rd European multi-colloquim of parasitology. Semptember 1980.

A REVIEW OF THE STATUS OF LEISHMANIASIS IN PAKISTAN FROM 1960 - 1986

M.A. Munir, M.A. Rab, J. Iqbal, A. Ghafoor,
M.A. Khan and M.I. Burney

Public Health Division
National Institute of Health
Islamabad
Pakistan

INTRODUCTION

Visceral leishmaniasis was first reported in Pakistan from Baltistan in the Northern Areas (Ahmed, Burney and Wazir, 1960), and following strict control measures it was controlled in that area. Nevertheless the disease reappeared in that area in the mid seventies (Burney et al, 1979), and it was once again brought under control by active measures. Since the beginning of the eighties cases started appearing again not only from the previously known areas, but also from the neighbouring regions of Azad Jammu and Kashmir, parts of Northern Punjab and from the adjacent NWFP regions. Cases have now been reported from areas of Rawalakot, Muzaffarabad and Poonch (Azad Jammu and Kashmir), Gujar Khan and Muree (Punjab), Terbella and Abbottabad (NWFP).

Cutaneous leishmaniasis on the other hand is reported from all over the country (Nasir, 1964). However it is mainly endemic in Baluchistan and in adjoining regions (Burney and Lari, 1986). Both types of cutaneous leishmaniasis i.e. zoonotic cutaneous leishmaniasis (ZCL) and anthroponotic cutaneous leishmaniasis (ACL) occur, however the latter is predominant (Rajper et al., 1983., Rab et al., 1986).

Very few epidemiological studies on leishmaniasis have so far been carried out in the country. Visceral leishmaniasis appears to be spreading southwards and no information regarding its vector(s) and reservoir host(s) is available. Such information is also lacking in the CL area. There is, therefore, an urgent need to carry out further detailed epidemiological investigations including studies on vectors and reservoirs before formulating effective control strategies.

VISCERAL LEISHMANIASIS

Visceral leighmaniasis remained a neglected problem in Pakistan, until the report of Ahmed, Burney and Wazir, (1960) was published. This was the first report on clinically diagnosed cases of VL in hospital at Skardu, the principal town of Baltistan, in the Northern areas. The report was also confirmed by Barnett and Suyemoto (1961), who visited the area in September, 1960. Later, in 1962, Ahmed and Burney, published the detailed accounts of their investigations in Baltistan. These reports of the early sixties were the main source of information regarding VL in Pakistan.

As a result of the surveys in the 1960's intensive control measures were undertaken in the infected localities. The methodology adopted involved the treatment of cases and application of DDT-spraying specifically to control the sandflies. A follow up study conducted in 1964 did not reveal any cases. In 1974 and 1975, new foci of VL were discovered in the Kharmang valley, and a number of cases were recorded. Following these surveys, specific control measures were instituted again in 1975. A detailed account of the studies carried out until 1975 was published by Burney *et al* (1979).

In 1979 an extensive survey of the entire Baltistan area was undertaken at one time (Burney *et al* 1981). All possible means of communication and publicity were applied. Many patients were examined at the hospital and peripheral dispensary records were thoroughly searched. No VL case was recorded and this was attributed to the control measures previously employed. After the 1979 survey, immunological screening remained the only practical approach. Hence, in the same year sero-epidemiological assessments were carried out (Burney *et al* 1981). The results as taken from the original publication are summarized as follows;

```
Total Number of Sera Examined   76
Total Number of Sera Positive   33 (43%)

Titre range:    IFT         1:20-1:180 (mean 1:39.3)
                CFT         1:80-1:128 (mean 1:26.2)

Higher Sero-positive rates by age:  up to 5 Yrs    50%
                                    6 - 10 Yrs     93%
                                    11 - 15 Yrs    69%
```

Based on the information of the 1979 survey, it was thought that the disease had been eliminated from the area. However, the picture changed when fresh cases of VL started appearing in the early eighties, not only from Baltistan, but also from Azad Kashmir, an area previously not known to be endemic for VL. As a response, further studies were carried out and are still continuing.

A report on the 16 cases of VL was presented to the International Conference of Pakistan Medical Association of Pathologists by Rab *et al* in 1986. These authors, apart from

TABLE I. REVIEW OF VL. SITUATION (1960-1986)

YEAR	LOCALITY	NO. OF CASES RECORDED	DIAGNOSTIC TESTS	AGE	SEX
1960	Khaplu valley	55	27- Cases were throughly examined and diagnosis confirmed on the basis: i) LD-bodies seen in bone marrow material. ii) Serologically using CFT	1 - 6 Yrs (80 %)	Male children showed higher infection rates than females
	Kharmang valley	05			
	Total	60			
1964	Follow up study of the above areas.		No cases recorded.		
1974	Kharmang valley	25	Confirmation on: i): LD-Bodies seen in Bone Marrow Material	< 15 Yrs less frequent in adolescent and adult age group.	–
1975	Kharmang valley	2	–	–	–
1979	Khaplu-valley Kharmang valley Shigar valley Rondu valley	NIL			
1983-85	Azad Kashmir Gilgit Agency Abbottabad Rawalpindi	9 cases 2 " 1 " 2 "	Confirmed on i) LD-bodies seen in Bone marrow material ii) Biopsy		Male:female ratio was 3.7:1
1986	Azad Kashmir/ Northern Areas	16	Confirmed on: i) LD-bodies seen in Bone marrow material ii) Serologically using IFAT.	10 months 6 years	Male:female ratio was 3:1
TOTAL CASES- (1960-1986)		101			

TABLE II RESULTS OF CL - SURVEYS CONDUCTED BETWEEN 1977 - 1986

YEAR	LOCALITY	PROVINCE	TOTAL NUMBER OF CASES RECORDED	NO.OF ACTIVE CASES	NO.OF RECENTLY CURED CASES	TYPE OF LESION	% OF CASES WITH MULTIPLE LESION	% CASES WITH SINGLE LESION	AV.NO.OF MULTIPLE LESION PER PERSON
1977	JHELUM	PUNJAB	32	-	32	WET	26(81.25%)	6(18.7%)	2 - 7 °°13
*1980 (Feb/Mar)	UTHAL	BALUCHISTAN	38	29	9	WET	30(78.94%)	8(21.05)	2 -11
**1982 (Feb/Mar)	UTHAL	BALUCHISTAN	220	10	12	-	-	-	-
***1982	UTHAL	BALUCHISTAN	117	60	57	WET	-	-	-
1982 (April)	DUKKI (Loralai)	BALUCHISTAN	177	-	-	-	-	-	-
1983 (NOV)	KOHLU	-do-	(0.9%)	4	-	-	-	-	-
1984 (May)	KHUZDAR	-do-	NIL	-	-	-	-	-	-
°1986	UTHAL	-do-	116	5	111	WET	5	-	-

*   - Survey carried out among the textile workers of Uthal Textile Mills.

** - School survey conducted in Uthal. School students examined.

*** - Survey conducted in Uthal. 2000 textile workers examined.

°   - Survey conducted in school children

°° - Thirteen Lesions seen only in one person.

recording cases, with the age and sex distribution of the disease, also cultured the parasite, and identified it by isoenzyme characterization as *Leishmania infantum* ss. A mortality rate up to 33% was recorded. Since most of the cases came from Azad Kashmir, a separate study for the assessment of antibody level in the local population is being carried out.

Another recently published report is that of Saleem et al (1986), who published a record of 14 cases of VL diagnosed at Armed Forces Institute of Pathology, Army Medical College and Military Hospital at Rawalpindi between 1983-85. Again the majority of the cases belonged to Azad Kashmir (6 from Poonch District and 3 from Muzaffarabad). One case was from Gilgit Agency (from an endemic area) and three cases (one from Abbottabad and two from Rawalpindi) were from the areas previously not known to be endemic for VL. The study also includes details of clinical/haematological findings as well as treatment.

The results recorded in various studies carried out between 1960 and 1986 are summarized in TABLE I.

Furthermore, in the present year cases are still being referred for the sero-diagnosis of VL. Up to the present we have diagnosed another 8 cases. The diagnosis has been confirmed serologically by using IFAT and on the basis of LD-bodies seen in the bone marrow. Further studies are continuing.

CUTANEOUS LEISHMANIASIS

Cutaneous leishmaniasis has been reported to occur all over the country in epidemic form (Nasir, 1964). The record of major epidemic out-breaks during (1935-1977) as published by Burney et al (1986) is presented in TABLE III.

Both anthroponotic CL (urban or dry type) and zoonotic CL (rural or wet type) occur in the region. (Rajper et al, 1983), Burney and Lari, 1986).

Attention was focused on cutaneous leishmaniasis, mainly in 1979, and thereafter various studies were carried out. A detailed review of the situation of CL from 1979 to 1984 has been published by Burney and Lari (1986). The known distribution records of CL indicate its existence in the extreme north (Gilgit Agency) on the one hand, and the coastal areas of Lasbella and Mekran in the extreme south in Baluchistan on the other hand. However, the disease has been found to be endemic in some areas of Baluchistan. The areas include Gambas, Maiwand, Kehan, Gangi, Tangi, Dera Bugti, surrounding areas of Kum, District Loralai, For Sandeman, Khuzdar and Lesbella.

Information regarding CL in the Baluchistan area as summed up from 1979 to 1984 by Burney and Lari (1986), and the results of the recently conducted study by Rab et al (1986) among school children in Uthal are summarized in TABLES II, III and IV.

TABLE III CUTANEOUS LEISHMANIASIS : DISTRIBUTION OF CASES ACCORDING TO AGE GROUP 1977-1984 [BURNEY & LARI 1986]

YEAR	LOCATION	PROVINCE	AGE	GROUP	PERCENTAGE
1980	UTHAL	BALUCHISTAN	34	16-48 Yrs	89%
			4	>12 Yrs	11%
1982	DUKKI	-do-	55	upto 5 Yrs	31%
			42	5-10 Yrs	24%
			30	11-20 Yrs	17%
			26	21-30 Yrs	15%
			17	31-40 Yrs	10%
			7	41-60 Yrs	4%
1986	UTHAL	-do-	5	5-10 Yrs	1% Active Lesion
			111	5-16 Yrs	27% With Scars

TABLE IV CUTANEOUS LEISHMANIASIS : DISTRIBUTION OF LESIONS ACCORDING TO ANOTOMICAL SITE [BURNEY & LARI 1986]

ANATOMICAL REGION	PERCENTAGE
FEET AND LOWER 1/3 LEG	64%
HANDS AND FORE ARM	26%
KNEE	5%
TRUNK	3%
FACE AND NECK*	–

* For the involvement of face and neck see Rab et al 1986

TABLE V MAJOR EPIDEMICS OF LEISHMANIASIS IN PAKISTAN

YEAR	CITY	PROVINCE	NO. CASES	TYPE CASES
1935	QUETTA	BALUCHISTAN	–	Earthquake victims.
1971-72	MULTAN	PUNJAB	2,500	OPD Nishtar Hospital
1974	–	BALUCHISTAN	892	Army Personnel
1975	–	-do-	502	-do-
1977	UTHAL	-do-	100	Textile workers

OPD = Out Patient Department

RESERVOIR STUDIES

1. VISCERAL LEISHMANIASIS

Only two attempts have so far been made to discover the animal reservoir involved in the transmission of VL. The first attempt was made by Ahmed, Wazir and Burney (1960) in Baltistan. They examined dogs and rodents from that area, and none of them was found to be positive. Another study in this regard has been carried out by Rab et al (1986) who examined sera from dogs using IHA, but again the results were negative.

2. CUTANEOUS LEISHMANIASIS

Baluchistan, parts of Sind, Punjab and NWFP provinces have distributional records of rodents, gerbils (Burney and Lari, 1986):

Rhombomys opimus
Meriones persicus
Meriones lybicus
Meriones crassus
Meriones hurrianae

Four of the above species, except *Meriones crassus*, have been incriminated as the reservoir of human infection with CL, in Afghanistan, Iran, USSR, Mongolia and India. (Durbrovsky, 1979; Krasnonos and Razakov, 1979 & Safyanova, 1979).

During the surveys conducted in Baluchistan between Jan 1982 and May 1984, the following rodents were trapped and identified. (Burney and Lari 1986).

Species	Count
Rattus rattus	1
Mus musculus	3
Tatera indica	5
Meriones lybicus	13
Meriones crassus	15

According to the authors, some of these rodents had lesions on toes or tails, but none of them were positive on examination of the material.

In 1986 Rab et al trapped the following rodent species from Uthal, Baluchistan:

Species	Count
Meriones hurrianae	9
Meriones spp	1
Tatera indica	1

None of these rodents showed clinical evidence of disease, but smears taken from their ear scrapings were positive for LD-bodies in one *Tatera indica*. According to the authors, histological sections and touch smears from spleen and liver were negative.

SANDFLY FAUNA

Professor H.C. Barnett during 1959 and 1960 carried out field investigations on sandfly fever and kalazar in Pakistan. During the period he collected many thousands of sandflies of the genera *Phlebotomus* and *Sergentomyia* for virus isolation. (Barnett and Suyemoto, 1961). Out of this collection Lewis (1967), examined 9,900 specimens and identified them to the species level. Later in June 1963, Dr. D.J. Lewis himself visited Pakistan and collected sandflies from Lahore,

Rawalpindi, Texla, Peshawar, Saidu Sharif, Behrain, Kalam, Abbottabad, Nathia Gali, Gilgit, Chilas, Akardu, Keris, Karachi and the neighbouring areas. In his paper on the Phlebotomine Sandflies of West Pakistan (Diptera: Psychodidae) 1967; Lewis states that as many as 11,100 specimens were collected, out of which the sandflies from Lahore, Gujrat and Mir Mohammad were distributed to him by Mr. W.A. McDonald.

This was the first inventory of sandflies from Pakistan. General notes on their bionomics, and the relation of sandflies to human diseases are also discussed in his paper. The following species were identified from the genus *Phlebotomus*. Some names have been updated according to Lewis (1978) [WHO/VBC/80.786, Page 68].

Sub genus *Phlebotomus*:	*papatasi*
Sub genus *Paraphlebotomus*:	*alexandri,* (*nuri sp.n, sergenti*)
Sub genus *Larrousius*:	*kandelkii* (= K burneyi sub sp.n of Lewis,1967 keshishiani major major)
Sub genus *Adlerius*:	*longiductus* (= Chinensis longiductus, of Lewis 1967)
Sub genus *Euphlebotomus*:	*argentipes*
Sub genus *Anaphlebotomus*:	*colabaensis*

In addition, 16 species of *Sergentomyia* were also identified.

VECTOR STUDIES

The vector of VL and CL has not yet been incriminated in Pakistan, but among the commonest found species of *Phlebotomus*, most are the proven vectors of VL and CL in various other countries. (WHO, Tech. Rep. Series, 701, 1984). Various attempts have been made to discover VL and CL vectors in Pakistan between 1960 - 1986 these are summarized as follows:

1.VISCERAL LEISHMANIASIS
After the discovery of Kala azar cases in Baltistan, the first attempt to study the vectors was made by Burney et al (1960). They made the night collections in the houses of VL patients and identified the following species:- *Phlebotomus chinensis*, *P. kandelakii*, and *P. major*. They were dissected but found negative for leishmanial promastigotes.

2 CUTANEOUS LEISHMANIASIS
According to Burney and Lari (1986), *P. papatasi* and *P. sergenti* are the commonest species of sandflies in Pakistan especially in the plains.

The only detailed survey to ascertain the vectorial significance of sandflies in Pakistan was conducted in 1975, in Baluchistan: Quetta, Sibi, Khuzdar, Kalat, Zhob and Bostan. During this survey 3450 specimens of sandflies were collected and identified as *P. papatasi* scopoli and *P. sergenti*. The habitats of the sand flies were described. None of the specimens were positive on dissection.

Recently Rab *et al* (1986), during their study on cutaneous leishmaniasis in Uthal Baluchistan, collected 432 sandflies from rodent burrows, but again none was positive for the *Leishmania* promastigotes on dissection.
Among the specimens collected:

212	*Ph papatasi*	(49.07%)
15	*Ph salehi**	(3.37%)
3	*S.africana*	(0.69%)
178	*S.clydei*	(41.20%)
23	*S.dentata*	(5.32%)
1	*S.squamipleuris*	(0.23%)

**Ph salehi* is a proven vector of ZC1 in India (See WHO Tech. Rep. Series, 704, 1984).

CONCLUSION

Based on the evidence provided by recent studies, the re-appearance of VL-cases from the previously known foci in Northern Areas and the occurrence of sporadic cases in the adjoining areas, specially Azad Kashmir, needs serious attention. It is important to determine the reasons for the recrudescence of infection. If the disease is made notifiable it would facilitate assessment of the size of the problem, case management, and prevention.

Our knowledge regarding the Vector(s) and Reservoir (s) is limited, therefore studies in this context are needed to:

(i) Confirm whether the disease in Baltistan is of the anthroponotic India VL-type or is the Mediterranean type of VL characterized by the existence of an animal reservoir.

(ii) To formulate effective control strategies.

Moreover isolation of parasites from human patients as well as from the vector(s) and the reservoir(s) and their precise characterization are needed.

The incidence, prevalence and distribution of cutaneous leishmaniasis on the other hand are better known but the Gilgit focus needs survey. As knowledge of vector population, reservoir(s) and ecological characteristics of transmission is meagre, the relationship between man, sandfly and reservoir(s) needs to be investigated.

REFERENCES

Ahmed, N., Burney, M.I. and Wazir, Y., (1960)
A preliminary report on the study of Kala-azar in Baltistan (West Pakistan). Armed Forces Med. J. Karachi 10,1

Barnett H.C. and Suyemoto, W. Field (1962)
Studies on sandfly fever and kalazar in Pakistan, in Iran, and in Baltistan (Little Tibet) Kashmir, Trans. N.Y. Acad. Sci. Ser. 2, 609

Burney, M.I. Wazir, Y. and Lari, F.A. (1979)
A longitudinal study of visceral leishmaniasis in Northern areas of Pakistan. Trop. Doctor, London 9,110.

Burney, M.I. Lari, F.A. and Khan, M.A. (1981)
Status of visceral leishmaniasis in northern Pakistan Trop.Doctor, 11:46

Burney, M.I. and Lari, F.A. (1986)
Status of cutaneous leishmaniasis in Pakistan, Pak. J. Med. Res.25,101.

Durbrovsky, Y.U.A. (1979)
Ecology of great gerbil, the carrier of the agent of zoonotic cutaneous leishmaniasis, WHO Travelling Seminar on Leishmaniasis control, USSR, Ministry of Health, Moscow 1-7.

Krasnonos, L.N. and Razakov, Sh A. (1979)
Epidemiology of leishmaniasis in USSR WHO Travelling Seminar on leishmaniasis control, USSR, Ministry of Health, Moscow, 1-27

Lewis, D.J. (1967)
The Phlebotomine Sandflies of West Pakistan (Diptera: Psychodidae). Bull. Br. Mus. Nat. Hist. Entom 19,57.

Nasir, A.S. (1964)
Sandflies as vector of human diseases in West Pakistan, Pak. J. Hlth; Karachi 14,26.

Rab, M.A. Azmi, F.H. and Hamid, J. (1986)
Visceral leishmaniasis in North of Pakistan, second international conference of Pakistan Association of Pathologists, Karachi, Pakistan. Dec.

Rab, M.A. Azmi, F.A. Iqbal. J. Hamid, J. Ghafoor, A. and Rashti. M.A.S. (1986)
Cutaneous leishmaniasis in Baluchistan: Reservoir host and sandfly vector in Uthal Lasbella, J.N.P.A. PP. 137, June.

Rajper, G.M. Khan, M.A. and Hafiz, A. (1983)
Laboratory investigation of cutaneous leishmaniasis in Karachi, J.M.P.A. pp. 248.

Safyanova, Y.M. (1979)
Epidemiology of Leishmaniasis in USSR, WHO Travelling seminar on leishmaniasis control, USSR, Ministry of Health, Moscow. pp. 1-35.

Saleem, N. Anwar, C.M. and Iftikhar, A.M. (1986)
Visceral leishmaniasis in children a new focus in Azad Kashmir, J.P.M.A., pp. 230

Lari, F.A. (1980)
Leishmaniasis in Pakistan. WHO, Travelling Seminar on leishmaniasis control, Moscow, USSR.

World Health Organization, (1984) The leishmaniasis, WHO Tech. Rep.series, 701.

ZOONOSES AND LEISHMANIASIS

Robert S. Bray

Department of Pure and Applied Biology
Imperial College of Science and Technology
London, SW7 2AZ
England

What causes leishmaniasis? The answer is manifold. It is caused by a <u>Leishmania</u>, by a sandfly, by the proximity of the sandfly and man, or sandfly and reservoir, by the susceptibility of man or reservoir or sandfly.

I am concerned today with the role of the reservoir, as the extra consideration in a zoonosis, in this net-work of causes of Leishmaniasis.

I would like to explore the various zoonotic situations in leishmaniasis to see if any patterns or rules emerge that are common to all zoonoses or may be added to the list of laws ruling the study of zoonoses.

So I shall say nothing that is new, much that is quite plain to you all, but occasionally, perhaps, I may illuminate a situation in a way not perceived before.

It was Garnham (1971) who pointed out that leishmaniasis like plague runs the gamut of the zoonotic fugue. Plague starts as an enzootic of <u>Yersinia pestis</u> transmitted by fleas among field rodents; Class 2 of Baker (1943). This situation may become an epizootic among the rodents and their carnivorous predators, it may then move via the flea to man and set up bubonic plague, while involving new rodents and fleas Class 4 & 5 of Baker (1943). Eventually, it may become transmitted from man to man by the human flea (septicaemic plague) Class 6 of Baker (1943) or finally leave the flea behind altogether and pass directly from man to man by droplet infection (pneumonic plague).

Visceral leishmaniasis as an enzootic involves <u>L</u>. <u>infantum</u>, canids and phlebotomine sandflies. Occasionally a sandfly infected from a canid bites a child and infantile kala-azar ensues; Class 3 of Baker (1943), but the infection stops there. At some point in history in Bengal and surrounding areas, the organism reached the blood of man in sufficient quantities to infect sandflies and the infection started to go from man to man via the sandfly. This situation of change from zoonosis to anthroponosis is apparently on-going in China where infantile zoonotic kala-azar and anthroponotic kala-azar exist side by side. That the full progression to the anthroponotic spread has not yet occurred in kala-azar is exemplified by the fact that it is not yet transmitted direct from man to man without the help of a vector and nor has the organism made the critical move beyond the blood where it is available to the sandfly to a part of the body from which it can be transmitted directly from man to man such as the lung or the intestinal tract. In fact Baker's (1943) Epidemic Series based on typhus fits leishmaniasis better than plague as it passes from the sporadic zoonosis to the epidemic, man vector man, situation then regresses, but never shows direct man to man transmission.

A progression is visible here whereby an organism striving for the greatest multiplication rate (usually presented in disease as virulence) tends to move evolutionarily in the direction of the most simple and direct transmission between hosts. The move will also tend towards the transmission which presents the least amount of hazard to the organism. It can be seen that droplet transmission maximises survival in terms of numbers and least exposure to hostile environments. The faeces are a less direct vehicle.

The progression of leishmaniasis along this road can be seen to have reached the man-vector-man stage from the reservoir-vector-reservoir and occasionally man stage in Bengal and its environs. I feel sure from the epidemiology of kala-azar in Kenya this too is a zoonosis but I doubt if it is yet an anthroponosis. There is little to be surprised at in the lability of these infections. Leishmania is assumed to have evolved from the Monoxenous Leptomonas of sandflies and moved from there into vertebrates such as rodents, canids and edentates with the sandfly remaining as the primary host. From there it is a short jump to an occasional infection of man. Then the shift in man from organs to blood is nothing to an organism which may in man and rodents occupy either the skin or the inner organs.

Now to look at some of the essential conditions which must prevail in order to set up a zoonosis. First the relationship between reservoir and sandfly. The reservoir should be the main host of the sandfly. In order to maintain an endemic of leishmaniasis in man it is essential to maintain an enzootic among the reservoirs as the primary existence of the Leishmania. So it follows that the relationship between reservoir and sandfly must be intimate. While it is not always true in all human disease situations that the reservoir is the main host of the vector (e.g. Glossina palpalis and Trypanosoma gambiense where a non-reservoir - the crocodile - is the favoured host of the tse-tse fly) it seems so far to be true of leishmaniasis (L. longipalpis may be the exception). It follows that a search for the main concentration of the vector may often lead to the habitat of the reservoir. An useful epidemiological lead!

When the relationship between vector and reservoir is close they are likely to be proximate in breeding and resting places also. Thus P. longipes is found in hyrax caves, P. dubosqi and P. papatasii are both found in rodent holes which is also where P. papatasii breeds. L. olmeca rests on the ground in the forest as do its rodent hosts. L. umbratilis rests in the boles of these trees that harbour sloths. P. ariasi rests in kennels. In fact this relationship can be so close that the adult fly will not easily leave the shared microhabitat to bite man unless the prevailing climatic conditions are right and man is close to the reservoir's environment. P. longipes in the cold season will not venture even one metre from the hyrax cave in order to bite man. Further south however in warmer weather its sibling species P. pedifer will rove freely around the village built on the rocks which make the caves for the rock-hyraxes.

A relationship between the reservoir and an activity of man will assist a zoonosis as in the famous case of the inexperienced Chinese fur-trappers, the Manchurian Marmots and the disasterous pneumonic plague outbreak of 1910. Such a relationship in the case of man and the dog is obvious in hunting and pet-keeping and both activities assist the development of an endemic of infantile kala-azar. In South America the addition of turkeys and chickens to this domestic situation anchors L. longipalpis even more firmly to the domestic environment.

All sorts of activities can concentrate man and reservoir into the domain of a zoonosis. These may be complicated moves of whole peoples for the purpose of feeding flocks or planting crops such as is the case with the people in the Sudan who move towards the Nile at certain times of the year and thus meet P. orientalis and its rodent hosts who harbour L. donovani. In the sahel savannah of the Senegal the monks of Keur Moussa irrigated and watered a few hectares for the growth of vegetables. Such richness in the near-desert brought in all the local savannah rats including the reservoirs of L. major. The rats brought with them P. dubosqi and the monks got cutaneous leishmaniasis.

In S.W. Ethiopia man left Ficus vasta growing to shade his coffee trees. Rock hyrax found the hollow Ficus to their liking and brought with them to their new environment P. longipes. Man visited the windless shade of the Ficus to tend his coffee bushes. Hence Ficus vasta cutaneous leishmaniasis. Irrigation in Tadjikistan created the conditions for the colonisation of the areas by Rhombomys opimus the major reservoir of cutaneous leishmaniasis.

Next it is necesary to examine the effect of susceptibility and immunity on the potentiality of a reservoir. The first and most important thing to be said here is the absolute necessity for a reservoir to maintain the infection in a state so that transmission is possible and that for as long as and when transmission can occur. This means not only that the parasite is kept in the skin or blood in sufficient quantities to infect sandflies but that it is represented in a similar way in the next transmission season which will be in 9 or 10 months time in many cases. In the savannahs and desert areas where most of the L. major infections occur transmission occurs for only a few months of the year. In these situations the immune system of the reservoir must react to the presence of the parasite in such a manner that while preventing it from doing any irrevocable damage it is not wiped out-a process which requires subtle fine-tuning of the immune system.

At the same time the reaction of the reservoir must be such that the parasite is presented to the sandfly so that feeding takes up the parasite. For instance the dog infected with L. infantum begins to become infective to sandflies about 3 years after the original infection. As might be expected, this is also the time when amastigotes begin to appear in the skin in large numbers. It is difficult for sandflies with their long legs and many hairs to feed on areas of skin which are particularly hairy. It is not co-incidental therefore that colonization of the dog's skin by amastigotes causes depilation leaving areas of hairless skin on which sandflies can easily feed.

The hyrax becomes infected in only one tiny bit of the skin with L. aethiopica. This highly confined place is at the very tip of the nose. Sandflies are attracted to their hosts by the exhaled carbon dioxide.

So the sandfly is attracted to the very tip of the nose of the hyrax where it both delivers the infection and picks it up. The role of the hyrax in the zoonosis is now only to maintain the infection there until the next time a sandfly bites whether this is next week or next year.

Rhombomys opimus lives between one and two years. It receives an infection of L. major from the burrow-inhabiting P. papatasii and perhaps P. caucasicus, largely in the ears, in the summer months of Southern Central Siberia. To be an effective reservoir it must first live long enough to survive until the next transmission period otherwise the infection among rodents and therefore man will die out. Rhombomys can do that. It must also either control, or allow the parasite to control, its immune reaction to the parasite, so that amastigotes survive in numbers in the lesion until the next summer. The ears are hairless and the favourite biting place of Phlebotomus.

It is essential, when studying the epidemiology of many zoonoses, including leishmaniasis, to understand that if the last evolutionary stage of transmission from man to man or man to reservoir has not been reached then man can only be infected from the reservoir. It follows that geographical spread of the disease can only occur by spread of the infected reservoir or in the case of long-lived insects by infected vectors. So the spread of rabies is governed by the existence of foxes, bubonic plague by Rattus rattus, occasionally other rodents and sometimes infected fleas. The spread of leishmaniasis is governed by the existence and spread of the reservoir, except in some forms of kala-azar. The other possible anthroponosis - L. tropica cutaneous leishmaniasis is dying out anyway. So blaming the Haj, or the Huns, Avars, Mongols, Tamarlane and the Moghuls for movement of L. major is only possible if all these wanderers take their gerbils with them. The movement of plague is equally under the same restrictions and epidemiology based upon the movements of Indian fakirs omits the need for Rattus rattus.

REFERENCES

Baker, A.C., 1943, The typical epidemic series. Am. J. trop. Med., 23:559-566.
Garnham, P.C.C., 1971, Progress in Parasitology. Tha Athlone Press, London.

RESERVOIRS OF VISCERAL LEISHMANIASIS

P. Abranches

Disciplina de Protozoologia
Instituto de Higiene e Medicina Tropical
Rua da Junqueira 96
1300 Lisbon
Portugal

INTRODUCTION

1. Definition of Reservoir
Reservoir is the animal which is the source of infection to man in an endemic area (Deane, 1956).

2. Classification and General Characteristics of Reservoir
It is not sufficient to incriminate an animal as a reservoir of human leishmaniasis only by its susceptibility to *Leishmania* sp. There are two kinds of reservoir, habitual reservoirs and accidental reservoirs. The latter are animals in which infection develops under unusual conditions rarely repeated. In reality, the designation of reservoir here is not appropriate. A better definition is accidental host. These animals do not play a significant role in the epidemiology of leishmaniasis.

A good reservoir must show the following characteristics: its distribution area must be superimposed on that of human leishmaniasis, it must have frequent contact with anthropophilic phlebotomine vectors, a mode of parasitism favourable to transmission by the bite of the insect, a high infection rate and chronic infection. In most good reservoirs the infection is symptomless or is not very harmful to the host.

Since Garnham (1965) it is usual to classify the reservoirs of leishmaniasis as sylvatic reservoirs, supporting primitive or natural endemic foci, and secondary reservoirs, closely linked with secondary endemic foci. Some proven secondary reservoirs, such as the dog, are domestic animals. The role of wild animals as either primary or secondary reservoirs is highly controversial. This is discussed later.

VERTEBRATE RESERVOIRS OF KALA-AZAR

In zoonotic endmeic areas, the visceral forms of leishmaniasis are generally associated with wild domestic Canidae and the cutaneous ones with wild rodents. There are many exceptions to this rule.

1. Man

Man is the only known reservoir in the Indian subcontinent and, probably also in North-east China (Len Yan Jia, 1982). In Kenya and the Emilia Romagna region of Italy, it is possible that the infection in man is sufficient for the disease to maintain itself. In the neo-tropical region, visceral leishmaniasis (VL) is predominantly zoonotic, but Deane (1956) and Alencar (1961) consider that man can play the role of reservoir.

In all other kala-azar endemic areas, man generally seems to be a final stage in the epidemiological cycle, as in the Mediterranean sub-region.

2. Canidae

2.1 Dog (*Canis familiaris* L. 1758). The dog is the most important reservoir of VL in prevalence and geographical distribution. It is the principal factor in the maintenance of endemicity all over the world, except India, part of China, Sudan and some rural foci in Central Asia.

2.2 Wild Canidae. Several types of canids were discovered parasitized. The first was the jackal *Canis aureus* L., 1758, found in Tadjikstan, in 1946 (Latyshev *et al.*, 1961), and later in other regions of Central Asia (Dursunova *et al.*, 1965; Lubova, 1973 cit. Kellina, 1981) and Iran (Nadim *et al.*, 1978; Hamidi *et al.*, 1982). The wolf *Canis lupus* L., 1758 was also discovered parasitized in Central Asia (Petrisceva, 1961); but among wild Canidae, the fox is the most representative, with several species and genera being affected. In central Asia, Iran and Europe the fox *Vulpes vulpes* L., 1758 was found parasitized (Maruashvili and Bardzhadze, 1966; Rioux *et al.*, 1968; Bettini *et al.*, 1980; Marin Iniesta *et al.*, 1982; Abranches *et al.*, 1983, 1985). In Africa (Sudan) the sand fox *Vulpes pallida* Cretzschmar, 1826 was discovered presumably infected (Kirk, 1956). Another fox, the fennec fox *Vulpes zerda* Zimmerman, 1980, died with Leishmaniasis in 1970, in the zoo of Chicago (Conroy *et al.*, 1970). This fox was probably captured in northern Africa (Sahara desert) a few years before. In South America some foxes *Dusicyon vetulus* Lund, 1842 were found infected in Ceara, Brazil (Deane, 1956, Alencar, 1961) and sixteen foxes of another species, *Dusicyon thous* L., 1776, in the Amazon region of Brazil (Lainson *et al.*, 1969, 1987; Silveira *et al.*, 1982).

TABLE 1. WILD CANIDAE RESERVOIRS OF KALA-AZAR

COMMON NAME	SPECIES	NUMBER	GEOGRAPHICAL DISTRIBUTION
Jackal	Canis aureus	5(?)	Central Asia, (Tadjikstan, + other places)
		5(+2by IFAT)	Iran
Wolf	Canis lupus	1	Central Asia
Fox	Vulpes vulpes	3	Central Asia
		1	Iran
		10	Europe: France(2) Italy(1) Spain (3) Portugal(4)
Fox(?)	Vulpes pallida(?)	1(?)	Sudan(?)
Fox(Fennec fox)	Vulpes zerda	1	North of Africa (Sahara Desert)(?)
Fox	Dusicyon vetulus	11	Brazil: Ceara
Fox	Dusicyon thous	16	Brazil: Amazonia

TABLE 2. RODENT RESERVOIRS OF KALA-AZAR

COMMON NAME	SPECIES	NUMBER	GEOGRAPHICAL DISTRIBUTION
?-Ground Squirrel	Xenus rutilus(?)	1(?)	Kenya(?)
?-Gerbil	Tatera nigricuada(?)	4(?)	Kenya(?)
Nile grass Rat	Arvicanthis niloticus	4	Sudan
Spiny Mouse	Acomys capirinus	2	Sudan
Black Rat	Rattus rattus	1	Sudan
Black Rat	Rattus rattus	4	Yugoslavia
		4	Italy
		1	Spain

TABLE 3. VERTEBRATE RESERVOIRS OF KALA-AZAR (EXCLUDING CANIDAE AND RODENTS)

COMMON NAME	SPECIES	NUMBER	GEOGRAPHICAL DISTRIBUTION
Serval Cat	Felis serval	1	Sudan
Genet	Genetta genetta	1	Sudan
Porcupine	Hystrix indica	1	Central Asia
Racoon Dog	Nycterentes procyanoides	1	China
Opossum	Didelphis albiventris	1	Baia (Brazil)

3. Rodents

The first discovery of these animals parasitized by visceralising strains of *Leishmania* was noted in Kenya, Africa, but the isolates were not like those producing human VL in the same region (Ngoka and Mutinga, 1978). In Sudan, the Nile grass rat *Arvicanthus niloticus* Desmarest, 1922, the spiny mouse *Acomys capirinus* Desmarest, 1891 and the black rat *Rattus rattus* L., 1758 found in different foci of the country were parasitised and some of them are habitual reservoirs (Hoogstraal and Heyneman, 1969).

In Europe, only quite recently has the role of rodents as reservoirs of kala-azar been emphasized, following the discovery of some parasitezed *R.rattus* in Yugoslavia (Petrovic et al., 1975). In Italy (Bettini et al., 1980; Pozio et al., 1981) and in Spain (Morillas Marquez et al., 1985) other infected *R.rattus* were discovered.

4. Other Animals

Apart from a few old reportings in Sudan, a felid, the serval cat *Felis serval* Scherber, 1776, and a viverrid, the genet *Genetta genetta* L., 1758, both carnivores, were found infected (Hoogstraal and Heynemann, 1969). All these animals are probably accidental hosts.

More recently, a porcupine, *Hystrix indica*, was found infected in Turkmenistan, USSR (WHO, 1980) and a racoon dog, *Nycterentes procyanoides*, in China (Xu Zhi Biao et al., 1984). The strain of *Leishmania* isolated from the latter had isoenzyme patterns indistinguishable from a marker strain of *L.infantum* zymodeme MON-1 (Xu Zhi Biao et al., 1984). In the state of Baia in Brazil, an opossum, *Didelphis albiventris*, was found naturally infected by an isolate identified as *L.donovani* (sensu lato) (Sherlock et al., 1984).

EPIDEMIOLOGICAL MEANING OF VERTEBRATE RESERVOIR PARASITISM

1. Man

In anthroponotic areas, like India, the form of human parasitism is suitable for transmission by phlebotomine bite. In fact, amastigotes circulate in peripheral human blood in

50 to more than 80% of patients and 5 to more than 20% of them develop late dermal lesions rich in amastigotes, i.e., post-kala-azar dermal leishmaniasis. In eastern Africa, parasitism is similar to the indian type but the parasitaemia and dermal lesions are less frequent.

2. Dog

Canine leishmaniasis is a severe disease, leading to the animal's death in almost all cases, even with treatment. It is generally a prolonged disease lasting, on average, two years.

Lanotte et al., (1979) has described four clinical epidemiological forms of the disease: two patent forms, treated and not treated, and two latent ones, pre-clinical and resolving. The first ones are similar, but in the treated form there is a period of remission of some months to a year. The latent forms are symptomless and prolonged, about ten months. They are almost all pre-clinical. Because of this, in the majority of epidemiological surveys, about 50% of the infected dogs do not show evident symptoms. The latent regressive forms do not exceed 10% of the total.

Canine Leishmaniasis is viscero-cutaneous and in superficial layers the amastigotes are found either in lesions or apparently healthy skin. The latter characteristic has a significant epidemiological meaning because of the habits of the phlebotomine vector, which prefers to bite healthy skin, often the nose owing to the absence of hair and high concentration of carbon dioxide in expired air (Bray, 1982). Infection of phlebotomine gut is in danger if the sandfly bites a sore, as this is not only incompatible with leishmanial parasites development in the insect, but also may lead to its death (Adler and Theodor, 1931).

Though it is evident that canine leishmaniasis is the principal pillar of the endemicity of the disease in a great part of the world, the incidence of human disease does not always develop in parallel with the prevalence of infection in the dog. The main example of this is the island of Ustica, near Sicily, where 37% of dogs were found infected, but no human cases have been reported (Mansueto et al., 1982). Our own experience confirms this. The reasons for this are complex and related to zoophilic preferences of the insect vector in most cases.

There is, however, an important characteristic of canine leishmaniasis that is suitable for disease control but rarely used. This phenomenon was experimentally proved by Rioux et al. (1972) and Lanotte et al. (1979) and is related to the fact that phlebotomine sandflies are infected at significant rates, only when fed on patent cases. This characteristic provides the use of clinical surveys as a method of control of kala-azar, as has been done in the USSR (WHO, 1980). Nevertheless, the fact that the dog only becomes infective at an advanced stage of disease does not reduce the epidemiological importance of pre-clinical cases, since they represent latent reservoirs that may evolve into infective hosts in the course of a year of more (Bettini and Gradoni, 1966).

3. Wild Canidae

Since Garnham (1965) it is usual to consider that the infection of these animals is symptomless in most of them, reflecting a well balanced relation between the host and the parasite and, in consequence, old infections. Nevertheless, we think that the apparently symptomless course of infection in wild animals is misunderstood and only a consequence of a wild life. Indeed the fox, (whose behaviour we know well), is an animal with fixed hunting territory. A diseased fox in a very competitive biotope will be ousted by a healthy vigorous competing animal, and will die. Under these conditions there is little probability of finding animals with severe advanced disease symptoms, as most of them die before this can happen.

In spite of the usual course of infection in wild animals there are some examples of severe disease in nature and experimentally. In Iran, two of the jackals captured by Nadim et al. (1978) and Hamidi et al. (1982) had advanced disease. The same was seen in several foxes studied by Rioux et al. (1970) with a fox infected, probably, in North Africa. On the other hand the studies of experimental infection of Deane and Deane (1955) and Rioux et al. (1968, 1971) seem to confirm the data of natural fox infections showing that the disease in foxes and jackals is very similar to that of the dog.

This symptomology contradicts the concept of ancient leishmaniasis in sylvatic Canidae with the possibility of synanthropic animals becoming infected through the dog, as was suggested by Soviet scientists (WHO, 1980) and Rioux et al. (1968). However it is possible that in some endemic areas a semi-autonomous sylvatic cycle is established.

Probably this occurs if there is in the area a potential exophilic vector like *Phlebotomus ariasi* in Cevenes and Arrabida. In the rural area of Arrabida studied by us, the prevalence of canine leishmaniasis is 8.8% and vulpine infection 5.6% (Abranches et al., 1985). In the area, Pires (1984) found three infected *P.perniciosus* and two infected *P.ariasi*. Pires (in press) also observed that the first sandfly species was found predominantly (96%) in shelters associated with human activity, while the second was captured almost entirely in sylvatic biotopes (97.2%).

It is possible that wild Canidae have different roles as reservoirs, according to the particular endemic area. For example, Lainson et al. (1987) believe that the fox *Dusicyon thous* is the primary reservoir in the Amazon region where kala-azar is sporadic, while the fox, *D.vetulus* is a secondary reservoir in Ceara, as Deane (1956) has already suggested.

The problem is complex and controversial, and has not been solved yet.

4. Rodents

In Sudan several rodents were found parasitized with *L.donovani* (s.l.). One of them, the Nile grass rat *A.niloticus* has been considered a good reservoir (Hoogstraal and Heyneman, 1969).

In Mediterranean Europe, some *R.rattus* were found infected, but only in Tuscany, Italy has its role as a reservoir been studied. Experimental inoculation was performed by Gradoni et al. (1983) who verified that the infection was symptomless and self-limiting. On the other hand, the two potential vectors in the region, *P.perniciosus* and *P.perfiliewi* were able to feed on that rodent (Gradoni et al., 1983) and the first species was able to transmit the infection by bite (Pozio et al., 1985).

These studies prove the possibility that *R.rattus* may be an habitual reservoir of leishmaniasis in Tuscany, but its actual role is not yet solved.

5. Other Animals

The remaining infected vertebrates referred to here may be accidental hosts. Insufficient data exists on this subject. Sometimes the inoculation route is unusual, (for example, ingesting parasitized rodents).

EVOLUTION OF ANIMAL PARASITISM

ACTUAL SITUATION OF NATURAL FOCI OF DISEASE

Rodents have evolved since the Eocene period and they probably acquired leishmaniasis before carnivores did, though only forms of disease that are cutaneous in man.

According to Lanotte et al. (1981) the greater part of the zoonotic cutaneous leishmaniasis in the old world is caused by the more ancient *Leishmania* species such as *L.major*, which have rodents as reservoirs. They are less often reservoirs of the *L.donovani* and *L.tropica* complexes which have probably evolved more recently, perhaps in the Pleistocene (Lanotte et al., 1981).

The visceral types evolved later and the Canidae would have been introduced into the cycle at the beginning of this evolution, perhaps by the ingestion of infected rodents.

With the reasoning presented here, it is difficult to accept that wild Canidae like the jackal and fox, are primary reservoirs of leishmaniasis. On the other hand, *R.rattus* is not an autochtonous species in Europe being introduced in the Middle Ages.

The origin and identification of real natural foci remains puzzling and their actual existence controversial.

REFERENCES

Abranches,P.,Conceição-Silva,F.M.,Ribeiro,M.M.S.,Lopes,F.J. and Teixeira Gomes, L. (1983). Kala-azar in Portugal. IV : The wild reservoir : The isolation of a *Leishmania* from a fox. Trans. R. Soc. Trop. Med. Hyg. 77 : 420.

Abranches, P., Conceição-Silva, F.M. and Silva-Pereira, M.C.D. (1984). Kala-azar in Portugal. V: The sylvatic cycle in the enzootic endemic focus of Arrábida. J. Trop. Med. Hyg., 87 : 197.

Adler, S. and Theodor, D. (1931). Investigations on Mediterranean kala-azar. I - Introduction and Epidemiology. Proc. R. Soc., Series B, Biological Sciences (London), 108 : 447.

Alencar, J. E. (1961). Profilaxia do Calazar no Ceará, Brasil. Rev. Inst. Med. Trop. São Paulo, 3 : 175.

Bettini, S. and Gradoni L. (1986). Canine leishmaniasis in the Mediterranean area and its implications for human leishmaniasis. Ins. Sci. App.7:241

Bettini, S., Pozio, E. and Gradoni, L. (1980). Leishmaniasis in Tuscany (Italy) : (II) *Leishmania* from wild Rodentia and Carnivora in a human and canine leishmaniasis focus. Trans. R. Soc. Trop. Med. Hyg., 74:77.

Bray, R. S. (1982). The zoonotic potential of reservoirs of Leishmaniasis in the old World. Ecology of Disease, 1 : 257.

Conroy, J. D., Levine, N. D. and Small, E. (1970).Visceral leishmaniasis in a fennec fox (*Fennecus zerda*). Path. Vet., 7 : 163.

Deane, L. M. (1956). Leishmaniose visceral no Brasil. Estudos sobre reservatórios e transmissores realizados no Estado do Ceará. Tése. Serviço Nacional de Educação sanitária. Rio de Janeiro.

Deane, L. M. and Deane, P. M. (1955). Observações preliminares sobre a importância comparativa do homem, do cão e da raposa (*Lycalopex vetulus*) como reservatórios da *Leishmania donovani* em área endêmica de Calazar, no Ceará. O Hospital, 48 : 61.

Dursunova, S. M., Karapetyian. A. B. and Ponirovsky, E. N. (1965). (Some data of investigation of visceral leishmaniasis in the Turkman SSR) (Summary in English). Med. Parasit. and Parasit. Dis., 34 : 303.

Garnham, P. C. C. (1965). The leishmanias, with special reference to the role of animal reservoirs. Amer. Zool., 5 : 141.

Gradoni, L., Pozio; E., Gramiccia, M., Maroli, M. and Bettini, S. (1983). Leishmaniasis in Tuscany(Italy). VII : studies on the role of the black rat, *Rattus rattus*, in the epidemiology of visceral leishmaniasis. Trans R. Soc. Trop. Med. Hyg., 77 :427.

Hamidi, A. N., Nadim, A., Edrissian, G. H., Tahvildar-Bidruni, Gh. and Javadian, E. (1982). Visceral leishmaniasis of jackals and dogs in northern Iran. Trans. R. Soc. Trop. Med. Hyg., 76 : 756.

Hoogstraal, H. & Heyneman, D. (1969). Leishmaniasis in the Sudan Republic. 30 - Final epidemiological report. Amer. J. Trop. Med. Hyg., 18 : 1091.

Kellina, O. I. (1981). Problems and current lines in investigations on the epidemiology of leishmaniasis and its control in the U.S.S.R.. Bull. Soc. Path. Exot., 74 : 306.

Kirk, R. (1956). Studies in leishmaniasis in the Anglo-Egyptian Sudan. XII. Attempts to find a reservoir host. Trans. R. Soc. Trop. Med. Hyg., 50: 169.

Lainson, R., Shaw, J. J. and Lins, Z. C. (1969). Leishmaniasis in Brazil. IV. The fox, *Cerdocyon thous* (L.) as a reservoir of *Leishmania donovani* in Pará State, Brazil. Trans. R. Soc. Trop. Med. Hyg., 63 : 741.

Lainson, R., Shaw, J. J., Silveira, F. T. and Braga, R. R. (1987). American visceral leishmaniasis : on the origin of *Leishmania (Leishmania) chagasi*. Trans. R. Soc. Trop. Med. Hyg., 81 : 517.

Lanotte, G., Rioux, J.-A., Maazoun, R., Pasteur, N., Pratlong, F. and Lepart, J. (1981). Application de la méthode numérique à la taxonomie du genre *Leishmania* Ross, 1903. Ann. Parasit. Hum. Comp., 56 : 575.

Lanotte, G., Rioux, J.-A., Perieres, J. and Vollhardt, H. (1979). Ecologie des leishmanioses dans le sud de la France. 10. Les formes évolutives de la leishmaniose viscérale canine. Elaboration d'une typologie bio--clinique à finalité épidémiologique. Ann. Parasit. Hum. Comp. 54: 277.

Latyshev, N. I., Kryukova, A. P. and Povalishina, T. P. (1951). (Essays on the Regional Parasitology of Middle Asia. I - Leishmaniasis in Tadjikistan. Materials for the Medical geography of Tadjik SSR (résultats of expeditions in 1945-47)). Prob. Reg. Exp. Parasit. & Med. Zool., Moscow, 7 : 35. (Summary in Trop. Dis. Bull., 51 : 37, 1954).

Leng Yan-Jia (1982). A review of kala-azar in China from 1949 to 1959. Trans. R. Soc. Trop. Med. Hyg., 76 : 531.

Mansueto; S., di Leo, R., Miceli, M. D. and Quartararo, P. (1982). Canine leishmaniasis in three foci in western Sicily. Trans. R. Soc. Trop. Med. Hyg. , 76 : 565.

Marin Iniesta, F., Marin Iniesta, E. and Martin Luengo; F. (1982). Papel de perros y zorros como reservatório de leishmaniosis en la region murciana. Resultados preliminares. Rev. Ib. Parasit., 42 : 307.

Maruashvilli, G. M. and Bardzhadze, B. G. (1966). (Natural focality of Visceral leishmaniasis in Georgia). Med. Parasit. & Parasit. Dis., 35 : 462. (summary in english).

Morillas Marquez, F., Benavides Delgado, I., Gonzalez Castro, J., Reyes Magana, A. and Valero Lopes (1985). Découverte de *Leishmania* sp. dans les *Rattus rattus* de la province de Grenade (Espagne). Ann. Parasit. Hum. Comp., 60 : 768.

Nadim. A., Navid-Hamidi, A., Javadian, E., Tahvildari Bidruni, Gh. and Amini, H. (1978). Present status of kala-azar in Iran. Amer. J. Trop Med. and Hyg., 27 : 25.

Ngoka, J. M. and Mutinga, M. J. (1978). Visceral Leishmaniasis animal reservoirs in Kenya. East Afr. Med. J., 55 : 332.

Petrisceva, P. A. (1961). (Methods of study and the profilaxis of the leishmaniasis and sadfly fever). Madgiz, Moscow.

Petrovic, Z., Bordjoski, A. and Savin, Z. (1975). Les résultats de recherches sur le réservoir de *Leishmania donovani* dans une région endémique du kala-azar. Proceedings of Second European Multicolloquy of Parasitology. Trogir. Págs. 97-98.

Pires, C. A. (1984). Les phlebotomes de Portugal. I - Infestation naturelle des *Phlebotomus ariasi* Tonnoir, 1921 et *Phlebotomus perniciosus* Newstead 1911, par *Leishmania* dans le foyer zoonotique de Arrábida (Portugal). Ann. Parasit. Hum. Comp., 59 : 521.

Pires, C. A.. Os flebotomos de Portugal (*Diptera, Psychodidae*). III - Endofilia e exofilia de *Phlebotomus perniciosus* e *P. ariasi* no foco de kala-azar da região da Arrábida. Actas do III Congresso Ibérico de Entomologia (Granada). 1987. (Para publicação).

Pozio, E., Gradoni, L., Bettini, S. and Gramiccia, M. (1981). Leishmaniasis in Tuscany (Italy). V. Further isolation of *Leishmania* from *Rattus rattus* in the province of Grosseto. Ann. Trop. Med. Parasit., 75 : 393.

Pozio, E., Maroli, M., Gradoni, L. and Gramiccia, M. (1985). Laboratory transmission of *Leishmania infantum* to *Rattus rattus* by the bite of experimentally infected *Phlebotomus perniciosus*. Trans. R. Soc. Trop. med. Hyg., 79 : 524.

Rioux, J.-A., Albaret, J. L., Houin, R., Dedet, J. P. and Lanotte, G.(1968). Ecologie des leishmanioses dans le sud de la France. 2. Les réservoirs selvatiques. Infestation spontanée du Renard (*Vulpes vulpes* L.). Ann. Parasit. Hum Comp., 43 : 421.

Rioux, J.-A., Lanotte, G., Croset, H. and Dedet, J. P. (1972). Ecologie des leishmanioses dans le sud de la France. 5. Pouvoir infestant comparé des diverses formes de leishmaniose canine vis-à-vis de *Phlebotomus ariasi* Tonnoir, 1921. Ann. Parasit. Hum Comp., 47 : 413.

Rioux, J.-A., Lanotte, G., Destombes, P., Vollhardt, Y. and Croset, H. (1971). leishmaniose expérimentale du Renard *Vulpes vulpes* (L.). Rec. Med. Vet. Ecole d'Alfort, 147 : 489.

Sherlock, I. A., Miranda, J. C., Sadigursky, Y. M. and Grimaldi, G. Jr. (1984). Natural infection of the opossum *Didelphis albiventris (Marsupialia, Didelphidae)* with *Leishmania donovani* in Brazil. Mem. Inst. Oswaldo Cruz, 79 : 511.

Silveira, F. T., Lainson, R., Shaw, J. J. & Póvoa, M. M. (1982). Leishmaniasis in Brazil : XVIII. Further evidence incriminating the fox *Cerdocyon thous* (L.) as a reservoir of Amazonian visceral leishmaniasis. Trans. R. Soc. Trop. Med. Hyg., 76 : 830.

W.H.O. (1980). TDR/Leish-sem./80.3. Report of a training seminar on epidemiological methods for the leishmaniasis. Moscow, Baku, Samarkand.

Zhi-Biao, Xu., Le Blancq, S., Evans, D. A. and Peters, W. (1984). The characterization by isoenzyme electrophoresis of *Leishmania* isolated in the people's Republic of China. Trans. R. Soc. Trop. Med. Hyg., 78 : 689.

EFFECTIVENESS OF CONTROL MEASURES AGAINST CANINE LEISHMANIASIS IN THE ISLE OF ELBA, ITALY

L. Gradoni[1], M. Gramiccia[1], F. Mancianti[2] and S. Pieri[3]

[1] Laboratorio di Parassitologia
  Istituto Superiore di Sanita, Rome
[2] Dipartimento di Patologia Animale
  Universita di Pisa, Pisa
[3] Unita Sanitaria Locale 26
  Portoferraio, Isola d'Elba

INTRODUCTION

The dog is the domestic reservoir of Mediterranean visceral leishmaniasis (VL). Therefore, the application of measures aimed at controlling canine leishmaniasis should represent the main strategy to prevent human infections. Unfortunately, the antimonial drugs which are successfully used for the treatment of human VL are poorly effective in the radical treatment of canine leishmaniasis. Killing of infected dogs is usually considered the only effective measure to control or to prevent epidemics in man (WHO, 1984). However, in Mediterranean foci where a canine leishmaniasis seropositivity prevalence of 15-20% is commonly found (Bettini and Gradoni, 1986), the elimination of all serologically positive dogs is not achievable.

Recent clinical, serological and entomological findings have provided evidence that antimonial drugs could represent an additional control measure against canine leishmaniasis (Gradoni et al., 1986, 1987, and in preparation).
These findings may be summarizes as follows:
(i) Treatment of asymptomatic cases, which were found to be non-infective to sandflies (Adler and Theodor, 1932; Rioux et al., 1972) yielded high recovery rates (47%) or prevented the progression of disease towards patency (47% of cases).
(ii) Treatment of oligosymptomatic cases yielded low recovery rates, but a strong reduction in the infection rate of phlebotomine vectors which were fed on them.

(iii) Treatment of symptomatic cases yielded very low recovery rates and, in addition, a high infection rate in vectors, even after several courses of the drug.

A control strategy based on the treatment of asymptomatic and oligosymptomatic cases, and on the removal of symptomatic dogs has been applied to evaluate the effectiveness of these combined measures.

MATERIALS AND METHODS

A large sample of the dog population of the isle of Elba was the object of this study. In a previous survey, the prevalence of canine leishmaniasis averaged 19.1% (range 2.5-39.6%) (Mancianti et al., 1986). Control measures were applied in 6 communes, out of the 8 on the island, which showed the highest frequencies of the disease (range 17.3-39.6%).

Clinical examination of dogs, specimen collection, and indirect immuno-fluorescence test (IFAT) were carried out as previously reported (Gradoni et al., 1980; Pozio et al., 1981).

Both clinical examination and specimen collection were carried out at the veterinary clinic of Portoferraio or by visiting farms or peripheral districts of towns.

Drug treatment consisted of one or more courses of meglumine antimoniate (Glucantime) (one course: 100/kg/day, 10 days of treatment (dt) + 10 days off treatment (+ 10 dt)).

Prevalence of the infection was estimated through tests carried out between two transmission seasons. A transmission season was defined as the period of higher density of the local vector, _Phlebotomus perniciosus_, i.e. from June to September (Maroli and Bettini, 1977).

A cohort study was carried out according to criteria shown in Figure 1. Cohort I was represented by dogs born within two transmission seasons. They were mainly puppies or young dogs examined during passive case detection at the veterinary clinic.

Cohort II was represented by adult dogs (average 4.7 years) examined and found negative before each transmission season. They were examined mainly during active case detection. The only data taken into consideration were those from tests carried out after a serological latency period. The analysis of the results showed that this latency period lasted 4 months at the most.

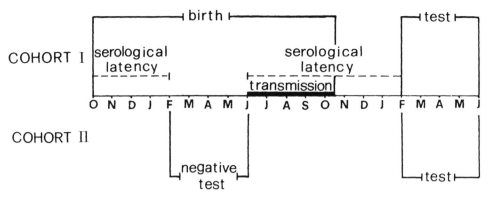

FIGURE 1. CRITERIA FOR DEFINITION OF COHORTS I AND II AND PERIOD OF TEST

RESULTS

More than 2,000 tests were carried out on 1,500 dogs examined from 1984 to 1987. Control measures were applied before the transmission seasons 1985 and 1986 (Table I). Eighty-five infected dogs were treated with 1-3 courses of meglumine antimoniate and 77, mainly symptomatic, were killed.

Table I. MEASURES APPLIED FOR CANINE LEISHMANIASIS CONTROL IN THE ISLE OF ELBA

PERIOD	TREATED			KILLED
	1 course	2 courses	3 courses	
OCT 1984-MAY 1985	40	14	1	42
OCT 1985-MAY 1986	21	6	3	35
TOTAL	85			77

Data on canine leishmaniasis prevalence in the six communes involved were obtained for years 1985, 1986 and 1987 (Table II).The IFAT-positive dogs varied from 22.2% in 1985 to 14.2% in 1987. Before the application of control measures the frequency of infected dogs showing a clinically patent leishmaniasis (oligosymptomatic and symptomatic cases) was 14.4%. This percentage was reduced to 7.2% in 1986 and to 5.2% in 1987.

Table II. Prevalence of canine leishmaniasis in the Isle of Elba from 1985 to 1987

Year	Dogs examined	IFAT-POSITIVE DOGS			TREATED	Recovered
		Asymptomatic	Oligosymptomatic	Symptomatic		
1985	631	46(7.3%)	39(6.2%)	52(8.2%)	3(0.5%)	2(0.3%)
1986	375	25(6.7%)	15(4.0%)	12(3.2%)	32(8.5%)	9(2.4%)
1987	404	18(4.5%)	12(3.0%)	9(2.2%)	18(4.5%)	20(4.9%)

Incidence of new cases after the transmission seasons 1984, 1985 and 1986 was estimated through the cohort study (Table III). In cohort I the incidence decreased from 11.6% before control measures were applied, to 2.9% after 1986. In the same period, incidence in cohort II decreased from 15.4% to 5.4%. The average incidence was 12.4% after 1984, 9.4% after 1985 and 4.6% after 1986. The reduction obtained from 1984 to 1986 was found to be highly significant by the chi-square test.

Table III. Incidence of canine leishmaniasis in cohorts I and II from 1984 to 1986.

Cohort	1984	1985	1986
I	12/106(11.3%)	6/121(4.9%)	2/69(2.9%)
II	6/39(15.4%)	22/176(12.5%)	8/147(5.4%)

DISCUSSION

The control measures were adopted on the basis of findings obtained through both serological and clinical methods. The serological method (IFAT) was found to be highly sensitive, as confirmed by 100% of parasitological correlation which has been previously found (Mancianti et al., 1986), as well as by the data obtained through the hundreds of case studies carried out for incidence estimates. Through this technique, it was apparently possible to reveal all prepatent cases during the annual surveys. Clinical examination was more subjective and obviously it did not reveal asymptomatic cases. However, it was useful in giving an appraisal of the severity of signs and symptoms and in deciding if an infected dog was to be treated or killed.

The cohort study was used for the first time in an investigation on canine leishmaniasis. For its application, however, the transmission and the serological latency periods had to be known. In the Mediterranean foci, where the sandfly season lasts no longer than 4-6 months, tests for incidence evaluation may be carried out over a 3-4 month period without confusion from infection by a new generation of new cases. Thanks to the high number of case studies carried out during the three years, we had the opportunity to determine to a good approximation the maximum period of serological latency (in relation to the IFAT test only) which we have shown to last about four months from the end of the sandfly season. The majority of new seropositives, however, were detected 1-2 months after this season. Two different cohorts showed the same incidence trend over three years. However, incidence in cohort I (puppies and young dogs) was always lower than in cohort II. This finding could be explained by the different sampling method used, which usually was passive case detection for cohort I and active detection for cohort II.

The presence of new canine infections and, hence, the risk of human cases, appeared to be striclty correlated with the prevalence of patent cases only. In fact, after two years of control the overall prevalence of IFAT-positive dogs did not vary greatly, but the group represented by oligosymptomatic and symptomatic cases showed a 64% reduction. This value equals the observed reduction in average incidence (63%).

The year by year decrease in the prevalence of patent cases was presumably due not only to the exclusion of dogs that had been killed, but also to the treatment of prepatent cases which did not develop signs of the disease. On the other hand, the percentage of dogs which recovered after treatment increased from 0.3% in 1985 to 4.9% in 1987.

REFERENCES

Adler S. & Theodor O. 1932
   Proc. Roy. Soc London Series B 110 402-412

Bettini S & Gradoni L, 1986
   Ins Sci Appl 7 241-245

Gradoni L, Pozio, E , Bettini S & Gramiccia M 1980
   Trans Roy Soc Trop Med Hyg 74, 421-422

Gradoni L, Gramiccia M, Mancianti, F, Maroli M, Pieri S & Maroli M, 1986
   Atti XIV Congr Soc Ital Parassitologi Pisa 21st-24th May 1986 Parassitology

Gradoni L, Maroli M, Gramiccia M, & Mancianati F, 1987
   Med Vet Entomol 1, In Press

Mancianati F, Gradoni L, Grammiccia M, Pieri S & Marconcini A, 1986
   Trop Med Parasitol 37, 110-112

Maroli M & Bettini S, 1977
   Trans Roy Soc Trop Med Hyg 71, 315-321

Pozio E, Gradoni L, Bettini S & Gramicia M, 1981
   Acta Trop 38, 383-393

Rioux. J.A, Lanotte G, Groset H & Dedet J.P, 1972
   Ann Parasitol Hum Comp 47, 413-419

WHO 1984   The Leishmaniases
   Techn Rep Ser 701 WHO Geneva

THE INCIDENCE OF CANINE LEISHMANIASIS IN NORTHERN GREECE: AN EPIZOOTIOLOGICAL STUDY OF THE DECADE 1977-1987

V.I. Kontos and A.G. Spais

Clinic of Medicine, College of Veterinary Medicine
Aristotelian University Thessaloniki
11 St. Voutyra Str.
546 27 Thessaloniki
Greece

INTRODUCTION

In Greece human visceral leishmaniasis has been known for many years. Since 1885, a disease with an unknown aetiology called "ponos", had characteristics similar to those of leishmaniasis [1,2]. From the beginning of this century the disease was diagnosed in dogs in the area of Athens [3] and later in several other areas in Southern Greece [1,4,5,6,7]. In all cases the research on canine leishmaniasis was carried out in parallel with that on human leishmaniasis. So far as the leishmaniasis situation in N. Greece is concerned, there are limited data concerning only one area [8].

In the present study an effort was made to investigate the extent of canine leishmaniasis in N. Greece generally and particularly in the Thessaloniki district during the last ten years.

MATERIALS AND METHODS

Animals
During the past ten years (1977-87), 11,501 dogs presenting at the clinic of Medicine of our Faculty for different reasons were taken as our study material. Most of these dogs came from the Thessaloniki area, less from other parts of N. Greece and few from other areas of the country.

The diagnosis of leishmaniasis was based on the detection of the protozoon microscopically in smears made from material aspirated from lymph nodes, the isolation of the protozoon from the same material or other tissues in cases where the dogs died or were killed. All these examples were cultured on the biphasic medium 3N [9].

Strain Identification
Ten of the *Leishmania* strains isolated during our study were sent for identification to the Department of Parasitology, the Kuvin Centre for the Study of Infectious and Tropical Diseases, Hebrew University-Hadassah Medical School, Jerusalem, Israel (Director Prof. Schnur) via the Pasteur Institute of Athens. The identification was based on the determination of the Excreted Factor (EF) and on the results obtained by the polyacrylamide gel electrophoresis (PGE) method using the specific enzymes MDH, GPI, G-6-PDH and 6-P-GDH [10,11].

Sera
Three hundred and five sera (305) were collected from dogs showing no signs of leishmaniasis, during the 1979-1981 period. These randomly selected sera were examined for antibodies against *Leishmania* by the indirect immunofluorescent assay (IFAT) [9]. Fifty six more sera were collected from dogs suspected to be infected by *Leishmania*, but where this diagnosis had not been confirmed a microscopical examination was made.

RESULTS

In the ten years of our study, leishmaniasis was diagnosed in 185 (1.6%) out of 11,501 dogs visiting out clinic. The annual distribution is presented in Table 1.

The ten strains that were identified as *Leishmania donovani* were found to be identical. By the method of the determination of the excreted factor, it was also found that all belong to the serotype B_2. By the PGE method, it was found that they had the characteristics of different types depending on the enzyme used. Thus, they belong to type VII when the enzyme MDH was used, to type I with the enzyme GPI, to type II with the enzyme G-6-PDH and to type III with the enzyme 6-P-GPH.

TABLE 1 ANNUAL DISTRIBUTION OF CANINE LEISHMANIASIS CASES DURING THE DECADE 1977-1987.

Year	No of dogs examined	No of dogs with leishmaniasis
1977-1987	900	13
1978-1979	914	18
1979-1980	1223	25
1980-1981	1724	13
1981-1982	1209	17
1982-1983	1443	13
1983-1984	837	16
1984-1985	674	17
1985-1986	1212	27
1986-1987	1365	26
Total	11501	185 (1.6%)

Thirty three (33) out of 305 randomly collected dog sera were found to be positive (10.8%) by the IFAT with titres ranging from 1/160 to 1/2560. This positivity could not be related statistically to the area these dogs were coming from, their functional role, the type of their hair or their sex or age.

Twenty two out of the 56 sera collected from dogs suspected to be infected by *Leishmania* were found to be positive (39%) in titres ranging from 1:160 to 1:2560 by the IFAT.

DISCUSSION

The protozoan responsible for the disease of the dog population in N. Greece proved to be *L. infantum* of a single type. Moreover, all of our strains were identical to other strains examined simultaneously at the same laboratory in Israel and which had been isolated from people and dogs with visceral leishmaniasis from Greece and elsewhere [10,11]. Nevertheless, it seems that there are also other strains in the Mediterranean countries. In Italy 8 out of 11 strains isolated from dogs, foxes (*Vulpes vulpes*) and rats (*Rattus rattus*) were shown to be identical to ours, whereas the remaining three strains were not. Two of these strains were isolated from dogs and the other from a fox [12].

From the cases diagnosed as leishmaniasis during the last decade (185 dogs out of 11501 examined, incidence 1.6%) and from our serological survey carried out during the 1979-1981 period (33 positive out of 305 dog sera examined, prevalence 10.8%) it is apparent that the number of infected animals is large.

In similar surveys conducted in other Mediterranean countries, it was found that in Italy, for instance, the incidence was from 2.9% to 23.9% [13,14], in Southern France 4.4% [15], in Algeria 11.4% [16], and in Tunisia 6.2% [17]. Thus, it is obvious that the spread of the *Leishmania* infection is wide, although it does not always show clinical symptoms.

All the above findings show that there is a major problem of leishmaniasis. The disease is not related to the area where the animals are living (country or city), the purpose for which they are kept, the type of their hair, their sex or age.

Our findings could be interpreted as indicating a major public health problem. But at least for one area, it is not really a serious human problem. The cases of visceral leishmaniasis that present at the AHEPA hospital are very few (Sclavounnnou-Tsouroutsoglou, personal communication, 1986). This is consistent with older information concerning the whole country [18].

Although an extensive epidemiological survey has not yet been undertaken, the 10.8% prevalence of infection of the dogs should not be taken as criterion for the extent of human visceral leishmaniasis in the Thessaloniki area. Of course it would be desirable and very interesting to carry out two surveys, epizootiological and epidemiological, at the same time in order to determine the relationship between canine and human visceral leishmaniasis in the area.

CONCLUSION

In conclusion therefore, from a total number of 11,501 dogs which were presented with various complaints at the Small Animal Clinic of the Aristotelian University's Veterinary College during the past decade (1977-1987), visceral leishmaniasis was diagnosed in 185 of them (1.6%). The diagnosis of this protozoan disease is based essentially on the demonstration of the parasite in the smears made of material aspirated from lymph nodes and in a number of cases on the IFAT and on culture. Ten of the isolated parasite strains were found to be similar to each other and were identified as belonging to the species *L. infantum*.

In addition, an epidemiological survey was conducted during the three year period 1979-1981, which involved dogs living in the greater territory of Thessaloniki. A total number of 305 blood sera was collected from asymptomatic dogs and screened for *Leishmania* antibodies using the indirect immunofluorescence assay (IFAT). The results of this survey showed that 33 dogs (10.8%) were serologically positive for *Leishmania* and that no correlation could be demonstrated between the infection rate and the area that affected dogs came from, their functional role, the type of their hair coat, sex or age.

ACKNOWLEDGEMENTS

The authors are grateful to the Greek Ministry of Agriculture for the financial support which made this study possible.

REFERENCES

1. J. Caminopetros, 1934 Actuelles donnees epidemiologiques et experimentales sur les leishmanioses en Grece, Bull. path. exot., 25:450.

2. A. Aravantinos, 1942 Particular Diseases and Their Treatments, Athens.

3. S.P. Cardomastis, 1912 Leishmaniose du chien en Grece, Bull. path. exot., 21:88.

4. J. Caminopetros, 1934 Lesions cutanees du chien revetent les caracteres du Bouton d'Orient, Bull path. exot., 27:527.

5. J. Caminopetros, "Le Kala-azar. Recherches epidemiologiques et experimentales sur son mode de transmission", S.A. Eleptheroudakis, ed., Athenes (1976).

6. S. Adler and O. Theodor, 1932 Investigations of Mediterranean Kala-azar VI. Canine visceral leishmaniasis,
   Proc. Roy. Soc. B., 110:402.

7. S. Adler and O. Theodor, 1934 Investigations of Mediterannean Kala-azar VII. Further observations on canine visceral leishmaniasis,
   Proc. Roy. Soc. B., 116:494 ().

8. A. M. Papadakis,1956 Parasitology, Athens.

9. V.I. Kontos, 1986 A contribution to the study of Leishmaniasis in dogs. Clinical, Terminological and Experimental Investigations, Doctorate Thesis, Scientific Anniversary of the Department of Veterinary Science, Thessaloniki.

10. L.F. Schnur, M.L. Chance, F. Ebert, S.C. Thomas and W. Peters, 1981 The biochemical and serological taxonomy of visceralizing *Leishmania*,
    Ann. Trop. Med. Parasit., 75:131

11. N. Tzamouranis, L.F. Schnur, A. Garifallou, E. Pateraki and C. Serie, 1984 Leishmaniasis in Greece I. Isolation and identification of the parasite causing human and canine visceral leishmaniasis,
    Ann. Trop. Med. Parasit., 78:363

12. M. Gramiccia, R. Maazoon, G. Lanotte, J.A. Rioux, S. Leblanco, D.A. Evans, W. Peters, S. Bettini, L. Gradoni and E. Pozio, 1982 Typage enzymatique de onze souches de *Leishmania* isolees, en Italy continentalle, a partir des formes viscerale murines, canines et vulpines. Mise en evidence d'un variant enzymatique chez le renard (*Vulpes vulpes*) et le chien,
    Annal. Parasit., 57:527.

13. L. Gradoni, E. Pozio, M. Gramiccia, M. Maroli and S. Bettini, 1983 Leishmaniasis in Tuscany (Italy): VII Studies on the role of the black rat, *Rattus rattus*, in the epidemiology of visceral leishmaniasis,
    Trans. Roy. Soc. Trop. Med. Hyg., 77:427.

14. E. Pozio, L. Gradoni, S. Bettini and M. Gramiccia, 1981 Leishmaniasis in Tuscany (Italy): VI Canine leishmaniasis in the focus of Monte Argentario (Grosseto),
    Acta Tropica, 38:383.

15. G. Lanotte, J.A. Rioux, H. Croset and Y. Vollhardt, 1974 Ecologie des leishmanioses dans le sud de la France. 7. Depistage de l'enzootie canine par les methodes immunoserologiques,
    Annal. Parasit. hum. Comp., 49:41.

16. J.P. Dedet, 1979 Les leishmanioses en Afrique du nord,
    Bull. Inst. Past., 77:49.

17. J.P. Dedet, F. Ben Osman, A. Chadli, H. Groset and J.A. Rioux, 1973 La leishmaniose en Tunisie. Frequence actuelles de l'enzootie d'apres enquete sero-immunologique,
    Ann. Parasit., 48:653.

18. O. Marselou-Kinte, T. Stephanou, M. Violaki and D. Avramides, 1980 Leishmaniasis in Greece during the decade 1970-1979. Proceedings of the 9th National Conference of Microbiology, Athens.

STUDIES ON THE ROLE OF THE GROUND SQUIRREL (*Citellus citellus*): IN THE EPIDEMIOLOGY OF LEISHMANIASIS

V.I. Kontos[1], G.S. Koptopoulos[2], S. Th. Haralabidis[3] and A.G. Spais[1]

[1]Clinic of Medicine, [2]Lab. of Microbiology and Parasitology, [3]Lab. of Applied Elminthology and Entomology, College of Veterinary Medicine
Aristotelian University Thessaloniki
11 St. Voutyra Str.
546 27 Thessaloniki
Greece

INTRODUCTION

The ground squirrel or spermophil (*Citellus citellus*) is a very common rodent in the fields around Thessaloniki. From preliminary work conducted 50 years ago [1,2] it is known that this rodent is sensitive to experimental infection and can be used in the diagnosis of visceral leishmaniasis. This old observation, when related to the frequent appearance of visceral leishmaniasis in dogs around Thessaloniki [3] led to the present research studies to confirm the possible sensitivity of the ground squirrel to *Leishmania* infection and to determine its role in the epidemiology and ecology of the protozoan.

MATERIALS AND METHODS

Ground Squirrels
256 ground squirrels were trapped in three different areas around Thessaloniki, during the months of April and May 1985. Most of them were young as determined by the body weight. Thirty nine (39) were collected from a rural area (area A), 152 from a marshy area in the delta of the river Axios (area B) and the remaining 65 were trapped in a rural and industrial area, where there are a lot of irrigated fields (area C). In these areas leishmaniasis was diagnosed in

dogs. All squirrels were anaesthetized with the aid of a fluothane mask and a sufficient quantity of blood was taken from the heart. They were then killed and the spleen was removed.

Blood Smears
Blood smears were made from all squirrels and stained by Giemsa's method.

Smears from Spleen
The spleen was cut transversely in the middle and a few impressions from the cut surfaces were made on a glass slide. They were also stained using Giemsa.

Cultures
All cultures were made in the biphasic medium 3N [3]. In summary, two tubes with this medium were used per squirrel. The first was inoculated with 1 ml of freshly collected blood. A little piece of spleen was placed into the second tube. Blood cultures were made from 207 squirrels and spleen cultures from 200.

Serological Examination
129 sera were examined for *Leishmania* antibodies by ELISA. 10 were from squirrels trapped in area A, 52 from area B and the remaining 67 from area C. These squirrels were among those from which smears and cultures were also made.

As antigen a *L. infantum* promastigote culture was used. The parasites were washed 10x with PBS at pH 7.2, homogenised for 45 sec in an Ultra Turrax mixer (20,000 revs min^{-1}) and then centrifuged at 3000 g for one hour at 4ºC. The supernatant was concentrated 10x (PEG) 20,000) and after its titration it was used as soluble antigen in the ELISA [4].

As conjugate an anti-mouse IgG antibody (Pel-Freeze, Arkansas, USA) was used conjugated [5] to alkaline phosphatase (Sigma). The ELISA procedure followed was as described previously [6]. Known reference negative and positive sera were included as controls.

Experimental Infection
Seven squirrels from area B were not sacrificed after the sedation and blood collection, but were kept in separate boxes and were fed with concentrated food pellets for mice. Care was taken to avoid any contact with *Phlebotomous* spp. The cultures and the smears made from them were negative for *Leishmania*.

After three months of staying in and adaptation to the laboratory they were used as experimental animals. Six were infected with promastigotes of a strain isolated from a dog one month prior to inoculation and it was identified as *L.infantum* [3]. Four squirrels were infected by the intraperitoneal route (IP) and the other two intradermally in two sites, in the lobe of an ear and in the tail. The total quantity of the infectious material used in all cases was 1 ml of the liquid phase of the culture, very rich in promastigotes. The seventh squirrel was used as control and it was inoculated (IP) with 1 ml of the liquid phase of a non-infected 3N culture medium. All were observed daily for the appearance of any dermal lesion, for their appetite and liveliness. After they had died, smears and cultures were made from the blood, spleen, liver, lungs and bone marrow.

RESULTS

No *L. infantum* was seen in the smears or isolated from the cultures made from the wild squirrels examined.

Three out of the 129 sera assayed by ELISA were considered as positive. They had antibodies to the $OD_{405\ nm}$ of 0.762 and 0.986 (the positive control serum had 0.836). The first two were from squirrels from area B and the last from area C. All the other sera and the negative reference one had an $OD_{405\ nm}$ up to 0.408.

The results of the experimental inocultaion of the six squirrels and the control are presented in Table 1. The inoculated animals showed almost no abnormalities during the 7 months post inoculation (PI). Squirrel number C_2 was sacrificed in the third month PI. No *Leishmania* was seen in smears made from blood and spleen or isolated in cultures. After the 7th month a focal hair fall started to appear, as well as dermal hyperkeratosis. At the same time a reduction of the appetite and loss of weight were noticed. Between the 8th and 16th months all the squirrels died. *Leishmania* was observed in the smears and isolated in cultures made from the pathological material taken from these. In the smears of the blood a great number of free living amastigotes were also seen.

TABLE 1 EXPERIMENTAL INFECTION OF GROUND SQUIRRELS (SPERMOPHILS)

No	Inoculation route	Strain	Inoculation (months)	Death (months)	Parasites in smears	Parasites in culture
C_1	I.C	L.i prom	8	14	+	+
C_2	I.C	L.i.prom	–	3*	–	–
C_3	I.P	L.i.prom	7	9	+	+
C_4	I.P	L.i.prom	9	13	+	+
C_5	I.P	L.i.prom	9	16	+	+
C_6	I.P	L.i.prom	7	8	+	+
C_7	–	–	–	24*	–	–

I.C - intracutaneous
I.P - intraperitoneally
L.i.prom - *Leishmania infantum* promastigote
* - sacrificed.

DISCUSSION

The experimental infection of the six squirrels with *L.infantum* has confirmed the previous observation of many years ago, that these animals are very sensitive to this parasite. It is interesting that the appearance of the symptoms (focal fall of hair, dermal lesions, loss of weight) is similar to that of dogs. In our experience the parasites are very easily seen in blood smears of squirrels, whereas it is difficult to see them in blood smears of dogs. With the sensitivity of this experimental model it is difficult to explain that we did not find or isolate *Leishmania* in the smears and cultures taken during this epizootiological study. Most probably this was due to the young age of the squirrels. We now know from the experimentally infected animals that it takes a long time to detect the parasite or to reproduce the disease (Table 1). Three months after their inoculation with a great number of parasites there were no leishmanias in the smears or in the cultures: the disease was reproduced only after 7 months. Similar observations were made in dogs naturally or experimentally infected.

The antibodies detected in the three sera by the ELISA should be considered as specific although the conjugate used was heterologous but from a closely related animal species (mouse). On the basis of the experimental and serological findings it is obvious that the ground squirrel can be naturally infected. The two positive sera were from squirrels living in the marshy area B and the other in area C where there are a lot of irrigated fields. It seems that there is a connection between this serum positivity and the conditions of the environment, because this kind of environment is the most suitable for the intermediate host and natural transmitter of leishmanias, the *Phlebotomus* spp.

CONCLUSIONS

In conclusion therefore, ground squirrels (Spermophils, *Citellus citellus*) are abundant in the rural and suburban areas of Thessaloniki, where canine visceral leishmaniasis is prevalent. The experimental and epizootiological survey undertaken suggests that the ground squirrel may act as a reservoir host of canine leishmaniasis.

Six ground squirrels were inoculated IP or ID with a suspension of promastigotes from a culture strain of *L.infantum* isolated from a dog. All inoculated animals developed lesions similar to those seen in the generalized form of canine leishmaniasis, and died 8 to 16 months post inoculation. The protozoan was readily detected in their tissues by light microscopy and by culture.

Two hundred and sixty spermophils collected in three locations were screened for *L.infantum* by direct smear microscopy and culture in biphasic 3N medium. In addition, thir sera were screened for antibodies by ELISA. All smears and cultures were negative, however, serology was positive in three animals.

ACKNOWLEDGEMENTS

The authors are grateful to the Greek Ministry of Agriculture, the financial support of which made this study possible.

REFERENCES

1. G. Blanc and J. Caminopetros, 1930 Sensibilite du spermophile de Madecoine (*Citellus citellus*) au kala-azar medeterraneen,
   C.R. Acad. Scien., 21:800.

2. E. Brumt and H. Gailliard, 1935 Grand sensibilite du spermophile d'Europe, *Citellus citellus*, au virus du la;a-azar Chinois,
   C.R. Soc. Biol., 5:21.

3. V.I. Kontos, 1986 A contribution to the study of Leishmaniasis in dogs. Clinical, Terminological and Experimental Investigations. Doctorate Thesis, Scientific Anniversary of the Department of Veterinary Science, Thessaloniki.

4. S. Th. Haralabidis, 1984 The immunodiagnosis of parasitic diseases and the immunoenzyme assay ELISA (enzyme-linked immunosorbent assay),
   Scientific Yearbook of the Veterinary Faculty of the Aristotelian University of Thessaloniki, 22:75.

5. E. Engrall and P. Perlmann, 1974 Enzyme-linked immunosorbent assay ELISA. III. Quantitation of specific antibodies by enzyme-labeled anti-immunoglobulin in antigen-coated tubes,
   J. Immunol., 109:129.

6. S. Th. Haralabidis, 1984 Immunodiagnosis of giardiasis by ELISA and studies on cross reactivity between the anti-*G.lamblia* antibodies and some heterologous parasitic antigens and fractions,
   Ann. Trop. Med. Parasit., 78:295.

FIELD APPLICATION OF A DIRECT AGGLUTINATION TEST FOR VISCERAL LEISHMANIASIS

P.A. Kager[1], J. Leeuwenburg[2], R. Muigai[2], S. Kiugu[2], D.W. Iha[2], J.K. Mwaniki[2], D.K. Koech[2] and A.E. Harith[3]

[1]University of Amsterdam, Amsterdam, The Netherlands
[2]Kenya Medical Research Institute, Nairobi, Kenya
[3]Royal Tropical Institute, Amsterdam, The Netherlands

INTRODUCTION

The definitive diagnosis of visceral leishmaniasis (VL) is based on the demonstration of the parasite.

Serological tests are useful for epidemiological studies in endemic areas and for screening individual patients where more invasive techniques may not be possible. The serological techniques should be simple, specific and cheap, and be applicable in the adverse conditions that prevail in many areas where leishmaniasis is endemic.

Several tests for the serological diagnosis of VL are available (IFAT, CFT, ELISA) but they do not meet the requirements of a field test as mentioned above.

A recently developed direct agglutination test (DAT), Harith et al. (1986) is promising in meeting these requirements. We report on the application of this test both in the laboratory and in the field.

MATERIALS AND METHODS

Antigen
The antigen was prepared in the Laboratory of Tropical Hygiene, Royal Tropical Institute Amsterdam, as previously described (Harith et al., 1986). Basically it consists of promastigotes of *L.d.donovani*, strain 1-S, treated with trypsin, fixed with formalin and stained with Coomassie Brilliant Blue.

Test Performance
Serial dilutions of the sera in 0.9% saline with 1% foetal bovine serum were made in V-shaped wells of microtitre plates. 50 µl of antigen suspension was added. Results were read visually against a white background after 18 hr, and a titre of 1:3200 or more considered a positive result.

Sera
I. Laboratory work in Amsterdam and Nairobi
A. - 31 Kenyan VL patients, (21 before, during or up to 1 month after treatment, 10 from 4 to 14 months after cure).
    - 27 Zairian trypanosomiasis patients.
    - 10 European and 10 African healthy controls.
    - 45 patients with various communicable diseases (10 mansonian schistosomiasis (Kenya) 10 leprosy (* Surinam, 1 Vietnam, 1 Indonesia) 7 tuberculosis (treated), 10 giardiasis, 8 toxoplasmosis (all Netherlands)).
B. 280 persons from Perkerra area, near Marigat, Baringo District, Kenya, a focus of VL, inclusive of 3 cured VL patients, houshold members, neighbours and 2 patients with VL, admitted to the district hospital.
C. 507 Kenyans (various areas):
    -177 with visceral leishmaniasis
    - 4 with cutaneous leishmaniasis
    - 39 with malaria
    - 5 with brucellosis
    - 12 with hydatid disease
    - 6 with infertility and antisperm antibodies
    -264 controls

II. Field application
D. In 1985 a field laboratory was set up in tents in Perkerra area, Baringo District, Kenya. Sera were stored at about 4ºC in a refridgerator working on gas. 200 sera from the area and from the adjacent Loboi area where recently VL had been demonstrated were tested locally. Sera of 4 VL patients admitted to the district hospital were included.
E. In 1986 the facilities of the Division of Vector Borne Diseases in Marigat were used. 100 sera, all from clusters around VL patients, were tested, and filter paper eluates were evaluated.
F. In 1986 19 VL patients from Baringo District, Kenya, diagnosed and treated between 1981 and 1986, could be traced and examined in the field. Results of 5 more patients from the area, examined and tested in 1984 and 1985 were added.

RESULTS

I. The results of group A sera are shown in Figure 1 and the results of group B sera, together with group C sera, are shown in Table 1.

TABLE 1 DIRECT AGGLUTINATION TEST FOR VISCERAL LEISHMANIASIS IN 280 SERA FROM BARINGO DISTRICT, KENYA AND IN 507 SERA FROM VARIOUS AREAS IN KENYA.

Sera	no.	≤ 800	1600	3200	> 3200
B. VL*	2				2
ex VL**	3		1	1	1
malaria	37	37			
brucellosis	5	5			
splenomegaly	97	96	1		
healthy	136	135		1	
	280	273	2	2	3
C. VL*	177				177
CL***	4	4			
malaria	39	39			
brucellosis	5	5			
hydatid disease	12	12			
infertility	6	6			
controls	264	264			
	507	330			177
total	787	603	2	2	180

(reciprocal of titre)

* VL visceral leishmaniasis
** Resp. 36, 36 and 3 months post cure
*** CL cutaneous leishmaniasis

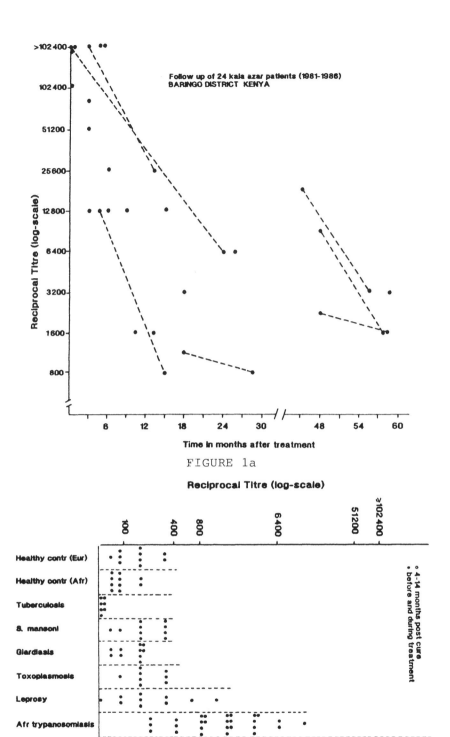

FIGURE 1a

FIGURE 1b

FIGURE 1 a,b & c DIRECT AGGLUTINATION TEST FOR VISCERAL LEISHMANIASIS

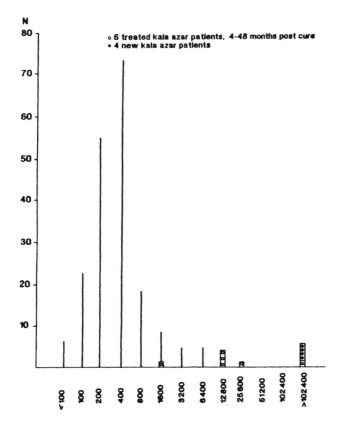

FIGURE 1c

Based on the data from the field (an area free from trypanosomiasis and Chagas' disease) the sensitivity and specificity of the test were 100% and 99% respectively. The 2 ex-VL patients, both 36 months after cure had titres of 1:1600 and 1:3200 and were excluded from the calculations. The predictive value of a positive and negative test were high, 100 and 99% respectively.

In the laboratory, sensitivity, specificity and predictive value of a negative and positive test were all 100% in the Kanya population, C, but in the patients with specific diseases, A, Figure 1a, 30% of trypanosomiasis cases gave a positive reaction.

II. The test proved easy to perform under field circumstances (temperatures from 18 to 37°C; relative humidity from 32 to 70%). The results for group D are shown in Figure 1b. In group E, out of the 100 sera tested, the results were as follows:

N°	RECIPROCAL OF TITRE	COMMENT
87	≤ 1600	
4	3200	
3	6400	2 ex VL, 1 splenomegaly
6	≥ 12800	4 ex VL, 2 new VL

Thirteen filter paper eluates tested locally gave comparable results (VL patients were clearly detected) but comparison of 93 filter paper eluates and corresponding sera later in Amsterdam showed generally lower titres in the eluates (though VL cases were still clearly detected). Finaly, the results for group F are shown in Figure 1c.

CONCLUSIONS

The DAT developed by Harith et al. (1986) is simple and cheap and can be used under field circumstances. The sensitivity and specificity of this DAT are high (about 92 and 99%) in the absence of trypanosomiasis. The predictive value of a negative and positive test (depending much on the prevalence of the disease) need further study and assessment in endemic areas , but in the work reported here (partly in the laboratory and partly in the field) score favourably. The use of filter paper blood and of whole blood need further study before fruitful conclusions can be drawn.

REFERENCE

Harith, A.E., Kolk, A.H.J., Kager, P.A., Leeuwenburg, J., Muigai, R., Kiugu, S. and Laarman, J.J. 1986, A simple and economical direct agglutination test for serodiagnosis and sero-epidemiological studies of visceral leishmaniasis,
Trans. R. Soc. Trop. Med. Hyg., 80:583.

LEISHMANIASIS IN THE LOWLANDS OF BOLIVIA (LEISHBOL) : PART 1. AN OVERVIEW OF THE INTEGRATED PROJECT FOR THE CHARACTERIZATION, VIGILANCE AND CONTROL OF LEISHMANIASIS

M. Recacoeolas[1], G. Villarroel[1], H. Bermudez[1],
R. Urjel[1], J.C. Dujardin[2], and D.le Ray[2]

[1]Dpto. de Atencion Midica
Centro Nacional de Enfermedades Tropicales (CENETROP)
Casilla 2974
Santa Cruz
Bolivia

[2]Institute of Tropical Medicine
Prince Leopold (IMTA)
Laboratory of Protozology
155, Nationalstraat
B-2000 Antwerpen
Belgium

INTRODUCTION

The republic of Bolivia is located in a central position in South America: it has borders with Brasil, Peru, Chile, Argentina and Paraguay. The country consists of the Andean cordillera, of high altitude, in the west, with interandean valleys which, towards the north and east, decrease progressively in altitude to reach the large eastern and sub-tropical and tropical lowlands that are part of the Amazon region.

In Bolivia, knowledge of tegumentary leishmaniasis is fragmentary and incomplete since the pre-colonial period. Its actual distribution in the country covers 9 departments as far as reported human cases are concerned (Figure 1). All sub-tropical and tropical regions of the country are enzootic and endemic.

Leishmaniasis is a disease which has been studied with priority in the "Centro Nacional de Enfermedades Tropicales" (CENETROP) since 1976. The information obtained has been one of the reasons why the government health authorities of Bolivia decided recently to consider leishmaniasis as a priority disease. The creation of new areas of colonization, the opening of new ways of communication, mine and oil

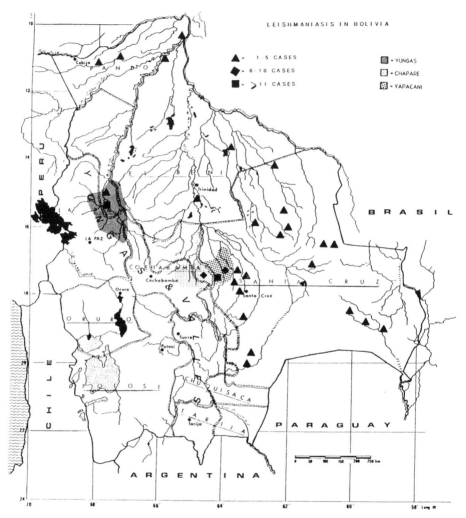

Fig.1- Distribution of 241 cases of human tegumentary (CL and MCL) leishmaniasis in Bolivia as recorded by Recacoechea (1983).

prospecting, forest exploitation, and other events have increased the number of persons exposed to the disease.

The present multidisciplinary project (see Figure 2) was started in 1984. It includes four sub-projects closely related and involves three collaborating institutions: CENETROP, IMTA and IBBA. The pilot area covers about 300 km^2, (see Figures 3 & 4) with a total population of 1,380 persons. Seventy percent of the population is scattered on isolated plots along both sides of the railway. The other 30% are concentrated in a few hamlets near the railway.

The pilot project has four components:
1. Community health
2. Human leishmaniasis: diagnosis, treatment and epidemiology
3. The sylvatic cycle: vector and reservoirs
4. The parasite: characterization of the causative agents.

Community Health

The first subproject has as its objective the development of a community health care system based on local human resources: the community health representatives (CHR), who are designated by the community see (Villarroel *et al*, in this chapter).

After less than three years, 9 CHRs, one for each health sector (Figure 4), are in charge of the diseases prevailing in the area (including leishmaniasis), of the vaccinations, oral rehydration units and the other national health programmes. CHRs also supervise the 3 new community pharmacies. Supervision of CHRs and their tasks has been performed by a project-appointed resident doctor.

At present it appears that the CHRs could become integrated into the National Health Services, with minimal supervision.

Human Leishmaniasis

The objectives of this second subproject are: to identify the magnitude of the endemic leishmaniasis problem; to perform a longitudinal survey of the population; and to carry out early, specific diagnosis and treatment (Recacoechea *et al*, in this chapter). The two sectors of the pilot area which have been studied so far are shown in Figure 4. In the first sector, more than one thousand residents were followed up clinically for one and a half years. The population belonged to the group with scattered households. In the second sector, 250 people in semi-concentrated settlements, were surveyed clinically and serologically for 3 years.

The overall clinical prevalence of leishmaniasis was found to be 2%, with an incidence of 1.4% annually. Clinical and serological results were in general agreement. The seroconversion rate for *L.mexicana* was about 2 fold higher than for *L.braziliensis*. It should be added that a high

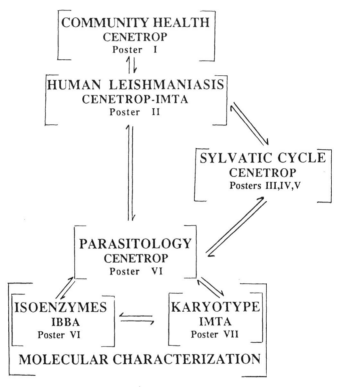

Fig.2- Diagramme of the "LEISHBOL" project, showing the inter- and intra-relationships amongst the objectives and the participating institutions

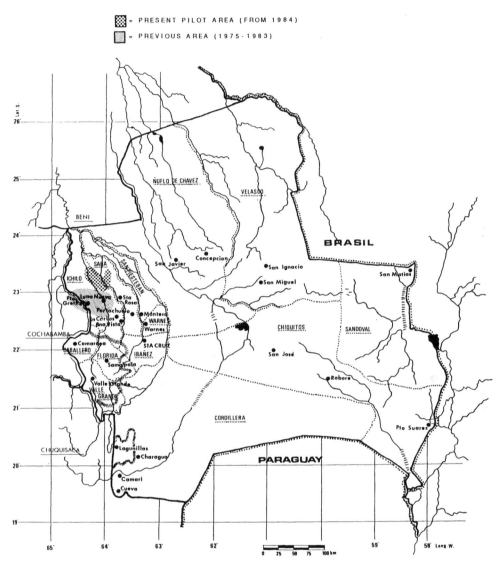

Fig.3- Location of the integrated "LEISHBOL" project being developed since 1984 in the Lowland tropical rain forest of Yapacani in the department of Santa Cruz.

serological prevalence of Chagas' infection (40%) was encountered. The pilot area appears to be a recent focus of active transmission, according to the prevalence of active and recently healed cases, and the scarcity of mucosal cases.

Our present conclusion is that surveillance of leishmaniasis by the community and by the CHRs has proven to be effective for the early detection of cases, as wellas for the treatment of patients on the spot. We therefore intend to extend these studies to other areas.

The Sylvatic Cycle

This third subproject aims to identify the sanfly species, determine the variations in population density over the year, and to characterize the vector species (Bermudez et al (Part IV), in this chapter).

Two field stations were set up (Figure 4). A team of three collectors stayed in the field all the year round. Trapping of wild mammals was initiated. In all 23 species of Phlebotomines were observed, including 18 *Lutzomya* and 3 *Brumptomya*, *Lutzomya yucumensis* being prevalent in all the capture sites. The monthly density of *Lu.yucumensis* is variable: it peaks at the onset and end of the rainy season. Overall density is lower in the parts of the primary forest which became marshy or flooded at the peak of the rainy season. Altitudinal density from ground level towards the forest canopy was, surprisingly, found to increase steadily up to 15 m (the highest altitude checked so far).

Dissection for the presence of flagellates was performed on 5,537 sandflies. Only five of them had promastigotes: 4 *Lu.yucumensis* and 1 *Lu. carrerai carrerai*. Subinoculations into hamster have not yet proven positive or negative. During this work a key was developed for the rapid and specific identification of the sandlfies in the field. The key is based on the external characters of the thorax and has proved to be reliable and is now used daily by the field workers.

The Parasite

The objectives were to isolate, to characterize and to identify *Leishmania* from patients, wild animls and vectors originating from the lowlands (see Urjel et al, in this chapter). Sixteen human stocks have so far been isolated, 5 from the Yapacani pilot area and 11 fromn other regions; and biological and molecular characterization has begun. Morphometry of amastigotes, and measurments of the size and rate of lesion development in hamster paws are in progress.

Enzyme analysis and pulsed field gradient karyotyping were used for 11 isolates. Both methods were in complete agreement with each other. Only one isolate was found to be *L.mexicana amazonensis*, while the 10 other isolates were all *L.b.braziliensis* and displayed a high individual variability.

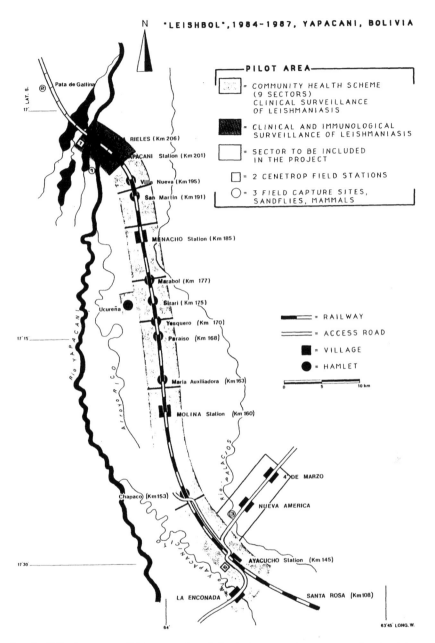

Fig.4- Pilot area of Yapacani subject to spontaneous colonization, showing the subdivision into 9 health sectors for community health and for specific surveillance, and the location of field stations and trapping sites.

The rarity of *L.m.amazonensis* in Yapacani is in contradiction with the serological survey of the population at risk. From the karyotyping data, nuclear DNA repetitive probes are being developed, for comparison with kDNA probes and for the development of non-radioactive dot blot test for use in the field.

GENERAL CONCLUSIONS

Our project LEISHBOL has convinced us that a multidisciplinary approach combining both field and laboratory aspects of leishmaniasis is feasible. We have shown that the Yapacani endemic area of primary forest submitted to spontaneous colonization is at the first stage of transmission. Both *L. mexicana* and *L.braziliensis* are detectable in Bolivian lowlands and, most probably, *Lu.yucumensis* is the main vector.

For the population at risk, a community health system relying on community representatives appears to be the most efficient system at the present stage of colonization. Such a health system can cope with the local priorities, it can put into action the Ministry health policy, and it is suitable to become part of the national health service. So far as the specific problem of leishmaniasis is concerned, our project is still at a very early stage. It offers a basis for in-depth specific reserach acceptable by the population at risk, in the present pilot area as well as in other ecological regions.

ACKNOWLEDGEMENTS

This project was supported by EEC contract STD-M.022-B and UNDP/WB/WHO/TDR/ grant 780.555. We are most indebted to Simone De Doncker, Diane Jacquet, Lucndrix and Sabine Desager for the preperation of Figures and typing the manuscripts most expediently.

LEISHMANIASIS IN THE LOWLANDS OF BOLIVIA (LEISHBOL): PART II. COMMUNITY HEALTH CARE FOR SPONTANEOUS SETTLERS IN ENDEMICTROPICAL FOREST

G. Villarroel, M. Recacoechea and S. Balderrama

Centro Nacional de Enfermedades Tropicales (CENETROP)
Casilla 2974
Santa Cruz
Bolivia

INTRODUCTION

Development of new colonization areas is increasing in the tropical Lowlands of Bolivia. They are located easterly on the Amazonian side of the Andes Cordilleras and are covered mainly by primary rain forest. Most of the colonization process is spontaneous with no planning whatsoever. As a consequence of spontaneous migration and settling, no basic health care is available in most instances. Therefore it was felt necessary to implement specific studies on leishmaniasis straight away by a community health care (CHC) project.

A pilot area, Yapacani (department of Santa Cruz), was identified in the endemic tropical forest. The CHC project has been progressively designed as a function of the resident population, and it relies on local human resources, called community health representatives (CHR). The latter were volunteers identified by their own community.

METHODOLOGY

A 300 km^2 pilot area was delimited (Figure.1) in Yapacani, whare a new railway line was under construction. A census of residents was carried out by local leaders with the help of a project-appointed resident medical doctor. Primary health care (PHC) was organized on a community basis.

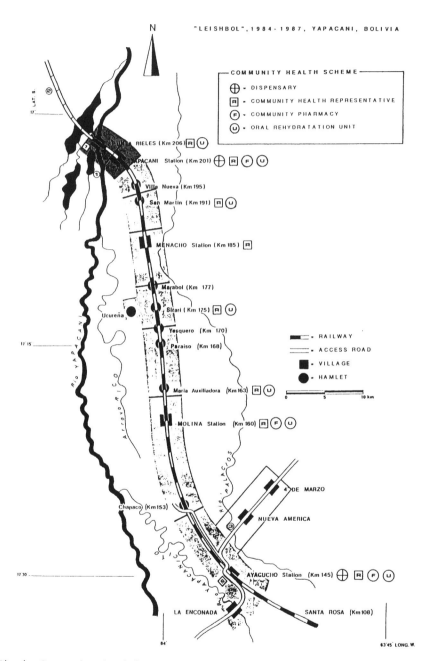

Fig.1- Community health care scheme developed over the last three years (1984-1987) in the Yapacani pilot area for surveillance, and studies on leishmaniasis.

RESULTS

The census (Table 1) identified 1,380 persons, predominantly dispersed and isolated (eg see Figure 2), and originating generally from the Altiplano and the andean valleys.

TABLE 1 CENSUS OF THE POPULATION IN THE YAPACANI PILOT AREA

+ Population :	1,380 persons		density = 4.6 inh/km
	semi-concentrated	= 29%	
	dispersed	= 71%	
+ Origin :	altiplano, valleys	= 73%	
	Santa Cruz Dpt	= 21%	
	others (tropical)	= 6%	
+ Activities :	agriculture	= 88.7%	rice, yuca, vegetables...
	hunting	= 0.9%	self-subsistance, sale
	others	= 10.4%	timber, etc...
+ Social life :	unions and cooperatives	= 79.1%	
	none	= 20.9%	
+ Mobility :	in the area	= 4.9%	
	emigration	= 11.6%	

Agriculture was their main activity and most of them were organized in unions and cooperatives. The mobility of the population was found to be important.

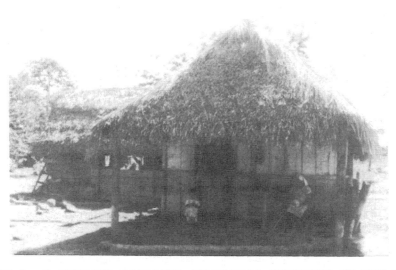

FIGURE 2. A TYPICAL ISOLATED SETTLER'S DWELLING IN THE PILOT AREA IN YAPACANI

Initial health conditions, as reflected by morbidity and mortality, are described in Table 2. Infectious diseases were very prevalent.

TABLE 2. HEALTH CONDITIONS AT THE ONSET OF THE PROJECT IN THE YAPACANI PILOT AREA

+ Morbidity

Prevailing causes (sequence according to frequency) were :

1. diarrhea and malnutrition
2. intestinal parasites
3. acute respiratory infections
4. dental caries
5. dermatologic diseases
6. tetanus, neonatal
7. child infectious diseases (whooping cough, measles,...)
8. leishmaniasis
9. occupational injuries
10. TBC, pulmonar
11. delivery, complications

+ Mortality

Prevailing causes (sequence according to frequency) were :

1. dehydration (diarrhea)
2. acute respiratory infections
3. tetanus, neonatal
4. whooping cough, measles (complications)
5. accidents
6. delivery

The initial human health resources found locally are shown in Table 3. Only two local drugstores existed and these had at best a limited supply of medicines, and referral hospitals were almost out of reach. CHRs were therefore trained for activities related to (i) management of the prevalent diseases, for referral of serious illness cases; (ii) for active search of specific diseases (Leishmaniasis, TBC, and Malaria);(iii) for immunizations, intentinal deparasitization and,(iv) management of oral rehydratation units. All of which are part of the national health policy.

TABLE 3. PRE-EXISTING HUMAN HEALTH RESOURCES IN THE YAPPACANI PILOT AREA

+ Locally

. "syringe"shotpersons
. empirical midwifes and husbands
. medicine men, curers

+ Referral hospitals

. Santa Rosa Hospital, by railway (37 km, 3x a week, irregular)
. San Carlos Hospital, by road (temporary pathway = 11 km,
   + permanent pathway = 36 km)

+ Medicines supply

local drugstores at Ayacucho and Yapacani Station
(drugs supplied for auto-medication)

To date (see Table 4), 9 CHRs and 3 community pharmacy managers are in operation. Specific tasks have been identified. Technical integration of the activities of the CHRs in the national rural health network is currently in progress. The pilot area of Yapacani is now covered to about 80% of its effective area, and therefore 80% of the projects objectives have been accomplished.

CONCLUSIONS

At this stage of the project a community health system was shown to be best developed by local community health representatives who are designated by their own communities. A resident health auxiliary acts as an area coordinator, and both are under the supervision of a hospital doctor. This health system appeared to be well adapted to an area of recent colonization with a highly scattered population.

TABLE 4   LEISHBOL OBJECTIVES AND ACHIEVEMENTS TO DATE

	To date	Target
+ Human resources		
1. community health representatives (CHR)*	9	15
2. Community pharmacy managers	3	5
3. auxiliary nurse (local scheme manager)	0	1
+ Supportive structures		
1. CHR's stations	9	15
2. CHR's portable, first-line pharmacies	9	15
3. Oral Rehydration Units (ORH)	8	15
4. Acute Respiratory Infections Units	0	15
5. Community Pharmacies (CP)	3	5
6. Medical consultories	2	2
+ Coordination and logistics		
1. Technical integration of the scheme into national rural health network	60%	
2. National health priorities	80%	
3. Supplies and consumables to CHRs	80%	
+ Effective coverture		
Over the whole pilot area	84%	

* Tasks of the CHR :
 . treatment of prevailing morbidity, referral of serious cases
 . clean-delivery assistance
 . vaccinations
 . management of ORUs
 . simplified morbidity records
 . detection and sampling of TBC, leishmaniasis, malaria

LEISHMANIASIS IN THE LOWLANDS OF BOLIVIA (LEISHBOL): PART III. STATUS OF THE DISEASE IN AN AREA OF SPONTANEOUS AGRICULTURAL COLONIZATION

M.Recacoechea[1], G.Villarroel[1], S.Balderrama[1], R. Urjell, S. De Doncker[2], D. Jacquet[2] and D. Le Ray[2]

[1]Centro Nacional de Enfermedades Tropicales (CENETROP)
Casilla 2974
Santa Cruz
Bolivia

[2]Institute of Tropical Medicine Prince Leopold (IMTA)
Laboratory of Protozoology
155, Nationalestraat
B-2000 Antwerpen
Belgium

INTRODUCTION

The present development of planned and unplanned areas of colonization in the primary forest of Bolivia, together with mining, oil prospection and the opening of new roads, etc., has increased considerably the risk of infection by leishmanias. We have established that leishmaniasis is endemic in 5 of the 9 states of Bolivia (Recacoechea, 1983).

The objectives of our study on leishmaniasis were to identify the magnitude of the endemic, to perform a longtitudinal survey of the population at risk, to correlate clinical manifestations with cellular and humoral immunity and to carry out specific diagnosis and treatment with GlucantimeR.

METHODS

This study took place in Yapacani (provinces of Ichilo and Sara, department of Santa Cruz), a new area of spontaneous agricultural colonization in the lowlands of Bolivia (see Recacoechea et al, in this chapter). The 1380 inhabitants assessed (see Villarroel et al., in this chapter) are distributed over a 300-km^2 area and they fall into two categories: 253 persons live in hamlets as a semi-concentrated population (Figure 1a) while the other 1,127 subjects are scattered in isolated settlements (Figure 1b).

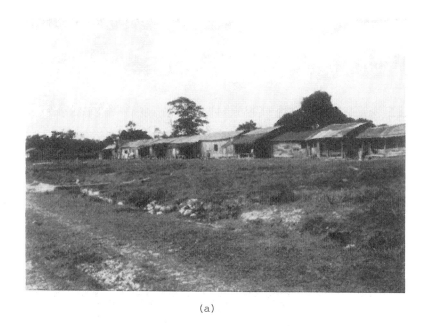

(a)

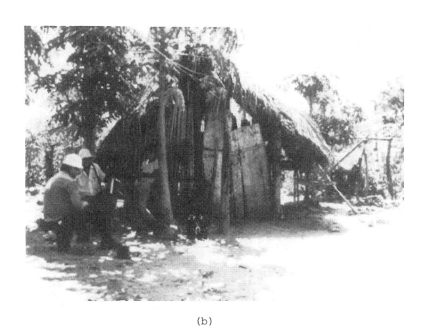

(b)

Fig. 1- Semi-concentrated (a) and isolated (b) dwellings of spontaneous settlers in the colonization area of Yapacani

Table 1. Prevalence and incidence of tegumentary leishmaniasis in the 9 health sectors of the Yapacani pilot area

SECTORS	POPULATION	PREVALENCE		INCIDENCE (retrospective)	
		Lesions (scars) > 1-yr-old	%	Lesions(active&scars) < 1-yr-old	%
1.1 Under serological surveillance					
Punta Rieles	157	5	3,18	2(2*CL)	1,27
Yapacani Station	96	2(1*MCL)	2,08	0	0
Subtotal	253	7(1*MCL)	2,77	2(2*CL)	0,79
1.2 Without serological surveillance					
Villanueva	80	0	0	0	0
San Martin	111	5	4,50	1	0,90
Menacho	183	4	2,19	5	2,73
Sirari	256	1	0,39	2(1*CL)	0,78
Yeskero	133	7	5,26	6(4*CL)	4,51
Molina	176	1	0,57	3(1*CL)	1,70
Ayacucho	188	2	1,06	0	0
Subtotal	1127	20	1,77	17(6*CL)	1,51
GRAND TOTAL	1380	27(1*MCL)	1,96	19(8*CL)	1,38

*MCL = mucocutaneous lesion
*CL = active cutaneous lesion

The first population, semi-concentrated in Punta Rieles and in Estacion Yapacani (Figure 2), was the object of a clinical and immunological surveillance while the second population scattered between Estacion Yapacani and Ayacucho underwent only clinical surveillance. Surveillance was performed by the local community leaders backed up by a project-appointed resident medical doctor.

RESULTS

Figure 2 shows the actual distribution of cases in the 9 health sectors. Overall prevalence Table 1 of leishmaniasis (defined as the number of persons with lesions and scars >1 year old) was 1,96%, while yearly incidence (defined as active lesions or scars <1 year old) concerned 1,38% of the population.

No new cases (Table 2) were detected in the partly concentrated population during 3 years of surveillance, while in the dispersed area 4 new cases developed over 1·5 years of surveillance. Only one muco-cutaneous case was detected in the whole area.

TABLE 2 THE ACTUAL INCIDENCE OF TEGUMENTARY LEISHMANIASIS IN POPULATIONS EITHER SEMI-CONCENTRATED (SC) OR DISPERSED (D) IN THE YAPACANI AREA

SECTORS	POPULATION Type	POPULATION Nr	SURVEILLANCE PERIODE	NEW CASES
Punta Rieles to Yapacani St.	SC	253	3 yrs	0
Villanueva to Ayacucho	D	1127	1 1/2 yr	4

The preliminary overall antibody prevalence (Table 3) (as measured by a precipitation-in-gel test) in 225 persons of the relatively concentrated population is high (12%) for *L.m.amazonensis* and *L.b.brasiliensis*, but when we considered the prevalence in *Trypanosoma cruzi*-negative residents (138) only, serological prevalence was reduced to 3.6% for *L.m.amazonensis* and to 2.1% for *L.b.brasiliensis*.

The incidence according to seroconversion during longitudinal surveillance was 1.4% for *L.m.amazonensis*, and 0% for *L.b.braziliensis* (Table 4). While the incidence according to seroconversion during longitudinal surveillance was 1.4% for *L.m.amazonensis*, and 0% for *L.b.braziliensis* (Table 4).

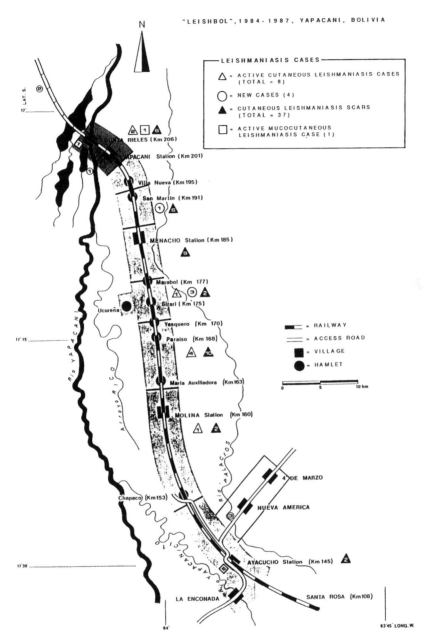

Fig.2- Repartition of the clinical cases of leishmaniasis in the 9 community health sectors of the "LEISHBOL" project in Yapacani.

Table 3. Prevalence of antibodies to T.cruzi and to Leishmania in the Yapacani population

SECTOR PUNTA-RIELES YAPACANI ST.	3.1. OVERALL ANTIBODY PREVALENCE (n=225)		
	T.CRUZI % (n)	L.MEX.AMAZ. % (n)	L.B.BRAZ. % (n)
Norte (n=75)	29,3 (22)	10,6 (8)	5,3 (4)
Sur (n=67)	34,3 (23)	10,4 (7)	11,9 (8)
Est. Y (n=83)	45,7 (38)	15,6 (13)	14,4 (14)
TOTAL (n=225)	36,8 (83)	12,4 (28)	11,5 (26)

SECTOR PUNTA-RIELES YAPACANI ST.	3.2. PREVALENCE IN CRUZI-NEGATIVES (n=138)	
	L.MEX.AMAZ. % (n)	L.B.BRAZ. % (n)
Norte (n=51)	3,9 (2)	1,9 (1)
Sur (n=43)	6,9 (3)	2,3 (1)
Est. Y (n=44)	- (0)	2,2 (1)
TOTAL (n=138)	3,6 (5)	2,1 (3)

Table 4. Incidence of T.cruzi and Leishmania according to seroconversion during longitudinal surveillance of the Yapacani population

SECTOR PUNTA RIELES YAPACANI ST.	SURVEILLANCE PERIOD (n persons)	SEROCONVERSION			
		T.CRUZI		CRUZI-NEGATIVES	
		- to +	+ to -	L.MEX.AMAZ. - to +	L.B.BRAZ. - to +
	8 months (59 p.)	2	6	1	0
	14 months (22 p.)	0	0	0	0
	22 months (59 p.)	0	5	1	0
TOTAL persons %	140	3 2,1%	11 7,9%	2 1,4%	0 -

COMMENTS AND CONCLUSIONS

The Yapacani pilot area is a recent focus of active transmission as shown by the frequency of cutaneous cases as compared to the scarcity of mucosal involvment. The prevalence of *T.cruzi* interfered markedly with leishmanial serology as the *L.mexicana* antigens can cause false positivity. Nevertheless overall agreement was observed between clinical and serological data.

A correlation study between clinical, serological and Montenegro (IDR) data will be carried out for tracing asymptomatic cases. Surveillance of leishmaniasis in recent, dispersed colonization areas appeared to be best secured by a community health scheme with community health representatives (CHRs). The latter are responsible for early detection, sampling, treatment (with Glucantime R), follow-up of treatment and of the evolution of lesions, reporting of cutaneous cases and referral of serious cases.

On the basis of present experience, clinical and immunological surveillance should be developed, with special attention to symptomatic patients and to asymptomatic, Montenegro-positive and/or seroconverted cases. Surveillance will be expanded to other foci and studies on risk factors will be included.

REFERENCE

Recacoechea, M. (1983). Estado de conociemientos sobre la leishmaniasis tegumentaria americana en Bolivia. Bol. Inf. CENETROP, 9: 6-12.

LEISHMANIASIS IN THE LOWLANDS OF BOLIVIA (LEISHBOL): PART IV. FIELD IDENTIFICATION KEY FOR *LUTZOMYA* SPP. BASED ON THORACIC EXTERNAL CHARACTERS

H. Bermudez, A. Rivero, J.L. Claure, B. Montalvan and S. Rocha

Centro Nacional de Enfermedades Tropicales (CENETROP)
Casilla 2974
Santa Cruz
Bolivia

INTRODUCTION

The only systematic study of the phlebotomine faune of Bolivia carried out so far was performed in the Andean region of Los Yungas near La Paz (Velazco, 1973) and 11 species of *Lutzomy* were recorded. Recently we have initiated a multidisciplinary project on leishmaniasis in the Lowlands of Bolivia (Recacoechea et al., in this chapter) in the primary rain forest of Yapacani, department of Santa Cruz, a region undergoing rapid conolization.

Sandfly trapping by a permanent team of three people at each of two sites has taken place since 1984 (Bermudez et al., in this chapter) and has included dissection for species identification and establishment of flagellate infections (Figure 1). More than 5,000 dissections were performed and 18 species of *Lutzomya* were recorded.

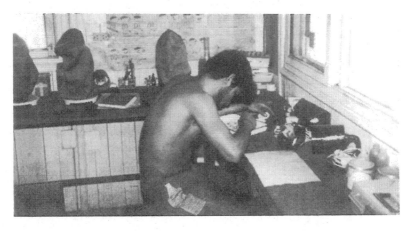

FIGURE 1 THORACIC IDENTIFICATION OF SANDFLIES AT THE FIELD STATION IN THE YAPACANI AREA

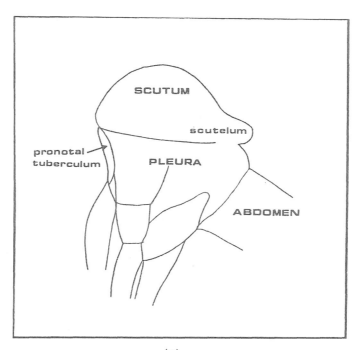

(a)

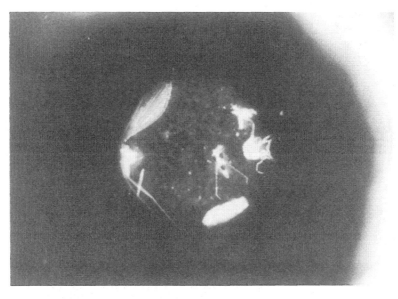

(b)

FIGURE 2 (a) SCHEMATIC DRAWING OF PHLEBOTOMINE THORAX (LATERAL VIEW, LEFT SIDE) AND, (b) FIELD DISSECTION FOR EXAMINATION OF FEMALE GENITALIA

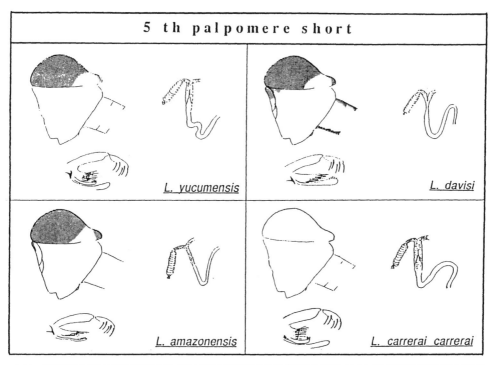
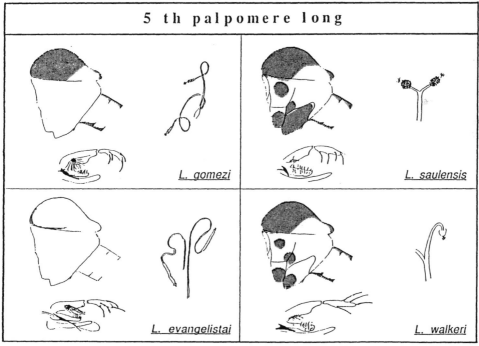

FIGURE 3 IDENTIFICATION KEY OF LUTZOMYA spp. PRESENT IN THE YAPACANI PRIMARY RAIN FOREST, SHOWING THORACIC (SEE INSERT) AND GENITALIA CHARACTERS   (continued)

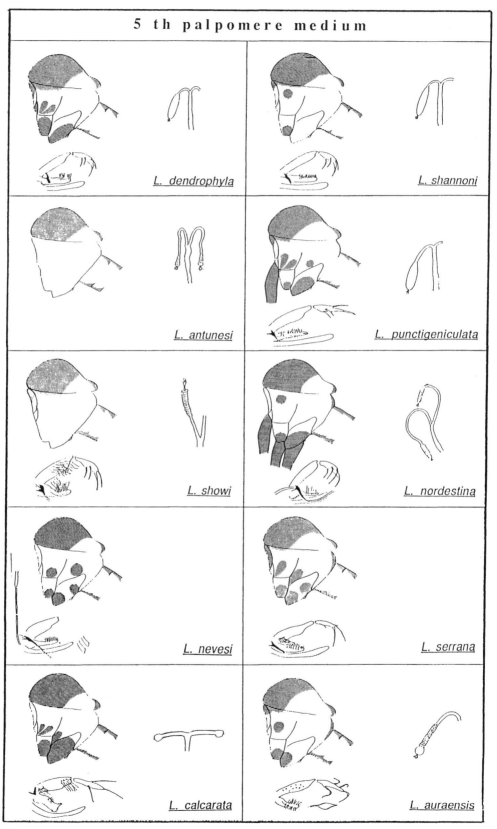

FIGURE 3 (continued)

RESULTS AND DISCUSSION

In Considering the need for rapid identification of the species prior to mass dissection, particular attention was paid to external morphology as a possible alternative to the morphology of genitalia. Stereomicroscope observation of sandflies, dry or in fluid (saline, alcohol, etc.) on a microscope slide or in a cavity slide, was systematically carried out (Figure 2a & b). External characteristics of the thorax (Figure 2a) were recorded, in particular color, shape, size, number and location of the sclerites on mesonotum and pleura. Correlation of those characters with the morphology of male and female genitalia proved to be positive and a pictorial key was developed accordingly (Figure 3).

Thoracic identification, as compared to dissection of genitalis proved to be efficient for rapid identification of all the 18 species of *Lutzomya* encountered in the Yapacani area. It was much faster (over 600 sandflies/man/hour) and it was shown to be easily mastered by non-specialized field workers. By avoiding compulsory dissection, it does not interfere with subsequent decision relating to bloodmeal identification and pathogen isolation (viruses, leishmaniae, etc.). Preliminary controls performed with Dr. D. Young at the Gainesville Reference Collection of neotropical sandflies indicated that thoracic characters are more accurate than genitalia characters for species identification of *Lutzomya*. Further evaluation of thoracic characters will be done with other species of sandflies from other biotopes and other foci of leishmaniasis.

REFERENCE

Velazco J., 1973, The phlebotomine sandflies of the "Los Yungas" region of Bolivia. M.Sc. Thesis, Louisiana State University, 204 pp.

LEISHMANIASIS IN THE LOWLANDS OF BOLIVIA (LEISHBOL): PART V. MONTHLY DENSITY OF LUTZOMYA YUCUMENSIS, *LU.DAVISI* AND *LU.CARRERAI CARRERAI* IN THE RAIN FOREST OF YAPACANI, DEPARTMENT OF SANTA CRUZ

H. Bermudez, A. Rivero, B. Montalvan, J.L. Claure
and S. Rocha

Centro Nacional de Enfermedades Tropicales (CENETROP)
Casilla 2974
Santa Cruz
Bolivia

INTRODUCTION

A survey of the phlebotomine fauna of the Lowlands of Bolivia was initiated in 1984 within the frame of a multidisciplinary project on leighmaniasis (Recacoechea et al., in this chapter). Eighteen different species of *Lutzomya* were identified (see Bermudez et al., in this chapter).

The present study aimed at the monitoring of seasonal and altitudinal density of prevalent species. Sandfly trapping was carried out on an all-the-year-round basis in the primary rain forest of Yapacani (see Recacoechea et al., in this chapter for details).

SEASONAL DENSITY

Two trapping sites were selcted. The first one, "marshy", was located at the edge of a railway contractor camp close to the Yapacani River, in the lowest part of the region (Figure 1) and it was prone to flooding at the peak (January) of the rainy season. The second one, "dry", was situated 10 km North from the first site in a slightly elevated part of the forest (Figure 2) and it was never flooded. On both sites trapping was done with a light-baited Shannon trap erected at ground level. Results were recorded as the monthly average number of females/trap/hour.

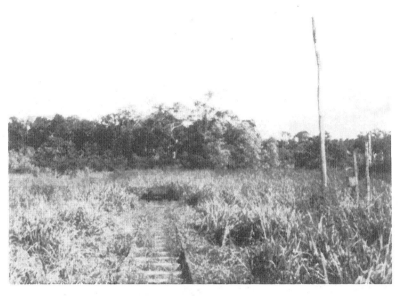

FIGURE 1   MARSHY TRAPPING SITE N° 1 AT THE EDGE OF THE PRIMARY FOREST

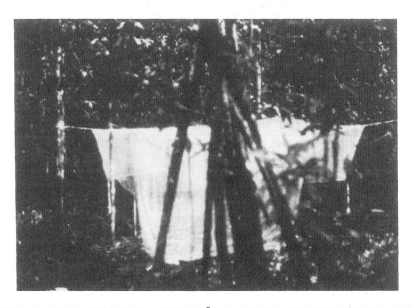

FIGURE 2   DRY TRAPPING SITE N° 2 (WITH SHANNON TRAP) IN THE PRIMARY RAIN FOREST

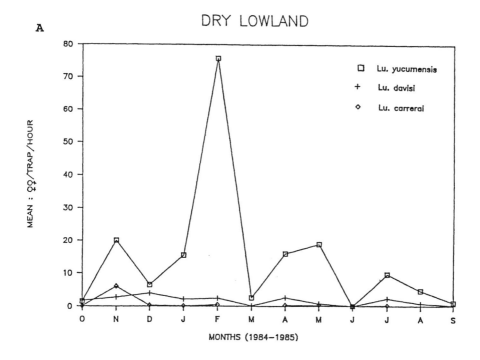

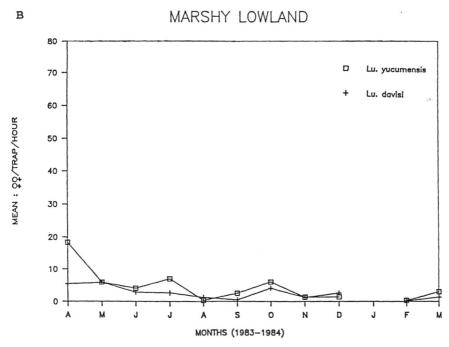

FIGURE 3 MONTHLY DENSITY OF SANDFLIES PREVALENT AT (A) MARSHY LOW LOWLAND SITE (N° 1) AND (B) DRY LOWLAND SITE (N° 2)

RESULTS

1.1 Marshy Trapping Site (N°. 1)

Trapping was carried out from 19.00 to 24.00 hrs daily from April 1983 untill March 1984. Eleven species of sandflies were encountered and most of them were sporadic. Two species were prevalent throughout the year: *Lu.yucumensis* and, to a lesser extent *Lu.davisi* (Figure 3b). Density of *Lu.yucumensis* was constant but low, with an average of 0.16 to 7 females/trap/hr.

1.2 Dry Trapping Site (N°. 2)

Trapping was performed from 20.00 to 24.00 hrs daily from October 1984 till September 1985. Three *Lutzomya* species showed a yearly prevalence: *Lu.c.carrerai* and the same two species prevalent on site N°.1 (Figure 3a). *Lu.yucumensis* had the highest prevalence which fluctuated markedly and culminated at various periods, mainly in February (75.71 females/trap/hr) at the end of the rainy season.

2. Altitudinal density

As almost no blood-fed and/or mated females were encountered during trapping, altitudinal trapping was performed in an attempt to collect indications for breeding site(s). CDC light traps (Figure 4) were set at 0.4, 5, 10 and 15 m above ground level in the dry trapping site N°. 2, from March till September 1986. Results were recorded as the average number of females/trap/night. *Lu.yucumensis* and *Lu.davisi* were the only two species found consistently at all levels. For both species density increased with altitude (Figure 5).

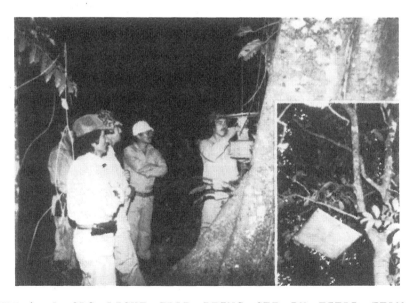

FIGURE 4   A CDC LIGHT TRAP BEING SET BY FIELD TEAM AND (IN INSERT) A CDC TRAP IN A TREE FOR THE ALTITUDINAL DENSITY STUDIES

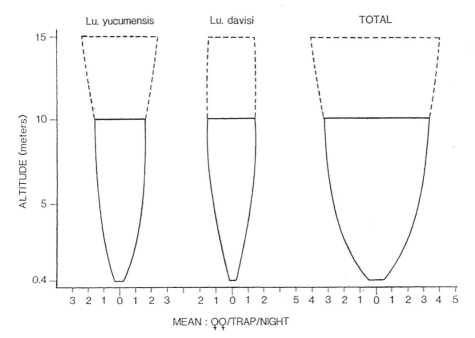

FIGURE 5 ALTITUDINAL SANDFLY DENSITY STUDIES: RESULTS FROM CDC TRAPS AT DRY TRAPPING SITE (N° 2)

CONCLUSIONS

Out of 18 *Lutzomya* spp. endemic in the primary rain forest of Yapacani, only 3 were prevalent all the year round, i.e. *Lu.yucumensis*, *Lu.davisi* and *Lu.c.carrerai* in decreasing order of density. Overall sandfly density was higher in the "dry", not prone to flooding, forest.

Seasonal density appeared to be higher at the onset of, and by the end of the rainy season, depending on the species and the location considered. As for diferences in altitudinal density these increased steadily from ground to 15 m in our study.

With respect to human leishmaniasis, further data on seasonal density, anthropophily and vectorial capacity are needed before any firm conclusion can be drawn. At this stage, occupational risk could be higher for hunters ("dry" forest) rather than for fishermen ("marshy" forest), and with respect to enzootic leishmaniasis, trapping further up to the canopy, bloodmeal analysis and dissection for mated females and infected sandflies should be developed. Present data suggest that cyclical transmission could possibly take place in, or near the canopy.

LEISHMANIASIS IN THE LOWLANDS OF BOLIVIA (LEISHBOL): Part VI. FLAGELLATE INFECTION IN SANDFLIES FROM THE RAIN FOREST OF YAPACANI

H. Bermudez, R. Urjel, A. Rivero, J.L. Claure and B. Montalban

Centro Nacional de Enfermedades Tropicales (CENETROP)
Casilla 2974
Santa Cruz
Bolivia

INTRODUCTION

Continuous trapping of sandflies has been carried out since 1984 in the primary rain forest of Yapacani (Bermudez et al., in this chapter) using Shannon and CDC traps. More than 5,000 sandflies were dissected and examined for gut infection with flagellates to identify potential vectors of Leishmania.

RESULTS AND DISCUSSION

In Table 1 it can be seen that four *Lu.yucumensis* and one *Lu.c.carrerai* species of sandfly were found to harbour leishmanial promastigotes. The former showed a suprapylarian infection, the latter hosted a peripylarian colonization. Furthermore, two sandflies (one *Lu.dendrophyla* and one *Lu.shannoni*) had hypopylarian trypomastigotes. Positive sandflies were all trapped during the dry season, between March and September.

Positive gut preparations were inoculated *in vitro* and/or *in vivo*. Fungal superinfection interfered with *in vitro* isolation. In hamster infections no lesions have, as yet, developed and observations continues.

In conclusion, we have tentatively indentified both *L.braziliensis* and *L.mexicana* and suggest that both are present in the tropical rain forest of Yapacani. However unequivocal evidence has still to come from the successful isolation of stocks. Putative vectors which are the locally predominant species include *Lu.yucumensis* and *Lu.c.carrerai* whose blood-feeding preferences should be studied.

Infection was found during the dry season when sandfly density is lower, and the multiparous/nulliparous female ratio is probably higher, a fact which could explain the higher infection rate.

Table 1 Sandflies species trapped in the Yapacani forest, dissected (N°) and found infected (+) by suprapylarian (●) and peripylarian (○) promastigotes or by hypopylarian typomastigotes (□).

1985

SANDFLY SPECIES	JAN N°	JAN +	FEB N°	FEB +	MAR N°	MAR +	APR N°	APR +	MAY N°	MAY +	JUN N°	JUN +	JUL N°	JUL +	AUG N°	AUG +	SEPT N°	SEPT +	OKT N°	OKT +	NOV N°	NOV +
Lu. yucumensis	264				152	1●	528		473	1●			129		93		138		900	1	102	
Lu. davisi	31				8		50		12				6		2		5		42		29	
Lu. c. carreirai	2						15	1○	5										5		3	
Lu. calcaraia													1				1		3		1	
Lu. dendrophyla			33																			
Lu. shannoni																						
Lu. auraensis									1													
Lu. antunesi																						
Lu. gomezi																						
Lu. nevesi													1				1					
TOTAL	297	0	33	0	160	1●	593	1○	491	1●	-		137	0	95	0	145	0	950	1	135	0

dry season

1986

SANDFLY SPECIES	MAY N°	MAY +	JUN N°	JUN +	JUL N°	JUL +	AUG N°	AUG +	SEPT N°	SEPT +	OCT N°	OCT +	TOTAL N°	TOTAL +
Lu. yucumensis	967	1●	172		77		184		336	1●	247		4762	4●
Lu. davisi	107		106		9		20		108		101		636	0○
Lu. c. carreirai	7		4		1				1		1		44	1○
Lu. calcaraia	7		3		1		3		3		3		26	
Lu. dendrophyla	3						2	1○					38	1○
Lu. shannoni	4						4	1○					8	1○
Lu. auraensis	6		1		1				1				10	
Lu. antunesi	3		3						1				6	
Lu. gomezi	4												4	
Lu. nevesi													2	
TOTAL	1108	1●	289	0	89	0	213	2○	450	1●	352	0	5537	7(5)

dry season

130

LEISHMANIASIS IN THE LOWLANDS OF BOLIVIA (LEISHBOL): PART VII. PRELIMINARY CHARACTERIZATION OF ELEVEN *LEISHMANIA* ISOLATES

R. Urjel[1], M. Recacoechea[1], Ph. Desjeux[2], H. Bermudez[1], G. Villarroel[1], S. Balderrama[1], J. Carrasco[1], O. Aguilar[1], J.Cl. Dujardin[3] and D. Le Ray[3]

[1]CENETROP, Casilla 2974, Santa Cruz, Bolivia
[2]IBBA, Casilla 824, La Paz, Bolivia
[3]ITMA, Nationalestraat 155, 2000 Antwerp, Belgium

INTRODUCTION

In the context of the LEISHBOL project in Yapacani in the Lowlands of Bolivia (see Recacoechea et al.(Part 1), in this chapter) a parasitological technique for *in vivo* isolation was evaluated. Identification of the isolates used exploited biological and molecular characteristics, as well as, parasitological and serological information (eg Recacoechea et al.(Part 3), in this chapter).

MATERIAL AND METHODS

1. Parasites

Direct examination of smears from clinically suspected patients was performed using the matchstick sampling technique (Urjel et al., 1983). Biopsies from positive patients, positive sandfly digestive tracts and biopsies from wild animals were inoculated in vivo into hamsters (hindpaws and nose, 2 hamsters per sample) and infections followed-up for at least one year.

When lesions developed in the hamsters parasites were isolated *in vitro* in Noguchi-Wenyon soft agar blood medium. Eleven human isolates were obtained, five of which were from the pilot area of Yapacani (Table 1).

TABLE 1. STOCKS AND STRAINS CONSIDERED FOR MOLECULAR CHARACTERIZATION

Reference stocks		Lowlands isolates
Species	Code	*Leishmania* sp. code
L.b.braziliensis	MHOM/BR/75/M-2904	MHOM/BO/84/CENP-001
L.b.guyanesis	MHOM/BR/75/M-4147	MHOM/BO/84/CENP-002
L.b.panamensis	MHOM/BR/75/M-4037	MHOM/BO/85/CENP-003
L.m.amazonensis	IFLA/BR67/PH-8	MHOM/BO/85/CENP-004
L.m.mexicana	MNYC/BZ/62/M-379	MHOM/BO/85/CENP-005
L.m.pifanoi	MHOM/VE/77/L-20	MHOM/BO/85/CENP-006
		MHOM/BO/85/CENP-007
		MHOM/BO/85/CENP-008
		MHOM/BO/85/CENP-009
		MHOM/BO/85/CENP-010
		MHOM/BO/85/CENP-011

2. Biological characterization

Development of the lesion in the hindpaw of the hamster (Lainson, 1983) was studied by measuring the thickness of the lesion with a calliper gauge during its evolution (slow or fast). Morphometry of the amastigotes was performed according to Shaw and Lainson (1979).

3. Molecular characterization

3.1. Enzyme electrophoresis

Electrophoresis was carried out on cellulose acetate (Tibayrenc & Le Ray, 1984, adapted from Lanham et al., 1981) for thirteen enzymes (Table 2).

TABLE 2. ENZYMES USED IN THIS STUDY

EC 1.1.1.-37,MDH	EC 1.4.1.2.,GDH NADP+
EC 1.1.1.-40,ME	EC 2.5.1.1.,GOT
EC 1.1.1.-42,ICD	EC 2.7.5.1.,PGM
EC 1.1.1.-44,6 PGDH	EC 3.4.11.1.,PEP 1
EC 1.1.1.-49,G6PD	EC 4.2.1.3.,ACON
EC 1.2.1.2,GDH NAD+	EC 5.3.1.8.,MPI
EC 5.3.1.9.,GPI	

3.2 Pulse Field Gradient Electrophoresis (PFGE)

The procedure used by Dujardin et al., (in this chapter) was exploited for karyotyping the various isolates.

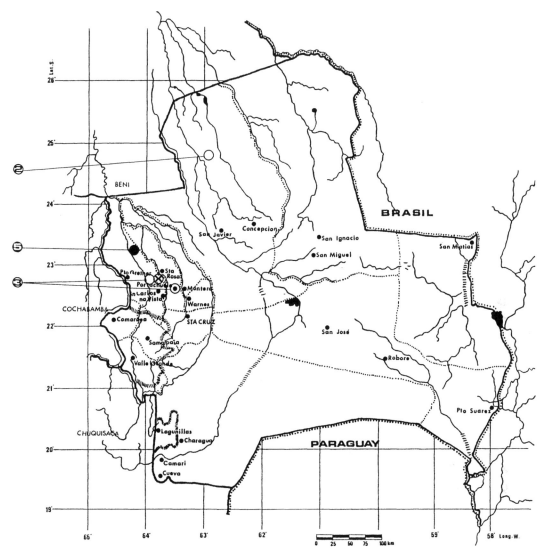

Fig. 1 : Map of the department of Santa Cruz showing the origin of the 11 isolates characterized ● = Yapacani pilot area, 5 isolates all L.b.braziliensis; ○ = Lowlands out of Yapacani pilot area, 5 isolates: 4 L.b.braziliensis,1 L.m.amazonensis (⊗) ; 1 L.b.braziliensis from the department of Pando not indicated.

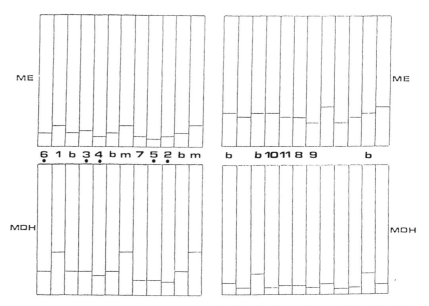

Fig.2 : Enzyme variability amongst isolates from the Lowlands as observed with ME and MDH: • = Yapacani isolates; b= L.b.braziliensis reference stock M-2904; m = L.m.amazonensis reference stock PH-8.

RESULTS

Isolation

Sixteen stocks (44%) were isolated out of 36 positive human cases. Out of 5 positive sandflies and 65 suspect wild animals, no isolation has succeeded as yet.

Identification

Eleven isolates were considered (see Table 1). For biological characterization, only the overall aspect of the lesions has been studied so far. A high variability was observed amongst Lowlands isolates. Some isolates induced typical small "*L.b.braziliensis*"-type lesions. In one instance, a large ulcerated lesion developed. Several stocks provoked lesions of interderminate size. Quantification of lesion size and rate of development is in progress.

Using PFGE karyotyping 10 isolates were identified as *L.b.braziliensis* and one (stock CENP 001) as *L.m.amazonensis* (Figure 1). Pronounced variability was observed amongst the *L.b.braziliensis* isolates. Enzymatical identification confirmed those results and similarly, variability was observed amongst the *L.b.braziliensis* isolates (Figure 2) for ME and MDH.

CONCLUSION

Only human isolates proved positive *in vivo*. A 44% isolation rate was achieved. However, a higher sensitivity (Weigle et al., 1987) and a quicker result could be obtained by direct *in vitro* isolation.

By using enzyme electrophoresis and PFGE karyotyping, 10 isolates were identified as *L.b.braziliensis*, and 1 and *L.m.amazonensis*. Both biological and molecular characters of the *L.b.braziliensis* isolates from the Lowlands showed pronounced variation in contrast to the isolates from the Yungas in the Andean Valleys (see Dujardin et al.,in this chapter). In relation to this observation, the characterization of the isolates needs to be confirmed with clone populations. Contrary to the serological results (Recacoechea et al.(Part 3), in this chapter) the frequency of *L.m.amazonensis* isolates versus *L.b.braziliensis* isolates was very low.

For field identification of isolates it should be important to develop rapid and easy techniques which could at least permit one to distinguish between *L.braziliensis* and *L.mexicana* complexes in biopsy samples. We are developing *in situ* morphometry of amastigotes and DNA hydridization tests (Barker, 1986), using a non-radioactive probe in order to overcome possible selection during isolation.

REFERENCES

Barker, D.C., Butcher, J., Gibson, L.J. and Williams, R.H. (1986): Characterization of *Leishmania* sp. by DNA hybridization probes.
A laboratory manual.UNDP/World Bank/WHO (TDR), 57 pp.

Lainson, R. (1983): The American leishmaniases: some observations on their ecology and epidemiology.
Trans. Roy. Soc.Trop.Med.Hyg., 77(5), 569-596.

Lanham, S.M., Grendon, J.M., Miles, M.A., Povoa, M. and De Souza, A.A. (1981): A comparison of electrophoretic methods for isoenzyme characterization of Trypanosoma cruzi. I: Standard stocks of Trypanosoma cruzi zymodemes from northeast Brazil.
Trans.Roy.Soc.Trop.Med.Hyg., 75(5), 742-750.

Shaw, J.J. and Lainson, R. (1976): Leishmaniasis in Brazil. XI. Observations on the morphology of Leishmania of the braziliensis and mexicana complexes.
J. Trop. Med. Hyg., 79, 9-13.

Tibayrenc, M and Le Ray, D. (1984): General classification of the isoenzymic strains of Trypanosoma (Schyzotrypanum) cruzi and comparis with T.(S)c.marinkellei and T.(Herpetosoma) rangeli
Ann. Soc. belge Med. trop., 64, 239-248.

Urjel, R., Recacoechea, M., La Fuenta, C. and Orellana, H. (1983): A simple method for the collection of material from cutaneous and mucocutaneous leishmaniasis lesions.
Trans.Roy.Soc.Trop.Med.Hyg., 77, 882.

Weigle, K.A., De Davalos, M., Heredia, P., Molineros, R., Saravia, N.G. and D'Alessandros, A. (1987): Diagnosis of cutaneous and mucocutaneous leishmaniasis in Colombia: a comparison of seven methods.
Am. J.Trop.Med.Hyg., 36(3), 489-496.

LEISHMANIASIS IN THE LOWLAWNDS OF BOLIVIA (LEISHBOL):

Part VIII. CHARACTERIZATION AND IDENTIFICATION OF BOLIVIAN ISOLATES BY PFG KARYOTYPING

J.Cl. Dujardin (1), N. Gajendran (2), R. Hamers (2), G. Matthijsen (2), R. Urjel (3), M. Recacoechea (3), G. Villarroel (3), H. Bermudez (3), Ph. Desjeux (), S. De Doncker (1) and D. Le Ray (1)

(1) ITMA, Protozoology, 155 Nationalestraat, 2000 Antwerp, Belgium (2) VUB, 65 Paardenstraat, 1640 St. Genesius Rode, Belgium. (3) CENETROP, Casilla 2974 Santa Cruz, Bolivia

INTRODUCTION

Within the frame of molecular identification of Leishmania species, karyotyping by Pulsed Field Gradient Gel Electrophoresis (PFG) (Schwartz et al., 1983) has been applied (Spithill and Samaras, 1985; Comeau et al., 1986; Garveyand Santi, 1986; Giannini et al., 1986; Scholler et al., 1986). In this new kind of electrophoresis, the combination of two perpendicular asymetrical electrical fields activated alternatively, induces the resolution of the nuclear genome in chromosome-sized DNA molecules, and makes it possible to obtain a karyotype of the organism being studied.

In the present work, we have combined PFG and beta-tubulin hybridization for the study of reference strains of New World Leishmania belonging to the main complexes, braziliensis and mexicana. Karyotypic stability was studied in relation to life cycle. Intra- and inter-specific differences were observed. Specific profiles as well as marker chromosomes were preliminarily identified and they were assessed on a series of field isolates from Bolivia (Lowlands, Alto Beni, Yungas). Karyotypic data were found to agree internally as well as externally with isoenzyme data, for both identification and classification.

MATERIALS AND METHODS

PFG Technique

The tank used in our study is derived from the one of Carle and Olson (1984) and contains 2 cathodes (N, W) made up with 15 Pt wires connected to diodes, and 2 anodes consisting of point electrodes. Electrophoresis was performed in a 10 x 15 x 0.5 cm agarose gel (1 to 1.5%) in 0.5 TBE buffer at a temperature of 1-18°C during 24 hours at a voltage of 15 V/cm. The yeast Saccharomyces cerevisiae was used for sizing DNA molecules up to 700 kb.

Parasites and Preparation of Samples

International reference stocks and Bolivian isolates used in this study (Table 1) were cultivated as promastigotes on blood agar (Tobie, 1950) or in GLSH (Le Ray, 1975) and harvested at early plateau phase, by day 2. The procedure for embedding the parasites into blocks was adapted from Van der Ploeg et al. (1984).

Southern Blotting and Hybridization

All procedures were adapted from Maniatis ( ) and blotting was made on Amersham Hybond N filter. The beta-tubulin cDNA probe used was pTb Tc-2 (Tomashow et al., 1983) and was received from Dr. N. Agabian.

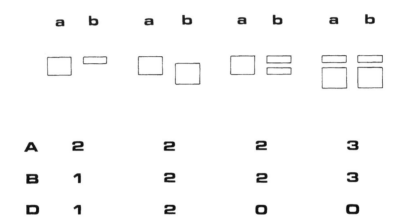

Fig. 1. Evaluation of A, B and D for the calculation of a difference index (DI), when differences in fluorescence or resolution are observed.

Karyotype Banding Patterns

Position of chromosome-sized bands and hybridization with beta-tubulin gene probe were the two criteria used for comparing karyotypes.

For identification patterns, all the different bands observed in the various isolates were taken into account. They were grouped in six classes I to VI, from low to high size. Within each class the bands were given an identification number multiple of 10 : from 10 to X, from low to high size.

An attempt at the quantification of differences between karyotypes was made by introducing a difference index : DI = D/(A+B-D) with D standing for the number of bands differing amongst organisms a and b, A the number of bands in organism a and B the number of bands in organism b. The strongly fluorescent bands were given a double value and D was estimated as follows.

Table 1 : Leishmania stocks used in this study

Species	Designation
a. L. major	MHOM/SU/73/5-ASKH (3)
b. L. donovani infantum	MHOM/BL/67/ITMAP 263
c. L. braziliensis complex	
-L. b. braziliensis	MHOM/BR/72/M 1670 (1)
	MHOM/BR/75/M 2904 (2)
	MHOM/BR/75/M 2903 (3)
-L. b. guyanensis	MHOM/BR/78/M 5378 (4)
	MCHO/BR/78/M 5378 (3)
	MHOM/BR/75/M 4147 (3)
-L. b. panamensis	MCHO/PA/OO/M 4039 (4)
	MHOM/PA/67/Boynton (3)
	MHOM/BR/69/M 1142 (3)
	MHOM/PA/71/LS 94 (3)
d. mexicana complex	
-L. m. amazonensis	MPRO/BR/77/M 1845 (1)
	IFLA/BR/67/PH 8 (5)
	MPRO/BR/71/M 649 (1)
	MHOM/BR/73/M 2269 (3)
	MHOM/BR/69/M 1132 (3)
-L. m. mexicana	MNYC/BZ/62/M 379 (3)
	00/CR/00/Zeledon (3)
-L. m. aristedesi	MORY/PA/68/GML 3 (3)
-L. m. garnhami	MHOM/VE/76/JAP 78 (3)
-L. m. pifanoi	MHOM/VE/57/LL 1 (3)
e. Bolivian isolates Alto Beni and Yungas	
-L. b. braziliensis	MHOM/BO/82/LPZ 13 (2)
	MHOM/BO/82/LPZ 17 (2)
	MHOM/BO/83/LPZ 355 (2)
	MHOM/BO/84/LPZ 440 (2)
	MHOM/BO/84/LPZ 662 (2)
	IYUC/BO/84/LPZ 704 (2)
-Leishmania sp.(Lowlands)	MHOM/BO/84/CENP 001 (5)
	MHOM/BO/84/CENP 002 (5)
	MHOM/BO/85/CENP 003 (5)
	MHOM/BO/85/CENP 004 (5)
	MHOM/BO/85/CENP 005 (5)
	MHOM/BO/85/CENP 006 (5)
	MHOM/BO/85/CENP 007 (5)
	MHOM/BO/85/CENP 008 (5)
	MHOM/BO/85/CENP 009 (5)
	MHOM/BO/85/CENP 010 (5)
	MHOM/BO/85/CENP 011 (5)

(1) Dr. M. Chance, Department of Parasitology, Liverpool School of Tropical Medicine, Liverpool;
(2) Dr. Ph. Desjeux, Instituto Boliviano de Biologia de Altura, La Paz;
(3) Dr. D. Evans, Department of Medical Protozoology, London School of Hygiene and Tropical Medicine, London;
(4) Dr. J. J. Shaw, The Wellcome Parasitology Unit, Instituto Evandro Chagas, Belem;
(5) Dr. R. Urjel, Laboratory of Parasitology, CENETROP, Santa Cruz de la Sierra, Bolivia.

RESULTS

Karyotypic Stability

Various populations from the stock L. mexicana amazonensis M 1845 (Fig. 2) were analyzed in order to check whether maintenance conditions like cloning, nature of the culture medium, passage in vivo, long maintenance in vitro and day of harvesting could affect the karyotype. High and low pulses showed the same profiles for each population, but for population B (Fig. 3) where the third band (II.40, 330 kb) was lacking. It is noteworthy that this band reappeared in the lines derived from population B and in line C, which was subisolated from population A.

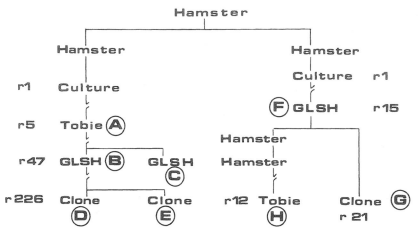

Fig. 2. Flow diagram of L. mexicana amazonensis M 1845 maintained by culture in vitro on blood agar (lines A, H) or in semi-defined medium (lines B, D, E, G), by long term cultivation and cloning (D and E) and ensuing promastigote-induced infection of hamster (H).

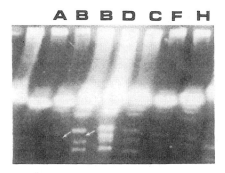

Fig. 3. Karyotype (30s pulses, 250 mA, migration for 19 hrs, 15°C) of different lines of L. mexicana amazonensis M 1845 : all karyotypes identical but for line B where the third lowest band (330 kb, II.40) is absent (arrow). Conditions : 30 s, 250 mA 19 hrs migration, 15°C).

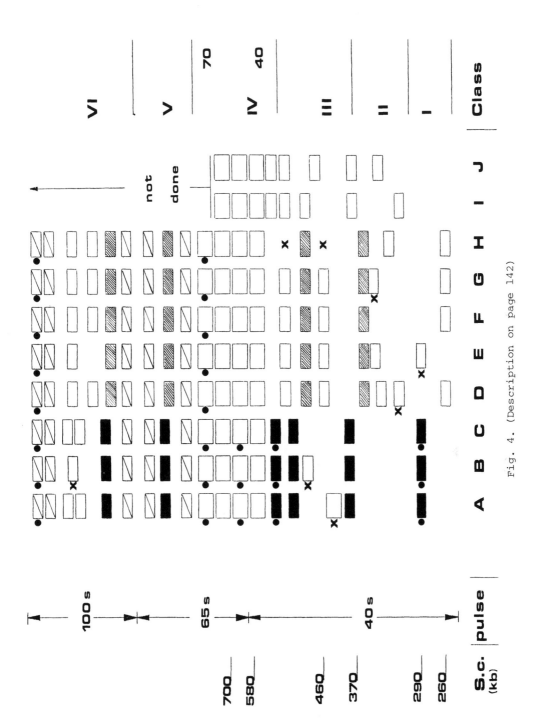

Fig. 4. (Description on page 142)

Fig. 4. Total karyotype representative of the subspecies.
S.c. = Sacharomyces cerevisiae used for sizing up to 700 kb. Pulse duration used for resolving a given class of the karyotype is quoted.
Subspecies : A = L. b. braziliensis (2); B = L. b. guyanensis (3); C = L. b. panamensis (3); D = L. m. amazonensis (5); E = L. m. mexicana (3); F = L. m. aristedesi (1); G = L. m. garnhami (1); H = L. m. pifanoi (1); I = L. major (1); J = L. donovani infantum (1), (number of isolates used between brackets).
Classification of chromosomes according to class and number goes from low to high size (see material and methods).
Specific markers : ■ = braziliensis complex; ▨ = mexicana complex; ✗ = subspecies.
▱ = bands common to both complexes; ● = bands with beta tubulin gene (hybridization not done with L. major and L. donovani).

Karyotypic Variation and Specific Markers

Isolates belonging to different subspecies of the L. mexicana and L. braziliensis complex were studied; isolates of L. major and L. donovani were also included as recommended by Momen et al. (1985).

In general. approximately 20 bands could be resolved with the method described herein. Considering the differences observed in staining intensity, this number is certainly an underestimate. Some bands (Fig. 4) were not well separated (IV. 40-70, 580 to 800 kb). Five bands were found always at the same position in all the isolates of the L. braziliensis and L. mexicana complexes and they were all of high molecular size (classes V and VI). Beside these bands, the following specificities were observed:

Complexes L. braziliensis and L. mexicana. In all the strains of the L. braziliensis complex, 6 bands (low and high sizes) were found at the same position, while 4 bands (low and high sizes) were apparently specific to the L. mexicana complex (Fig. 4).

Subspecies. Within the 2 complexes, at least one subspecies-specific band was observed, generally in the low size area. For L. braziliensis complex, this candidate marker band was found in class III, while in the L. mexicana complex, it was present in both classes I and II.

Tubulin Hybridization Patterns

After Southern blotting of the PFG gels and hybridization with a beta tubulin probe, it was observed that in the L. braziliensis complex, the probe hybridized with 5 bands situated in low and high position. In the L. mexicana complex, only 2 of those bands (all of high molecular size) contained the beta-tubulin gene. There was no variation in hybridization pattern within the 2 complexes (Fig.4).

Molecular Tree

Molecular relationships among New World Leishmania were evaluated by a difference index (DI), and a tree was constructed from the DIs (Fig. 5).

Differences between the complexes were higher than differences between subspecies belonging to the same complex. In the L. mexicana complex, L. mexicana mexicana was the most remote subspecies (DI = 0.25). L. m. garnhami and L. m. aristedesi were the closest subspecies (DI = 0.03). In the L. braziliensis complex, L. braziliensis braziliensis and L. braziliensis panamensis were found to be closely related (DI = 0.14).

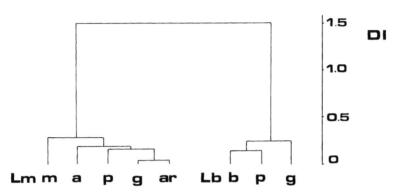

Fig. 5. Molecular relationships between subspecies in the L. braziliensis and L. mexicana complexes according to difference index.

Bolivian Isolates

The value of candidate chromosome markers identified in international reference stocks and strains was tested blindly on isolates coming from different areas of Bolivia, the Yungas and Alto Beni on one side, and the Lowlands on the other side. Independently, isoenzyme typing was performed at IBBA.

The isolates from the Yungas and Alto Beni, were all tentatively identified as L. braziliensis braziliensis according to their DNA pattern, and this was confirmed by enzyme analysis.

Five of the 11 uncloned isolates from the Lowlands originated from the pilot area of Yapacani. All 5 presented a braziliensis complex pattern. Subspecies identification was possible for 2 of them which were shown to be L. b. braziliensis. The other 3 isolates presented variations in DNA pattern which were never observed before in the international reference isolates (Fig. 6) and they were considered as "atypical" for the time being.

In the 6 other isolates, 1 L. mexicana amazonensis, 3 typical L. braziliensis braziliensis and 2 atypical L. braziliensis subspecies were identified. Isoenzymatically, the identity of L. mexicana amazonensis was confirmed and the other 10 isolates were identified as L. braziliensis braziliensis, but with a high variability too in enzyme pattern.

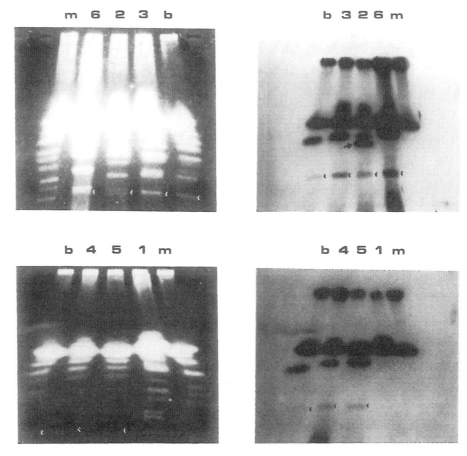

Fig. 6. PFG and beta-tubulin hybridization pattern of isolates from the Lowlands of Bolivia : L. mexicana amazonensis M 1845 (m) and L. braziliensis braziliensis M 1670 (b) used as references. Position of first chromosome and beta-tubulin hybridization pattern allows clear identification of complex(∢: isolates 2-6 = L. braziliensis, 1 = L. mexicana. L. braziliensis braziliensis marker (third chromosome) observed only in isolates 6 and 3 (third chromosome : broad banding indicates presence of two fused bands); isolates 2,4 and 5 : third band in a position never observed elsewhere, isolate 2 beta-tubulin hybridization pattern unusual (←—) (pulse 35s, I : 300 mA, electrophoresis : 16 hrs, T : 18°C).

DISCUSSION

The PFG set-up used in this study is derived from the one described by Carle and Olson (198). Use of diodes for cathodes reduced electrical distortion and induced a more linear migration. Further improvement could be provided by FIGE (Carle and Olson, 1986) where separation occurs in one-dimensional electrical fields periodically inverted.

Leishmania DNA submitted to pulses of 30 to 120 seconds segregated into about 20 bands ranging from 280 to over 2000 kb, a fact consistant with data from previous authors (Giannini et al., 1986; Scholler et al., 1986; Comeau et al., 1986). In our set-up, 4 strongly fluorescent bands belonging to class IV, (nr 0-70, molecular size estimated between 580 and 800 kb) did not segregate properly, a limiting factor for some of the results presented herein.

For reference and comparison purposes, a comprehensive system for identification of individual karyotype was developed. Banding patterns of all the Leishmania stocks were taken into account and every individual band was given a class and number value according to molecular size. By doing so, any band can be specified and entered in any computer program in the form of a 1 or 0 matrix, and room is left for further introduction of bands.

Karyotypic Stability

Scholler et al. (1986) and mainly Comeau et al. (1986) described variations in ethidium bromide staining patterns between clones from the same population. In the present study, variation during maintenance in vitro and in vivo and cloning of two reference stocks was limited to one single chromosome (third band, Fig. 3) in only one line out of eight. This observation, as compared to the high karyotypic variability among uncloned isolates from the Bolivian Lowlands, illustrates the utility of comparing stocks and derived clone populations.

The disappearance of this chromosome in a line during maintenance and its reapparition in derived lines could suggest the presence of two cell populations fluctuating in time. Alternatively, chromosomal recombination like the one reported in T. brucei by Van der Ploeg et al. (1984) could be considered. In the present Leishmania lines however, when chromosomal disappearance occurred, no size variation of another chromosome was noticed.

Notwithstanding these small variations, karyotype was found to be sufficiently stable to allow comparisons at taxonomic level.

Karyotypic Variation and Specific Markers

In previous studies, Giannini et al. (1986) and Scholler et al. (1986) provided evidence in favour of distinct similarities at species and subspecies level, while Comeau et al. (1986) insisted more on the karyotype plasticity of Leishmania.

For identification of complexes by considering the position of the bands, 6 marker chromosomes were tentatively identified in the L. braziliensis complex, and 4 markers were apparently specific to the L. mexicana complex. With beta-tubulin hybridization, a specific set of 5 bands was found to contain the gene in the braziliensis complex, and another set of 2 in the mexicana complex.

For identification of subspecies, at least one candidate marker band was observed. In some subspecies, only one isolate was

was studied and further evaluation is needed. Subspecies markers were always of low size (less than 500 kb) and they belong to class I and II for L. mexicana subspecies and to class III for L. braziliensis subspecies (Fig. 4).

Beside these markers, 5 bands were shared by all the isolates of the 2 New World complexes. The distribution of this set within, and beyond the genus Leishmania is still an open question.

Evaluation of Markers

Evaluation of the markers described above was done on 17 unknown isolates coming from different regions of Bolivia (Yungas, Alto Beni and Lowlands). Complex identity of all the isolates by karyotyping was easily achieved, in complete agreement with enzyme analysis. Subspecies identification however was less clear cut in some instances. All the 11 clone isolates from Alto Beni and the Yungas had the karyotype specific for L. b. braziliensis, but only half of the (uncloned) isolates from the Lowlands did so, even though all of them but one belonged clearly to the braziliensis complex. In the Lowlands, karyotypes never observed elsewhere were encountered and the same situation prevailed with enzyme analysis. Furthermore, variation in the development of lesions in hamsters was also observed for the Lowlands isolates (Urjel, unpublished). Cloning is obviously needed before any further study of this variation can be undertaken.

Molecular Trees

In the present work, preliminary molecular trees (Fig. 5) were built up by using a difference index (DI) based on the relative molecular size (position). But these could be modified when the IV 40-70 bands could be better resolved.

Beverley et al. (1987) compared nDNA restriction fragment patterns of several subspecies of Leishmania. Differences between the major lineages could not be assessed due to the lack of identity among them. Our karyotype data showed obvious similarities between complexes, and DI between the braziliensis and mexicana complexes was found higher than DI between subspecies in the two complexes.

Within the mexicana complex, L. m. mexicana was the most remote subspecies, and L. m. aristedesi and L. m. garnhami the most closely related organisms. These results are in contradiction with enzyme analysis data (Desjeux et al., 1984), where L. m. pifanoi was the most remote subspecies with a nought similarity index. In the braziliensis complex, L. b. panamensis and L. b. braziliensis were shown to be the closest subspecies, at the difference of the relationships index from other techniques (Desjeux et al., 1984; Beverley et al., 1987) which suggested that L. b. panamensis and L. b. guyanensis were the more related. We think that these results could be improved by a better resolution on the IV 40-70 bands, however these differences in the results have to be investigated further.

Comparison of kDNA sequences could not discriminate L. m. mexicana from L. m. pifanoi (Barker and Butcher, 1983). Here karyotype data from the same isolates clearly show differences between those subspecies. Discrepancies among conclusions from different analyses point out the necessity to integrate different approaches on different parts of the genome. As far as karyotype data are concerned, relation between homology of chromosome positions and homology of nucleotide sequences is an open question.

CONCLUSION

PFG karyotyping appears to offer a good tool with many applications to the field of Leishmania research. It can be of use for identification of complex and subspecies. Further improvement in resolution and extension of karyotyping to more isolates should confirm the value of the chromosome markers. Genomic organization of Leishmania can be studied by probe hybridization. Specific bands can be eluted, tested as nDNA probes whenever repetitive, and hybridized for homology comparison. Finally, karyotyping appears to present new information on phylogenetic relationships up tp the complex rank.

ACKNOWLEDGEMENTS

We would like to thank Drs M. Chance, J.J. Shaw and P.C.C. Garnham for giving reference stocks, Dr N. Agabian for providing the beta-tubulin probe, E. Witthoeck for excellent technical assistance and Mrs S. Desager for skillful typing of this work. This investigation received financial support from the EEC (Contract TSD-M.002-B) and from the FGWO (Contract 3.0082.85).

REFERENCES

Barker, D. C. and Butcher, J., 1983, The use of DNA probes in the identification of leishmanias : discrimination between isolates of the Leishmania mexicana and L. braziliensis complexes, Trans. Roy. Soc. Trop. Med. Hyg., 77, 285-297.

Beverley, S. M., Ismach, R. B. and McMahon Pratt, D., 1987, Evolution of the genus Leishmania as revealed by comparison of nuclear DNA restriction fragment patterns, Prov. Nat. Acad. Sci. USA, 84, 484-488.

Carle, G.F. and Olson, M.V., 1984, Separation of chromosomal DNA molecules from yeast by orthogonal field alternation gel electrophoresis. Nucleic Acids Res., 12, 5647-5664.

Comeau, A. M., Miller, S. I. and Wirth, D. F., 1986, Chromosomal location of four genes in Leishmania, Mol. Biochem. Parasitol., 21, 161-169.

Desjeux, P., Le Pont, F., Mollinedo, S. and Tibayrenc, M., 1984, Las leishmania de Bolivia. I. Leishmania braziliensis braziliensis en los departementes de La Paz y Beni. Primeros aislamientos de cepas humanas y su caracterizacion enzimatica, IBBA Anuario 1983-1984, 155-162.

Garvey, E. P. and Santi, D. V., 1986, Stable amplified DNA in drug-resistant Leishmania exists as extrachromosomal circle, Science, 233, 535-540.

Giannini, S. H., Schittini, M., Keithly, J. S., Warburton, P. W., Cantor, C. R. and Van der Ploeg, L. H. T., 1986, Karyotype analysis of Leishmania species and its use in classification and clinical diagnosis, Science, 232, 762-765.

Le Ray, D., 1975, Structures antigéniques de Trypanosoma brucei (Protozoa, Kinetoplastida). Analyse immunoélectrophorétique et étude comparative, Ann. Soc. belge Méd. Trop., 55, 158-160.

Momen, H., Grimaldi, G., Pacheco, R. S., Jaffe, C. L., McMahon Pratt, D. and Marzochi, M. C. A., 1985, Brazilian Leishmania stocks phenotypically similar to L. major, Am. J. Trop. Med. Hyg., 34, 1076-1084.

Scholler, J. K., Reed, S. G. and Stuart, K., 1986, Molecular karyotype of species and subspecies of Leishmania, Mol. Biochem. Parasitol., 20, 279-293.

Schwartz, D. C., Safran, W., Welsh, J., Haas, R., Goldenberg, M. and Cantor, C. R., 1983, New techniques for purifying large DNAs and studying their properties and packaging, Cold Spring Harbor Symp. Quant. Biol., 47, 189-195.

Spithill, T. W. and Samaras, N., 1985, The molecular karyotype of L. major and mapping of alpha and beta tubulin gene families to multiple unlinked chromosomal loci, Nucleic Acids Res., 13, 4155-4169.

Tomashow, L. S., Milhausen, M., Rutter, W. S. and Agabian, N., 1983, Tubulin genes are tandemly linked and clustered in the genome of Trypanosoma brucei, Cell, 32, 35-43.

Tobie, E. J., Von Brand, T. and Mehlman, B., 1950, Cultural and physiological observations on Trypanosoma rhodesiense and Trypanosoma gambiense, J. Parasit., 36, 48-54.

Van der Ploeg, L. H. T., Cornelissen, W. W. C. A., Michels, P. A. M. and Borst, P., 1984, Chromosome rearrangements in Trypanosoma brucei, Cell, 39, 213-221.

THE DISTRIBUTION AND AETIOLOGY OF DIFFUSE CUTANEOUS LEISHMANIASIS IN THE NEW WORLD

Bryce C. Walton[1] and Oscar Velasco[2]

[1]WHO, PAHO (Retired)
Gettysburgh
PA. USA

[2]Institute of Health and Tropical Diseases
Mexico D.F.
Mexico

INTRODUCTION

Diffuse cutaneous leishmaniasis (DCL) is an unusual manifestation of cutaneous leishmaniasis in which the skin lesions do not ulcerate, but grow and proliferate as nodules and plaques which slowly but relentlessly spread to cover the entire body, with the exception of the scalp, axillae, inguinal fold, palms of the hands and soles of the feet. It was demonstrated simultaneously but independently in the highlands of Africa [1] and in Venezuela [2], that the condition involves the failure of the patient to elaborate a cell-mediated immune response to the parasite antigen. Apparently there also is a parasite influence involved in this disease manifestation, in that not all species or subspecies of *Leishmania* which produce cutaneous leishmaniasis produce DCL. To date, to the best of our knowledge, all parasites which have been identified by molecular biology methodologies have been either *L.aethiopica* in the Old World, or one of the members of the *L.mexicana* complex in the New World [3]. The great majority of New World cases are reported from Venezuela, Brazil, and the Dominican Republic, with only very few scattered cases from a few other South American countries. All Old World cases are from the African continent; most are from the Ethiopian/Kenyan highlands, although cases have also occurred in Namibia and Tanzania [3]. Hence, at the present time, the generally held concept is that this is a very rare condition, caused in patients with a special immunological status by a very few species/subspecies of *Leishmania* which have a very restricted distribution, and constitutes a very small proportion of the infections; the usual disease manifestation of these leishmanias is an ordinary ulcerating cutaneous lesion.

The purpose of this report is to signal the existence of many more cases of DCL, with a much wider distribution in the New World than has hitherto been recognized, and to suggest that the condition may also be produced by species/subspecies of New World *Leishmania* other than the *L.mexicana* complex.

MATERIALS AND METHODS

Two sets of criteria for classification of cases as DCL were used in compiling the list for charting geographic distribution. In studies of current patients there was strict adherence to the criteria generally accepted as defining the condition:

1. Non-ulcerative lesions, nodules or plaques with areas of depigmentation containing parasites.

2. Anergy to leishmanial antigen, usually demonstrated by a negative intradermal test with leishmanin (Montenegro test).

3. Slow but unrelenting spread of lesions.

4. Essentially complete resistance to antimony and other chemotherapeutic agents.(Clinical improvement can occur, but eventual relapse always occurs).

5. No evidence of visceralization, and no mucosal lesions (see note in Discussion).

6. Characteristic histopathology ; vacuolated macrophages 'foam cells', with large numbers of amastigotes.

For literature reports and other situations where some of these parameters could not be determined, proven leishmaniasis cases with clinical features consistent with DCL, and the absence of suspicion of post kala azar dermal leishmaniasis, was accepted as a probable case.

Some of these cases reported here resulted from information kindly supplied by colleagues who have not yet published case reports; their collaboration is acknowledged and greatly appreciated. In Mexico, suspect cases were located in a survey by a team working in endemic areas and singled out for confirmatory studies, which included biopsy of the lesion, isolation and identification of the parasite, and skin testing with leishmanin as a minimum. In the surveillance program of the Institute for Tropical Diseases, suspect cases located by Primary Health Care and other medical facilities in the endemic areas, were referred to the capital for the confirmatory studies. In the Dominican Republic suspect cases were detected by active search in conjunction with the Leprosy Surveillance and Control program of the Institute of Dermatology, (H. Bogaert-Diaz, personal communication) and similar studies were done in that institution.

RESULTS

Geographical Distribution

The geographical distribution of DCL in the Americas is shown in Figure 1. The range is from the state of Texas in the North, where a single case was reported from San Benito (4), to Brazil in the South, where *L.m.amazonensis* is apparently the causative agent [3]. Multiple cases in the same locality occur only in the original focur in Venezuela, in Brazil, Mexico, the Dominican Republic, and three probable cases in siblings in Honduras.

The focus in the Dominican Republic [5] is of particular interest in several ways. It is the only insular focus in the hemisphere and has a relatively large number of cases in spite of the fact that no ordinary cutaneous leishmaniasis is known from the island, and only a very few cases, scattered in time and over other islands have been reported in the Caribbean. The apparent vector is *Lutzomyia christophei* which is the only anthropophilic sandfly in that country and has a distribution limited to only a few localities [6].

Probably the most significant aspect of this distribution map is the number of cases and relatively widespread distribution in Mexico, since most of the information is exceedingly recent [7,8]. The first cases were reported from Coahuila [9] in the north and soon thereafter from Tabasco in the south [10]. The northern focus is now known to be confluent with the area in Texas in the United States from which the only autochthonous cases of CL are known from that country [7]. Indeed, the single U.S. case of DCL was in a patient who had also visited the neighbouring Mexican states of Taulipas and Nuevo Leon, and it was at first suspected that the infection might have been acquired there [11], but it is now believed that the source of infection was in Texas. The greatest number of cases now, however, come from the southern regions in the states of Oaxaca, and Tabasco. The total number of probably and confirmed DCL cases currently stands at 23, placing it among the areas of highest prevalence in the hemisphere.

In Central America DCL is shown in the neighboring countries of Nicaragua and Honduras. The former is from a recent journal report [12] but the initial report from Honduras [18] appeared quite early in the emerging story of DCL. However, more recently three siblings, sisters aged 7 and 3 (twins) were admitted to a hospital in Tegucigalpa for treatment of CL. The lesions did not exhibit the classical appearance of DCL, but they were extensive, non-ulcerative and progressive lesions which were essentially non-responsive to antimony treatment. *Leishmania* were isolated in blood agar culture from all 3 patients. All three were nonreactors to leishmanin and there were no mucosal lesions or indication of visceralization. Thus, 5 of the 6 defining criteria for DCL were exhibited. Unfortunately, so far it has not been possible to obtain a biopsy to verify the histopathological appearance. It is of interest that the initial case in 1968 came from the Caribbean coastal region, while the 3 recent cases are from the central highlands, which are close to, and ecologically similar to, the Nicaraguan locality.

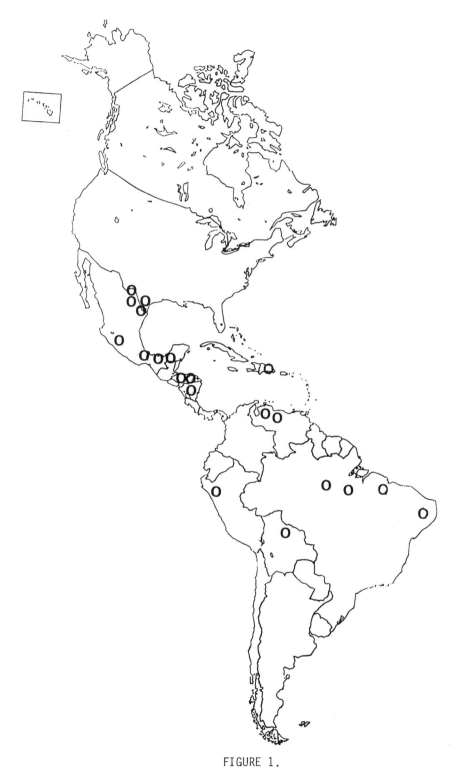

FIGURE 1.

DISTRIBUTION OF DIFFUSE CUTANEOUS LEISHMANIASIS

There has been little or no information regarding new cases from Venezuela in recent years, and apparently it remains a rarity there, as it was at the time of the original pioneering investigations of Convit et al , representing only an exceedingly small proportion of the total cases of cutaneous leishmaniasis. Similarly, Bolivia, the country which produced the first case report from the hemisphere, [14] apparently has had no cases recognized since.

The single case indicated in the Andean region of Peru is a patient studied by Professor Miranda and colleagues at Trujillo, who has both the history and appearance of classical DCL and the case meets all criteria for DCL. There is a history of over 20 years development of the disease, which could easily be confused with lepromatous leprosy.

No confirmed cases have been reported from Colombia. Hoever, in their meticulous search of local records and publications, Werner and Barreto [15] encountered descriptions of cases in that country which are very suggestive of DCL.

Aetiological agents

L.m.pifanoi. Soon after the description of DCL as an entity in the New World, the disease was believed to be produced by a parasite different and distinct from that causing CL in the area and it was described as a separate species *Leishmania pifanoi* [16]. By original definition, it was the parasite that caused DCL and hence for a period any parasite causing DCL was caused *L.pifanoi* [e.g. 13]. After the advent of biochemical characterization it was shown to possess the characters of the *L.mexicana* complex, and is now generally designated as *L.m.pifanoi*[3]. However, few DCL isolates have been characterized by isoenzyme patterns, kDNA analysis, or monoclonal antibodies, so it is not certain that this parasite is limited to the focus in northern Venezuela.

L.m.amazonensis. In Brazil all isolates from DCL cases identified by the methods of molecular biology have proven to be *L.m.amazonensis*. There is no doubt that this subspecies possesses the special characteristics which can produce this condition, and it has even been suggested that it has an exceptionally high rate of association, producing DCL in 30% of infections in one small series of cases followed in Brazil [17].

***L.mexicana* ssp. 1.** The Dominican Republic parasite has many characteristics of the *L.mexicana* group, including having a "suprapylarian" growth in sandflies (J.J. Shaw, personal communication), and clearly is assignable to that complex. However, it has significant differences in biological and exo-antigen characteristics [18] from most members of the complex, and is separable on the basis of isoenzyme electrophoretic patterns from other *L.mexicana* subspecies (D. Evans, personal communication). The unique insular location, unusual sandfly vector and distinctive disease pattern, as well as its biochemical characters, clearly separate it from the other subspecies.

***L.mexicana* ssp. 2.** The parasite causing DCL in Mexico could well be a form different from *L.m.mexicana*. However, the only evidence for this at the present time is epidemiological. By far the greatest number of cases of CL in Mexico come from the Yucatan peninsula, the type locality for this subspecies, where the known vector, *Lu.olmeca.olmeca*, is the predominant anthropophilic sandfly. However, only 2 cases are reported from the south-western transition zone in Campeche and no case of DCL has ever been reported from Quintana Roo on the eastern half of the peninsula in spite of the thousands of recorded cases of CL [8]. On the other hand, in the nearby states of Oaxaca, Tabasco, Veracruz, and part of Campeche, which have ecologies quite distinct from the forests of the Yucatan peninsula, and outside of the known distribution of *Lu.o.olmeca*, relatively few cases of DCL are known, but a significant number of DCL cases occur. Likewise, in the northern focus in the Texas border states, few cases of DCL are reported, but the DCL rate is over 40%. (Walton & Velasco, unpublished). This suggests that the parasite in those areas possesses the as yet undefined characteristic which produces this condition, but *L.m.mexicana* in its type locality does not. A few isolates from DCL cases have been typed by isoenzyme electrophoresis, but do not show any difference in patterns from *L.m.mexicana* (D. Evans, personal communication).

L. peruviana. This parasite is not a member of the *L.mexicana* complex, but is usually considered a member of the *L.braziliensis* group on the basis of isoenzyme patterns, although it is distinct biologically in not producing MCL, and geographically by its high altitude range in the Andes. However, an isolate from the proven DCL case in Pagash, Peru has been unequivocably identified by isoenzyme characterization by Dr. Romero {Alexander von Humboldt Institute of Tropical Medicine] as *L.peruviana*. (H. Miranda, personal communication). This is the first suggestion that a member of the *L.braziliensis* complex possesses the characteristic that causes this condition.

L.b.panamensis. A possible corroboration of the occurrence of DCL caused by the *L.braziliensis* group might result from the suspect DCL cases in Honduras. Isolates were made from all 3 siblings by C. Ponce in Tegucigalpa, and two of these stocks survived transport to the U.S., and one to England. They were characterized by isoenzyme patterns in 2 laboratories (R. Kreutzer, Youngstown, Ohio and D. Evans, London) and shown to be *L.b.panamensis,* although there were variants in some enzymes.

DISCUSSION

In defining DCL, some authors include the statement that there is."no visceralization, and no mucosal involvement". However, because amastigotes can readily be found in macrophages in stained smears of nasal swabs from DCL patients in Mexico and the Dominican Republic, we have modified this criterion to read "no evidence of mucosal lesions".

Post kala azar dermal leishmaniasis (PKDL) can closely mimic DCL, and has been confused with it. A report of DCL in a Japanese patient [19] is a case in point, where the patient's prior military service in China suggests the more probable aetiology of *L.donovani*. However, PKDL is extremely rare in the Western Hemisphere, and not likely to be a source of confusion, although a case of DCL in Mexico was erroneously diagnosed as PKDL [20]. The two conditions are easily differentiated by histopathology.

The histopathology of cutaneous leishmaniasis due to *L.aethiopica* shows a spectrum of response between classical CL and DCL [3] and a similar situation in New World forms which produce DCL would not be unlikely. Although the characteristic histopathology of DCL has not been confirmed in the three young sisters in Honduras, it has not been ruled out, since biopsies are not available. Even if the biopsies should show an uncharacteristic picture, the condition of these patients is clearly very close to DCL, and the possibility of producing DCL must be considered for this parasite, particularly in an area where *L.mexicana* has never been reported.

Paradoxically, the exceedingly rare entity, DCL, can be an epidemiological indicator of the presence of the relatively more common ordinary cutaneous leishmaniasis. The people most likely to acquire leishmaniasis are accustomed to endure the inconvenience and pain of minor ills and injuries, and not likely to seek medical attention (which is often not readily available) for a small skin ulcer. With relatively benign lesions of the type usually caused by the *L.mexicana* group, self healing usually occurs before medical attention is sought, or the aetiology is not suspected by the physician before healing occurs, and the infection goes undiagnosed and unreported. However, the enduring and progressive nature of DCL forces the patient to seek attention and the physician to persevere to reach a diagnosis, so the first recognized leishmanial infection in the area results. After clinical suspicion is established and the infection is known to occur in the area, the more benign ordinary ulcerating lesions are diagnosed, as well. This was the course of events in Coahuila and Tamaulipas in the north of Mexico. More recently, in the state of Michoacan in west-central Mexico the first case of DCL was recognized [8]. It will be interesting to see how soon simple CL lesions will be encountered. The situation in regard to the Dominican Republic seems to be different, in that no ordinary CL lesions seem to occur. None have been encountered in spite of an intensive search by informed and capable investigators over a period of several years.

REFERENCES

1. Bryceson, A.D.M., 1970. Diffuse cutaneous leishmaniasis in Ethiopia. III. Immunological studies.
   Trans Roy Soc Trop Med Hyg $\underline{64}$: 380

2. Convit, J., Pinardi, M.E. and Rondon, A.J., 1971. Diffuse cutaneous leishmaniasis: a disease due to an immunological defect of the host.
   Trans Roy Soc Trop Med Hyg $\underline{66}$: 603

3. World Health Organization. 1984. The Leishmaniases: Report of a WHO Expert Committee.
   Tech Report Series 701.

4. Simpson, M.H., Mullins, J.F. and Stone, O.J., 1968. Disseminated anergic cutaneous leishmaniasis. Arch Dermatol 97:301-

5. Bogaert-Diaz H., Rojas, R.F., De Leon, A., Martinez, D. and Quinones M., 1975. Leishmaniasis tegumentaria americana: reporte de los primeros tres casos. Forma anergica en tres hermanos. Rev Dominicana Dermatol 9:19

6. Fairchild, G.B. and Trapido, H., 1950. The West Indian Species of Phlebotomus (Diptera-Psychodidae) Ann Entomol Soc Am 43:405

7. Walton, B.C., 1985. Evaluacion de la situacion del foco de lieshmaniasis cutanea/cutanea diseminada en los estados de la frontera Mexicano/Estadounidense. Reporte, OPS, Washington, D.C.

8. Velasco, O., 1987. Las leishmanisis en Mexico. Rev Lat-amer Microbiol 29:119

9. Marquez, F.1966. Leishmaniasis cutanea disemin adaanergica Med Cut 3:287

10. Martinex, J.L., Alvarez, G. and Biagi, F. 1968. Presencia de la leishmaniasis cutanea generalizada en Mexico. Rev Invest Salud Publica (Mex) 27:107

11. Simpson, M.H., Mullins J.F., and Stone, O.J. 1968. Disseminated anergic cutaneous leishmaniasis. Arch Dermatol 97:301

12. Missoni, E. and Morelli, R., 1984. J. Trop Med Hyg 87:159

13. Corrales-Padilla, H. and Lainez H., 1968. Leishmaniasis cutanea diseminada(Revision del tema e informe del primer caso en Honduras) Med Cutan (Barcelona) III:119.

14. Prado Barrientos, L. 1948. Un caso atipico de leishmaniose cutaneo mucosa (espundia) Mem Inst O Cruz 46:417

15. Werner, J.K. and Barreto, P., 1981. Leishmaniasis in Colombia: A Review. Am J Trop Med Hyg 30:751

16. Medina, R. and Romero, J., 1962. Leishmania pifanoi N.Sp. El agente causal de la Leishmaniasis tegumentaria difusa. Arch Venezolanos Med Trop Parasitol Medica 4:349

17. Lainson, R. 1981. Epidemiologia e ecologia de leishmaniose tegumentar na Amazonas. Hileia Medica (Belem) 3:35

18. Schnur, L.F., Walton, B.C. and Bogaert-Diaz, H., 1983.
    On the identity of the parasite causing diffuse cutaneous leishmaniasis in the Dominican Republic.
    Trans Roy Soc Trop Med Hyg $\underline{7}$:756

19. Takahashi, S. and Sata, T., 1981.
    Disseminierte kutane Leishmaniose.
    Der Hautartzt $\underline{32}$:459

20. Welsch, O., 1971.
    Leishmaniasis in Nuevo Leon.
    Vi Congr Mex Dermatologia:78

EPIDEMIOLOGICAL STUDIES ON CUTANEOUS LEISHMANIASIS IN THE STATE OF RIO DE JANEIRO, BRAZIL. DOMESTIC AND PERIDOMESTIC SANDFLY FAUNA

R.P. Brazil, B.G. Brazil, M.C. Gouvea, D.C. De Almeida, S.M.P. De Oliveira and J.A. De Menezes

Department of Parasitologia - JCB - CCS
Universidade Federal Do Rio De Janiero
Cidade Universitaria - 21941 -
Rio De Janeiro
Brazil

INTRODUCTION

Cutaneous leishmaniasis is an important public health problem in most states of Brazil (Deane and Grimaldi, 1985). In the past, cutaneous leishmaniasis was mainly associated with primary forest but now it is also found in areas where primary forest does not exist. The great and varied extent of the country which has different types of vegetation and also rapid urbanisation of the area makes the epidemiology of cutaneous leishmaniasis complex (Gomes, 1986).

In the state of Rio De Janeiro where less than 1% of the original tropical forest is left, cutaneous leishmaniasis is sporadic and small outbreaks of the disease are found in suburban and rural areas (Guimaraes, 1955; Coutinho et al., 1985).

In this report the sandfly fauna of suburban and rural areas of Rio De Janeiro was studied. A comparative analysis of sandflies captured indoors and outdoors was made to clarify the transmission of cutaneous leishmanisis to man and domestic animals.

MATERIALS AND METHODS

Studies were carried out in two areas where several cases of cutaneous leishmaniasis have been found (Figure 1). The district of Itaipu in the municipality of Niteroi is close to the urban zone of the city of Niteroi. Itaipu possesses basic water supplies and public illumination; however the district remains rural in character. The locality of Catimbau-Grande belongs to the municipality of Rio Bonito and lies 80 km north of the city of Rio De Janeiro. The area is rural and there is no electricity supply; and agriculture is the main activity.

To date, 56 cases of cutaneous leishmaniasis from both areas have been diagnosed with 44 isolates made by one of us (J.A.M.), and natural infections of horses and dogs have also been diagnosed. All the isolates have been characterised by monoclonal antibodies as *Leishmania b. braziliensis* (Menzes et al., in press).

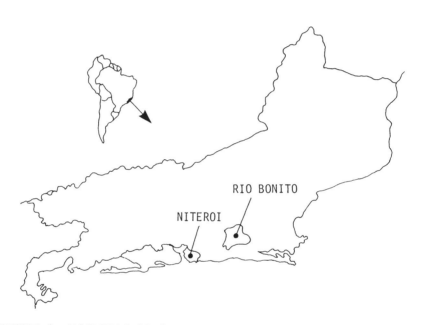

FIGURE 1   LOCATION OF STUDY AREAS IN RIO DE JANEIRO STATE

Sandflies were captured during 1986 and the beginning of 1987 using CAC light traps. Traps were set in chicken houses, horse and pig shelters, and catches were made directly on these animals. Indoor captures were made from walls or on inhabitants by manual catching. Captures were carried out between 1800 and 2100 h and occasionally between 1800 and 0600 h. Sandflies were taken to the laboratory in tubes with 70% ethyl alcohol, mounted and classified according to Martins *et al.* (1978). In some cases live sandflies were brought to the laboratory in plaster-bottomed and net-covered cups for subsequent dissection.

RESULTS

As seen in Tables 1 and 2, 97 hours of catching resulted in the capture of 2,918 sandflies of 10 species from both areas. *Lutzomyai (N) intermedia* was the predominant species, followed by *Lutzomyia migonei*.

During the search for natural infection of sandflies with *Leishmania* we dissected and examined 471 (444 *Lu. intermedia*, 25 *Lu. migonei* and 2 *Lu. fischeri*) females caught indoors in houses where cutaneous leishmaniasis was diagnosed. The results were all negative.

TABLE 1 DOMESTIC AND PERIDOMESTIC SANDFLY FAUNA IN ITAIPU AREA, MUNICIPALITY OF NITEROI, RIO DE JANEIRO STATE

Species	DOMESTIC								PERIDOMESTIC					
	Males		Females		Total	Total %	Freq per h	Males		Females		Total	Total %	Freq per h
	N°	%	N°	%				N°	%	N°	%			
Lu. (N.) intermedia	90	10.3	422	48.3	512	58.6	5.9	367	34.6	526	49.6	893	84.3	10.2
Lu. migonei	150	17.1	209	23.9	359	41.0	4.1	80	7.5	33	3.1	113	10.6	1.3
Lu. (P.) fischeri			2	0.2	2	0.2	0.02	3	0.3	40	3.8	43	4.1	0.5
Lu. (P.) pessoai			1	0.1	1	0.1	0.01			1	0.1	1	0.1	0.01
Lu. pelloni								2	0.2			2	0.2	0.02
Lu. firmatoi								2	0.2	2	0.2	4	0.3	0.04
Lu. (M.) schreiberi								1	0.1	1	0.1	2	0.2	0.02
Lu. (Barretomyia) sp										1	0.1	1	0.1	0.01
TOTAL	240	27.4	634	72.5	874	99.9	10.03	455	42.9	604	57.0	1059	99.9	12.2

Obs: Hours of captures: 10
Total of sandflies: 1933

TABLE 2 DOMESTIC AND PERIDOMESTIC SANDFLY FAUNA IN CATIMBAU GRANDE AREA., MUNICIPALITY OF RIO BOMITO, RIO DE JANEIRO STATE.

Species	DOMESTIC								PERIDOMESTIC					
	Males		Females		Total	Total %	Freq per h	Males		Females		Total	Total %	Freq per h
	N°	%	N°	%				N°	%	N°	%			
Lu. (N.) intermedia	17	10.1	72	42.5	89	52.6	8.9	400	49.1	94	11.4	494	60.4	49.4
Lu. migonei	6	3.6	9	5.3	15	8.9	1.5	182	22.3	16	1.9	198	24.2	19.8
Lu. (P.) fischeri			5	2.9	5	2.9	0.5	1	0.1	10	1.2	11	1.3	1.1
Lu. (L.) longipalpis	44	26.0	15	8.9	59	34.9	5.9	68	8.3	39	4.8	107	13.1	10.7
Lu. (M.) schreiberi								3	0.3	3	0.3	6	0.7	0.6
Lu. (Barretomyia) sp	1	0.6			1	0.6	0.1							
TOTAL	68	40.3	101	59.6	169	99.9	16.9	654	80.1	162	19.6	816	99.7	81.6

Obs: Hours of captures: 10
Total of sandflies: 985

DISCUSSION

It is well known that in several urban and suburban foci of American cutaneous leishmaniasis, domestic animals play an important role in the maintenance of infection (Alencar, 1959; Bonfante-Garrido, 1972; Aguilar et al., 1982; Brazil et al., 1987). The probable anthropophilic vector should be found in the peridomestic environment. Our results show that Lu. ntermedia is the sandfly that is the most adapted to the peridomestic environment. The same behaviour has been shown by several other authors in south-east Brazil (Fpratini, 1953; Gomes, 1980; De Souza et al., 1981; Lima, 1981). This sandfly is the most prevalent in foci of cutaneous leishmaniasis of Sao Paulo, Rio De Janeiro and Espirito Santo states. The conclusive proof that Lu. intermedia is the vector or the sole vector of Leishmania braziliensis braziliensis in both areas. The recent isolation of L.b.braziliensis from Lu.(p)hirsuta by Rangel et al. (1985) from the remains of primary forest in Alem Poraiba (MG) along the border of Rio De Janeiro state would support the view that Lu.hirsuta is the vector of L.b.braziliensis among wild reservoirs in the forest of south-east Brazil. However, less than 1% of the original atlantic forest remains in the state of Rio De Janeiro and outbreaks of cutaneous leishmanisis are still occuring in areas without primary forest.

In both areas studied the original atlantic forest has been depleted for agricultural development and urbanisation. The sandfly fauna in both are similar in the domiciliary areas showing that species such as Lu. intermedia and Lu. migonei are well adapted to this new environment. Lu. intermedia is so well adapted that it can be regarded as a syanthropic species as suggested by Gomes et al. (1986).

Although the sandfly fauna is shown to be very similar in foci of cutaneous leishmaniasis in the states of Sao Paulo, Rio De Janeiro and Espirito Santo, species seem to have different abilities to adapt to the man-made environment. In Sao Paulo Lu.(N.)whitmani was among the anthropophilic species found in primary forest (Barreto, 1943) but it lacked the ability to persist in rural or suburban areas (Gomes et al., 1986). In the states of Bahia and Minas Gerais Lu.whitmani is well adapted to the peridomestic environment and there is strong evidence that it is the vector of L.b.braziliensis (Vexenat et al., 1986). The highly anthropophilic Lu.migonei in both areas studied together with Lu.intermedia suggests that this species may be responsible for transmission of cutaneous leishmaniasis among man, equines and dogs.

ACKNOWLEDGEMENTS

We wish to express our thanks to Dr R. Ward (LSTM) for his help, and to the Fundacao Univertaria Jose Bonifacio and FINEP for financial support.

REFERENCES

Alencar, J.E., 1959, Um caso de leishmaniase tegumentar em equus asinus. XVI Congr. Basic Higiene, Niuteroi, Brazil.

Aguilar, C.M., Fernandez, E., Fernandez, R. and Deane, L.M., 1987, Study of an outbreak of cutaneous leishmaniasis in Venezuela. The role of domestic animals. Mem. Inst. Oswaldo Cruz, 79:181.

Barreto, M.P., 1943, Observacoes sobre a biologia em condicoes naturais dos flebotomos do estado de Sao Paulo. Thesis, Faculdade de Medicina - USP.

Bonfante-Garrido, R., Torres, R., Morillo, N. and Melendez, R., 1972, Leishmaniasis tegumentaria Americana em perros de guamacire. VI Jor. Venez. Microb., Barquisimeto, Venezuela.

Brazil, R.P., Nascimento, M.D.S.B. and Macau, R.J., 1987, Infeccao natural do porco (*Sus scrofa*) por *Leishmania* em foco recente de leishmaniose tegumentar na ilha de Sao Luiz, Maranhao. Mem. Inst. Oswaldo Cruz, 82:145.

Coutinho, S.G., Nunes, M.P., Marzochi, M.C.A. and Tramontano, N.C., 1985, A survey for American cutaneous and visceral leishmaniasis among 1,372 dogs from areas in Rio De Janeiro (Brazil) where the human disease occurs. Mem. Inst. Oswaldo Cruz, 80:17.

Deane, L.M. and Grimaldi, J.R.G., 1985, Leishmaniasis in Brazil. In Human Parasitic Diseases Vol. 1, K.P. Chang and R.S. Bray Ed., Elsevier Press, Amsterdam.

De Souza, M.A., Sabroza, P.C., Marzochi, M.C.A., Coutinho, S.G. and Dr Souza, W.J.S., 1981, Leishmaniose visceral no Rio De Janeiro. 1. Flebotomineos da area de procedencia de casos humanos autoctone. Mem. Inst. Oswaldo Cruz, 76:161.

Forattini, O.P., 1953, Nota sobre criadouros natorais de flebotomes em dependecias peridomiciliares no estado de Sao Paulo. Arq. Fac. Hig. S. Paulo, 7:157.

Forattini, O.P., Pattoli, D.B.G., Rabello, E.X. and Ferreira, O.A., 1972, Infeccao natural de flebotomineos em foco enzootico de leishmaniose tegumentar no estado de Sao Paulo, Brazil. Rev. Saude Publica, S. Paulo, 6:731.

Gomes, A de C, 1980, A spectos ecologicos da leishmaniose tegumentar Americana. 1. Estudo esperimental da frequencia de flebotomineos em ectopos artificais com referencia especial a *Psychodopygus intermedius*.

Gomes A. de C., 1986, Ecological aspects of American cutaneous leishmaniasis. 4. Observations on the endophilic behaviour of the sandfly and the vectorial role of *Psychodopygus intermedius* in Ribeira Valley region of the Sao Paulo state, Brazil. Rev. Saude Publica S. Paulo, 20:280.

Lima, L.C.R., Marzochi, M.A.A. and Abroza, P.C., 1981, Flebotomineos em area de ocorencia de leishmaniose tegumentar no Bairro de Campo Grand, Rio De Janeiro. Rev. Bros. Macar., 33:67.

Martins, A.V., Williams, P. and Falcao, A.L., 1978, American sandflies (Diptera: Psychodidae, Phlebotominae). Academia Brasileira De Ciencias, Rio De Janeiro.

Rangel, E.F., Ryan, L., Lainson, R. and Shaw, J.J., 1985, Observations on the sandlfy (Diptera: Psychodidae) fauna of Alem Paraiba state of Minas Gerais and the isolation of a parasite of the *Leishmania braziliensis* complex from *Psychodopygus hirsutus hirsutus*. Mem. Inst. Oswaldo Cruz., 80:373.

Rangel, E.F., Souza, N.A., Wermelinger, E.D. and Barbosa, A.F., 1984, Infeccao natural de *Lutzomyia intermedia* Lutz and Neiva, 1912 em area endemica de leishmaniose tegumentar no estado do Rio De Janeiro. Mem. Inst. Oswaldo Cruz, 79:395.

Vexenat, J.A., Barreto, A.C., Cuba, C.C. and Marsden, P., 1986, Caracteristicas epidemiologicas da leishmaniose tegumentar Americana em uma regiao endemica do Estado da Bahia III. Fauna Flebotominica. Mem. Inst. Oswaldo Cruz, 81:293.

EVALUATION OF THE CANINE RESERVOIR OF VISCERAL LEISHMANIASIS : A METHODOLOGICAL REVIEW

R. Houin

Labo de Parasitologie et de Mycologie
Centre Hospital et Uni. de Cereteil
6, Rue Du General Sarrail
94010 Cereteil
Cedex
France

INTRODUCTION

Most of the leishmaniasis being zoonoses, the definition of their foci cannot rely on the exclusive study of the human cases. Contrarily to what happens in anthroponoses, such as the indian kala-azar, they are scattered in the population. This makes them quite difficult to collect, as their scarcity does not attract the attention of the medical organizations. Moreover, when they are diagnosed and when reliable statistics are available, the human cases often do not reflect the true structure of the focus, as man is only a reflection of the zoonose, which can affect wide areas without consequence for him.

When the reservoir is a wild animal, as is the case in *L.major* foci, its study needs preliminary investigations on the local fauna, and an evaluation of the susceptible animals, both experimentally and naturally. It happens quite frequently that such animals, though sensitive to the parasite, do not play the role of reservoir: the evolution of their disease, or of their ethology do that the necessary conditions are not fulfilled for a further transmission. Actually, this is frequently the case for man, but it may be so, as well, for other animals, and it is sometimes quite difficult to determine if an animal, even trapped in a known focus, and naturally infected, is a reservoir, or simply the victim of a zoonosis belonging to another species.

In the case of zoonotic visceral leishmaniasis, due to *L. infantum* (and also *L. chagasi*), the life cycle involves an additional factor, a domestic reservoir, the dog. Its importance is obvious in what concerns the transmission to man: its behaviour makes it the step between the wild reservoir (canids such as foxes or jackals) and man. Most of the transmitting sandflies bite both dog and man, finding them in the same biotopes, which permits the transmission from the first to the second. The knowledge of the epizootology of leishmaniasis in the canine population is, therefore, a major step in the understanding of the epidemiology of visceral leishmaniasis in man.

Since the beginning of the century, and especially Charles Nicolle's work at the Institute Pasteur in Tunis, this aspect of the mediterranean leishmaniasis has been constantly investigated. Canine leishmaniasis is perfectly described, following veterinary studies in many countries around the mediterranean basin, but also in other regions, such as Brazil. The disease is considered, in these areas, as a major dog pathology and is well known by the local veterinarians, who diagnose and treat the cases found during their normal activities. This allows them to supply the epidemiologists with valuable information, which complete the data obtained from the human cases, to detect the foci of visceral leishmaniasis, and evaluate their extension.

Nevertheless, such results remain limited: even if the canine disease is more frequent than the human one, it is only one of the canine pathologies in the areas concerned. Veterinarians can hardly focus on it and, in some cases, the clinical diagnosis may be difficult; the necessary biological confirmation is not always possible, due to the lack of trained laboratories or, more often, to the relatively high price of such investigations. Moreover, the number of dogs examined by the veterinarians often remains low in areas where the income of the population is not high enough to afford medical care for domestic animals. For all these reasons, the data obtained from the normal activities of the veterinary services, though capital, remain insufficient for scientific evaluation of the foci.

Early, in the history of visceral leishmaniasis, a further step was climbed, by studies on dogs in pounds. Such animals are easily available for research including their sacrifice. Histological examinations, and also parasite isolations can be performed in excellent conditions. This kind of investigation brought valuable information on the canine disease, and also on the parasite itself, and helped greatly to prepare efficient media for the isolation of new strains.

However, from an epidemiological point of view, such data remain far from the expected goal, i.e. the knowledge of the behaviour of the parasite in the canine population. Pound dogs are a very small part of this population, and cannot reflect what happens in other "classes" of dogs. These animals are collected in important cities, and cannot give any information on what happens in rural areas; these dogs are generally wandering stray dogs, whose conditions of life cannot reflect what happens in other classes such as house-dogs or field dogs, which live much more closely to man, and can provide a better reservoir for the parasite.

For these reasons, and even if important information are made available through these channels, specific investigations on the whole canine population, in the suspected foci, are necessary; they are only able to give the best views on the structure of the reservoir population. Together with the study of the vector, they explain the local mechanisms of the transmission, and open the way to prophylactic measures.

CHOOSING THE POPULATION FOR STUDY

Before any field investigation, it is extremely important to define where and when the relatively heavy effort of such a study has to be focused. Concerning dog leishmaniasis, the time, at least in a year, is not important as the disease is relatively slow in its evolution. However, important differences can be observed from one year to another, and long term studies are necessary for understanding the dynamics of the enzooty.

Even if the available techniques allow the screening of an important number of dogs, the choice of the investigated places is extremely important. Preliminary information comes from both medical and veterinary sources. This must be carefully analysed to determine the places where the parasite is most probably transmitted. Some elements can also come from analogies with already known foci, and, of course, from data concerning the vector(s), if available.

The next step of the choice needs good physical maps of the area. In some countries, excellent 1/100.000 maps are available: they are the best, but 1/500.000 maps can also give all the necessary information to place into the ecological conditions what is known of the distribution of the disease and, further, to choose the places to investigate. Sometimes, such maps are difficult to obtain, being more-or-less considered as military information. If they cannot be purchased from the health authorities, an alternative solution is aeronautical charts, which are excellent physical maps. In most countries, such 1/500.000 maps exist (even if not sold inside the country) and, anyway, a 1/100.000 chart of the whole planet is available: even if some details are lacking, such as scale, this map is much better than road maps which must be avoided.

On such convenient maps are marked the places where proved cases of human and canine diseases have been found (not too old, maximum 4-5 years). This may give an initial idea of the suspected kind of landscape where the disease is transmitted: urban or rural, and, in this case, valleys or hills. It may also happen that no difference appears, which can indicate that the disease is widespread, or that the available information is scarce, or epidemiologically not valuable. Hence, the first investigation will try to precise this kind of information, choosing the places among the different kinds of landscapes, and including both suspected transmitting places and also probably non-transmitting ones. As much as possible during the first campaign, all the main landscapes will be screened.

COLLECTION OF DOGS

In such investigations, all kinds of dogs are of interest: this means that the cooperation of dog owners is mandatory. Depending on the administrative structure of the country concerned, different means can be followed to obtain their cooperation: in some cases, the official veterinary services will be the most active; in other cases, the local administration will be the best agents to convince the population to bring the dogs for examination. Anyway, both of them have to be informed, as do the regional and national authorities. The consequence is that all the results will have to be available for them, which will allow some prophylactic and therapeutic consequences. The dog owners will be informed of these consequences, and it is also important that they can take the opportunity of this investigation to meet veterinaries and, if necessary, obtain information or other advantages for their dogs. In the case of the cited survey in Turkey, the possibility of a free vaccination against rabies was linked with the screening.

This work has to be initiated long before the date of the visit of the team, which must be clearly indicated. This allows the local representatives to explain the expected benefits to the population, and the dog owners to discuss and inform themselves. Informaiton in the local newsmedias is also very helpful, and improves results.

THE TEAM

Even if it is possible to do, on a limited scale, such work along with the local veterinarian, it is better, for large investigations, to assemble parties of 3/4 persons. One at least must be previously trained in bleeding dogs, another one in correct manipulation of blood in the field. These two people must also be able to perform lymph nodes puncturation and inoculation of culture media in field conditions.

One or two other assistants are useful, for handling and maintaining dogs, and for discussions with the owners, collection of information on the screened animals, and conviction of the most reluctant about the inocuity and the interest of the operation. If rabies exists in the area concerned, all of the participants must be vaccinated in due time.

MATERIALS AND METHODS

The quqlity of the investigation will depend greatly on the materials, generally used far from the laboratory: a careful preparation, and the use of convenient package, able to keep the material fully operational in hard field conditions, is an important part of the work. Two distinct operations have to be prepared:(i) bleed the dogs for serological examination, (ii) obtain lymph from clinically suspect dogs, for parasite detection and identification.

The first operation, when opening the session, is to collect the necessary information about the dogs. This secretarial work is extremely important for the interpretation of the results. The items generally asked are the name of the dog and of the owner, his address (for results), the sex, race and age of the animal, where it was born and if it travelled, its kind of occupation (house-keeping, hunting, companionship) and, finally, clinical observations, if there are some. If possible, a photograph is made of the dog showing possible manifestations of leishmaniasis. After completion of the questionnaire, a numbered ticket is given to the owner for the sampling itself.

For serological investigastions, the main difficulty is the frequent haemolysis of dog blood, which can trouble some of the tests. For the other ones, as for example I.F.I., when it is possible to use whole blood, one can collect it on filter paper, as dots, simply dired, and later, in the laboratory, eluted in definite conditions depending on the absorption of the paper, to reconstitute dilutions of the serum components. This method is very useful in difficult field conditions, but it permits the use of only some of the test and limits the value of the investigation.

To obtain pure dog sera, it is generally necessary to separate immediately the plasma and the red cells, before the coagulation. Even if some rather expensive materials (vacutainers) decrease the risk of haemolysis, it is a good precaution to centrifuge the blood immediately. The coagulation is then white an the serum will be perfect for investigations.

Dogs generally accept quite well the bleeding, if their owner is present and secures them. However, it is a good precaution to close their mouth with a harmless bond. A blouse belt is excellent for this use. A first knot is made under the mouth, a second behind the neck. Then, the dog can be handled and, except when too heavy, placed onto a table for operating comfortably. It must sit on ots posterior legs and, if possible, extend one of the anteriors forth to the operator. Hair is cut with a curved scissor, and the skin is cleaned with 70% alcohol. A garrot is placed above the elbow. It must be tight enough to stop the veinous circulation, but not too much as blood must continue to come through the arteries. The needle is introduced into the vein, and the blood comes by itself, without any aspiration, directly into a tube adapted to the centrifuge (usually 10 ml).

After centrifugation, the blood coagulates. It is then necessary to seperate the coagulum from the sides of the tube, to allow a good retraction. Later (generally in the evening, or next morning) the serum is taken off; as it generally cntains some few red blood cells, it is centrifuged again, and stored in a fresh place, after addition of 1 drop of 4/1000 sodium azide, for preservation.

For lymph nodes puncturation, the dog is lying on a side to expose its posterior legs, as the most infected lymph nodes, in canine leishmaniasis, are located behind the knees. Cultivation on blood added media being the target of the operation, maximum sterility is required. The surface of the skin is washed with soap, the hair is cut and the skin is carefully disinfected with 70% alcohol. It is better to do a local anaesthesia with, for example novocain, around the lymph node, before entering the needle. A syringe, which can contains several microliters of a sterile medium (Locke or simple saline) allows a strong aspiration of the lymph and cells out of the node. It is also possible to add the dilutant after the collection of the biological sample.

The following step, inoculation into a culture medium, must be performed immediately, and with the maximum possible precautions for sterility. The medium can be NNN (which can be kept 2/3 weeks in the field if stored in a refrigerator or in a cool place), or any *Leishmania* culture medium. The inoculation must be performed in a closed room, without wind, to avoid dust and contaminants, in front of a flame (gas or alcohol), following strictly the rules of asepsy. The tubes are then stored in a cool place (as near as possible to 27ºC) until they are transported to the laboratory.

Finally, the last drops remaining in the needle or syringe are used to prepare smears for direct examination.

THE USE OF THE COLLECTED MATERIAL

Herein is not the place to describe the different serological techniques used to determine the level of the anti-leishmanial antibodies. A high degree of standardization and, if possible, an automization of the process is necessary to obtain comparable results throughout important collections of sera.

Then, the results can be studied from the epidemiological point of view. Maps are completed and will be used to prepare further surveys. It is of great interest to use for the interpretation a computerized program, such as "EPI-INFO", available from the C.D.C., which allows all the comparisons with automatic statistical treatment.

In what concerns the research of parasites in lymph nodes, its main interest is the isolation of the strains from the considered focus. It is no longer necessary to insist on the importance of the exact identification of the parasite, through modern techniques, such as isoenzyme analysis, DNA studies. All of them need isolates, which are sent to reference centres.

CONCLUSIONS

Field investigation is sometimes considered by those who do not practice it, as tourism or butterflies collection! Actually, it is in some cases, but then no scientific result can be expected. On the contrary, the collection in the field of serious data, including statistically valuable numbers of samples, taken in correct conditions, needs a maximum of strictness. It is often particularly difficult to comply with all the required precautions in field conditions, when the "laboratory" is quite far from what is generally associated with that name, and when the team is submitted to physical efforts and, in some cases, poor living conditions.

However, the results of such investigations are necessary to understand the structures of the foci. Even if, nowadays, the available tools are not yet strong enough to obtain decisive results in the prophylaxis of zoonotic foci, the progress of the applications of molecular biology to *Leishmania*, as well as the development of immunology, allow us to expect, in the near future, that efficient weapons will be available. Then, the knowledge of the natural circulation of the parasite will be the basis of their application and, finally, of the control of leishmaniasis.

REFERENCES

DE ALENCAR BARROS VASCONCELOS, I. (1983) La leishmaniose viscerale en Turquie. Enquete serologique chez le chien et etude isoenzymatique d'une souche isolee. Memoire de REA Tours, 102pp.

DEANE, L. (1956) Leishmaniose viscerale no Brasil; estudos sobre reservatorios e transmissores realizados no estado do Ceara. Thesis Medicina, Sao Paulo, 162pp.

LANOTTE, G., RIOUX, J.A., CROSET, H. & VOLLHARDT, Y. (1978) Ecologie des leishmanioses dans le sud de la France. 9- Les methodes d'echantillonnage dans le depistage et l'analyse de l'enzootoe canine. Ann. Paras. hum. comp. 53, 33-45.

RIOUX, J.A. et al., (1969) Epidemiologie des leishmanioses dans le sud de la France. Monographie INSERM no 37, Paris, 223pp.

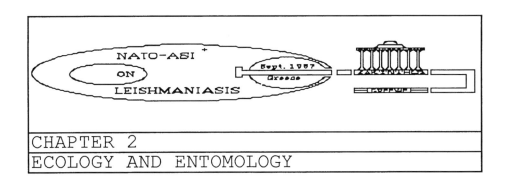

CHAPTER 2
ECOLOGY AND ENTOMOLOGY

THE ECOLOGY AND ENTOMOLOGY OF THE LEISHMANIASES

R. Killick-Kendrick

MRC External Scientific Staff
Department of Pure and Applied Biology
Imperial College at Silwood Park
Ascot
Berks SL5 7DE

Pavlosky's concept of landscape epidemiology underpins all studies on the ecology of *Leishmania*. The Trinity of vector-parasite-reservoir host can be considered as one entity neatly fitting its habitat. In foci which are well studied, characteristic features of the landscape are often recognised which act as markers revealing places where the parasite is circulating. Examples are: **Acacia forests** in the Sudan in foci of visceral leishmaniasis (VL) caused by *Leishmania donovani* transmitted by *Phlebotomus orientalis*; **termite hills** in VL foci of East Africa where the vectors of *L. donovani* are sandflies of one or more species of the subgenus *Synphlebotomus*; **two species of oak trees** at particular altitudes in the VL focus in the Cevenne, France, where *L. infantum* is transmitted by *P. ariasi*; and **chenopod plants** in foci of zoonotic cutaneous leishmaniasis (ZCL) in Saudi Arabia and elsewhere where the sandrat *Psammomys obesus*, is the reservoir host of *L. major* and *P. papatasi* is the vector. The marker features of the landscape are a consequence of the climate and soil but, while recognizable in these and some other foci of the leishmaniases in the Old World, they are generally obscured in the extraordinarily complex habitat of the Neotropical rain forests.

One essential feature of each focus is the vector which, like all animals, has requirements which determine its distribution and the niches it occupies in the habitat. There appears to be a restriction of leishmanial parasites to certain species or groups of species of sandflies which is one factor in variations of the foci. For example, in the Mediterranean Basin, species of the subgenus *Larroussius* are the only proven vectors of *L. infantum*; in all foci of ZCL, the proven vectors of *L. major* are all in the small subgenus *Phlebotomus*; species of *Psychodopygus* of the New World are important vectors of leishmaniae of the subgenus *Viannia*; and the only proven vector of *L. tropica* is *P. sergenti*.

Whether or not a particular species of sandfly carries a given *Leishmania* does not, of course, depend solely upon its ability to support the growth of the parasite, but also upon its feeding preferences; it must be in close, regular contact with animals which are reservoir hosts of the parasite. Laboratory experiments may shoe that a *Leishmania* grows well in a sandfly and can even be transmitted experimentally by the bite of the fly but, without some basic understanding of the biology of the insect, a final conclusion cannot be reached about its role as a vector in nature based solely on laboratory experiments.

Until recently, very few studies were made on the biology of sandflies. The demonstration of a sex pheromone of male *Lutzomyia longipalpis* discovered by Ward and colleagues illustrates the value of moving into this virtually untouched field. For the first time, there is convincing evidence of morphologically indistinguishable sibling species of a sandfly separable, in this instance, by pheromones of the tergal glands of the males. Presumably this is one mechanism inhibiting gene flow between sympatric populations of the sibling species in nature.

Studies on cuticular hydrocarbons of sandflies by Phillips and collaborators have also shown differences which are highly significant, between closely related populations of sandflies, notably between *P. ariasi* from peridomestic and silvatic habitats. The interpretation of these observations in genetic terms is, however, not yet possible.

The biology of sandfly larvae in nature is little understood and the preimaginal stages of very few species of sandflies have been found. Results of a study in Sardinia by an Italian team led by Bettini in which thousands of sandflies of three species have been caught in emergence traps are, therefore, remarkable. Some of the findings pose intriguing questions. The extraordinarily high proportions of males in the catches remain unexplained and the rate of parous females of species not previously thought commonly to display autogeny was unexpected. These interesting observations emphasise the need for further studies on the breeding places of sandflies which, if better known, may be a point of attack for control.

Encouraging results on a new method of reducing populations of sandflies came from work by Maroli and Lane who have experimented in the field in Italy with permethin impregnated nets. Although, by itself, no claim is made that this will totally prevent transmission, it may play an important part in integrated control.

In the broad field of epidemiology, the contributions of Dye on mathematical models of leishmaniasis have brought the shortcomings in the knowledge of the biology of sandflies, and variations between vector species, into sharp focus. Most importantly, Dye questions the value of gathering time-consuming data which are so variable that repetition is difficult or impossible. The need for predictive models is nevertheless undeniable, especially to compare risks at different times or places and in planning and assessing the effect of control measures.

The age of descriptive epidemiology, however, is by no means finished, even in some countries where, in the past, field research on leishmaniasis was enormously productive and much is already known. This is illustrated by a review of the leishmaniases of Kenya where, until recently, VL was known in several foci but cutaneous leishmaniasis was thought to be rare or absent. The review by Lawyer and collaborators reveals that not only is *L. major* now known to be present in that country, but that, quite unexpectedly, *L. tropica* has recently been shown also to be autochthonous.

This work once again underlines the remarkable strength of biochemical typing of isolates of *Leishmania* in unraveling knots in the descriptive epidemiology of the leishmaniases. The ability unequivocally to state that parasites found in vectors or suspected reservoir hosts are indistinguishable from those from patients is a mainstay in incriminating the sandfly and vertebrates responsible for the maintenance and circulation of the parasite. This has long been evident in field studies on African sleeping sickness and nagana, the diseases for which biochemical typing of parasitic protozoa was pioneered by Godfrey. But the need is greater in leishmaniasis than in African trypanosomiasis. There are 20 named species of *Leishmania* generally accepted at the moment, spread unevenly over countries of four continents. Of these, five have never been found in man and are, apparently, of no medical importance. Other species have been found but have yet to be described and named. About 60 species of sandflies of three different genera are known or suspected vectors of one or other form of leishmaniasis, and more species are coming under suspicion as new places are explored or well studied foci are re-examined. There are still important foci where little is known of possible vectors and new species of sandflies are being regularly discovered. The list of reservoir hosts is being added to at an increasing rate, and the precise role of some animals, such as *Rattus* spp., is not yet clear. With this complexity, the need for biochemical typing of parasites encountered in investigations of the components of a focus is obvious. it is regrettable, therefore, that well established centres where, for many years, isolates have been typed as a service to field workers are finding increasing difficulty in obtaining funds to continue this vital activity. Sources of national funding are drying up and international funding bodies, while often paying lip service to the immense value of biochemical typing, appear to be increasingly reluctant to support the efficient and highly experienced centres in developed countries which are still pressed to type isolates sent to them by research workers in foci in the Third World where the leishmaniases are an important public health problem, but where the facility does not yet exist.

A word of warning is sounded in a study by Minter and colleague of sandflies in an apparently silent focus of VL in Cyprus. Vector species are present in spite of extensive and regular aerial spraying of insecticides for agricultural purposes. At the moment, canine leishmaniasis appears to be rare or absent but, with the movement of people to Cyprus from known active foci in Greece and Turkey, the risk of the importation of infected dogs followed by new outbreaks in the human population appears to be high. Dogs imported from Greece to the UK occasionally develop the first signs of leishmaniasis long after the obligatory six-months period of quarantine and, while this represents no risk of the establishment of the enzootic in that country (because of the absence of sandflies) the same cannot be said of Cyprus.

The current state of the art in studies on the ecology of the leishmaniases and sandflies is encouraging. Descriptive epidemiology has been so strengthened by the biochemical typing of *Leishmania* that analysis of many foci are complete and firm evidence of the roles of vector species and reservoir hosts is now available in many places. A number of poorly known foci are being actively studied for the first time, and new patterns in the kaleidoscopic variations of transmission are becoming visible. Studies on the biology of sandflies have made great strides pointing to new possibilities of control. One of the greatest stimuli to this progress is undoubtedly the selection by the UNDP/World Bank/WHO Special Programme for Research and Training in Tropical Diseases of the leishmaniases as one of six major tropical diseases, the impact of which could be much reduced by an integrated international effort.

SANDFLY BREEDING SITES

Sergio Bettini

Department of Parasitology
University of Cagliari
Cagliari
Italy

INTRODUCTION

The importance of identifying larval breeding sites of Phlebotomine sandflies is twofold. Firstly, if any possible type of larval control is to be undertaken, the knowledge of the exact location of larval breeding sites is essential. Secondly, the study of sandlfy species in their preimaginal habitat may supply basic information on the life cycle, physiology, population dynamics, physico-chemical composition of the breeding soil, etc.

For these reasons, from the beginning of this century scientists have spent much time looking for larval breeding places, but it must be said, often with little success. Though the biology and habitat of species belonging to the Old World have many aspects different from those of the New World, the methods used to identify the larval breeding sites are substantially similar. On the other hand, the habitats where larvae have so far been found are notably heterogeneous, varying from burrows of desert rodents to the floor of the rain forest.

By examining the results of different authors who succeeded in collecting only a few specimens, often after a time-consuming search, one is puzzled and doubtful about the authenticity of the breeding site identified; possible the technique used was not ideal.

The problem rests with the behavioural traits of the ovipositing sandflies: if eggs are laid one by one on a large soil surface, then the finding of a low density of larvae, or emerged adults, is sufficient to recognize a breeding site. If, on the other hand, eggs are laid in batches in well defined habitats, then specimens ought to be collected by the hundreds, or thousands.

This is well illustrated by the strikingly different results obtained by us in two investigations on *P. perniciosus* larval breeding sites, one in Tuscany (Pozio *et al.*, 1983) and the other in Sardinia. In Tuscany, with 140 emergence traps, only 24 specimens were caught in two years, while in Sardinia with 9 traps, thousands of emerged sandflies were collected.

To identify larval breeding sites, a useful approach is to survey the area with oiled papers. A high density of adults and a high percentage of males displaying unrotated genitalia suggest proximity to a larval breeding site.

If the physico-chemical characteristics of the soil where larvae or emerged adults are detected are known, this information is useful to exclude other types of soil as potential breeding places.

Other characteristics generally required by adult sandflies and their preimaginal stages, such as protection from sunshine and rain, closeness to livestock or to wild animals (rodents in their burrows, etc), should also be taken into consideration when searching for larval breeding sites.

REVIEW AND COMMENTS ON PRECEDING WORK

Reviews on larval breeding sites of sandflies are given by Hanson (1961) and Killick-Kendrick (in press). On the basis of these papers and of recent information, we present in Table I and II all findings concerning the identification of larval breeding sites in the Old and New Worlds.

In the Old World, the first worker to search for sandfly larvae was Grassi (1908) in Italy, who found larvae of *P. apatasi* in a cellar in Rome. From that time, many workers detected larvae and pupae in different regions, from Europe to India. In the New World, sandfly larvae were first found by Ferreira *et al.* (1938) in Brazil. In 1957, Hertig and Johnson in Panama began a series of important surveys for the identification of larval breeding sites of the sandfly species in the Canal Zone. Most of the work was carried out with techniques to recover larvae and pupae. Methods for trapping emerging adults were also used in some of the work. In all cases, however, the number of specimens collected was, with a few exceptions, rather low. Hanson (1961) in a 4 year period collected 2,258 larvae and pupae from 370 soil samples in Panama. According to Perfil'ev (1968), 1,00 emerged *P.tobbi* were caught from chicken coops covered with fine-mesh netting.

Even by using emergence traps, the number of specimens caught was never high. Therefore, our catches with emergence traps, 3,631 specimens in three years, from a surface of one m^2, and 27,405 from the whole breeding site in 1986, are exceptional.

TABLE I. IDENTIFICATION OF OLD WORLD LARVAL BREEDING SITES AFTER 1961 (FOR REFERENCES TO EARLIER PAPERS, SEE HANSON (1961))

Species	Technique used	No. specimens collected	Area of collecting	Reference
P. papatasi	Oiled papers at rodent burrow entrance	6.2 adults per burrow entrance	Saudi Arabia	Buttiker & Lewis (1979)
P. papatasi (?)	Macfadyen's funnels		Iran	Seyedi-Rashti & Nadim (1972)
P. duboscqi	Hand collection from	5 larvae	Senegal	Dedet et al. (1980)
P.p. perfiliewi	Emergence traps	19 adults	Tuscany, Italy	Pozio et al. (1983)
P. perniciosus	Emergence traps	5 adults	Tuscany, Italy	Pozio et al. (1983)
P. ariasi	Hand collection from rotton goat manure	6 larvae	Cevennes, S. France	Killick-Kendrick (in press)
P. ariasi	Emergence traps	6 adults	Cevennes, S. France	Killick-Kendrick (in press)
P. papatasi P. argentipes S. babau	Hand collection from soil, etc	50 larvae & 6 pupae	Bilhar, India	Dhiman et al. (1983)
P. argentipes	Emergence traps from scrapings of cow shed floor	12 adults	India	Hati (1983)

TABLE II IDENTIFICATION OF NEW WORLD LARVAL BREEDING SITES AFTER 1961. (FOR REFERENCES TO EARLIER PAPERS, SEE HANSON (1961)).

Species	Technique used	No. specimens collected	Area of collecting	Reference
B. hamata	Flotation	117 larvae & pupae	Panama Canal Zone	Rutledge & Mosser (1972)
L. micropyga	Flotation	2 larvae	Panama Canal Zone	Thatcher (1968)
L. dysponeta	Flotation	6 larvae	Panama Canal Zone	Thatcher (1968)
L. trapidoi	Emergence traps*	90 adults	Panama Canal Zone	Ellenwood (1975)
L. pessoana	Emergence traps*	13 adults	Panama Canal Zone	Ellenwood (1975)
L. panamensis	Emergence traps*	33 adults	Panama Canal Zone	Ellenwood (1975)
L. insolita	Emergence traps*	31 adults	Panama Canal Zone	Ellenwood (1975)
L. gomezi	Emergence traps*	28 adults	Panama Canal Zone	Ellenwood (1975)
L. rorotaensis	Emergence traps*	42 adults	Panama Canal Zone	Ellenwood (1975)

* Collected using an aspirator.

The techniques used for detecting larval breeding sites are summarized in Table III. The advantages and disadvantages of the methods are the following.

The main advantages of collecitng larvae and pupae are:
(a) the larval microhabitat can be found and studied,
(b) larval morphology can immediately be studied without breeding adults in the laboratory.

The main disadvantages are:
(a) very few larvae and pupae are usually obtained, unless large amounts of soil are examined or processed,
(b) only a low percentage of the collected larvae and pupae survive and emerge to be identified as adults,
(c) it is time-consuming,
(d) the larval breeding sites are often difficult to reach, as in rodent burrows where larvae are commonly in chambers located deep inside the burrows.

The main advantages of collecting adults are:
(a) labour is reduced to a minimum,
(b) the breeding site is not altered by trapping, thus collecting can be carried out throughout the entire emergence period for several years,
(c) adults can be collected either dead (in oiled containers) or alive with oil-free trapping containers,
(d) some parameters of the biology of adult sandflies (sex ratio, autogeny, quiescence) can be studied.

Table III.   Methods employed for detecting larval breeding sites of *Phlebotomine* sandlflies.

I   Search for larvae and pupae
 1. Examination of soil samples
 2. Separation from soil by flotation
 3. Separation from soil with Berles's funnels (or modifications such as Macfadyen's funnels)

II   Search for adults
 1. Emergence from soil samples
 2. Through emergence traps
    (a) with oiled containers
    (b) with oil free containers
    (c) without containers
    (collecting with mouth aspitrators)
 3. Through oiled papers at entrance of rodent burrows (or with trapping cylinders)
 4. When the breeding site is located indoors, the openings of the construction may be sealed and traps set on them.

There seems to be no serious disadvanteges in collecting adults; the only possible one is that, if an important breeding site is found, for instance by using method II 4 reported in Table III, the number of specimens collected may be so high as to create a real problem in mounting and identifying them.

RESULTS

We present here the results of a survey carried out from 1983 to 1986 which may well illustrate the advantages of the methods employed. Data for 1983-84 and for 1985 have already been published (Bettini et al., 1986; Bettini and Atzeni, 1986).

In 1982, the town of Soleminis, 15 km north of Cagliari, was found to be a canine leishmaniasis focus (Bettini et al., 1983). On its outskirts, P.perniciosus, P.p.perfiliewi and S. minuta were caught with oiled papers (about 90 specimens of P.perniciosus / m^2 of paper) (Bettini et al., 1983). There, we decided to work toward the identification of the larval breeding sites of P.perniciosus, the proven vector of Leishmania infantum s.s (Bettini et al., 1986).

After a series of negative trials with emergence traps, in September 1983 we collected the first adults in an abandoned cement construction on the outskirts of Soleminis.

The traps were described by Bettini et al. (1986). One trap covered a soil surface of about 0.1 m^2. Since the breeding site measured about 25 m^2 in surface, nine traps covered approximately 1/27 of the entire breeding surface. The oiled containers were changed at least twice a week, and the specimens caught were cleared and mounted.

The methods of setting the traps to avoid entrance of adults into the traps, and the discussion on such an extremely improbable event are reported by Bettini et al. (1986).

The larval breeding site consisted of an uneven clay soil of 5.3 x 4.7 m in surface and 1.4-1.9 m in height, where vegetation was practically absent. Three large openings were present in two of its walls.

Trapping was carried out from 1983 to 1985 with the same methods except for the period of the year when trapping was started.

Due to the intense building activity in the area surrounding our breeding place, in February 1986 we were told by the landowner that at the end of the year the cement construction would be demolished. We therefore decided to seal the three openings of the construction and to place two traps at each opening so that all sandflies emerging from the breeding site wouls be caught when trying to escape.

Table IV gives the results of trapping from 1983 to 1985. In 1983, 4 out of 7 traps were negative, probably because of the short time of permanence on the breeding site. In 1983 and 1984 the traps were placed after the onset of emergence, thus the number of specimens caught was lower than in 1985. The species collected were P. perniciosus, P.p.perfiliewi and S.minuta. P.perniciosus was always the predominant species.

Table IV. Results of collecting with emergence traps from 1983 to 1985

	1983	1984	1985
N°. of traps employed (positive)	7 (3)	9 (7)	9 (8)
Period of collecting	Sept 5-22 (3 weeks)	July 23-Oct 14 (12 weeks)	June 7-Oct 16 (20 weeks)
No. of specimens collected:			
P. perniciosus	352 (81.3%) (males 72.6%)	1156 (95.8%) (males 78.4%)	2223 (95.6%) (males 83.5%)
P.p. perfiliewi	58 (18.7%) (males 96.5%)	16 (1.3%) (males 81.2%)	9 (0.4%) (males 88.9%)
S. minuta	0	35 (2.9%) (males 77.1%)	92 (4.0%) (males 78.3%)

In the three years the sex ratio was markedly and constantly in favour of males, for all three species. In 1985, the only year in which the traps were set before the onset of emergence, the trend appeared to be bimodal suggesting quiescence during the hot period of the season and that all emerged adults originate from eggs laid the prededing year (Bettini et al., in preparation).

The trend of the sex ratio of *P.perniciosus* is uniform throughout the three years. Also the frequency of emerged gravid females is evenly distributed throughout the collecting seasons (Bettini et al., in preparation).

Gravid females of *P.perniciosus* were found at a constant rate (1.4, 5.2 and 2.7%) for the years 1983, 1984 and 1985 respectively. A higher percentage (10%) was found in 1985 for *S. minuta*. This indicates that the local population of these two species shows facultative autogeny (Bettini et al., in preparation).

As it is difficult to compare data obtained with different techniques, the results of 1986, which deal with the trapping of sandflies trying to escape from the sealed construction, were analysed separately.

The numbers of *P. perniciosus*, *P.p. perfiliewi* and *S. minuta* caught in the six traps set at the three sealed openings of the construction were 23,338, 1,309 and 2,758 respectively. The frequency of gravid females of *P. perniciosus* (4.0%) which is within the limits found in the previous years (1.4-5.2%) confirms the autogenous trait of the local population of this species (Bettini et al., in preparation).

The trend of *P. perniciosus* caught in 1986 shows a bimodal trend as in the previous years. The percentage of males varies throughout the emergence season but maintains a high average, above 70%. The peak of gravid females coincides with the period of lower emergence.

Regarding *S. minuta*, the results differ from those obtained in 1984-85. The sex ratio was nearly 50:50 and the rate of gravid females reached 38%. This is not surprising.as emerged *S. minuta* might have fed on reptiles, thus giving rise to a second generation inside the construction.

Soil analysis on 17 samples obtained in 1983 and 1984 from the breeding site was also carried out (Bettini and Melis, in press). A high clay content (30%) which maintains a sufficient moisture in the sandfly larval habitat, is the only peculiar characteristic of the breeding site soil. The organic matter content averaged 3.07%. No correlation was found between organic content of soil samples and numbers of sandflies emerging, nor with the presence of gravid females in places where traps had been placed. An important characteristic of the breeding site as a whole is that the construction itself provided a protection from sunshine, rain and wind, maintaining the constant physical parameters of the breeding site.

It should also be mentioned that neither from repeated examination nor from flotation trials of numerous soil samples could we detect larvae or pupae. Only 3 larvae and 1 pupa were found in less than 1 g of debris collected at the bottom of the soil fissures 10-15 cm below the soil surface. After careful direct observation *in situ*, 2 more larvae were found (Bettini et al., 1986).

CONCLUSIONS

It may therefore be concluded that the use of emergence traps is useful and practical for the identification of larval breeding sites and for the study of sandfly biology.

REFERENCES

Bettini, S., and Atzeni, M.C., 1986, Osservazioni su un focolaio larvale di Flebotomini in Sardegna dal 1983 al 1985. Parassitologia (in press)

Bettini, S., and Melis, P., 1987, Leishmaniasis in Sardinia. III. Soil analysis of phlebotomine sandflies larval breeding sites. Med. Vet. Entom. (in press).

Bettini, S., Contini, C., Atzeni, M.C., and Tocco, G., 1986, Leishmaniasis in Sardinia. I. Observations on a larval breeding site of *Phlebotomus perniciosus*, *Phlebotomus perfiliewi perfiliewi* and *Sergentomyia minuta* (Diptera: Psychodidae) in the canine leishmaniasis focus of Soleminis (Cagliari). Ann.Trop.Med.Paras.,80, 307-315.

Bettini, S., Contini, C., Maroli, M., Tocco, G., and Sigon, M., 1983, Nota preliminare sullo studio dei vettori della leishmaniosi in Sardegne. Parassitologia, 25, 206-209.

Buttiker, W., and Lewis, D.J., 1979, Ecological studies at Holuf, Eastern Saud Arabia, in relation to dermal leishmaniasis. Tropen Parasit., 30, 220-229.

Dedet, J.P., Desjeux, P., and Derouin, F., 1980, Ecologie d'un foyer de leishmaniose cutanee dans la region de Thies (Senegal, Afrique de l'ouest). 4. Infestation spontanee et biologie de *Phlebotomus duboscqi* Neveau-Lemair, 1906. Bull. Soc. Path. exot., 73, 266-276.

Dhiman, R.C., Shetti, P.S., and Dhanda, V., 1983, Breeding habitats of phlebotomine sandflies in Bilhar, India. Indian J. Med. Res., 77, 29-32.

Grassi, G.B., 1908, Intorno ad un nuovo flebotomo. Rc. R. Accad. Lincei S., 17, 681-682.

Hanson, W.J., 1961, The breeding places of Phlebotomus in Panama (Diptera, Psychodidae). Ann. Ent. Soc. Amer., 54, 317-322.

Hati, H.K., 1983, Reviews on current status of leishmaniasis: vector biology. Proc. Indo-UK Workshop Leish.

Killick-Kendrick, R., 1987, Breeding places of *Phlebotomus ariasi* in the Cevennes focus of leishmaniasis in the south of France. Parassitologia (in press)

Perfil'ev, P.P., 1968, Fauna of the USSR. Diptera, vol. III, No.2. Phlebotomidae (sandlfies). Academy of Sciences of the USSR, new series No.93. English translation from Russian, Israel Program for Scientific Translations Jerusalem, 1968.

Pozio, E., Gradoni, L., Bonarelli, R., Squitieri, N., Bettini, S., Maroli, M., and Cocchi, M., 1980, Indagine sui focolai larvali dei flebotomi in Provinvia di Grosseto. Atti XII Congr. Naz. Ital. Entomol., Rome, II, 395-400.

Rutledge, L.C., and Ellenwood, D.A., 1975, Production of phlebotomine sandflies on the open forest floor in Panama: the species component. Environ. Ent., 4, 71-77.

Rutledge, L.C. and Mosser, H.L., 1972, Biology of immature sandflies (*Diptera: Psychodidae*) at bases of trees in Panama. Environ. Ent., 1, 300-309.

Seyedi-Rashti, M.A., and Nadim, A., 1972, The use of Macfadyen's technique for the collection of sandlfy larvae. Bull. Soc. Path. exot., 65, 881-884.

Thatcher, V.E., 1968, Arboreal breeding sites of phlebotomine sandlfies in Panama. Ann Ent. Soc. Amer., 61, 1141-1143.

LEISHMANIASIS RESEARCH IN KENYA: PARASITE-VECTOR-HOST ASSOCIATIONS *

P. Lawyer[1,2], J. Githure[1], Y. Mebrahtu[1,2], P. Perkins[1,2,3], R. Muigai[1], and J. Leeuwenburg[1]

[1] Kenya Medical Research Institute, P.O. Box 54840, Nairobi Kenya
[2] U.S. Army Medical Research Unit-Kenya, Box 401, A.P.O. New York 09675
[3] Current address: Department of Entomology, Walter Reed Army Institute of Research, Washington, DC 20307-5100, USA.

* The opinions and assertions contained herein are the private views of the authors and are not to be construed as official or as reflecting the views of the U.S. Army, the U.S. Department of Defense or the Government of Kenya

Introduction

Clinically speaking, there are 2 types of leishmaniasis in Kenya, visceral leishmaniasis, or kala-azar, caused by *Leishmania donovani*, and cutaneous leishmaniasis caused by *L. aethiopica*, *L. major*, *L. tropica* (a recent discovery), and *L. donovani* (post kala-azar dermal leishmaniasis). These will each be discussed from a historical perspective, then from a perspective of current research on *Leishmania* parasite-vector-host associations.

Visceral Leishmaniasis (Kala-azar)

Historical Overview

Kala-azar Foci. Although Forbes (1933) was the first to demonstrate parasitologically the presence of visceral leishmaniasis (*L. donovani*) in an indigenous Kenyan, kala-azar was virtually unknown in Kenya prior to the second world war. It was not until Cole et al. (1942) and Anderson (1943) described a kala-azar epidemic among Kenyan soldiers of the King's African Rifles that attention was drawn to the importance of the disease in Kenya. It was suggested that kala-azar was introduced into Kenya by soldiers returning from neighboring countries of Sudan and Ethiopia (Anderson, 1943). After the war several cases were reported from different parts of the

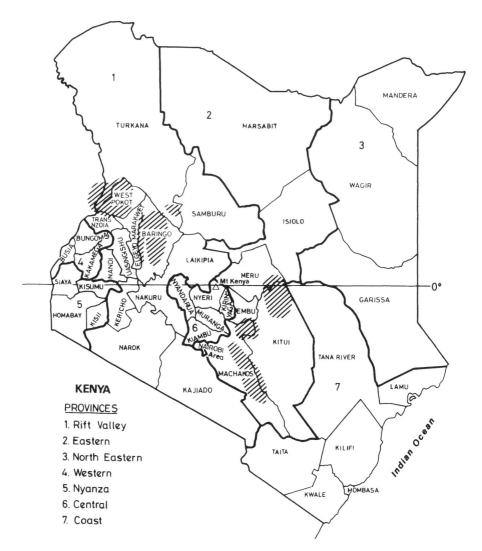

Fig. 1. Map showing approximate locations of visceral leishmaniasis foci in Kenya

country, but the disease remained sporadic in nature until a severe outbreak occurred in northern Kitui District (Fendall, 1961; Figure 1). This outbreak started in October 1952 and has persisted at endemic levels with periodic epidemics ever since (Mbugua & Siongok, 1981).

Foci of kala-azar were discovered in Baringo and West Pokot Districts of Rift Valley Province in 1955 and 1956, respectively, but in these areas the disease has never reached epidemic proportions (McKinnon & Fendall, 1955; Wijers & Minter, 1962; Leeuwenburg et al., 1981; Figure 1).

In 1959 an outbreak of kala-azar occurred in Meru District, directly north of and across the Tana River from the Kitui District focus (Wijers & Minter, 1966), and from 1972-1980 epidemic conditions existed in the Athi River Valley, Machakos District (Wijers & Kiilu, 1984). Between 1978 and 1981, a minor epidemic occurred in Masinga location (Machakos District) which lies between the Kitui and Athi River Valley foci (Mutinga, 1985). The disease in this area may have been introduced from neighboring foci. The construction of a series of dams along the Tana river attracted people from the Kitui and Athi River Valley foci who were seeking employment and irrigated land. On the other hand, it may have been a matter of new host populations migrating into an area where the disease was already present but unknown.

From the time kala-azar was recognized as an endemic disease in Kenya, it has shown rapid spread. Cases continue to be reported throughout the arid lowlands, both north and south of the equator (Figure 1). The most recent outbreak in Kenya began in July-August 1986, in the Nadome area of southern Turkana District, with many clinically acute cases of the disease and an estimated 60 to 100 deaths (unpublished). This is in contrast to the usual picture of clinically chronic disease and few deaths.

Vectors. Attempts to find the vector(s) of kala-azar in Kenya were started in 1953 by Heisch, and have continued to the present day (Heisch, 1955; Heisch & Guggisberg, 1953; Heisch et al., 1956, 1962; Wijers, 1963; Wijers & Minter, 1962; Minter, 1962; Minter et al., 1962; Minter, 1963; Minter & Wijers, 1963; Wijers & Minter, 1966; Wijers & Ngoka, 1974; Mutinga & Ngoka, 1978; Beach et al., 1982; Wijers & Kiilu, 1984; Perkins et al., 1987). Sand fly species of the *Synphlebotomus* group, i.e. *Phlebotomus martini*, *P. vansomerenae*, and *P. celiae*, were suspected because of their close relationship to known vectors of visceral leishmaniasis in the Old World (Heisch et al. 1956). Heisch et al. (1962), working in Kitui District, reported a probable natural infection of *L. donovani* in what they thought was *P. martini*. Although the parasite strain was proven to be pathogenic to man and was subsequently identified as *L. donovani* 15-16 years after initial isolation (Schnur & Zuckerman, 1977; Chance et al., 1978), the identity of the sand fly was not confirmed. This is because the *Synphlebotomus* group females, all 3 species of which are present in that area, are morphologically inseparable. Nonetheless, *Phlebotomus martini* remained the primary suspect because it was the only species of the *Synphlebotomus* group encountered in all endemic areas (Mutinga & Ngoka,1978). It was not until 1986, however, in Baringo District where *P. martini* is the only representative of the *Synphlebotomus* group, that Perkins et al. (1987) found 2 *P. martini* females infected with *L. donovani*, providing further evidence to incriminate this species as a vector of kala-azar.

Reservoirs. The search for reservoirs of kala-azar has occupied researchers since the onset of epidemics during and after the second world war, with a wide variety of potential reservoirs being examined (Heisch, 1954, 1963; Ngoka & Mutinga, 1978). Mutinga et al. (1980), working in the Machakos focus, examined 288 sickly dogs and found 2 infected with *Leishmania*-like flagellates. One of these isolates was later characterized as *L. donovani*. Since this is the only confirmed instance of *L. donovani* in a dog reported in Kenya, it would probably be quite wrong to conclude that dogs are the reservoirs of kala-azar in Kenya. The search continues for further evidence of *L. donovani* in dogs and in other potential reservoir animals. Humans themselves are prime suspects. Minter et al. (1962) fed 58 wild-caught *P. martini* on 3 kala-azar patients who had positive blood cultures. They reported that 28 of these flies were infected with "leptomonads" 72 hours postfeeding, implicating humans as potential reservoirs of the disease. In addition, Chulay et al. (1985) showed that 75% of patients with kala-azar had demonstrable parasitemia by blood cultures or animal inoculation.

Current Research

Vector studies. Studies of potential kala-azar vectors continue in the Baringo District kala-azar focus. Daily sand fly collections using 4 trapping methods (light trap, paper trap, mouth aspirator, and flitting) are made from various habitats at 10 kala-azar case sites within a 25 km radius of our field camp at the Perkerra irrigation scheme. A typical case site consists of one or more thatched huts built on the edge of thorn-bush and open country. The huts consist of a circular framework of poles interwoven with small branches. These are sometimes plastered on the outside with mud or dung. The compounds are usually surrounded by a thorny fence of cut *Acacia* branches, and are often subdivided by a separate fence, inside which the goats, sheep, and cattle sleep at night. Chickens and dogs are usually present, as well. Ubiquitous sand fly resting habitats in and around the case sites include the huts themselves, termite hills, animal burrows, tree holes, and rock crevices. Four species of *Phlebotomus* are collected in and around the case sites, 2 of them routinely (*P. martini* and *P. duboscqi*) (Table 1.). *Phlebotomus martini* is the most common of these. Ten *Sergentomyia* species are found in this area, *S. schwetzi* being the most abundant. Several species of both genera are known to bite humans (asterisk), however, only *Phlebotomus* species have been incriminated as *Leishmania* vectors. In our studies, more than 500 *Leishmania*-like isolates, with an average of about 30 per month in 1987, have been obtained from over 13,000 sand flies dissected. Of these, 262 or about 54% have been successfully cultured and preserved in the Nairobi *Leishmania* Bank. So far only 13% of the isolates have been characterized by cellulose acetate electrophoresis (CAE); 2 of these were *L. donovani* from *Phlebotomus martini* (Perkins et al., 1987). Characterization of the remaining isolates by CAE is now our first priority.

In August 1987, sand flies representing 16 species were collected from kala-azar case sites in the Nadome epidemic focus in southern Turkana District (Table 2.). These case sites are located on rugged lava flows containing many deep holes and fissures which provide cool resting sites for sand fly species during the hottest part of the day. A few termite hills are also present. Seven *Phlebotomus* species were collected from these sites; they include *P. saevus*, 2 representatives of the *Synphlebotomus* group (*P. vansomerenae* and *P. martini*), 3 species that are usually considered to be cave dwellers (*P. longipes, P. pedifer*, and *P. elgonensis = aculeatus*), and *P. duboscqi* (an animal burrow dweller). The most abundant of these *Phlebotomus* species is *P. saevus*. Nine *Sergentomyia* species were collected from this focus, of which *Sergentomyia clydei* comprises about 60% of all flies collected (Table 2). The presence of *P. martini* in this focus is consistent with the hypothesis that it is the principal vector of kala-azar in Kenya, but other species may also play a role. Efforts will continue in this most recent kala-azar focus to identify potential vectors.

Reservoir studies. The search continues for further evidence to either incriminate or exonerate the dog as a reservoir of kala-azar in Kenya. In an ongoing mammal trapping program, which began in 1983 in both the Baringo and Masinga foci, 2,080 rodents, 5 mongooses, 3 genet cats, and 44 dogs, have been trapped and attempts made to isolate parasites from cutaneous lesions, healthy skin, and visceral organs. To date, 146 *Leishmania*-like isolates have been made from rodents, the majority of which are as yet uncharacterized. However, 21 rodent isolates from Baringo District have been characterized as *L. major* (Githure et al., 1986).

To augment the reservoir mammal trapping program, we are developing an enzyme-linked immunosorbent assay (ELISA) for identifying host blood meals in wild caught sand flies. Based on preliminary results, bloodmeal sources for *P. martini* include human, dog, chicken, rabbit, and cow. We are also investigating the ability of laboratory-reared *P. martini* and *P. duboscqi* to pick up *Leishmania* amastigotes by feeding on kala-azar patients. So far none have turned up positive. Interestingly enough,

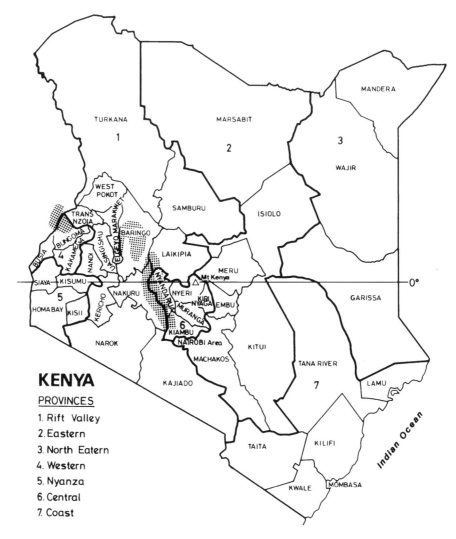

Fig. 2. Map showing approximate locations of cutaneous leishmaniasis foci in Kenya

however, about 10% of the patients subjected to this xenodiagnosis develop papulonodular lesions, similar to those seen in post kala-azar dermal leishmaniasis (PKDL), at the sites of the sand fly bites 1 to 2 weeks after the experimental feed. When biopsied, these lesions are found to be full of

Table 1 - Sand flies associated with kala-azar case sites in Baringo District, Rift Valley Province, Kenya

Phlebotomus sp.	% of Total	*Sergentomyia* sp.	% of Total
*martini	12	*schwetzi	33
*duboscqi	3	antennata	18
*pedifer	<1	*clydei	16
rodhani	<1	bedfordi	10
		africana	2
	15	squamipleuris	2
		*adleri	2
		inermis	1
		dureni	<1
		affinis	<1
n=14,652			
*known to bite humans			85

amastigotes. Evidently the inflammatory skin reaction caused by the bites of the sand flies, attracts circulating macrophage to the site of irritation. Some of these may be infected with *Leishmania*, and after metastasizing at the bite site, cause the lesions. What role this phenomenon plays in the transmission cycle of the disease in nature is unknown.

Table 2 - Sand flies associated with kala-azar case sites in Nadome area, Turkana District, Rift Valley Province, Kenya

Phlebotomus sp.	% of Total	*Sergentomyia* sp.	% of Total
*saevus	2	*clydei	59
*vansomerenae	2	squamipleuris	11
*martini	1	antennata	10
*longipes	<1	africana	5
*pedifer	<1	*schwetzi	4
*aculeatus	<1	affinis	2
*duboscqi	<1	adleri	1
		inermis	<1
	6	bedfordi	<1
n=1376			
*known to bite humans			94

Table 3 - Sand flies associated with suspected case sites of *Leishmania tropica* in central Rift Valley Province, Kenya (preliminary data)

Phlebotomus sp.	% of Total	*Sergentomyia* sp.	% of Total
*vansomerenae	2	bedfordi	41
*celiae	2	suberecta	25
*martini	1	*graingeri	8
*saevus	1	*garnhami	8
*longipes	<1	*multidens	5
*guggisbergi	<1	*schwetzi	2
sp. (unidentified)	<1	antennata	1
		*adleri	<1
	7	squamipleuris	<1
		sp. (unidentified)	<1
n-521			
*known to bite humans			93

Cutaneous Leishmaniasis

Leishmania aethiopica. Cutaneous leishmaniasis due to *Leishmania aethiopica* was first discovered in Kenya in 1969 (Mutinga & Ngoka, 1970). It is primarily a zoonotic disease with sporadic occurrence in humans living on the forested eastern slopes of Mt. Elgon, in Bungoma District (Mutinga and Ngoka, 1970; Kungu et al., 1972; Sang et al., 1983; Figure 2). Movement of people into forested areas in search of more or better agricultural land has brought them in contact with the sand fly vectors. *Leishmania aethiopica* parasites were isolated from a cave dwelling sand fly *Phlebotomus pedifer* (Mutinga, 1971, 1975; Kaddu and Mutinga, 1981). Mutinga and Odhiambo (1986) demonstrated that *Phlebotomus pedifer* is able to transmit *L. aethiopica* parasites from infected humans to clean hamsters by bite, incriminating this species as a competent vector of the disease in Kenya. Two other cave dwelling species, *Phlebotomus longipes* and *Phlebotomus elgonensis* (*=aculeatus*) are also listed as suspected vectors (Sang et al., 1983; Ngoka et al., 1975). In addition to humans, reservoirs of the disease include rock and tree hyraxes (*Dendrohyrax arboreus* and *Procavia johnstoni*) and the giant rat (*Cricetomys* sp.) (Mutinga, 1975).

Leishmania major. Heisch and colleagues, while searching for reservoirs of kala-azar in Baringo and West Pokot Districts of Kenya, accidentally isolated what they thought were *L. donovani* promastigotes from a ground squirrel (*Xerus rutilus*) and 2 gerbils (*Tatera robusta*) (Heisch, 1957: Heisch et al, 1959). The authors described these as avirulent strains of *L donovani* because, when inoculated into the skin of man, they formed nodules containing *Leishmania* but did not visceralize. These isolates were later characterized by Chance et al. (1978) as *L. major.* Beach et al. (1982) discovered the sand fly *Phlebotomus duboscqi*, a vector of *L. major* in Senegal (Dedet et al., 1978), breeding in Baringo District. Beach collected 12 female *Phlebotomus duboscqi* from an animal burrow and allowed them to feed on his hand (Beach et al., 1984). The flies were subsequently dissected and one was found to be infected with *L. major.* At each site where the infected sand fly probed, small lesions developed which were typical of those caused by *L. major,* thus incriminating this sand fly species as a vector of the parasite in Baringo District. More isolations of *L. major* from *P. duboscqi* have been made by our field team and the search continues for other possible vectors of in the Baringo District focus. Laboratory experiments are underway to chronicle the development of *L. major* in *P. duboscqi* and compare the parasite's pattern of development in this sand fly species with that in other, nonvector species.

The search for animal reservoirs of leishmanias in Baringo District have resulted in the isolation of *L. major* from 5 different species of rodents (*Tatera robusta, Arvicanthis niloticus, Taterillus emini, Mastomys natalensis*, and *Aethomys kaiseri*) (Githure et al., 1984, 1986). The latter 3 species represent newly recorded hosts. In addition, *L. major* was recently isolated from a naturally infected vervet monkey (*Cercopithecus aethiops*) from Kiambu District, adjacent to the Machakos District kala-azar focus (Binhazim et al., in press). This finding represents the first recorded case of a natural infection of *L. major* in a nonhuman primate. Experiments have recently been conducted to determine the suitability of East African primates as animal models for cutaneous leishmaniasis caused by *L. major* (Githure et al., 1987). Vervet monkeys, Sykes monkeys, and baboons showed a self cure phenomenon about 3 months post infection and have been recommended for use in immunological investigations.

Following the discovery of a rodent-fly-rodent cycle of transmission for *L. major* in Baringo District, case finding surveys were conducted. *Leishmania major* was isolated from lesions on the face and arms of 3 patients (Muigai et al., 1987). These represent the first records in Kenya of human cutaneous leishmaniasis due to *L. major*.

Leishmania tropica. Prior to 1985, *Leishmania tropica* had not been reported in Kenya. However, in 1985 and 1986, 9 leishmanial strains, isolated from cutaneous papulonodular lesions on 3 patients, were characterized by CAE using 7 enzymes. The strains were indistinguishable from a *Leishmania tropica* reference strain and all 9 strains were noninfective to Balb/c mice (Mebrahtu et al., 1987). Since the 3 patients were Americans, there was much skepticism as to whether or not these cases were autochthonous. However, 2 of the patients, a boy aged 9 years and his sister aged 12 were born and raised in Kenya. The boy had never left the country, but the girl had left 7 years previous to the onset of the disease for a short visit to the U.S.A. The 3rd patient, a 34-year-old male, and close acquaintance of the other 2, had lived in Kenya for about 22 years and had not travelled outside of the country for 8 years previous, except for a 10-day visit to Zaire in 1984. During the 6 months prior to the onset of symptoms, all 3 patients had visited or lived in areas of Samburu, Laikipia, Nakuru, Narok, and Nyandarua Districts, in Rift Valley and Central Provinces. These were not only the first cases of *L. tropica* reported in Kenya but the first in Sub-saharan Africa as well.

Kreutzer et al. (1987) independently characterized a 1979 Kenyan isolate, originally from our laboratory, as *L. tropica*. At our request, Dr. Kreutzer graciously provided us with the isolate histories. With this information we were able to find corresponding stabilates in the Nairobi *Leishmania* Bank, which were subsequently characterized by CAE using 8 enzymes. The isolate, which had been obtained from a Canadian girl who was visiting her parents and grandmother in Central and Rift Valley Provinces, was indistinguishable from an *L. tropica* reference strain and from the 3 autochthonous *L. tropica* isolates described earlier. This finding prompted us to search our *Leishmania* bank for other cutaneous lesion isolates obtained from patients in the same general area. Four other *Leishmania* isolates from 3 indigenous Kenyans and 1 more Canadian (the girl's grandmother), were characterized by CAE and compared with 5 Old World *Leishmania* reference strains using 8 enzymes. The respective enzyme migration patterns obtained were indistinguishable from those of the *L. tropica* reference strain. These are the first reports of autochthonous cutaneous leishmaniasis due to *L. tropica* in indigenous Kenyans. When the known and suspected cases are plotted on a map, they all fall within the same highland region of Central and Rift Valley Provinces (Figure 2). A detailed report of this study is in preparation and will be published soon.

In November of 1986 we began field studies to search for the source and possible vectors of *L. tropica* in Kenya. Sand fly species collected so far are listed in Table 3. These include all 3 members of the *Synphlebotomus* group and *Phlebotomus saevus* (closely related to *Phlebotomus sergenti*, the vector of *L. tropica* in the Old World). *P. longipes*, a vector of *L. aethiopica*, is also present.

Leishmania donovani. Post kala-azar dermal leishmaniasis (PKDL), caused by *L. donovani*, occurs in 2-4% of kala-azar patients after successful cure of visceral leishmaniasis (Rashid et. al.,1985). One aspect of our xenodiagnosis protocol is to determine if *Leishmania* amastigotes in lesions resulting from this form of cutaneous leishmaniasis are accessible to biting sand flies. If so, patients who return to their homes with unsuccessfully treated PKDL may serve as additional reservoirs to infect more sand flies.

Conclusion

As we continue our research on leishmaniasis in Kenya it seems that more questions than answers are encountered. Although there is compelling evidence to incriminate certain sand fly species and reservoir mammals in the transmission cycle of the various leishmanias, there is still much uncertainty. Our Nairobi *Leishmania* Bank now contains over 900 stabilates of *Leishmania* isolates from patients, wild and domestic mammals, reptiles, and sand flies. Identification of these will undoubtedly allay some of the uncertainties pertaining to the epidemiology of leishmaniasis in Kenya. There is no question, however, that the leishmaniases are an important group of diseases in Kenya, and that their control and treatment will be enhanced by continued research for a better understanding of parasite-vector-host associations.

Acknowledgements

The authors wish to thank the scientifiic and technical staff of the Kenya Medical Research Institute (KEMRI) and the U.S. Army Medical Research Unit-Kenya (USAMRU-K) who have supported and participated in the various studies described herein.

Aspects of this work were made possible through Research Grant No. DAMD 17-85-G-5000 from the U.S. Army Medical Research and Development Command, Fort Detrick, Maryland 21701 and through the UNDP/World Bank/WHO Special Programme for Research and Training in Tropical Diseases.

This paper was published with the approval of the Director of the Kenya Medical Research Institute.

References

Anderson, T.F. (1943). Kala-azar in East African Forces. *East African Medical Journal*, 20, 172.

Beach, R.F., Mutinga, M.J., Young, D.G. & Kaddu, J.B. (1982). Laboratory colonization of *Phlebotomus martini* Parrot 1936 (Diptera: Psychodidae), a vector of visceral leishmaniasis in Kenya. *Proceedings of the 3rd Annual Medical Scientific Conference, KEMRI & KETRI*, pp. 189-190.

Beach, R., Kiilu, G., Hendricks, L., Oster, C. & Leeuwenburg, J. (1984). Cutaneous leishmaniasis in Kenya: transmission of *Leishmania major* to man by bite of a naturally infected *Phlebotomus duboscqi*. *Transactions of the Royal Society of Tropical Medicine & Hygiene*, 78, 747-751.

Beach, R., Young, D.G. & Mutinga, M.J. (1982). *Phlebotomus* (*Phlebotomus*) *duboscqi* from Kenya: a new record. *Transactions of the Royal Society of Tropical Medicine & Hygiene*, 76, 707-708.

Binhazim, A.A., Githure, J.I., Muchemi, G. & Reid, G.F.D. (1987). The isolation of *Leishmania major* from a naturally infected vervet monkey, *Cercopithecus aethiops* from Kiambu District, Kenya. *Journal of Parasitology*, in press.

Chance, M.L., Schnur, L.F., Thomas, S.C. & Peters, W. (1978). The biochemical and serological taxonomy of *Leishmania* from the Aethiopian zoogeographical region of Africa. *Annals of Tropical Medicine & Parasitology*, 72, 533-542.

Cole, A.C.E., Coosgrare, P.C. & Robinson, G. (1942). A preliminary report of an outbreak of kala-azar in a battalion of King's African Rifles. *Transactions of the Royal Society of Tropical Medicine & Hygiene*, 36, 25.

Chulay, J.D., Odoyo, M.A. & Githure, J.I. (1985). *Leishmania* parasitemia in Kenyan visceral leishmaniasis. *Transactions of the Royal Society of Tropical Medicine & Hygiene*, 79, 218-222.

Dedet, J.P., Derouin, F. & Cornet, M. (1978). Infestation spontan'ee de *Phlebotomus duboscqi* par des promastigotes de *Leishmania* au Senegal. *Compte rendu de l' Acad'emie des Sciences, Paris*, Series D, 286, 301-302.

Fendall, N.R.E. (1961). The spread of kala-azar in Kenya. *East African Medical Journal*, 38, 417.

Forbes, J. (1933). A case of kala-azar from Elgeyo Reserve. *East African Medical Journal*, 10, 363.

Githure, J.I., Beach R.F & Lightner, L.K. (1984). The isolation of *Leishmania major* from rodents in Baringo District, Kenya. *Transactions of the Royal Society of Tropical Medicine & Hygiene*, 78, 283.

Githure, J.I., Reid, G.F., Binhazim, A.A., Anjili, C.O., Shatry, A.M. & Hendricks, L.D. (1987). The suitability of East African primates as animal models of cutaneous leishmaniasis. *Experimental Parasitology*, in press.

Githure, J.I., Schnur, L.F., Le Blancq, S.M. & Hendricks, L.D. (1986). Characterization of *Leishmania* spp. and identification of *Mastomys natalensis, Taterillus emini* and *Aethomys kaiseri* as new hosts of *Leishmania major. Annals of Tropical Medicine & Parasitology*, 80, 501-507.

Heisch, R.B. (1954). Studies in leishmaniasis in East Africa. I. The epidemiology of an outbreak of kala-azar in Kenya. *Transactions of the Royal Society of Tropical Medicine & Hygiene*, 48, 449.

Heisch, R.B. (1955). The vector of an outbreak of kala-azar. *Nature*, London, 175, 433.

Heisch, R.B. (1957). The isolation of *Leishmania* from a ground squirrel in Kenya. *East African Medical Journal*, 34, 183.

Heisch, R.B. (1963). Is there an animal reservoir of kala-azar in Kenya? *East African Medical Journal*, 40, 359.

Heisch, R.B. & Guggisberg, C.A.W. (1953). Notes on the sandflies (*Phlebotomus*) of Kenya. *Annals of Tropical Medicine & Parasitology*, 47, 44-50.

Heisch, R.B., Grainger, W.E. & Harvey, A.E.C. (1959). The isolation of *Leishmania* from gerbils. *Journal of Tropical Medicine and Hygiene*, 62, 158-159.

Heisch, R.B., Guggisberg, C.A.W. & Teesdale, C. (1956). Studies in leishmaniasis in East Africa. II: The sandflies of the Kitui kala-azar area in Kenya, with description of six new species. *Transactions of the Royal Society of Tropical Medicine & Hygiene*, 50, 209-226.

Heisch, R.B., Wijers, D.J.B. & Minter, D.M. (1962). In pursuit of the vector of kala-azar in Kenya. *British Medical Journal*, 1, 1456-1458.

Kaddu, J.B.& Mutinga, M.J. (1981). *Leishmania* in Kenyan phlebotomine sandflies - I. *Leishmania aethiopica* in the midgut of naturally infected *Phlebotomus pedifer*. *Insect Science & Its Application*, 2, 245-250.

Kreutzer, R.D., Souraty, N. & Semko, M.E. (1987). Biochemical identities and differences among *Leishmania* species and subspecies. *American Journal of Tropical Medicine & Hygiene*, 36, 22-32.

Kungu, A., Mutinga, M.J. & Ngoka, J.M. (1972). Cutaneous leishmaniasis in Kenya. *East African Medical Journal*, 49, 459.

Leeuwenburg, J., Mutinga, M.J. & Koech, D.K. (1981). Report on a leishmanin skin test survey. *Proceedings of the 2nd Annual Medical Scientific Conference, KEMRI & KETRI*, pp. 141.

Mebrahtu, Y., Oster, C.N., Shatry, A.M., Hendricks, L.D., Githure, J.I., Rees, P.H., Perkins, P.V. & Leeuwenburg, J. (1987). Cutaneous leishmaniasis caused by *Leishmania tropica* in Kenya. *Transactions of the Royal Society of Tropical Medical Hygiene*, in press.

Mbugua, G.G. & Arap Siongok, T.K. (1981). Epidemiology of Kala-azar in Kitui and Meru Districts. *Proceedings of the 2nd Annual Medical Scientific Conference, KEMRI & KETRI*, pp. 132-136.

McKinnon, J.A.,& Fendall, N.R.E. (1955). Kala-azar in the Baringo district of Kenya: a preliminary communication. *Journal of Tropical Medicine & Hygiene*, 58, 205.

Minter, D.M. (1962). *Phlebotomus* (*Phlebotomus*) *celiae* sp. nov. (Diptera: Psychodidae), a new sandfly from Kenya. *Annals of Tropical Medicine & Parasitology*, 56, 457.

Minter, D.M. (1963). Studies on the vector of kala-azar in Kenya III. - Distributional evidence. *Annals of Tropical Medicine & Parasitology*, 57, 19-23.

Minter, D.M. & Wijers, D.J.B. (1963). Studies on the vector of kala-azar in Kenya IV. - Experimental evidence. *Annals of Tropical Medicine & Parasitology*, 57, 24-31.

Minter, D.M., Wijers, D.J.B., Heisch, R.B. & Manson-Bahr, P.E.C. (1962). *Phlebotomus martini* - a probable vector of kala-azar in Kenya. *British Medical Journal*, 2, 835.

Muigai, R., Githure, J.I., Gachihi, G.S., Were, J.B.O., Leeuwenburg, J. & Perkins, P.V. (1987). Cutaneous leishmaniasis caused by *Leishmania major* in Baringo District, Kenya. *Transactions of the Royal Society of Tropical Medicine & Hygiene*, 81, 600-602.

Mutinga, M.J. (1971). *Phlebotomus longipes*, a vector of cutaneous leishmaniasis in Kenya. *Transactions of the Royal Society of Tropical Medicine & Hygiene*, 65, 106.

Mutinga, M.J. (1975). The animal reservoir of cutaneous leishmaniasis on Mount Elgon, Kenya. *East African Medical Journal*, 52, 142-151.

Mutinga, M.J. (1975). *Phlebotomus* fauna in the cutaneous leishmaniasis focus of Mount Elgon, Kenya. *East African Medical Journal*, 52, 340-357.

Mutinga, M.J. (1986). Leishmaniasis in Kenya. *Medicus*, 4, 11-22.

Mutinga, M.J. & Ngoka, J.M. (1970). Culture, isolation and description of cutaneous leishmaniasis in Kenya. A preliminary report. *Proceedings of the East African Medical Research Council Scientific Conference*, 4, 72.

Mutinga, M.J. & Ngoka, J.M. (1978). Incrimination of the vector of visceral leishmaniasis in Kenya. *East African Medical Journal*, 55, 337-340.

Mutinga, M.J., Ngoka, J.M., Schnur, L.F. & Chance, M.L. (1980). Isolation and identification of leishmanial parasites from domestic dogs in the Machakos district of Kenya and possible role of dogs as reservoirs of kala-azar in East Africa. *Annals of Tropical Medicine & Parasitology*, 74, 139.

Mutinga, M.J. & Odhiambo, T.R. (1986). Cutaneous leishmaniasis in Kenya - II: Studies of vector potential of *Phlebotomus pedifer* (Diptera: Phlebotomidae) in Kenya. *Insect Science & Its Application*, 2, 171-174.

Ngoka, J.M., Madel, G. & Mutinga, M.J. (1975). *Phlebotomus (Larroussius) elgonensis* sp. nov. (Diptera, Phlebotomidae), a new sandfly from Kenya. *East African Medical Journal*, 52, 132-141.

Ngoka, J.M. & Mutinga, M.J. (1978). Visceral leishmaniasis animal reservoirs in Kenya. *East African Medical Journal*, 52, 132.

Perkins, P.V., Githure, J.I., Mebrahtu, Y., Kiilu, G., Anjili, C., Ngumbi, P.S., Nsovu, J., Oster, C.N., Whitmire, R.E., Leeuwenburg, J., Hendricks, L.D. & Koech, D.K. (1987). The isolation of *Leishmania donovani* from *Phlebotomus martini* collected in Baringo District, Kenya. *Transactions of the Royal Society of Tropical Medicine & Hygiene*, in press.

Rashid, J.R., Chunge, C.N., Oster, C.N., Wasunna, K.M., Muigai, R. & Gachihi, G.S. (1986). Post-kala-azar dermal leishmaniasis occuring long after cure of visceral leishmaniasis in Kenya. *East African Medical Journal*, 63, 365-371.

Sang D.K., Mbugua, G.G. & Arap Siongok, T.K. (1983). Cutaneous leishmaniasis and *Phlebotomus longipes* on Mount Elgon. *East African Medical Journal*, 60, 826.

Schnur, L.F. & Zuckerman, A. (1977). Leishmanial excreted factor (EF) serotypes in Sudan, Kenya, and Ethiopia. *Annals of Tropical Medicine & Parasitology*, 71, 273-294.

Wijers, D.J.B. (1963). Studies on the vector of kala-azar in Kenya II. Epidemiological evidence. *Annals of Tropical Medicine & Parasitology*, 57, 8-18.

Wijers, D.J.B. & Kiilu, G. (1984). Studies on the vector of kala-azar in Kenya, VIII. - The outbreak in Machakos District; epidemiological features and a possible way of control. *Annals of Tropical Medicine & Parasitology*, 78, 597-604.

Wijers, D.J.B.,& Minter, D.M. (1962). Studies on the vector of kala-azar in Kenya I.- Entomological Evidence. *Annals of Tropical Medicine & Parasitology*, 56, 462-472.

Wijers, D.J.B. & Minter, D.M. (1966). Studies on the vector of kala-azar in Kenya V. - The outbreak in Meru district. *Annals of Tropical Medicine & Parasitology*, 60, 11-21.

Wijers, D.J.B. & Ngoka, J.M. (1974). Studies on the vector of kala-azar in Kenya VII: Western Tharaka (Meru district). *Annals of Tropical Medicine & Parasitology*, 68:,21-31.

SANDFLIES AND DISEASE IN CYPRUS; 1944 - 1985

Donald M Minter

Department of Entomology
London School of Hygiene & Tropical Medicine
Keppel Street (Gower Street)
London WC1E 7HT, England

U R Eitrem

Department of Infectious Diseases and National Bacteriological
Central Hospital   Laboratory, S - 105 21
S - 371 85 Karlskrona, Sweden   Stockholm, Sweden

INTRODUCTION

The only previous sandfly survey of Cyprus was that of Adler (1946), in which about 2 000 sandflies were collected, from all parts of the island, in the period 10 August - 9 September, 1944. This report mainly deals with a partial re-survey of the island 41 years later, from 26 June - 26 July, 1985.

With an area of 9 250 square kms, Cyprus is the third largest island in the Mediterranean Sea. It lies only some 70 kms south of mainland Turkey (whose forces occupied the north of the island in 1974) and about 103 kms west of the shores of Lebanon: Egypt lies 240 kms to the south. The population (circa 750 000) are mainly of Greek (80%) and Turkish (20%) origin, who now respectively live in southern and northern areas of the island. United Nations forces for more than a decade have guarded the cease-fire line which still divides the island.

Visceral leishmaniasis (VL), never considered endemic, was first reported from Cyprus in 1935, but was apparently never common, although its occurence was (and continues) poorly documented (Omran, 1961; Zahar, 1980); Adler (1946) stated that most VL occured in the Kyrenia range in the north of the island, although, since the disease was not notifiable, he had no quantitative information. VL apparently disappeared as a result of the successful malaria eradication campaign which ended about 1950. Canine leishmaniasis, with cutaneous infection, was formerly common (Adler, 1946; Steele et al., 1960), particularly in coastal areas, but virtually disappeared as a result of destruction of unlicensed dogs in the successful echinococcosis control campaign of 1970 - 1975. In 1969 there were 46 000 dogs registered (15 - 20% infected with Echinococcus granulosus); by 1975 there were fewer than 6 000 and probably numbers have not significantly risen since then. Human cutaneous leishmaniasis (CL) was never reported in Cyprus and sandfly fever (SF) was unknown, prior to the first report by Niklasson & Eitrem (1985).

Sandfly fever is caused by members of the genus Phlebovirus, family Bunyaviridae. Eight Phleboviruses cause human disease: Sicilian, Naples and Toscana viruses infect man in the Mediterranean region. None were known to occur in Cyprus before 1985. Serological evidence of SF was first detected among Swedish UN troops serving on the island in 1984 (Niklasson & Eitrem, 1985). Seven of 15 Swedish soldiers with self-limiting febrile illness (in a battalion of about 350 men, serving a 6-month summer tour in Cyprus) were positive for Sicilan SF virus antibodies. Further (unpublished) studies by indirect immunofluorescent antibody test (IFAT) in 1985 showed that 15 (4.4%) of 341 Swedish soldiers were infected with SF (Naples or Sicilian serotype) in Cyprus during a six-month summer tour in 1985. In 13 of these soldiers a significant four-fold rise in antibody titre was demonstrated. Two SF virus strains (one probably of Sicilian and one probably of Naples serotype) were isolated from two acutely ill soldiers (Eitrem et al, 1986). Fifty sera of native Cypriots were tested by IFAT and a high proportion were found to have antibodies against SF virus, of Naples and Sicilian serotypes (unpublished observations).

SF has other names: e.g. Phlebotomus fever, papatasi fever, three-day fever. Sandflies were suspected as vectors in 1909; this was proved in 1952. The disease, described a century ago, has a variable presentation, but self-limiting fever of abrupt onset, with pains in limbs, head and eyes, are common features. Sometimes conjunctivitis, facial congestion and occasional relative bradycardia occur. Respiratory and gastrointestinal symptoms are absent.

Vectors of SF are phlebotomine sandflies, notably Phlebotomus (Phlebotomus) papatasi. Viruses are transmitted vertically by sandflies, from eggs and larvae to adults. Viruses overwinter in the sandflies, probably in diapausing larvae; adult flies are active only between April and October each year in the Mediterranean.

The first sandfly survey of Cyprus by Adler in 1944 was concentrated on the northern coast and the Kyrenia range inland, with most other localities in the central Troodos mountains. The survey revealed a characteristic east Mediterranean fauna of 7 Phlebotomus spp. and three of Sergentomyia, with some endemic forms (Table I). From 1944 to 1984 there were a few casual records of sandflies (1971 and 1980; unpublished), which included only four of the ten species recorded in 1944. The partial re-survey of 1985 was concentrated in the southeast of the island, with only few collections elsewhere and virtually none in the north of the island, which is nowadays inaccessible to visitors from the Cyprus Republic in the south. One brief overnight visit was made under UN auspices in July, 1985, to the Kyrenia (=Girne) and Belle Paise (=Bellabayis) area.

MATERIALS and METHODS

Phlebotomine Sandflies

Sandflies were collected by electric or mouth suction aspirators in buildings, and outdoors by transparent plastic sheets coated lightly with castor oil. Some oiled sheets were clipped up into a cylinder and provided with a chemical camping light, as effective makeshift light-traps. Two CDC light traps were also used outdoors; one with a normal tungsten bulb, the other with either a UV or a white fluorescent tube.

The nomenclature of Artemiev & Neronov (1984) is adopted for species of the genus Phlebotomus, except that P. mascittii is here provisionally retained in the subgenus Larroussius. The three Sergentomyia species of Cyprus listed by Adler (1946) are more difficult to allocate, as separate status for these forms presently seems unjustified. They are here treated conservatively, pending further study, as S. fallax (fallax group) for "P. fallax var. cypriotica", S. antennata gp (fallax group) for the former "P. azizi" and S. minuta (minuta group) for "P. parroti".

Virus isolation 630 domiciliary Phlebotomus papatasi were cryopreserved for virus isolation (in 18 pools by different locality and collection date).

RESULTS

I. Viruses

i) Virus isolation From one pool of 59 female Phlebotomus papatasi a SF virus was isolated, but this is not yet fully identified.

II. Phlebotomine sandflies

i) Possible site(s) of SF infection in Swedish military personnel.
No sandflies at all were found in either buildings or sandbagged bunkers in the Swedish battalion base-camp near Larnaca, smaller unit camps elsewhere, or in the forward positions occupied by Swedish troops along the UN ceasefire line. All such places were routinely and regularly treated with insecticides by the Swedish military. A cave close to one Swedish Company HQ contained an empty and rusted insecticide aerosol can, but no sandflies.

Due to suspected cases among Swedish soldiers, attention then turned to a coastal resort on the SE coast (= sector 3, Table I), where most of the men spend local leave. Until a few years ago this was a small fishing village, but recently it has undergone rapid expansion and urban development, including the conversion of a former monastery in the old village centre into residential accomodation for religious meetings. Many new hotels and blocks of self-catering hotel-apartments were built to accomodate tourists, notably in areas on the growing periphery of the one-time village. During evening visits Phlebotomus papatasi were collected from the monastery bedrooms and in bedrooms of houses and apartments in the village centre (mainly rented by tourists). P. papatasi were most numerous, particularly in bedrooms, in several of the recently-built peripheral blocks of hotel-apartments on the stony hillside (many still amid builder's rubble). Tourist residents were mainly Scandinavian or German. P. papatasi were especially numerous in apartments directly overlooking the undisturbed hillside, with nearby dry-stone sheep-folds either still in use, or lately abandoned. A former quarry in the village centre, near the monastery, was full of rubble and urban rubbish, and overgrown by trees and bushes; the site appeared very suitable as a breeding-place for P. papatasi. A few hundred metres from infested apartment blocks at the periphery of the village, the various sheep-folds (with rich deposits of dung) probably filled the same role. SF virus, as noted above, was recovered from a pool of P. papatasi collected in a bedroom of an apartment block in just this situation, and a febrile tourist in another had the clinical characteristics of SF.

ii) Urban/suburban sandflies: Nicosia, Larnaca and Limassol areas
(= sectors 4 and 3, Table I). A Health Inspector collected 34 P. papatasi in the bedroom of his house in Nicosia during the 1985 visit. A few P. papatasi were found in occasional houses in the old part of Larnaca town (near the Chrysopolitissa church), but none were found in church crypts or in underground tombs elsewhere in the town. P. sergenti did not occur in any of the collections of 1985, but in a small collection of 46 sandflies in alcohol at the Nicosia laboratory of the Cyprus Agricultural Department,

TABLE I   Phlebotomine sandflies of Cyprus: summary, 1944 - 1985

KEY TO SYMBOLS

Sectors 1 = north coast and Kyrenia range
         2 = south-central highland area (Troodos), over 200 m
         3 = southern littoral, below 200 m
         4 = eastern lowlands, below 200 m, Nicosia to E coast
         5 = north-western lowlands, below 200 m

Habitat   D = domestic
          P = peridomestic
          S = sylvatic

Diseases SF = sandfly fever
          CL = cutaneous leishmaniasis
          HVL = human visceral leishmaniasis
          CVL = canine leishmaniasis

Sandfly species	Cyprus proved (+)/ possible(?) vector of	1944 (Adler)			1971-1984			1985		
		Record (+/-)	Sector	Habitat	Record (year)	Sector	Habitat	Record	Sector	Habitat
I. Genus Phlebotomus										
P. (Phlebotomus) papatasi	+SF	+	1-5	D,P	+ (1980: biting)	3	D,P	+	1,3,4	D,P
P. (Paraphlebotomus) sergenti	?CL	+	1,2	D,P	+ (1984: biting)	3	P	-		
P. (Paraphlebotomus) alexandri	?HVL	+	1,2	D,P	-			-	(*)	
P. (Larroussius) galilaeus	?	+	1(rare)	D	+ (1971: light traps)	1	P,S	+	1,3,4	D,P
P. (Larroussius) tobbi	?HVL	+	1,2,3	D,P	-			+	2	D,P
P. (Larroussius)** mascitti	?	+	1(rare)	P	-			-	(*)	
P. (Adlerius) kyreniae	?CVL	+	1	D,P	-			-	(*)	
II. Genus Sergentomyia										
S. fallax (fallax group)	nil	+	1 - 4	D,P	-			+	3,4	P,S, rarely D
S. antennata gp (fallax group)	nil	+	1,2,5	D,P	-			+	1,3,4	P,S, rarely D
S. minuta (minuta group)	nil	+	1 - 4	D,P	+ (1971: light traps)	3	P,S	+	1,3,4	P,S, rarely D

(*) species recorded only from Sector 1 (N. coast & Kyrenia range), essentially not surveyed in 1985.
** = subgenus Transphlebotomus of Artemiev & Neronov, 1984

a single male P. sergenti was found, with 44 P. papatasi and 1 S. antennata gp. (det. DMM). This collection, labelled as "annoying people", was made in August of 1984 at the outdoor Curium stadium, near Episkopi, to the west of Limassol. This new record of 1984 is included in Table I. In a short daytime visit to Curium in July of 1985, no sandflies were found in empty ancient underground storage cisterns, nor on oiled sheets with chemical lights, left in the cisterns overnight.

iii) Phlebotomine sandflies in rural village locations of Larnaca District.
Several villages in the dry, low-lying littoral hinterland west of Larnaca (= sector 3 of Table I) were visited in the evening hours; bedrooms and bathrooms were searched for sandflies with the consent of the owners (to whom they were a well-known biting nuisance; called "silent mosquitoes", in Greek, to distinguish them from Culicines). A more intensive study was made, for several days, of one among a cluster of peasant smallholdings in Menoyia village.

Aspirators were used for evening indoor collections, and CDC light traps and castor oil sheets (with or without chemical lights) were left to catch outdoor sandflies. The results, in Table II below, show clearly that P. papatasi was the main species, particularly in bedrooms. The few P. galilaeus collected were found in bedrooms and in peridomestic areas: only 3 P. tobbi were found (outdoors); the small numbers of this species at the time (July) probably reflects their late seasonality in the Mediterranean. The three Sergentomyia species were found mainly outdoors, especially in hollow olive trees among wheat stubble.

iv) Other localities visited in 1985 No sandflies were found (during a brief daytime visit) in the crypt of the church, or in the domestic quarters, of the ancient (founded 327 A D) Stavrovouni monastery, situated on the summit (688 m) of an isolated peak 20 km due west of Larnaca. (Sector 2 of Table I.)
Paphos: Tombs of the Kings (sector 3): Oiled sheets with chemical lights left overnight in several tombs and natural rock cavities yielded only one male, S. minuta gp. (Sector 3, Table I).
Lysos: two specimens of S. antennata gp were the only sandflies collected overnight by oiled sheets with chemical lights left in a dry stone wall and an empty stone store in a field, shaded by a fig-tree. This sector 2 site, altitude about 550 m, is about 1 km above the village of Lysos, along the road leading from Polis to Stavros tis Psokas, in the north-west of the Troodos range.
North Cyprus: Kyrenia area Only a short overnight visit was possible, under UN auspices. In the village of Arapkoy (= Klepini), about 8 km east of the port of Kyrenia (= Girne), P. papatasi and P. galilaeus were found in bedrooms and P. galilaeus, S. fallax, S. minuta and S. antennata gp were caught on oiled sheets left outdoors overnight near houses. One male S. antennata gp was found on oiled sheets left overnight in a small cave on the northern flanks of the Kyrenia range (about 250 m above sea level).
Oiled sheets and chemical lights left overnight in uninhabited rocky scrub with pines (c. 800 m alitude), above the village of Bellapais (= Bellabayis), yielded one specimen each of S. fallax and S. antennata gp.

v) Species not encountered in Cyprus since 1944. These are indicated in Table I by an asterisk; the three species concerned (all from sector 1) are as follows:-
P. (Paraphlebotomus) alexandri
P. (Larroussius) mascittii
P. (Adlerius) kyreniae

The recent record (see ii) above; Curium stadium) of P. (Paraphlebotomus) sergenti indicates that this species is still extant in Cyprus.

TABLE II   Phlebotomine sandflies of a rural Cyprus village (Menoyia; Larnaca District), from a farm house and peridomestic animal houses (sheep, pigeons and poultry): July, 1985

Phlebotomine species	Numbers collected	Overall % (n = 609)	% *Phlebotomus* (n = 382)	Notes
P. papatasi	361	60	95	Predominantly in bedrooms
P. galilaeus	18	3	<5	Mainly peridomestic; occasionally indoors
P. tobbi	3	0.5	<1	Mainly peridomestic ?
S. antennata gp	110	18	-	Essentially peridomestic, especially in hollow olive trees; rarely indoors.
S. fallax	84	14	-	
S. minuta	33	5	-	

III. Recent reports of Leishmaniasis in Cyprus

Cyprus government veterinarians in Nicosia had seen no canine leishmaniasis cases for many years and no recent cases of human infections were known to Health Inspectors in the southern part of the island. However, a recent case of VL in a 10-month old Cypriot child (from Apesha village, about 12 kms north of Limassol, altitude 550 m, in sector 2) was diagnosed in Athens (mid-1987) by ELISA test in high titre, with rapid response to antimonial treatment (V. Syriopoulou & K. Tzanetou, pers. comm.).

In the brief visit to the Kyrenia area in 1985, we were reliably but unofficially informed of at least one recent case of infantile VL in the north of the island; and one of indigenous CL in a child, treated by a dermatolgist.

DISCUSSION

The sandfly fauna of Cyprus apparently has survived the insecticide era since 1944 substantially unscathed (Table I). Only three species of sandflies recorded in 1944 were not encountered since (see above); all three were then reported only from the north coast - Kyrenia range area, substantially unsurveyed since. The Malaria Eradication Campaign of the 1950's, based on household spraying, was successfully concluded; but insecticides are still widely used, both domestically for nuisance insects and in agriculture (six aerial applications of a dimethoate formulation are made to all olive-growing areas - including Menoyia and neighbouring village areas - between June and October each year). The managements of newer coastal resort hotels and apartments we visited used a variety of proprietary insectides for mosquito and sandfly control, but clearly to little avail so far as sandflies were concerned. It remains to be determined if P. papatasi from Cyprus are resistant or tolerant to modern insectides: limited tests made on individual Cyprus colony insects to date, however, have not shown raised esterase levels indicative of resistance (Eitrem: unpublished observations).

CONCLUSIONS

1) Swedish UN soldiers, together with other expatriates, are probably infected with SF viruses (Naples and Sicilian serotypes) whilst resident in coastal summer resorts. Summer case rates in non-immune Swedish UN troops were 4.4%. The vector of SF in Cyprus is proved to be the ubiquitous P. (Phlebotomus) papatasi, common in houses in rural and urban areas, and particulary evident in new hotels and apartment blocks built on the periphery of former coastal villages, lately developed to serve the thriving tourist industry. Native Cypriots are probably infected in infancy in towns and villages in many parts of the island.

2) Although still apparently very uncommon, human leishmaniasis still exists in Cyprus and requires further investigation; of particular interest are the parasites which give rise to the cutaneous lesions reported (? Leishmania infantum ?). It is unknown if canine leishmaniasis continues to any significant extent, after its virtual elimination as an indirect result of dog destruction during the echinococcosis campaign, 1970-1975.

Acknowledgements

U R Eitrem is grateful to the Medical Board of the Swedish Armed Forces for financial support of visits to Cyprus and to the officers and men of the 1984 and 1985 Swedish UN battalions for their interest and practical help.

We also wish to acknowledge the indefatigable assistance of Mr R C Page, who participated at his own expense in the 1985 fieldwork in Cyprus.

References

Artemiev, M M & Neronov, V M (1984). Distribution and ecology of sandflies of the Old World (genus Phlebotomus). [In Russian.] Moscow, pp. 207.

Adler, S (1946). The sandflies of Cyprus (Diptera). Bulletin of entomological Research, 36, 497-511.

Eitrem, U R, Niklasson, B & Minter, D M (1986). Sandfly Fever and Sandflies in Cyprus. Proceedings of the Ninth International Congress of Infectious and Parasitic Diseases, (Munich, 20-26 July), Abstract No 809.

Lupaşçu, G, Duport, M, Dănescu, P & Cristescu, M (1977). Éthologie et phénologie des phlébotomes vecteurs potentiels de la leishmaniose en Roumanie. Colloques Internationaux du Centre National de la Recherche Scientifique, No. 239 (Ecologie des Leishmanioses), 191-194.

Niklasson, B & Eitrem, R (1985). Sandfly Fever among Swedish UN troops in Cyprus. Lancet, 1 (No 8439: May 25), 1212.

Omran, A R (1961). The ecology of leishmaniasis. In: Studies in Disease Ecology, ed. J M May, New York, Hafner Publishing Company, Inc., pp 331-388.

Steele, J H, Polydorou, K, Orphanides, A, Crowther, R & Markides, A A (1976). Zoonoses in Cyprus past and present including a comment on the public health.
International Journal of the Zoonoses, 3, 65-76.

Zahar, A R (1980). Studies on leishmaniasis vectors/reservoirs and their control in the Old World: Part III. Middle East. WHO, Geneva: unpublished document, WHO/VBC/80.776, pp. ii + 78.

APPENDIX

KEY TO THE SANDFLIES OF CYPRUS

(Based on Adler, 1946 and Léger, Pesson & Madulo-Leblond, 1986
[Bull. Soc. Path. Exot., 79, 514 - 524], with modifications)

Erect hairs on tergites 2 - 6. Cibarium unarmed. Group of setae on antero-inferior edge of mesanepisternum. Male style with 4 or 5 spines. Spermatheca annulated............................ genus Phlebotomus

Recumbent hairs on tergites 2 - 6. Cibarium with armature. No setae on mesanepisternum. Male style with 4 spines (terminal or subterminal) and small subterminal non-deciduous seta. Spermatheca not annulated, tube-like... genus Sergentomyia

Phlebotomus MALES

1. style with 4 spines; coxite with internal lobe and setae 4
   style with 5 spines; lobe of coxite small or lacking 2

2. 3 short terminal spines, 2 median: distinctive tri-lobed paramere...
   .... P. (Phlebotomus) papatasi
   2 long terminal spines, 3 median: paramere not tri-lobed...........
   3

3. penis sheath with divided tip; apical point larger than lateral point.
   (Antennal formula: 2/III - VII; 1/VIII - XV): ....
   .... P. (Larroussius) tobbi

   penis sheath tapered, with rounded tip: ....
   .... P. (Larroussius)* mascittii

   penis sheath spatulate, concave & terminates in long curved hook with distal serrations; genital filaments emerge from distal third.
   (Antennal formula: 2/III - VIII; 1/IX - XV): ....
   .... P. (Larroussius) galilaeus

   penis sheath with small subterminal tubercle; genital filaments emerge from penis tip. (Antennal formula: 2/III - V; 1/VI - XV): ....
   .... P. (Adlerius) kyreniae

4. 2 long spines of style terminal and 2 median; coxite has internal lobe with setae.......
   lobe of coxite short, slender; AIII long (c. 0.2 mm), about equal to epipharynx: ....
   ....P. (Paraphlebotomus) sergenti

   lobe of coxite flattened like a water-sprinkler; AIII short (c. 0.1 mm), much shorter than epipharynx: ....
   ....P. (Paraphlebotomus) alexandri

---

(* = subgenus Transphlebotomus of Artemiev & Neronov, 1984)

Phlebotomus FEMALES

1. Spermatheca completely segmented

    (i) head not on long neck:
    4 - 5 annuli, apical segment enlarged; pharynx with network of strong scales: AIII long (c. 0.2 mm), longer than IV + V, about equal to epipharynx: .... P. (Paraphlebotomus) sergenti
    AIII short (c. 0.1 mm), less than IV + V, about half length of epipharynx; spermathecal segments equal: .. .. P. (Paraphlebotomus) alexandri

    8 - 12 subequal annuli; pharynx armed with fine-toothed scales: .... P. (Phlebotomus) papatasi

    (ii) head on long neck (subgenus: Larroussius):
    spermathecal ducts with enlarged asymmetrical bases:.... .... P. (Larroussius) tobbi
    spermathecal ducts with large basal diverticula, shaped like a crumpled hat: .... P. (Larroussius) galilaeus

2. Spermathecal capsule incompletely segmented (in the form either of a striated cylinder or of a tapered capsule)

    (i) spermatheca tubular, densely striated and without neck, opens into ducts greatly dilated proximally: pharyngeal teeth large and irregular, like a network of scales .... P. (Larroussius)* mascitti

    (ii) spermatheca a cigar-shaped capsule, with definite neck and few overlapping triangular striations, opens into narrow ducts: pharyngeal teeth wedge-shaped, regular and of medium size .... P. (Adlerius) kyreniae

Sergentomyia MALES

non-deciduous seta of style long, location more or less median: ... . S. minuta (minuta group)

non-deciduous seta of style very short and subterminal:............ .... S. fallax (fallax group)

non-deciduous seta of style at about 0.7:......................... .... S. antennata gp (fallax group)

Sergentomyia FEMALES

80 - 90 cibarial teeth in a straight line. Pigmented area broad laterally. Pharynx with few teeth: .... S. minuta (minuta group)

16 - 32 cibarial teeth on an arc:
    16 - 20 uniform teeth; posterior pharynx expanded, flask-shaped .... S. fallax (fallax group)
    28 - 32 teeth; posterior pharynx not expanded: .... S. antennata (fallax group)

THE EFFECT OF PERMETHRIN IMPREGNATED NETS ON PHLEBOTOMUS

(DIPTERA: PSYCHODIDAE) IN CENTRAL ITALY

M. Maroli[1] and R.P. Lane[2]

1. Laboratorio di Parassitologia, Istituto Superiore di Sanità, Viale Regina Elena, 299. 00161 Rome, Italy
2. Department of Entomology, London School of Hygiene and Tropical Medicine, Keppel Street, London WC1 England

SUMMARY

Permethrin impregnated nets over CDC light traps and as window-net in a stable were used in four localities of Central Italy to test the effectiveness against Phlebotomus perfiliewi (Diptera: Pshychodidae). The results on CDC light traps of pooled catches for each replicate of the four localites show that there is a very significant difference between the catches in the treated and untreated traps (untreated = 1,312, treated = 750 : X^2 = 152.63 p << 0.001). The data of window-net experiment also clearly indicated the effectiveness of permethrin in reducing the flies entering the building (1,696 untreated, 185 treated; X^2 = 366 p << 0.001).

INTRODUCTION

The use of repellents as protection against attacks by biting insects has been extensively investigated, particularly in respect of personal protection. However there has been recent interest in repellent impregnated nets or clothes to protect an enclosed space. This latter strategy is particularly useful for the control of sandflies in the many areas where the disease occurs sporadically and widespread spraying is not cost effective.

The synthetic pyrethroid permethrin has been the subject of much study since it has a low mammalian toxicity and is remarkably persistent in treated clothing. The protective action of permethrin has been attributed to its toxic rather than its repelent action (when compared to other compounds such as DEET) (Bredeen et al., 1982). Among the arthropods which have been tested are blackflies (Lindsay & Mc Andless, 1978)), chiggers, Trombicula spp.(Bredeen et al., 1982), bodylice (Nassif & Kamel, 1977), mosquitoes (Schreck et al., 1978) and ticks (Mount & Snoddy, 1983). Permethrin has been tested against sandflies in two previous studies: in Panama Schreck et al. (1982) found that permethrin impregnated jackets did not provide the protection expected against attack from four species of anthropophilic Lutzomyia species. Laboratory studies on topical application of permethrin to the skin of rabbits have been carried out by Wirtz et al. (1986). These studies were not entirely satisfactory for the control of sandflies.

Impregnated jackets are of little use since sandflies will not bite through clothing as other biting flies will and secondly, permethrin has a low vapour pressure and therefore does not produce a repellent barrier around an individual and thus protect non-treated areas such as hands and face. Furthermore, permethrin is not acceptable when applied directly to the skin of man. The benefit of this and other similar compounds in the control of phlebotomine sandflies therefore lies in the use of impregnated nets to provide a protective barrier preventing access to an enclosed area such as a building or bed. Sandfly bed-nets have a smaller mesh size than conventional bed nets and are therefore most uncomfortable to sleep under. The use of a larger mesh size would improve the acceptability of nets to control sandfly biting. The objective of this study is to test the effectiveness of permethrin impregnated into large-mesh nets against a common anthropophilic sandfly in central Italy: Phlebotomus perfiliewi. This species is one of the most abudant sandflies in Italy and is strongly suspected as transmitting cutaneous leishmaniasis (Maroli et al., in press) and phleboviruses there (Verani et al., 1980). P. perfiliewi is strongly phototropic, as many as 3,000 individuals can be caught by a single CDC light trap in a night (Maroli, unpublished), and is therefore ideally suited for sampling when individual attractiveness of human baits needs to be minimised. In this study, permethrin impregnated nets over CDC light traps were used in four localities in central Italy and also window nets in one locality. Small numbers of P. perniciosus, a vector of visceral leishmaniasis, were also present in the localities sampled.

MATERIALS AND METHODS

Two sets of experiments were carried out; the first used impregnated nets over CDC light traps and the second used the same nets as window nets in a small building housing rabbits. In both experiments, cotton nets of 1.5 cm mesh size were impregnated with 1.0 g. permethrin (formulated as 10% emulsifiable concentrate by IG.ECO, Italy) per square metre of cloth following the method described in Majori et al. (1987). The experiments were carried out on farms in four localities in central Italy where P. perfiliewi is the dominant sandfly species, one in Tuscany and three in Abruzzi. They were:
TUSCANY: Baccinello, Groseto Province (Renzi Farm) an area of rolling hills and mixed agriculture. The general area has been described by Maroli and Bettini (1977).
ABRUZZI: Spoltore, Pescara Province (Di Muzio Farm) is also an area of mixed farming and is described in Maroli et al. (in press).

St. Nicolo al Tordino, Teramo Province in the Tordino Valley was on the perimeter of a control programme against sandfly vectors outlined in Coraddetti (1954) and is the site of the work given in Maroli (1983).

Palmoli, Chieti Province, a hilltop town 700m altitude. Amongst lightly wooded, mixed agricultural land with numerous small farms. The trapping sites were around two adjacent farms (Taddeo and Maroli Farms) 2Km from the village.

Light Trap Experiments. To eliminate the differences between individual attractiveness of human baits, light traps were used as 'baits'. Cylindrical nets 36cm diameter and 50cm long were put over standard CDC light traps (Hausherr's Machine Works, New Jersey) which completely covered the trap and its holding cage (fig.1.). Light traps were used in pairs, one with an untreated net and the other with a treated net. The traps were set close to one another (e.g. either side of a building and usually out of line-of-sight). The position of the

Table 1

The effect of permethrin impregnated nets over CDC light-traps on phlebotomine sandflies in four different localities in central Italy.

Locality	replicate	Traps with untreated nets			Traps with treated nets			Significance levels between totals
		males	females	total	males	females	total	
Baccinello	i	113	91	204	76	8	84	
	ii	39	25	64	18	0	18	
	iii	76	30	106	63	1	64	
	total			374			166	$\chi^2 = 87.86$ $P \ll 0.001$
Spoltore	i	4	3	7	0	0	0	
	ii	10	28	38	0	1	1	
	iii	1	2	3	1	2	3	
	total			48			4	$\chi^2 = 0.38$ $P \ll 0.001$
St.Nicolo' al Tordino	i	2	4	6	0	2	2	
	ii	1	6	7	1	0	1	
	total			13			3	$\chi^2 = 0.38$ $0.05 < P < 0.10$
Palmoli	i	88	429	517	67	249	316	
	ii	48	207	255	20	157	177	
	iii	13	90	103	12	80	92	
	total			875			586	$\chi^2 = 56.77$ $P \ll 0.001$
Totals (48 trap nights)				1,312			750	$\chi^2 = 152.63$ $P \ll 0.001$

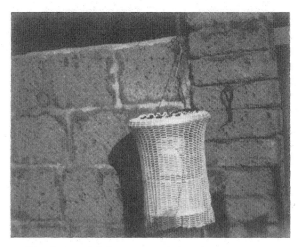

Fig.1 CDC light-trap with wide-mesh net.

traps was reversed from one night to another to eliminate the effect of differences between trap sites. Three replicate pairs of traps were used (total six traps) at each of the four localities described above except St. Nicolo al Tordino where only two replicate pairs were used. These experiments were carried out during July and August 1986.

Window Net Experiment. This experiment was carried out at one locality only: Palmoli in Abruzzi for seven successive nights between 13th and 19th of August 1986 inclusive. Nets covered the single window (1m x 1.5m) of a small rabbit breeding building (8m x 4m) in which 20 rabbits were kept. The door was sealed with adhesive tape each night. A CDC trap was used to sample sandflies in the building. Treated and untreated nets were used over the window on alternate nights.

Samples of all trap catches were mounted and the species identified.

RESULTS AND DISCUSSION

The results of the pooled catches for each replicate at each of the four localities in the light-trap experiment are given in Table 1. Overall, there is a very significant difference between the catches in the treated and untreated traps, clearly indicating that permethrin has a marked 'repellent' effect.

However, permethrin does not deter the flies from entering the traps completely. When flies were abudant, e.g. at Palmoli, a reasonable number of flies still entered traps, although they were all dead when collected the following morning.

There was some difference between the localities in the abundance of flies despite the experiments being made within a few weeks, number of flies caught in some localities was low. However when pooled there is a significant difference between treated and untreated trap catches.

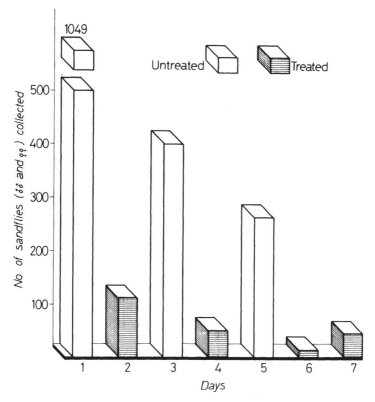

Fig.2. Catches of phlebotomine sandflies in building with window-nets, alternately untreated and treated, at Palmoli, over seven successive night.

The proportion of males and females also differed: at Baccinello the ratio of males to females was 1:56 in the untreated traps and 16.4 in the treated traps, indicating that females were repelled more than males. However, this difference was not found in the other localities, where females were more abundant. The preponderance of males at Baccinello may be because this site was sampled first and at the beginning of the 'sandfly season' when males predominate.

The results of the window-net experiment also clearly indicated the effectiviness of permethrin (table 2) in reducing the number of flies entering the building. When the number of flies caught each night a treated net was used over the window is expressed as a proportion of the previous night's catch (untreated) the reduction in the numbers of flies caught varied between 88% and 96%, an enormous and highly significant reduction ($p \ll 0.001$).

In this experiment it is not possible to discriminate between those flies caught in the CDC traps which had bred in the building from those which had passed through the nets. The effect of the permethrin on the behaviour of the flies immediately after exposure is unknown. Throughout the period of the experiment there was a trend of diminishing catches when both the treated and untreated nets were used (fig.2). This is possibly due to trapping-out by both the light trap and the toxicity of the permethrin.

In conclusion, wide mesh nets impregnated with permethrin significantly reduce the number of P. perfiliewi entering traps and buildings. Further work on the period of survival of those flies passing through treated nets is required, especially to determine the effect on subsequent feeding activity.

Table 2

Number of sandflies collected in CDC light-trap in stable with impregnated window nets (untreated and permethrin-treated nets used on alternate nights).

Date	untreated net			treated nets			% previous untreated catches
	males	females	total	males	females	total	
13 Aug.	47	1002	1049	–	–	–	
14 Aug.	–	–	–	5	102	107	10.67
15 Aug.	10	382	392	–	–	–	
16 Aug.	–	–	–	0	47	47	12.30
17 Aug.	7	248	255	–	–	–	
18 Aug.	–	–	–	0	10	10	4.03
19 Aug.	–	–	–	0	21	21	8.46
Totals	64	1632	1696	5	180	185	

χ^2 between overall totals = 366 $P \ll 0.001$.

ACKNOWLEDGEMENTS

We wish to thank the British Council, Consiglio Nazionale delle Ricerche and WHO (VBC) for their generous financial support and IG.ECO, Italy for supplying the permethrin impregnated nets.

REFERENCES

1. G.C. Breeden, C.E. Schreck, A.L. Soresen, 1982. Permethrin as clothing treatment for personal protection against chigger mites (Acarina: Trombiculidae). Am. J. Trop. Med.., 31: 589.

2. A. Corradetti, 1954. The control of Leishmaniasis through Phlebotomus control in Italy. Rend. Ist. Sup. Sanità, suppl., 1: 57.

3. I.S. Lindsay, J.M. McAndless, 1978. Permethrin treated jackets versus repellent treated jackets and hoods for personal protection against black flies and mosquitos Mosq. News, 38: 350.

4. G. Majori, G. Sabatinelli, M. Coluzzi, 1987. Permethrin impregnated curtains for malaria vector control. Med. & Vet. Entomol., 1 (in press).

5. M. Maroli, 1983. Laboratory colonization of Phlebotomus perfiliewi (Parrot). Trans. Roy. Soc. Trop. Med. & Hyg, 77: 876.

6. M. Maroli & S. Bettini, 1977. Leishmaniasis in Tuscany (Italy): (I). An investigation on phlebotomine sandflies in Grosseto Province. Trans. Roy. Soc. Trop. Med. & Hyg, 71: 315.

7. M. Maroli, M. Gramiccia, L. Gradoni, 1987. Natural infection of sandfly Phlebotomus perfiliewi Parrot, 1930 with Leishmania infantum Nicolle, 1908 in a cutaneous leishmaniasis focus of the Abruzzi region (Italy). Trans. Roy. Soc. Trop. Med. & Hyg., 81 (in press).

8. E.C. Mount, E.L. Snoddy, 1983. Pressurized sprays of permethrin and deet on clothing for personal protection against the lone star tick and the American dog tick (Acari: Ixodidae). J. Econ. Entomol., 76: 529.

9. M. Nassif, O. Kamel, 1977. A field trial with Permethrin against body lice, Pediculus humanus in Egypt, 1976. Pest. Sc., 8: 301

10. C.E. Schreck, N. Smith, D. Weidhass, K. Posey, D. Smith, 1978. Repellents vs. toxicants as clothing treatments for protection from mosquitoes and other binting flies. J. Econ. Entomol., 71: 919

11. C.E. Schreck, D.L. Kline, B.N. Chaniotis, N. Wilkinson, T.P. McGovern, D.E. Weidnass, 1982. Evaluation of personal protection methods against phlebotomines sandflies including vectors of Leishmaniasis in Panama Am. J. Trop. & Hyg., 31: 1046.

12. P. Verani, M.C. Lopes, L. Nicoletti, M. Balducci, 1980. Studies on Phlebotomus transmitted virus in Italy: (I) Isolation and characterization of a sandfly fever Naples like In "Arboviruses in Mediterranean Countries", Zbl. Bakt. suppl. 9: 195.

13. R.A. Wirtz, E.D. Rowton, J.A. Hallam, P.V. Perkins, L.C. Rutledge, 1986. Laboratory testing of repellents against the sandfly Phlebotomus papatasi (Diptera: Psychodidae). J. Med. Entomol., 13, 64.

CUTICULAR HYDROCARBON ANALYSIS AS A TOOL IN SANDFLY IDENTIFICATION

Angela Phillips, Shaden Kamhawi, P.J.M. Milligan and
D.H. Molyneux

Department of Biological Sciences
University of Salford
Salford M5 4WT, UK

INTRODUCTION

It has been recognised over the last twenty years that many important groups of insect vectors which were initially thought to be single species are, in fact, complexes of sibling species. Characteristically, these species are morphologically indistinguishable or separable only by minor characters involving detailed morphometric examination. Identification of the sibling species becomes a necessity in studies involving the vector, as often important differences are shown to exist between these species, eg. in their vectorial capacity, feeding preferences etc. (for example see Milligan et al., 1986). Since the determination of the Anopheles gambiae species complex (Davidson, 1964; Coluzzi and Sabatini, 1967) and Simulium damnosum s.l (Vajime and Dunbar, 1975), there has been increasing evidence that many other groups of Anopheles (e.g. Baimai et al., 1984), Simulium (e.g. Shelley et al., 1987) and now also Phlebotomus and Lutzomyia (present study) are complexes of very closely related species.

The determination of the existence of sibling species was originally based on the reproductive incompatibility between samples of the 'same' species, as noted by workers in the field. Later, studies on the polytene chromosomes of Anopheles ovarian nurse cells and larval Simulium salivary gland cells determined the presence of species specific differences in the banding pattern of these chromosomes (Coluzzi and Sabatini, loc.cit.; Green, 1972; Vajime and Dunbar loc.cit.). More recently studies on isoenzyme variants have demonstrated the presence of distinct electromorphs characteristic of particular cytogenetically defined species (for A.gambiae s.l see Miles 1979; for Simulium damnosum s.l see Meredith and Townson, 1981). Presently the development of DNA probes for the identification of a variety of species complexes is underway (see Townson et al., in press; Gale and Crampton, 1987; Ready, this volume).

In addition to these techniques the analysis of insect cuticular hydrocarbons by gas liquid chromatography (GLC), a method previously used in plant taxonomy (Eglinton and Hamilton, 1963) has been successfully applied to the discrimination of vector sibling species. Examples include A.gambiae s.l (Carlson and Service, 1980; Hamilton and Service, 1983), A.culicifacies (Milligan et al., 1986) and Simulium damnosum s.l (Carlson and Walsh, 1981; Phillips et al., 1985).

Until recently the identification of sandflies was not thought to pose problems as most species were clearly separable on morphological grounds. However, in some species groups, e.g. the Psychodopygus squamiventris series, females are not distinguishable whereas the males are separable by morphological characteristics (Ready and da Silva, 1984). A similar problem is found in Phlebotomus pedifer, P.longipes and P.aculeatus, Lutzomyia shannoni vexator and L.verrucarum species groups (Sang, 1987). There is also increasing evidence for the existence of sandfly sibling species which are difficult to identify and require the application of new methods of identification.

The problem of cryptic sandfly species was recently highlighted in a report of the World Health Organisation's Expert Committee on Leishmaniasis (WHO, 1984) which recommended the use of biochemical and genetic techniques for the elucidation of such problems. Isoenzyme analysis and cuticular hydrocarbons were specifically mentioned in the recommendations.

This paper reports our recent work on the application of GLC and Gas Chromatography/Mass Spectrometry (GC/MS) to the study of various species of sandflies which are proven vectors of Leishmaniasis.

MATERIALS AND METHODS

Cuticular hydrocarbons were extracted from sandflies by immersing them in 10 ul of n-hexane for 10 mins. Exact details of the method can be found in Kamhawi et al. (1987). For the analysis of compounds contained within the tergal glands of sandflies, dissection of the relevant abdominal segments was usually undertaken, followed by extraction of the compounds with n-hexane. Details of this latter method are given in Lane et al. (1985) and Phillips et al. (1986). For all extracted cuticular hydrocarbons, analysis of their relative quantities was made by gas chromatography. Quantitative differences in hydrocarbons thus determined were used to separate the species. Qualitative differences, i.e. the presence of a particular hydrocarbon in one species and not in another, were initially demonstrated by GLC, while their identity was determined by GC/MS. All studies on tergal gland compounds were performed on the GC/MS to ensure the correct identification of the peaks.

RESULTS

Lutzomyia longipalpis

It has long been recognised that the sandfly Lutzomyia longipalpis, a proven vector of visceral Leishmaniasis, has two distinct forms in the male (Mangabeira, 1969). These forms are characterised by pale patches on the abdominal tergites (Ward et al., 1983, 1984; Lane and Ward, 1984). The form known as the "one spot" has a single pale patch on the 4th abdominal tergite whilst the "two spot" form has such patches on tergites 3 and 4. In general one spot forms are more widely distributed in certain areas of Brazil, however, one and two spot forms are sympatric, for example, in Ceara, N.E. Brazil. Scanning Electron Microscope studies of these pale patches indicated that the areas were glandular in appearance consisting of small papules with central pores (Lane and Ward, loc.cit.). This finding prompted the analysis of the contents of the segments using GC/MS. Details of the results of these investigations have been reported by Lane et al. (loc.cit.) and Phillips et al. (loc.cit.). Table 1 gives details of the chemical components extracted from various populations of L.longipalpis males examined to date. Initial analysis of one spot populations originating from Lapinha Cave, Minas Gerais, Brazil, showed the single spot contained concentrations of a homofarnesene-like hydrocarbon of molecular weight 218 ($C_{16}H_{26}$). This compound was present in two peaks which had very similar mass spectra, suggesting the presence of isomers. Further work is required to clarify the relationship between these two very similar compounds. Two spot forms of L.longipalpis from Morada Nova, Ceará, Brazil, had an entirely different chemical, a diterpenoid of molecular weight 272 ($C_{20}H_{32}$) which was present in males of this population.

Phillips et al. (loc.cit.) then analysed sympatric one and two spot flies from Sobral, Ceará. One spot populations contained the homofarnesene-like compound and two spot populations, the diterpenoid. The number of pale patches, therefore, seemed to indicate which type of compound they contained. However, further analysis of males of one spot populations from other areas of Brazil, including recent foci of visceral Leishmaniasis in Santarém and Marajó Island, showed surprisingly that the one spot form from these sites contained the diterpenoid (see Table 1). Ward et al. (1983) suggested that the two spot Ceará populations were the likely vectors of visceral leishmaniasis (caused by Leishmania chagasi), in view of the absence of visceral leishmaniasis in areas where one spot populations were present. The observations that two spot forms were more anthropophilic and peridomestic led Ward et al. (loc.cit.) to suggest that differences in susceptibility to L.chagasi might occur with the polymorphism of the males. Present results, however, indicate that any epidemiological association between susceptibility to Leishmania in L.longipalpis must be linked to the chemicals present in the males rather than to the number of tergal spots. Santarém and Marajó Island populations (one spot) have been clearly demonstrated to be vectors of visceral leishmaniasis (Lainson et al., 1984; Ryan et al., 1984) and have the same diterpenoid as two spot forms from the endemic area of Ceará.

Studies on populations from Jacobina, Bahia, Brazil, have suggested the presence of a third type of compound. These flies have two spots producing one peak with a molecular weight of 218. It is similar to the homofarnesene-like compound, of Lapinha Cave flies in that it has the same molecular weight. However, it has a consistently shorter retention time, produces only one peak and exhibits differences in its fragmentation pattern. All this information leads us to suggest that it is a different compound. Crossing experiments between Jacobina two spot females and Sobral two spot males, yielded a hatch rate of less than 20%. The resulting males, which had two spots, were analysed by GC/MS and demonstrated that the progeny had inherited the chemical characteristics from the mother (i.e. one peak of molecular weight 218), suggesting that the maternal genes for this compound had been inherited Ward et al. (in press).

TABLE 1

Lutzomyia longipalpis. Analysis of compounds extracted from the pale abdominal tergites

Origin of population	No. of spots	Molecular weight of compounds extracted from spots (and number of peaks)
BRAZIL		
Lapinha Cave, Minas Gerais	1	218 2 peaks (possibly isomers)
Sobral (one spot), Ceará	1	218 2 peaks "
Sobral (two spot) Ceara	2	272
Morada Nova, Ceará	2	272
Marajó Island, Pará	1	272
Santarém, Pará	1	272
Ibirite, Minas Gerais	1	272
Jacobina, Bahia	2	218 1 peak
BOLIVIA		
Chijchipa	1	218 2 peaks (possibly isomers)
COLOMBIA		
L'Aquila	1	218 2 peaks "

Studies on the L.longipalpis complex clearly demonstrate the need for further chemical analysis and exact identification, as the application of such tools will provide an essential basis for the future understanding of fly biology and Leishmania epidemiology as applied to what is clearly a species complex.

Psychodopygus squamiventris series

Representatives of this complex, P.wellcomei and P.complexus, are sympatric in the endemic areas of mucocutaneous Leishmaniasis due to L.braziliensis braziliensis in Brazil (Serra dos Carajas) (Lainson et al., 1973). The females are isomorphic (Ready and da Silva, 1984; Lane and Ready, 1985) but males can be distinguished by morphology of genitalia. It is considered on epidemiological grounds that P.wellcomei is the vector. P.squamiventris s.str. similarly has females isomorphic with P.wellcomei and P.complexus. Ryan et al. (1986) undertook the first study on sandfly cuticular hydrocarbons. Using females derived from isofemale broods, a high degree of separation of P.wellcomei and P.complexus was achieved. Earlier attempts to separate the females of these species, using isoenzyme techniques (Ready and da Silva, loc.cit.) and multivariate statistical analysis of a number of morphometric parameters (Lane and Ready, loc.cit.) were unsuccessful. More recently Phillips et al. (in preparation) in an analysis of female P.squamiventris s.str (similarly obtained from isofemale reared flies) has revealed qualitative differences between this species and specimens of P.wellcomei and P.complexus. P.squamiventris s.str has the following cuticular components which are not present in P.wellcomei and P.complexus; namely 11-methyltricosane, 13-methylnonacosane and n-triacontene.

Phlebotomus ariasi

Recently Kamhawi et al. (1987) reported the analysis of cuticular hydrocarbons of P.ariasi from a focus of visceral Leishmaniasis in the Cévennes region of France. Evidence was provided for the existence of two populations of flies in this area; a domestic population and a sylvatic one. The study was undertaken as a blind trial and flies were supplied in six tubes giving no indication as to origin. Our results allocated five of the six tubes to one of two groups whilst the sixth tube was shown to contain flies of both groups. It was subsequently admitted that flies in this tube had been deliberately mixed. All flies from the mixed tube could be allocated to either the domestic or sylvatic collections. Evaluation of the possible epidemiological significance of these findings and the application of other techniques to P.ariasi populations from these two sites remain to be undertaken. However, Rioux et al. (1969) had previously suggested that different populations of P.ariasi could be present in the Cévennes. It is apparent from the analysis of the cuticular hydrocarbons that differences do occur between flies caught in domestic and sylvatic sites. The degree of isolation between these sites is currently under investigation.

Phlebotomus perfiliewi perfiliewi

Studies on the vector sandfly P.perfiliewi perfiliewi in Italy have indicated that hydrocarbon analysis is able to distinguish populations of flies from different geographical locations and has, in the case of P.p.perfiliewi, confirmed the earlier differences described by Ward et al. (1981) between flies from the Adriatic and Tyrrhenian coasts of Italy. Ward et al. (loc.cit.) reported differences in allelic frequencies of phosphoglucomutase in flies from different sides of the Appenines. Tyrrhenian flies showed significantly less polymorphism than Adriatic flies, which possessed an additional allele which was not observed in Tyrrhenian populations.

Initial results from two laboratory colonies of P.p.perfiliewi were inconclusive but wild-caught material from three locations, from East and West of the Appenines and from Calabria in Southern Italy was obtained (supplied by Drs M Maroli and R Lane). The results of hydrocarbon analysis indicated a clear separation of flies from Marche (Adriatic coast) and Tuscany (Tyrrhenian coast) whilst flies from Calabria were again distinct. Several explanations have been proposed for the differences seen and the results add weight to the theory that the Appenines form a barrier to the movement of flies (Phillips et al., in preparation).

Phlebotomus papatasi

This widely distributed vector of cutaneous Leishmaniasis was subjected to hydrocarbon analysis, using material colonised by Dr R Killick-Kendrick and Dr R Lane. Although the use of laboratory reared material in experimental work must be treated with extreme caution, this initial study was undertaken to obtain a general profile of this species. Five populations derived from Puma (India), Saudi Arabia, Iraq, Cyprus and Bihar (India) were examined. The results indicated that differences do exist between these populations, with the sample from Bihar being considerably different from the others examined.

Wild-caught material is required from different sites before conclusive results can be obtained for P.papatasi but initial results indicate that there is less intra-specific variation in the populations of this fly, which are allopatric, than has been found in our studies on P.p.perfiliewi and P.ariasi.

CONCLUSION

Our studies have shown that species-specific differences in the cuticular hydrocarbons of closely related vector species is commonplace and can be effectively utilised as a means of identification (Phillips and Milligan, 1986). The usefulness of any character in identification, however, must depend upon the degree to which it is affected by factors such as diet, age and environmental conditions. It is well known that insects synthesise their cuticular hydrocarbons de novo and precise biochemical pathways exist to explain how this is achieved (e.g. Lockey, 1985). There is also evidence that dietary alkanes can be incorporated into the wax layer (Nelson et al., 1971; Blomquist and Jackson, 1973). However, in grasshoppers which consume large quantities of plant material containing alkanes, the contribution of these alkanes to the cuticular complement of hydrocarbons is estimated as negligible (Howard and Blomquist, 1982). The alteration and variation of the cuticular hydrocarbons with age is another explanation of the results seen. Extensive studies on laboratory reared mosquitoes have shown that age affects only the total hydrocarbon content. Species separation by this technique is based on differences in specific peaks, never an overall reduced quantity in one species compared to another. A recently emerged fly contains the same compounds as a week old fly but in reduced amount. In mosquitoes two hours after emergence, the full complement of compounds is present at a concentration that remains stable for at least two weeks. Studies on laboratory reared P.ariasi demonstrated the presence of age differences (between 1- and 7-day old flies). However, the peaks which were determined as characteristic for sylvatic and domestic populations were unaffected by this age difference.

The temperature and humidity of the environment might also be expected to influence the cuticular hydrocarbon composition, but no significant differences in the type or amount of hydrocarbons present has been seen in specimens of the same species taken from very different habitats (e.g. desert, savanna and forest zones). This is consistent for all vector species studied to date. Therefore, age of fly, diet and environmental conditions are not thought to greatly influence the composition of the cuticular wax. It is important to note, however, that sampling of specimens can introduce bias and care must be taken to ensure that the description of distinct populations is not the result of the discreet sampling of a continuous distribution.

The species specificity of hydrocarbons cannot be explained solely by their role as waterproofing compounds. The list of functions attributed to hydrocarbons in insects does, however, suggest that their expression and production is precisely controlled; they function as caste recognition cues, pheromones, aphrodisiacs etc. (Howard and Blomquist, loc.cit.).

Our studies on a range of vector species have suggested that hydrocarbons may also function as surface compounds in the identification of potential mates. Recent work on Anopheles gambiae s.l. suggests that there is close association between karyotype and the expression of a particular hydrocarbon profile (Phillips et al., 1987). However, although hydrocarbon specificity can be used as a taxonomic tool, the interpretation of the biological significance of this specificity is speculative at present.

The future of cuticular hydrocarbon analysis for sandfly identification will involve the continuation and extension of existing studies and the initiation of studies on other vector species complexes where identification of the vector is necessary to determine vectorial status and to investigate the epidemiology of disease transmission.

Further work on the genetic basis of hydrocarbon expression and their biological function as mate recognition markers is currently under way.

REFERENCES

Baimai, V., Green, C.A., Andre, R.G., Harrison, B.A. and Peyton, E.L. 1984. Cytogenetic studies of some species complexes of Anopheles in Thailand, S.E.Asia. S.E.Asian J.Trop.Med.Pub.Hlth. 51:536-546

Blomquist, G.J. and Jackson, L.L. 1973. Incorporation of labelled dietary n-alkanes into cuticular lipids of the grasshopper Melanoplus sanguinipes. J.Insect Physiol. 19:1639-1647

Carlson, D.A. and Service, M.W. 1980. Identification of mosquitoes of Anopheles gambiae species complex A and B by analysis of cuticular components. Science 207:1089-1091.

Carlson, D.A. and Walsh, J.F. 1981. Identification of two West African black flies (Diptera: Simuliidae) of the Simulium damnosum species complex by analysis of cuticular paraffins. Acta.trop.(Basel) 38:235-239.

Coluzzi, M. and Sabatini, A. 1967. Cytogenetic observaions on species A and B of the Anopheles gambiae complex. Parassitologia 9:73-88

Davidson, G. 1964. Anopheles gambiae, a complex of species. Bull.WHO. 31:625-634

Eglinton, G. and Hamilton, R.J. 1963. The distribution of alkanes in: "Chemical Plant Taxonomy", T. Swain ed. pp. 187-217. Academic Press.

Gale, K.R. and Crampton, J.M. 1987. DNA probes for species identification of mosquitoes in the Anopheles gambiae complex. Med.and Vet.Entomol. 1(2):127-136

Green, C.A. 1972. Cytological maps for the practical identification of females of the three freshwater species of the Anopheles gambiae complex. Ann.trop.Med.Parasit. 66:143-148

Hamilton, R.J. and Service, M.W. 1983. Value of cuticular and internal hydrocarbons for the identification of larvae of Anopheles gambiae Giles, Anopheles arabiensis Patton and Anopheles melas Theobald. Ann.trop.Med.Parasit. 77:203-210.

Howard, R.W. and Blomquist, G.J. 1982. Chemical ecology and biochemistry of insect hydrocarbons. Ann.Rev.Entomol. 27:149-172

Kamhawi, S., Molyneux, D.H., Killick-Kendrick, R., Milligan, P.J.M., Phillips A., Wilkes T.J. and Killick-Kendrick, M. 1987. Two populations of Phlebotomus ariasi in the Cévennes focus of leishmaniasis in the south of France revealed by analysis of cuticular hydrocarbons. Med. and Vet. Entomol. 1:97-102.

Lainson, L., Shaw, J.J. Ward, R.A. and Fraiha, H. 1973. Leishmaniasis in Brazil. IX. Considerations on the Leishmania braziliensis complex: importance of the sandflies of the genus Psychodopygus (Mangabeira) in the transmission of Le.braziliensis in north Brazil. Trans.R.Soc.trop.Med.Hyg. 67:184-196.

Lainson, R., Shaw, J.J., Ryan, L., Ribeiro, R.S.M. and Silveira, F.T. 1984. Presente situacao de leishmaniose visceral na Amazonia, com especial referencia a um novo surto da doenca ocorrido em Santarém, Estado do Pará, Brasil. Boletim Epidem.SESP. No. Especial Julho 8pp.

Lane, R.P. and Ward, R.D. 1984. The morphology and possible function of abdominal patches in males of two forms of the leishmaniasis vector Lutzomyia longipalpis (Diptera: Phlebotominae). Cah.ORSTOM., ser.Ent.med.et Parasitol. XXll No. 3: 245-249

Lane, R., Phillips, A., Molyneux, D.H., Procter, G. and Ward, R. 1985. Chemical analysis of the abdominal glands of two forms of Lutzomyia longipalpis: site of a possible sex pheromone? Ann.trop.Med.Parasit. 79:225-229.

Lane, R. and Ready, P.D. 1985. Multivariate discrimination between Lutzomyia wellcomei the vector of mucocutaneous leishmaniasis and Lutzomyia complexus. Ann.trop.Med.Parasit. 79:469-472.

Lockey, K.H. 1985. Insect cuticular lipids. Comp.Biochem.Physiol. 81B:267-273

Mangabeira, O. 1969. Sobre a sistematica e biologia dos Phlebotomus do ceara. Revta bras.Malar Doenc.trop. 21:3-26.

Milligan, P.J.M., Phillips A., Molyneux, D.H., Subbarao, S.K. and White, G.B. 1986. Differentiation of Anopheles culicifacies Giles (Diptera: Culicidae) sibling species by analysis of cuticular components. Bull.ent.Res. 76:529-537.

Meredith, S.E.O and Townson, H. 1981. Enzymes for species identification in the Simulium damnosum complex from West Africa. Tropenmed.Parasit. 32:123-129.

Miles, S.J. 1979. A biochemical key to adult members of the Anopheles gambiae group of species (Diptera:Culicidae). J.Med.Ent. 15:297-299.

Nelson, D.R., Sukkestad, D.R. and Terranova, A.C. 1971. Hydrocarbon composition of the integument, fat body, haemolymph and diet of the tobacco hornworm. Life Sci. 10:411-419.

Phillips, A., Walsh, J.F., Garms, R., Molyneux, D.H., Milligan, P. and Ibrahim, G.H. 1985. Identification of adults of the Simulium damnosum complex using hydrocarbon analysis. Tropenmed.Parasit. 36:97-101

Phillips, A. and Milligan, P. 1986. Cuticular hydrocarbons distinguish sibling species of vectors. Parasit.Today. 2:180-181.

Phillips, A., Ward, R., Ryan, L., Molyneux, D.H., Lainson, R. and Shaw, J.J. 1986. Chemical analysis of compounds extracted from the tergal "spots" of Lutzomyia longipalpis from Brazil. Acta trop. (Basel) 43:271-276.

Phillips, A., Milligan, P.J., Coluzzi, M., Toure, Y., Broomfield, G. and Molyneux, D.H. 1987. Studies on the chromosomal forms of Anopheles gambiae s.str. and A.arabiensis using cuticular hydrocarbon analysis. Abstract 3rd International Conference on Malaria and Babesiosis. 7-11th September 1987, Annecy, France. International Laveran Foundation.

Phillips, A., Maroli, M., Kamhawi, S., Milligan, P.J. and Lane, R. (in prep.). Intraspecific variation in the cuticular hydrocarbons of Italian Phlebotomus perfiliewi (Diptera:Psychodidae).

Phillips, A. and Molyneux, D.H. (in prep.). Marker cuticular hydrocarbons in female Psychodopygus squamiventris s.str. (Diptera:Psychodidae).

Ready, P.D. and da Silva, R.M.R. 1984. An alloenzymic comparison of Psycholopygus wellcomei - an incriminated vector of Leishmania braziliensis in Pará State, Brazil - and the sympatric morpho-species Ps.complexus (Diptera, Psychodidae). Cah.ORSTOM ser.Ent.Med.parasit. 22:3-8.

Ready, P.D. (this volume). DNA polymorphisms as genotypic markers for Phlebotomus vectors of Leishmania.

Rioux, J.A., Golvan, Y.J., Croset, H., Tour, S., Houin, R., Abonnenc, E., Petitdidier, M., Vollhardt, Y., Dedet, J.P., Albaret, J.L., Lanotte, G. and Quilici, M. 1969. Epidémiologie des leishmanioses dans le Sud de la France. Monographie INSERM, No. 37.

Ryan, L., Silveira, F.T., Lainson, R. and Shaw, J.J. 1984. Leishmania infections in Lutzomyia longipalpis and L.antunesi (Diptera:Psychodidae) on the Island of Marajó, Para State, Brazil. Trans.R.Soc.trop.Med.Hyg. 78:547-548.

Ryan, L., Phillips A., Milligan, P., Lainson, R., Molyneux, D.H. and Shaw, J.J. 1986. Separation of female Psychodopygus wellcomei and P.complexus (Diptera:Psychodidae) by cuticular hydrocarbon analysis. Acta trop.(Basel) 43:85-89

Sang, D. 1987. Studies on cutaneous Leishmaniasis in Kenya. PhD thesis. University of Liverpool.

Shelley, A.J., Luna dias, A.P.A., Moraes, M.A.P. and Procunier, W.S. 1987. The status of Simulium oyapockense and Simulium limbatum as vectors of human onchocerciasis in Brazilian Amazónia. Med.Vet.Entom. 1(3):219-234

Townson, H.J., Post R. J. and Phillips A. (in press). Biochemical approaches to blackfly taxonomy, in: "Blackflies: Ecology and Population Management". K.C. Kim and R.W. Merritt eds. Penn State Press.

Vajime, C. G. and Dunbar, R. W. 1975. Chromosomal identification of eight species of the subgenus Edwardsellum Near and including Simulium (Edwardsellum) damnosum Theobald (Diptera: Simuliidae). Tropenmed. Parasit. 26:111-138

Ward, R.D., Phillips, A., Burnet, B. and Brisola, C.M. (in press). The Lutzomyia longipalpis complex: reproduction and distributiuon. In: Biosystematics of Haematophagous Insects. (ed. M. Service). Oxford University Press.

Ward, R.D., Bettini, S., Maroli, M., McGarry, J.W. and Draper, A. 1981. Phosphoglucomutase polymorphism in *Phlebotomus perfiliewi perfiliewi* Parrot (Diptera:Psychodidae) from central and northern Italy. Ann.trop.Med.Parasit. 75:653-661.

Ward, R.D., Ribeiro, A.L., Ready, P.D., and Murtagh, A. 1983. Reproductive isolation between different forms of *Lutzomyia longipalpis* (Lutz and Neiva) (Diptera: Psychodidae), the vector of *Leishmania donovani chagasi* Cunha and Chagas and its significance to Kala-azar distribution in South America. Mem.Inst.Osw.Cruz. 78:269-280.

Ward, R.D., Ribeiro, A.L., Ryan, L., Falcão, A.L. and Rangel, E.F. 1985. The distribution of two morphological forms of *Lutzomyia longipalpis* (Lutz and Neiva, 1912) (Diptera: Pyschodidae). Mem.Inst.Osw.Cruz. 80:145-148

World Health Organisation, 1984. The Leishmaniases. Report of a WHO Expert Committee, technical report series 701.

BIOASSAYS AS AN INDICATOR OF PHEROMONE COMMUNICATION IN

LUTZOMYIA LONGIPALPIS (DIPTERA: PSYCHODIDAE)

R.D. Ward, I. Morton, V. Lancaster, P. Smith and A. Swift

Department of Medical Entomology
Liverpool School of Tropical Medicine
Pembroke Place, Liverpool L3 5QA, U.K.

INTRODUCTION

The sandfly Lutzomyia longipalpis is the vector of Leishmania donovani chagasi, the causative organism of visceral leishmaniasis in Central and South America. The males have pale tergal spots on the abdomen, with some bearing one pair on the 4th segment, whilst others have partial or full development of an additional pair of spots on the 3rd segment. These spots are the sites of pheromone emission from glands which lie beneath the cuticle (Lane & Ward, 1984; Lane et al., 1985). Different populations produce different pheromones and these appear to act as sexual recognition signals which ensure mating between conspecific members of the Lu. longipalpis complex (Ward, 1983; 1986).

We have noted that when feeding our colonies of phlebotomines in the laboratory, male flies are strongly attracted to hosts and court blood-seeking females. Similarly in the field (Colombia), one of us (RDW) has observed large congregations of agitated, jostling males on the haunches of a dog infected with kala-azar. In the laboratory and in the natural circumstances described, male behaviour includes frequent wing vibration, which apart from sound production, may also function to disperse pheromones. These observations suggested that males produce the pheromone on the host to attract females for courtship and mating. The present paper describes two laboratory bioassays to determine if the pheromone functions in the way suggested. Some preliminary investigations into the stability of these semiochemicals are also described.

MATERIALS AND METHODS

The Olfactometer

The sandflies used were from a colony first established in 1973 with adults collected from Morada Nova, Ceará, Brazil. The males of this population have two complete pairs of pale tergal patches on abdominal segments III and IV and the pheromone is thought to be a diterpenoid with the molecular structure $C_{20}H_{32}$. The olfactometer was constructed with three 20cm^3 Barraud cages, joined by two 23cm lengths of 4.5cm diameter clear perspex tubes (Figs. 1 & 2). A current of air (34-37cm/sec) was drawn through the apparatus by a six-volt motor and fan, mounted in a 10cm diameter perspex tube, placed adjacent to cage 'A' (Fig. 2). The motor was powered by a single R20B dry cell battery mounted in a plastic food container.

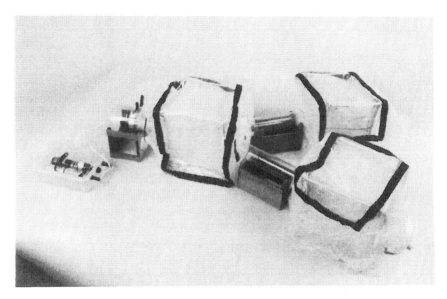

Fig. 1. A 3-cage olfactometer for testing the response of female
Lutzomyia longipalpis to (1) hamsters and male flies and
(2) hamsters and extracts of male pheromone gland.

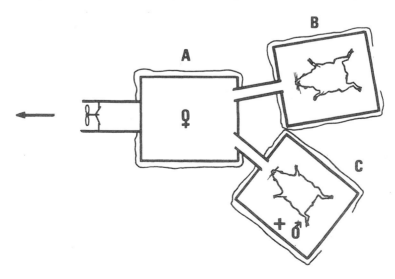

Fig. 2. Diagram of three-cage olfactometer.
A = Response cage   B = Control cage
C = Experimental cage

In the first series of experiments, virgin flies were obtained by isolating almost mature pupae in 2 x 4cm snap-cap vials and, following eclosion, the sexes were maintained in separate cages for 3-6 days. The flies were maintained in a 12:12 hour light/dark cycle. In six experiments, batches of 33-85 females (total of 384) were placed in cage 'A' and left at the beginning of the scotophase for an acclimatization period of 1 hour under reduced lighting conditions at $26^{\circ}C$ and 80% RH. During this period Clingfilm seals on the connecting tubes denied the insects access to cages 'B' and 'C'. In each experiment between 30 and 109 virgin males (total of 437) were placed in either cage 'B' or 'C'. Following the acclimatization period, an anaesthetised Syrian hamster was placed in each of the cages 'B' and 'C' and the Clingfilm seals were then broken, allowing random movement of the insects within the apparatus. These conditions were maintained for one hour in darkness and then the numbers of females that were in each of the three cages were recorded.

In a second series of experiments conditions were similar to those described above. In six experiments, a range of 31-99 virgin female flies (total of 417) were released into cage 'A'. However, males were replaced by an extract of the tergal glands absorbed onto a 2cm diameter filter paper disc. The extract was prepared by dissecting out the 3rd and 4th tergal segments of 8 males, which were then placed in 200µl of spectrophotometric grade hexane for 10 minutes. The extract disc was placed on the abdomen of one of the hamsters and a control disc moistened with 200µl of hexane was placed on the abdomen of the other animal.

Disc contacts

A series of disc contact bioassays was then developed to provide direct observations of sandfly behaviour in the presence of pheromone. We also wanted to examine the response of flies to different pheromone concentrations and determine if it remained biologically active following storage for a number of days. Sandflies used in the experiments were from the Morada Nova colony and from Sobral, Ceará, Brazil. Both populations have the diterpenoid-like pheromone. The sexes were maintained for 6-7 days in separate cages, provided with concentrated sucrose and held under a 12:12 light/dark regime at $26^{\circ}C$ and 80% RH. The bioassay was carried out using a $20cm^3$ cage containing 20 or 30 test flies and two anaesthetised Syrian hamsters, laid side by side on their backs. A pheromone extract disc was placed on the abdomen of one hamster and a control disc on the other (Fig. 3.). The number of contacts that flies made with each disc was then recorded during 30 minutes. Experiments were conducted 4 hours before the scotophase under conditions of $24^{\circ} \pm 1^{\circ}C$ and 60 $\pm$ 5% RH in a room illuminated with fluorescent lights.

To examine the effects of different pheromone extract concentrations, experimental discs prepared with 1 male/200µl of hexane and 8 males/200µl of hexane were compared with control solvent discs. Six experiments were carried out at each concentration. To study the effects of pheromone disc storage, fresh discs prepared with extracts of 2 males/200µl of hexane were compared with similar preparations that had been stored at $23^{\circ}C \pm 3^{\circ}C$ in closed vials for 1 and 6 days. In the six experiments, for each storage interval, the extract discs were compared with solvent discs. The response of males to extract made of 8 males in 200µl of hexane was also tested in a third series of experiments in which 30 males/ 6 trials were used.

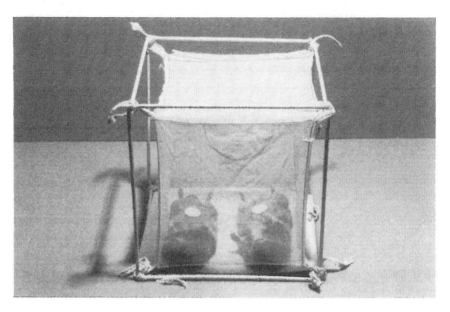

Fig. 3. Pheromone and control discs on the abdomens of hamsters during a bioassay.

RESULTS

The Olfactometer

In the first series of experiments over five times more female flies were attracted to the hamster when in the presence of male flies (Table 1; Fig. 4). Some of those females which are recorded as having failed to respond were blood-fed (12/123) and had therefore visited cage 'B' or 'C' and returned to cage 'A' during the experiment. At the end of the experiment over half of the males had also moved into cage 'A', although under 2% had moved into the other cage containing a hamster. In the second series of experiments, over eight times as many female flies were attracted to the hamster when in the presence of male tergal gland extract than to the hamster with the control solvent disc (Table 2; Fig. 5). In this experiment 163 females (39.1%) were recorded as failing to respond, although this included 41 which had fed and returned to cage 'A' during the experimental period.

Disc contacts

Most disc contacts were made by flies repeatedly hopping on and off discs. Long resting periods and intermittent wing vibration were observed when females were in contact with, or close to, the pheromone source. In the experiments to compare concentrations, the pheromone discs ranged from 3-8 times more attractive to females than control discs. Twice as many contacts were made with discs prepared from the extracts of 8 males than with those which included only 1 male (Table 3; Fig. 6a & b). Increased concentration of pheromone, despite raising the percentage pheromone disc contacts, did not show statistically significant differences between the two preparations at the 5% level.

Table 1. Response of female Lutzomyia longipalpis (Morada Nova colony) in an olfactometer to a hamster in the presence of male flies

No. females in response cage (A)	No. males in experimental cage (B or C)	No. females attracted to a hamster	No. females attracted to a hamster and male flies
68	94	0	36
62	78	3	26
33	40	1	9
82	86	13	42
85	109	9	70
54	30	14	38
384	437	40	221

Host vs Host + Males
(*N*=384)

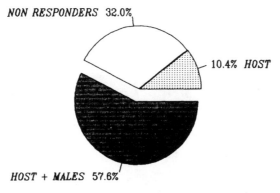

Fig. 4. Response of female Lutzomyia longipalpis in an olfactometer to hamsters with and without the presence of male flies

Table 2. Response of female Lutzomyia longipalpis (Morada Nova colony) in an olfactometer to a hamster in the presence of male tergal gland extract

No. females in response cage	No. of females attracted to a hamster with hexane on filter paper disc	No. of females attracted to a hamster with hexane gland extract on filter paper disc
99	12	45
90	5	52
89	1	54
77	1	46
31	2	19
31	7	10
417	28	226

Extract vs Solvent
Discs on Hosts (N=417)

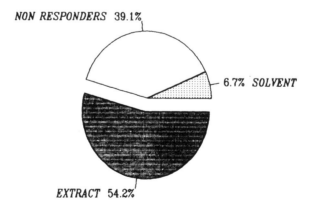

Fig. 5. Response of female Lutzomyia longipalpis in an olfactometer to hamsters in the presence of a male pheromone gland extract disc and a control solvent disc

In the second series of experiments to examine the effect of disc storage, the responses of females was 8-10 times greater than to the control discs. Pheromone discs that had been stored for 6 days were significantly ($P<0.05$) more attractive to females than freshly prepared discs (Table 3; Fig. 6c, d & e). In the experiment to test male response to male gland extract there was no significant difference, with 154 contacts on the pheromone disc and 156 on the control. The greater number of adults used (30) and territorial skirmishes on and around the discs probably account for the large number of disc contacts recorded.

DISCUSSION

Olfactometers were developed to produce quantitative and objective measurements of insect responses to odours. They have been used, for example, to investigate the responses of fruit flies to fermenting fruit and of male houseflies to pseudoflies moistened in solvent extracts of females (Wright, 1966; Rogoff et al., 1964). Bioassays of pheromone discs similar to that described in the present work, have been used to investigate the biological activity of pheromones of the Queensland fruitfly Dacus tryoni (Fletcher, 1969).

The attraction of sandflies to pheromones has only been studied previously in Israel where Schlein et al. (1984) found that Phlebotomus papatasi females appear to produce an aggregation pheromone. Chaniotis (1967) observed that Lutzomyia vexator occidentis adults of both sexes are attracted to hosts and speculated that these may act as meeting sites for sexual behaviour. Similarly, Beach et al. (1983) commented that sexual behaviour in some sandflies in Kenya was most intensive in the presence of a blood source. Other observations have, however, described sexual activity on the surface of rocks by P. orientalis (Molyneux & Ashford, 1983) and when adults of P. ariasi were attracted to a light source (Baudrimont, 1946). The function of these male aggregations, whether on hosts or inanimate objects, may be similar to the leks observed in the Queensland fruitfly Dacus tryoni (Tychsen & Fletcher, 1971). The immediate increase in flight activity and subsequent wing fluttering observed in these experiments, following the introduction of hosts and pheromone discs into cages, are typical responses to sex attractants. Females rested on and around the discs for long periods, suggesting that the pheromone apart from acting as an attractant with host odour, may also be an arrestant similar to some cockroach pheromones (Roth, 1969). The pheromone/host odour was effective in attracting females over relatively short distances up to 60cm and it remains to be determined if they are active over a much wider range. The results also show that discs impregnated with tergal gland extract are biologically active for at least six days. The bioactivity is enhanced by storage possibly due to some oxidative process. For example, the males of the yellow-headed spruce sawfly Pikonema alaskensis respond to the oxidation products of the female pheromone (Bartelt & Jones, 1983). Although males are not preferentially attracted to hosts in the presence of male extract, it is not known if pheromone concentration in the lek regulates release rates of the semiochemical, as it does in the Caribbean fruitfly Anastrepha suspensa (Nation, 1987).

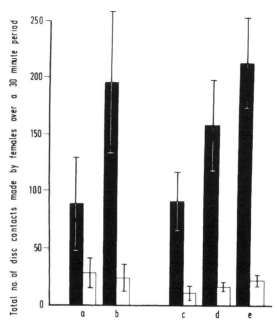

Fig. 6. The number of contacts made by 20 female Lu. longipalpis over a 30-minute period to pheromone gland extract discs of different concentrations - a = 1 male/200μl hexane   b = 8 males/200μl hexane and discs of different ages - c = 0 hours   d = 1 day   e = 6 days. Pheromone discs (black); Control discs (white) and vertical lines are standard errors.

Table 3. The number of contacts by female Lu. longipalpis with discs containing male tergal gland extract at different concentrations and after storage for different periods. Tergal segments were extracted in 200μl of hexane

Males/extract	Age of disc	Replicates	No. of contacts Extract (%)	Control (%)	P
1	0	8	88 (77)	27 (23)	NS
8	0	6	196 (89)	23 (11)	<0.05
2	0	7	91 (87)	11 (13)	<0.05
2	1 day	6	159 (91)	16 (9)	<0.01
2	6 days	6	214 (91)	22 (9)	<0.01

REFERENCES

Bartelt, R.J. and Jones, R.L., 1983, (Z)-nonadecenal, a pheromonally active air oxidation product of (Z,Z)-9, 19 dienes in the yellow headed spruce sawfly, J. Chem. Ecol., 9: 1333.

Baudrimont, A., 1946, Nouvelles observations sur la presence de Phlebotomus Tonnoir, 1921 a Saint Sauveur (Haute Pyrenees), Arch. Soc. Linn. Bordeaux, 95: 1-4.

Beach, R., Young, D.G. and Mutinga, M.J., 1983, New phlebotomine sandfly colonies: Rearing Phlebotomus martini, Sergentomyia schwetzi and Sergentomyia africana (Diptera: Psychodidae), J. Med. Entomol., 20: 579.

Chaniotis, B.N., 1967, The biology of California Phlebotomus (Diptera: Psychodidae) under laboratory conditions, J. Med. Entomol., 20: 221.

Fletcher, B.S., 1969, The structure and function of the sex pheromone glands of the male Queensland fruit fly, Dacus tryoni, J. Insect Physiol., 15: 1309.

Lane, R. and Ward, R.D., 1984, The morphology and possible function of abdominal patches in males of two forms of the leishmaniasis vector Lutzomyia longipalpis (Diptera: Phlebotominae), Cah. O.R.S.T.O.M. ser. Ent. Med. et Parasitol., 22: 245.

Lane, R., Phillips, A., Molyneux, D.H., Procter, G. and Ward, R.D., 1985, Chemical analysis of the abdominal glands of two forms of Lutzomyia longipalpis: site of a possible sex pheromone?, Ann. Trop. Med. Parasit., 79: 225-229.

Molyneux, D.H. and Ashford, R.W., 1983, The biology of Trypanosoma and Leishmania, parasites of man and domestic animals, Taylor and Francis, London.

Nation, J.L., 1987, Chemical and behavioural ecology of pheromone releases by male Carribean fruit flies, Abstract - 4th Meeting of the International Society of Chemical Ecology, Hull University.

Rogoff, W.M., Beltz, A.D., Johnsen, J.O. and Plapp, F.W., 1964, A sex pheromone in the house fly Musca domestica, J. Insect Physiol., 10: 239.

Roth, L.M., 1969, The evolution of male tergal glands in the Blattaria, Ann. Entomol. Soc. Amer., 62: 176.

Schlein, Y., Yuval, B. and Warburg, A., 1984, Aggregation pheromone released from the palps of feeding female Phlebotomus papatasi (Psychodidae), J. Insect Physiol., 30: 153.

Tychsen, P.H. and Fletcher, B.S., 1971, Studies on the rhythm of mating in the Queensland frut fly Dacus tryoni, J. Insect Physiol., 17: 2139.

Ward, R.D., 1986, Mate recognition in a sandfly (Diptera: Psychodidae), J. Roy. Army Cps., 132.

Ward, R.D., Ribeiro, A.L., Ready, P. and Murtagh, A., 1983, Reproductive isolation between different forms of Lutzomyia longipalpis (Lutz & Neiva), (Diptera: Psychodidae), the vector of Leishmania donovani chagasi Cunha & Chagas and its significance to kala-azar distribution in South America, Mems. Inst. Oswaldo Cruz, 78: 269.

Wright, R.H., 1966, An insect olfactometer, Canad. Entomol., 98: 282.

WHY MEASURE THE VECTORIAL CAPACITY OF SANDFLIES?

Christopher Dye

Department of Entomology
London School of Hygiene & Tropical Medicine
Keppel Street, London WC1E 7HT

INTRODUCTION

Lysenko & Beljaev [1], among others, have recently proposed that the malariologist's concept of Vectorial Capacity will occupy a central place in future quantitative studies of leishmaniasis. The Vectorial Capacity should have an important role to play because the malarias and the leishmaniases have much in common, particularly in their mode of transmission. The vectors are flies which have cycles of bloodfeeding and egg-laying. The parasite has a latent period in the fly which may be quite long relative to the fly's life expectancy. Further, although the leishmaniases are noted for their broad taste in vertebrate hosts, some species of Leishmania in some places have, in common with human Plasmodium species, just one principal vertebrate host which is infectious to the vector. Indian and Kenyan Le. donovani are examples.

However, in adopting, and adapting, this collection of ideas, phlebotomists must first be aware of the limitations. Turning to the malaria literature, they will find numerous references to the classic theoretical work of Macdonald [2] and Garrett-Jones [3-6]. My aim in this paper is to outline the strengths and weaknesses of this body of work - particularly of Garrett-Jones' approach to 'epidemiological entomology'- and the consequences for its application to the leishmaniases.

VECTORIAL CAPACITY: A FRAMEWORK FOR 'EPIDEMIOLOGICAL ENTOMOLOGY'

After Macdonald had drawn attention to the importance of some entomological components, notably mosquito survival rate, Garrett-Jones set out to measure them. To assess the rate of transmission by a vector, and hence the success of vector control, he proposed estimating the Vectorial Capacity, C. He defined [3] C as the average number of inoculations with a specified parasite, originating from one case in unit time, that the population would distribute to man if all the vector females biting the case became infected. The index is essentially the maximum daily case reproductive rate of the parasite. Macdonald's model provided a method of estimation:

$$C = ma^2 p^n / -\log_e p \qquad (1)$$

simply uses the entomological components of his expression for the basic reproductive rate, R. Here m is the number of flies per person, p is the daily survival rate of an adult female, and n is the latent period of the parasite in that female. a is the daily biting rate of a fly on any host multiplied by the probability that the host is man. The latter is measured by the Human Blood Index (HBI). Though equation (1) was conceived for anopheline mosquitoes, it could apply equally to a sandfly which transmits <u>Leishmania</u> among the individuals of one kind of vertebrate host.

This clarification of the relationship between entomological variables has been of enormous conceptual value. For example, it is now very widely understood why insecticidal attack on adult survival rate should be a particularly effective way of reducing transmission [7].

In its quantitative role, however, the Vectorial Capacity has been less useful than expected. It was hoped, first of all, that estimates of Vectorial Capacity would conform closely with Garrett-Jones' definition. But the real goal was to use Vectorial Capacity, together with the per capita rate of human recovery, r, to calculate the basic reproductive rate of the parasite [6],

$$R = C/r \qquad (2)$$

It would then be clear what reduction in C was required to force R below (or equal to) 1, whereupon the parasite would die out of the community.

As malaria eradication was never achieved in countries like Nigeria where the measurements were made, estimates of C and R were not put to that test. Nonetheless, the utility of such estimates must now be held in considerable doubt. Much recent work has questioned the assumptions which underpin equations (1) and (2). Furthermore, whilst considerable progress has been made in parameter estimation since the 1960's - notably of the survival rate of adult flies [8] - accuracy still cannot always, or even usually, be guaranteed.

ASSUMPTIONS WHICH UNDERPIN THE VECTORIAL CAPACITY

The first column in Table 1 shows some of the important assumptions which are made in using equation (1) to calculate Vectorial Capacity. Most have been questioned in malariology [9,10]; the second column lists the ways in which they are known to be, or are probably, violated by sandflies. Sometimes, simple modifications to equation (1) can accommodate known departures from the usual assumptions, without serious loss of tractability (ref. in 10). Often, they cannot. Note also that the definition of Vectorial Capacity inherently assumes that all flies biting a case become infected. In fact, individuals with <u>Leishmania</u> parasites have very variable abilities to infect sandflies [11]. The efficiency of transmission from vertebrate to invertebrate must be accounted for somewhere in transmission models.

Table 1. Assumptions behind estimation of the Vectorial Capacity by equation (1), with examples of how they are violated by sandflies.

Assumption	Violation
Parasite has one identifiable type of invertebrate host	Cryptic kinds of vector [12,13,14]
Parasite has one type of infectious vertebrate host	Two or more kinds of vertebrate become infectious with one kind of parasite [15]
Daily survival rate of vectors is constant with respect to time, age and infection	Survival rate may decline in presence of parasite [16], and may be best considered per feeding cycle [17]
Individual flies in a population take bloodmeals from vertebrate host at random	Biting rate depends on characteristics of individual hosts eg location, age/size etc
Flies take a fixed number of bloodmeals per unit time	Number of attempted bloodmeals increases with presence of parasite [18,19]
Susceptible vertebrates always acquire infection (and become infectious) after a bite by a fly harbouring infective forms	Is the probability of infection usually less than one? [20]

Table 2. On the problems of estimating parameters and variables in equation (1).

Parameter/variable	Comment
Man-biting rate (light/sticky trap/resting catches give indices of fly abundance [17, 21-25]	Measurements are at best proportional to the true biting rate.
Human Blood Index (bloodmeal analyses [24, 26, 27])	Difficult to sample fed flies representatively in different habitats
Duration of feeding cycle [28]	Relatively easy to measure when cycles coherent eg in stable weather
Survival rate [17, 29]	Must be measured relatively accurately as C is sensitive to change in p.
Latent period of parasite (refs. in 20)	Relatively easy to measure, but beware temperature sensitivity

ACCURACY OF ESTIMATES

Table 2 indicates the relative tractability of parameters and variables in equation (1). Numbers in the first column refer to some of the studies which have attempted to measure the parameters and variables of sandfly transmission. Comments in the second column are stimulated mainly by experience in malariology [9,10].

MACDONALD'S MODEL

The problems arising from violated assumptions and difficult measurements apply with equal force to the parasitological component of Macdonald's model. There is still no good estimate of r, the per capita recovery rate, which adequately encompasses the temporal distribution of infectiousness of a case of falciparum malaria. As the clinical manifestations of infection with Leishmania are generally more variable than those of Plasmodium, we can expect r to be even less tangible for the leishmaniases.

IMPLICATIONS: THREE KINDS OF ENTOMOLOGICAL MEASUREMENTS

These last three sections make it plain that equation (1) gives an approximation to Garrett-Jones' Vectorial Capacity which is most unlikely to fulfil its original purpose: to act as an index of transmission which leads to an estimate of the basic reproductive rate.

How then can we improve confidence in, and the utility of, entomological measurements which are based on untested assumptions and made with unknown errors? I shall try to explain by identifying entomological measurements with three levels of utility:

1. Little progress will be made with isolated measurements of Vectorial Capacity and its components at one time and one place. The relative magnitude of survival rate and latent period does give a guide to the sensitivity of C to changes in p. But single measures of survival and biting rates will be of limited generality - given the difficulties mentioned above, estimates could not be confidently applied to the same vector at another time or place.

2. Comparative measurements more usefully show the _potential_ for differences in transmission from species to species, from time to time, or from place to place. But because entomological and parasitological variables are not usually linearly related (ref. 30 for an example in leishmaniasis), significant variation in the Vectorial Capacity may or may not induce variation in the incidence or prevalence of infection.

3. In general, entomological measurements will be most informative when made hand in hand with parasitological, demographic and clinical observations. By standardizing and matching measurements, we hope to create a coherent framework which tests the reliability of those measurements, and which provides epidemiological explanations and predictions with known confidence. It should also help with the allocation of scarce resources in field monitoring.

Dynamic population models, which aim at precision and reality, will provide the most sophisticated form of matching. In leishmaniasis, these are likely to be as elusive as the animal reservoir of Indian kala-azar. Nonetheless, we must work in that direction because entomological observations will always be more useful when made in an epidemiological context.

As yet, it is hard to find quantitative 'epidemiological entomology' in the leishmaniasis literature. However, two studies of Kenyan and Indian kala-azar go some way towards illustrating the value of making entomological observations in context.

The first uses temporal data. Southgate[31] compared seasonal changes in the abundance of the sandfly Phlebotomus martini and kala-azar cases in the Kitui District of Kenya. He found a strong correlation between the two time series when the first was lagged by six months. He thus showed that entomological measurements really were a good index of transmission, and that the incubation period was about six months.

The second uses spatial data. Examining the incidence of kala-azar cases in a group of villages near Calcutta, Kermack & McKendrick[32] found that the chance of infection arising in a household was proportional to the square root of the number of occupants, n. To explain this, they conjectured that sandflies moved randomly throughout the villages, and that people lived in houses which could be thought of as cylinders (or at least objects of the same height and shape) in which the number of occupants was proportional to volume. If the chance of a sandfly entering a house depends on the surface area of its walls (which governs the number of windows and doors), then the probability that an infection arises in the house will indeed vary proportionally with root n. Matched entomological data could give additional confidence in sandfly measurements, and help to test the idea. A significant regression of incidence against sandfly density would reject the hypothesis. Did the density of sandflies per household in fact vary with root n?

CONCLUSIONS

Estimates of the Vectorial Capacity (and its components) are based on observations which are technically difficult to make, and which commonly rely on untested assumptions. They cannot be trusted to measure precisely the rate of parasite transmission by a vector population.

The performance of entomological measurements is better judged by standardizing and matching against coincident parasitological, demographic and clinical observations. They then become part of a framework whose coherence tests the propriety of its components. It further gives epidemiological explanations, and makes predictions with known confidence.

Dynamic mathematical models provide the most sophisticated framework for interpreting the interplay between vectors, parasites and vertebrate hosts. But any more modest comparison which tests the expected relation between vectors and parasites promises to be of greater value than either set of observations alone.

REFERENCES

1. A.J. Lysenko and A.E. Beljaev, Quantitative epidemiology, in: "The Leishmaniases, Volume 1," W. Peters and R. Killick-Kendrick, eds., Academic Press, London (1986).
2. G. Macdonald, "The Epidemiology and Control of Malaria," Oxford University Press, London (1957).
3. C. Garrett-Jones, Prognosis for the interruption of malaria transmission through assessment of the mosquito's vectorial capacity, Nature 204:1173 (1964).
4. C. Garrett-Jones, The human blood index of malaria vectors in relation to epidemiological assessment, Bull. World Health Org. 30:241 (1964).
5. C. Garrett-Jones and B. Grab, The assessment of insecticidal impact on the malaria mosquito's vectorial capacity, from data on the proportion of parous females, Bull. World Health Org. 31:37 (1964).
6. C. Garrett-Jones and G.R. Shidrawi, Malaria vectorial capacity of a population of Anopheles gambiae, Bull. World Health Org. 40:531 (1969).
7. D.J. Bradley, Epidemiological models - theory and reality, in: "Population Dynamics of Infectious Diseases," R.M. Anderson, ed., Chapman and Hall, London (1982).
8. P.R. Holmes and M.H. Birley, An improved method for survival rate analysis from time series of haematophagous dipteran populations, J. Anim Ecol. 56:427 (1987).
9. L. Molineaux and G. Gramiccia, "The Garki Project," World Health Organization, Geneva (1980).
10. C. Dye, Vectorial Capacity: must we measure all its components?, Parasit. Today 2:203 (1986).
11. J.-A. Rioux, G. Lanotte, H. Croset and J.-P. Dedet, Écologie des leishmanioses dans le sud de la France 5. Pouvoir infestant comparé des diverses formes de leishmaniose canine vis-à-vis de Phlebotomus ariasi Tonnoir, 1921, Ann. Parasit. 47:413 (1972).
12. R.D. Ward, A.L. Ribeiro, P.D. Ready and A. Murtagh, Reproductive isolation between different forms of Lutzomyia longipalpis (Lutz & Neiva), (Diptera:Psychodidae), the vector of Leishmania donovani chagasi Cunha & Chagas and its significance to kala-azar distribution in South America, Mem. Inst. Oswaldo Cruz 78:269 (1983).
13. R. Lane and P.D. Ready, Multivariate discrimination between Lutzomyia wellcomi the vector of mucocutaneous leishmaniasis and Lutzomyia complexus, Ann. trop. Med. Parasit. 79:469 (1986).
14. D.M. Minter, Phlebotomus (Phlebotomus) celiae sp. nov. (Diptera, Psychodidae), a new sandfly from Kenya, Ann. trop. Med. Parasit. 56:457 (1962).
15. W. Peters and R. Killick-Kendrick, "The Leishmaniases," Academic Press, London (1986).
16. R.W. Ashford, M.A. Bray, M.P. Hutchinson and R.S. Bray, The epidemiology of cutaneous leishmaniasis in Ethiopia, Trans. Roy. Soc. Trop. Med. Hyg. 67:568 (1973).
17. C. Dye, M.W. Guy, D.B. Elkins, T.J. Wilkes and R. Killick-Kendrick, The life expectancy of phlebotomine sandflies: first field estimates from southern France, Med. & Vet. Ent. 1:417 (1987).
18. R. Beach, G. Kilu and J. Leeuwenburg, Modification of sandfly biting behaviour by Leishmania leads to increased parasite transmission, Am. J. Trop. Med. Hyg. 34:279 (1985).
19. R. Killick-Kendrick, A.J. Leaney, P.D. Ready and D. Molyneux, Leishmania in phlebotomid sandflies. IV. The transmission of Leishmania mexicana amazonensis to hamsters by the bite of experimentally infected Lutzomyia longipalpis, Proc. Roy. Soc. London B 196:105 (1977).
20. R. Killick-Kendrick, The transmission of leishmaniasis by the bite of the sandfly, J. Roy. Army Med. Corps 132:134 (1986).

21. W.A. Foster, Studies on leishmaniasis in Ethiopia III: Resting and breeding sites, flight behaviour, and seasonal abundance of Phlebotomus longipes (Diptera:Psychodidae), Ann. trop. Med. Parasit. 66:313 (1972).
22. J.-A. Rioux, R. Killick-Kendrick, J. Perieres, D.-P. Turner and Lanotte, Écologie des leishmanioses dans le sud de la France 13. Les sites de "flanc de coteau", biotopes de transmission privilégiés de la leishmaniose viscérale en Cévennes, Ann. Parasit. 55:445 (1980).
23. J.-A. Rioux, J. Perieres, R. Killick-Kendrick, G. Lanotte, and M. Bailly, Écologie des leishmanioses dans le sud de la France 17. Échantillonage des phlebotomes par le procédé des pièges adhesifs. Comparison avec la technique de capture sur appât humain, Ann. Parasit. 57:631 (1982).
24. A.K. Hati, Current status of leishmaniasis - vector biology, in: "Proceedings of the Indo-UK Workshop on Leishmaniasis," Indian Council for Medical Research, Delhi (1983).
25. J.C. Beier, B.M. El Sawaf, A.I. Merdan, S. El Said and S. Doha, Sandflies (Diptera:Psychodidae) associated with visceral leishmaniasis in El Agamy, Alexandria Governorate, Egypt I. Population ecology, J. Med. Entomol. 23:600 (1986).
26. W.A. Foster, P.F.L. Boreham and C.H. Tempelis, Studies on leishmaniasis in Ethiopia. IV: Feeding behaviour of Phlebotomus longipes (Diptera: Psychodidae), Ann. trop. Med. Parasit. 66:433 (1972).
27. M.W. Guy, R. Killick-Kendrick, G.S. Gill, J.-A. Rioux and R.S. Bray, Ecology of leishmaniasis in the south of France 19. Determination of the hosts of Phlebotomus ariasi Tonnoir, 1921 in the Cévennes by bloodmeal analyses, Ann. Parasit.Hum. Comp. 59:449 (1984).
28. R. Killick-Kendrick, T.J. Wilkes, J.-A. Rioux, C. Dye and E. Guilvard, Ecology of leishmaniasis in the south of France 22. Field observations on gonotrophic concordance and variations in the length of the gonotrophic cycle of Phlebotomus ariasi Tonnoir,1921 in the Cévennes,unpub.
29. A.V. Dolmatova, Geography, biology and ecology of sandflies (Phlebotominae) in the USSR, unpublished (1967).
30. C. Dye, The epidemiology of canine visceral leishmaniasis in southern France: classical theory offers another explanation of the data, Parasitology in press.
31. B.A. Southgate, The structure of foci of visceral leishmaniasis in north-eastern Kenya, in: "Écologie des Leishmanioses," Colloques Internationaux du CNRS, Paris (1977).
32. W.O. Kermack and A.G. McKendrick, Mathematical analysis of Dr. Napier's statistics of house infection in kala-azar, Ind. J. Med. Res. 19:343 (1931).

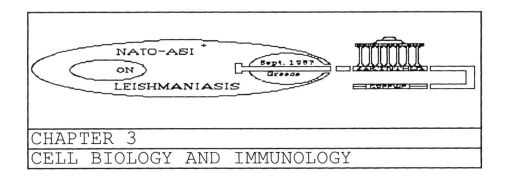

CHAPTER 3
CELL BIOLOGY AND IMMUNOLOGY

CELL BIOLOGY AND IMMUNOLOGY OF LEISHMANIASIS

F.E.G. Cox

Department of Biophysics, Cell and Molecular Biology
King's College London
26-29 Drury Lane
London   WC2B 5RL

The spectrum of diseases that collectively constitute leishmaniasis ranges from simple cutaneous lesions that heal spontaneously to mucocutaneous conditions with metastatic spread or visceral involvement in which spontaneous recovery is rare. In man, these forms of disease can be loosely assigned to particular species or subspecies of Leishmania but correlations are not absolute suggesting that the outcome of the infection depends on the immune response of the host as much as it does on the nature of the invading organism. This concept is well supported by experimental evidence and it is clear that in mice three species, Leishmania donovani, L. major and L. mexicana mexicana, cause infections that are determined by the genotype of the host. Research pioneered by Jenefer Blackwell, and reported upon in these proceedings, has actually shown that the outcome of the infections caused by all three species is determined by genes occurring at or near the murine H-11 locus (Roberts, Kaye, Milon and Blackwell). At another level, L. major infections self cure in CBA or C3H mice but are fatal and visceralize in BALB/C mice. The importance of these findings is that they show that susceptibility or resistance to leishmaniasis can be controlled by the host and, provided that the immune system can be directed against the invader, that vaccination against this disease is possible.

Vaccination itself is discussed elsewhere in this volume and many attempts have been made to vaccinate susceptible strains of mice against the commonly used species of Leishmania. Experimentally, vaccination is possible but unfortunately only if the vaccine is given intravenously or intraperitoneally whereas if given subcutaneously the same vaccine exacerbates infections and even reverses the effects of previous successful vaccinations. Because of this problem, there is no simple way in which a vaccine can be developed and it is unlikely that these can be one until the whole pattern of immunity to leishmaniasis, including the various regulatory circuits involved, have been thoroughly worked out. The majority of presentations in this session were devoted to unravelling the mysteries of the immune response to this disease.

From an experimental viewpoint, the infection is usually initiated by injecting promastigotes into the skin. Promastigotes grow well in vitro and become infective to host macrophages during the stationary phase of the culture, (Howard, Sayers and Miles). Infection of host macrophages involves recognition and internalization without stimulating

phase of the culture, (Howard, Sayers and Miles). Infection of host macrophages involves recognition and internalization without stimulating an oxidative burst. Attachment involves surface molecules of the promastigote as ligands and one or more receptor sites on the macrophage. One receptor that fulfills all the required criteria is that which recognises the inactivated form of complement factor 3, CR3, (Cooper, Wozencraft, Roach and Blackwell). The next requirement is for a promastigote surface molecule that might bind with a macrophage receptor. The surface antigens of promastigotes and amastigotes have received a vast amount of attention (Anthony, Sacci and Williams) and the list of those so far recognised is almost endless. Nevertheless, there are a few immunodominant antigens of which a glycoconjugate, gp63, ubiquitous on promastigotes and conserved in amastigotes, is important in the present context as it is increasingly expressed as the promastigotes reach the stationary infective phase in vitro and can act as a ligand for CR3. However, there is also another candidate molecule, a surface glycolipid, and the possible roles of each are discussed by Cooper et al.

Having gained access to the host macrophage, the parasites multiply and initiate either a fulminating infection or a short-lived infection followed by recovery and immunity to reinfection. Immunity to leishmaniasis is cellular and not humoral and can now be partly explained in terms of our increasing knowledge of the events that occur during the overall immune response particularly the regulatory cells and molecules involved. it is not clear whether or not infected macrophages act as antigen presenting cells (APC) but what is clear is that some kind of APC releases IL-1 which activates T cells with the L3T4+ phenotype. What happens then is again unclear but it is likely that such cells release a variety of mediators including interferon-gamma (IFN-τ) and colony stimulating factor (CSF) which activate further macrophages which in turn produce IL-1 , tumour necrosis factor (TNF) and reactive oxygen intermediates that are thought to be involved in both parasite killing and pathology (Cox). The role of L3T4+ cells is therefore a central one and this viewpoint is argued by McElrath, Murray and Cohn and by Louis and his colleagues (Pedrazzini, Kindler, Vassalli, Marchal, Milon and Louis). Louis suggests that there are two subsets of L3T4+ cells that are functionally heterogeneous, one favouring exacerbation and one favouring resolution, the actual outcome of the infection depending on the balance between them. Whether these subsets correspond with recently described subsets of helper T-cells, Th-1 and Th-2, is not clear. There is also increasing evidence that Lyt2+ cells may also be involved in the resolution of leishmanial infections as their depletion exacerbates the infections (Pedrazzini et al.). Roberts et al. also urge re-evaluation of the role of Lyt2+ cells.

Immunity to leishmaniasis, then, involves T-cells of probably two phenotypes and in order to understand how they function it is necessary to understand how they are activated and this is discussed by Kaye, Monroy-Ostria, Roach and Blackwell who have found that the T-cell response is brought about by an elevation of Class II molecules on resident and inflammatory macrophages and that this process involves IFN-τ. IFN-τ can render macrophages parasiticidal but in the case of leishmaniasis, it is only effective early during an infection (Kiderlen). Nevertheless, the potential use of IFN-τ cannot be ignored in light of the fact that one of the defects of susceptible BALB/C mice is a failure to produce IFN-τ (Farrell, Nolan, Croop and Kirkpatrick). Farrell's group also draws attention to populations of macrophages that suppress T-cell proliferation through the production of prostaglandins suggesting that these molecules also have a role in determining the outcome of leishmanial infectious.

Gradually as our overall understanding of the immune response becomes more comprehensive, it should be possible to consider the rational design of vaccines. Among others, two well studied surface molecules have been considered as possible candidates, gp63 and excreted factor (EF). A vaccine against gp63 should block macrophage invasion but the problem has been that the intravenous route of immunization is not acceptable. However, if L. mexicana gp63 is presented in liposomes it does confer protection if given subcutaneously to CBA mice but not BALB/C (Alexander and Russell). Excreted factor by itself produces a good antibody response but not a cell mediated response so therefore has little potential as a vaccine. EF is an excreted polysaccharide and certain other carbohydrate-rich molecules including carbohydrate-lipid containing fractions (CLF) have been shown to elicit cell mediated response and may be more promising than EF (Londner, Rosen, Frankenburg, Seviever and Greenblatt).

In summary, it is clear that the immunological processes involved in leishmaniasis are complex but that there is nothing involved that does not obey the rules of classical immunology. Gradually everything is falling into place and it is now apparent exactly what the problems are and what questions have to be asked. However, our understanding of the immune process in leishmaniasis is based on experiments in laboratory animals, mainly mice, carefully selected for their ability to respond (or not) to leishmanial antigens. A cautious approach to vaccination against human leishmaniasis is urged by Schnur who summarises past failures and future problems. Bearing these comments in mind and drawing on the wealth of experimental data available the way forward would seem to recognise the central role of L3T4+ T-cells, or their human equivalents, and to devise methods of redirecting the immune responses away from suppression and pathology towards leishmanicidal activity and immunity. In this context, the interacting roles of IFN-τ, TNF, CSF and prostaglandins cannot be ignored and as these molecules are involved in many diseases it might not be too optimistic to hope for some general purpose immunomodulators that would turn the balance of the immune response in favour of the host. Such universally available substances would reduce the possible costs which presently make anti-leishmania vaccines and drugs prohibitively expensive. The proceedings of this meeting do point to new strategies for both the control and amelioration of leishmaniasis possibly by the use of drugs that affect the regulation of the immune response in combination with more traditional vaccines and recombinant or synthetic cytokines. The future of vaccines is not quite as dismal as Schnur suggests but who to vaccinate and when is also a problem for the epidemiologists.

STUDIES OF IMMUNE MECHANISMS IN H-11-LINKED GENETIC SUSCEPTIBILITY TO MURINE VISCERAL LEISHMANIASIS

Morven Roberts, Paul M Kaye, Genevieve Milon[*] and Jenefer M Blackwell

Department of Tropical Hygiene, London School of Hygiene and Tropical Medicine, Keppel Street, London WC1E 7HT, UK

INTRODUCTION

Previous studies have shown that congenic B10.129(10M) and C57BL/10ScSn (B10) mice, which differ only at H-11 and closely linked genetic loci, develop profoundly different disease phenotypes (noncure/nonhealing versus cure/healing) following infection with L. donovani[1,2], L. major[2] or L. mexicana[3], independently of the dose, route or stage of parasite inoculated. This was the first time that the same host resistance gene (or tight linkage group) had been shown to have parallel effects on all leishmanial infections (reviewed in reference 4). In immunological[2] terms the influence of H-11 was different too since, unlike Scl-controlled nonhealing responses to L. major[5] or H-2-controlled noncuring responses to L. donovani[6], sublethal irradiation of mice prior to infection failed to have a clear or consistent prophylactic effect. Although B10.129(10M) mice produced transient delayed-type hypersensitivity (DTH) reactions to parasite antigen early in L. major infection, the results overall suggested that this mouse strain possesses an inherent defect in ability to mount and/or sustain a good cell-mediated immune response effective at the level of macrophage antileishmanial activity in vivo. The ability to transfer both cure and noncure phenotypes in reciprocal radiation bone marrow chimaeras suggested that the primary cell population responsible for this defect was of haematopoietic origin. Studies presented here concentrate on in vitro functional analysis of the cell populations responsible for induction and maintenance of a cellular immune response, in particular to determine how early in infection the gene(s) manifests its effects on the development of specific immune responses, and to determine the secondary effects of this on the frequency and phenotype of the specific T cells generated as infection progresses.

MATERIALS AND METHODS

Mice

C57BL/10ScSn (or B10) ($H-2^b$, $H-11^a$) and B10.D2/n ($H-2^d$, $H-11^a$) mice were purchased at 4-6 weeks from Harlan Olac Ltd (Bicester, Oxon, UK)

---

[*]Address: Institut Pasteur, 28 Rue du Dr Roux, 75724 Paris Cedex 15

and maintained at the LSHTM. B10.129(10M) ($H-2^b$, $H-11^b$) mice were bred at the LSHTM from stock originally imported from the Jackson Laboratories (Bar Harbor, Maine, USA). Mice were used between 8-12 weeks of age and were age (+ 1 week) and sex matched within each experiment. C57BL/6 ($H-2^b$, $H-11^a$) mice used as recipients for DTH transfer were bred and maintained at the Institut Pasteur. B10 and B10.129(10M) mice used in these experiments were shipped from the LSHTM to Institut Pasteur 2 weeks prior to infection.

Parasites

Amastigotes of L. donovani LV9 were isolated from infected hamsters as described[7]. For infection in vivo mice were inoculated intravenously via the lateral tail vein with $2x10^7$ amastigotes.

In vitro bioassay for IL-2 responsiveness

An in vitro bioassay for IL-2 responsiveness in splenic T cells from infected mice was performed as described[8]. Total white cell populations were isolated over 21 days of infection from B10 versus B10.129(10M) mice. Cells were plated in quadruplicate at $5x10^5$/0.1ml RPMI in 96-well flat-bottomed plates (Flow Laboratories, Irvine, Ayshire, UK) and incubated with or without recombinant human IL-2 (50ng/ml SL2; Sandoz Ltd, Basle, Switzerland obtained from Dr M. Feldmann at the Charing Cross Sunley Research Centre, London, UK) for 18 hours at $37^{\circ}C$. Cells were harvested after a 6 hour pulse with tritiated thymidine (1uCi/well; 25Ci/mmol stock, Amersham International, Amersham, Bucks, UK).

Parasite-specific proliferation assays

Splenic adherent cells (SAC) were prepared from uninfected B10 and B10.129(10M) mice for use as antigen presenting cells (APC). Spleens were passed through a fine sieve, washed and red cells lysed with NH_4Cl/Tris pH7.2. White cell populations were washed (x3) in Hanks Balanced Salt Solution (HBSS) and incubated (1 hour; $37^{\circ}C$) in RPMI/5% heat-inactivated foetal calf serum in tissue culture flasks coated with 1% gelatin. Flasks were rinsed with warm HBSS to remove non-adherent cells and incubated at $4^{\circ}C$ to release the adherent cell population. Released adherent cells were harvested, irradiated (2000 rads), washed in RPMI and maintained at $37^{\circ}C$ in polypropylene tubes (Falcon) until required.

T cell responders were isolated and purified as described[8,9]. Responders were plated in triplicate at $2x10^5$/well in 96-well plates with different concentrations (10^5, $5x10^4$, $2x10^4$) of APC. Live amastigotes were added as antigen and titrated (10^6/well maximum) for each responder:presenting cell ratio. Plates were incubated for 96 hours at $37^{\circ}C$ and cells harvested following a 12 hour pulse with tritiated thymidine (1uCi/well; 5Ci/mmol stock).

Mixed Lymphocyte Reactions (MLR)

Irradiated (2000 rads) splenic white cell populations (stimulators) were prepared from uninfected and day 10 infected B10 and B10.129(10M) mice and titrated in triplicate (10^6/well maximum) against unirradiated splenic T cells (responders; $2x10^5$/well) from B10 or B10.D2/n mice. Plates were incubated for 90 hours at $37^{\circ}C$ and cells harvested following a 10 hour pulse with tritiated thymidine (1uCi/well; 5Ci/mmol stock).

Activation of macrophages for antileishmanial activity

Splenic adherent cells from uninfected B10 and B10.129(10M) mice obtained by 2 hour adherence to 13mm plastic coverslips (Lux Thermanox, Flow Laboratories) were infected with amastigotes for 1 hour at a ratio of 5 parasites:1 host cell. Noningested parasites were removed and relative uptake of parasites by macrophages from B10 versus B10.129(10M) mice assessed microscopically from methanol fixed, giemsa stained coverslips. Further coverslips were incubated with or without recombinant murine interferon gamma ($rIFN\gamma$, 25 units/ml, Genetech, obtained from Dr M. Feldmann) for 72 hours at $37^{\circ}C$ prior to fixation and staining. Parasites per 100 macrophages (Mean+SD) and percent macrophages infected were determined from quadruplicate coverslips, at least 1000 macrophages scored per coverslip.

Immunocytochemistry on liver cryosections

Expression of major histocompatibility complex (MHC, H-2) class II molecules (Ia) was monitored during infection for the two mouse strains on liver cryosections immunostained as described[10] using the anti-IA monoclonal antibody M5/114[11].

Limiting dilution analysis of T cells mediating DTH transfer

Limiting dilution analysis of $L3T4^+$ versus $Lyt-2^+$ T cells (purified from livers of day 16-100 infected mice) mediating antigen-specific transfer of DTH to C57BL/6 mice was carried out as described[12]. The subinflammatory dose of parasite antigen transferred with T cells was 3×10^5 LV9 stationary phase promastigotes. The number of specifically reactive T cells/organ was determined by interpolation at the 37% level of negative transfers using the minimum squares method.

RESULTS

Acquisition of IL-2 responsiveness

The ability of spleen cells from infected B10 and B10.129(10M) mice to respond to IL-2 in vitro is shown in figure 1. This bioassay, used

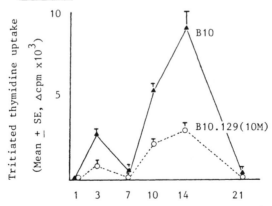

Figure 1. Measurement of in vivo T cell activation by the in vitro responsiveness to rIL-2 of splenic T cells isolated from B10 (▲) and B10.129(10M) (o) mice at different days after infection. Data (mean+SE) expressed as Δcpm [(cells + IL-2) - (cells - IL-2)].

here to detect activation of T cells in vivo, measures functional high affinity IL-2 receptor (IL-2R) expression independently of the presence of low affinity IL-2R and without bias for T cell subpopulations of different phenotypes[8]. For both strains of mice, a primary peak of IL-2 responsiveness was observed 3 days after infection with a second peak of higher magnitude at 11-14 days post infection. As we observe elsewhere[13], these waves of IL-2R expression are very similar to those observed in cloned populations in vitro suggesting synchronous T cell activation, the increased intensity of the second wave presumably reflecting an expanded range of available parasite antigens as well as an increase in the size of the responding T cell pool. Although similar patterns of IL-2 responsiveness were observed for the two mouse strains, the magnitude of the response in B10.129(10M) mice was lower throughout. Subsequent experiments were therefore designed to determine whether the B10.129(10M) strain was defective in antigen presenting cell function.

Antigen presenting cell function

Initially we compared the relative abilities of splenic adherent cells isolated from naive (i.e. uninfected) B10 and B10.129(10M) mice to act as APC in antigen-specific secondary proliferative assays using T cells isolated from day 6 infected B10 mice (figure 2). At 10^5 cells/well, B10.129(10M) SAC stimulated T cell proliferation but were clearly much less efficient than the equivalent numbers of B10 SAC. At lower numbers (5×10^4, 2×10^4/well), B10.129(10M) SAC failed to stimulate T cell proliferation. Hence there appeared to be a primary defect in the ability of adherent cells from naive B10.129(10M) mice to act as APC in this in vitro assay.

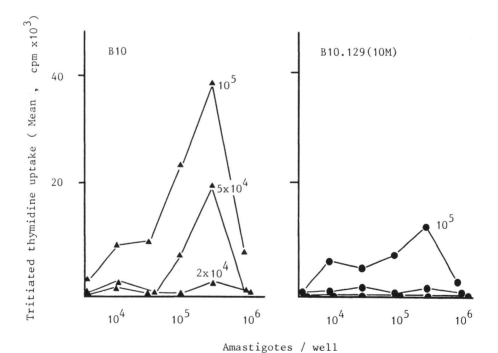

Figure 2. The ability of different numbers (as indicated) of splenic adherent cells from naive (uninfected) B10 (▲) and B10.129(10M) (●) mice to present amastigote antigen to splenic T cells from day 6 infected B10 mice in a standard secondary proliferation assay.

For these experiments it was important to establish that no primary MLR occurred between cells isolated from the two strains of mice. As had been well documented by other workers[14], the minor histocompatibility difference between B10 ($\underline{H-11^a}$) and B10.129(10M) ($\underline{H-11^b}$) mice failed to stimulate a primary MLR (figure 3a). In view of the defect in APC function in the B10.129(10M) mice shown above, we next considered whether this defect would also manifest itself in terms of the ability of cells from the two mouse strains to generate MLRs across an $\underline{H-2}$ barrier. As before, irradiated spleen cells from naive B10.129(10M) ($\underline{H-2^b}$) mice were less efficient than cells from B10 ($\underline{H-2^b}$) mice in stimulating MLR in unirradiated B10.D2/n ($\underline{H-2^d}$) spleen T cell populations (figure 3b). Within each mouse strain, irradiated splenic cells from day 10 infected mice stimulated higher MLRs (figure 3b) than cells from uninfected mice. Although recognition during MLR involves both class I and class II molecule expression, the 4-5 day MLR assay used here would preferentially measure class II molecule stimulated MLR[15]. Hence, the enhanced MLRs observed after infection most likely reflect upregulation of class II expression. As with stimulator cells from uninfected mice, the MLR elicited by B10.129(10M) stimulators was always lower than for equivalent numbers of B10 cells. Although class II molecule expression was enhanced in cryosections of livers from infected mice, it was not possible to quantify this accurately for the two strains. Nor were we able to detect gross differences in IA expression on splenic adherent cells using immunostaining techniques on coverslip preparations.

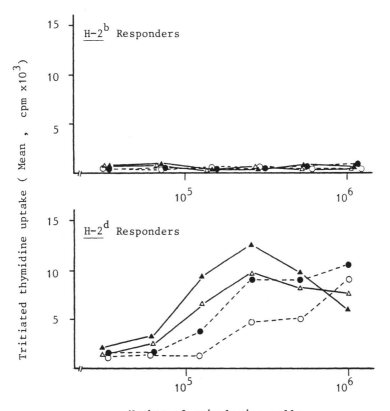

Number of stimulating cells

Figure 3. The ability of irradiated spleen cells from uninfected (open symbols) or infected (closed symbols) B10 (△,▲) or B10.129(10M) (○,●) mice to stimulate a primary MLR across (a) $\underline{H-11}$ or (b) $\underline{H-2}$ barriers.

rIFNγ activation for macrophage antileishmanial activity

Results obtained with APC from infected mice could be interpreted either as the reduced ability of cells from B10.129(10M) mice to respond to equivalent amounts of IFNγ in terms of upregulation of class II expression, or as reduced stimulation by macrophage activating lymphokines because of the lower primary activation of T cells observed. An inability to repond to IFNγ would also have important implications for antileishmanial activity of macrophages in vivo. In macrophage activation experiments performed in vitro using rIFNγ we observed that, although splenic macrophages from both mouse strains showed equivalent amastigote ingestion (47 ± 29 amastigotes/100 macrophages for B10 mice; 36 ± 9 for B10.129(10M)), rIFNγ-treated macrophages (160 ± 17) for B10.129(10M) mice failed to show any reduction in amastigote numbers relative to control (186 ± 47) at 72 hours post infection in vitro. rIFNγ-treated macrophages (70 ± 6) from B10 mice showed a significant ($p<0.002$) reduction in parasite numbers compared to control macrophages (170 ± 36). The same pattern was observed for the percent macrophages infected (data not shown). These results suggest that, in addition to their inability to act as APC, naive resident splenic macrophages from B10.129(10M) mice also fail to become leishmanicidal following rIFNγ activation in vitro.

Antigen-specific T cells in the livers of infected mice

In view of previous observations of an excess of antigen-specific T cells in the draining lymph nodes of nonhealing BALB/c mice infected with L. major[12], we were curious to determine what effect the early defect in antigen presenting cell function/T cell activation following L. donovani infection in B10.129(10M) mice would have on the later generation of antigen-specific T cells at the primary site of infection i.e. the liver. At day 16 post infection, the total number of hepatic T cells capable of mediating antigen-specific DTH transfer (table 1) was 3-fold higher in B10.129(10M) than B10 mice, the proportions of $L3T4^+$ versus $Lyt-2^+$ cells also differing for the two strains. A 3-fold increase in antigen-specific T cells in B10 mice at 30 days post infection was accompanied by a complete reversal in phenotype, from 100% $L3T4^+$ at day 16 to 100% $Lyt-2^+$ at day 30. This reversal in phenotype immediately preceeds the period of maximum resolution of parasite load in the liver in this self-curing mouse strain (data not shown). For B10.129(10M) mice, a drop in antigen-specific hepatic T cells was observed at day 30 with a subsequent rise later in infection accompanying the massive hepatosplenomegaly normally observed (data not shown). A 50:50 division of $L3T4^+:Lyt-2^+$ phenotypes was maintained throughout in the livers of infected B10.129(10M) mice. Hence, although the early defect in antigen presenting cell function/T cell activation pathways did not prevent the ultimate generation of large numbers of

Table 1. Limiting dilution analysis of T cells mediating DTH transfer from livers of infected B10 and B10.129(10M) mice.

DAY	B10		B10.129(10M)	
	T cells/liver	Phenotype	T cells/liver	Phenotype
16	30	100% L3T4	100	50% L3T4 50% Lyt-2
30	100	100% Lyt-2	40	50% L3T4 50% Lyt-2
100	232	34% L3T4 74% Lyt-2	450	50% L3T4 50% Lyt-2

antigen-specific T cells in B10.129(10M) mice, it did influence the kinetics and relative phenotypes of the T cells found at the primary site of infection.

DISCUSSION

Results presented here show that the primary defect associated with H-11-linked susceptibility to leishmanial infections in B10.129(10M) mice is measurable both at the level of reduced primary T cell activation early in infection in vivo, and as the reduced ability of splenic adherent cells from naive mice to act as antigen presenting cells in vitro for primed T cells. While the latter could be interpreted as a defect in antigen processing, the results for allopresentation suggest that the general inefficiency in presenting cell function may reflect differences in baseline levels of MHC class II molecule (Ia) expression. This in turn suggests that different levels of macrophage priming and/or activation are maintained in resident splenic macrophage populations in naive mice in vivo, a factor which might have broader implications for infections other than Leishmania and could be measured more precisely in terms of other well characterised priming and activation markers[16] in addition to a more precise quantification of Ia expression. To what extent these differences in baseline levels of macrophage priming or activation reflect the direct action of the minor histocompatibility locus (H-11) itself is at present unclear. Recent reports[17,18] in the literature suggest that minor histocompatibility loci coincide with endogenous retrovirial insertions into the mouse genome, which affect transcription and translation of genes encoding host molecules, e.g. Ia[17]. Hence, the differences in presenting cell function may reflect qualitative +/- quantitative differences in Ia expression. Further molecular and genetic studies will be required to determine whether the primary macrophage differences observed between B10 and B10.129(10M) mice, and their secondary effects on leishmanial infections in vivo, are attributable to H-11 itself or to tightly linked passenger genes carried over in production of the congenic strains. Whatever the result, it is clear that this single gene (or tight linkage group) difference, measurable in the naive mouse, has a profound effect upon the generation of an antigen-specific cellular immune response.

The primary macrophage defect observed early in infection in B10.129(10M) mice is clearly magnified as infection with L. donovani progresses. The reduced ability to respond to IFNγ in terms of leishmanicidal activity leads to a high parasite/antigenic load, massive hepatosplenomegaly, and eventually to high absolute numbers of antigen specific T cells in the infected organs. The high proportion of L3T4$^+$ T cells maintained throughout infection is consistent with the earlier observations in Scl-controlled nonhealing to L. major infection in BALB/c mice[12], suggesting that the generation of an excess of antigen-specific T cells of the helper phenotype may be a common endpoint for noncuring/nonhealing responses under separate genetic control. The predominance of Lyt-2$^+$ cells in the curing (B10) strain at the time of maximum resolution of parasite load lends support to current pleas[12,13] for a re-evaluation of the role of this subpopulation of T cells in mediating protection against leishmanial infections generally.

ACKNOWLEDGEMENTS

This work was supported by grants from the Medical Research Council, the Wellcome Trust and the Institut Pasteur. JMB is a Wellcome Trust Senior Lecturer.

REFERENCES

1. L. J. DeTolla, L. H. Semprevivo, N. C. Palczuk and H. C. Passmore, Genetic control of acquired resistance to visceral leishmaniasis in mice, Immunogenetics 10:353 (1980).
2. J. M. Blackwell, C. Hale, M. B. Roberts, O. M. Ulczak F. Y. Liew, and J. G. Howard, An H-11 gene has a parallel effect on Leishmania major and L. donovani infections in mice Immunogenetics 21:385 (1984).
3. J. M. Blackwell and J. Alexander, Different host genes recognise and control infection with taxonomically distinct Leishmania species in : "Taxonomy and Phylogeny of Leishmania" ed. J.A. Rioux, Louis-Jean (in press).
4. J. M. Blackwell, Genetically controlled host responses to leishmaniasis,in:"Ecology and genetics of host-parasite interactions" D. Rollinson and R. M. Anderson, Acad. Press, London (1985).
5. J. G. Howard, C. Hale, and F. Y. Liew, Immunological regulation of experimental cutaneous leishmaniasis. IV. Prophylactic effect of sublethal irradiation as a result of abrogation of suppressor T cell generation in mice genetically susceptible to Leishmania tropica, J. Exp. Med. 153:557 (1981).
6. J. M. Blackwell and O. M. Ulczak, Immunoregulation of genetically controlled acquired responses to Leishmania donovani infection in mice: demonstration and characterisation of suppressor T cell in noncure mice. Infect. Immun. 44:97 (1984).
7. J. Y. Channon, M. B. Roberts and J. M. Blackwell, A study of differential respiratory burst activity elicited by promastigotes and amastigotes of Leishmania donovani in murine resident peritoneal macrophages. Immunology 53:345 (1984).
8. P. M. Kaye, Acquisition of Cell Mediated Immunity to Leishmania 1.Primary T-cell activation detected by IL-2 receptor expression Immunology 61:345 (1987).
9. M. H. Julius, E. Simpson, and L. A. Herzenberg, A rapid method for the isolation of functional thymus derived murine lymphocytes Eur. J. Immunol. 3:645 (1973)
10. P. M. Kaye, Inflammatory cells in murine visceral leishmaniasis express a dendritic cell marker, Clin. Exp. Immunol. (1987) in press.
11. A. Battacharya, M. E. Dorf, and T. A. Spencer, A shared allo-antigenic determinant on Ia antigens encoded by IA and IE subregions, evidence for I region gene duplication, J. Immunol. 127:2488 (1981).
12. G. Milon, R. G. Titus J. C. Cerottini, G. Marchal, J. A. Louis Higher frequency of Leishmania major specific L3T4$^+$ T cells in susceptible BALB/c mice as compared to resistant CBA mice. J. Immunol. 136:1467 (1986).
13. P. M. Kaye, M. B. Roberts, and J. M. Blackwell, Analysing the immune response to L. donovani infection, Ann. Inst. Past. Forums in Immunol. in press.
14. B. Loveland and E. Simpson, The non-MHC transplantation antigens, neither weak nor minor. Immunology Today 7:223 (1986).
15. E. Simpson, and P. Chandler, Analysis of cytotxic T cell responses in "Handbook of Experimental Immunology" vol 2 Cellular Immunology ed. D.M. Weir, Blackwell Scientific, Oxford.(1986)
16. T. A. Hamilton, and D. O. Adams, Molecular mechanisms of signal transduction in macrophages, Immunology Today 8:151 (1987).
17. D. Meruelo, A. Rossomando, M. Offer, J. Buxbaum, and A. Pellicer, Association of endogenous viral loci with genes encoding murine histocompatibility and lymphocyte differentiation antigens, Proc. Natl. Acad. Sci. USA. 80:5032 (1983).
18. E. Simpson, Non-H-2 histocompatibility antigens: can they be retroviral products? Immunology Today 8:176 (1987).

CHARACTERIZATION OF LEISHMANIA DONOVANI INFECTIVE

(METACYCLIC) PROMASTIGOTES FROM AXENIC CULTURES

M. Keith Howard, Gillian Sayers and Michael A. Miles

Wolfson Unit/Department of Medical Protozoology
London School of Hygiene and Tropical Medicine
Keppel Street
London   WC1E 7HT   U.K.

INTRODUCTION

The infection of the female sand fly by Leishmania is initiated when the sand fly takes a bloodmeal from an infected mammal. Once in the midgut the amastigote transforms into the promastigote form of the parasite - a process which may or may not involve cell division (1,2). The promastigotes divide rapidly within the bloodmeal before being released into the gut lumen with the breakdown of the peritrophic membrane: division continues within the midgut. The motile parasites are free to migrate in an anterior or posterior direction within the gut lumen (1,3) although the bulk of the infection usually migrates anteriorly. This movement is associated with both a change in morphology (1) and infectivity (4) as the parasites cease division.

The form of promastigote responsible for the transmission of the infection from sand fly to mammal has been somewhat controversial. Sacks (4) have shown that parasites present in the sand fly midgut on day 3 of infection can initiate infection in mice. It is also known that sand flies without organisms in the mouthparts can transmit the infection when taking a bloodmeal (4). However, the morphology of the parasites, present in the oesophagus and pharynx of the sand fly is very characteristic (1,5) and it is tempting to associate this change in morphology with the acquisition of infectivity even if the blocking of the stomodeal valve by attached parasite is also required for transmission (6).

It is difficult both to maintain sand fly colonies in the laboratory and to study the relatively small number of parasites obtained from infected sand flies. Nevertheless, it may be possible to characterize the infective form of promastigote since it has been shown to exist in the stationary phase of axenic cultures (7,8). We have developed a culture system which stimulates the majority (85%) of the promastigotes to transform into the infective form. Here we summarize some of the initial characteristics of these promastigotes.

MATERIALS AND METHODS

Parasites: Leishmania donovani (MHOM/ET/67/HU3) amastigotes were isolated from the spleen of golden hamsters (9) and inoculated at a density of 5×10^7/ml into 20ml volumes of Grace's medium (without haemolymph: GIBCO); incorporating 5% foetal calf serum (FCS), 2mM pyruvate, 2mM glutamine, penicillin (200 U/ml), streptomycin (200 μg/ml), 5-fluorocytosine (1mg/ml Sigma), 2% amino acids (modified, Flow), 1% nonessential amino acids (Flow), 100mM L-proline (Sigma), and approximately 0.75% of a mixture of salts based on the composition of triatomine bug urine (sodium urate 10mg/ml, uric acid 10mg/ml, cysteic acid 50mg/ml, all Sigma) to give the complete medium a pH of approximately 5.5. Cultures were maintained in 75cm^2 flasks (Nunc) at 28°C in 5% CO_2. Every fourth day half of the culture volume was removed, by centrifugation (4000g, 15 min, 4°C). The parasite pellet was re-suspended in an equal volume of fresh medium and returned to the culture. Parasites for experiments were used after between 10-16 days in this culture system.

Lectin agglutination and assessment of resistance to killing by normal human serum were performed essentially as by Sacks et al. (8) with minor modifications.

Infectivity was tested in vitro as described by Sacks et al. (8) except that the P388D macrophage-like cell line replaced peritoneal macrophages (10) and in vivo using a technique similar to that of Hodgekinson and Herman (11).

RESULTS

Morphology: A clear distinction could be seen between the morphology of the dividing promastigotes (logarithmic phase) and the non-dividing (stationary phase) promastigotes. Logarithmic phase promastigotes were approximately 12 microns in body length with a flagellum of equal length. As the culture aged the promastigote body length decreased and the length of the flagellum increased (10). The resultant short-form parasites were highly motile with irregular, intense bursts of activity.

Complement-mediated lysis: Both logarithmic and stationary phase promastigotes were sensitive to lysis by factors in normal human serum. Heat-inactivation (30 mins, 56°C) and a requirement for magnesium ions implicated complement in the killing action. Stationary phase cells were more resistant to killing by normal human serum than logarithmic phase cells.

The survival of both logarithmic and stationary phase promastigotes exposed to given serum concentration was enhanced by either increasing the parasite cell density or decreasing the incubation temperature (10).

Lectin agglutination: Sacks et al. (8) have shown that stationary phase promastigotes of L. major are less susceptible to agglutination by peanut agglutinin and castor bean agglutinin than were the exponentially growing cells. Doran and Herman (12) have also found differential binding of RCA to logarithmic and stationary phase promastigotes of L. donovani. We observed that logarithmic phase cells were agglutinated by 32μg/ml PNA whereas 85% of the stationary phase promastigotes were not (10).

Infectivity: The P388D macrophage-like cell line killed all logarithmic phase promastigotes within 72 hours of ingestion. Under the same conditions 85% of stationary phase promastigotes survived and transformed into the amastigote stages.

When infectivity was assessed in vivo, using the BALB/c mouse model, the infectivities of dividing promastigote populations were between 19.8 and 23.5 LDU (13) whereas the infectivity of stationary phase promastigotes was 14 times greater at 273.9. Additionally, stationary phase promastigotes consistently produced greater parasite burdens than logarithmic phase parasites at any infecting dose capable of initiating an infection (10).

CONCLUSIONS

An axenic culture system has been devised in which up to 85% of L. donovani promastigotes are infective and they have a characteristic morphology and motility, an increased resistance to killing by normal human serum and a reduced ability to bind the lectin, peanut agglutinin.

The availability of metacyclic promastigotes from cultures will allow the development of genetic and immunological probes for the analysis of the differentiation and gene expression of infective promastigotes both in vitro and in the sand fly vector.

ACKNOWLEDGEMENTS

We thank the Wolfson Foundation for financing this research: MAM is a Wellcome Trust Senior Lecturer.

REFERENCES

1. R. Killick-Kendrick. Biology of Leishmania in phlebotomine sand flies. In "Biology of the Kinetoplastida" (W.H.R. Lumsden and D.A. Evans, eds.) Vol. 2, pp.395-460. Academic Press, New York/San Francisco/London (1979).

2. D.T. Hart, K. Vickerman and G.H. Coombs. Transformation in vitro of Leishmania mexicana amastigotes to promastigotes: nutritional requirements and the effect of drugs. Parasitology 83, 529-541 (1981).

3. L.L. Walters, G.B. Mode, R.B. Teoh and T. Burtage. Host-parasite relationship of Leishmania mexicana mexicana and Lutzomyia abonnenci (Diptera:Psychodidae) Am.J.Trop.Med.Hyg. 36(2), 294-314 (1987).

4. D.L. Sacks and P.V. Perkins. Development of infective stage Leishmania promastigotes within phlebotomine sand flies. Am.J.Trop.Med.Hyg. 34(3), 456-459 (1985).

5. A. Warburg and Y. Schlein. Scanning electron microscopy of Leishmania major in Phlebotomus papatasi. Z. Parasitenkd. 72, 423-431 (1986).

6. R. Beach, G. Kulu and J. Leeuwenburg. Modification of sand fly biting behaviour by Leishmania leads to increased parasite transmission. Am.J.Trop.Med.Hyg. 34, 278-282 (1985).

7. M.S. Giannini. Effects of promastigote growth phase, frequency of subculture and host age on promastigote-initiated infections with Leishmania donovani in the golden hamster. J. Protozool 21, 521-525 (1974).

8. D.L. Sacks, S. Hieny and A. Sher. Identification of cell surface carbohydrate and antigenic changes between noninfective and infective developmental stages of Leishmania major promastigotes. J.Immunol. 135(1), 564-569 (1985).

9. J.Y. Channon, M.B. Roberts and J.M. Blackwell. A study of the differential respiratory burst activity elicited by promastigotes and amastigotes of Leishmania donovani in murine resident peritoneal macrophages. Immunology 53, 345-355 (1984).

10. M.K. Howard, G. Sayers and M.A. Miles. Leishmania donovani metacyclic promastigotes: Transformation in vitro, lectin agglutination, complement resistance, and infectivity. Exp. Parasitol 64, in press.

11. V.H. Hodgkinson and R. Herman. In vivo assay of viability of amastigotes of Leishmania donovani. J.Parasitol 66(2), 245-249 (1980).

12. T.I. Doran and R. Herman. Characterization of populations of promastigotes of Leishmania promastigotes. J.Protozool 28, 345-350 (1981).

13. D.J. Bradley and J. Kirkley. Regulation of Leishmania populations within the host. I The variable course of Leishmania donovani infections in mice. Clin.Exp.Immunol 30, 119-129 (1977).

DIFFERENT EPITOPES OF THE MACROPHAGE TYPE THREE COMPLEMENT RECEPTOR (CR3) ARE USED TO BIND LEISHMANIA PROMASTIGOTES HARVESTED AT DIFFERENT PHASES OF THEIR GROWTH CYCLE

Andrea Cooper, Anne O Wozencraft[*], Tamara I A Roach and Jenefer M Blackwell

Department of Tropical Hygiene, London School of Hygiene and Tropical Medicine, London WC1E 7HT, U.K.

INTRODUCTION

A number of studies[1-4] have demonstrated that monoclonal antibodies (MAbs) directed against the type three complement receptor (CR3) block the binding and ingestion of Leishmania promastigotes by host macrophages. This receptor is known to recognise the inactivated form of complement factor 3 (iC3b)[5] and to mediate direct lectin-like attachment of particles such as yeast zymosan[6]. Binding via these different sites on CR3 may have important implications for parasite survival since ligation via the lectin-binding site stimulates release of antimicrobial reactive oxygen intermediates whereas ligation of iC3b does not[6]. In our earlier studies[1] we had demonstrated that the anti-CR3 MAb M1/70, Fab-anti-C3, and the nucleophile sodium salicyl hydroxamate (Saha), which inhibits the covalent binding of C3 to an activator surface, all inhibited the serum-independent uptake of L. donovani promastigotes to equivalent degrees. This suggested that binding of promastigotes to CR3 was complement mediated, and was supported by our subsequent demonstration of Saha-inhibitable deposition of macrophage derived C3 on the promastigote surface[7]. We also observed a strong correlation between the increased infectivity of stationary phase promastigotes of L. donovani, their enhanced C3 binding capacity, and their M1/70-inhibitable CR3-mediated attachment to host macrophages[3]. Overall we concluded that, for L. donovani, complement-dependent CR3-mediated entry into host macrophages might play an important role in determining initial infectivity of the parasite. What remained unclear was (a) whether the use of different epitopes on CR3, or different macrophage receptors, by logarithmic (log) versus stationary phase organisms of different species of Leishmania might contribute to their initial infectivity and/or their particular tissue tropism in the host; and (b) how these differences might relate to the various morphological[8-10] and molecular[9-12] changes observed for promastigotes examined at different phases of their growth cycle either in the sandfly vector or in culture. In the present study a direct comparison of macrophage binding inhibition using two anti-CR3 MAbs, M1/70[13] and 5C6[14], in conjunction with Saha, is made for L. donovani and

---

[*]Present address: Department of Biophysics, Cell and Molecular Biology, King's College (Chelsea), London SW3 6LX, U.K.

L. major promastigotes harvested at different phases of their growth cycle. No obvious inter-specific differences which might explain tissue tropism are observed, but dramatic differences in ability to inhibit binding of peanut agglutanin (PNA) positive late log/early stationary phase promastigotes versus PNA negative late stationary phase promastigotes were obtained using the two different MAbs and Saha. The results suggest that, despite their ability to bind more C3, the entry of the more infective PNA negative organisms into host macrophages might involve direct lectin-like binding to CR3. If binding is complement mediated it must involve C3 bound covalently to the parasite surface by amide linkages not inhibitable by Saha. The results obtained are related to the work of others on molecular changes[11,12] which accompany the transformation from noninfective logarithmic phase to infective stationary phase (metacyclic) promastigotes.

MATERIALS AND METHODS

Parasite isolation and culture in vitro

Amastigotes of L. donovani (LV9) and L. major (LV39 and NIH173) were isolated from hamster spleens or BALB/c footpads as previously described[15,16]. All three strains were seeded at 5×10^6 amastigotes/ml in RPMI containing 20% heat inactivated foetal calf serum (FCS), 20mM L-glutamine, 10mM sodium pyruvate, 100 U/ml penicillin, 100μg/ml streptomycin and 75μg/ml gentamicin, and allowed to transform at $24°C$ for 72 hours. Primary subcultures (5x100ml per parasite strain) were then seeded with 1×10^6/ml motile flagellated transformed promastigotes obtained by differential centrifugation at 650g, non transformed parasites remaining in the supernatant. Cultures were counted daily using a Helber bacteriological counting chamber. For use in experiments parasites were harvested by centrifugation at 650g and washed (x2) in RPMI without FCS. The proportion of promastigotes binding the lectin PNA was determined by fluorescence microscopy following incubation with TRITC labelled PNA (Sigma L-3766) at 50μg/ml for 30 minutes.

Promastigote infectivity in vivo

Promastigotes harvested at days 2,4,6,9,11 and 13 of culture in vitro were used to infect mice either intravenously (i.v.) via the lateral tail vein (2×10^7/mouse; 6-8 week old male C57BL/10ScSn) or subcutaneously (s.c.) into the footpad (10^6/mouse; 6-8 week old female BALB/c). The sex and strain of mice was chosen according to previous observations[17] of susceptibility to infection with L. donovani versus L. major given i.v. or s.c. Mice infected i.v. were killed after 14 days and parasite loads determined from liver impression smears (log_{10}LDU/liver) as described[15]. For s.c. infected mice, footpad thickness was measured weekly for 6 weeks using a direct reading vernier calliper. To allow direct comparison of s.c. infectivity of promastigotes harvested at different phases of the growth cycle, only the week 4 footpad thicknesses are shown. Beyond this point footpads become necrotic and accuracy of measurements may be affected by secondary infections in the lesions.

Promastigote infectivity in vitro

Promastigote infectivity (uptake and 72 hour survival) for murine resident peritoneal macrophages infected in vitro, and binding inhibition assays, were carried out as described previously[1,3]. The rat anti-mouse CR3 MAb M1/70 was prepared from hybridoma supernatants by ammonium sulphate precipitation and dialysis against phosphate buffered saline (PBS). A stock solution at 0.4mg/ml was used at a dilution of 1:5 in inhibition assays. Control P3NS1 myeloma supernatants treated in the same manner produced no inhibition of parasite binding. Affinity purified rat anti-mouse CR3 MAb 5C6 (2.8mg/ml) was a generous gift from Hugh Rosen of the Sir William Dunn School of Pathology, Oxford, and was used at 1:400. Both MAbs were used at saturation. Saha was prepared as described[1].

RESULTS

Growth curves and PNA binding capacity

Figure 1 shows the different growth curves obtained for L. donovani versus L. major promastigotes over 13 days of culture and their ability to bind the lectin PNA. Despite the apparent plateau in the growth curves after day 4, cultures of both species of Leishmania contained many dividing parasites through 7 (LV9) to 9 (LV39 and NIH173) days. PNA positivity peaked (70-80%) for both species at day 6 of culture in vitro. Parasites remained >75% viable (acridine orange/ethidium bromide fluorescence viability assay[15]) through 11 days of culture. At day 13, viability was maintained at >75% in L. major cultures but dropped to <60% for L. donovani. The differences in the growth curves for L. donovani versus L. major were repeatable over 4 separate experiments.

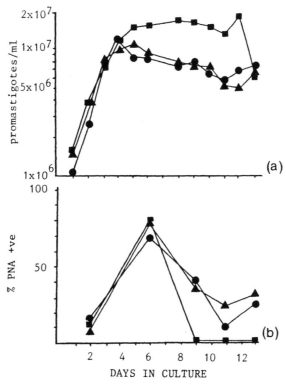

Figure 1. Parasites per ml (a) and percent PNA positive parasites (b) in in vitro cultures of L. donovani (LV9■) and L. major (LV39●; NIH173▲) maintained for 13 days after seeding cultures at 1×10^6/ml with freshly transformed promastigotes. Results are shown for one representative culture. Parasites from replicate cultures were harvested at different time points for infectivity and macrophage experiments.

Promastigote infectivity in vivo

Figure 2 compares i.v. and s.c. infectivity for L. donovani LV9 and L. major LV39 promastigotes harvested at various times during their growth cycle. Results obtained for L. major NIH173 mimicked those for LV39 except that the NIH173 strain produced larger footpad lesions throughout. L. donovani amastigotes and promastigotes failed to produce any increase in footpad thickness over 6 weeks following s.c. inoculation. Similarly, infectivity of L. major promastigotes was much reduced (approximately 100-fold) compared to numerically equivalent

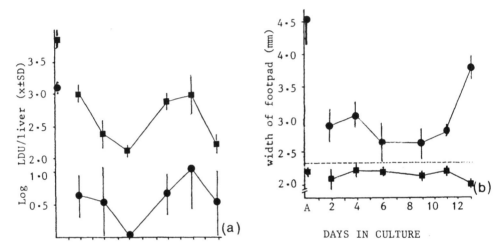

Figure 2. Infectivity in vivo for L. donovani LV9 (■) and L. major LV39 (●) amastigotes (A) or promastigotes (harvested at different times in the growth cycle) inoculated (a) i.v. (2×10^7 parasites/mouse; 3-4 mice per group), or (b) s.c. in the footpad (10^6 parasites/mouse; 4-5 mice per group). Parallel results were obtained for L. major NIH173 and L. major LV39.

inocula of L. donovani promastigotes. Promastigotes of both species thus maintained their expected tissue tropism. Amastigotes of both strains of L. major inoculated i.v. were as infective as the most infective L. donovani promastigotes. Hence the viscerotropic nature of the NIH173 strain noted by previous workers[17] probably relates to their use of amastigote inocula and is not peculiar to that strain of L. major. As with previous studies[19], peak PNA positivity in the promastigote cultures in vitro (day 6, figure 1) coincided with the lowest infectivity in vivo (day 6, figure 2) for both species of parasite inoculated either i.v. or s.c.

Promastigote infectivity in vitro and macrophage binding inhibition

Figure 3 (a and b) compares the inhibition of parasite binding obtained with the two anti-CR3 MAbs, M1/70 and 5C6, and with Saha for promastigotes of L. donovani LV9 and L. major LV39 harvested at various times during the growth cycle. The patterns of inhibition were similar for the two species of parasite. Inhibition with M1/70 was generally high throughout and increased further after day 6 when late stationary phase PNA negative parasites (see figure 1) appeared in the cultures. Inhibition with 5C6 followed closely the curve (see figure 1) for PNA positive parasites in the cultures, the drop in 5C6 inhibition observed in late stationary phase cultures being paralleled by a decrease in Saha inhibition. Results obtained for L. major NIH173 were essentially the same as those for L. major LV39.

The proportion of bound parasites surviving 72 hours in macrophages in vitro (figure 3, c and d) followed a similar pattern to that observed for infectivity in vivo (see figure 2). As we had previously noted[3], the survival of late stationary phase promastigotes of L. donovani LV9 was not dramatically higher than the less infective log/early stationary phase (day 6) parasites. For L. major, on the other hand, day 11 late stationary parasites showed markedly enhanced survival consistent with earlier observations of Sack and coworkers[9].

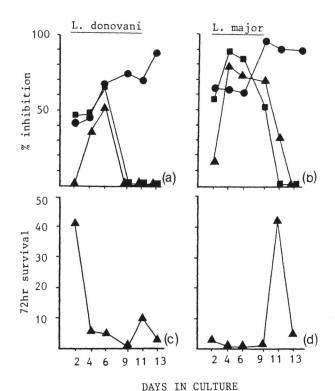

Figure 3. Inhibition of parasite binding (a and b) and 72 hour survival (c and d) for L. donovani LV9 (a and c) and L. major LV39 (b and d) promastigotes harvested at different times in the growth cycle and used to infect murine resident peritoneal macrophages in vitro. Inhibitors used were the anti-CR3 MAbs, M1/70 (●) and 5C6 (▲), and the nucleophile Saha (■). Parallel results were obtained for L. major NIH173 (not shown) and L. major LV39.

DISCUSSION

As with earlier studies[3,9], results presented here demonstrate marked differences in infectivity of promastigotes of L. donovani and L. major harvested at different points of the growth cycle. Results with L. donovani did not mimick exactly those obtained in our earlier study[3] but confirm the recent observation of Da Silva and Sacks[19] that infectivity correlates more precisely with reduced expression of a PNA specific binding site on the promastigote membrane. In the work presented earlier, Wozencraft and Blackwell[3] used promastigotes from day 7 of a primary culture to seed the subcultures used for infectivity studies. This presumably selected for PNA positive log phase promastigotes with lower infectivity from days 3 through 6 of the new subculture. In contrast, newly transformed day 3 promastigotes used to seed the first subcultures for the infectivity studies presented here were PNA negative and still amastigote-like in their infectivity in vivo. The appearance of PNA positive promastigotes correlated with an increase in dividing parasites in the cultures and peaked after the total numbers of parasites had ceased to increase. Many dividing forms were still observed in these cultures suggesting an initial balance between promastigote death and generation of new parasites in early stationary phase cultures. The proportion of PNA positive parasites in the cultures dropped dramatically after dividing forms had ceased to be observed. Da Silva and Sacks[19] and Howard and coworkers[10] also demonstrated a relationship between PNA binding and promastigote division for both L. major and L. donovani. We also noticed repeatedly that cultures of L. major promastigotes plateaued at a lower cell density than did L. donovani cultures, with dividing forms present in the cultures further into the apparent stationary phase of the growth cycle. This may represent some adaptation to development within different sandfly species. It was the only difference observed between cutaneous L. major and visceral L. donovani species.

In studies of promastigote binding to murine resident peritoneal macrophages in vitro, similar patterns of binding inhibition were observed for L. donovani and L. major using the two anti-CR3 MAbs and Saha. Hence there were no obvious differences in the use of CR3 as a receptor for entry into host macrophages which might explain the differences in tissue tropism for the different Leishmania species. However, dramatic differences were observed in the ability of the different soluble inhibitors to block binding and ingestion of parasites harvested at different phases of the growth cycle. Significant among these was (a) the marked correlation between 5C6 inhibition and the expression of the PNA lectin binding site on the parasite surface, with a parallel drop in Saha inhibition as PNA negative parasites appeared in the cultures; and (b) a high level of M1/70 inhibition observed throughout which increased as the number of PNA negative parasites increased in the cultures. In previous studies both M1/70[5] and 5C6[14] have been shown to inhibit binding of iC3b-coated erythrocytes to CR3, but it is not known whether either MAb binds directly to the iC3b binding site or whether inhibition is caused by binding of the MAbs to epitopes adjacent to this site on the receptor molecule. 5C6, but not M1/70, also inhibits CR3-mediated adhesion of macrophages to bacterial plastic[14] suggesting that the two MAbs do recognise distinct epitopes on CR3. One interpretation of our findings is that the binding of PNA negative late stationary phase organisms to CR3 is not complement mediated and that M1/70, but not 5C6, blocks direct lectin-like binding of the promastigotes to CR3. The binding of PNA positive promastigotes, on the other hand, appears to be mediated by Saha inhibitable covalently bound iC3b on the parasite surface. The precise correlation between 5C6 inhibition and the presence of PNA positive parasites suggests that the acceptor site for the iC3b mediating binding to CR3 may coincide with the PNA binding site on the parasite surface. The observation that PNA negative parasites may bind to the lectin binding site of CR3 is perhaps counter-intuitive since it suggests that the more infective parasites ligate the site on CR3 known to trigger the release of toxic reactive oxygen intermediates[6]. Other workers have suggested, however, that membrane bound acid phosphatase on promastigotes may inhibit the macrophage respiratory burst[20], as does the major surface glycolipid molecule (D. Sacks, personal communication). This interpretation of our results fails to take account of our own earlier observation[3] of an increase in C3 deposition on the surface of late stationary phase promastigotes which correlates with the enhanced CR3-mediated binding to macrophages in vitro. Hence we need to examine further the nature of the molecular changes which accompany the generation of PNA negative promastigotes in late stationary phase cultures.

In earlier studies[21,22] two distinct molecules on the promastigote surface have been implicated as ligands for macrophage receptors. Handman and Goding[21] suggested that a major surface glycolipid on L. major promastigotes mediated binding to host macrophages, while Russell and Wilhelm[22] implicated the major surface glycoprotein (Gp63-65) as the ligand for macrophage attachment both because it is a major C3 acceptor molecule and because it appeared to bind directly to the macrophage mannose-fucose receptor also thought to mediate promastigote binding to macrophages[1,15]. Thus both molecules may be important in phagocytosis of promastigotes by macrophages and both alter their nature or expression during the growth cycle[11,12]. Sacks and Da Silva[11] suggest, for example, that the PNA binding site of promastigotes of L. major resides in a subterminal galactose residue of the surface glycolipid molecule and that further glycosylation of this residue results in loss of PNA specific binding in late stationary phase parasites. Changes in PNA binding capacity observed here and by others[10] may reflect changes in glycosylation of the equivalent glycolipid molecule of L. donovani promastigotes. More recently, Sacks and coworkers (Puentes et al.[23]) have shown that the glycolipid of L. major is also a major C3 acceptor molecule. Their results shown that PNA positive parasites activate the alternative complement pathway and bind C3 by O-ester covalent linkages inhibitable by nucleophiles like Saha, 10-15% of the total C3 bound being in the form iC3b. PNA negative parasites, on the other hand, activate the classical complement pathway with most C3 bound noncovalently to the parasite surface. These results are consistent with our hypothesis that PNA positive parasites bind to CR3 by Saha inhibitable covalently bound iC3b, whereas PNA negative parasites do not. Further work is required to determine whether the form of the glycolipid molecule on PNA negative parasites mediates direct lectin-like binding to CR3.

Kweider and coworkers[12] have also observed enhanced expression of the major surface glycoprotein (Gp63-65) of L. brasiliensis and L. mexicana as promastigotes proceed from log to stationary phases of the growth cycle. In their studies pretreatment of stationary phase parasites with an anti-Gp65 MAb severely reduced parasite survival in host macrophages in vitro, suggesting that the molecule contributes directly to increased infectivity. The covalent binding of C3 to Gp63 has been shown to consist of a mixture of amide and ester linkages[24], the nucleophile Saha having the ability to disrupt the ester but not the amide linkages. Hence an alternative interpretation for our failure to observe Saha inhibition in PNA negative late stationary phase promastigotes may be because of preferential binding of C3 to Gp63 via amide linkages. Inactivation of amide linked C3b to iC3b would provide a ligand for CR3, although it is not clear why the MAb 5C6 fails to inhibit this binding. The ability of the Gp63-65 molecule to act as a direct ligand for CR3 and/or for the macrophage mannose/fucose receptor also requires further clarification, but it more likely that the importance of the GP63-65 molecule in parasite/macrophage interactions relates more to intracellular survival than to interactions at the macrophage surface. Overall, the results of our study suggest that changes in expression of the glycolipid molecule may be important in determining the different epitopes of CR3 used in binding PNA positive versus PNA negative parasites and may thus play an important role in determining infectivity in the host.

ACKNOWLEDGEMENTS

This work was supported by grants from the Medical Research Council and the Wellcome Trust. JMB is a Wellcome Trust Senior Lecturer. We are grateful for the continued interest and support of Dr Siamon Gordon and his colleagues at the Sir William Dunn School of Pathology in Oxford, without which this work would not have been possible.

REFERENCES

1. J. M. Blackwell, R. A. B. Ezekowitz, M. B. Roberts, J. Y. Channon, R. B. Sim, and S. Gordon, Macrophage complement and lectin-like receptors bind Leishmania in the absence of serum. J. Exp. Med. 162:324 (1985).
2. D. M. Mosser and P. J. Edelson, The mouse macrophage receptor for C3bi (CR3) is a major mechanism in the phagocytosis of Leishmania promastigotes. J. Immunol. 135:2785 (1985).
3. A. O. Wozencraft and J. M. Blackwell, Increased infectivity of stationary-phase promastigotes of Leishmania donovani: correlation with enhanced C3 binding capacity and CR3-mediated attachment to host macrophages. Immunology 60:559 (1987).
4. M. E. Wilson and R. D. Pearson, The role of CR3 and mannose receptor in the attachment and ingestion of Leishmania donovani by human mononuclear phagocytes. Infect. Immun. (in press 1987).
5. D. I. Beller, T. A. Springer, and R. D. Schrieber, Anti Mac-1 selectively inhibits the mouse and human type three complement receptor. J. Exp. Med. 156:1000 (1982).
6. G. D. Ross, J. A. Cain, and P. J. Lachmann, Membrane complement receptor type three (CR3) has lectin like properties analogous to bovine conglutin and functions as a receptor for zymosan and rabbit erythrocytes as well as a receptor for iC3b. J. Immunol. 134:3307 (1985).
7. A. O. Wozencraft, G. Sayers, and J. M. Blackwell, Macrophage type 3 complement receptors mediate serum-independent binding of Leishmania donovani. J. Exp. Med. 164:1332 (1986).
8. R. Killick-Kendrick, Biology of Leishmania in phlebotamine sandflies, in: "Biology of the Kinetoplastida" vol.2. W. H. R. Lumsden and D. A. Evans, eds, Academic Press, London (1979).
9. D. L. Sacks, S. Hieny, and A. Sher, Identification of cell surface carbohydrate and antigenic changes between non-infective and infective developmental stages of Leishmania major promastigotes. J. Immunol. 135:564 (1985).
10. M. K. Howard, G. Sayers, and M. A. Miles, Leishmania donovani metacyclic promastigotes : transfomation in vitro, lectin agglutination, complement resistance and infectivity. Exp. Parasitol. (in press, 1987).

11. D. L. Sacks and R. da Silva, The generation of infective stage Leishmania major promastigotes is associated with the cell surface expression and release of a developmentally regulated glycolipid. Submitted for publication.
12. M. Kweider, J-L. Lemesre, F. Darcy, J-P Kusnierz, A. Capron, and F. Santoro, Infectivity of Leishmania braziliensis promastigotes is dependent on the increasing expression of a 65,000-dalton surface antigen. J. Immunol. 138: 299 (1987).
13. T. Springer, G. Galfre, D. S. Secher, and C. Milstien, Mac-1: a macrophage differentiation antigen identified by a monoclonal antibody. Eur. J. Imm. 9:301 (1979).
14. H. Rosen and S. Gordon, Monoclonal antibody to the murine type three complement receptor inhibits adhesion of myelomonocytic cells in vitro and inflammatory cell recruitment in vivo. J. Exp. Med. (in press, 1987).
15. J. Y. Channon, M. B. Roberts, and J. M. Blackwell, A study of the differential respiratory burst activity elicited by promastigotes and amastigotes of Leishmania donovani in murine resident peritoneal macrophages. Immunology 53:345 (1984).
16. J. Alexander and K. Vickerman, Fusion of host cell secondary lysosmes with the parasitophorous vacuoles of Leishmania mexicana infected macrophages. J. Protozool. 22:502 (1975).
17. B. A. Mock, A. H. Fortier, M. Potter, J. Blackwell, and C. A. Nacy, Control of systemic Leishmania major infection: identification of subline differences for susceptibility to disease. Curr. Top. Microbiol. Immunol. 122:115 (1985).
18. D. J. Bradley and J. Kirkley, Regulation of Leishmania populations within the host: variable course of Leishmania donovani infection in mice. Clin. Exp. Immunol. 30:119 (1977).
19. R. da Silva and D. L. Sacks, Metacyclogenesis is a major determinant of Leishmania promastigote virulence and attenuation. Infect. Immun. (in press, 1987).
20. A. T. Remaley, D. B. Kuhns, R. E. Basford, R. H. Glew, and S. S. Kaplan, Leishmania phosphatase blocks neutrophil O_2^- production. J. Biol. Chem. 259:11173 (1984).
21. E. Handman and J. W. Goding, The Leishmania receptor for macrophages is a lipid containing glycoconjugate. EMBO J. 3:2301 (1985).
22. D. G. Russell and H. Wilhelm, The involvement of the major surface glycoprotien GP63 of Leishmania promastigotes in attachment to macrophages. J. Immunol. 136:2613 (1986).
23. S. M. Puentes, D L. Sacks, R. da Silva and K. A. Joiner, Complement binding by two developmental stages of Leishmania major promastigotes varying in expression of a surface glycolipid. Submitted for publication.
24. D. G. Russell, The macrophage-attachment glycoprotein GP63 is the predominant C3-acceptor site on Leishmania mexicana promastigotes. Eur. J. Biochem 164:213 (1987).

IMMUNODOMINANT EPITOPES OF THE LEISHMANIA SURFACE MEMBRANE

Ronald L. Anthony, John B. Sacci, Jr., and
Kristina M. Williams

Department of Pathology, University of Maryland
School of Medicine
Baltimore, Maryland 21201, USA

INTRODUCTION

The many different antigens which comprise the surface membrane of leishmania play contrasting roles in parasite-host cell interactions. Some of these antigens influence virulence and infectivity (Kink and Chang, 1987; Kweider et al., 1987; Sacks et al. 1987), others contribute to pathogenecity (Bordier et al., 1982; Anthony et al., 1985) and still others elicit immunosuppressive or immunoprophylactic responses (Slutzky and Greenblatt, 1977; Rodrigues et al., 1986). Thus, successful development of a vaccine against the various species of leishmania which infect man is contingent upon the identity of the defined membrane sub-units which induce protection without causing deleterious side-effects.

METHODS

The advent of cell-fusion technology for the construction of hybridomas synthesizing exquisitely specific monoclonal antibodies has provided the immunoparasitologist with the tools needed for the antigenic dissection of parasite membranes. Use of the monoclonals in sensitive immunoassays now permits precise characterization of isolates to the sub-species level (McMahon-Pratt et al., 1982, 1985), and the identification of specific epitopes associated with parasite differentiation (Handman and Hocking, 1982; Handman et al., 1984). Concomitantly, reactivity of monoclonal antibodies with Western blots of parasite extracts resolved by SDS-PAGE has culminated in the identification of at least 20 externally displayed membrane proteins with molecular sizes ranging between 10-200 kilodaltons (kd) (Gardiner and Dwyer, 1983; McMahon-Pratt et al., 1985). Even more important, the use of monoclonal antibodies as ligands on immnoaffinity chromatography columns has allowed for the recovery of defined antigens from crude unfractionated extracts of promastigotes (Kahl and McMahon-Pratt, 1987; Sacci et al., 1987). Some of these purified molecules have been biochemically characterized as membrane bound enzymes (Bordier, 1987), glycoconjugates (Handman and Goding, 1985; Turco et al., 1984) and glycolipids (Handman et al., 1986). Functionally, they have been implicated as membrane receptors essential in intracellular communication (Chang, 1983; Chang and Fong, 1983), excreted factors (Slutzky et al., 1979; Jaffe and Sarfstein, 1987; Hernandez, 1983), moieties necessary for virulence (Kink and Chang, 1987; Kweider et al., 1987) and immunologic targets (Berman and Dwyer, 1981; Williams et al., 1986b; Slutzky and Greenblatt, 1977).

RESULTS AND DISCUSSION

The most ubiquitous of the leishmania membrane antigens, covering the entire surface of the promastigote (Figure 1A), is the 10-20kd, polydisperse molecule which was first visualized in SDS-PAGE electropherograms of purified pellicular membranes of L. donovani by Dwyer (1980). It was subsequently observed in immuno-autoradiographs of SDS-PAGE patterns of Iodo-Gen labeled promastigotes and amastigotes of L. tropica (Gardiner and Dwyer, 1983) and characterized by Turco et al. (1984) as a glycoconjugate. Electrophoretically, the polydisperse molecule migrates to an extremely anodic zone; it stains weakly with conventional protein stains but is positive with periodic acid-Schiffs reagent.

McMahon-Pratt et al. (1985) and Williams et al. (1986a) have generated a number of murine monoclonal antibodies which recognize the glycoconjugate in Western blots (Figure 1B) and they have demonstrated their species-specificity by radioimmune binding assays and indirect immunofluorescent antibody assays, respectively. Rodrigues et al. (1986) confirmed that the molecule acts as a T-cell mitogen in immunized and infected mice but that it shares cross-reactive determinants with other Genera of the Family Trypanosomatidae. This striking variability in the of spectrum reactivity of the monoclonal antibodies suggested that this polydisperse substance displays multiple epitopes which are involved in host-parasite interactions (Table 1).

The epitope recognized by monoclonal L2D3 is common to all members of the genus whereas the determinants reactive with monoclonals T9D3 and U7D5 are common only to species of the L.mexicana and L.donovani complexes. A similar antigenic homology between these two species has been uncovered by Reed et al. (1987).

Table 1. Epitopes of the 10-15kd Surface Molecule of Leishmania

Epitope	L	T	U
Recognized by monoclonal antibody:			
L2D3 (IgM)	x		
T9D3 (IgG-2b)		x	
U7D5 (IGG-3)			x
Species-differentiation	no	yes	yes
Surface membrane expression:			
Promastigotes	yes	yes	yes
Amastigotes	yes	yes	yes
Infected macrophages	yes	no	no
Excreted into media	yes	yes	yes
Inhibition of internalization	yes	no	no
Mitogenic	yes	no	yes

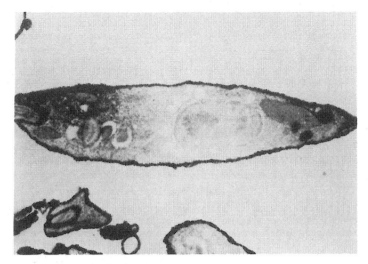

Fig. 1a. Immunoelectron micrograph confirming the presence of the 83L-2D3/a reactive epitope on the surface membrane of L. b. panamensis. Magnification, 15,900X.

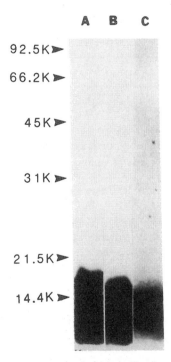

Fig. 1b. Western blot identification of the low-molecular-weight, surface membrane antigen of L. mexicana subsp. mexicana promastigotes recognized by monoclonal antibodies 83T-9D3 (lane A), 83U-7D5 (lane B), and 83L-2D3 (lane C).

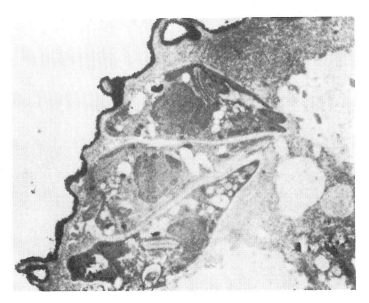

Fig. 2a. The 83L-2D3/a reactive antigen (→) on the surface membrane of mouse peritoneal macrophages infected with L. b. panamensis (WR-470) in vitro, longitudinal section. Magnification, 5800X.

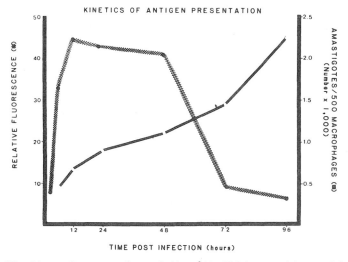

Fig. 2b. Kinetics of expression of the 83L-2D3/a reactive antigen on the surface membrane of mouse peritoneal macrophages infected with L. b. panamensis in vitro.

These differences in specificity were established by flow cytometric analyses of the intensity of the fluorescent signal emitted by each of 5000 living promastigotes subsequent to their incubation in the presence of the FITC-labeled monoclonal antibody.

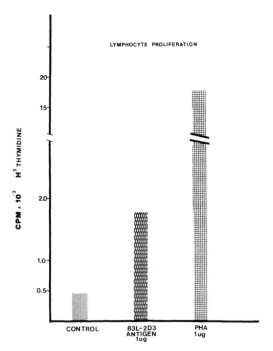

Fig. 3a. Immunoproliferative response of immune mouse splenocytes to the L2D3 antigen. PHA = + control; Fresh media = - control.

Williams et al. (1986b) observed that the epitopes recognized by each of the 3 antibodies are conserved throughout parasite differentiation into the amastigotes. However, the genus-specific epitope, recognized by L2D3, is peculiar in that it is resistant to lysosomal degradation and is subsequently displayed on the surface membrane of the infected macrophage (Figure 2A). The epitope appears at the macrophage

surface within 6 hours after infection and, as measured by flow
cytometry, continues to accumulate for an additional 42 hours (Figure
2B). As the parasite load continues to increase, the macrophages
apparently lose their capacity to process additional antigen and
reactivity declines rapidly. By 72 hours post infection most of the
antigen is either shed into the medium or internalized as a normal
consequence of membrane turnover.

Williams et al. (1986c) also demonstrated that opsonization of the
promastigote membrane with the monoclonal antibody to the "L" epitope
prevents internalization of the parasite by the macrophage. Since Balb/c
macrophages do not express receptors for the Fc portion of IgM, this
obvious adherence but ensuing paralysis cannot be attributed to the
cytophilic mechanisms reported by Farah et al. (1975). Steric and/or
antibody-specific blockage of the triggering sequence required for
phagocytosis seems more plausible.

The glyconjugate has now been recovered from CHAPS extracts of
promastigotes by using the different monoclonal antibodies as ligands in
immunoaffinity chromatography columns and the purified fractions have
been examined for their mitogenic activity on both immune and non-immune
mouse lymphocytes (Figure 3A). The increased stimulation of cells from
the immune animals implies that the epitope is acting as a antigen-specific mitogen. Rodrigues et al. (1986) reported that this response
depended upon T-helper cells and antigen presenting cells and was
restricted by a major histocompatibility complex Class II gene product.
More recent assays with human lymphocytes from active cases of
leishmaniasis (performed in collaboration with Dr. Nancy Saravia at The
International Center for Medical Investigation -Tulane University, Cali
Colombia) confirm these findings. Of the human cases examined to date,

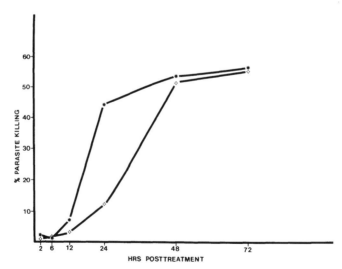

Fig. 3b. Capacity of media supporting L2D3 stimulated splenocytes to
enhance killing of intracellular amastigotes by macrophages in
vitro. (●) = + control; (○) = L2D3.

the stimulation index of one patient's lymphocytes to the purified glycoconjugate far exceeded that which was obtained when an unfractionated, crude promastigote extract was used as the mitogen (unpublished data). As anticipated, media harvested from lymphocyte cultures, stimulated with the glycoconjugate recovered on the L2D3 affinity column, contained lymphokines which activated the intracellular killing mechanisms of macrophages in vitro (Figure 3B).

The second immunodominant membrane antigen, common to all major species of leishmania which infect man, is the 63kd glycoprotein which was initially described by Bouvier et al. (1985). This molecule was subsequently purified by Etges et al. (1985) and characterized as a protease by Bordier (1987). Russell and Wilhlem (1986) have proceeded to demonstrate that this major membrane component also plays an essential function in the binding of promastigotes to macrophage surfaces and in initiating phagocytosis. Kink and Chang (1987) found increasing concentrations of gp63 in tunicamycin resistant variants of L. mexicana amazonensis of increased virulence.

Other investigators have failed to identify this defined molecule in parasite membrane extracts but they have described a composite of molecules, common to all species of the genus, in the 58-68kd range. The recognition of this composite by sera from patients infected with L. donovani (LePay et al., 1983; Ramasay, et al., 1983), L. d. chagasi (Reed et al., 1987), and L. major (Handman, et al., 1984) establishes their role as potent immunogens in human disease. Although the molecules appear to be structurally similar among the major species of leishmania, Reed et al. (1987) have reported on the use of a very similar antigen for the specific serodiagnosis of L. donovani chagasi. Interestingly, Kwieder et al. (1987) found that the gp63 on isolates of L. mexicana and L. braziliensis were not common to isolates of L. donovani chagasi. As stressed by Gardiner et al. (1984), the variability in complexity of the pattern and in the molecular size of the resolved components can be

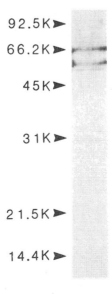

Fig. 4a. Western blot characterization of membrane antigens recognized by monoclonal antibody 83U-9B3.

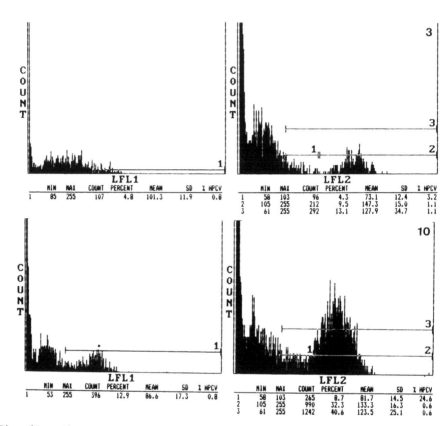

Fig. 4b. Flow cytometric analysis of the expression of the epitope recognized by monoclonal antibody U9B3 on 3 day log versus 10 day stationary phase promastigotes of L. mexicana mexicana.

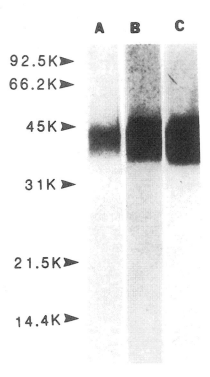

Fig. 5a. Western blot identification of the 42-kDa surface membrane antigen of L. mexicana subsp. mexicana promastigotes recognized by monoclonal antibodies.

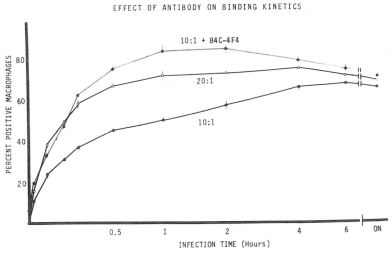

Fig. 5b. Effect of monoclonal antibody to 42kd antigen (84C-4F4) on promastigote-macrophage binding kinetics. Percent positive macrophages refers to the number of cells emitting a fluorescent signal per total number of cells passing through that particular channel.

attributed, in most instances, to the extent of endoproteolysis which occurs during specimen preparation, use of different detergents for extraction, and the lack of uniform conditions for reduction. Colomer-Gould et al. (1985) established that the major 65kd glycoprotein, common to the genus and highly immunogenic in human disease, migrates as a 50kd moiety under non-reducing conditions and as a composite of bands between 50kd and 65kd after incomplete reduction. After partial proteolysis, the 65kd molecule is degraded into a 48-33-22kd triplet. Likewise, Kink and Chang (1987) demonstrated that pretreatment of wild-type or tunicamycin resistant isolates of L. mexicana with tunicamycin increased the electrophoretic mobility of gp63.

We have generated a monoclonal antibody (U9B3) which is strongly reactive with purified gp63 (a gift from Dr. Bordier) in a solid phase ElISA. However, in a Western blot of a Triton-X extract of L. m. mexicana promastigotes, U9B3 recognized two major proteins of 66kd and 58kd and a minor component of 56kd (Figure 4A). A similar triplet, which covers the entire surface of the promastigote, has been visualized by Chang and Fong (1983) in immunoblots of 35-S methionine labeled organisms and by Colomer-Gould et al. (1985) in non-reduced extracts of L. mexicana amazonensis. It has been suggested that these protein molecules, because of their increased glycosylation and resistance to enzymatic degradation, are part of a protective shield which protects the amastigote in the lysosomal compartment of the macrophages. Kweider et al. (1987) demonstrated that the increasing expression of gp65 on promastigote surface membranes represents a vital mechanism for ensuring survival of leishmania within macrophages. Flow cytometric analysis of the kinetics of expression of the epitope recognized by U9B3 (Figure 4B) supported those earlier observations. The expression of gp63 or gp65, continued to increase with the age of the culture; e.g. during differentiation of the non-infectious to the infectious promastigote. By late stationary phase, 10 days post passage, 40% of the viable parasites were reactive with the monoclonal.

The third immunodominant antigen on the leishmania surface membrane is the 42kd glycoprotein which was first described by Handman et al. (1984). They identified the molecule by immunoprecipitation of radioiodinated amastigote antigens with sera from mice that had been hyperimmunized with live promastigotes of L. major. Subsequently, Sadick and Raff (1985) reported that hyperimmunization of rabbits with a mixture of freeze-thawed promastigotes and amastigotes of L. tropica resulted in the formation of antibodies which were reactive with a promastigote-specific 42kd molecule. McMahon-Pratt et al. (1985) succeeeded in generating monoclonal antibodies to this glycoprotein and, in addition to reporting on its species-specificity, provided evidence that it plays a integral role in the induction of protective immunity in the susceptible Balb/c mouse.

We have also generated several monoclonal antibodies to the 42kd surface moieties of L. m. mexicana, L. m. amazonensis and L. b. braziliensis (Williams et al., 1986c) (Figure 5A). Unexpected, however, was the resolution of a 35-45kd doublet when affinity purified material was blotted against the L. b. panamensis antibody. The reactive epitope is externally oriented on the surface membrane of living promastigotes, as revealed by dual parameter flow cytometric analysis, and it elicits a profound antibody response in human disease (Sacci et al., 1987).

Williams et al. (1986c) reported that opsonization of viable promastigotes with monoclonal antibodies to this 42kd antigen significantly enhances their binding to mouse macrophages in vitro (Figure 5B).

We suspect that the opsonic reactivity of these antibodies is a consequence of the formation of immune complexes which have a strong avidity for the FcR1 and FcR2 immunoglobulin receptors displayed on the Balb/c mouse macrophage membrane. Such Fc receptor-mediated adherence of opsonized parasites could serve to counterbalance any inhibition through antibody (Fab) mediated blocking of the surface ligand.

CONCLUSIONS

The specificity and functional attributes of many additional surface membrane antigens of leishmania have been published. Notably, the 20-60kd lipid containing glycoconjugate which has been described by Handman and Goding (1985) as a leishmania receptor for macrophages and which confers parasite survival within macrophages (Handman et al., 1986); the carbohydrate-rich factors isolated by Slutzky and Greenblatt (1977); the 116kd cell surface carbohydrate peculiar to infective developmental stages of L. major promastigote identified by Sacks et al. (1985). The list is now extensive. We contend, nevertheless, that future efforts must strive for standardization of methods of antigen analysis and, since it is often difficult or impossible to compare findings from different laboratories, the free-exchange of reagents, parasites and monoclonal antibodies should be encouraged. The identification of the antigens of diagnostic and vaccine relevance then will follow quickly.

REFERENCES

Anthony, R. L., Williams, K. M., Sacci, J. B., and Rubin, D. C., 1985, Subcellular and toxonomic specificity of monoclonal antibodies to New World Leishmania, Am. J. Trop. Med. Hyg., 34:1085.
Berman, J. D., and Dwyer, D. M., 1981, Expression of Leishmania antigen on the surface membrane of infected human macrophages in vitro, Clin. Exp. Immunol., 44:342.
Bordier, C., Garavito, R. M., and Armbruster, R., 1982, Biochemical and structural analyses of microtubules in the pellicular membrane of Leishmania tropica, J. Protozool., 29:560.
Bordier, C., 1987, The promastigote surface protease of Leishmania, Parasitol. Today, 3:151.
Bouvier, J., Etges, R.J., and Bordier, C., 1985, Identification and purification of membrane and soluble forms of the major surface protein of Leishmania promastigotes, J. Biol. Chem., 260:15504.
Chang, K.P., 1983, Cellular and molecular mechanisms of intracellular symbiosis in Leishmaniasis, Internat. Rev. Cytol., Supplement 14:267.
Chang, K.P., and Fong, D., 1983, Cell-biology of host-parasite membrane interactions in Leishmaniasis, in: Cytopathology of Parasitic Disease, Pitman Books, London.
Colomer-Gould, V., Quintao, L.G., Kiethly, J., and Nogueira, N., 1985, A common major surface antigen on amastigotes and promastigotes of Leishmania species, J. Exp. Med., 162:902.
Dwyer, D., 1980, Isolation and partial characterization of surface membranes from Leishmania donovani promastigotes, J. Protozool., 27:176.
Etges, R.J., Bouvier, J., Hoffman, R., and Bordier, C., 1985, Evidence that the major surface proteins of three Leishmania species are structurally related, Mol. Biochem. Parasitol., 14:141.
Farah, R.S., Samra, S.A., and Nuwayri-Salti, N., 1975, The role of the macrophage in cutaneous leishmaniasis, Immunology, 29:755.

Fong, D., and Chang, K.P., 1982, Surface antigen change during differentiation of a parasitic protozoan, Leishmania mexicana: Identification by monoclonal antibodies, Proc. Natl. Acad. Sci., 79:7366.

Gardiner, P.R., and Dwyer, D.M., 1983, Radioiodination and identification of externally disposed membrane components of Leishmania tropica, Mol. Biochem. Parasit., 8:283.

Gardiner, P.R., Jaffe, C., and Dwyer, D.M., 1984, Identification of cross-reactive promastigote cell surface antigens of some leishmanial stocks by I-125 labeling and immunoprecipitation, Infect. Immun., 43:637.

Handman, E., and Hocking, R.E., 1982, Stage-specific, strain-specific and cross-reactive antigens of Leishmania species identified by monoclonal antibodies, Infect. Immun., 37:28.

Handman, E., Jarvis, H.M., and Mitchell, G.F., 1984, Leishmania major: identification of stage-specific antigens and antigens shared by promastigotes and amastigotes, Parasite Immunology, 6:223.

Handman, E., and Goding, J.W., 1985, The leishmania receptor for macrophages is a lipid containing glycoconjugate, EMBO Journal, 2:329.

Handman, E., Schnur, L.F., Spithill, T.W., and Mitchell, G.M., 1986, Passive transfer of leishmania lipopolysaccharide confers parasite survival in macrophages, J. Immunol., 137:3608.

Hernandez, A.G., 1983, Leishmanial excreted factors and their possible biological role, in: Cytopathology of Parasitic Disease, Pitman Books, London.

Jaffe, C.L., and Sarfstein, R., 1987, Species-specific antibodies to L. tropica (minor) recognize somatic antigens and exometabolites, J. Immunol., 139:1310.

Kahl, L.P., and McMahon-Pratt, D., 1987, Structural and antigenic characterization of a species- and promastigote-specific Leishmania mexicana amazonensis membrane protein, J. Immunol., 138:1587.

Kink, J.A., and Chang, K.P., 1987, Biological and biochemical characterization of tunicamycin-resistant Leishmania mexicana: mechanism of drug resistance and virulence, Infect. Immun., 55:1692.

Kweider, M., Lemesre, J.L., Darcy, F., Fusnierz, J.P., Capron, A., and Santoro, F., 1987, Infectivity of Leishmania braziliensis promastigotes is dependent on the increasing expression of a 65,000-dalton surface antigen, J. Immunol., 138:299.

Lepay, D.A., Nogueira, N., and Cohn, Z., 1983, Surface antigens of Leishmania donovani promastigotes, J. Exp. Med., 157:1562.

McMahon-Pratt, D., and David, J.R., 1981, Monoclonal antibodies that distinguish between New World species of Leishmania, Nature, 291:581.

McMahon-Pratt, D., Bennett, E., and David, J.R., 1982, Monoclonal antibodies that distinguish subspecies of Leishmania braziliensis, J. Immunol., 129:936.

McMahon-Pratt, D., Bennett, E., Grimaldi, G., and Jaffe, C.L., 1985, Subspecies- and species-specific antigens of Leishmania mexicana characterized by monoclonal antibodies, J. Immunol., 134:1935.

Ramasay, R., Kar, S.K., and Jamnadas, H., 1983, Cross-reacting surface antigens on Leishmania promastigotes, Internat. J. Parasitol., 13:337.

Reed, S.G., Badaro, R., and Lloyd, R.M.C., 1987, Identification of specific and cross-reactive antigens of Leishmania donovani chagasi by human infection sera, J. Immunol., 138:1596.

Rodrigues, M.M., Xavier, M.T., Previato, L.M., and Barconski, M.A., 1986, Characterization of cellular immune response to chemically defined glycoconjugates from Leishmania mexicana subsp. amazonensis, Infect. Immun., 51:80.

Russell, D.G., and Wilhelm, H., 1986, The involvement of the major surface glycoprotein (gp63) of Leishmania promastigotes in attachment to macrophages, J. Immunol., 136:2613.

Sacci, J.B., Christensen, H.A., Vasquez, A., and Anthony, R.L., 1987, Serodiagnosis of New World Leishmaniasis by using a genus-specific antigen in enzyme linked immunosorbent assays, Diag. Microbiol. Infect. Dis., 6:229.

Sacks, D.L., Hieny, S., and Sher, A., 1987, Identification of cell surface carbohydrate and antigenic changes between noninfective and infective developmental stages of Leishmania major promastigotes, J. Immunol., 135:564.

Sadick, M.D., and Raff, H.V., 1985, Differences in expression and exposure of promastigote and amastigote membrane molecules in Leishmania tropica, Infect. Immun., 47:395.

Slutzky, G.M., and Greenblatt, C.L., 1977, Isolation of a carbohydrate-rich immunologically active factor from cultures of Leishmania tropica, FEBS Letter, 80:401.

Slutsky, G.M., El-on, J., and Greenblatt, C.L., 1979, Leishmanial excreted factor:protein bound and free forms from promastigote cultures of Leishmania tropica and Leishmania donovani, Infect. Immun., 26:916.

Turco, S.J., Wilkerson, M.A., and Clawson, D.R., 1984, Expression of an unusual acidic glycoconjugate in Leishmania donovani, J. Biol. Chem., 259:3883.

Williams, K.M., Sacci, J.B., and Anthony, R.L., 1986a, Characterization and quantitation of membrane antigens of New World Leishmania species by using monoclonal antibodies in Western blot and flow microfluorometric assays, J. Protozool., 33:490.

Williams, K.M., Sacci, J.B., and Anthony, R.L., 1986b, Identification and recovery of Leishmania antigen displayed on the surface membrane of mouse peritoneal macrophages infected in vitro, J. Immunol., 136:1853.

Williams, K.M., Sacci, J.B., and Anthony, R.L., 1986c, Flow cytometric analysis of the effects exerted by monoclonal antibodies on binding and uptake of Leishmania mexicana subsp. mexicana promastigotes by murine peritoneal macrophages, Infect. Immun., 52:36.

ANTIGENS RECOGNIZED BY SERA FROM PATIENTS WITH VISCERAL LEISHMANIASIS

Charles L. Jaffe,[1] Shmuel Argov,[2] Mariano Zalis,[1] Nurit Rachamim,[1] Margalit Krup[2] and Yehuda Shoenfeld[2]

[1]Department of Biophysics – MacArthur Center for Molecular Biology of Tropical Diseases Weizmann Institute of Science, Rehovot Israel and [2]Research Unit of Autoimmune Diseases Dept. of Medicine D', Soroka Medical Center Beersheva Israel

INTRODUCTION

Visceral leishmaniasis is a fatal disease, generally caused by the parasite Leishmania donovani. This disease is typified by anemia, irregular fever and hepatosplenomegaly[1,2]. Patients with visceral leishmaniasis are immunosuppressed and fail to mount delayed-type skin hypersensitivity reactions to leishmanial antigen. However, hyperglobulinemia is a characteristic feature of the disease and globulin levels as high as 5g per 100 ml have been noted. Although leishmanial specific antibodies are present most of the antibody is not parasite specific and is thought to result from polyclonal B cell stimulation.[1-3]

Sera from patients with visceral leishmaniasis recognize from 5 to more than 20 different components in Leishmania depending on the technical protocols utilized to assay antibody reactivity.[4-7] However certain antigens are commonly recognized by a majority of sera, though differences between the patterns of individual patients can be noted.[7] These patterns are similar to those seen with infected dog sera(C.L.J., unpublished data) and polyclonal rabbit sera.[4] While both specific- and cross- species antigens can be identified,[6-8] the functions for most serum-reactive parasite antigens are unknown.

Autoantibodies are present in many parasitic diseases, malaria, Chagas', leprosy, African trypanosomiasis and leishmaniasis.[9-13] Antibodies aganist laminin, rheumatoid factors and tublin have noted in patients with cutaneous and/or visceral types of disease.[13-15] In one study[13] greater than 68% of the visceral leishmaniasis patients had circulating immune complexes and 93% had rheumatoid factors. Antibodies against host proteins may be associated with much of the pathogenicity seen in visceral leishmaniasis.

In this paper we examine some of the antigens recognized by parasite specific- and auto-antibodies. Their use in diagnosis of visceral leishmaniasis is discussed.

MATERIAL AND METHODS

Leishmania. Promastigotes were grown in Schneider's Drosophila medium containing 10% fetal calf serum and antibiotics.[16] The following isolates were used in all subsequent studies: L. donovani (MHOM/ET/67/HU3 and MHOM/BR/??/EDMAEL); L. major (MHOM/IL/79/Perlstein); L. tropica (MHOM/IL/ ??/JerichoI), L. mexicana amazonensis (MHOM/BR/??/LTB0016).

Antigens. Crude parasite membranes were prepared from $1-5 \times 10^{10}$ promastigotes as described[17] by nitrogen cavitation and differential centrifugation. Briefly, washed parasites were resuspended at 4°C in lysis buffer containing several proteolytic inhibitors. The cells were disrupted in a Parr cell disruption bomb (10 min at 1500 psi) and the homogenates separated into three fractions by successive centrifugation at 4,350 and 39,000 x g in a Sorval SS-34 rotor. The second fraction, that pelleting at 39,000 x g was used throughout this study designated as crude membranes.

When needed whole cell lysates were obtained by resuspending washed promastigotes in 1-2 ml lysis buffer as above and sonicating the cell suspension for 10-15 s in a water bath sonicator. The lysates were snap frozen and stored at -70° until use. Protein concentration was determined by the Bio-Rad Protein assay.

RNP, Sm, SSA and SSB were kindly provided by H. Slor, Dept. of Genetics, University of Tel-Aviv, Ramat Aviv, Israel. Histones, ssDNA, dsDNA, poly(I) and poly(dT) were obtained from Sigma Chemical Co.

Antibodies. The production and characterization of many of the monoclonal antibodies employed in this study have been described and are referenced in Table VI. Antibodies T8-T10 and A9-A12 were raised in BALB/c mice to membranes prepared from respectively, L. major (LRC-L251) and L. aethiopica (MHOM/ET/71/L100). AMAS-1 and AMAS-2 were produced from mice injected i.v. with irradiated (50 Krads) amastigotes of L. major (LRC-L251). Finally, monoclonal antibodies 170-1 and 170-2 were generated by injecting BALB/C mice with a 170 kDa band recognized in Western Blots by T11 (ref 17). The band was cut from the nitrocellulose paper, dissolved in DMSO, mixed with Freunds incomplete adjuvant and injected s.c. into the mice. The spleen cells were fused with a NS-1 (P3-X63 Ag8) mouse plasmacytoma cell line to generate hybridoma cells. The fusions were carried out as previously described.[17] Hybridoma culture supernatants were used for all immunoassays. Ascites fluid containing antibodies D2 and D13 were produced by injecting the cloned hybrid cell line (10^6 to 10^7 cells, i.p.) into pristane primed BALB/c mice.

Sources of human sera are summarized in Table II. Dog sera were obtained in Israel by C.L.J. and were assayed by tissue biopsy and ELISA (unpublished results).

Immunoassays. All immunoassys carried out were enzyme-linked immunosorbent assays (ELISA). Polyvinylchloride microtiter plates were coated overnight with crude parasite lysates (50 to 80νg/ml) and subsequently blocked with 2% fetal calf serum in 50mM phosphate-buffered saline, pH 7.2 (PBS). Alternatively, nitrocellulose paper was spotted with pure

L. donovani proteins gp70-2 or dp72 (150 or 300ng, respectively) for dot-blot assay. The competitive ELISA[8] and dot-blot[18] assays were carried out as previously described. Assays using other antigens were performed using precoated microtiter plates provided by H.Slor, Dept. Genetics, Tel-Aviv University, Israel. The plates were incubated for 2 h at room temperature with the various human sera (1/500 dilution), washed 4 times with 0.1% Tween-20 in PBS (2X washing buffer) and alkaline phosphatase conjugated protein A (1/2000 dilution in 2X washing buffer containing 1%BSA) added. After 1 h at 37o the plates were washed 4 times with 2X washing buffer and the substrate p-nitrophenol phosphate added. All the reactions were stopped after 1h and the absorbance read at 405nm.

Affinity resin. Ascites fluid to hybridoma clones D2 and D13 were raised in BALB/c mice and purified by hydroxylapatite chromatography.[19] The purified antibodies were dialyzed verus 0.2M sodium bicarbonate buffer and coupled to a p-nitrophenyl derivative of ϵ-caprioc/β-alanine Sepharose 4B (Pharmacia).[20] The amount of protein coupled to the resin was 5mg/ml.

Purification of the L.donovani proteins. Membranes (2mg) from either Edmael or LV9 were solubilized for 1 h at 4°C in 30 mM Tris-HCl, pH 8.2 containing 0.5% (w/v) sodium deoxycholate (DOC) and proteolytic inhibitors. The material was centrifuged at 39,000 x g for 0.5 h and the supernatant removed. The supernatant was incubated batchwise with the affinity resin(s) in a 50 ml tube for 2 h at 4°C. Following three washes of the affinity resin by centrifugation for 5 min at 1500 x g the bound protein was eluted from the matrix with 50 mM diethylamine, pH 11.5. The column was re-equilibrated by washing with 30 mM Tris-HCl, pH 8.2, 0.1% DOC.

SDS-polyacrylamide gel electrophoresis (PAGE) and western blotting. SDS-PAGE was carried out in 5-12% gradient gels and silver stained for protein.[21,22] Proteins from polyacrylamide gels for western blotting[23] were transferred electrophoretically (2 h, 40 V) onto 45νm nitrocellulose paper without fixing. The nitrocellulose was quenched with 0.3% Tween-20/PBS and washed twice with washing buffer. Following a 2 h incubation at room temperature with the appropriate antibodies (human at a 1/1000 dilution and a 1/4 dilution of hybridoma culture supernatant), the blots were rinsed 4 x with washing buffer and probed for 1 h a suitable second antibody. ^{125}I-rabbit F(ab')$_2$ anti-mouse IgG (Zymed) and a radioiodinated sheep F(ab')$_2$ anti-human IgG (Amersham) were used. Finally the nitrocellulose paper was rinsed for times in washing buffer and air dried. The strips were exposed to X-Ray film at -70°C using an intensifying screen (Dupont).

RESULTS AND DISCUSSION

Human visceral leishmaniasis patient sera show titers on leishmanial antigens of 10^{-5} (ref. 8). When western blots with these sera are carried out on membranes of L. donovani reactions can be observed with many different components, molecular weights (M_r) from 14300 to >150000.[4-7] Sera from patients with other diseases also show reactions with parasite antigen but at higher serum concentrations.[6,7,31] A similar pattern of reaction is also seen with infected dog sera (data not shown). A band of approximately 55-60 kDa is seen with most patient sera from both visceral and cutaneous leishmaniasis (ref. 7,31 and unpublished data). This probably corresponds to the major radioiodinatable glycoprotein, gp63, which can be immuno-precipitated by leishmaniasis patient serum.[4]

It has been shown that sera from patients with visceral leishmaniasis recognize particular proteins not identified by sera from patients with cutaneous disease or other parasitic diseases.[7;8] In addition, parasite antigens identified by species specific monoclonal antibodies to L. donovani are also recognized by visceral leishmaniasis patient sera (ref. 6). A highly specific and sensitive competitive ELISA[8] was developed using three of these L. donovani specific monoclonal antibodies D2, D13 and D14. Titers against these antigens equal or exceed 10^{-3}. No false positives were found with this assay using any other disease examined, including Chagas' disease.

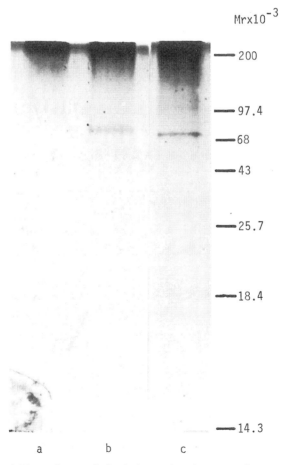

Figure 1. Purification of Leishmania donovani proteins by affinity chromatography on monoclonal antibody resins. Silver stain of SDS-PAGE of purified proteins from Edmael. Lane a, SDS-PAGE sample buffer. Lane b, Material eluted from D2 affinity resin. Lane c, Material eluted from D13 affinity resin.

In order to developed a quicker, more easily standardized assay, as well as examine the function of these proteins, the antigens recognized by D2 and D13 were purified. The proteins reacting with the two monoclonal antibodies were isolated by affinity chromatography on resins to which the purified antibodies were coupled. Occasionally, the proteins were further purified by size exclusion-high performance liquid chromatography. The purified proteins had molecular weights of approximately 70 kDa by SDS-PAGE (figure 1, lanes b and c) and were still antigenically active by both western and dot blotting (data not shown). Though the proteins demonstrate similar molecular weights by PAGE they are not identical. Antibody D2 did not react with the protein purified on the D13 column and visa versa. Peptide mapping of [^{35}S]-methionine labelled proteins displayed different patterns and the binding of antibody D2 to antigen, unlike antibody D13, was sensitive to periodate oxidation.[24]

Direct ELISA's on crude parasite antigen have been used for the diagnosis of visceral leishmaniasis,[25-27] though false positive reactions were found when sera from other diseases were tested at high concentrations. However, dilutions of patient sera to 10^{-3} produced good results in two different studies.[25,27] At this dilution false positives were observed

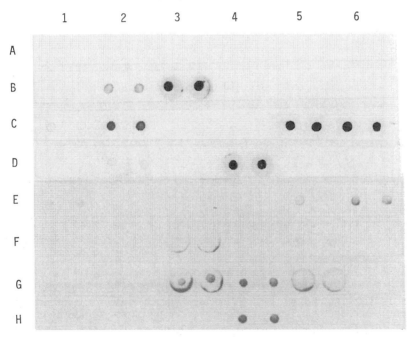

Figure 2. Dot-blot ELISA for visceral leishmaniasis of purified Leishmania donovani proteins gp70-2 and dp72. Rows A-D, gp70-2 (D2 affinity resin). Rows E-H, dp72 (D13 affinity resin). Serum - Visceral leishmaniasis B2-B4, C1,C2,C5,C6,D2,D4,E1,E5,E6,F3,F5,G2-G4,H4. African trypanosomiasis A1,A2,F1,F2. Malaria A4. Systemic lupus erythomatosus A5. Chagas' disease A6,C4,F6,G5,H2,H3. Leprosy B5,B6,E4,G1,H5,H6. Cutaneous leishmaniasis C3,D3,D5,D6,E2,E3. Endemic controls B1,D1,F4,G6,H1.

Table I. Results of direct ELISA using gp70-2

A. Visceral Leishmaniasis Sera

Origin	Serum tested	# positive	% positive	#False negative	%False negative
Brazil	22	19	86.4	3	13.6
Colombia	3	2	66	1	33
India	6	6	100	0	0
Africa	9	9	100	0	0
Total	40	36	90.0	4	10.0

Source[+] - 1,2,3,4,5,6 & 13

B. Sera from Normal Patients and Other Diseases

Sera	Serum tested	#False positive	%False positive	Source[+]
Cutaneous				
(old world)	5	0	0.0	14
(new world)	19	1	5.3	2,6
Chagas'	18	0	0.0	1
Malaria	6	0	0.0	3,8
Leprosy	4	0	0.0	7
African trypanosomiasis	5	0	0.0	12
SLE[*]	2	0	0.0	10
Schistosomiasis	3	0	0.0	9
Endemic normal	13	0	0.0	1,3
Non-endemic normal	3	0	0.0	
Other	8	0	0.0	3,5
Total	86	1	1.2	

[*] Systemic lupus erythematosus

[+] Key: 1 Drs. Rodolfo Teixeira and Roberto Badaro, Hospital Prof. Edgard Santos, Salvador Brazil; 2 Dr. Mauro Marzochi, Fundacao Oswaldo Cruz, Rio de Janeiro, Brazil; 3 Dr. C.P. Thakur, Patna Medical College, Bihar, India; 4 Dr. Richard Pearson, University of Virginia, Charlottesville, VA; 5 Dr. Frank Neva, LPD, NIH, Bethesda, MD; 6 Dr. Nancy Saravia, CIDEM-Tulane University, Cali, Columbia; 7 Dr. Patricia Rose, Hansen's Disease Control Program, Georgetown, Guyana; 8 Dr. Ian McGregor, England; 9 Dr. Allain Dessein, Centre D'Immunologie INSERM-CNRS, Marseille, France; 10 Dr. Peter Schur, Peter Bent Brigham Hospital, Boston, MA; 11 Dr. David Mirelman, Weizmann Institute of Science, Rehovot, Israel; 12 Dr. de Raadt, Trypanosomiasis Unit, W.H.O., Geneva, Switzerland;

Table II. Results of direct ELISA using dp72

A. Visceral Leishmaniasis Sera

Origin	Serum tested	# positive	% positive	#False negative	%False negative
Brazil	13	13	100	0	0
Columbia	2	2	100	0	0
India	3	3	100	0	0
Africa	3	3	100	0	0
Total	21	21	100	0	0

Source[+] - 1,2,3,4,5,6 & 13

B. Sera from Normal Patients and Other Diseases

Sera	Serum tested	#False positive	%False positive	Source[+]
Cutaneous				
(old world)	4	0	0.0	14
(new world)	13	3	23.0	2,6
Chagas'	15	1	6.6	1
Malaria	5	0	0.0	3,8
Leprosy	4	1	25.0	7
African trypanosomiasis	4	0	0.0	12
Amoebiasis	2	0	0.0	11
SLE[*]	1	0	0.0	10
Schistosomiasis	3	0	0.0	9
Endemic normal	14	0	0.0	1,3
Non-endemic normal	2	0	0.0	
Other	4	0	0.0	3,5
Total	71	5	7.0	

[*] Systemic lupus erythematosus
[+] See Table 1 for key.

---

13 Dr. M. Miles, London School of Hygiene and Tropical Medicine, London, England; 14 Dr. Justin Passwell, Chaim Sheba Medical Center, Tel Aviv, Israel.

only with sera from mucocutaneous leishmaniasis or Chagas' disease.[27-30]

A dot-blot ELISA on nitrocellulose paper was developed using the two pure proteins.[18] A composite figure of the results obtained using the two different proteins is shown in figure 2. Using one protein (150 ng of gp70-2 purified on the D2 affinity resin) 90% (36/40) of the kala azar sera were correctly diagnosed and only 1.2% (1/86) of the non kala azar sera were misdiagnosed. With the second protein (300ng of dp72 purified on the D13 affinity resin) 100% (21/21) of the kala azar sera tested were properly identified and 7.0% (5/71) of the other sera were misread. All sera were assayed at 1/100 dilutions. The data are summarized in tables I and II. None of the 18 sera from patients with Chagas' disease reacted on gp70-2 even though several of these sera when tested on crude antigen by ELISA[8,31] showed titers of 10^{-4}.

All assays were carried out in duplicate without any previous knowledge of the sera type. Each dot matrix included as negative controls a standard normal human and Chagas' sera. Visceral leishmaniasis sera was also included as a positive control. While the reaction intensity varies between different visceral leishmaniasis serum no fluctuation was noted upon repeated testing of a single serum. Interestingly one cutaneous leishmaniasis reacted with both antigens. All of the other sera misdiagnosed by dp72 were correctly identified by gp70-2. Together more than 95% of the human sera were correctly diagnosed.

This assay should also be useful for the rapid screening of canine visceral leishmaniasis. Infected dogs also produce antibodies against dp72 which can be detected either by competitive ELISA (Table III; C.L.J. paper in preparation, and McMahon-Pratt, personal communication) or by dot-blot on the pure proteins (C.L.J., unpublished results).

Table III. Serodiagnosis of canine visceral leishmaniasis[a]

Dog	Direct ELISA[b] Dilutions		Competitive ELISA[c]	
	10^{-2}	10^{-3}	MAb 13/14	MA b2
D2	>2.00	1.361	75.6	0.0
D3	0.184	0.042	3.0	0.0

[a] Dog sera were collected in Israel. Lymph node biopsy on D2 was positive for parasites which were typed as L. donovani by Dr. L. Schnur LRC, Jerusalem Israel.

[b] Absorbance 405^{nm}.

[c] % Inhibition

Table IV. Antibodies to nuclear antigens in leishmaniasis

Antigen	Percent Positive*	
	Cutaneous	Visceral
ds-DNA	0	0
ss-DNA	7	4
poly(I)	7	20
poly(G)	21	17
Histone	29	7
Sm	7	83
RNP	14	86
SSA	25	36
SSB	25	73

* Values (Abs_{405nm}) 2 S.D. above the mean of sera (1/200 dilution) from 15 healthy subjects was considered positive. A total of 12-14 cutaneous and 23 visceral leishmaniasis patient sera were examined. All leishmaniasis sera tested had specific antibody to parasite antigen.

When compared to other assays which use crude parasites as antigen several advantages are apparent. First pure proteins are employed. Standardized protein preparations can be easily monitored both biochemically and antigenically; thus ensuring reproducibility from batch to batch. The pure proteins are antigenically stable. They can be freeze dried without lose of activity and can be stored at 4°C on nitrocellulose for at least 1/2 year. Elimination of antigen and asssay variability between laboratories should facilitate interpretation and comparison of test results.

In addition to parasite specific antibodies, high levels of antibodies to haptens, foreign proteins and autoantigens are present in patients with visceral leishmaniasis.[13-15,36,37] Among the possible explanations for the appearance of high levels of non-leishmanial specific antibodies is the polyclonal activation of B cell clones which normally produce low amounts of natural antibodies against cellular components. Such mitogenic factors have been demonstrated in leishmanial antigen preparations.[14,36,38] The discharge of host cell antigens upon cell lysis and parasite release may also lead to the production of immunoglobulins against autoantigens. Finally molecular mimicry of epitopes on host cellular components by a pathogen may result in production of autoantibodies to crossreactive epitopes. Evidence for this mechanism has been seen with virus,[39] and bacteria.[40-42]

Sera from patients with visceral and cutaneous leishmaniasis were screened against several nuclear antigens (Table IV). All sera showed positive titers on leishmanial antigen by ELISA (data not shown). Reactions with cutaneous patient sera were observed on most of the antigens examined with the exception of ds-DNA. About 25% of the sera recognized poly(G), histone, SSA and SSB. However, when the binding of sera from patients with visceral leishmaniasis was examined strong reactions, more than 4 standard deviations above the mean found for healthy individuals, were observed on RNP, Sm and SSB for >75% of the sera. Titers observed were greater than > 1:500 for these same antigens. Reactions on the remaining antigens were similar to those observed with cutaneous patient sera. The binding of individual patient sera to RNP and Sm are shown in figure 3. Healthy endemic normal subjects showed higher baseline binding to antigens than controls from nonendemic regions. This later finding may be due to long term exposure to infectious agents which stimulate the production of antibodies, even though the subjects are asymptomatic.

Binding to Sm antigen could be completely inhibited in a competitive ELISA by preincubating the visceral leishmaniasis patient sera with either Sm or RNP prior to assaying (data not

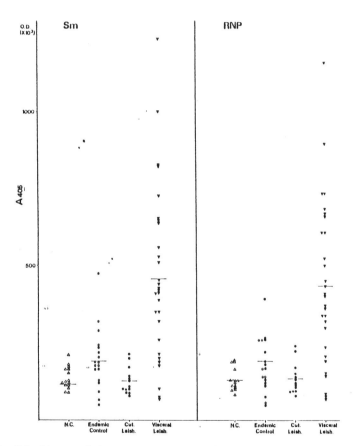

Figure 3. Binding of human serum to RNP and Sm antigens. A direct ELISA[35] was carried out using nonendemic control serum (N.C.,$\triangle$); control serum from an area endemic for visceral leishmaniasis (O); serum from patients with cutaneous leishmaniasis (O) and visceral leishmaniasis (▼). Sera were incubated with the antigens 2h. After washing, the plates were reacted with alkaline phosphatase conjugated to goat antihuman IgG and then developed with p-nitrophenyl phosphate.

Table V. Reactions of anti-leishmanial monoclonal antibodies on RNP and Sm

	Monoclonal antibodies	Reference	Specificity[a]	Reactivity[b] on antigens RNP	Sm
1	T2	46	Lm & ± Lt	<0.1	–
2	T3	46	Lm & ± Lt	<0.1	–
3	T4	46	Lm	<0.1	–
4	T8		Lm,Ld & ± Lt	<0.1	–
5	T9		Lm,Ld & ± Lt	<0.1	–
6	T10		Lm	<0.1	–
7	D2	6	Ld	<0.1	–
8	D9	6	Ld	<0.1	–
9	D10	6	Ld	<0.1	<0.1
10	D12	6	Ld	<0.1	–
11	D13	6	Ld	<0.1	<0.1
12	D14	6	Ld	<0.1	–
13	X1	6	all Leishmania	<0.1	–
14	X4	17	all Leishmania	<0.1	<0.1
15	X5	6	all Leishmania	<0.1	<0.1
16	A9		La,Ld & Lt	<0.1	–
17	A10		La,Lm & Lt	<0.1	–
18	A11		La,Lm & Lt	<0.1	<0.1
19	A12		La,Ld &Lt	<0.1	<0.1
20	170-1		all Leishmania	1.26	1.12
21	170-2		all Leishmania	1.43	1.41
22	AMAS-1		amastigotes-Lm	<0.1	<0.1
23	AMAS-2		amastigotes-all Leish.	<0.1	<0.1

[a] Reactivity on leishmanial membranes or lysates. Lm-L. major Lt-L. tropica Ld-L. donovani La-L. aethiopica.

[b] $ABS_{405-490nm}$

shown). No inhibition of binding to Sm antigen was found with ssDNA, poly(I) or poly(G). Likewise, binding to Sm, RNP, SSA or SSB antigen coated plates could be inhibited by membrane preparations of all Leishmania tested, L. major, L. donovani, L. tropica and L. mexicana amazonensis. Binding inhibition by membranes to RNP is shown in (data not shown). These results intimate that crossreacting determinants are present on Leishmania and these four nuclear antigens. In fact, as shown in table V, two monoclonal antibodies 170-1 & -2 against a pan- leishmanial membrane component crossreact with RNP and Sm; while monoclonal antibodies produced against pure Sm (data not shown) bind to parasite membrane antigen. The nature of this crossreactive parasite determinant is presently under investigation.

The presence of circulating immune complexes and antibodies to host components (rheumatoid factors), cellular components, DNA[13-15,36,37] and parasite mitogenic factors[14,38] suggests that polyclonal B cell stimulation is an important mechanism in the development of hypergammaglobulinemia and autoantibodies. These results parallel findings in other parasitic diseases such as malaria,[44] schistosomiasis[44] and African Trypanosomiasis.[45] However, antibodies to ssDNA and the polynucleotides with similar antigenic determinants are the predominant autoanti bodies observed with the latter parasitic diseases. The low level of anti-ssDNA antibodies found in patients with visceral leishmaniasis suggests that an additional mechanism may be involved. As is the case for M.leprae[11] or M.tuberculosis[40] and DNA, our results indicate that host and parasite antigens are immunogenically crossreactive and share similar antigenic determinants. Molecular mimicry should be taken into account as a possible mechanism for the induction of autoantibodies in visceral leishmaniasis.

ACKNOWLEDGEMENTS

This work was suported in part by the John and Catherine T. MacArthur Foundation, Keren Yeda, and the US-Israel Binational Science Foundation.

REFERENCES

1. P.D.Marsden (1979) New Eng.J.Med. 300:350.
2. R.D.Pearson, D.A.Wheeler, L.H.Harrison and H.D.Kay (1983) Rev.Inf.Dis. 5:907.
3. J.Mauel and R.Behin (1982) "Leishmaniasis: Immunity, immunopathology and immunodiagnosis." In: Immunology of Parasitic Infections (S.Cohen and K.S.Warren, eds.), pp.299-355, Blackwell Sci.Publ., Oxford, England.
4. D.A.Lepay, N.Nogueira and Z.Cohn (1983) J.Exp.Med 157:1562.
5. D.M.Dwyer (1981) "Structural, chemical and antigenic properties of surface membranes isolated from Leishmania donovani." In: The Biochemistry of Parasites (G.M. Slutzsky, ed.), pp.9-28, Pergamon Press, New York.
6. C.L.Jaffe, E.Bennett, G.Grimaldi and D.McMahon-Pratt (1984) J.Immunol. 133:440.
7. S.G.Reed, R.Badaro and R.M.C.Lloyd (1987) J.Immunol. 138:1596.
8. C.L.Jaffe and D.McMahon-Pratt (1987) Trans.Roy.Soc.Trop. Med.Hyg. 81:587.
9. G.O.Oyeyinka (1986) Nature 319:543.
10. J.N.Wood, L.Hudson, T.M.Jessell and M.Yamamoto (1982) Nature 296:34.
11. C.J.Thorns and J.A.Morris (1985) Clin.exp.Immunol. 61:323.
12. J.A.M.S.Anthoons, E.A.E.Van Marck and P.L.J.Gigase (1986) 72:443.
13. J.L.Avila, M.Rojas and M.Rieber (1984) Inf.Imm. 43:402.
14. M.W.J.Bohme, D.A.Evans, M.A.Miles and E.J.Holborow Immunology 59:583.
15. R.D.Pearson, T.Evans, D.A.Wheeler, T.B.Naida, J.E.De Alencar and J.S.Davis (1986) Ann.Trop.Med.Parasitol. 80:465.
16. C.L.Jaffe, G.Grimaldi and D.McMahon-Pratt (1984) "The

cultivation and cloning of Leishmania." In: Genes and Antigens of Parasites, A Laboratory Manual(C.Morel, ed.), pp.47-92, UNDP/WORLD BANK/WHO, Brazil.
17. C.L.Jaffe and R.Sarfstein (1987) J.Immunol. 139:1310.
18. M.Zalis and C.L.Jaffe (1987) J.Immunol.Methods 101:261.
19. L.H.Stanker, M.Vanderlaan and H.Juarez-Salinas (1985) J. Immunol.Methods 76:157.
20. M.Wilchek and T.Miron (1987) Biochemistry 26:2155.
21. U.K.Laemmli (1970) Nature 227:680.
22. W.Wray, T.Boulikas, V.P.Wray and R.Hancock (1981) Anal. Biochem. 118:197.
23. H.Towbin, T.Staehelin and J.Gordon (1979) Proc.Natl.Acad. Sci.U.S.A. 76:4350.
24. C.L.Jaffe and M.Zalis (1988) Mol.Biochem.Parasitol. 27:53.
25. K.M.DeCock, A.N.Hodgen, J.Y.Channon, T.K.Arap Siongok, S.B.Lucas and P.W.Rees (1985) J.Infect.Dis. 151:750.
26. M.Ho, J.Leeuwenburg, G.Mbugua, A.Wamachi and A.Voller (1983) Am.J.Trop.Med.Hyg. 32:943.
27. A.Jahn and H.J.Diesfeld (1983) Trans.R.Soc.Trop.Med.Hyg. 77:451.
28. R.Badaro, S.G.Reed, A.Barral, G.Orge and T.Jones (1986) Am.J.Trop.Med.Hyg. 35:72.
29. M.C.S.Guimaraes, B.J.Celeste, E.A.deCastilho, J.R.Mineo and J.M.P.Diniz (1981) Am.J.Trop.Med.Hyg. 30:942.
30. M.G.Pappas, R.Hajkowski AND W.T.Hockmeyer (1983) J.Immunol.Methods 64:205.
31. J.H.Passwell, R.Shor, H.Trau, J.Shoham and C.L.Jaffe (1987) J.Immunol. 139: In press.
32. B.D.Stollar (1977) Ann.Rheum.Dis.Suppl. 36:102.
33. Y.Shoenfeld, J.Rauch, H.Massicotte, S.K.Datta, J.Andre-Schwartz, B.D.Stollar and R.S.Schwartz (1983) N.Engl.J.Med 308:414.
34. Y.Shoenfeld, A.El-Roeiy, O.Ben-Yehuda and A.I.Pick (1987) Clin.Immunol.Immunopathol. 42:250.
35. P.J.Maddison, R.P.Skinner, P.Vlachoyiannopoulos, D.M. Brennand and D.Hough (1985) Clin.exp.Immunol. 62:337.
36. B.Galvao-Castro, J.A.Sa Ferreira, K.F.Marzochi, M.C.Marzochi, S.G.Coutinho and P.H.Lambert (1984) Clin.exp. Immunol. 56:58.
37. P.A.Krager, C.Van Der Plas-Van Dalen, P.H.Rees, F.M.Helmerhorst and A.E.G.Kr. Von Dem Borne (1984) Trop.geogr. Med. 36:143.
38. J.Weintraub, M.Gottlieb and F.I.Weinbaum (1982) Exp. Parasitol. 53:87.
39. M.B.A.Oldstone (1987) Cell 50:819.
40. Y.Shoenfeld, Y.Vilner, A.R.M.Coates, J.Rauch, G.Lavie, D.Shaul and J.Pinkhas (1986) Clin.exp.Immunol. 66:255.
41. A.El-Roiey, O.Sela, D.A.Isenberg, R.Feldman, B.C.Colaco, R.C.Kennedy and Y.Shoenfeld (1987) Clin.exp.Immunol. 67:507.
42. R.Sumazaki, T.Fujita, T.Kabashima, F.Nishikaku, A.Koyama, M.Shibasaki and H.Takita (1986) Clin.exp.Immunol. 66:103.
43. M.Zouali, P.Druilhe and A.Eyquem (1986) Clin.exp.Immunol. 66:273.
44. B.R.Ott, N.P.Libbey, R.J.Ryter and W.M.Trebbin (1983) Arch.Intern.Med. 143:1477.
45. B.M.Greenwood (1974) Lancet 1:434.
46. C.L.Jaffe amd D. McMahon-Pratt (1983) J. Immunol. 131:1987.

INTERACTIONS BETWEEN LEISHMANIASIS AND MALARIA

F.E.G. Cox

Department of Biophysics, Cell and Molecular Biology
King's College London
26-29 Drury Lane
London   WC2B 5RL

INTRODUCTION

Most of what we know about immunity to leishmaniasis has been derived from carefully controlled experiments involving a single species of parasite in laboratory animals free from any other infection. However, in nature leishmaniasis is likely to occur concurrently with a wide range of other infections and it is now becoming clear that the immunological responses to one organism can result in a complex interplay capable of affecting the outcome of either or both the interacting infections. The distribution of leishmaniasis coincides with that of malaria over much of its range to such an extent that it was once though that leishmaniasis was a manifestation of malaria. These two diseases must therefore frequently occur together and the possible interactions between them have many important implications. The immunological responses to both leishmaniasis and malaria are complex and it is only within the past few years that it has become possible to begin to understand the intricacies of these responses and the mechanisms for their control. In this paper, I propose to indicate some of the ways in which the immunological responses to both leishmaniasis and malaria can interact and to discuss the consequences of these interactions in the context of both diseases and their control by chemotherapy and vaccination.

LABORATORY MODELS

Our understanding of immunity to both leishmaniasis and malaria is confused not by too little knowledge but by too much. A variety of different experimental hosts are available for study and, in these, different species of Leishmania cause different patterns of disease and, in mice, the most widely used hosts, the outcome of the infection is determined by the genetic background of the host (Howard et al., 1980; Bradley, 1977). Similarly for malaria; some ten species or subspecies of Plasmodium can infect laboratory mice (Killick-Kendrick and Peters, 1978) and, as in leishmaniasis, the patterns of infection vary in mice of different genetic backgrounds (Stevenson, et al., 1984) although this variation is not as clear-cut as it is in leishmaniasis. The plethora of information that has accumulated has been used for extrapolations between species of experimental host and man. Such extrapolations tend to be simplistic and potentially confusing but nevertheless common patterns of events do emerge and these form the basis of this paper. For convenience, and because of the vast amount of well-documented information available, this paper will be largely restricted to infections with Leishmania major and four species of Plasmodium, P. berghei, P. yoelii, P. vinckei and P. chabaudi in mice. Essentially, P. berghei and P. yoelii infect reticulocytes and immunity is largely antibody-mediated whereas P. vinckei and P. chabaudi inhabit mature red blood cells and immunity is largely antibody-independent (Grun and Weidanz, 1981).

IMMUNITY TO MICROPARASITES

Leishmania spp. and Plasmodium spp. are microparasites like bacteria and viruses and, as such, multiply within their hosts presenting an immediate threat unless controlled in some way. Control is effected by specific and non-specific mechanisms which are themselves regulated by a number of polypeptide molecules (see Old, 1987). Immediate control of life-threatening infections caused by parasites is usually incomplete and, because parasites have evolved many ways of evading the immune response, the infectious organisms persist at low levels in the host providing both a potential danger from recrudescent infections and a source of antigens that continually stimulate the immune system and its control mechanisms. Many of the molecules involved are non-specific in their action and may cause inappropriate or misdirected responses and thus contribute to the pathology of the disease. Thus we have a situation in which an invading organism is recognised as foreign and stimulates an immune response which inhibits the multiplication of the invader but also contributes to the pathology associated with the disease.

The events involved in antigen recognition and the elicitation of humoral and cell-mediated specific immune responses are well understood and damage to cells and tissues caused by antigen-antibody complexes, complement and molecules secreted by macrophages, neutrophils and other cells are recognised as representing the undesirable consequences of well-intentioned immune mechanisms. What is less clear, however, is what happens in the various regulatory circuits and it is only recently that any progress has been made in this area even in single parasite infections. In dual infections, the host has to contend with a complex of interacting immune responses and their respective regulatory circuits and these will be discussed later.

IMMUNITY TO MALARIA

Humans and experimental animals do recover from malaria but the actual mechanisms involved are far from clear. Acquired immunity is directed against the erythrocytic stages and antibody is thought to be involved in preventing merozoites from entering red blood cells. In actual fact, the evidence for antibody involvement is largely circumstantial and attention has now focused on other mediators (see Clark, et al., 1987). The overall events that occur when a malarial infection is brought under control are as follows. For a time, the infection of red cells, multiplication therein and invasion of fresh cells continues unabated. Antigen is processed by macrophages and induces a T-cell dependent B-cell response and the production of specific antibody. Malaria parasites also act as B-cell mitogens causing proliferation of these cells and the production of large amounts of non-specific antibody (Rosenberg, 1978). Specific antibody binds with malarial antigens forming antigen-antibody complexes which, with or without complement, contribute to the pathology of the disease (Cohen and Lambert, 1982).

It is, however, antibody independent activity that is most important from the point of view of possible interactions with other organisms. The best understood model is Plasmodium chabaudi adami in mice in which recovery occurs in the absence of antibody or antibody-producing cells (Grun and Weidanz, 1981) and this observation has formed the basis for studies on other subspecies of P. chabaudi and the related species P. vinckei and its subspecies. Immunity to these parasites can be induced non-specifically following exposure to Mycobacterium bovis (BCG), Corynebacterium parvum (Propionibacterium acnes) or a variety of other immunomodulators (see Cox, 1982). The central cells involved appear to be macrophages which when stimulated by BCG, Lipopolysaccharide (LPS), colony stimulating factor (CSF) and possibly antigen-antibody complexes, release a number of mediators (Nathan, 1987). One of these is tumour necrosis factor (TNF) which plays a major role in the effector arm of non-specific immune responses stimulating further macrophages, which in turn release TNF, IL-1 and reactive oxygen intermediates (ROI), and also neutrophils which also produce a variety of substances including reactive oxygen intermediates.

Reactive oxygen intermediates are formed as part of the respiratory burst characteristic of phagocytic cells and are able to kill intracellular parasites. These molecules are also released externally and are thought to kill intraerythrocytic parasites as the red cells squeeze through the sinusoids of the liver and spleen (Dockrell, et al., 1986). The actual killing involves a process of lipid peroxidation (Buffington et al., 1986). Unfortunately these externally released substances also damage host cells and largely contribute to the pathology associated with malaria (Clark et al., 1987). The central roles in this whole process are played by primed macrophages which release TNF and IL-1, which have many functions in common and enhance the release of reactive oxygen intermediates by macrophages, and gamma-interferon which itself stimulates the release of TNF (Old, 1987). Superimposed on the antibody-dependent and antibody-independent activities is first an increase and than a decrease in generalised phagocytic activity (Cox et al., 1964) and overall immunodepression (Wedderburn, 1974).

IMMUNITY TO LEISHMANIASIS

It is not appropriate here to say much about leishmaniasis which has been reviewed a number of times recently. The essential features in the context of the present paper are that the parasites inhabit macrophages and elicit strong antibody and DTH responses neither of which seems to be implicated in protective immunity (Liew, 1986). Immunity can be induced in various ways and involves L3T4$^+$ T-cells which produce, among other molecules, gamma-interferon. Intracellular parasite killing involves ROI (Locksley and Klebanoff, 1983) thus the likely sequence of events is the stimulation of T-cells to produce gamma-interferon and colony stimulating factor (CSF) which in turn activate macrophages to release ROI and probably TNF. In BALB/c mice, there is a natural tendency to limit the infection but this is abrogated by the activation of specific suppressor cells (Howard et al., 1981). Leishmaniasis, like malaria, is also accompanied by polyclonal B-cell activation and immunodepression (see Cohen, 1982). In addition, there is inhibition of the respiratory burst (Buchmuller-Rouiller and Mauel, 1987). Anaemia also occurs during leishmaniasis.

There are a number of similarities between the immune responses in malaria and leishmaniasis and these suggest that similar mechanisms may be involved in recovery from infection. C3H, CBA or C57BL mice are resistant to leishmaniasis whereas BALB/c are not (see Albright and Albright, 1984) and this is also true for certain malaria parasites (Stevenson et al., 1984) suggesting a similar genetic predisposition to resistance and susceptibility. Mice pre-treated with various immunomodulators, such as BCG and P. acnes, become resistant to both leishmaniasis and malaria (Cox, 1982) and ROI are involved in parasite killing in both infections (Thorne and Blackwell, 1985).

Bearing in mind the characteristics of malaria and leishmaniasis, it is possible to identify various points at which the actual cells and molecules involved impinge and to speculate on how the two infections might interact. First consider the possible effects of leishmaniasis on a superimposed malaria infection. The leishmanial parasites trigger the production of gamma-interferon and other molecules that activate macrophates to produce ROI which can act extracellularly to kill malaria parasites within the red cells. In this way leishmanial parasites act like BCG to stimulate macrophages and could thus inhibit a superimposed malarial infection. Leishmaniasis - induced anaemia would have a similar effect by depriving the malaria parasites of preferred host cells. On the other hand, leishmaniasis - induced immunodepression could benefit the malaria parasites. It is, however, necessary to know much more about the actual antigens involved as Leishmania major depresses the immune response to some antigens but not others (Colle et al., 1983), and in malaria the suppression of immune responses to some antigens does not necessarily correlate with the outcome of infections with Plasmodium chabaudi (Stevenson and Skamene, 1986). There is also the possibility that immunodepression might ameliorate some of the pathological effects of malaria which may have an immunopathological basis (Grau et al., 1986).

From the point of view of leishmaniasis, similar principles apply. Macrophage activation resulting from stimulation by malaria parasites or antigen-antibody complexes could adversely affect leishmaniasis and malaria-induced immunodepression would favour the superimposed infection. Such speculation is subject to the reservations mentioned above and it is probable that this overall analysis will prove to be too simplistic and will be affected by the ways in which particular cells and the production of mediators are switched on and off by parasite products and other intracellular signals. For example L. major - infected macrophages produce reduced amounts of IL-2 (Cillari et al., 1986) and there is evidence that B-cells and/or their products are required for the activation of T-cells in infections with L. major (Scott et al., 1986). In this context, it is important to remember that many immunological processes are initiated specifically yet act non-specifically often affecting both invading organisms and host tissues in the crossfire and upsetting the delicate regulatory networks that keep potentially dangerous responses in check.

Our understanding of the complex interactions that exist between malaria and leishmaniasis revolves around a number of cells and molecules of which the most important appear to be T lymphocytes with the inducer/helper L3T4+ phenotype which play a central role in the activation of macrophages. There are at least two kinds of such cells, now designated TH1 and TH2 (Mossmann and Coffman, 1987). TH1 cells produce gamma-interferon, lymphotoxin (LT), IL-2 and IL-3 and are therefore probably the most important cells in antibody-independent interactions. TH2 cells produce IL-3, IL-4 and IL-5 and thus their role is mainly associated with antibody-dependent reactions largely involving polyclonal B-cell stimulation, antigen-antibody complexes and complement-mediated damage. Another cell of prime importance is the suppressor Ts cell which is responsible for modulating immune responses and there may be several different kinds of such cells. Finally, macrophages have diverse activities and there is increasing evidence that there are several functionally distinct forms of these cells also. Neutrophils (Salmon et al., 1986) and platelets may also be involved in the immune responses to interacting infections.

IMPLICATIONS OF MALARIA - LEISHMANIASIS INTERACTIONS

The implications of interactions between malaria and leishmaniasis lie not merely in alterations in the outcome of the two infections but also in the ways in which chemotherapy or immunological interactions are implemented. Vaccination inevitably involves the perturbation of all the component parts of the immune system including the regulatory circuits and whereas a specific vaccine might achieve the intended end it might equally exacerbate a superimposed infection or cause the recrudescence of a latent one. Similarly, the administration of a particular drug might affect the immune respond to a completely different infection. Chloroquine, the most widely used antimalarial drug, has immunodepressive effects (Bygbjerg et al., 1986) and whereas in the treatment of malaria this disadvantage is outweighed by potent antimalarial activity and the possible amelioration of immunopathological damage these advantages do not extend to leishmaniasis. In conclusion, although it is convenient to consider particular diseases in isolation in reality they are likely to be part of a complex of infections and the interaction between leishmaniasis and malaria is but one example of a number of possible situations that cannot and should not be ignored. Our understanding of the interactions between various cells and molecules in dual infections must depend on our understanding of what happens in single parasite infections thus it is important that those working on leishmaniasis and malaria, and also their infections, do not lose sight of what others are doing.

Albright, J.F. and Albright, J.W., 1984, in: "Immunobiology of Parasites and Parasitic Infections," J.J. Marchalonis, ed., Plenum, New York.
Bradley, D.J., 1977, Regulation of Leishmania populations within the host. II. Genetic control of acute susceptibility of mice to Leishmania donovani infection, Clin. Expl. Immunol., 30:130.
Buchmüller-Rouillier, Y. and Mauel, J., 1987, Impairment of the oxidative metabolism of mouse peritoneal macrophages by intracellular Leishmania spp., Infect. Immun., 55:587.
Buffington, G.D., Cowden, W.B., Hunt, N.H. and Clark, I.A., 1986, Bleomycin-detectable iron in plasma from Plasmodium vinckei vinckei-infected mice, FEBS Letters, 195:65.
Bygbjerg, I.C., Theander, T.G., Anderson, B.J., Flachs, H., Jepsen, S. and Larsen, P.B., 1986, In vitro effects of chloroquine, mefloquine and quinine on human lymphoproliferative response to malaria antigens and other antigens/mitogens, Trop. Med. Parasit., 37:245.
Cillari, E., Liew, F.Y. and Lelchuk, R., 1986, Suppression of interleukin-2 production by macrophages in genetically susceptible mice infected with Leishmania major, Infect. Immun., 54:386.
Clark, I.A., Cowden, W.B. and Butcher G.A., 1987, Cell-mediated immunity in protection and pathology of malaria, Parasitology Today, 3:300.
Cohen, S., 1982, Survival of parasites in the immunocompetent host, in:

"Immunology of Parasitic Infections," S. Cohen and K.S. Warren, eds., Blackwell, Oxford.

Cohen, S. and Lambert, P.H., 1982, Malaria, in: "Immunology of Parasitic Infections," S. Cohen and K.S. Warren, eds., Blackwell, Oxford.

Colle, J.H., Truffa-Bachi, P., Chedid, L. and Modabber, F., 1983, Lack of a general immunosuppression during visceral Leishmania tropica infection in BALB/c mice: augmented antibody response to thymus-independent antigens and polyclonal activation, J. Immunol., 131:1492.

Cox, F.E.G., 1982, Non-specific immunity against parasites, Clinics in Immunol. Allergy, 2:705.

Cox, F.E.G., Bilbey, D.L.J. and Nicol, T., 1964, Reticulo-endothelial activity in mice infected with Plasmodium vinckei, J. Protozool., 11:229.

Dockrell, H.M., Alavi, A. and Playfair, J.H.L., 1986, Changes in oxidative burst capacity during murine malaria and the effect of vaccination, Clin. Exp. Immunol., 66:37.

Grau, G.E., del Giudice, G. and Lambert, P.H., 1987, Host immune response and pathological expression in malaria: possible implications for malaria vaccines, Parasitology, 94 (Supplement): S123.

Grun, J.L. and Weidanz, W.P., 1981, Immunity to Plasmodium chabaudi adami in the B-cell deficient mouse, Nature, 290:143.

Howard, J.G., Hale, C. and Chan-Liew, W.L., 1980, Immunological regulation of experimental cutaneous leishmaniasis. 1. Immunological aspects of susceptibility to Leishmania tropica in mice, Parasite Immunol. 2:303.

Howard, J.G., Hale, C. and Liew, F.Y., 1981, Immunological regulation of experimental cutaneous leishmaniasis. IV. Prophylactic effect of sublethal irradiation as a result of abrogation of suppressor T-cell generation in mice genetically susceptible to Leishmania tropical, J. Exp. Med., 153:557.

Killick-Kendrick, R. and Peters, W., eds., 1978, "Rodent Malaria," Academic Press, London.

Liew, F.Y., 1986, Cell-mediated immunity in experimental cutaneous leishmaniasis, Parasitology Today, 2:264.

Locksley, R.M. and Klebanoff, S.J., 1983, Oxygen dependent microbicidal systems of phagocytes and host defense against intracellular parasites, J. Cell Biochem., 22:173.

Mossmann, T.R. and Coffman, R.L., 1987, Two types of mouse helper T-cell clone. Implications for immune regulation, Immunology Today, 8:223.

Nathan, C.F., 1987, Secretory products of macrophages, J. Clin. Invest., 79:319.

Old, L.J., 1987, Polypeptide mediator network, Nature, 326:330.

Rosenberg, Y.J., 1978, Autoimmune and polyclonal B-cell responses during murine malaria, Nature, 274:170.

Salmon, D., Vilde, J.L., Andrieu, B., Simonovic, R. and Lebras, J., 1986, Role of immune serum and complement in stimulation of the metabolic burst of human neutrophils by Plasmodium falciparum, Infect. Immun., 51:801.

Scott, P., Natovitz, P. and Sher, A., 1986, B lymphocytes are required for the generation of T-cells that mediate healing of cutaneous leishmaniasis, J. Immunol., 137:1017.

Stevenson, M., Lemieux, S. and Skamene, E., 1984, Genetic control of resistance to murine malaria, J. Cell. Biochem., 24:91.

Stevenson, M. and Skamene, E., 1986, Modulation of primary antibody responses to sheep erythrocytes in Plasmodium chabaudi - infected resistant and susceptible mouse strains, Infect. Immun., 54:600.

Thorne, K.J.I., and Blackwell, J.M., 1983, Cell-mediated killing of protozoa, Adv. Parasitol., 22:43.

Wedderburn, N., 1974, Immunodepression produced by malarial infection in mice, Ciba Foundation Symp., 25:137.

MODULATION OF CELL-MEDIATED IMMUNITY IN EXPERIMENTAL CUTANEOUS LEISHMANIASIS

F. Y. Liew

Department of Experimental Immunobiology, The Wellcome Research Laboratories, Langley Court, Beckenham, Kent BR3 3BS U.K.

INTRODUCTION

It is now generally accepted that cell-mediated immunity plays a causal role in acquired resistance to leishmaniasis. This is based on an impressive range of clinical and experimental evidence (Table 1). Patients with active visceral leishmaniasis failed to respond to L. donovani antigens in delayed-type hypersensitivity (DTH) skin test (Rezai et al, 1978) and in lymphocyte proliferation assay in vitro (Ho et al, 1983). The patients developed a positive skin test and resistance to challenge with L. donovani following successful antimony therapy (Carvalho et al, 1981). Resistant strains of mice rendered relatively T cell deficient by adult thymectomy followed by irradiation and reconstitution with syngeneic bone marrow cells are less able to control L. major infection and have delayed healing (Preston et al, 1972). Athymic mutants of the highly resistant CBA and C57BL/6 mice are totally unable to control L. major infection which progresses and visceralises. Normal resistance can be fully restored by reconstituting these T cell deficient mutants with syngeneic T cells (Mitchell et al, 1980). Acquired protective immunity to L. major (Preston and Dumonde, 1976) and L. donovani (Rezai, Farrell and Soulsby, 1980) in resistant or susceptible mice ban be adoptively transferred by T cells but not by B cells (Liew, Hale and Howard, 1982; Liew, Howard and Hale, 1984). Treatment of resistant C3H mice from birth with anti-IgM antibody rendered them defective in antibody response and also susceptible to L. major infection. However, lesion progression in these treated mice can be arrested and the disease outcome reversed by adoptive transfer of T cell alone from normal C3H donors (Scott, Natovitz and Sher, 1986) without any restoration of humoral antibody formation.

There now appears to be a broad consensus that T cells conferring protective immunity belong to the subset bearing $Lyt-1^-2^+$ phenotype. This is supported by experimental evidence from several laboratories using adoptive transfer and replacement studies with the murine L. major (Liew et al, 1982; Liew et al, 1984) and L. mexicana (Gorczynski, 1985) models. Lymphokines such as macrophage activating factor (MAF) and interferon-gamma (IFN-γ) produced by specifically sensitized T cells are deemed to be essential for the activation of infected macrophages to eliminate intracellular amastigotes (Mauel and Behin, 1982).

This paper will discuss the various factors regulating the induction and manifestation of the protective T cell response leading to the control or otherwise of the disease progression in experimental cutaneous leishmaniasis.

Table 1.   Evidence for a Causal Role of Cell-mediated Immunity in Leishmaniasis

Clinical

1. Patients with VL fail to develop DTH to
   L. donovani   Rezai et al, 1978
   or
   specific lymphocyte proliferation   Ho et al, 1983
2. Patients recovered from VL develop DTH and
   resistance to challenge   Carvalho et al, 1981

Experimental

3. ATxXBM resistant mice are less able to
   control L. major infection   Preston et al, 1972
4. Athymic resistant mice are unable to control
   L. major infection but gain resistance when
   injected with T cells   Mitchell et al, 1980
5. Acquired immunity transferable with T cells
   - convalescent   Preston et al, 1976
                                                                  Rezai et al, 1980
   - prophylactic   Liew et al, 1982, 1984
6. C3H mice rendered susceptible by anti-μ
   treatment regain resistance when
   transferred with T cells   Scott et al, 1986
7. Resistance correlated with IFN-γ, MAF in vivo   Sadick et al, 1986
                                                                  Liew et al, 1987

IMPAIRMENT OF PROTECTIVE IMMUNITY

The most striking immunological feature of fatal disseminating L. major infection which develops uniformally in genetically highly susceptible BALB/c mice, is profound leishmanin-specific suppression of CMI in the presence of normal antibody response. Such anergy, however, is not due to any intrinsic failure of BALB/c mice to develop CMI against the parasite. BALB/c mice can be rendered resistant to L. major infection by prior sublethal whole body γ-irradiation (Howard, Hale and Liew, 1981), treatment from birth with anti-IgM antibody (Sacks et al, 1984), injection with anti-L3T4 antibody (Titus et al, 1985) or cyclosporin A (Behforonz, Wenger and Mathison, 1986; Solbach et al, 1986). These recovered mice develop a classical tuberculin-type of DTH and their splenic and lymph node T cells can adoptively transfer resistance in otherwise susceptible BALB/c recipients (Liew and Dhaliwal, 1987).

The protective T cells like those found in the recovered resistant strains of mice (Liew et al, 1982) are $Lyt-1^-2^+$ and produce MAF when cultured with leishmanial antigens in vitro. The prophylactic effect of sublethal irradiation or anti-IgM treatment can be reversed by the injection into these treated BALB/c mice with T cells from normal syngeneic or, even more dramatically, T cells from mice with progressive L. major injection (Howard et al, 1981). At a population level, the disease-promoting T cells (operationally called suppressor T cells) from mice with progressive disease are functionally opposite to the protective T cells obtained from recovered mice (here referred to as Tr cells) (Table 2). The suppressor T (Ts) cells which also express the $Lyt-1^+2^-$ phenotype do not mediate DTH or produce MAF; instead they can suppress the expression of DTH of Tr cells (Liew and Dhaliwal, 1987). Thus, L. major infection of susceptible mice leds to the preferential induction of Ts cells which prevent the generation and expression of protective CMI. The mechanism leading to such preferential induction and the manner of interaction between Ts and Tr cells are at present unknown.

EXPERIMENTAL VACCINATION

Genetically susceptible BALB/c mice develop substantial resistance to L. major infection following repeated intravenous (i.v.) or intraperitoneal (i.p.) immunisation with lethally irradiated, heat-killed or sonicated promastigotes (Howard et al, 1982). The protective immunity which lasts for more than 150 days and extends to L. mexicana, L. amazonensis and L. panamenesis is passively transferable with splenic or lymph node T cells into normal or sublethally irradiated syngeneic recipients (Liew et al, 1984). Repeated i.v. immunisation with killed promastigotes induces an antibody response in the isotype sequence M → G1/G3 → G2a/G2b → A with substantially higher titres than are found in response to the infection itself. Splenectomy before immunisation drastically reduces this antibody reponse without incurring any impairment of the extent of protection. Passive transfer of large amounts (up to 10ml) of hyperimmune serum (or isotype fractions thereof) throughout the first eight weeks of infection fail to arrest disease progression during this period. The effector T cells are of the $Lyt-1^+2^-$ phenotype, devoid of demonstrable cytotoxic activity.

Immunity is not stage specific and encompasses both amastigote and promastigote challenges. Similar prophylaxis can also be induced by immunisation with heterologous irradiated L. donovani promastigotes. The immunised donors show no detectable cutaneous DTH or its early memory recall in response to live or killed promastigotes or soluble L. major antigen preparation. Spleen, lymph and peritoneal exudate cells from protectively immunised donors similarly fail to transfer DTH locally or systemically. Thus protection against L. major induced by prophylactic i.v. immunisation with killed promatigotes appears to be conferred by T cells of the helper lineage that are distinguisable from T cells mediating either DTH or cytotoxicity.

The protective immunity induced by killed promastigotes is critically dependent on the route of immunisation. Injection of killed or sonicated promastigotes by the subcutaneous (s.c.), intradermal or intramuscular routes with or without a whole range of adjuvants, are not only ineffective in inducing protection, they often exacerbate disease development if given prior to infection (Liew, Hale and Howard, 1985). When mice given 4 x s.c. injections are subsequently immunised i.v. with 2×10^7 irradiated promastigotes, they fail to develop protection against a challenge infection with L. major promastigotes. Thus, s.c. injections are capable of blocking the prophylactic effect of i.v. immunisation. This inhibition can be achieved with a single s.c. injection, although rather less potently than with four, and is even effective against four repeated weekly i.v. immunisations. Once induced, the effect persists undiminished after 100 days. A weeker effect is also inducible by s.c. injection given after i.v. immunisation. The phenomenon extends to mouse strains genetically resistant as well as susceptible to L. major, L. mexicana and L. braziliensis infections. In congenic mice of BALB background, it is independent of the major histocompatibility (H-2) gene complex.

The induction of this blocking effect is leishmanial specific for although prevention of protection against L. major infection can be obtained with either homologous or L. donovani promastigotes, it does not follow s.c. administration of an immunogenic Trypanosoma cruzi epimastigote preparation. Multiple s.c. injections of irradiated L. major promastigotes do not inhibit the subsequent antibody response of any major isotype to i.v. immunisation but rather induce some priming. The same s.c. injections induced the early peaking, transient type of DTH, the Jones-Mote reactivity that can be transferred locally and systemically. Parallel CMI responses are also reflected in in vitro specific T cell proliferation assays.

Despite this evidence of a DTH/helper type of T cell response, transfer of splenic or lymph node T cells from 4 x s.c. immunised donors to normal recipients completely abrogates the protective response to i.v. immunisation. The inhibitory

Table 2. Different Populations of T Cells in Response to Cutaneous Leishmaniasis

Cells	Source	DTH	IL-3	MAF	Disease Outcome
Tr	Recovered mice	Tuberculin-type	-	++	Protective
Ts	Mice with progressive disease	Negative	+	-	Counter-protective
Ti	i.v. immunised mice	Negative	-	+	Protective
Tsc	s.c. immunised mice	Jones-Mote type	+	-	Counter-protective

T cells were defined by positive and negative in vitro selection experiments as possessing an $Lyt-1^+2^-$, $L3T4^+$ phenotype. T cells from s.c. (Tsc cells, Table 2) immunised donors were also shown, by mix transfer experiments, to counteract completely the protective effect of Ti (T cells from i.v. immunised mice) cells. They are as potent as Ts cells both in this capacity and in abrogating the prophylactic effect of sublethal irradiation. Like Ts cells, when freshly isolated, they produce little or no MAF when stimulated with leishmanial antigen in vitro (Liew, Hodson and Lelchuk, 1987).

FUNCTIONAL HETEROGENEITY OF $L3T4^+$ T CELLS

From the above, it appears that four functional distinct subsets of $Lyt-2^-$, $L3T4^+$ T cells can be induced during leishmanial infection or immunisation. These are the so called Ts, Tr, Ti and Tsc cells (Table 2). However, since all the T cell population described here belong to the $Lyt-2^-$ subsets, it has been argued that they are all infact the same cell and that protection or disease-promotion merely reflects the difference in the number of activated leishmanial-specific $Lyt-2^-$ cells present in the host at any given time. Thus, susceptibility in BALB/c mice is caused by the excessive activation of specific $Lyt-2^-$ $L3T4^+$ T cells (Milon et al, 1986) and the reduction of such cells with anti-L3T4 antibody in vivo brings about disease containment (Titus et al, 1985). This hypothesis argues that small numbers of specific $L3T4^+$ $Lyt-2^-$ cells are host-protective whereas excessive numbers of such cells are detrimental to the host (Titus et al, 1985). However, evidence against this interpretation and supporting the heterogeneity of $L3T4^+$ cells is accumulating. This is summarised in the following sections.

(a) Cell Titration Experiments

T cells freshly isolated from mice immunised s.c. with killed promastigotes either inhibit protective immunisation ($>10^7$ cells/recipient) or have no effect ($<10^7$ cells/recipient). No protection was observed at any dose (Liew, Hodson and Lelchuk, 1987). Conversely, freshly isolated T cells from mice given prophylactic i.v. immunisation are either protective ($>10^7$ cells/recipient) or ineffective ($<10^7$ cells/recipient). No exacerbation of disease was observed at any dose. In mix transfer experiments, increasing numbers of T cells from s.c. immunised donors progressively inhibit the protective effect of T cells from i.v. immunised donors. These results would argue against a quantitative effect of protective and counter protective T cells.

(b) IFN-γ/MAF Production

Freshly isolated T cells from protected recovered mice (Tr) or i.v. immunised mice (Ti) produce IFN-γ/MAF when stimulated in vitro with leishmanial antigens. In contrast, T cells from mice with progressive disease or after s.c. immunisation produce little of no MAF when similarly stimulated in vitro (Liew and Dhaliwal, 1987).

Even more direct evidence was obtained when mRNA of T cells from healed and nonhealed mice was analysed with an IFN-γ probe (Sadick et al, 1987). Messenger RNA was extracted from the draining lymph nodes and spleens from resistant C57BL/6 and nonhealer BALB/c mice infected with L. major. It was enriched for poly-A^+ message, and the presence of IFN-γ message probed by Northern analyses. In both lymph nodes and spleen, 50-100 fold greater amounts of message was present in the healer mice. IFN-γ message was present in amounts comparable to that of resistant mice when the cells from BALB/c mice which had healed following L. major infection and treatment with anti-L3T4 antibody in vivo. This suggests that the observed differences were not related to an intrinsic defect or the absence of T cells capable of responding to leishmanial antigen.

These data are in direct contrast to experiments using in vitro propogated T cell lines (Titus et al, 1984). Leishmanial specific $L3T4^+$, $Lyt-2^-$ T cell lines or clones, derived from BALB/c mice immunised s.c. with killed promastigotes together with Freunds' complete adjuvant, exacerbated L. major disease progression when transferred into syngeneic recipients. These T cell lines were found to mediate DTH, T cell help and produce MAF. However, long-term in vitro propogation and cloning are imperfect means of estimating homogeneity or otherwise of T cells, since large differences may exist in the ability of different T cells to grow in vitro. In addition, the possibility exists that continuous activation and growth factor stimulation may deregulate unipotential T cells to those capable of multiple biological activities.

(c) In Vivo Depletion of $L3T4^+$ T Cells

Mice injected with anti-L3T4 antibody are relatively deficient in $L3T4^+$ T cells. Susceptible BALB/c mice pretreated with two injections of 300μg of highly purified anti-L3T4 antibody are able to control an otherwise lethal L. major infection, with the majority of the mice achieving complete healing by 150 days post-infection with 2×10^6 promastigotes. The healed mice develop the classical tuberculin type of DTH and their T cells are capable of leishmanial-specific proliferation in vitro and produce MAF (Jacque Louis, per Comms.; Liew et al, in preparation) in a manner identical to mice recovered from infection as a result of prior sublethal irradiation. When BALB/c mice are profoundly depleted of $L3T4^+$ cells by adult thymectomy followed by repeated injection with anti-L3T4 antibody, they are no longer able to resist L. major infection. Furthermore, attempts to induce the disease-exacerbatinbg Tsc cells (with s.c. immunisation) or the protective Ti cells (with i.v. immunisationusing killed promastigotes) in these profoundly $L3T4^+$ cell-depleted mice are equally unsuccessful (Liew et al, in preparation). There results again argue for a qualitative difference between the protective and counter-protective T cells. It may be that the precursors of protective T cells and the disease-promoting T cells have different density of the cell surface L3T4 antigens.

(d) Delayed-type Hypersensitivity

The role of DTH in infectious disease is controversial. In leishmaniasis, a direct correlation was obtained in clinical visceral leishmaniasis (VL) in that patients with progressive VL are skin test negative against leishmanial antigens; whereas patients recovered from the disease following chemotherapy regained specific DTH. In experimental murine cutaneous leishmaniasis, BALB/c mice developed specific DTH at the early stage of L. major infection. This reactivity declines as the disease progresses. In contrast, resistant CBA mice develop and sustain a strong DTH reaction throughout the course of infection. BALB/c mice recovered from L. major infection as a result of prior sublethal irradiation or anti-L3T4 antibody treatment also develop strong DTH. However, BALB/c mice protectively immunised with i.v. doses of killed promastigotes not only failed to develop skin DTH, their splenic and lymph node T cells could adoptively suppress the induction and expression of leishmanial specific DTH in mice immunised intradermally with the same antigen (Dhaliwal, Liew and Cox, 1986). The intradermal (i.d.) or s.c. immunised mice developed exacerbated disease despite the fact that they expressed strong specific DTH (Dhaliwal and Liew, 1987). The results therefore are inconsistent with a protective role of DTH in cutaneous leishmaniasis.

DTH is a gross measurement of the infiltration of mononuclear cells at the site of antigen administration. It consists of a variety of cellular activation and interaction. Kinetically, it can be divided into the transient Jones-Mote reaction (which peaks at 15-18h after antigen injection) and the tuberculin-type of hypersensitivity (which peaks at 24-48h). Detailed analysis of kinetics of footpad swelling showed that the DTH in the i.d. immunised mice which expressed exacerbated disease belongs entirely to the Jones-Mote type of DTH whereas that of the resistant convalescent mice is the classical tuberculin DTH (Liew and Dhaliwal, 1987). These results suggest that: (a) the Jones-Mote reaction may be disease promoting whilst the tuberculin-type hypersensitivity is protective; (b) DTH is an additional criterium to differentiate the protective and disease-promoting T cells.

CONCLUSION

The subdivision of $L3T4^+$ T cells into four subsets (Table 2) is based largely on the differential ability of these cell populations to mediate DTH. In the absence of specific T cell clones for direct testing, it is quite possible that DTH may turn out to be an accompanying phenomenon which, like humoral antibody, has little relevence to the course of leishmania infection. In this case, Tsc cells would be identical to the disease-promoting Ts cells obained during progressive infection and Ti cells are infact the same protective T cell responsible for convalescent immunity.

One of the major unresolved questions in leishmaniasis is the mechanism by which the disease-promoting cells interact with the protective cells. Recent results show that the supernatant of spleen cells from mice with progressive disease contains substances which inhibit the MAF activity presence in the supernatant of T cells from recovered mice (Liew et al, in preparation). The identity of the substance and the mechanism of inhibition is being investigated. Elucidation of cellular interaction in this field may open up the possibility of pharmacological and immunological intervention of the disease outcome.

Another area of research which is receiving a great deal of attention is the mechanism by which the disease promoting T cells and the protective T cells are preferentially induced under different conditions. Since these cells are stimulated by s.c. or i.v. immunisation respectively with the same antigen, it is likely that antigen-presentation must play a crucial role. This is supported by the finding that the Lsh gene is expressed in the Kuppfer cells (Crocker et al, 1984). Understanding of the means by which these different subsets of T cells are preferentially activated will help in rational design of effective vaccines.

Since the original proposal by Mirkovich et al (1986) that colony stimulating factor may be important in generating 'safe target' for continuous leishmanial growth, evidence is accumulating that IL-3 or GM-CSF may play an important role in the outcome of cutaneous leishmaniasis. Repeated injections of GM-CSF (Solbach et al, 1987) or continuous infusion of recombinent IL-3 by an inplanted diffusion chamber (Louis et al, 1987) could lead to exacerbated L. major infection in BALB/c mice. On a cell to cell basis, splenic T cells from susceptible strains of mice infected with L. major produce significantly higher levels of IL-3 compared to those from resistant strains of mice when stimulated with leishmanial antigens in vitro (Lelchuk, Graveley and Liew, 1987). Furthermore, disease promoting T cells produce high levels of IL-3, whereas host protective T cells produce little or no IL-3 when stimulated with leishmania antigens in vitro (R. Lelchuk, R. Graveley and F. Y. Liew, in preparation). These data suggest that IL-3 may be a mediator by which disease-promoting T cells manifest their effect. It does so probably by their presumptive ability to attract to the site of infection immature macrophages which can serve as targets of infection (Gergens and Marr, 1979) but are incapable of responding to MAF (Hoover and Nacy, 1984).

ACKNOWLEDGEMENT

I would like to thank my colleagues: Dr. J. G. Howard, Mrs. Christine Hale, Dr. J. S. Dhaliwal, Dr. Rosalia Lelchuk and Miss Stephanie Millott for their valuable contributions.

REFERENCES

Behforouz, N. C., Wenger, C. D. and Mathison, B. A. Prophylactic treatment of BALB/c mice with cyclosporin A and its analog B-5-49 enhances resistance to Leishmania major. J. Immunol. 136:3067 (1986).

Carvalho, E. M., Teixeira, R. and Johnson, W. D. Cell-mediated immunity in American visceral leishmaniasis: reversible immunosuppression during acute infection. Infect. Immun. 33:498 (1981).

Dhaliwal, J. S., Liew, F. Y. and Cox, F. E. G. Specific suppressor T cells for delayed-type hypersensitivity in susceptible mice immunised against cutaneous leishmaniasis. Infect. Immun. 49:417 (1985).

Gergens, R. L. and Marr, J. J. Growth of L. donovani amastigotes in a continuous macrophage-like cell culture. J. Protozol. 26:453 (1979).

Gorczynski, R. M. Immunization of susceptible BALB/c mice against Leishmania braziliensis. II. Use of temperature-sensitive avirulent clones of parasite for vaccination purposes. Cell Immunol. 94:11 (1985).

Ho, M., Koech, D. K., Iha, D. M. and Bryceson, A. D. M. Immunosuppression in Kenyan visceral leishmaniasis. Clin. Exp. Immunol. 51:207 (1983).

Hoover, D. L. and Nacy, C. Macrophage activation to kill L. tropica: defective intracellular killing of amastigotes by macrophages elicited with sterile inflammatory agents. J. Immunol. 132:1487 (1984).

Howard, J. G., Hale, C. and Liew, F. Y. Immunological regulation of experimental cutaneous leishmaniasis. IV. Prophylactic effect of sublethal irradiation as a result of abrogation of suppressor T cell generation in mice genetically susceptible to Leishmania tropica. J. Exp. Med. 153:557 (1981).

Howard, J. G., Nicklin, S., Hale, C. and Liew, F. Y. Prophylactic immunisation against experimental leishmaniasis. I. Protection induced in mice genetically vulnerable to fatal Leishmania tropica infection. J. Immunol. 129:2206 (1982).

Howard, J. G., Liew, F. Y., Hale, C. and Nicklin, S. Prophylactic immunisation against experimental leishmaniasis. II. Further characterisation of the protective immunity against fatal L. tropica infection induced by irradiated promastigotes. J. Immunol. 132:450 (1984).

Lelchuk, R., Graveley, R. and Liew, F. Y. Susceptibility to murine cutaneous leishmaniasis correlates with the capacity to generate interleukin-3 in response to leishmania antigen in vitro. Cell Immunol. (In Press).

Liew, F. Y. and Dhaliwal, J. S. Distinct cellular immunity in genetically susceptible BALB/c mice recovered from Leishmania major infection or after subcutaneous immunisation with killed parasites. J. Immunol. 138:4450 (1987).

Liew, F. Y., Hale, C. and Howard, J. G. Immunologic regulation of experimental cutaneous leishmaniasis. V. Characterisation of effector and specific suppressor T cells. J. Immunol. 128:1917 (1982).

Liew, F. Y., Howard, J. G. and Hale, C. Prophylactic immunisation against experimental leishmniasis. III. Protection against fatal Leishmania tropica infection induced by irradiated promastigotes involves Lyt-1^+2^- T cells that do not mediate cutaneous DTH. J. Immunol. 132:456 (1984).

Liew, F. Y., Singleton, A., Cillari, E. and Howard, J. G. Prophylactic immunisation against experimental leishmaniasis. V. Mechanism of the anti-protective blocking effect induced by subcutaneous immunisation against Leishmania major infection. J. Immunol. 135:2101 (1985).

Liew, F. Y., Hale, C. and Howard, J. G. Prophylactic immunisation against experimental leishmaniasis. IV. Subcutaneous immunisation prevents the induction of protective immunity against fatal Leishmania major infection. J. Immunol. 135:2095 (1985).

Liew, F. Y., Hodson, K. and Lelchuk, R. Prophylactic immunisation against experimental leishmaniasis. VI. Comparison of protective and disease-promoting T cells. J. Immunol. (In Press).

Louis, J. A., Pedrazzini, Th., Titus, R. G., Muller, I., Farrell, J. P., Kindler, V., Vassali, P., Marchal, G. and Milon, G. Subsets of specific T cells and experimental cutaneous leishmaniasis. Ann. Inst. Pasteur/Immunol. (In Press).

Mauel, J. and Behin, R. Leishmaniasis. In Immunology of Parasitic Infections. S. Cohen and K. S. Warren Eds. Blackwell Scientific Publications. P. 299-355 (1982).

Milon, G., Titus, R. G., Cerottini, J-C., Marchal, G. and Louis, J. A. Higher frequency of Leishmania major-specific $L3T4^+$ T cells in susceptible BALB/c as compared with resistant CBA mice. J. Immunol. 136:1467 (1986).

Mirkovich, A. M., Galelli, A., Allison, A. C. and Modabber, F. Z. Increased myelopoiesis during Leishmania major infection in mice: generation of 'safe target', a possible way to evade the effector immune mechanism. Clin. Exp. Immunol. 64:1 (1986).

Mitchell, G. F., Curtis, J. M., Handman, E. and McKenzie, I. F. C. Cutaneous leishmaniasis in mice: disease patterns in reconstituted nude mice of several genotypes infected with Leishmania tropica. Aust. J. Exp. Biol Med. Sci. 58:521 (1980).

Mitchell, G. F., Curtis, J. M., Scollay, R. G. and Handman, E. Resistance and abrogation of resistance to cutaneous leishmaniasis in reconstituted BALB/c nude mice. Aust. J. Exp. Biol. Med. Sci. 59:539 (1981).

Preston, P. M., Carter, R. L., Leuchars, E., Davies, A. J. S. and Dumonde, D. C. Experimental cutaneous leishmaniasis. III. Effects of thymectomy on the course of infection of CBA mice with Leishmania tropica. Clin. Exp. Immunol. 10:337 (1972).

Preston, P. M. and Dumonde, D. C. Experimental cutaneous leishmaniasis. V. Protective immunity in subclinical and self-healing infection in the mouse. Clin. Exp. Immunol. 23:126 (1976).

Rezai, H. R., Ardehali, S. M., Amirhakimi, G. and Kharazmi, A. Immunological features of Kala-azar. Am. J. Trop. Med. Hyg. 27:1079 (1978).

Rezai, H. R., Farrell, J. and Soulsby, E. L. Immunological responses of L. donovani infection in mice and significance of T cell in resistance to experimental leishmaniasis. Clin. Exp. Immunol. 40:508 (1980).

Sacks, D. L., Scott, P. A., Asofsky, R. and Sher, F. A. Cutaneous leishmaniasis in anti-IgM-treated mice: enhanced resistance due to functional depletion of a B cell-dependent T cell involved in the suppressor pathway. J. Immunol. 132:2072 (1984).

Sadick, M. D., Locksley, R. M., Tubbs, C. and Raff, H. V. Murine cutaneous leishmaniasis: Resistance correlates with the capacity to generate interferon-γ in response to leishmania antigens in vitro. J. Immunol. 136:655 (1986).

Sadick, M. D., Heinzel, F. P., Shigekane, V. M., Fisher, W. L. and Locksley, R. M. Cellular and humoral immunity to Leishmania major in genetically susceptible mice after in vitro depletion of $L3T4^+$ T cells. J. Immunol. 139:1303 (1987).

Scott, P., Pearce, E., Natovitz, P. and Sher, A. Vaccination against cutaneous leishmaniasis in a murine model. I. Induction of protective immunity with a soluble extract of promastigotes. J. Immunol. 139:221 (1987).

Solbach, W., Forberg, K., Kammerer, E., Bogdan, C. and Rollinghoff, M. Suppressive effect of cyclosporin A on the development of Leishmania tropica-induced lesions in genetically susceptible BALB/c mice. J. Immunol. 137:702 (1986).

Solbach, W., Greil, J. and Rollinghoff, M. Anti-infectious responses in Leishmania major infected BALB/c mice injected with recombinant granulocyte-macrphage colony-stimulating factor. Ann. Inst. Pasteur/Immunol. (In Press).

Titus, R. G., Lima, G. C., Engers, H. D. and Louis, J. A. Exacerbation of murine cutaneous leishmaniasis by adoptive transfer of parasite-specific helper T cell populations capable of mediating Leishmania major specific delayed-type hypersensitivity. J. Immunol. 133:1594 (1984).

Titus, R. G., Ceredig, R., Cerottini, J. C. and Louis, J. A. Therapeutic effect of anti-L3T4 monoclonal antibody GK1.5 on cutaneous leishmaniasis in genetically susceptible BALB/c mice. J. Immunol. 135:2108 (1985).

THE LOCAL T CELL RESPONSE IN EXPERIMENTAL LEISHMANIASIS

M.J. McElrath, H.W. Murray, and Z.A. Cohn

The Rockefeller University
The Cornell University Medical Center
New York, N.Y.
USA

INTRODUCTION

Leishmania protozoa infect mononuclear phagocytes, replicate in parasitophorous vacuoles, and cause either visceral or cutaneous disease in a susceptible host. Inbred mouse strains provide useful experimental models in understanding the cell mediated immune response that controls susceptibility or resistance to leishmanial infection. Systematic analysis of T lymphocyte subsets have implicated the L3T4+ T cell in both protective and suppressive immunity in leishmania infection [1,2]. We have chosen mouse strains that are acutely susceptible to infection but differ in their capacity to develop acquired resistance. These include BALB/c and C57BL/6 mice in *L. mexicana amazonensis* cutaneous infection, and athymic (nu/nu) and euthymic (+/+, nu/+) BALB/c mice in *L donovani* visceral infection. We have analyzed the cell types that accumulate at the local site of infection, skin and liver, using immunocytochemistry. We provide evidence that failure to mount a local T cell response is associated with prolonged susceptibility in the Leishmania-infected animal.

MATERIALS AND METHODS

BALB/c (+/+) mice were obtained from the Rockefeller University Laboratory Animal Research center breeding colony and Charles River Breeding Laboratories, Wilmington, MA. Heterozygous euthymic (nu/+) and homozygous athymic (nu/nu) BALB/c mice were purchased from Life Sciences, St. Petersburg, FL. C57BL/6 mice were received from Charles River Laboratories. Mice weighed 18-25 g when infected.

Leishmania mexicana amazonensis promastigotes were cultivated in Schneider's *Drosophila* medium to stationary phase, and 10^7

in 0.1 ml phosphate buffered saline (PBS) were injected introdermally into the depilated tailbase of BALB/c (+/+) and C57BL/6 mice. *L. donovani* amastigotes were isolated from the spleen of an infected Syrian golden hamster, and 10^7 in 0.2 ml PBS were injected into euthymic (+/+, nu/+) and athymic (nu/nu) BALB/c mice.

At weekly intervals three animals from each group were sacrificed, and cutaneous lesions and infected livers were removed, but into small portions, and fixed in either paraformaldehyde-lysine-periodate or 10% formalin. Tissue was processed for immunoperoxidase staining or routine histology as previously described (3). Hybridoma culture supernatants containing rat monoclonal antibodies were used to identify mouse leukocytes. Nonspecific staining was monitored at each step, and positive controls were compared with each study group (3). A Nikon Microphot FX light microscope was used to visualize immunoperoxidase staining and for photography.

RESULTS

Cutaneous lesions were palpable after two weeks of *L.mexicana amazonensis* infection, and progressively enlarged over 8-10 weeks in the BALB/c amd C57BL/6 mouse. Parasite load and cellular response was similar in the two mouse strains. Amastigotes were visible in large parasitophorous vacuoles of dermal macrophages, identified by the resident macrophage marker (F4/80), the C3Bi receptor antigen (M1/70), and MHC class II Ia antigen (B21.2). Granulocytes, particularly eosinophils, accumulated throughout the infected dermis.

The skin lesions of the C57BL/6 mice began to heal by 12 weeks of infection and resolved by 25 weeks. T cell influx of both the L3T4 (GK1.5) and Ly2 (53-6.72) phenotype was demonstrated by immunoperoxidase staining at 12 weeks, coincident with clinical healing. Intracellular amastigotes were scarce and T cell accumulation was marked by 22 weeks of C57BL/6 dermal infection. Basal keratinocytes of the epidermis expressed Ia antigen by immunoperoxidase staining with B21.2 between 12-15 weeks of infection but by 22 weeks this staining pattern had disappeared. Dissemination of leishmania infection to liver was minimal, and was associated with granulomas containing many L3T4+ and Ly2+ T cells.

The BALB/c skin lesions continued to expand over the course of infection and never healed. The cutaneous lesion contained heavily infected macrophages, eosinophils, and fibroblasts. By 18 weeks of infection hepatic dissemination was marked. Granulomas consisted primarily of infected F4/80+ macrophages; only a small number of T cells were demonstrated along the periphery.

L.donovani infection

Visceral infection in BALB/c euthymic (nu/+, +/+) and athymic mice was demonstable in liver sections by one to two weeks of infection. Hepatic infection in the two euthymic groups, nu/+ and +/+, was similar, peaking at 4 weeks and resolving by 8 weeks (4). Progressive infection over 8 weeks led to death in many of the athymic nu/nu mice.

Amastigotes were visible only in carbon-labelled Kupffer cells (KC) in both euthymic and athymic mice. Granulomas formed around infected KC, and contained inflammatory monocytes (C3Bi receptor positive by Ml/70 staining), granulocytes, and lymnphocytes in the euthymic mice. An L3T4+ T cell reponse was marked at the peak of infection, and diminished with resolution. Influx of Ly2+ T cells persisted over the 8 weeks of infection. The congenitally athymic mice formed ill-defined granulomas, composed primarily of infected KC. Immunoperoxidase studies failed to demonstrate L3T4+ or Ly2+ T cells in the nu/nu infected livers.

DISCUSSION

We have performed a longitudinal analysis of the local cellular response in cutaneous and visceral experimental leishmaniasis. Using mouse strains that vary in their ability to control infection, we have been able to correlate certain cellular responses with a favorable disease outcome. Our studies indicate that T cell migration into the infected tissue, dermis or liver, is associated with acquired resistance to leishmanial intracellular parasitism.

The macrophase is generally considered the effector cell in leishmania destruction. Its antimicrobial activity appears to be regulated by T cell derived soluble products, particularly gamma interferon, through generation of reactive oxygen intermediates. Gamma interferon may also be associated with expression of gene products, including gamma IPI0 (5), that promate chemotaxis of inflammatory cells. Local infiltration of sensitized T cells may be necessary to activate macrophages and to recruit new ones. Influx of inflammatory monocytes into local hepatic infection may be essential for parasite killing because the Kupffer cell is oxidatively unresponsive to gamma interferon.

The lack of local T cell influx into the nu/nu BALB/c livers in *L.donovani* infection can be explained by the congenital absence of T cells in these mice. Failure of T cell migration in the euthymic mice infected with *L m.amazonensis* cannot be attributed to a central absence of T cell subsets. Appropriate numbers are found in spleen and peripheral blood of infected BALB/c mice over the course of infection (3). We are presently performing immunization procedures to presensitize T cells and stimulate a local T cell response, which will hopefully clarify the mechanism of the T cell migratory defect.

REFERENCES

1. F.Y. Liew, C. Hale, and J.G. Howard. Prophylactic immunization against experimental leishmaniasis. III. Protection against fatal *Leishmania tropica* infection induced by irradiated promastigotes involve Lyt-1+2- T cells that do not mediate cutaneous DTH.
J. Immunol. 132:456 (1984).

2. G. Milon, R.G. Titus, J.-C. Cerottini, G. Marchal, and J.A. Louis. Higher frequency of *Leishmania major*-specific L3T4+ T cells in susceptible BASLB/c as compared with resistant CBA mice.
J. Immunol. 136:1467 (1986).

3. M.J. McElrath, G. Kaplan, A. Nusrat, and Z.A. Cohn. Cutaneous Leishmaniasis. The defect in T cell influx in BALB/c mice.
J. Exp.Med. 165:546 (1987).

4. M.J. McElrath, Manuscript in preparation.

5. A.D. Luster, J.C. Unkeless and J.V. Ravetch. Gamma-Interferon transcriptionally regulates an early-response gene containing homology to platelet proteins.
Nature. 315:672 (1985).

THE ROLE OF SPECIFIC T CELL SUBSETS IN THE IMMUNOLOGICAL CONTROL OF EXPERIMENTAL CUTANEOUS LEISHMANIASIS

Th. Pedrazzini, V. Kindler, P. Vassalli, G. Marchal,
G. Milon and J.A. Louis

The WHO Immunology Research and Training Centre, Institute of Biochemistry, University of Lausanne, Epalinges Switzerland, the Department of Pathology, University of Geneva, Switzerland and the Cellular Immunophysiology Unit Pasteur Institute, Paris, France

The murine model of infection with L.major represents an important system for the analysis of the cellular parameters which entail susceptibility or resistance to infection with L.major. Indeed, depending on the genetic background of the mice, the entire spectrum of the clinical manifestations observed in human leishmaniasis can be seen. After s.c. infection with L.major, resistant mice (e.g. CBA) develop locally small lesions which resolve spontaneously whereas in susceptible mice (e.g. BALB/c) these lesions are much more severe, do not heal and viserali-sation occurs (1,2).

Several studies have shown that the expression of disease in experimentally induced murine leishmaniasis depends upon the activity of macrophages the host cells in which L.major replicates (3,1). Furthermore, the virulence of Leishmania could be related to surface molecules involved in its binding to and survival in mononuclear phagocytes (4). A considerable body of evidence from various laboratories also strongly indicates that specific T cell responses generated during infection play a crucial role both in the resolution and progression of cutaneous leishmaniasis (reviewed in 5,6,7). This manuscript will review only the work performed in our laboratories pertaining to the assessment of the possible role of T cell responses in favouring susceptibility or resistance to infection with L.major in mice.

Importance of L3T4$^+$ T cells: in vivo analysis

In an attempt to evaluate the role of L3T4$^+$ T cells in susceptibility or resistance to infection with L.major, we have studied the course of infection in mice in which the pool of L3T4$^+$ cells had been reduced by administration of anti-L3T4 monoclonal antibodies. It was observed that virtual elimination (>95%) of L3T4$^+$ T cells by intensive treatment with anti-L3T4 mAbs resulted in the development of severe uncontrolled lesions in resistant mice and exacerbated the lesions of susceptible mice (8). These results clearly show that L3T4$^+$ cells play a major role in the resolution of L.major-induced lesions. Interestingly, although the elimination of only 60-70% of L3T4$^+$ cells from lymphoid tissues still led to an exacerbation of lesions in genetically resistant CBA mice, this treatment reversed completely the exquisite susceptibility of BALB/c mice to infection with L.major (9,10). These results strongly indicate that L3T4$^+$ T cells can also be detrimental to the host. In a second approach, the number and phenotype of parasite-specific T cells triggered in lymphoid tissues as a result of infection was compared in susceptible and resistant mice. T cells were scored by determining their ability to transfer locally a delayed-type hypersensitivity reaction to viable L.major promastigotes and their frequencies determined by classical limiting dilution analysis. Results have shown that the frequency of specific T cells was significantly higher (up to 50 times) in the lymph nodes draining the lesions of susceptible mice than in resistant mice as assessed various times after infection. Furthermore, in susceptible BALB/c mice 90% of these specific T cells (i.e. able to mediate DTH) expressed the L3T4$^+$ cell surface phenotype (11). Therefore, using a DTH assay to detect L.major-specific T cells, it appears that the immune response of susceptible mice to infection with L.major is characterized by the generation of high numbers of specific L3T4$^+$ T cells. Although it is realized that our DTH assay might not detect all specific T cells, these results together with observations showing that reduction of L3T4$^+$ cells in vivo by treatment with anti-L3T4 mAb renders genetically susceptible mice resistant to infection with L.major led us to speculate that the protective role of specific L3T4$^+$ T cells may depend upon the actual number of such cells that are generated during infection (10,11). Alternatively, it is possible that the L3T4$^+$ response is qualitatively different between susceptible and resistant mice. According to this hypothesis, two types of specific L3T4$^+$ T cells are generated during infection with L.major: one cell type having mainly a protective effect (preferentially induced in resistant mice), another type favouring the development of lesions (preferentially induced in susceptible mice). The outcome of infection would then be dependant upon the balance between these functional subsets (6).

Indirect evidence which could suggest the triggering in lymphoid tissues of two functionally distinct parasite-specific L3T4$^+$ T cell populations has recently been obtained. We have observed that the cutaneous lesions of BALB/c mice treated with two injections of anti-L3T4 mAb (GK 1.5), given on days 10 and 11 after initiation of infection, resolve completely around 60 days after infection. At that time, the absolute number of L3T4$^+$ T cells in the lymph nodes of these mice was found to be similar to that seen in normal mice. Compared to control mice similarly infected but not treated with mAb GK 1.5, the L3T4$^+$ lymph node cells of mice given two injections of anti-L3T4 mAb provided similar helper activity as tested in a secondary anti-DNP antibody response in vitro using DNP-L.major as the immunogen. In sharp contrast, the frequency of L3T4$^+$ T cells able to transfer locally DTH reaction was drastically reduced in lymph nodes of these mice (Th. Pedrazzini, G. Milon, G. Marchal, J. Louis. In preparation). Despite this reduction in the number of T cells able to transfer DTH reactions in their lymph nodes, mice cured as a result of treatment with anti-L3T4 Mab developed DTH reactions after challenge with live parasites. However, the kinetics of these DTH responses were drastically different from that observed in control infected mice. Cured mice showed DTH responses which peaked 24 hours after challenge and were maintained until 48 hours, kinetics typical of a tuberculin-type of DTH responses. The DTH reactions in infected mice peaked much earlier, around 12 hours after challenge, and disappeared after 24 hours. These results suggest that different types of DTH reactions are induced in infected mice and cured mice as a result of anti-L3T4 Mab administration. It is tempting to speculate that these two forms of DTH responses are mediated by distinct subsets of L3T4$^+$ cells. Moreover, the proliferation in vitro of lymph node cells from infected mice is caracterized by, beside the specific response, a high non specific, polyclonal activation of cells in the absence of antigen or in the presence of an irrelevant antigen. In contrast, the proliferation of lymph node cells from cured mice is highly specific. Furthermore, these cells are capable of producing MAF upon antigenic stimulation whereas cells from mice infected only are not able to show any MAF production. These results, taken together, strongly suggest that two different L3T4$^+$ T cell subpopulations are triggered during cutaneous leishmaniasis in mice. Our current belief is that one of these two subsets could be detrimental to the host whereas the other subpopulation could be protective. Whether or not these two types of L3T4$^+$ cells belong to one or the other distinct L3T4$^+$ subsets (T_{h1}, T_{h2}) which have been recently described remains to be determined (12).

Importance of Lyt-2$^+$ T cells: in vivo analysis

Depletion of Lyt-2$^+$ cells in vivo by administration of anti-Lyt-2 mAb before and during infection with L.major resulted in the exacerbation of lesions in both susceptible and resistant mice (8). However, it is important to emphasize that resistant mice severely depleted of Lyt-2$^+$ T cells were still capable to heal their lesions. Furthermore, compared to susceptible mice, higher numbers of specific Lyt-2$^+$ T cells, able to mediate DTH reactions, were present in lymph nodes draining the lesions of resistant mice just before the onset of resolution of lesions. These results suggest that specific Lyt-2$^+$ cells, although not being the main protective cells, also contribute to the immunological control of experimental leishmaniasis.

L.major-specific L3T4$^+$ T cells that exacerbate cutaneous leishmaniasis

Because of the central role of T cells in resistance and susceptibility to infection with L.major, efforts were made in our laboratory to derive homogeneous populations and clones of parasite-specific T cells in vitro, to characterize these cells phenotypically and functionally and to study their effect on the course of cutaneous leishmaniasis. Following a protocol described in detail elsewhere, L3T4$^+$ T cells populations and clones specific for L.major antigens were derived and functionally characterized (13,14). Recent studies have revealed that, after activation by L.major antigen in vitro, these L3T4$^+$ T cells release, in addition to macrophage activating factors (MAF), considerable amounts of hemopoietic stimulating factors, namely multilineage colony stimulating factors (Interleukin 3, IL3) and granulocyte macrophage colony stimulating factors (GM-CSF) (10 and unpublished observations). Interestingly, all L3T4$^+$ T cell lines and clones tested so far were shown, after adoptive transfer i.v. in syngeneic recipients, to exacerbate the course of cutaneous leishmaniasis (15). This effect was neither the consequence of the production of specific antibodies by the host as a result of adoptive transfer of "helper" T cells nor the result of the induction of suppressor cells by the host (10). On the basis of a study showing that significant numbers of the i.v. injected L3T4$^+$ T cells localized rapidly into the lesion site, we proposed that these cells exacerbate the development of lesions by continuously recruiting, to the site of infection, blood-derived phagocytes, the host cells required for the growth of Leishmania (9,11). This hypothesis has now been experimentally substantiated (10). Furthermore, since after activation these L3T4$^+$ T cells release molecules capable of modulating the proliferation and the differentiation of hemopoietic progenitor cells, it is possible that these factors increase the pool of circulating phagocytes recruitable to the lesions thus favouring the multiplication of the parasites. This contention is supported by recent observations which have shown that treatment of susceptible BALB/c mice with rIL-3 resulted in the development of more severe lesions(Figure 1) (V. Kindler, Th. Pedrazzini, P. Vassalli and J. Louis, in preparation).

Although the exacerbation of cutaneous leishmaniasis by these L3T4+ T cells can already be explained by their capacity to release molecules capable of a) increasing the pool of circulating phagocytes and b) recruiting these phagocytes to the site of lesions, recent observations indicate that, in addition, the incubation of some of these hemopoietic colony-stimulating molecules (IL-3 and GM-CSF) with cultures of macrophages infected with L.major promotes the growth of intracellular L.major in vitro (V. Kindler, J. Louis and P. Vassalli, in preparation).

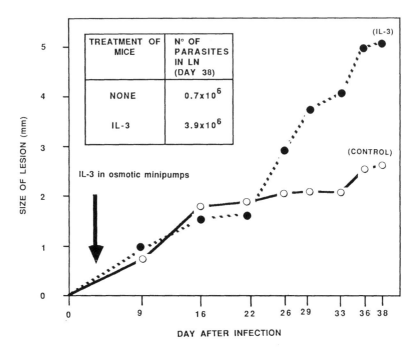

Figure 1: Effect of recombinant bacterial murine interleukin 3 on cutaneous leishmaniasis in BALB/c mice. BALB/c mice were implanted i.p. with osmotic minipumps containing either PBS (control) or recombinant interleukin 3 (40 µg)(Il-3) 3 days after s.c. infection with 2×10^6 L.major promastigotes. The size of lesions was monitored and the number of parasites in the draining lymph nodes estimated using a limiting dilution technique (16).

Inasmuch as, in titration experiments, these L3T4+ T cells either exacerbate the development of lesions or had no effect on the course of disease, it is likely that they represent a functionally homogenous population of L3T4+ T cells capable of promoting the growth of parasites in vivo. So far, we have not been able to derive and maintain in vitro homogenous populations of specific-L3T4+ T cells having a protective activity against cutaneous leishmaniasis. This failure could indicate that "protective" and "deletorious" L3T4$^+$ T cells have different requirement for growth, at least in vitro.

It is clear that studies aimed at delineating either the specificity, the functional activities or the parameters of activation of these two types of parasite-specific L3T4$^+$ T cells will be greatly facilitated by the possibility to maintain them in vitro.

Acknowledgments

This work has been supported by grants from the Swiss National Science Foundation, the UNDP/World Bank/WHO Special Programme on Tropical Diseases, the CNRS and the Pasteur Institute. The excellent technical assistance of K. Hug and A. Porret is gratefully acknowledged.

References

1. Behin, R., J. Mauel, and B. Sordat. Leishmania tropica: Pathogenicity and in vitro macrophage function in strains of inbred mice. Exp. Parasitol. 48 : 81 (1979).

2. Handman, E., R. Ceredig, and G.F. Mitchell. Murine cutaneous leishmaniasis: Disease patterns in intact and nude mice of various genotypes and examination of some differences between normal and infected macrophages. Aust. J. Exp. Biol. Med. Sci. 57 : 9 (1979).

3. Nacy, C.A., A.H. Fortier, M.G. Pappas, and R.R. Henry. Susceptibility of inbred mice to Leishmania tropica infection: Correlation of susceptibility with in vitro defective macrophage microbicidal activities. Cellular immunol: 77 : 298 (1983).

4. Handman, E., L.F. Schnur, T.W. Spithill and G.F. Mitchell. Passive transfer of leishmania lipopolysaccharide confers parasite survival in macrophages. J. Immunol. 137 : 3608 (1986).

5. Liew, F.Y. In: R.M. Steinman and R.J. North: eds. Mechanisms of host resistance to infectious agents, tumors and allografts. The Rockefeller University Press. N.Y. p.305 (1986).

6. Mitchell, G.F. Host-protective immunity and its suppression in a parasitic disease: murine cutaneous leishmaniasis. Immunology Today. 5 : 224 (1984).

7. Mitchell, G.F. and E. Handman. T-lymphocytes recognise Leishmania glycoconjugates. Parasitol. Today. 1 : 61 (1985).

8. Titus, R.G., G. Milon, G. Marchal, P. Vassalli, J.C. Cerottini and J.A. Louis. Involvement of specific Lyt-2$^+$ T cells in the immunological control of experimentally induced murine cutaneous leishmaniasis. Eur. J. Immunol. In press (1987).

9. Titus, R.G., R. Ceredig, J.C. Cerottini and J.A. Louis. Therapeutic effect of anti-L3T4 monoclonal antibody GK 1.5 on cutaneous leishmaniasis in genetically-susceptible BALB/c mice. J. Immunol. 135 : 2108 (1985).

10. Louis, J.A., S. Mendonça, R.G. Titus, J.C. Cerottini, A. Cerny, R. Zinkernagel, G. Milon and G. Marchal. The role of specific T cell subpopulations in murine cutaneous leishmaniasis. In: Progress in Immunology VI (B. Cinader and R.G. Miller, eds). Academic Press, N.Y. p.762 (1986).

11. Milon, G., R.G. Titus, J.C. Cerottini, G. Marchal and J.A. Louis. Higher frequency of Leishmania major-specific L3T4$^+$ T cells in susceptible BALB/c as compared with resistant CBA mice. J. Immunol. 136 : 1467 (1986).

12. Mosmann, T.R., H. Cherwinski, M.W. Bond, M.a. Giedlin and R.L. Coffman. Two types of murine helper T cell clone. I. Definition according to profiles of lymphokines activities and secreted proteins. J. Immunol. 136 : 2340 (1986).

13. Louis, J.A., G. Lima, J. Pestel, R. Titus and H.D. Engers. Murine T-cell responses to protozoan and metazoan parasites: Functional analysis of T-cell lines and clones specific for Leishmania tropica and Schistosoma mansoni. Contemporary topics in Immunobiology. 12 : 201 (1984).

14. Louis, J.A., R.H. Zubler, S.G. Coutinho, G. Lima, R. Behin, J. Mauel and H.D. Engers. The in vitro generation and functional analysis of murine T cell populations and clones specific for a protozoan parasite, Leishmania tropica. Immunological Reviews. 61 : 215 (1982).

15. Titus, R.G., G.C. Lima, H.D. Engers and J.A. Louis. Exacerbation of murine cutaneous leishmaniasis by adoptive transfer of parasite-specific helper T cell populations capable of mediating Leishmania major-specific delayed-type hypersensitivity. J. Immunol. 133 : 1594 (1984).

16. Titus, R.G., M. Marchand, T. Boon and J.A. Louis. A limiting dilution assay for quantifying Leishmania major in tissues of infected mice. Parasite Immunol. 7 : 545 (1985).

PARAMETERS OF T CELL ACTIVATION IN MURINE LEISHMANIASIS

Paul M. Kaye, Amalia Monroy-Ostria, Tamara I.A. Roach
and Jenefer M. Blackwell

Department of Tropical Hygiene, London School of Hygiene
and Tropical Medicine, Keppel St., London. WC1E 7HT U.K.

INTRODUCTION

Immunity to Leishmania has been shown in many studies to predominantly reflect the induction of specific cell mediated immune responses. Protective responses as generated in resistant mouse strains are accompanied by the generation of antigen specific T cell populations bearing the L3T4$^+$ phenotypic marker and able to produce soluble mediators (lymphokines) capable of inducing normally quiescent macrophages to a state of leishmanicidal activity.[1] Recently, however, attention has also focussed on the possible role of Lyt2$^+$ T cells.[2,3] The situation has been further complicated by the additional demonstration that there may be functional variability between T cells in vitro vs. in vivo. Thus, macrophage activating T cells clones can exacerbate disease in cell transfer experiments.[4] In spite of the numerous studies on lymphocyte responses during Leishmania infection, many vital questions evidently remain unanswered.

We have been studying the influence of host genetics on the outcome of infection with L.donovani. By conventional genetic approaches, loci both within the major histocompatibility complex (MHC) and distinct from it (e.g. Lsh, H-11) have been shown to have profound effects on the course of infection.[5] These studies, performed over a number of years, have now provided an invaluable base with which to address the question of how such distinct immune responses occur. An understanding of the induction phase of different immune responses will be vital not only in unravelling the complex immunoregulation occurring during murine infection but in its future application to human vaccine design.

In this paper, we describe some of our recent studies aimed at this goal.

MATERIALS AND METHODS

Mice and Parasites

A panel of congenic strains on the C57BL/10 (B10) background, expressing alternate alleles at Lsh, H-2 and H-11 were used in these studies. C57BL/10ScSn (Lsh^s;H-2^b;H-11^a), B10.D2/n (Lsh^s;H-2^d;H-11^a)

and B10.RIII(7INS) ($Lsh^s; H-2^r; H-11^a$) were obtained from Harland Olac Ltd. (Bicester, Oxon, U.K.). B10.129(10M) ($Lsh^s; H-2^b; H-11^b$) were bred at LSHTM. $B10.L-Lsh^r$ were produced as previously described[5] and mated to B10 to produce $(B10xB10.L-Lsh^r)F_1$ heterozygotes. These are phenotypically Lsh^r. BALB/c ($H-2^d$) were obtained from Harland Olac. Amastigotes of Leishmania donovani LV9 were prepared from the spleens of infected Syrian hamsters as previously described.[6]

Cell preparations

Spleen cell suspensions were prepared from naive and infected mice by mincing through nylon mesh sieves. T cells were purified by adherence and nylon wool filtration and spleen adherent cells (SAC) by adherence to plastic followed by recovery with 5mM EDTA. For further details, see references 6+7.

Primary T cell activation

An in vitro bioassay for the detection of IL2 receptor (IL2R) bearing cells was used as previously described.[6] Briefly, spleen cell populations were cultured overnight in the presence or absence of recombinant IL2 in medium containing 0.5% syngeneic normal mouse serum. ^{3}H-TdR uptake over a 6 hour pulse was assessed by scintillation counting.

Proliferative assays

Whole spleen suspensions ($5x10^5$/well) or purified T cells ($2x10^5$/well) supplemented with graded numbers of 2000R irradiated SAC were cultured with varied concentrations of L. donovani amastigotes or nitrocellulose bound antigen for 96 hours at 37 C in complete culture medium (Dutch modified RPMI + 5% FCS, $5x10^{-5}$M 2-ME, 25 g/ml gentamycin, 100 U/ml penicillin, 100 g/ml streptomycin, glutamine and pyruvate). Proliferation was assessed by ^{3}H-TdR uptake.

Quantitation of MHC Class II Expression

I-A expression on spleen adherent populations isolated during infection and on 3 day rested peritoneal macrophage populations induced with recombinant interferon gamma in vitro was determined by either immunocytochemistry or a cell ELISA using biotin avidin detection systems as described elsewhere.[7] Immunohistochemistry of cryosectioned liver was performed as described in reference 8

Preparation of nitrocellulose bound antigens

Parasites were lysed and boiled in Laemmli sample buffer (125mM Tris HCl, 25% glycerol, 5% 2-mercaptoethanol) and protein antigens resolved on a 7-20% linear gradient SDS-polyacrylamide gel (Hoeffer vertical slab unit, overnight at 55 V.) Amastigotes were loaded at an equivalent of $3x10^7$ per lane and molecular weight markers were run alongside antigen preparations.

After electrophoresis, gels were preequilibrated in western blot buffer (25mM Tris, 192mM Glycine, 20% v/v methanol, pH 8.2) for 30 min. with three changes and then blotted to nitrocellulose for 3 hours at 70 V with cooling (Bio-Rad Transblot). Dried blots were cut into lanes and divided equally into 10-20 0.5 cm fractions along the length of the lane . The molecular weight range encompasses by each fraction was determined from a standard curve plotted from the Coomassie blue stained markers. Individual fractions were then solubilized with DMSO, and reconstituted in particulate form with carbonate buffer, pH 9.6, as described by Abou-Zeid et.al.[9] After 3 washes in RPMI, particles were resuspended in 1 ml and stored at -20 C. Serial ($\log_3$) dilutions were performed in proliferative assays.

RESULTS

Detection of T cell activation

In addition to the methods already available for analysing T cell responses, the ability to directly and non-selectively analyse early activated populations was considered important for addressing the mechanisms behind the genetic control of responsiveness to L. donovani. Though the different T cell subsets may have different requirements for their full functional activation, they share the common feature of expressing high affinity receptors for IL2 as a consequence of the triggering of their antigen specific receptors. In order to determine this expression with a suitable degree of sensitivity, a bioasssay for IL2 responsiveness was developed.[6] This was found to be sufficiently sensitive, under both bulk culture and limiting dilution conditions, to detect activated T cells as early as 18-24 hours after infection in B10 mice. Furthermore, the technique facilitated the phenotypic characterisation of these responder populations.

Features of the primary response to L. donovani

One of the first notable findings using this system was the striking kinetics of IL2 receptor expression in vivo. The response peaked sharply at day 3 but had declined to negligible levels by day 7. Limiting dilution analysis confirmed that this was due to a decrease in the frequency of receptor bearing cells and not due to the generation of suppressive influences affecting the in vitro assay stage. Therefore, the polyclonal T cell response in vivo retained all the hallmarks of IL2R expression on cloned populations in vitro.

When we examined a series of H-2 congenic strains bearing r, b and d haplotypes and representative of early cure, cure and non-cure infection profiles respectively, a clear correlation in the quantitative expression of IL2R emerged.[2] Thus, there was a clear dichotomy between high responder B10.RIII(7INS) and low responder B10.D2/n mice, with B10 falling somewhat variably between the two. Significantly, no such differences were observed in the response of these strains to Listeria. At 18 hours baseline proliferation in the absence of added exogenous IL2

Table 1. Early T cell activation in H-2 congenics.

Strain	^{3}H-thymidine uptake (cpm x 10^{-3})			
	Control		Day 3 infected	
	-IL-2	+IL-2	-IL-2	+IL-2
B10RIII(7INS)	1155+160	1764+443	4229+906	8322+1646
B10.D2/n	1351+160	2378+220	1012+67	4891+36

5×10^5 spleen cells were cultured overnight with or without rIL-2 (50ng/ml) and pulsed with ^{3}-thymidine. Data are mean + S.D. of 3 mice per group.

was minimal compared to respective controls. However, by day 3 levels of proliferation rose in early cure B10.RIII(7INS) mice, to a level equivalent to that seen in B10.D2/n mice after the addition of IL2 (Table I). This response could be further amplified by exogenous IL2 illustrating that endogenously produced growth factor may limit T cell expansion.

In parallel to these studies, experiments were performed with a series of strains bearing non-MHC linked genes known to affect the host response to infection. The introduction of the Lsh^r allele onto the B10 background appeared to have no effect upon the magnitude of this early level of T cell activation[2] whereas mice bearing the $H-11^b$ allele associated with the non-curing response of B10.129(10M) mice showed markedly deficient responses (Roberts et.al., this volume).

In relation to the cell surface phenotypic composition of these responding populations, no significant differences have yet been demonstrated between B10, B10.D2/n, B10.RIII(7INS) or $(B10 \times B10.L-Lsh^r)F_1$ mice, with activation occuring in both $L3T4^+$ and $Lyt2^+$ subsets. A population transiently expressing both these markers has also been identified.[6]

Studies with these strains have branched out in two main directions, influenced by the nature of the genetic differences involved. On the one hand, differences between H-2 congenics are likely due to the role of H-2 encoded antigens as determinants of T cell antigen recognition. Hence, these studies have progressed towards an understanding of the complexity of leishmanial antigens. The known influence of Lsh and that suspected for H-11 lies at the level of the macrophage and has therefore swayed our studies towards analysing the regulation of accessory cell function in these mice.

Antigen recognition and H-2 polymorphism

We have recently adopted the technique of T cell blotting to enable us to dissect the developing T cell response in relation to defined antigen specificities. While these studies are still at a preliminary stage, and have not yet been modified to analyse early $IL2R^+$ populations, analysis of the profiles of antigen stimulation generated by using a secondary proliferative response to compare strains differing at H-2 does illustrate a number of points (Figure 1): 1) T cells recognize a number of antigens, distributed across the entire molecular weight range. 2) recognition does not correlate with the absolute amount of protein antigen detected in the respective fractions (by Coomassie blue staining). 3) For some antigens, the response in mice bearing whole haplotyope differences is equivalent, but for others high and low responder status can be assigned. 4) individual antigens show further characteristics of Ir gene control in that responder status is dependent on antigen dose (e.g. F 47-39).

Role of non MHC genes

If polymorphism at H-2 determines differential responsiveness in terms of T cell antigen specificity, what is the contibution of other genetic elements?

The data on IL2R expression indicated that initial levels of T cell activation were not influenced, either quantitatively or qualitatively, by Lsh. However, in a series of experiments analysing the secondary proliferative responses in these mice, there was a clear enhancing effect of this gene, both in terms of the magnitude of the response and

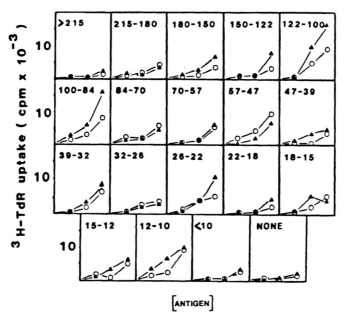

Figure 1. Proliferative responses of H-2 congenic strains to fractionated L.donovani amastigotes.

Spleen cells from 7 day infected B10.D2/n (O) and B10.RIII(7INS) (▲) were cultured with L. donovani amastigote antigens, fractionated by SDS-PAGE and immobilised on nitrocellulose as described. ^{3}H-TdR uptake was determined at 96hr. Figures in blocks represent approx. molecular weight encompassed by respective fractions.

the antigen concentration required to achieve it.[7] Secondary responses in vitro, like primary responses in vivo, are dependent on accessory cell function, though the precise requirements may be different. As the priming during the early response was determined to be identical, differences now observed are more likely to reflect secondary changes in accessory cell function.

A number of lines of experimental evidence confirm this suggestion: 1) SAC isolated from naive B10 and (B10xB10.L-Lsh^r)F$_1$ mice stimulate equivalent responses in populations of L.donovani primed B10 T cells and in mixed lymphocyte reactions across H-2 (Figure 2). 2) SAC from infected F$_1$ mice have heightened activity both on a cell per cell basis (Figure 2b) and in terms of antigen concentration compared to similarly infected B10 SAC. 3) This correlates with elevated levels of I-A on SAC within the first week of infection in F$_1$ but not B10 mice (31+5% to 53+6% vs. 33+4% to 36+5% respectively). 4) This enhancement of I-A on F$_1$ splenic macrophages is reflected in the hyper-responsiveness of peritoneal macrophages to gamma interferon in vitro (Table II). These data also illustrate that under these conditions, L. donovani have no negative effects on I-A expression and indeed enhance it in B10 mice.

In contrast to this finding, the influence of the H-11^b allele appears directed towards reduced accessory cell function (Roberts et.al., this volume).

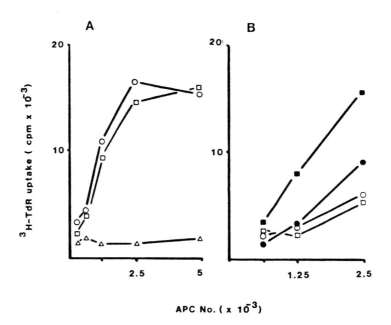

Figure 2. Accessory Cell Function of Lsh^r and Lsh^s spleen adherent cells. SAC from naive (open symbols) and 7 day infected (closed symbols) B10 (O ●) and (B10xB10.L-Lsh^r)F_1 (□ ■) mice were used to stimulate A) BALB/c ($H-2^d$) T cells and B) L. donovani primed B10 T cells. ^{3}H-TdR uptake was assessed at 96hr. In A), BALB/c SAC (Δ) were used as controls.

Table II. Class II Regulation in Lsh^r and Lsh^s Macrophages.

Strain	AM	IFN	% I-A Expression
C57Bl/10	-	-	<1
	+	-	<1
	-	+	24+13
	+	+	53+7
(B10xB10.L-Lsh^r)F_1	-	-	<1
	+	-	<1
	-	+	92+4
	+	+	87+5

Peritoneal macrophages were cultured for 3 days then infected with amastigotes (AM) at a 2:1 ratio and cultured with or without 15U/ml recombinant murine gamma-interferon (IFN). I-A was determined on triplicate coverslips by immunoperoxidase staining with MAb M5/114.

DISCUSSION

How do these finding relate to the induction of cell mediated immunity to L. donovani ?

Following infection, parasites are taken up by members of the mononuclear phagocyte system and their antigens acquired by various members of the accessory cell compartment. These may or may not represent equivalent populations, dependent upon factors such as parasite tropisms and site of innoculation. This " black box " of antigen presentation requires much finer dissection, especially in terms of the recognized heterogeneity of accessory cells for the activation of discrete T cell functions (reviewed in reference 10). The process of T cell activation is dependent upon the formation of a trimolecular complex between the clonally distributed T cell receptor, antigen and major histocompatibility complex encoded products expressed on the surface of accessory cells (Class I and Class II antigens for Lyt2 and L3T4 T cell populations respectively). Formation of such complexes has recently been shown to require an initial direct interaction between MHC and processed antigenic determinants[11] and hence the likelihood of a T cell response to any given determinant is related to the affinity of this interaction. Numerous studies have also shown that the affinity for a given peptide varies amongst the polymorphic MHC encoded molecules, providing a rational explanation for the existance of low and non-responder strains against various peptide antigens. Thus individual determinants are said to be under the control of MHC encoded immune response (Ir) genes.[12] However, as the complexity of the antigen increases, so a multiplicity of determinants may exist and increase the possibility that for any given haplotype, a responder determinant will be present. The response to complex microorganisms, not surprisingly therefore, often lacks direct evidence for Ir gene control. A striking feature of the response to L. donovani infection in B10 background mice is the exaggerated Ir genetics. Thus H-2 congenic mice show marked differences in parasite burden and the ability to resolve infection.[13] Furthermore, the non-cure response in B10.D2/n mice is dose dependent[14] and dominant in some heterozygous conditions. (Though this would classically indicate Is genetics, in leishmaniasis the distiction may merely be one of nomenclature). This situation suggested that a limited number of immunodominant antigens may be of importance in determing disease outcome. This hypothesis was further strengthened by the differential levels of T cell activation (as detected by IL2R expression) in a pattern correlating with degree of resistance. To date, we have only analysed the antigen specificity of the T cell response in these H-2 congenics in relation to the more selective secondary in vitro proliferative response. However, even these data clearly illustrate the significant contribution of MHC polymorphism to the recognition pattern of T cells. Interestingly, the response to whole amastigotes in such assays does not show as clear cut segregation of responses compared with either the IL2R assay or the response to many of the antigen fractions (data not shown). This somewhat paradoxical situation may however reflect differing conditions for activation (e.g. antigen concentrations in vitro vs. in vivo). Defining the repertoire of the 24hr. $IL2R^+$ population may well be more fruitful. It should be emphasised that the proliferative T cell response may also be rather innappropriate, being primarily a function of growth factor production. In light of the vexed question of T cell phenotype in leishmaniasis, these studies require extension to address the functional features (e.g. lymphokine production) of the cells responding to given antigens.

In addition to MHC differences, other features of accessory cell function (e.g. antigen handling) may give rise to selection of the expanded T cell repertoire.[10] However, we have initially concentrated on the ability of unfractionated accessory cells to present L. donovani and the ensuing regulatory events within the accessory cell compartment. This area has been of particular interest, forming the backbone behind mechanisms of T cell mediated immunosuppression. Hence, it was proposed[15] that extensive parasite growth in susceptible macrophages and a decrease in the expression of Class II antigens leads to the preferential induction of T suppressor cells. Evidence for such a mechanism has been slow to appear and down regulation of MHC antigens has only recently been convincingly demonstrated in BALB/c derived macrophages infected with large numbers of L. donovani amastigotes in vitro.[16] In our own studies, we have little evidence to support this concept either from in vitro studies or by analysis of Class II expression in tissue sections. High levels of expression are demonstrable on infected Kupffer cells in situ.[8] Even more strikingly, chronically infected B10.D2/n mice have greatly elevated expression of both I-A and I-E on the majority of splenic macrophages (Kaye et.al. in prep). Current views on T cell heterogeneity do not however, require such a mechanism and indeed are complemented by the results described above. Recent studies by Locksley et. al.[17] suggest that the functional dichotomy of L3T4$^+$ cells may relate to the recently characterised T_{H1} and T_{H2} helper cell subsets.[18] Both of these require Class II restricted antigen recognition but are distinct in their lymphokine profiles. Whereas both produce lymphokines which upregulate Class II expression (IFN-γ and IL-4 for T_{H1} and T_{H2} respectively) only IFN-γ in isolation can drive macrophages to leishmanicidal activity.[19] Thus the elevated levels of Class II in B10.D2/n mice in the absence of reduction in parasite burden may reflect T_{H2} activation. In vivo monoclonal antibody therapy showing the prophylactic effect of anti-I-E antibody in this mouse strain[20], may fuel speculation about the restriction specificity of such cells.

Expansion of T cell responses is accomplished by elevation of Class II on resident and inflammatory macrophage populations. Our data clearly illustrate that this function is influenced by the presence of the Lsh^r allele apparently resulting in heightened responsiveness to interferon. Thus, although accessory function is initially the same and equivalent T cell responses are generated, accelerated activation may follow the preferential expansion of the accessory cell pool under conditions where lymphokine production is still limited. This may well contribute to the early cure associated with resistant strains and complement their enhanced anti-microbial activity. Though the molecular and biochemical mechanisms involved in this effect are at present unclear, the case for identifying a human counterpart would appear as sound as ever.

ACKNOWLEDGEMENTS

This work was supported by grants from the Medical Research Council and the Wellcome Trust. JMB is a Wellcome Trust Senior Lecturer. AMO was supported by ENCB, COFAA, IPN and CONACYT, Mexico.

REFERENCES

1. F. Y. Liew, Cell mediated immunity in experimental cutaneous leishmaniasis Parasitology Today 2:262 (1986)
2. P. M. Kaye, M. B. Roberts and J. M. Blackwell, Analysing the immune response to L.donovani infection. Ann.Inst.Past. Forums
3. G. Milon, R. G. Titus, J.C. Cerottini, G. Marchal, J. A. Louis Higher frequency of Leishmania major specific L3T4$^+$ T cells in

susceptible BALB/c mice as compared to resistant CBA mice. J.Immunol 136:1467 (1986)
4. R. G. Titus, G. C. Lima, H. D. Engers and J. A. Louis, Exacerbation of murine cutaneous leishmaniasis by adoptive transfer of parasite specific helper T cell populations capable of mediating Leishmania major specific delayed type hypersensitivity J.Immunol. 133:1594 (1984)
5. J. M. Blackwell, Genetic Control of discrete phases of complex infections: Leishmania donovani as a model Progress Leukocyte Biol 3:31 (1985)
6. P. M. Kaye, Acquisition of cell mediated immunity to Leishmania I. Primary T cell activation detected by IL2 receptor expression. Immunol. 61:345 (1987)
7. P. M. Kaye, N. A. Patel and J. M. Blackwell, Acquisition of cell mediated immunity to Leishmania II. Lsh gene regulation of accessory cell function. Immunology submitted
8. P. M. Kaye, Inflammatory cells in murine visceral leishmaniasis express a dendritic cell marker. Clin Exp.Immunol (1987) in press
9. C. Abou-Zeid, E. Filley, J. Steele and G. A. W. Rook, A simple new method for using antigens separated by polyacrylamide gel electrophoresis to stimulate lymphocytes in vitro after converting bands cut from Western blots into antigen bearing particles. J.Immunol.Methods 98:5 (1987)
10. P. M. Kaye, Antigen Presentation and the response to parasitic infection Parasitology Today 3:293 (1987)
11. E. R. Unanue and P. M. Allen, The basis for the immunoregulatory role of macrophages and other accessory cells Science 236:551 (1987)
12. R. H. Schwartz, Immune response genes of the murine MHC Adv.Immunol. 38:31 (1986)
13 J. M. Blackwell, Leishmania donovani infection in heterozygous and recombinant haplotype mice Immunogenetics 18:101 (1983)
14. O. M. Ulczak and J. M. Blackwell, Immunoregulation of genetically controlled acquired responses to Leishmania donovani infection in mice: the effects of parasite dose, cyclophosphamide and sublethal irradiation. Parasite Immunol. 5:449 (1983)
15. R. M. Gorczynski and S. MacRae, Analysis of subpopulations of glass adherent mouse skin cells controlling resistance/susceptibility to infection with Leishmania tropica and correlation with the development of independent proliferative signals to $Lyt1^+/Lyt2^+$ T lymphocytes. Cell Immunol 67:74 (1982)
16. N. E. Reiner, N. G. Winnie and W. R. MacMaster, Parasite-accessory cell interactions in murine leishmaniasis.II Leishmania donovani suppresses macrophage expression of Class I and Class II major histocompatibility complex gene products J.Immunol 138:1926 (1987)
17. R. M. Locksley, F. P. Heinzel, M. D. Sadick, B. J. Holaday and K. D. Gardner Jr., Murine cutaneous leishmaniasis: Susceptibility correlates with differential expansion of Helper T cell subsets Ann.Instit.Past. Forums in Immunol. in press
18. T. R. Mossmann and R. L. Coffman, Two types of mouse helper T cell clone Immunology Today 8:223 (1987)
19. M. Belosevic and C. A. Nacy, Gamma-interferon and other lymphokines cooperate in the induction of resistance to Leishmania major infection by macrophages. Fed.Proc 46:4147 (1987)
20 J. M. Blackwell and M. B. Roberts, Immunomodulation of murine visceral leishmaniasis by administration of monoclonal anti-Ia antibodies: Differential effects of anti-I-A and anti-I-E antibodies.Eur.J.Immunol in press

A POSSIBLE ROLE FOR PROSTAGLANDINS IN REGULATION OF DISEASE IN MURINE

CUTANEOUS LEISHMANIASIS

Jay P. Farrell, Thomas J. Nolan,
William L. Croop, and Carl E. Kirkpatrick
Department of Pathobiology
University of Pennsylvania
Philadelphia, Pennsylvania 19104-6050

Following intradermal inoculation of Leishmania major promastigotes, various strains of inbred mice develop either of two distinct disease patterns. A majority of inbred strains develop small, ulcerating lesions at the cutaneous injection site. These lesions spontaneously resolve over a period of several weeks or months. In contrast, BALB/c mice develop severe local lesions, as well as multiple metastic lesions, with death the invariable outcome of infection.[1,2] Genetic susceptibility is controlled by cells of the hematopoietic system since lethally irradiated BALB/c mice, when reconstituted with bone marrow from genetically resistant B10.D2 mice, develop an infection pattern characteristic of the cell donor[3]. BALB/c mice can be altered to heal a infection by prior sublethal (550 rad) irradiation.[5] Reconstitution of these mice with normal Ly1$^+$ T cells reverses the prophylactic effect of irradiation.[5] BALB/c mice treated in vivo with antibodies directed against the L3T4$^+$ subset of T cells also heal infection.[6] These, as well as other studies, suggest that Ly1$^+$, L3T4$^+$ cells play a central role in either the nonhealing or exacerbation of L. major infections in BALB/c mice. However, neither the reason that BALB/c mice, in contrast to healing strains, develop disease-promoting T cells nor their mode of action in the promotion of disease has yet been determined.

In addition to studies showing a role for T cells in the nonhealing process, work done in this laboratory has shown that infected BALB/c mice also develop a population of splenic macrophages which suppress both antigen-and mitogen-induced T cell proliferation through the production of prostaglandins.[7] Similar studies have demonstrated that an indomethacin-sensitive macrophage from infected BALB/c mice suppresses interleukin-2 production.[8] More recently, we have shown that BALB/c mice treated in vivo with indomethacin develop smaller primary lesions and fewer metastatic lesions than control mice suggesting that prostaglandins may play a role in disease exacerbation in these animals.[9] In this paper we extend these observations to how prostaglandin production may be activated during infection and how the production of prostaglandins may correlated with inflammatory responses associated with cutaneous leishmaniasis.

MATERIALS AND METHODS

Mice: Five-week old female BALB/cByJ, B10.D2nSnJ and C57Bl/6J mice were obtained from The Jackson Laboratory (Bar Harbor, ME)

Parasites: L. major (MRHO/SU/59/Neal P) was used in these studies. Promastigote cultures were maintained in Schneider's Drosophila medium

(GIBCO, Grand Island, NY) containing 10% fetal bovine serum and passaged weekly.

Antigen: Parasite antigen consisted of heat-killed (56°C/30 min) L. major promastigotes.

Infections: Two to five million stationary-phase promastigotes were injected into the shaved skin above the tail. This inoculum routinely leads to the development of a primary lesion within 2 weeks. These mice did not develop visceral infections until 15 to 20 weeks of infection when low numbers of amastigotes were sometimes observed in impression smears.

Reagents: Indomethacin (Sigma Chemica Co., St. Louis, MO) was disolved in absolute ethanol at 10mg/ml. Appropriate dilutions were made in RPMI 1640.

Radioimmunoassay for PGE_2: Supernates from cell cultures were assayed for PGE_2 using a rabbit antibody to PGE_2 (Sigma) that cross-reacted by 3.2% with PGE_1. PGE_2 standard and $^3H[PGE_2]$ were obtained from Sigma and New England Nuclear Products (Boston, MA), respectively.

Cells and culture conditions: Medium for cell cultures consisted of RPMI 1640 buffered with sodium bicarbonate and 15mM HEPES. In addition, 10 fetal bovine serum (FBS), 100 U/ml penicillin G-potassium and 100 µg/ml streptomycin were added to the medium.

Spleen or draining lymph node cells, in the presence or absence of antigen ($1x10^6$ heat-killed promastigotes), were cultured for varying lengths of time. Supernates were collected by centrifugation (2000 x g) for 20 minutes and stored at -70°C until used. In some cases, supernates were purified by ultrafiltration in Amicon Centricon-10 microconcentrators and restored to their original volume with RPMI.

Resident peritoneal cells, or peritoneal exudate cells recovered from mic on day 3 following IP inoculation of $1x10^7$ heat-killed promastigotes, were adhered to plastic for 2-4 hours, washed and cultured in medium containing 10% FBS. The macrophage content of both resident and exudate populations was determined by quantitating cells capable of ingesting latex beads.

Colony Stimulating Factor (CSF) Assay: Colony stimulating factor levels in culture supernates were determined by a previously published technique.[10] Briefly, whole bone marrow was cultured at a concentration of $5x10^4$ cells/0.2ml in 96 well plates. Test or control supernates were added to cultures (10% of total volume) which were incubated at 37°C for 90 hours, pulsed for 6 hours with ^3H thymidine and harvested for counting by liquid scintillation. CSF activity is expressed as stimulation index (SI) where S.I.= mean CPM of sample containing test supernates/mean CPM of sample containing medium only. Colony Forming Unit-Culture (CFU-C) Assays were performed according to established techniques.[11] Briefly, triplicate cultures of $1x10^5$/ml bone marrow cells or $1x10^6$ spleen cells were plated in 35mm culture dishes in Alpha MEM (GIBCO) containing 0.3% wt/vol. Difco Bacto Agar, 10% FBS, 5% horse serum, and 10% L-cell conditioned medium. Colonies (>40 cells) were counted after 7 days of incubation at 37°C in 5% CO_2.

Hydrogen Peroxide Assays: Peritoneal exudate cells were cultured at $2x10^6$ cells/ml for 2 hours to allow adherence of macrophages, washed, and stimulated with phorbol myristate acetate (1µg/ml). Supernates were assayed for H_2O_2 content by standard protocols.[12]

Assay for I-A on macrophages: Peritoneal exudate macrophages were assessed for I-A expression at 48 hours after IP inoculation of L. major antigens by immunofluorescence using the monoclonal anti-I-A^d (MK-D6), kindly provided by Dr. Carol Cowing, and FITC-conjugated $F(ab')_2$ fragments of goat anti-mouse Ig.

Statistical Analysis: Student's T-test or the Mann-Whitney U test were used to evaluate data for signficance.

RESULTS

Production of PGE_2 During Infection

Spleen cells were obtained from normal BALB/c mice and infected mice at

1, 3, and 7 weeks after parasite inoculation. Cells were cultured for 48 hours and supernates were harvested for the determination of PGE_2 levels. The results, as shown in Figure 1, demonstrated increased PGE_2 production by spleen cells from infected mice when compared to control values. Increased levels of PGE_2 by spleen cells were noted as early as one week after parasite

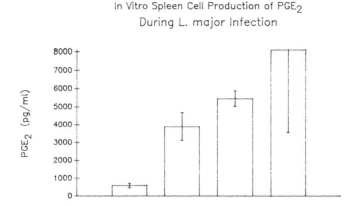

Fig. 1. PGE_2 production by 2×10^6 spleen cells in 48hr. Mean ± SD of 4 to 6 mice.

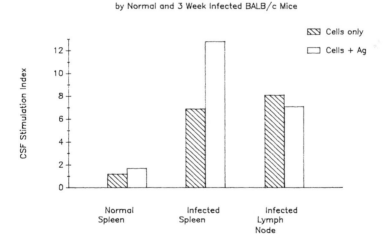

Fig. 2. CSF production by pooled cells of 4 mice after 5 days in culture.

inoculation and increased with time of infection. It should be noted that in other experiments, elevated levels of PGE_2 were not observed until several weeks after parasite inoculation, but again progressively increased with time of infection.

Colony Stimulating Factor Production

In order determine if L. major infection is accompanied by altered production of colony stimulating factors (CSF), 3 or 4 BALB/c mice were sacrificed at 3 weeks of infection and their spleens and lymph nodes recovered for use in CSF assays. Total spleen or lymph node cells were cultured in vitro in the presence or absence of L. major antigens for a period of 5 days. The supernates from these cultures were then added at a 10% concentration to cultures of normal bone marrow cells and bone culture cell proliferation was assessed by incorporation of ^{3}H thymidine. The results (Fig. 2) show that supernates from both spleen and lymph node cells from infected mice contain significantly higher (6-7 fold) levels of CSF than supernates from normal spleen cell cultures. The addition of antigen to cultures of spleen cells, but not lymph node cells, increased CSF production in this particular experiment. No significant effect of antigen was noted in cultures of normal spleen cells.

Colony Forming Units - Culture (CFU-C)

The number of colony forming units in the bone marrow and spleen of normal and 3 week infected mice were compared in a soft-agar culture assay. No differences were seen with respect to bone marrow CFU-C between normal and infected mice. There was a moderate (4 fold), but significant increase in splenic CFU-C in infected mice (Table 1). The addition of indomethacin (1μ/ml) did not significantly alter the number of CFU-C in cultures from either normal or infected mice.

Table 1. Colony Forming Units at 3 Weeks of Infection

Tissue	Indomethacin[a]	CFU/10^6 cells[b]
Normal Bone Marrow	−	1680
Normal Bone Marrow	+	1100
Infected Bone Marrow	−	1060
Infected Bone Marrow	+	1010
Normal Spleen	−	8
Normal Spleen	+	5
Infected Spleen	−	35
Infected Spleen	+	42

a. 1 uM
b. Colony Forming Units (Mean of Triplicate Cultures)

In Vivo Recruitment of Macrophages Following Antigen Stimulation

Groups of BALB/c and B10.D2 mice were infected with L. major. At 2 and 5 weeks of infection, groups of mice (3/gp) were inoculated IP with 1x10^7 heat-killed L. major promastigotes. On day 3 following IP inoculation of antigen, peritoneal exudate cells (PEC) were harvested, enumerated, and assessed for H_2O_2 production following stimulation with PMA. The results, as seen in Table 2, show that significantly higher numbers of PEC were recruited in BALB/c mice than in B10.D2 mice at 2 wks in infection. These results were reversed at week 5 of infection, at which time only B10.D2 mice yielded high PEC numbers compared to controls.

The production of H_2O_2 following PMA stimulation was signifcantly elevated compared to controls in cultures of cells from both BALB/c and B10.D2 cells at 2 weeks of infection. H_2O_2 production at 5 weeks of infection was signficantly higher in cultures of B10.D2 cells compared to BALB/c cells, and significantly elevated in cell cultures from both strains of infected mice when compared to uninfected controls.

Table 2. In Vivo Recruitment and Activation of Macrophages in Mice Infected with L. major

Week Post-Infection	Number of Cells (X 10^6)[a]		Micromoles H_2O_2[b]	
	BALB/c	B10.D2	BALB/c	B10.D2
Control	11.7 (3.0)	8.3 (2.0)	3.9 (1.0)	3.0 (4.5)
2 wk	27.3 (8.0)[c]	13.3 (4.0)	9.1 (6.5)	9.6 (1.9)[c]
5 wk	14.5 (2.0)	21.2 (11.0)[c]	17.4 (4.1)[c]	28.0 (1.7)[c]

a. Peritoneal exudate cells recovered 3 days after IP injection of 1 X 10^7 killed promastigotes. Mean (SD).
b. Micromoles of H_2O_2/10^6 PEC after PMA stimulation. Mean (SD)
c. Significantly different from control.

In a separate experiment, PEC were harvested following antigen stimulation in BALB/c and C57BL/6 mice at 2, 4, and 6 weeks of infection. PEC were adhered to coverslips for 2 hours to enrich for macrophages and assessed for the percentage of I-A$^+$ cells by immunofluorescence. The results (Table 3) show that the percentage of I-A$^+$ cells in C57BL/6 mice were significantly elevated over controls at each time point tested. In contrast, the percentage of IA$^+$ macrophages in the PEC of infected BALB/c mice was elevated only in animals assayed at 4 weeks of infection, with values returning to control levels at 6 weeks of infection. It should be noted that no significant differences were seen in the percentage of macrophages in peritoneal exudates from the two strains of mice (data not shown).

Table 3. In Vivo Recruitment of I-A$^+$Cells

Weeks Post-Infection[a]	C57BL/6[b] Control	C57BL/6 Infected	BALB/c Control	BALB/c Infected
2	5%	31%	6%	11%
4	5%	32%	4%	29%
6	12%	34%	6%	6%

a. Mice inoculated ID with 1 X 10^6 L. major promastigotes.
b. % I-A$^+$ macrophages within a 48hr PEC population following IP inoculation of 1 X 10^6 killed promastigotes.

Factor Production by Cells from Infected Mice

Since spleen and lymph node cells from infected mice were shown to produce colony stimulating factors, the possibility that they also produced factors capable of stimulating PGE_2 production was examined. Supernates were collected from spleen and lymph node cells from 3-week infected mice and cultured for 5 days in the presence of L. major antigen. Supernates were dialyzed to remove PGE_2 and added to either cultures of resident peritoneal macrophages to test for the stimulation of PGE_2 production or to bone marrow cultures to determine levels of colony stimulating factor. The results (Fig. 3) show that supernates from normal spleen cells, cultured in the presence or absence of antigen, contain only low levels of CSF and failed to stimulate the production of PGE_2 by resident peritoneal macrophages. In contrast,

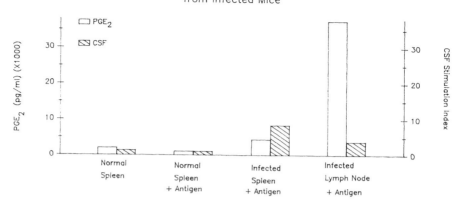

Fig 3. Supernates from cultures added to bone marrow (CSF Assay) or macrophages (PGE Assay).

supernates from antigen-stimulated spleen and lymph node cell from 3-week infected mice contained significantly elevated levels of CSF. Supernates from antigen-stimulated spleen cells induced only a 2 fold increase in PGE_2 production by macrophages, but lymph node supernates stimulated PGE_2 production by almost 20 fold.

DISCUSSION

The studies presented in this paper have focused on the early events affecting inflammatory responses in L. major infected mice. Clearly, infection in genetically susceptible BALB/c mice is accompanied by the development of a population of splenic macrophages which secrete elevated levels of PGE_2. Enhanced PGE_2 production was noted during the early weeks of infection and appears to accompany the splenic hyperplasia which occurs in this strain of mouse. It should be noted that the time course of elevated PGE_2 production by spleen cells varies from experiment to experiment and may depend upon the numbers and infectivity of promastigotes in inocula, which would influence the subsequent progression of lesion development.

Infection in BALB/c mice is also accompanied by an increase in spleen, but not bone marrow, colony forming cells assayed 3 weeks after parasite inoculation. This observation is in agreement with a previous study in which increased spleen, but not bone marrow CFU-C were noted at approximately 6 weeks of infection with peak CFU-C formation occurring at about 12 weeks of infection.[13]

Increases in splenic myelopoiesis may be associated with the increased formation of colony stimulating factors produced by spleen and lymph node cells from infected mice. Our results show that CSF activity, as measured in a bone marrow proliferation assay, increased 6 to 7 fold in mice infected for 3 weeks. It is interesting to note that the CSF produced in infected mice had a stimulating effect on normal BALB/c bone marrow cells, even though neither we, nor others[13], found evidence of a significant increase in bone marrow myelopoiesis during infection. It is possible that other regulatory interactions are limiting in vivo hematopoiesis to the spleen. Alternatively, stimulated bone marrow stem cells may be transported to the spleen prior to differentiation into mature cells of the granulocyte-macrophage lineage.

Attempts were also made to analyze antigen-specific inflammatory responses following intraperitoneal injection of killed Leishmania promastigotes. The data comparing susceptible BALB/c and resistant B10.D2 mice suggest that BALB/c mice mount an earlier inflammatory response than do B10.D2 mice, with respect to the number of peritoneal exudate cell recovered on day 3 after antigen inoculation. Significantly elevated PEC numbers were noted in BALB/c mice at 2 weeks of infection, while responses in B10.D2 cells remained normal until later in infection. Inflammatory cells from both strains of mice showed an increased capacity to released H_2O_2 after PMA stimulation, but H_2O_2 from B10.D2 cells was generally higher. It should be noted that the production of H_2O_2 does not necessarily correlate with the ability of macrophage to exert effector functions such as tumor cell cytotoxicity or microbicidal activity. An analysis of the percentage of inflammatory macrophages expressing surface I-A antigen does suggest differences between macrophages in susceptible and resistant mice. In resistant C57 BL/6 mice, increased I-A expression was observed in mice infected for 2, 4 or 6 weeks, in contrast to BALB/c mice in which inflammatory exudates contained a higher percentage of I-A$^+$ cells at 4 weeks, but not at 6 weeks of infection. The loss in the capacity of infected BALB/c mice to recruit I-A$^+$ cells between 4 and 6 weeks of infection may correlate with previous observations which show that the capacity of these mice to mount a delayed-type hypersensitivity response to parasite antigens is lost at a similar time.[7]

The major stimuli for induction or suppression of Ia expression by macrophages are gamma-IFN and prostaglandins, respectively. Recently studies suggest that T cells from L. major infected BALB/c mice do not secrete significant amounts of gamma-IFN,[14]. Thus, a primary stimulus, for Ia expression (gamma-IFN) is missing while a inhibitor of Ia expression (PGE_2) is present in infected BALB/c mice.

The different factors which control an inflammatory response are complex. Multiple hemopoeitic colony-stimulating factors have been described, many of which can be produced by several cell types and exert multiple biological activities.[15] The production of PGE_2 by macrophages is also regulated by multiple factors[16] and may, itself, regulate hematopoieois.[17] We have attempted to determine if antigen stimulated spleen or lymph node cells produce factors which influence hematopiesis and/or PGE^2 production. Dialized supernates from antigen-stimulated spleen and lymph node cells from infected mice contained factors which induced a moderate increase in bone marrow cell proliferaton. These same supernates were able to induce normal macrophages to secrete elevated levels of PGE_2. Interestingly, the supernates from lymph node cell populations stimulated PGE_2 production to a much greater extent than did supernates from spleen cells, despite the fact that we have found little evidence that PGE_2 levels produced by lymph node cells are dramatically elevated during infection (data not shown). It is possible that lymph nodes do not contain sufficient numbers of macrophages to produce detectable PGE_2, even though the stimuli for PGE_2 production is present. Alternatively, other regulatory molecules may be present which block the production of PGE_2 by these cells.

Our results, taken in the context of previous studies, suggest that L. major infections in BALB/c mice are accompanied by increased splenic myelopoiesis, increased production of CSF and factors capable of stimulating PGE_2 production, and an increased capacity to mount an early inflammatory response to parasite antigens, but a decreased capacity to produce factors such as gamma-IFN which regulate macrophage effector functions. The apparent restriction of both hematopoiesis and PGE_2 production to the spleen in infected mice is especially interesting. Increased macrophage numbers in the spleen, possibly stimulated by CSF produced in response to leishmanial antigens, could lead to increased production of interleukin-1, a known stimulus for PGE_2 production.[16] The activation of PGE_2, therefore, could be a direct response by the host to regulate macrophage production. The apparent failure of infected BALB/c mice to produce gamma-IFN, a antagonist to the induction of PGE_2 production by Il-1, could play a major role in the events which characterize the inflammatory response in this strain of mouse.

REFERENCES

1. Howard, J.G., C. Hale and W.L. Chan-Liew. 1980. Immunological regulation of experimental cutaneous leishmanisis: I. Immunogenetic aspects of susceptibility to Leishmania tropica in mice. Parasite Immunol. 2:303.
2. DeTolla, L.J., P.A. Scott and J.P. Farrell. 1981. Single gene control of resistance to cutaneous leishmaniasis in mice. Immunogenetics 14:29.
3. Howard, J.G., C. Hale and F.Y. Liew. 1980. Genetically determined susceptibility to Leishmania tropica infection is expressed by haematopoietic donor cells in mouse irradiation chimaeras. Nature 288:161.
4. Howard, J.G., C. Hale and F.Y. Liew. 1981. Immunological regulation of experimental cutaneous leishmaniasis. IV. Prophylactic effect of sublethal irradiation as a result of abrogation of suppressor T cell generation in mice susceptible to Leishmania tropica. J. Exp. Med. 153:557.
5. Liew, F.Y., C. Hale and J.G. Howard. 1982. Immunological regulation of experimental cutaneous leishmaniasis. V. Characterization of effector and specific suppressor T cells. J. Immunol. 128:1917.
6. Titus, R.G., R. Ceredig, J.C. Cerottini, and J.A. Louis. 1985. Therapeutic effect of anti-L3T4 monoclonical antibody GK1.5 on cutaneous leishmaniasis in genetically-susceptible BALB/c mice. J. Immunol. 135:2108.
7. Scott, P.A. and J.P. Farrell. 1981. Experimental cutaneous leishmaniasis: I. Non-specific immunodepression in BALB/c mice infected with Leishmania tropica. J. Immunol. 127:2395.
8. Cillari, E., F.Y. Liew and R. Lelchuk. 1986. Suppression, of interleuken-2 production by macrophages in genetically susceptible mice infected with Leishmania major. Inf. Imm. 54:386.
9. Farrell, J.P. and C. E. Kirkpatrick. 1987. Experimental cutaneous leishmaniasis, II. A possible role for prostaglandins in excerbation of disease in Leishmania major - infected BALB/c mice J. Immunol. 138:902.
10. M. B. Prystowsky, M.F. Naukukas, J.N. Ihle, E. Goldwasser, and F.W. Fitch. 1983. A microassay for colony-stimulating factor based on thymidine incorporation. Amer. J. Path. 114:149.
11. Bradley, T.R. and D. Metcalf. 1966. The growth of mouse bone marrow cells in vitro. Aust. J. Exp. Biol. Med. Sci. 73:2472.
12. Pick, E. and Y. Keisari. 1980. A simple colorimetric method for the measurement of hydrogen peroxide produced by cells in culture. J. Immunol. Meth. 38:161.
13. Mirkovich, M.A., A. Balelli, A.C. Allison, and F.Z. Modabber. 1986. Increased my elopoiesis during Leishmania major infection in mice: gen eration of "safe targets" is a possible way to evade the effector immune mechanism. Clin. Exp. Immunol. 64:01.
14. Sadick, M.D., F.P. Heinzel, V.M. Shigekane, W.L. Fisher, and R.M. Locksley. 1987. Cellular and humoral immunity to Leishmania major in genetically susceptible mice after in vivo depletion of L3T4$^+$T cells. J. Immunol. 139:1303.
15. Nicola, N.A. and M. Vadas. 1984. Hemopoietic colony-stimulating factors. Immunol. Today 5:76.
16. Browning, J.L. and A. Ribolini. 1987. Interferon blocks interleukin-1 induced prostaglandin release from human peripheral monocytes. J. Immunol. 138:2857.
17. Kurland, J.I., R.S. Bockman, H.E. Broxmeyer, and M.A.S. Moore. 1978. Limitation of excessive myelopoiesis by the intrinsic modulation of macrophage-derived prostaglandin E. Science 199:552.

USE OF A DOT-ELISA PROCEDURE FOR THE DETECTION OF SPECIFIC

ANTIBODIES IN CUTANEOUS LEISHMANIASIS

Luis Guevara, Lourdes Paz, Elizabeth Nieto and
Alejandro Llanos
Instituto de Medicina Tropical "Alexander von
Humboldt"- Universidad Peruana Cayetano Heredia
P.O. Box 5045, Lima-100 Peru

INTRODUCTION

American Tegumentary Leishmaniasis is a disease endemic on the America continent from northern Mexico to Argentina. This disease is of major importance in Peru, with over 2700 new cases being reported annually to Peruvian Ministry of Health, a figure which most probably is an underestimate[1].

In Peru exist two forms of leishmaniasis, cutaneous and mucocutaneous. The cutaneous form is called Uta and occurs on the Andes Mountains (600-3000 m.o.s.l.) and in the interandean valleys[2].

Several serological techniques have been developed for the diagnosis of leishmaniasis, including indirect immunofluorescence [6,7,8] ELISA[9,10], and dot-ELISA[11,12,13]. However, these techniques have been of limited value for the diagnosis of cutaneous leishmaniasis, due to the low level of antibodies generally encountered in this disease.

In 1983, Guimaraes[14] reported an enzyme-linked immunosorbent assay for Ig G and Ig M antibodies to be used for the diagnosis of cutaneous leishmaniasis.

To improve the serological diagnosis of this disease, we have reported an improved dot-Elisa which has been used in the serological diagnosis of mucocutaneous leishmaniasis[15]. This dot-Elisa test is very simple, inexpensive and can be performed in field studies where appropiate laboratory conditions are lacking.

At present, we report the application of this test to the diagnosis of Andean cutaneous leishmaniasis.

MATERIAL AND METHODS

Antigen preparation

Leishmania braziliensis braziliensis promastigotes were used as a source of antigen. The parasites were cultured as reported by Romero[2], and harvested after 7-8 days. The parasites were washed three timeswith cold phosphate-buffered saline (PBS pH 7.2) and resuspended at 5×10^7 parasites /ml. 1ul volumes containing

5×10^4 parasites, equivalent to 326 ng of protein measured by the method of Lowry[16], were dotted onto the dull side of 5 mm nitrocellulose filter discs (Schleicher and Schuell) placed in the wells of flat-bottomed microtiter plates (Falcon), using a 10ul Hamilton syringe. Antigen was fixed by drying at 56°C for 20 minutes.

The microtiter plates containing sensitized discs were then stored at -20°C in a tightly closed plastic box until used.

Sera

Several groups of patients were studied: Set 1 was made up of 34 patients with cutaneous leishmaniasis confirmed by parasite isolation from lesions. All patients were classified as Andean cutaneousleishmaniasis on clinical and epidemiological grounds. Set 2 was made up of patients with other diseases endemic to Peru: brucellosis (3), typhoid fever (3), tuberculosis (3), Hansen'n disease (3), histoplasmosis (2), toxoplasmosis (1)and malaria(3). All serum samples were from patients whose diseases had been established by isolation of the causative agent and were obtained from the serum bank of the Instituto de Medicina Tropical "Alexander von Humboldt". Set 3 was made up of 8 samples from normal healthy personsfrom endemic areas and 8 samples from normal person neverexposed to leishmanial infection. Three positive serum to Chagas disease and Bartonellosis were considered separately.

Dot-Elisa assay

Sentized discs were allowed to reach room temperature. Positive and negative control sera, antigen and conjugate control were included in each experiment. Antigen discs were blocked with 75 ul of 8% non-fat dry milk-PBS-0.5% Tween-20 added to each well and incubated for 30 minutes. After aspirating off blocking solution, 75 ul of serum diluted in 2% nonfat dry milk-PBS-0.05% Tween 20 was added to each well and incubated for 30 minutes. Diluted sera were aspirated off and the discs washed three times with 100 ul of PBS-0.05% Tween20.

Alkaline Phosphatase labelled goat anti-human Ig G conjugate (gamma chain specific from SIGMA) diluted at 1:300 in 2% non fat dry milk-PBS-0.05% Tween 20 was dispensed into each well and incubated at room temperature for 30 minutes. The optimal dilution of conjugate was found by block titration of twofold dilution of the conjugate. Conjugate was aspirated off and the wells were incubate with 100 ul of 1.15 M NaCl solution, for exactly 30 seconds. The NaCl solution was discarded and thewells washed again with PBS-0.05% Tween 20 as described above. The indicator reagent was made up of 5 mg Nitro Blue Tetrazolium, 2.5 mg of 5-Bromo-4-Chloroindolyl Phosphate 50 ul of N-N' Dimethylformamida dissolved in 7.5 ul of alkaline phosphatase b-ffer at pH 9.5. Each well received 100ul of this reagent. Readings were made visually 15 minutes later. Development of a dark blue spot on discs when compared with negative control serum was considered positive.

Statistical Analysis

The serological analysis titers obtained for all sera could be cocnstructed dichotomously as either positive or negative by using two different cutoff dilutions for this test, 1/800 and 1/1600. This allowed a construction of 2x2 contingency tables with frequencies of true-positive, true-negative, false positive and false negative results with respect to the disease (table 3).
Standard diagnostic indexes such as sensitivity, specificity

were calculated by using formulas previously described[17]

RESULTS

A representative picture of the cutoff level with positive and negative controls are showed in fig. 1

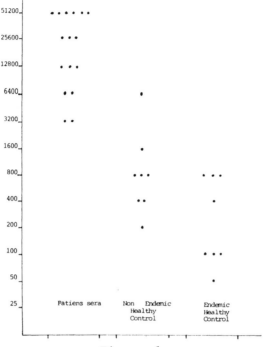

Figure 1.

32 patient sera (94.1%) reacted in the dot-Elisa at reciprocal titer of 800 and 1600, and positive titers ranged up to 1600 to over 25600. Two positives sera did not reach the cutoff level. From 8 control negative sera from endemic areas, one (12.5%) had a titer of 50, three (37.5%) 100, one (12.5%) of 400 and three (37.5%) of 800. of the 8 control negative sera from non edemic area, one (12.5%) had a titer of 200, two (25%) of 400, three (37.5%) of 800, one (12.5% of 1600 and one (12.5%) had high titer of 6400. The frequencies of titers obtained with dot-Elisa at two different cutoff leves in set 1, is showed in table[1]. Flase results, both positive and negative were low using the high cutoof level 1/1600. Small variation is observed at 1/800 cutoff level.

Table 1.

FREQUENCY OF RESULTS

Cutoff titer *	POSITIVE		NEGATIVE	
	True	False	True	False
800	32	4	32	2
1600	32	2	34	2

Frequency of test results obtained with the dot-Elisa at two different cutoff levels for the serological diagnosis of cutaneous leishmaniasis.

*: Specimens reacting at a titer greater than or equal to the cutoff level were considered positive.

These frequencies were used to display the diagnostic test index with 95% confidence limits, and are showed in table 2.

Table 2.

Cut off titer	Index (%) (95% confidence limit)	
	Sensitivity	Specificity
800	94.12 [80 - 99]	88.89 [74 - 97]
1,600	94.12 [80 - 99]	94.44 [81 - 99]

On other hand, in table 3, is showed the cross-reactivity in the dot-Elisa with sera from patients with other diseases than leishmaniasis. Chagas disease and Bartonellosis are more reactive.

Table 3.

DISEASE	N° SERAS	RECIPROCAL TITER	
		1:800	1:1600
Brucelosis	3	2/3	0/3
Thyphoid	3	0/3	0/3
Tuberculosis	3	0/3	0/3
Hansen	3	0/3	0/3
Histoplasmosis	2	0/2	0/2
Toxoplasmosis	1	0/1	0/1
Malaria	3	1/3	1/3
Chagas	3	3/3	2/3
Bartonellosis	3	2/3	1/3

DISCUSSION

Leishmaniasis is an endemic problem in Peru, and up to now there is no serological test available to use in the field. The conventional serological tests, lack sensitivity due to the low amount of antibodies produced during the parasite infection[6,18,11,12,13]. However, more sensitive techniques have been developed[7,10], and have made possible the detection of very small amount of antibodies.

In the present study, we report development of a dot-Elisa for cutaneous leishmaniasis. In this assay, we have developed a sensitive and specific test using Alkaline Phosphatase which detect antibodies in patients with cutaneous leishmaniasis up to titers of 1/26000. In our opinion, the gain of sensitivity may be due to two factors: -The use of an alkaline phosphatase conjugate as a second antibody, together with a substrate which has high sensitivity. -We have optimized the sistem of washing the discs in a manner which greatly reduces background as well as the number of false positives. In this aspect, we have found the step of washing with 1.15 M NaCl to be of great importance. However, We have observed a cross reaction with serum from patients with Chagas disease, but since we don't have regions that coexist both diseases

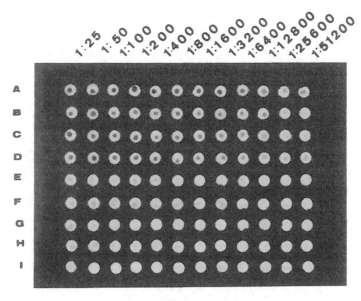

Figure 2. A representative dot-Elisa test.

CONCLUSIONS

We have improved a dot-Elisa test for the detection of antibodies in cutaneous leishmaniasis. The sensitivity an specificity at cutoff titer of 800 is 94.12% and 88.89%. At 1600 cutoff level, the sensitivity is the same but the specificity is improved to 94.44%.

This test is very simple, low cost can be used in field trials for epidemiological purposes and may be used for patients follow-up.

REFERENCES

1. H. Lumbreras and H. Guerra, Leishmaniasis in Peru, in: "Leishmaniasis", K-P Chang and R.S. Bray ed. Elsevier, Amsterdam (1985).
2. G. G. Romero, M. Arana, M. López, Y. Montoya, R. Bohl, M. Campos, J. Arévalo and A. Llanos, Characterization of Leishmania species from Peru, Trans. R. Soc. Trop. Med. Hyg. 81:14 (1987).
3. L. D. Hendricks and N. Wright, Diagnosis of cutaneous leishmaniasis by in vitro cultivation of saline aspirates in Schneider Drosophila medium, Amer. J. Trop. Med. Hyg., 28:962 (1979).
4. A. Herrer, V. E. Thatcher and C. M. Johnson, Natural infection of Leishmania and Trypanosomes demonstrated by skin culture, J. Parasitol, 52:954 (1966).

5. A. Herrer, H. A. Christensen and R. J. Beumer, Reservoir hosts of cutaneous leishmaniasis among Panamenian forest mammals, Am. J. Trop. Med. & Hyg. 22:585 (1973).
6. B. C. Walton, W. H. Brooks and J. Arjona, Serodiagnosis of American Leishmaniasis by indirect fluorescent antibody test, Am. J. Trop. Med. Hyg., 21:296 (1972).
7. C. A. Cuba-Cuba, P. D. Marsden, A. C. Barreto, R. Rocha, R. R. Sampaio and L. Patzlaff, Diagnóstico parasitológico e inmunológico de Leishmania tegumentaria americana, Bol. Of. Pan. Sal. 89:195 (1980).
8. M. G. Pappas, P. B. Mc Greevy, R. Hajkowski, L. D. Hendricks, C. N. Oster and W. T. Hockmeyer, Evaluation of promastigotes antigens in the indirect fluorescent antibody test for American cutaneous leishmaniasis, Am. J. Trop. Med. Hyg., 32:1260 (1983).
9. M. Hommel, Enzymoimmunoassay in Leishmaniasis, Trans. R. Soc. Trop. Med. Hyg., 70:15 (1976).
10. M. Hommel, N. Peters, J. Ranque, M. Quilici and G. Lanotte, The micro-elisa technique in the serodiagnosis of visceral leishmaniasis, Am. Trop. Med. Parasitol., 72:213 (1978).
11. M. G. Pappas, R. Hajkowski and W. T. Hockmeyer, Dot-Enzyme-linked immunosorbent assay (dot-Elisa): a micro technique for the rapid diagnosis of visceral leishmaniasis, J. Immunol. Methods, 64:205 (1983).
12. M. G. Pappas, R. Hajkowski and W. T. Hockmeyer, Standarization of the dot-enzyme-linked immunosorbent assay (dot-Elisa) for human visceral leishmaniasis, Am. J. Trop. Med. Hyg., 33:1105 (1984).
13. M. G. Pappas, R. Hajkowski, D. B. Tang and W. T. Hockmeyer, Reduced false positive reactions in the dot-enzyme-linked immunosorbent assay for human visceral leishmaniasis, Clin. Immunol. Immunopathol., 34:392 (1985).
14. M. C. S. Guimaraes, B. J. Celeste, M. E. Camargo and J. M. P. Dimiz, Seroepidemiology of cutaneous leishmaniasis from riberia do Iguape Valley. Ig M and Ig G antibodies detected by means of an immunoenzymatic assay (ELISA), Rev. do Ins. Med. Trop. Sao Paulo, 25:99 (1983).
15. L. A. Guevara, L. T. Paz, F. E. Nieto and J. Arévalo, Improvement of a dot-Elisa, using alkaline phosphatase, for the detections of antibodies in mucocutaneous leishmaniasis, (1987, submitted).
16. O. H. Lowry, N. J. Rosebrough, A. L. Farr and R. J. Randall, Protein measurement with Folin phenol reagent, J. Biol. Chem., 193:275 (1951).
17. P. Griner, J. Raymond, A. Mushlin and P. Greenland, Selection and interpretation of diagnostic test and procedures, Ann. Int. Med. 94:553 (1981).
18. R. E. Duxbury and E. H. Sadum, Fluorescent antibody test for the serodiagnosis of visceral Leishmaniasis, Am. J. Trop. Med. Hyg., 18:525 (1964).

A NOVEL METHOD OF VACCINATION USING PARASITE MEMBRANE ANTIGENS

James Alexander

Immunology Division
University of Strathclyde
Glasgow G4 ONR, Scotland

David G. Russell

Department of Pathology
New York University Medical Centre
New York, N.Y.10016, U.S.A.

INTRODUCTION

There have recently been a large number of vaccination studies using mouse models of cutaneous leishmaniasis. These have tended to use either whole attenuated organisms (Howard et al, 1982; Liew et al, 1985) or crude antigen preparations (Liew et al, 1985). Although these vaccine preparations increased resistance if inoculated intravenously (i.v.) or intraperitoneally (i.p.), they exacerbated infections if administered subcutaneously (s.c.). Intravenous or i.p. vaccination procedures are obviously not acceptable for use with humans. Ideally a vaccine should comprise a purified biochemically defined antigen administered by a cutaneous or intramuscular route without any risk of exacerbating naturally acquired infections. Two antigens have been suggested as potential candidates for successful vaccination, the plasma membrane glycoprotein gp63 and the glycoconjugate excreted factor (EF). Both antigens are involved in the attachment of the parasite to its host cell, the macrophage (Handman & Goding, 1985; Russell & Wilhelm, 1986), and are found in related forms in all species of Leishmania examined to date (Etges et al, 1985; Colomer-Gould et al, 1985; Handman et al, 1984). We describe here a novel means of presenting these antigens to the immune system and we have successfully vaccinated mice against L.mexicana by the s.c. route.

Materials and Methods

Parasites: L.mexicana (MNYC/BZ/62/M379), L.major (MRHO/SU/59/NEAL) and L.donovani (MHOM/ET/67/82) were used in these experiments. L.mexicana and L.major promastigotes were transformed from amastigotes harvested from BALB/c mice at 6 week intervals. They were grown in RPMI medium supplemented with 10% foetal calf serum and were used for experiments when in the infective stationary phase of the growth cycle. L.donovani amastigotes were isolated from liver homogenates excised from Golden Hamsters.

Antigen preparation and reconstitution into liposomes: The promastigote antigens gp63 and EF were isolated from L.mexicana crude membrane preparations as described previously (Russell & Wilhelm, 1986). Briefly antigens were extracted in 1% octyl glucoside in PBS with 50 µM Leupeptin and 50 µM TLCK from enriched plasma membrane fractions. These fractions had been obtained from parasites suspended in hypotonic buffer and disrupted using either a Braun Homogeniser (Melsunger FRG) or a Nitrogen bomb (Parr Co.,

Illinois). The soluble extract was passed over a concanavalin A-sepharose (Pharmacia) column. The EF ran through whilst the gp63 was bound to the column. The gp63 was further purified by anion exchange chromatography on DEAE sephadex. EF was isolated by incubation with W1C108.3-sepharose (W1C108.3, a monoclonal antibody against EF was kindly provided by Dr D. Snary).

Promastigote antigens were reconstituted into liposomes by a modification of the technique of Russell and Wilhelm (1986). Phospholipids isolated from Crithidia fasciculata were mixed with octyl glucoside in the presence of chloroform and cholesterol added to a final concentration of 15%. Alternatively, a mixture of 80% soyabean lecithin, 15% cholesterol and 5% dicetyl phosphate in chloroform was used. The mixture was dried to a thin film under N2 and incubated for 1 hr at $37°C$. The parasite antigens in PBS and detergent (1% octyl glucoside) were added to the lipid film (2 µg antigen to 1 mg phospholipid/cholesterol) and sonicated in an ice bath. The detergent was removed by overnight dialysis against PBS at $4°C$ and the resulting liposomes washed by centrifugation at 100,000 g for 1 hr at $4°C$.

Vaccination procedures: Groups of 6, ten week old CBA/Ca and BALB/c mice (OLAC.U.K.) were each inoculated with one of a variety of vaccine and control formulations (for details see Table 1). The vaccine preparations contained either 5 µg gp63 or 4 µg EF or both gp63 and EF or 10 µg crude membrane antigens reconstituted into 2.5 mg of liposomes in 50 µl PBS. After 4 weeks vaccination was repeated and the animals rested 4 weeks before subcutaneous challenge into the shaven rump with 5×10^4 L.mexicana promastigotes. Lesion diameter was measured at 2 weekly intervals. The therapeutic effect of adding complete Freund's adjuvant (CFA) to gp63/EF liposomes was also examined. Comparative antibody levels were measured by radioimmunoassay 4 weeks after infection and immediately before challenge infection (Russell & Alexander, 1987).

In a further experiment the potential of L.mexicana membrane antigens reconstituted into liposomes to protect against heterologous challenge was examined. Groups of at least 6, ten week old, BALB/c mice were vaccinated twice, at 2 week intervals with 8 µg antigen-liposomes i.p. or i.v. Two and three weeks later mice were infected s.c. with 10^6 L.major promastigotes or i.v. with 1.2×10^7 L.donovani amastigotes. Parasite growth was measured by lesion diameter (L.major), and by the number of L.donovani amastigotes in the spleen, liver and bone marrow.

Adoptive transfer experiments: T cells were obtained from the macerated spleens of CBA/Ca mice 16 weeks after infection with L.mexicana and passaged through nylon wool columns. The effluent cells contained 5% B lymphocytes as measured by direct immunofluorescence. T cell subsets were isolated by treatment with either anti Lyt-2(3.168) plus complement or anti L3T4 (RL 172.4) plus complement. (The monoclonal antibodies were kindly supplied by Dr P.M. Kaye, see Kaye (1987) for details). Mice were inoculated i.p. with 5×10 whole T cells or their T cell subsets (approximately 60% L3T4+ and 30% Lyt-2+) and infected immediately afterwards with 10 L.mexicana amastigotes.

RESULTS

Protective effect of antigen-liposome preparations: The results are summarised in Table 1. No matter what the route of vaccine administration all antigen-containing liposomes protected CBA/Ca mice against homologous challenge with L.mexicana promastigotes. No mice vaccinated with gp-liposomes developed lesions and only 1 mouse vaccinated with EF-liposomes. On the other hand, all but one of the control mice (liposomes alone) developed non-healing lesions. Surprisingly, the addition of CFA to gp63/EF-liposomes exacerbated lesion growth as did i.p. but not s.c. vaccination with CFA alone.

Table 1. The effects of various vaccine preparations on L.mexicana infections in CBA/Ca and BALB/c mice

Treatment	CBA/Ca			BALB/c		
	Lesion			Lesion		
	Size[a]	No.[b]	Ab[c]	Size[a]	No.[b]	Ab[c]
Control	5.3+0.71	6	0	11.2+2.71	6	0
Liposomes (s.c.)	4.6+0.71	6	-	7+3.66	5	-
(i.p.)	4.1+1.27	5	-	8.7+1.83	6	-
Crude Ag-lip[d] (s.c.)	0.8+1.33	2	51	9.5+1.14	6	151
(i.p.)	0.5+0.84	2	420	1.4+1.09	2	303
gp63-lip. (s.c.)	0	0	42	7.2+5.65	4	32
(i.p.)	0	0	408	7+3.21	5	186
EF-lip. (s.c.)	0.5+1.22	1	12	8+4.19	5	3
(i.p.)	0	0	-15	5.5+4.41	4	38
gp63/EF-lip. (s.c.)	0	0	21	8.8+2.71	6	62
(i.p.)	1.0+2.45	1	347	0.6+0.94	2	385
gp63/EF-lip. (s.c.) + CFA	10.2+2.53	6	12	8.3+4.17	5	123
(i.p.)	7.8+1.4	6	132	5.7+3.83	5	1080
CFA (s.c.)	5.1+1.14	6	-	10.8+2.11	6	-
(i.p.)	8.5+2.14	6	-	11.8+2.31	6	-
gp63/EF-lip. (i.v.)		1	348		5	236

(a) Mean lesion diameter (mm) ± S.D. 16 weeks post-infection in each group of 6 mice.
(b) Number of mice with lesions in each group of 6 mice, 16 weeks post-infection.
(c) Relative antibody titre (C.P.M.) above control before infection
(d) Lip = Liposomes

BALB/c mice developed quicker growing lesions than CBA/Ca mice and vaccination s.c. was only partially protective. However, vaccination i.p. was much more protective and only 2 of the gp63/EF liposome group and 2 of the crude antigen-liposome group developed lesions. No exacerbation of infection was noted following vaccination by any route. Anti-Leishmania antibodies were generally higher if animals were vaccinated i.p. rather than s.c. but otherwise there was no correlation with protection.

Heterologous protection: Normal BALB/c mice develop non healing lesions when infected s.c. with L.major (Table 2). Following i.v. or i.p. vaccination with L.mexicana membrane antigens reconstituted into liposomes a significant level of resistance was induced against L.major as measured by lesion size (Table 2). Lesions in vaccinated mice were flat and crusty by day 45 after infection while non-vaccinated mice had large nodules with small ulcerating centres.

Table 2. Growth of L.major in BALB/c mice[a]

	Vaccinated[b]	Non Vaccinated
Day 15	2.6+1.1	4.2+2.3
Day 30	5+1.2	8.2+2.1
Day 45	6.6+1.6	12+3.6

(a) Mean lesion diameter (mm) + S.D. following subcutaneous infection with 10^6 promastigotes.

(b) L.mexicana membrane antigen 8 μg reconstituted into liposomes i.v. 5 weeks and 3 weeks before infection.

A similar vaccine protocol in BALB/c mice conferred no measurable protection against intravenous infection with 1.2×10^7 L.donovani (Table 3).

Table 3. The number of L.donovani amastigotes in the spleen, liver and bone marrow of BALB/c mice[a]

Treatment	Spleen	Liver	Bone Marrow
Control	633+213	2257+581	724+194
Antigen-liposomes	598+197	1949+666	688+443

(a) Measured 50 days after infection; the number of amastigotes/1000 host nuclei + S.D.

Adoptive T cell transfers: As we have previously demonstrated (Russell & Alexander, 1987) T cells from CBA/Ca vaccinated with antigen-liposomes adoptively transfers resistance against L.mexicana to syngeneic recipients (Fig.1). On the other hand, T cells harvested from mice with exacerbated lesion growth following vaccination with CFA+antigen-liposomes, transferred increased susceptibility to recipient mice as measured by increased lesion growth compared with control mice. The recipients of T cells from non-vaccinated L.mexicana infected CBA/Ca mice developed lesions of similar size to control mice (Fig.2). Surprisingly T cells from infected non-vaccinated mice that were depleted of either Lyt-2+ or L3T4+ subsets adoptively transferred resistance to syngeneic recipients both as measured by lesion growth and by the number of animals developing lesions (Fig.2).

DISCUSSION

Vaccination against human cutaneous leishmaniasis using living organisms, although long practiced (Greenblatt, 1980), has now largely being discontinued because of the likelihood of individuals developing severe infections.

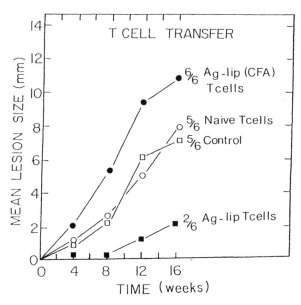

Fig.1. The growth of L.mexicana in CBA/Ca mice. Mice were inoculated i.p. with either PBS, naive T cells, T cells from mice with exacerbated lesion growth (Ag-liposomes with CFA) or T cells from resistant mice (Ag-liposomes). Numbers represent animals developing lesions.

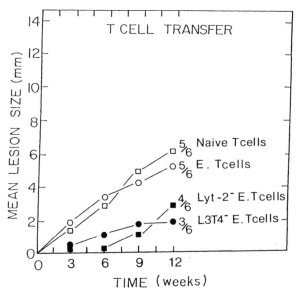

Fig.2. The growth of L.mexicana in CBA/Ca mice. Mice were inoculated i.p. with either naive T cells, educated (E) T cells from infected non-vaccinated mice, or T cells from infected mice treated with either anti Lyt-2 and complement or anti L3T4 and complement. Numbers represent animals developing lesions.

Recently, however, in a human field trial Mayrink et al. (1985) demonstrated the feasibility of a human vaccine using crude parasite antigens. Nevertheless, vaccine experiments in mice suggest that certain vaccine protocols (Liew et al. 1985) or certain parasite antigens (Mitchell & Handman, 1986) can exacerbate subsequent infections. Thus before large scale human vaccination can be envisaged it is essential not only to identify antigens that are protective but also to devise suitably safe means of administration. Until recently only one purified antigen, EF, had been used successfully for vaccination (Handman & Mitchell, 1985). However, mice were protected against L.major only if vaccinated i.p. with EF together with C.parvum. In this and a more detailed study (Russell & Alexander, 1987) we have also demonstrated that EF, as well as gp63, can protect mice against L.mexicana even when vaccinated s.c., as long as the antigens are reconstituted into liposomes. Not only is the immunogenicity of plasma membrane antigens greatly enhanced by reconstitution into liposomes (Hopp 1984) but the technique has also been used successfully to stimulate responses against viral antigens (Watari et al. 1987).

As both EF and gp63 are present in related forms in all species of Leishmania it is also possible that a single cross-protective vaccine could be developed. The inhibition of lesion growth in BALB/c mice infected with L.major following i.v. or i.p. vaccination with L.mexicana antigen-liposomes is certainly encouraging. However, vaccination i.v. or i.p. with the same preparation failed to protect BALB/c mice against i.v. infection with 1.2×10^7 L.donovani amastigotes. This is not perhaps surprising given the size and route of the infecting inoculum. By contrast naturally acquired L.donovani infections are initiated in the dermis with relatively few promastigotes and some time elapses before the parasites migrate to the viscera (Manson-Bahr, 1961). By by-passing the dermis we may circumvent any mechanisms of resistance which are operating exclusively in the cutaneous tissues. In support of this suggestion Manson-Bahr (1961) successfully vaccinated 3 volunteers against L.donovani using live promastigotes originating from a ground squirrel visceral infection: these organisms were later identified as L.major (Chance et al., 1978).

The protective immune response induced by vaccination with antigen-liposomes was not associated with antibody. Protection as demonstrated by adoptive transfer experiments was T cell mediated as was the exacerbated response induced by FCA. Although unfractionated T cells transferred from non vaccinated L.mexicana infected CBA/Ca mice to syngeneic recipients had little effect on the normal lesion growth pattern, this population depleted of either the Lyt-2+ or L3T4+ T cell subsets transferred resistance. This indicated that the non healing response in L.mexicana infected mice could be mediated by cells expressing both phenotypes. Indeed, such antigen specific T cell subsets have been identified in early L.donovani infections (Kaye 1987). Alternatively, the ratios of specific Lyt-2+ to L3T4+ cells could determine resistance. Titus et al. (1985) has proposed that this is the mechanism which determines resistance and susceptibility to L.major. However, as both resistance and susceptibility to L.major can be adoptively transferred with L3T4+ cells, Liew & Dhaliwal (1987) have suggested functional heterogeneity in this T cell subset. Functional heterogeneity is well established for both the Lyt2+ and L3T4+ subsets and adoptive transfer experiments have also implicated the role of both populations in anti-tumour immunity (Hamarka & Fujiwara, 1987). As either T cell subset from non healing CBA/Ca mice can adoptively transfer resistance to L.mexicana it will be interesting to determine which subset is associated with protection in vaccinated mice.

Finally these results describe several important improvements over previous vaccination studies. Firstly, the antigen-liposome preparations induced protection even following s.c. vaccination. Secondly, unless CFA was used, no exacerbation of infection was recorded. Thirdly, relatively small amounts of purified antigen were able to stimulate substantial protection against both homologous (L.mexicana) and heterologous (L.major) challenge infections. Finally, unlike other adjuvants, liposomes are physiologically neutral and therefore would be acceptable in the development of vaccines for use in humans.

CONCLUSIONS

CBA/Ca and BALB/c mice were vaccinated subcutaneously (s.c.), intraperitoneally (i.p.) or intravenously (i.v.) with Leishmania mexicana plasma membrane antigens reconstituted into liposomes. Liposomes contained either crude membrane antigen, the purified glycoprotein, gp63, and/or the glycoconjugate excreted factor (EF). Mice were vaccinated with between 4-8 μg antigen twice at an interval of 4 weeks. After a further 4 weeks mice were infected subcutaneously with 5x10 L.mexicana promastigotes. All the above vaccination procedures, including the s.c. route protected CBA/Ca mice against L.mexicana. Exacerbation of lesion growth was noted only when the vaccine incorporated Freund's Complete Adjuvant. Both protection and exacerbated lesion growth could be adoptively transferred with T cells. While T cells from non vaccinated L.mexicana infected CBA/Ca mice had little effect on the normal non healing lesion growth pattern in syngeneic recipients, resistance could be transferred with either the Lyt-2+ or the L3T4+ subsets from this population. Vaccination i.v. or i.p. but only weakly s.c. was found to inhibit L.mexicana growth in BALB/c mice. Significantly BALB/c mice vaccinated i.p. or i.v. with liposome reconstituted L.mexicana antigen had also increased resistance to subcutaneous L.major infection but not to i.v. infection with L.donovani. Most importantly antigen-containing liposomes did not cause the disease exacerbation observed in previous studies when vaccination was by the s.c. route.

REFERENCES

Chance, M.L., Schnur, L.F., Thomas, S. C. and Peters, W., 1978, The biochemical and serological taxonomy of Leishmania from the Aethiopian zoogeographical region of Africa, Ann.Trop.Med. and Parasitol., 72:533.

Colomer-Gould, V., Quintas, L. G., Keithly, J. and Noguiera, N.,1985, A common major surface antigen on amastigotes and promastigotes of Leishmania species, J.Exp.Med., 162:902.

Etges, R. J., Bouvier, J., Hoffman, R., and Bordier, L.,1985, Evidence that the major surface proteins of three Leishmania species are structurally related, Mol.Biochem.Parasitol., 14:141.

Greenblatt, C. H., 1980, The present and future for cutaneous leishmaniasis, in: "New Developments with Human Vaccines", A. Mizrahi, M. A. Klingberg and A. Kohn, eds., Alan R. Liss, New York.

Hamaoka, T., and Fujiwara, H., 1987, Phenotypically and functionally distinct T-cell subsets in anti-tumour responses, Immunol.Today 8:267

Handman, E., and Goding, J. W., 1985, The Leishmania receptor for macrophages is a lipid-containing glycoconjugate, EMBO J., 4:329.

Handman, E., and Mitchell, G. F., 1985, Immunization with Leishmania receptor for macrophages protects mice against cutaneous leishmaniasis, Proc. Natl.Acad.Sci.USA, 82:5910.

Handman, E., Greenblatt, C. H., and Goding, J., 1984, An amphipathic sulphated glycoconjugate of Leishmania characterization with monoclonal antibodies, EMBO J., 3:1206.

Hopp, T. P., 1984, Immunogenicity of a synthetic HBsAg. peptide:enhancement by conjugation to a fatty acid carrier, Mol.Immunol., 21:13.

Howard, J. G., Nicklin, S., Hale, C., and Liew, F.Y., 1982, Prophylactic immunization against experimental leishmaniasis: 1. Protection induced in mice genetically vulnerable to fatal Leishmania tropica infection, J.Immunol., 129:2206.

Kaye, P. M., 1987, Activation of cell-mediated immunity to Leishmania. 1. Primary T-cell activation detected by IL-2 receptor expression, Immunol., 61:345.

Liew, F. Y., and Dhaliwal, J. S., 1987, Distinctive cellular immunity in genetically susceptible BALB/c mice recovered from Leishmania major infection or after subcutaneous immunization with killed parasites, J.Immunol., 138:4450.

Liew, F. Y., Hale, C., and Howard, J. G. 1985, Prophylactic immunization against experimental leishmaniasis. IV. Subcutaneous immunization prevents the induction of protective immunity against fatal Leishmania major infection, J.Immunol., 135:2095.

Manson-Bahr, P. E. C., 1961, Immunity in Kala-azar, Trans.R.Soc.Trop.Med.Hyg. 55:550.

Mayrink, W., Williams, P., DaCosta, C. A., Magalpaes, P. A., Melr, M. N., Dias, M., Oliveira Lima, A., Michaelick, M. S. M., Ferriera Carvahho, E., Barros, G. C., Sessa, P. A., and De Alencar, J. T. A., 1985, An experimental vaccine against American dermal leishmaniasis: experience in the State of Espirito Santo, Brazil, Ann.Trop.Med. Parasitol., 79:259.

Mitchell, G. F. and Handman, E., 1986, The glycoconjugate derived from a Leishmania receptor for macrophages is a suppressogenic, disease promoting antigen in murine cutaneous leishmaniasis, Parasite Immunol. 8:255.

Russell, D. G., and Alexander, J., 1987, Effective immunization against cutaneous leishmaniasis with defined membrane antigens reconstituted into liposomes, J.Immunol., submitted.

Russell, D. G., and Wilhelm, H., 1986, The involvement of the major surface glycoprotein (gp63) of Leishmania promastigotes in attachment to macrophages, J.Immunol., 136:2613.

Titus, R. G., Ceredig, R., Cerottini, J. C., and Louis, J. A., 1985, Therapeutic effect of anti-L3T4 monoclonal antibody GK 1.5 on cutaneous leishmaniasis in genetically-susceptible BALB/c mice, J.Immunol., 135:2108.

Watari, E., Dietzschold, B., Szohan, G., and Heber-Katy, E., 1987, A synthetic peptide induces long term protection from lethal infection with Herpes simplex virus 2, J.Exp.Med., 165:459.

LEISHMANIA MAJOR: IMMUNE RESPONSES ELICITED BY CARBOHYDRATE-LIPID CONTAINING FRACTIONS (CLF)

Mauricio V. Londner, Graciela Rosen, Shoshana Frankenburg, Daniel Sevlever and Charles L. Greenblatt

Department of Parasitology and The Kuvin Centre for the Study of Infectious and Tropical Diseases, The Hebrew University-Hadassah Medical School, P.O.Box 1172 Jerusalem 91010, Israel

INTRODUCTION

Leishmania major, the causative agent of Old World cutaneous leishmaniasis, produces a self limiting disease that is followed by long lasting immunity.

The parasite has a highly glycosylated surface membrane. There is evidence that these carbohydrate-containing molecules are involved in important biological functions such as macrophage-promastigote recognition[1], infectivity[2], immunological response of the host[3,4,5] and protection against degradation by digestive enzymes[6]. Carbohydrate moieties are also important for serotyping Leishmania strains[7].

It is now established that cell mediated responses play a major role in the development of immunity and in the resistance to reinfection[8-10]. Studies performed on mouse models[11,12] and on cells of human origin[3] have shown that the whole promastigote, or extractions of the whole promastigote, induced T-cell dependent responses by immune individuals.

To date, only the living parasite has been used to elicit protection in humans[13]. In the research for antigenic molecules which could be used as possible vaccines, one obvious criteria for the measurement of the effectiveness of such molecules should be their capacity to elicit cell mediated responses. The group of antigens from Leishmania parasites which have probably been most widely studied are the excreted polysaccharides, such as the excreted factor (EF)[7,14]. These antigens, although they elicit a specific antibody response, do not appear to enhance cell mediated responses. This has been shown for L. major[9] and for L. donovani[15]. We have also shown that EF inhibits in vitro lymphoproliferative responses of immune cells in the presence of L. major promastigotes[3]. Attempts to vaccinate with EF alone have proven unsuccessful[5,13,16], but when bound to heterologous antibody it was partially protective[17]. Another antigen, which apparently contains EF and is a glycolipid, has been recently described[5]. This glycolipid has been used to protect C3H and Balb/c mice from infection with L. major, when injected with Corynebacterium parvum as adjuvant. Recently, two glycoconjugates from L. mexicana were shown to elicit cellular responses in immunized and infected mice[4]. Carbohydrate containing antigens from L. donovani have been reported by Sheppard, Scott and Dwyer[18] to stimulate the production of murine T-lines and clones.

We have recently isolated two carbohydrate-containing fractions from L. major and L. donovani promastigotes. Extraction with a mixture of hexane-isopropanol[19] yielded a precipitate and a lipid supernatant. These two fractions were shown to react with sera of rabbits immunized against L. major and L. donovani promastigotes and sera from mice convalescing from L. major infection. By means of a radioimmunoassay (RIA) antileishmanial activity could be demonstrated in sera from human beings infected with L. major and L. donovani[19]. This RIA was used effectively for an epidemiological study in a leishmania endemic area[20].

The present report provides purification and preliminary characterization of the antigens from these two fractions able to bind human immune sera. These antigens differed immunologically and chemically from EF.

We show that one of these antigenic fractions, CLF-1, elicits cell mediated responses in resistant immunized mice in vitro and in cells of human immune donors, in vitro. Furthermore, C3H mice vaccinated with CLF-1-containing liposomes showed a significant degree of protection to challenge. Thus, this antigen may play a role in the development of immunity to cutaneous leishmaniasis.

MATERIALS AND METHODS

Parasites

The two strains of parasites used in this study were: Leishmania major, LCR-L348 and L. donovani, LRC-L52 obtained from the World Health Organization's reference collection, Hebrew University-Hadassah Medical School, Jerusalem. The two strains were kept by regular transfer in Schneider's medium, to which 10% inactivated fetal calf serum, 100 μg/ml streptomycin, 100 u/ml penicillin and 1 mM glutamine were added. For in vivo studies, freshly isolated parasites from infected hamsters were used after one passage through culture medium.

Antisera

Sera from CL patients were obtained from the Kuvin Centre.

Preparation of Carbohydrate-Lipid Containing Fractions (CLF)

Promastigotes cultures with approximately 1×10^{10} cells per liter medium were harvested by centrifugation and washed three times with phosphate buffered saline (PBS), pH 7.2. The packed cells were then extracted three times (9 ml, 3 ml and 3 ml) with hexane-isopropanol 3:2 with some modifications of the original extraction method[19,20]. The volume of the total lipid fraction was reduced to dryness under a stream of nitrogen, and 3 ml hexane-isopropanol 3:2 were added. A white precipitate was removed by centrifugation, dried, washed twice with hexane, dried again and weighed. This fraction was called CLF-1. The supernatant was removed and extracted with 1 ml water. The water phase containing the antigen was washed twice with 1 ml hexane, evaporated, lyophilized and weighed. This fraction was called CLF-2. Protein was estimated by the method of Bradford[21] and the amount of hexoses by the method of Dubois et al.[22].

Preparation of Excreted Factor (EF)

EF was prepared as previously described[3].

Surface Membrane Labelling of Promastigotes

Iodination of surface membranes was carried out by the Iodo-Gen method[23] Galactose oxidase and [^{3}H] sodium borohydride were used to label surface galactose and galactosaminyl residues essentially as described by Gahmberg et al.[24]. Parasite labeling in the absence of galactose oxidase was performed in parallel.

After labeling, the cells were added to a sample of 1×10^{10} unlabeled promastigotes and antigen fractions were prepared as described above.

SDS-Polyacrylamide Gel Electrophoresis

Samples of 1 mg of CLF-1 or CLF-2 fractions, heated 5' at 100°C in the presence of 5% 2-mercaptoethanol, were applied on 11% gels as previously described[15].

Radioimmunoassay

The supernatant was tested by radioimmunoassay for lipid antigens[26]. Alternatively, for CLF-1, CLF-2 and fractions eluted from thin layer chromatography plates, the radioimmunoassay was performed as previously described[20] using 20-200 µg/ml antigen.

Biosynthetic Labeling of Promastigotes

Promastigotes from Schneider's culture in early stationary phase (4 days) were washed three times in PBS. 1.5×10^8 parasites in a volume of 20 ml were used for labeling with 50 uCi of D-[U-^{14}C] mannose (sp. act. 200-300 mCi/mmol), 50 uCi of D-[U-^{14}C] galactose (50-200 mCi/mmol) or 50 uCi of D-[U-^{14}C] glucose (270 mCi/mmol)(Amersham). The labeling was done in Dulbecco's glucose-free media supplemented with 5% dialyzed fetal calf sera, xantine (0.05 mM), adenosine (0.05 mM), hemin (5 mg/liter) and biotin (1 mg/liter) for 4 hrs at 28°C. Labeling of promastigotes with 500 uCi [^{32}P] ortophosphate (200 mCi/mmol) was performed for 5 hrs in phosphate-free Dulbecco as described above. Incorporation of [^{3}H] oleic acid was performed by adding 500 mCi [^{3}H] oleic acid (2-10 Ci/mmol) (Amersham) to 6×10^8 parasites in 13 ml RPMI containing 5% dialyzed FCS for 4 hrs at 28°C. Cells were radiolabeled with [U-^{14}C] myoinositol (30 nCi/ml, 270 mCi/mmol) (Amersham) as previously described[27]. After labeling, the cells were added to 1×10^{10} unlabeled promastigotes and antigen fractions were prepared as before.

Chromatographic Analysis

Thin layer chromatography (TLC) was performed on 0.25 mm silica gel plates (E. Merck, Darmstadt, Germany) activated at 100°C for 15 min. and developed in butanol:acetic acid:water 60:20:20. Differential staining was with orcinol-sulfuric acid reagent (Sigma) for carbohydrates, ninhydrin for primary amino groups and iodine for lipids. TLC plates were submitted to autoradiography at -70°C for 3-7 days after chromatography of radiolabeled fractions. For [^{3}H] labeled fractions the plates were sprayed with Amplify (Amersham) and autoradiographed for 4-7 days at -70°C. To test for activity in the solid phase RIA the bands were scraped off the plates with a razor blade and the material eluted with methanol:acetic acid 7:0.02, evaporated and further dissolved in water.

Antigen Blotting and Immunological Detection

Immunoblotting was performed as previously described[28].

Preparation of Liposomes

Liposomes were prepared from the remaining lipidic supernatant (organic phase) after the water extraction of CLF-2. The lipids, which did not contain antigens recognized by immune cutaneous leishmaniasis human sera, were dried in a rotary evaporator and kept overnight under vacuum in a desiccator. The liposomes (multilamellar vesicles) were formed by suspending the lipids in 0.15 M NaCl or CLF-1 in 0.15 M NaCl and incubating in a shaking bath at 37°C.

Lymphoblast Transformation

Blood was drawn from two donors immune to L. major and from two normal controls. Mononuclear cells were isolated on Ficoll-Hypaque gradients[29], and brought to a final concentration of 2×10^6 cells/ml in RPMI-1640 (Biolab, Jerusalem), supplemented with 5% autologous plasma. Triplicate samples of 0.1 ml cells/well were cultured in flat-bottomed microplates (Nunclon, Delta, Denmark). The antigens were added in various concentrations, as detailed in Results, in volumes of 25 µl. The plates were incubated for 6 days at 37°C in an atmosphere of air and 5% CO_2. Twenty four hours before harvesting, ^{3}H-thymidine (Nuclear Research Centre, Israel, 2 uCi/mmol) was added. The cells were harvested with an automatic cell harvester (Titertek) and the incorporated radioactivity was measured with a liquid scintillation counter (Packard Tricarb). Results are presented as counts per minute (cpm) or as stimulation indices (cpm of wells with antigen divided by cpm of control wells with cells only).

Measurement of DTH Responses

C3H mice were immunized against L. major by a subcutaneous injection in the base of the tail of 1×10^6 parasites isolated from an infected hamster. Forty to sixty days later, after the lesions on the tails cured, DTH was measured by a modification of the radiometric assay described by Lefford[30]. Briefly, a subcutaneous pulse of ^{3}H-thymidine (0.35 uCi/g body weight, 2 Ci/mmol) was injected into immunized and into normal mice. The radioactive thymidine was added in order to label monocyte and macrophage precursors accumulating at the DTH reaction site. Twenty four hours later, 20 ul of the tested antigens were injected into the left hind foot pad of the mice, and 20 ul of saline injected into the right hind foot pad. The antigens tested were FTS (10 µg/mouse) and CLF-1 (5-40 µg/mouse, according to optimal in vitro activity of the given batch). After 48 hrs the animals were sacrificed, and each foot was cut off, dissolved and counted as described[30]. The ratio of radioactivity of the left to the right pad of each individual mouse was expressed as the stimulation index.

Vaccination and Assessment of Lesions After Challenge

Liposomes containing 1 mg lipid and 120 µg CLF-1 per mouse were injected IP. Control animals received liposomes devoid of CLF-1. Ten days later, the mice received a second IP injection of CLF-1 containing liposomes (80 ug/mouse).

Immunized mice were challenged subcutaneously near the base of the tail ten days after the second antigen injection with L. major LRC-L348 promastigotes isolated two weeks earlier from infected hamsters. The parasites, 1×10^6 per mouse, were injected six days after the second passage in Schneider's medium (infective phase) and lesions were scored weekly, as previously described[21], with the following scoring method: 1 = small lesion (or resolving scar); 2 = larger swelling (<5 mm diameter); 3 = open lesion (5-10 mm diameter); 4 = open lesion (>10 mm diameter).

Statistical Analysis

Statistical analysis was performed using the Student's test, or the Chi square test with the Yate's correction.

RESULTS

Extraction of the Antigens

Extraction of whole promastigotes with hexane-isopropanol 3:2 produced two immunologically active fractions: a precipitate and a supernatant lipid fractions[19]. There was antigenic activity present in the precipitate (which was water soluble probably as a result of miscelle formation) and activity in the lipid supernatant. This led us to modify the extraction procedure. Two immunologically active fractions against CL immune human sera were obtained: the precipitate described above[19] (CLF-1) and a water extract (CLF-2) containing the active components of the lipid fraction. It is worth noting that the remaining lipid fraction did not recognize antibodies from immune sera of patients with CL, indicating that the antigens in the original active lipid fraction can be selectively extracted with water. The binding index (cpm immune/cpm normal) for CL human sera decreased from 2.6 to 1.4 after the water extraction of the lipidic supernatant. Before dialysis, CLF-1 and CLF-2 were found to contain a lipidic bulk and 4% protein. Hexoses comprised 4% of CLF-1 and 5% of CLF-2.

The autoradiographic pattern of CLF-1 after surface labeling of promastigotes and SDS-gel electrophoresis showed the presence of two bands of M.W. 63,000 and 205,000 (data not shown). These proteins were not found in CLF-2.

Table 1.   Thin Layer Chromatography of CLF-2

Fraction	RF	Sera Activity cpm(a) Immune	Normal	Index	Surface Labeling cpm(a) +GO	-GO
Origin	0	2032	1592	1.2	--	--
A	0.20	2948	907	3.2	3653	67
B	0.25	4768	1110	4.3	3456	220
C	0.39	6567	1263	5.2	ND	ND
D	0.43	2003	1001	2.0	226	128
E	0.48	2638	1050	2.5	170	180
F	0.51	1252	990	1.3	637	168
G	0.56	1034	1018	1.0	315	242
H	0.65	828	939	0.9	170	176

TLC of CLF-2. Layer: silica gel plates; solvent: butanol: acetic acid: water 60:20:20 (per vol). Chromatographic conditions are given in "Materials and Methods". Each band was scraped, eluted with methanol:acetic acid 7:0.02 (per vol) and evaporated. The residue was dissolved in water, filtered and immunological activity was measured by RIA. The index represents the cpm CL immune sera/cpm normal sera. [^{3}H] sodium borohydride surface labeling after treatment with (+GO) or without (-GO) GALACTOSE OXIDASE. ND: not determined.
(a) Calculated as 200 μg of applied material.

The protein content of these two fractions were mainly small peptides devoid of antigenic activity. These peptides migrated together with the glycolipids in the TLC plates. Glycolipids in both fractions were isolated from the peptides by gel chromatography on LH-20 equilibrated in butanol: acetic acid:water 60:20:20 (data not shown) and recovered in the void volume (MW>5000). The peptides were fractionated by the column. Alternatively, peptides were eliminated from CLF-1 or CLF-2 by dialysis.

Chromatographic Analysis of CLF-1 and CLF-2

Separation of the active glycolipids was achieved using butanol:acetic acid:water 60:20:20 as the developing solvent. Both fractions, with identical chromatographic pattern, resolved in eight bands. Their RF are given in Table 1. Compounds A, B, C and E with RF of 0.19, 0.25, 0.39 and 0.48 were able to bind immune sera from patients with CL (Table 1). A, B and C stained with orcinol (carbohydrate specific) while E was only visualized by Iodine (data not shown). Though a carbohydrate-containing antigen, E is probably under the limits of detection by the orcinol staining. Autoradiography after immuno-blotting of the TLC, confirm the immunological activity of the compounds tested by radioimmunoassay after elution of the TLC plates (data not shown).

Differences in the metabolic labeling of the antigens was observed. Compound A could be labeled biosynthetically with [^{14}C] galactose, [^{14}C] mannose, [^{14}C] glucose, [^{3}H] oleic acid and [^{32}P] phosphate. Compound B incorporated [^{14}C] galactose, [^{14}C] mannose, [^{14}C] glucose and [^{14}C] myo-inositol. Sometimes there was poor incorporation of [^{3}H] oleic acid and [^{32}P] phosphate observed in this antigen. Thus, antigenic glycolipid B differs from A in its inositol content and a lower incorporation of [^{32}P] phosphate and [^{3}H] oleic acid. Compound C was labeled with [^{14}C] galactose and [^{14}C] mannose, while E incorporated [^{14}C] mannose, [^{14}C] glucose, [^{3}H] oleic acid, [^{32}P] phosphate and [^{14}C] myo-inositol. In promastigotes labeled with [^{3}H] sodium borohydride following treatment with galactose oxidase (Table 1) suggesting the presence of terminal galactose residues in these cell surface molecules. D, F, G and H three phosphorylated glycolipids were unable to bind CL sera after solubilization of the compounds in water or in ethanol (data not shown) prior to the RIA under conditions where A, B, C and E were active upon solubilization with both solvents.

When the excreted factor (EF), a polysaccharide antigen of Leishmania,

Table 2. Response of Cells from Two Normal and Two Immune Human Donors to Stimulation with Various Antigenic Preparations

	Normal (S.I.[1] ± S.D.)		Immune (S.I. ± S.D.)	
	Donor 1	Donor 2	Donor 1	Donor 2
FTS - L. major	2.2±0.4	0.4±0.01	34.4±3.5	44.2±16.4
CLF-1 - L. major	1.4±0.8	0.8±0.2	43.9±1.6	57.1±24.3
CLF-1 - L. donovani	N.D.	0.7±0.09	35.5±8.7	96.1±45.9
CLF-2 - L. major	N.D.	0.2±0.28	0.3±0.07	1.5± 0.5

[1]S.I., stimulation index; FTS, freezed-thawed and sonicated promastigotes; CLF-1, carbohydrate-lipid containing fraction - 1; CLF-2, carbohydrate-lipid containing fraction - 2; N.D., not done.

purified from culture media was chromatographed under these conditions it did not migrate from the origin indicating the absence of components common to these antigens.

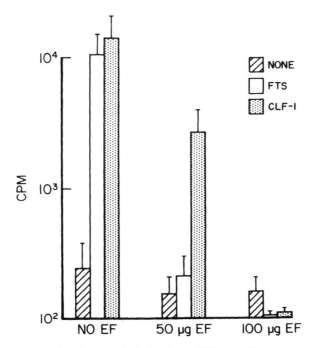

Fig. 1. Effect of excreted factor (EF) on the presence of immune lymphocytes to FTS (freeze-thawed and sonicated parasites) and to CLF-1 (carbohydrate-lipid containing fraction - 1).

Response of Cells from Normal and Immune Donors to Stimulation with Various Promastigote Extracts

Cells from normal and immune donors were assayed in a lymphoblast transformation test, using two antigens, CLF-1 and CLF-2, which have previously been shown to bind antibodies present in the serum of convalescent or immune donors. It was found that the CLF-1 extracted from L. major and from L. donovani produced a strong stimulation of cells from immune but not from normal donors (Table 2). Using optimal antigen concentrations, it was found that the response to the CLF-1 was of the same order of magnitude as the response to the FTS. The optimal antigen concentration varied from one batch to another, but usually ranged between 15-40 µg/well. The CLF-2 from L. major did not stimulate mononuclear cells from immune donors.

Effect of EF on the Response to CLF-1

We have previously shown that EF inhibits blast transformation of lymphocytes from immune donors in response to FTS[3]. The following series of experiments was performed in order to compare this response to the effect of EF on the CLF-1. It was found that EF significantly inhibited the blastogenic response to CLF-1. The inhibition of the response was measured at two EF concentrations. Fifty ug EF inhibited more strongly the response to FTS than to CLF-1, while 100 ug EF inhibited both similarly (Fig. 1).

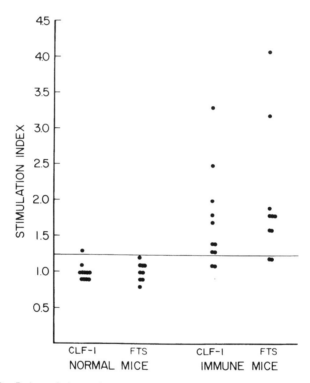

Fig. 2. Delayed type hypersensitivity of normal and immune C3H mice, in response to FTS (freeze-thawed and sonicated parasites) and to CLF-1 (carbohydrate-lipid containing fraction - 1). Each dot represents one mouse, and the horizontal line represents the average of the normal values + two standard deviation values.

DTH Response to CLF-1 In Vivo

In two independent experiments, which included a total of 80 C3H mice, it was demonstrated that mice cured from an L. major infection, when sensitized with L. major FTS or CLF-1 responded in a DTH test, after

Table 3. Vaccination of mice with CLF-1 containing liposomes

	Controls	Liposomes	Liposomes+CLF-1
Protected mice[1]/total mice	1/21	4/23	13/22
(Percentage - Statistical protection) significance	(5%)	-N.S.- (17%)	-p<0.001- (59%)

[1]Protected mice: Animals that did not show any lesion during the whole experimental period (70 days).

48 hrs, showing significantly higher stimulation indices than normal mice ($p<0.001$). There was no significant difference between the DTH level of FTS or CLF-1 sensitized mice. The results of one experiment are summarized in Fig. 2. Thus, it appears that immune mice recognize CLF-1, and respond to it in vivo in a classical DTH response.

Vaccination with CLF-1

Vaccination of C3H mice with CLF-1 containing liposomes caused 59% protection and vaccination of animals with PBS-containing liposomes or PBS only caused 17% and 5% protection, respectively (Table 3). The protected animals did not show any lesions during the whole experimental period (70 days). The unprotected animals in the vaccinated group did not differ significantly in their lesion score from the control mice. The largest lesions in the animals injected with CLF-1 liposomes and PBS liposomes, observed 6 weeks after infection, showed an average score of 1.5 ± 0.9 and 1.5 ± 1.0 respectively. These results summarize two independent experiments, with a total of 20-23 mice in each group.

DISCUSSION AND CONCLUSIONS

We have here provided evidence that the antigenic components recognized by immune human sera of CLF-1 and CLF-2 (two enriched fractions of non-proteic immunologically active compounds) are at least four different antigens (A, B, C and E) as detected by RIA and immunoblotting after TLC. Antigen A is a phosphorylated glycolipid while C was only revealed by autoradiography after biosynthetic radiolabeling with [^{14}C] galactose or [^{14}C] mannose. Inositol containing lipids from L. donovani have been analyzed by Kaneshiro et al.[27]. These authors found [^{14}C] inositol, diphenylamine positive spots with RF similar to the mannose-containing inositol sphingolipids already described in some yeast cells[31]. In this report we find that two of the antigens, B and E are inositol-containing glycolipids. The possibility that these two inositol-containing antigens are chemically and antigenically related remains to be determined.

Analysis of CLF-2 by TLC shows that it probably shares the same antigenic components recognized by antileishmania antibodies in CLF-1. However, differences have been found between CLF-1 and CLF-2: a) after surface iodination of promastigotes, SDS-polyacrylamide gel electrophoresis of CLF-1 shows two proteins (MW 63,000 and 205,000). These proteins present in CLF-1 in minute amounts are absent from CLF-2 (data not shown); b) CLF-1, but not CLF-2, stimulated the in vitro response of lymphocytes from immune but not from normal human donors. Furthermore, in vitro, CLF-1 elicited delayed type hypersensitivity response in L. major-immunized C3H mice.

It was of interest to differentiate these antigens from other well
characterized molecules which are antigenic: the negatively charged polysaccharides isolated from the cells[32-34] or released by the promastigotes
into the culture medium[32-34] (EF) which is able to bind immune rabbit sera
raised against whole promastigotes, and a surface glycoprotein (MW 63,000)
found to be the major antigen recognized by the sera of patients with visceral, cutaneous and mucocutaneous leishmaniasis[35,36]. Though the electrophoretic analysis demonstrated that this protein is present in CLF-1 in
minute amouts (data not shown), proteins of this M.W. are not expected
to migrate from the origin under the conditions employed to resolve these
antigens.

Immunological and chemical differences have already been demonstrated
between CLF-1 and EF[19]. While both antigens reacted with rabbit antileishmanial sera, they did not show lines of identity on Ouchterlony plates. No
anti-EF antibodies were detected in sera from patients with CL[37]. Furthermore the anti-EF monoclonal antibody W.I.C. 79.3 recognized neither CLF-1[19]
nor CLF-2 (data not shown). Different chemical properties had also been
found with regard to charge and molecular weight[19]. We found a different
behavior in the migration pattern of these antigens on TLC, either reflecting differences in their molecular weight[38] or in their hydrophobicity.

Both *in vitro* and *in vivo* it appears that FTS and CLF-1 elicit similar
cell mediated responses. The response of human mononuclear cells, and the
effect of EF on the response, were similar for FTS and CLF-1. Furthermore, *in vivo* there was no significant difference in the DTH response of
immunized mice to CLF-1 and FTS.

The protective effect of CLF-1 is shown in the vaccinating experiments.
The injection of CLF-1 within multilamellar liposomes prior to challenge
had a protective effect on 59% of the animals, as compared to the controls
that received liposomes without CLF-1, which had a protective effect on 17%
of the mice. Liposomes were chosen as carriers for the vaccinating agent
because, being particulate, they have a propensity (when injected parenterally) to concentrate in the reticuloendothelial system. In these experiments, multilamellar liposomes were prepared with lipids extracted from
whole promastigotes. With the experimental data obtained to this point, it
appears that CLF-1 has indeed a protective effect, which can possibly be
improved by changing parameters such as lipid concentration and/or composition, antigen presentation in the liposome, or liposome preparation.

We have presented data that show that CLF-1 can elicit a delayed type
hypersensitivity response in mice previously immunized against L. major.
There is now evidence that DTH in leishmaniasis does not always correlate
with immunity. DTH reactions have been associated with the ability of the
host to eliminate the parasites and to protect from reinfection[10,39,40].
However L_3T_4 T-cell lines, capable of transferring parasite-specific DTH
responses and of activating leishmanicidal activity of macrophages, were
shown to exacerbate the lesions, when transferred to infected resistant and
susceptible mice[41]. Howard et al.[42] have reported on an immunization schedule against L. major which, although achieving protective immunity, fails
to raise a DTH response. The antigenic fraction described here appears to
elicit both protective immunity and a DTH response in resistant mice. In
humans, the Montenegro test, which uses a crude extract of parasites, is
still widely used to evaluate previous contact with leishmania parasite.
The possibility of using a purified and chemically defined component for
injection into humans for diagnostic purposes would have many obvious
advantages.

Other antigens extracted form different species of leishmania parasites, which elicit humoral or cell mediated responses have been described[4,5,43,44]. But only one of these antigens[5], a glycolipid from L. major which was purified using a specific anti-EF monoclonal antibody (WIC 79.3), has been shown to have a protective effect on mice. We have shown that CLF-1 is different from EF, both immunologically and chemically.

We found cross reactivity between CLF-1 from L. donovani and L. major. This is in keeping with the presence of major shared antigens involved in protection to different forms of Leishmaniases. The many instances in which serological and clinical crossimmunity between leishmanial species has been described substantiates this hypothesis, both by the extensive serological crossreactivity observed in patient's sera, by the presence of natural cross protection[45-48] and by crossimmunization experiments using irradiated promastigotes[42,49].

ACKNOWLEDGMENTS

We thank Miss Maria E. Westerman for her excellent technical assistance. This study was supported by US NIH-NIAID Research contract N01-AI22668 (Epidemiology and Control of Arthropod-Borne Diseases in the Middle East).

REFERENCES

1. Chang, K.P. Mol. Biochem. Parasitol. 4: 67, 1981.
2. Sacks, D.L., Hieny, S. and Sher, A. J. Immunol. 135: 564, 1985.
3. Londner, M.V., Frankenburg, S., Slutzky, G.M. and Greenblatt, C.L. Parasite Immunol. 5: 249, 1983.
4. Rodriguez, M.M., Xavier, M.T., Previato, L.M. and Barcinski, M.A. (1986). Infect. Immun. 51: 80, 1986.
5. Handman, E. and Mitchell, G.F. PNAS 82 17: 5910, 1985.
6. Chang, K.P. Int. Rev. Cytol. (Suppl.) 14: 267, 1983.
7. Schnur, L.F., Zuckerman, A. and Greenblatt, C.L. Israel J. Med. Sci. 8: 933, 1972.
8. Turk, J.L. and Bryceson, A.D.M. Adv. Immunol. 13: 209, 1971.
9. Preston, P.M. and Dumonde, D.C. Clin. Exp. Immunol. 23: 126, 1976.
10. Liew, F.Y., Hale, C. and Howard, J.G. J. Immunol. 128: 1917, 1982.
11. Preston, P.M., Carter, R.L., Leuchars, E., Davies, A.J.S. and Dumonde, D.C. Clin. Exp. Immunol. 10: 337, 1972.
12. Mitchell, G.F., Curtis, J.M., Handman, E. and McKenzie, I.F.C. Aust. J. Exp. Biol. Med. Sci. 58: 521, 1980.
13. Greenblatt, C.L. Leishmaniasis, eds. Chang and Bary, p. 163, 1985.
14. Slutzky, G.M. and Greenblatt, C.L. Infect. Immun. 37: 10, 1982.
15. Ray, R. and Ghose, A.C. Aust. J. Exp. Biol. Med. Sci. 63: 411, 1985.
16. El-On, J., Schnur, L.F. and Greenblatt, C.L. Exp. Parasitol. 47: 254, 1979.
17. Handman, E., El-On, J., Spira, D.T., Zuckerman, A. and Greenblatt, C.L. J. Prozool. (Suppl.) 24: 21A, 1977.
18. Sheppard, H.W., Scott, P.A., and Dwyer, D.M. J. Immunol. 131: 1496, 1983.
19. Slutzky, G.M., Londner, M.V. and Greenblatt, C.L. J. Protozool. 32: 347, 1985.
20. Rosen, G., Londner, M.V., Greenblatt, C.L., Morsy, T.A. and El-On, J. Exp. Parasitol. 62: 79, 1986.
21. Bradford, M.M. Analytical Biochemistry 72: 248, 1976.
22. Dubois, M., Gilles, K.A., Hamilton, J.K., Rebers, P.A. and Smith, F. Anal. Chem. 28: 350, 1956.
23. Zingales, B. Genes and antigens of parasites. (Morel, C.M.,

ed.), UNDP/World Bank/WHO, pp. 333, 1984.
24. Gahmberg, C.G., Itaya, K. and Hakomori, S.I. Methods in membrane biology (Korn, E.D., ed.). Plenum Publishing Corp., New York, pp. 170, 1976.
25. Laemmli, U.K. Nature 227: 680, 1970.
26. Smolarsky, M. J. Immunol. Methods 38: 85, 1980.
27. Kaneshiro, E., Jayasimhulu, K. and Lester, R.L. J. Lipid Res. 27: 1294, 1986.
28. Towin, H., Schoenenberger, C., Ball, R., Braun, D.G. and Rosenfelder, G. J. Immunol. Methods 72: 471, 1984.
29. Boyum, A. Scand. J. Clin. Lab. Invest. 21 (Supplement 97): 77, 1968.
30. Lefford, M.J. Int. Arch. of Allergy and Applied Immunol. 47: 570, 1974.
31. Smith, S.W. and Lester, R. J. Biol. Chem. 249: 3395, 1974.
32. Slutzky, G.M. and Greenblatt, C.L. Biochem. Med. 21: 70, 1979.
33. Turco, S.J., Wilkinson, M.A. and Clawson, D.R. J. Biol. Chem. 259: 3883, 1984.
34. Handman, E., Greenblatt, C.L. and Goding, J.W. EMBO J. 3: 2301, 1984.
35. Etges, R.J., Bouvier, J., Hoffman, R. and Bordier, C. Mol. Biochem. Parasitol. 14: 141, 1985.
36. Colomber-Gould, V., Quintao, L.G., Keithly, J. and Nogueira, N. J. Exp. Med. 162: 902, 1985.
37. El-On, J., Zehavi, V., Avraham, H. and Greenblatt, C.L. Exp. Parasitol. 55: 270, 1983.
38. Stahl, E. Thin layer chromatography, A laboratory Handbook (Stahl, E. ed.), Springer-Verlag, Berlin-Heidelberg-New York, pp. 807, 1969.
39. Howard, J.G., Hale, C. and Liew, F.Y. J. Exp. Med. 153: 557, 1981.
40. Sacks, D.L., Scott, P.A., Asofsky, R. and Sher, F.A. J. Immunol. 132: 2072, 1984.
41. Liew, F.Y. Nature (London) 305: 630, 1983.
42. Howard, J.G., Nicklin, S., Hale, C. and Liew, F.Y. J. Immunol. 129: 2206, 1982.
43. Ghose, A.C. and Rowe, D.S. Biochemistry 14: 459, 1977.
44. Col mer-Gould, V., Quintao, L.G., Keithly, J. and Nogueira, N. J. Exp. Med. 162: 902, 1985.
45. Lainson, R. and Shaw, J.J. Trans. Royal Soc. Trop. Med. Hyg. 60: 533, 1966.
46. Lainson, R. and Shaw, J.J. J. Trop. Med. Hyg. 80: 29, 1977.
47. Alexander, J. and Phillips, R.S. Exp. Parasitol. 45: 93, 1978.
48. Perez, H.B., Aredondo, H.B. and Machado, R. Exp. Parasitol. 48: 9, 1979.
49. Howard, J.G., Liew, F.Y., Hale, C. and Nicklin, S. J. Immunol. 132: 450, 1984.

PREMUNITION, A POSSIBLE LIMITATION IN THE PREVENTION OF THE LEISHMANIASES BY VACCINATION

L.F. Schnur

The Hebrew University-Hadassah Medical School
Jerusalem, Israel

THE NATURE OF THE PROBLEM

The development of an effective vaccine against smallpox led to its rapid eradication. This success has led to increased optimism regarding the prevention of other infectious diseases, including leishmaniases. However, the prospect of achieving a similar success in the case of the leishmaniases, where sandfly vectors and, in many cases, animal reservoirs are involved, is nigh impossible. However, vaccination in conjunction with control of sandfly vectors and reservoir animals could lead to a substantial reduction in the occurrence of cases. In the advent of a vaccine against Indian visceral leishmaniasis, which is considered to be anthroponotic, successful control, even if not total eradication, should be possible, if an effective vector control programme is carried out simultaneously.

Prevention of disease by vaccination has two main aspects: the development of vaccines and the logistics of their application. The former must include a view to the latter, since the nature of a vaccine will affect its subsequent handling. Its stability and life-span must allow for its transportation, to quite remote places in deserts and rain forests in the case of some leishmaniases. Its being 'live' or 'dead' will dictate its mode of storage, delivery, application and subsequent follow-up, all of which will be complicated, owing to the nature of the distribution of the leishmaniases.

PROSPECTS FOR AN EFFECTIVE VACCINE

Regarding leishmaniases, it is well to remember that one is dealing with a group of quite separate disease syndromes, each of which is caused by a distinct and identifiable agent. The term leishmaniases has been used deliberately, since prevention, in this case, means preventing several very different disease syndromes; and prevention by vaccination presupposes either one 'universal vaccine' that protects against all the known types of causative agent, or a number of specific preparations, each of which protects against one of the agents. The information on vaccination afforded to us to date, a large part of which has been well summarized in recent reviews on vaccination (Greenblatt,1980,1985; Handman,1986; Gunders,1987), indicates that the development of a 'universal vaccine' is highly unlikely; though, cross-protection can be achieved between certain related strains. For example, Leishmania major cross protects against L.tropica, but, strangely, the reverse is not so. Related, here, means being antigenically similar, since cross-protection infers sharing protective determinants. The idea of needing to prepare a specific vaccine against almost every type of leishmanial species known in nature, of which there are so many, is formidable, even if it could be done.

THE NATURE OF VACCINATING PREPARATIONS

Vaccines are either 'live', when infective virulent or attenuated organisms are used, or 'dead', when whole killed organisms, parts of organisms or released products from organisms are used.

With some types of leishmanial organism, e.g., L.major, L.tropica and L.mexicana, naturally acquired and artificially induced infections usually lead to protection following self-cure; and, as stated, some engender cross-protection. Recovered cases only very rarely, experience re-infection with the same type of organism. Guirges,(1971), Killick-Kendrick et al.,(1985) and Rioux et al.,(1986) describe such rare instances. In some cases, i.e., leishmaniasis recidivans (LR), diffuse cutaneous leishmaniasis (DCL), mucocutaneous leishmaniasis (MCL) and visceral leishmaniasis (VL), cure does not follow without treatment. In some of these instances, e.g., visceral leishmaniasis, protection does apparently ensue after treatment. The potential of certain types of strains to cause great harm excludes their use as 'live' vaccines. In fact, no strain can be considered totally safe and the use of 'live' vaccines must include conscientious follow-up.

Attenuated strains have generally not been shown to induce protective immunity in man and animals (Kellina, cited Heyneman,1971; Schnur et al., 1983a) and it seems that a strain must be infective and virulent, in order to force a host's immune system to provide protection. Recently isolated organisms are recommended for 'live' vaccines (Handman et al.,1974; Greenblatt,1980; Greenblatt et al.,1980) to ensure takes and induce protection. The effectiveness of radio-attenuated organisms in causing protection has been recorded. Irradiated amastigotes of L.major protected CBA mice against a heterologous challenge with virulent L.mexicana mexicana (Alexander,1982) and irradiated promastigotes of L.major protected BALB/c mice against homologous challenge with virulent L.major (Howard et al., 1982), although this was not achieved in guinea pigs using irradiated L.enriettii (Lemma and Cole, 1974). The successes with radio-attenuated organisms is anomalous, as protection was achieved against leishmanial species to which the respective types of inbred mice were genetically susceptible, implying that what was determined genetically could be overruled. A similar experience has been described by Mitchell and Handman (1983,cited Handman,1986), where avirulent clones of L.major, meaning infective but not causing overt pathogenesis, protected against virulent ones, that is ones able to cause obvious signs of disease seen as measurable lesions: swellings, nodules and ulcers. In most studies like these, little attempt is made to examine stained tissue smears and make cultures to determine the degree of infection, compared with the degree of obvious pathology, as suggested by Hill et al., (1983) and described by Schnur et al.,(1973). It is imperative that challenge sites are checked parasitologically, by making smears and cultures, especially if they remain normal-looking. Large lesions can contain minimal numbers of parasites, e.g., human LR, just as normal-looking tissue can contain numerous parasites, e.g., the skin of dogs prior to the onset of the typical symptoms of canine visceral leishmaniasis. Another important aspect that is often overlooked is dissemination to other organs from the site of infection (Schnur et al., 1973; Leclerc et al.,1981). Experiments like those described by Alexander (1982), Howard et al.(1982) and Mitchell and Handman (cited, Handman 1986) leave the protected, challenged animals alive and it should be possible to rechallenge after more extensive periods to see if protection is permanent or of short duration. Total necropsy of animals (Schnur et al.,1973; Schnur and Jacobson, 1987) would show whether protection is sterile immunity or premunition, with living parasites being present.

Nowhere has it been categorically shown that 'dead' leishmanial preparations afford protection against challenge infections and would be useful in prevention. Some attempts in man have assumed protection as experimental challenge with infective parasites cannot be done (e.g., Mayrink et al., 1979; 1985) and some animal studies showed reduced challenge infections, compared with normal control infections (e.g., Holbrook et al.,1981), others have indicated enhanced challenge infections (e.g., Kurotchkin,1931; Schnur et al., 1983b). This whole aspect requires further systematic study, since 'dead' vaccines are preferred to using living, potentially harmful, organisms. However, the idea of non-living vaccines against leishmaniasis may be very fanciful and unachievable, if one considers the whole subject of infection, immunity and protection in leishmaniasis, where all cases of protection seem to result from immunological stimulation by living organisms through infection. The process is not a simple antigen-antibody phenomenon resulting in stable, sterile protective immunity, but one of necrosis and the gradual resolution of granulomatous lesions conferring protective cell-mediated immunity. There are even indications that the lifelong protective immunity that follows infection might be premunition, with residual parasites persisting after cure that constantly stimulate and induce this protection. This possibly indicates that the protective antigens, so ardently sought when contemplating the development of vaccines, are short-lived and only found in the presence of living amastigotes. This is a point that does not augur well for approaches based on isolating protective antigens by monoclonal antibodies and other means.

The following evidence and phenomena are presented as indicating that protection in leishmaniases is by premunition. All leishmaniases are persistent chronic diseases. In LR and MCL, relapses occur long after cure of the primary lesions seems to have been achieved. In DCL, parasites persist after therapeutic cure, causing relapses (Bryceson, 1970). In VL, parasites can survive therapy, causing post-kala-azar dermal leishmaniasis and amastigotes have also been seen in the bone marrow of patients following treatment (Napier,1946). 'Live' scars have been reported by several Soviet researchers (Kozevnikov,1941; Kozevnikov et al.,1947; Subarova,1957; Latysev, no date, all cited, Heyneman, 1971), who respectively found living parasites in 'healed' cutaneous lesions six months, four years and thirteen years after cure. Nadim, (1984) cites a case of recrudescence of a healed lesion acquired by a subject at the age of two. This healed, leaving the scar and adjacent tissue red for many years. At the age of 15 or 16 this redness disappeared. At the age of 55, the redness returned, worsened and the skin thickened, after the subject had been given cortico-therapy for asthma. Smears made four years later, at 59, contained numerous amastigotes. Similarly, Bryceson (pers. comm.) described a recent case of a man living in Britain who developed a very large facial leishmanioma. It seems that the subject's only possible contact with leishmanial parasites could have been in Malta, Sicily or Italy some 45 years before, where the patient served as a soldier during the Second World War. Three reports from France (Hauteville et al., 1980; Herne et al.,1980; Gastaut et al.,1981) describe VL appearing in three patients receiving immuno-suppressive therapy, one for chronic active hepatitis and two for leukaemia. This activation of latent VL is not new. In the three reports just mentioned and Nadim's report on reactivated CL (Nadim,1984), reactivation was caused by therapeutic immuno-suppression. Corkhill (1948a,1948b) recorded similar reactivation of VL caused by concomitant infections of malaria and relapsing fever, and by physical and emotional stress caused by battle experience. Finally, there is the ever increasing number of cases of recrudescent VL in people having subsequently contracted AIDS (Antunes et al.,1987). All these reports indicate the persistence of leishmanial parasites in cases that either never showed disease symptoms or had become cured and, supposedly, protected. The occurrence of asymptomatic VL has been reported by several authors from various endemic regions (Armstrong,1945; Prata, 1957; Sen Gupta,1962, all cited Heyneman,1971; Badaro et al.,1986; Leeuwenburg, Bryceson and Koech, pers. comm.) and asymptomatic subclinical cases are thought to outnumber clinical cases by 5:1 (WHO,1984). The longterm persistence of leishmanial parasites in the spleens of mice that have undergone infection, disease and self-cure, conferring protection to reinfection has also been reported (Leclere et al.,1981), where premunition is also implied. Giannini (unpublished, poster presented in Denver,1986) has shown that, in murine CL, there is rapid and persistent infection of the regional lymph nodes and Montilio (pers. comm.) has often found parasites in draining lymph nodes of cured and protected mice. The reported successes in protecting mice with radio-attenuated parasites (Alexander,1982; Howard et al.,1982) could also have been through premunition as live parasites were used as vaccine. More is the pity that smears and cultures were not made of skin, draining lymph nodes, spleen and bone marrow from protected animals to verify this. Recent reviewers of vaccination against leishmaniasis (Greenblatt,1980, 1985; Handman, 1986; Gunders, 1987) have tended to ignore premunition. In the past (Adler, 1964; Heyneman, 1971) it was viewed with greater seriousness.

EXISTING VACCINATING PREPARATIONS

The unattenuated promastigotic vaccines of the type used in Israel, the Soviet Union and Iran against CL are far from perfect, when compared to some of the other known vaccines. The process of vaccination mimics normal natural infection in terms of extent and duration, often lasting many months and even a year or more, but does permit the choice of site of infection and reduces infection to single lesions, provided vaccinees keep out of endemic regions until protected. Every vaccinee becomes a carrier and a potential source of contaminative infection, during the time he has an active lesion. If protection stems from premunition, vaccinees are, supposedly, infected for life. This might afford lifelong protection, but could lead to relapses, if vaccinees were to become compromised immunologically. Leishmanial parasites are immunosuppressive and Serebryakov et al.,(1972) noticed a further disadvantage. That infection of children with leishmanial parasites depressed their immune response to diphtheria, pertussis and tetanus triple vaccine for up to six months. As Greenblatt (1980) points out, this type of preparation ought only to be used on populations at high risk, and only when one is convinced that the vaccinees run no risk greater than developing a normal self-curing lesion. People displaying immune deficiencies or abnormalities should not be vaccinated. This means that relatively few people can benefit from such vaccines, since most people living in highly endemic areas will probably contract infections long before this type of vaccine confers protection. Finally, one must ask, if it is justified to cause more infections through vaccination than would occur through natural infection, as past vaccination programmes using 'live' vaccine have done (Peters and Killick-Kendrick, 1987).

VACCINATION AND THE HUMAN IMMUNE RESPONSE

The people most in need of vaccination are those likely to develop the more severe types of leishmaniasis, i.e., potential LR, DCL, MCL and VL cases. These are all types of infection associated with immunological deficiency or abnormality. It follows, therefore, that these are the last people one would want to vaccinate with 'live' vaccines. As a corollary of this, one may ask if people showing such immunological abnormality would be able to derive any benefit from 'dead' vaccines. Sensitization with leishmanial antigens might possibly exacerbate their defectiveness when confronting natural infection.

THE CURRENT SITUATION

The foregoing deliberations do not portend a rosy future for prevention of the leishmaniases by vaccination, despite the current enthusiasm. One sincerely hopes, for the sake of those who suffer most from leishmaniasis, that modern technologies will provide 'dead' vaccines that will function in the face of immune insufficiency. New 'live' or 'dead' preparations conferring protection, must also conform to acceptable medical and ethical standards, and conditions making their production, storage and delivery commercially possible.

REFERENCES

Adler, S.,1964, Leishmania, Adv. Parasit., 2:35.
Alexander, J., 1982, A radioattenuated Leishmania major vaccine markedly increases the resistance of CBA mice to subsequent infection with Leishmania mexicana mexicana, Trans.R.Soc. Trop. Med. Hyg.,76:646.
Antunes, F., Carvalho, C., Tavares, L., Botas, J., Forte, M., del Rio,A.M., Dutschmann, L., Costa, A., Abranches. P., Silva Pereira, C., Paiva, J.E.D., Carvalho Araujo, F., and Baptista, A., 1987, Visceral leishmaniasis recrudescence in a patient with AIDS. Trans. R. Soc. Trop. Med. Hyg., 81:595.
Badaro, R., Jones, T.C., Carvalho, E.M., Sampaio, D., Reed, S.G., Barral, A., Teixeira, R., and Johnson, Jr.,W.D., 1986, New perspectives on a subclinical form of visceral leishmaniasis, J. Inf. Dis., 154:1003.
Bryceson, A.D.M., 1970, Diffuse cutaneous leishmaniasis in Ethiopia. II. Treatment, Trans. R. Soc. Trop. Med. Hyg., 64:369.
Corkhill, N.L., 1948a, Activation of latent kala-azar and malaria by battle experience, Ann. Trop. Med. Parasit., 42:224.
Corkhill, N.L., 1948b, Activation of latent kala-azar by malaria and relapsing fever, Ann. Trop. Med. Parasit., 42:230.
Gastaut, J.A., Blanc, A.P., Imbert, C., Sebahoun, G., and Carcassonne, Y., 1981, Leishmaniose viscérale méditerranéenne de l'adulte au cours de la rémission complète d'une leucémie aiguë lymphoblastique, Nouv. Press. Med., 10:1332.
Greenblatt, C.L., 1980, The present and future of vaccination for cutaneous leishmaniasis, in:"New Developments With Human and Veterinary Vaccines," A.Mizrahi, I.Hertman, M.A.Klingberg, and A.Kohn, eds, Alan R. Liss, New York.
Greenblatt, C.L., 1985, Vaccination for leishmaniasis, in: "Leishmaniasis," K.-P. Chang and R.S. Bray, eds, Elsevier Science Publishers, Amsterdam.
Greenblatt, C.L., Spira, D.T., Montilio, B., and Gerichter, H., 1980, An improved protocol for the preparation of a frozen promastigote vaccine for cutaneous leishmaniasis. J. Biol. Stand., 8:227.
Guirges, S.Y., 1971, Natural and experimental re-infection of man with oriental sore, Ann. Trop. Med. Parasit., 65: 197.
Gunders, A.E., 1987, Vaccination: past and future role in control, in: "The Leishmaniases in Biology and Medicine (Volume II)," W.Peters and R.Killick-Kendrick, eds, Academic Press, London.
Handman, E., 1986, Leishmaniasis: antigens and host-parasite interactions, in:"Parasite antigens Towards New Strategies for Vaccines," T.W. Pearson, ed., Marcel Dekker, New York and Basel.
Handman, E., Spira, D.T., Zuckerman, A., and Montilio, B., 1974, Standardization and quality control of Leishmania tropica vaccine, J.Biol. Stand., 2:223.
Hauteville, D., Chagnon, A., Camilleri, G., and Herne, N., 1980, Leishmaniose viscérale méditerranéenne chez un leucémique en rémission, Nouv. Press. Med., 31:1713.

Herne, N., Hauteville, D., Verdier, M., Chagnon, A., Abgrall, J., and Raillat, A., 1980, Kala-azar méditerranéen chez deux adultes traités par immuno-suppresseurs, Rev. Med. Int.,1:237.

Heyneman, D., 1971, Immunology of leishmaniasis, Bull. Wld Hlth Org.,44: 499.

Hill, J.O., North, R.J.,and Collins, F.M., 1983, Advantages of measuring changes in the number if viable parasites in murine models of experimental cutaneous leishmaniasis, Inf. Immun.,39:1087.

Holbrook, T.W., Cook, J.A., and Parker, B.W., 1981, Immunization against Leishmania donovani: glucan as an adjuvant with killed promastigotes, Am. J. Trop. Med. Hyg., 30:762.

Howard, J.G., Nicklin, S., Hale, C., and Liew, Y., 1982, Prophylactic immunization against experimental leishmaniasis:I. Protection induced in mice genetically vulnerable to fatal Leishmania tropica infection, J.Immun.,129:2206.

Killick-Kendrick, R., Bryceson, A.D.M., Peters, W., Evans, D.A., Leaney, A.J., and Rioux, J.-A., 1985, Zoonotic cutaneous leishmaniasis in Saudi Arabia: lesions healing naturally in man followed by a second infection with the same zymodeme of Leishmania major, Trans. R. Soc. Trop. Med. Hyg.,79:363.

Kurotchkin, T.J.,1931, An attempt to immunize hamsters against kala-azar, Natl Med. J. China, 18:458.

Leclerc, C., Modabber, F., Deriaud, E., and Chedid, L., 1981, Systematic infection of Leishmania tropica (major) in various strains of mice, Trans. R. Soc. Trop. Med. Hyg., 75:851.

Lemma, A., and Cole, L., 1974, Leishmania enriettii: radiation effects and evaluation of radioattenuated organisms for vaccination. Expl Parasit., 35:161.

Mayrink, W., da Costa, C.A., Magalhães, P.A., Melo, M.N., Dias, M., Oliveiri Lima, A., Michalick, M.S., and Williams, P., 1979, A field trial of a vaccine against American dermal leishmaniasis, Trans.R. Soc. Trop. Med. Hyg., 73:385.

Mayrink, W., Williams, P., da Costa, C.A., Magalhães, P.A., Melo, M.N., Dias, M., Oliveira Lima, A., Michalick, M.S.M., Ferreira Carvalho,E., Barros, G.C., Sessa, P.A., and de Alencar,J.T.A.,1985, An experimental vaccine against American dermal leishmaniasis: experience in the State of Espirito Santo, Brazil, Trans. R. Soc. Trop.Med. Hyg.,79:259.

Nadim, A., 1984, Immunity to cutaneous leishmaniasis, Trans. R. Soc. Trop. Med. Hyg., 78: 848.

Napier, L.E., 1946,"The Principles and Practice of Tropical Medicine," MacMillan, New York.

Peters, W., and Killick-Kendrick, R., 1987, Editorial note added in proof, in:"The Leishmaniases in Biology and Medicine (Volume II)," W.Peters and R.Killick-Kendrick, eds, Academic Press, London.

Rioux, J.-A., Moreno, G., Lanotte, G., Pratlong, F., Dereure, J., and Rispail, P., 1986, Two episodes of cutaneous leishmaniasis in man caused by different zymodemes of Leishmania infantum s.l., Trans. R. Soc. Trop. Med. Hyg., 80:1004.

Schnur, L.F., and Jacobson, R.L., 1987, Appendix III Parasitological Techniques, in:"The Leishmaniases in Biology and Medicine (Volume I)," W.Peters and R. Killick-Kendrick, eds, Academic Press, London.

Schnur, L.F., Slutzky, G.M. and Greenblatt, C.L., 1983a, Naturally attenuated strains of Leishmania do not elicit a protective response in Syrian hamsters, Israel J. Med. Sci., 19:1112.

Schnur, L.F., Slutzky, G.M., and Greenblatt, C.L., 1983b, Appraisal of a dead polyvalent vaccine against leishmaniasis,J.Protozool.(Suppl.), 30:56A.

Schnur,L.F., Zuckerman, A., and Montilio, B.,1973, Dissemination of leishmanias to the organs of Syrian hamsters following intrasplenic inoculation of promastigotes, Expl Parasit., 34:432.

WHO,1984,"The Leishmaniases",Technical Report Series 701,WHO, Geneva.
Serebryakov, V.A., Karakhodzhaeva, S. Kh., Dzhumaev, M.D., 1972, On the effect of leishmanial vaccinations on the dynamics of immunity to diphtheria under conditions of second vaccination with adsorbed diphtheria-pertussis-tetanus (DPT) vaccine, Med.Parazitol. 41:303.

IMMUNOLOGICAL PROFILES IN INDIAN POST KALA-AZAR DERMAL LEISHMANIASIS

Jyoti P. Haldar[1*], Kshitish C. Saha[2] and Asoke C. Ghose[1]

[1]Immunology Division, National Institute of Cholera and Enteric Diseases (I.C.M.R.), Calcutta, India
[2]Dermatology Department, School of Tropical Medicine Calcutta, India

INTRODUCTION

Post kala-azar dermal leishmaniasis (PKADL) is sequal to some of the visceral leishmaniasis (kala-azar) patients. More than 10% of Indian kala-azar (KA) patients develop this nonulcerative skin lesions, containing Leishmania donovani, within one to two years after recovery from visceral infection by the parasite (Brahmachari, 1922). The apparent change in the viscerotropic properties of L. donovani to dermatotropism is believed to be induced by the immunoregulatory mechanisms operating in these treated KA patients (Adler, 1964). Presence of antileishmanial antibodies were demonstrated in the sera of PKADL patients with active dermal lesions (Mukherjee et al., 1968, Haldar et al., 1981). Attention has been focussed on the cell-mediated immune (CMI) response (Haldar et al, 1983) as CMI plays a major role in protection against leishmaniasis (Mauel and Behin, 1982). In the present study, we have attempted to look into both the cellular and humoral immune profiles of 14 Indian PKADL patients, followed up longitudinally before and after the period of treatment. For this, lymphocyte transformation tests have been carried out in vitro in the presence of Leishmania antigen and the results are correlated with those of skin test experiments in vivo. Furthermore, alterations in the serum IgG and IgM class specific antileishmanial antibody titers have been determined by standardized ELISA method. All these results are discussed with respect to our knowledge on the immunology of clinical leishmaniasis.

MATERIALS AND METHODS

Patients

Fourteen PKADL patients who came to the Dermatology Clinic of the School of Tropical Medicine, Calcutta were chosen for this study. Clinical diagnosis was confirmed by the demonstration of amastigotes in Giemsa-stained skin smears. Nine of these patients had dermal lesions relatively fresh as they developed them for a period ranging from a few months to about one year. Seven of them had suffered from KA in recent

*Present address: University of Pennsylvania School of Medicine,624,Scheie Eye Institute, 51 North 39th Street,Philadelphia,PA 19104,USA

years and were treated with antileishmanial drug. Two patients did not give any history of being treated for KA. All of them had mainly hypopigmented lesions on various parts of the body, although few nodular lesions (mainly on the face) were present in some of them. The remaining five patients were chronic PKADL cases and were suffering from the disease for the last 15-30 years. They gave a history of contracting KA in their early childhood. Dermal lesions of these patients varied from milder (hypopigmented patches and a few nodules) to more severe forms (extensive nodules on the face and other parts of the body). Blood samples were collected longitudinally from all the PKADL patients before and after the course(s) of treatment with antileishmanial drug. Control blood was collected from normal individuals living in Calcutta, a nonendemic area for leishmaniasis.

Preparation of Leishmania Antigen

L. donovani, obtained from the bone marrow culture of a KA patient, was cultured in a liquid culture medium (Ray and Ghose, 1980) for the growth of promastigotes. Crude soluble extracts of the promastigotes (Haldar et al., 1983) was used as soluble Leishmania antigen for antibody assay and lymphocyte transformation experiments. Detail methodology for the preparation of soluble Leishmania antigen has been described before (Ghose et al, 1980).

Determination of Antileishmanial Antibody

IgG and IgM class specific antileishmanial antibody titers in PKADL sera were determined by an enzyme-linked immunosorbant assay (ELISA) method described previously (Haldar et al., 1981).

Delayed Type Hypersensitivity (DTH) Reaction In Vivo

Fourteen PKADL patients and 20 normal controls were tested for DTH reaction in vivo to leishmanin. The reaction was tested by intradermal injection of 0.2 ml of leishmanin reagent containing 10^8 L. donovani promastigotes per ml of 0.5% phenol saline. The skin reactions were recorded after 48 hours. An induration area $\geq$ 5 mm in diameter was considered as a positive reaction.

Lymphocyte Transformation Test In Vitro

Peripheral blood from PKADL patients and normal controls was collected in heparinized tubes and the lymphocytes were isolated by Ficoll-Hypaque density gradient centrifugation method (Boyum, 1968). Cells, after washing four times, were suspended in culture medium which was RPMI-1640 with bicarbonate (Flow Laboratories) supplemented with 2 mM L-glutamine, 20 mM HEPES, penicillin (100 U/ml), streptomycin (100 µg/ml) and 10% heat inactivated fetal bovine serum. Cells (1×10^6/ml) were cultured at 37°C in triplicate in the presence of 10 µg of Leishmania antigen, unstimulated cells (without antigen) being cultured in parallel. One µCi of ^{3}H-thymididine (The Radiochemical Center, Amersham, England) was added to each culture after 120 hours and cells were harvested after another 24 hours of culture. Radioactive incorporation was measured by a liquid scintillation counter and stimulation index (SI) was expressed as: counts per minute (ΔCPM) for stimulated culture/counts per minute (ΔCPM) for unstimulated culture.

RESULTS

Humoral Immune Response

Immunoglobulin G and Immunoglobulin M class specific antileishmanial antibody titers in the sera of 14 PKADL patients were determined by ELISA method. The ELISA titers were ranged between 1/200 to 1/1600 for IgG and 1/50 to 1/400 for IgM isotypes. The serum samples of these patients were again assayed for antibody titer after chemotherapy. It was observed that IgG-ELISA titers in the serum of these patients decreased by 4 to 8 fold after treatment for a period ranging from 20 to 81 weeks (Table 1). However, this type of change was less demonstrated with respect to IgM-ELISA titers, which remained unchanged in most cases after the course of treatment (Table 1). It may be noted that a decrease in circulating IgG-antibody level in treated patients was accompanied with the substantial diminution of skin lesions.

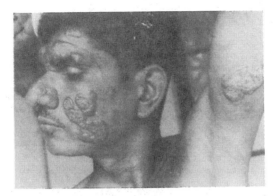

Fig. 1a. A chronic PKADL patient with extensive dermal lesions on the face.

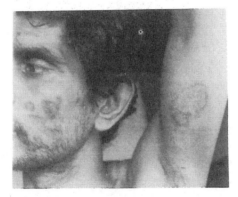

Fig. 1b. The same patient after repeated courses of chemotherapy. Note the substantial diminution of dermal lesions.

Cell-mediated Immune Response

Results of DTH skin reaction in vivo with leishmanin for each patient are presented in Table 1. These results indicated that 10 out of 14 PKADL patients, before commencement of chemotherapy, showed positive skin reac-

Table 1. Immunological Data on PKADL Patients

Patient	Age/Sex	IgG-ELISA titer (reciprocal)		IgM-ELISA titer (reciprocal)		DTH reaction to leishmanin (mm)		SI of lymphocyte culture with Leishmania antigen	
		Active	Treated[a]	Active	Treated[a]	Active	Treated[a]	Active	Treated[a]
Fresh group									
1	20/M	800	200 (30)	200	200 (30)	12	12 (30)	15.4	19.2 (30)
2	10/M	400	100 (28)	50	50 (28)	3	5 (28)	1.8	3.1 (28)
3	30/M	400	50 (38)	100	100 (38)	9	9 (38)	12.6	12.0 (38)
4	30/M	1600	200 (34)	400	100 (34)	6	7 (34)	6.8	8.0 (34)
5	27/M	800	200 (20)	100	100 (20)	9	8 (20)	9.5	9.3 (20)
6	18/M	1600	200 (39)	400	200 (39)	5	7 (39)	5.8	7.2 (39)
7	30/F	800	100 (31)	100	50 (31)	7	8 (31)	7.6	6.9 (31)
8	19/M	400	50 (38)	50	50 (38)	8	9 (38)	28.8	30.2 (38)
9	10/M	800	100 (42)	200	200 (42)	10	8 (42)	17.2	15.8 (42)
Chronic group									
10	42/F	1600	400 (43)	50	50 (43)	6	6 (43)	4.7	5.6 (43)
11	47/F	200	50 (55)	100	100 (55)	0	0 (55)	1.0	1.1 (55)
12	54/M	800	100 (47)	100	100 (47)	8	12 (47)	24.5	25.7 (47)
13	48/M	800	200 (57)	50	50 (57)	2	2 (57)	0.9	0.8 (57)
14	56/M	400	100 (81)	100	100 (81)	0	2 (81)	1.3	1.1 (81)
Mean ± s.e.m.						6.1 ± 0.96[b]	6.7 ± 0.87[b]	9.85 ± 2.37[b]	10.4 ± 2.47[b]
Normal controls (n=20)							0.60 ± 0.26		1.27 ± 0.18

[a] Figure in the parenthesis denotes weeks elapsed since the active phase (zero week) blood collection.

[b] Significant ($p < 0.005$) when compared with normal controls.

tivity against leishmanin, the induration area (diameter) ranged between 5-12 mm. Among 4 nonresponders (induration < 5 mm in diameter), only 1 demonstrated positivity (induration diameter 5 mm) after treatment. The remaining three patients (all had chronic lesions) did not show any positive DTH reaction in vivo against leishmanin, before and after the courses of treatment.

Results of lymphocyte transformation test (LTT) in vitro with the peripheral blood lymphocytes of 14 PKADL patients in the presence of 10 µg Leishmania antigen are also shown in Table 1. The majority (10 out of 14) of the patients exhibited a positive lymphoproliferative response (stimultion index >2) against the antigen. Results of LTT for each patient after chemotherapy are also presented in Table 1. It may be noted that three (all chronic cases) patients, lymphocytes of whom were not stimulated in the presence of Leishmania antigen, remained unresponsive to the antigen even after prolonged antimony therapy. However, dermal lesion in these patients diminished noticably after treatment. All, but one, patients who acquired the lesion relatively fresh, responded in antigen induced LTT equally well before and after chemotherapy. One of them, who did not respond before the treatment, responded weakly (SI > 3) after 28 weeks of treatment.

A reasonably good correlation was observed between the results of leishmanin skin test in vivo and the lymphoproliferative response in vitro. The Spearman's rank correlation between the two results was statistically significant ($p < 0.05$). All the 20 normal controls were unresponsive to Leishmania antigen when tested by DTH skin reaction in vivo and LTT in vitro. Thus, the results of DTH skin reaction and LTT for the PKADL patients were statistically significant ($p < 0.005$) when compared to those of normal controls.

DISCUSSION

PKADL is not a common leishmanial syndrome in different geographical foci of KA. It is rare in China and Brazil and only 1% of KA patients in East Africa are found to develop this skin lesion (Preston and Dumonde, 1976). However, it is relatively common in Indian KA patients, 10-20% of them being affected by this sequal. Indian PKADL is also long lasting as compared to the African one which heals within a short period (Wilcocks and Manson-Bahr, 1972). These patients are considered a good reservoir host for L. donovani in Indian subcontinent.

Immunological responses associated with PKADL were different in some respects from those associated with KA (Haldar et al., 1981; 1983). Individual variations in the serum antibody levels of PKADL patients were reported by Mukherjee et al. (1968) and Manson-Bahr (1967). In general, the amount of circulating antileishmanial antibodies in these patients were much lower when compared to that of KA patients (Haldar et al, 1981). DTH reactivity against leishmanin in Africa (Manson-Bahr et al., 1959) and Indian (Sengupta and Mukherjee, 1962) PKADL patients were both positive and negative. Variations in the histopathological profiles and skin test reactivities of these patients (Majumdar, 1967) suggest that PKADL might lie almost at any point of the leishmaniasis spectrum (Turk and Bryceson, 1971).

Data presented in this study suggest that the antileishmanial antibodies do not play a major role in protection against the parasite in PKADL cases. However, decrease in the circulating IgG antibody titers was recorded after the substantial diminution of skin lesions in treated patients. Thus, the circulating antibody levels might provide an idea of antigenic load and the degree of lesion in these patients. Serum antibody titers in KA patients, where the infection (and so the antigenic load) is more severe, were reported to be also higher (Ghose et al., 1980, Haldar et al., 1981). Chemotheraphy leading to the decrease of parasite load and recovery from visceral infection similarly resulted in the gradual decrease of circulating antileishmanial antibody levels in KA patients (Haldar et al., 1983).

Results of lymphoproliferative responses in the presence of *Leishmania* antigen indicate that majority of PKADL patients with active skin lesion have *Leishmania*-specific circulating lymphocytes. This is in contrast to that found in active KA patients (Carvalho et al., 1981, Ho et al., 1983, Haldar et al., 1983, Sacks et al., 1987). Some of the PKADL patients studied here failed to demonstrate positivity in their lymphocyte responsiveness to *Leishmania* antigen. They gave the history of contracting the KA 20-30 years ago and were harboring the parasite for so many years. None of these patients, however, showed any signs of the visceral infection during this period and were therefore immune to KA. Other patients who were definitely responsive against *Leishmania*, as evidenced by LTT and DTH skin reaction, also did not suffer from KA again. Thus, all these PKADL patients were immune to visceral but not to the dermatotropic form of the disease, caused by the same parasite. Therefore, the protection against *L. donovani* infection, especially in PKADL, can not be correlated with T-cell responsiveness with the antigen. This observation is interesting because the majority of the KA patients demonstrated *Leishmania*-specific positive lymphoproliferative response only after recovery from visceral infection (Carvalho et al., 1981, Ho et al., 1983, Haldar et al., 1983, Sacks et al., 1987). This positive CMI response against the parasite, however, does not protect some of the treated KA patients from a sequel dermal lesion.

We noted that 2 out of 14 patients studied here had no history of being treated for clinical infection of KA. Reports of subclinical and cryptic infection with *L. donovani* (Manson-Bahr, 1967, Van-Orshoven et al., 1979, Badaro et al., 1986) and spontaneous cure (Napier, 1946, Badaro et al., 1986) are not rare. It is possible that weak primary infection with the parasite conferred them immunity to the viscerotropic but not to the dermatotropic form of the disease. Various acquired factors within the host (such as nutritional status, superimposed infection which are quite common for people living in endemic areas) are likely to influence the course of the disease to some extent. Genetic differences among individuals should also be taken into account to explain the susceptibility, pathogenesis and subsequent recovery from *L. donovani* infection.

ACKNOWLEDGEMENTS

We thank Dr. S.C. Pal, Director, National Institute of Cholera and Enteric Diseases, Indian Council of Medical Research, Calcutta, for his constant encouragement during this study. We are indebted to Ms. Dolly A. Scott for her skillful preparation of this manuscript.

REFERENCES

Adler, S., 1964, Leishmania, p. 35, *in*: "Advances in Parasitology," vol. 2, B. Dawes, ed., Academic Press Inc., New York.

Badaro, R., Jone, T.C., Carvalho, E.M., Sampaio, D., Reed, S.G., Barral, A., Teixeira, R., and Johnson, W.D. Jr., 1986, New perspectives on a subclinical form of visceral leishmaniasis, *J. Infect. Dis.*, 154:1003.

Boyum, A., 1968, Isolation of mononuclear cells and granulocytes from human blood, Scand. J. Clin. Lab. Invest., 21(Suppl.):77.

Brahmachari, U.N., 1922, A new form of cutaneous leishmaniasis-dermal leishmanoid, Ind. Med. Gaz., 57:125.

Carvalho, E.M., Teixeira, R.S., and Johnson, W.D. Jr., 1981, Cell-mediated immunity in American visceral leishmaniasis: reversible immunosuppression during acute infection, Infect. Immun., 33:498.

Ghose, A.C., Haldar, J.P., Pal, S.C., Mishra, B.P., and Mishra, K.K., 1980, Serological investigations on Indian kala-azar, Clin. Exp. Immunol., 40:318.

Haldar, J.P., Saha, K.C., and Ghose, A.C., 1981, Serological profiles on Indian post kala-azar dermal leishmaniasis, Trans. R. Soc. Trop. Med. Hyg., 75:514.

Haldar, J.P., Ghosh, S., Saha, K.C., and Ghose, A.C., 1983, Cell-mediated immune responses in Indian kala-azar and post kala-azar dermal leishmaniasis, Infect. Immun., 42:702.

Ho, M., Koech, D.K., Iha, D.W., and Bryceson, A.D.M., 1983, Immunosuppression in Kenyan visceral leishmaniasis, Clin. Exp. Immunol., 51:207.

Majumdar, T.D., 1967, Post kala-azar dermal leishmaniasis, Dermatol. Inter., 6:174.

Manson-Bahr, P.E.C., 1961, Immunity in kala-azar, Trans. R. Soc. Trop. Med. Hyg., 55:550.

Manson-Bahr, P.E.C., 1967, Cryptic infections of humans in an endemic kala-azar area, East Afr. Med. J., 44:177.

Manson-Bahr, P.E.C., Heish, R.B., and Garnham, P.C.C., 1959, Studies on leishmaniasis in East Africa. IV. The Montenegro test in kala-azar in Kenya, Trans. R. Soc. Trop. Med. Hyg., 53:380.

Mauel, J., and Behin, R., 1982, Leishmaniasis: Immunity, Immunopathology and Immunodiagnosis, p. 299, in: "Immunology of Parasitic Infections", S. Cohen and K. Warren, ed., Blackwell Scientific Publications, Oxford.

Mukherjee, A.C., Neogy, K.N., and Sengupta, P.C., 1968, Passive haemagglutination in leishmaniasis, Bull. Cal. Sch. Trop. Med., 16:38.

Napier, L.E., 1946, "The Principles and Practice of Tropical Medicine," Macmillan, New York.

Preston, P.M., and Dumonde, D.C., 1976, Immunology of clinical and expermental leishmaniasis, p. 167, in: "Immunology of Parasitic Infections," S. Cohen and E.H. Sadun, ed., Blackwell Scientific Publications, Oxford.

Ray, R., and Ghose, A.C., 1980, Cultivation of leishmania donovani in vitro in a high yielding liquid culture medium, Ind. J. Med. Res., 71:203-206.

Sacks, D.L., Lal, S.L., Srivastava, S.N., Blackwell, J., and Neva, F.A., 1987, An analysis of T cell responsiveness in Indian kala-azar, J. Immunol., 138:908.

Sengupta, P.C., and Mukherjee, A.M., 1962, Intradermal test with Leishmania donovani antigen in post kala-azar dermal leishmaniasis, Ann. Biochem. Exp. Med., 22:63.

Turk, J.L., and Bryceson, A.D.M., 1971, Immunological phenomena in leprosy and related diseases, p. 209, in: "Advances in Immunology," vol. 13. F.J. Dixon and H.G. Kunkel, ed., Academic Press, London.

Van-Orshoven, B., Michielsen, A.P., and Vandepitte, J., 1979, Fatal leishmaniasis in renal transplant patient, Lancett ii:740.

Wilcocks, C., and Manson-Bahr, P.E.C., 1972, "Manson's Tropical Diseases," Bailliere Tindal, London.

EVALUATION OF NON-SPECIFIC IMMUNITY IN CANINE LEISHMANIASIS

Olga Brandonisio*, Maria Altamura*, Luigi Ceci**,
Salvatore Antonaci***, and Emilio Jirillo*

*Microbiologia Medica, **Clinica Medica Veterinaria
and ***Medicina Clinica
University of Bari Medical School, Policlinico
70124 Bari, Italy

INTRODUCTION

Leishmaniasis is a parasitosis which involves the immune system at humoral and cellular levels. In this respect, over the past few years many studies have emphasized the capacity of Leishmania parasites to cause immunodepression either in murine or human models[1].

Throughout the world, leishmaniasis spontaneously occurs in dogs and is sustained by several species of Leishmania[2]. However, in spite of the presence of this spontaneous disease, few studies have been conducted on the immune status of Leishmania-infected dogs. In particular, investigations have been made on the humoral arm of canine immune system[3], while the cellular compartment has been less explored, even if the chronicity of the disease may imply an involvement of cellular mechanisms.

In our area (Apulia, South Italy), canine leishmaniasis is widespread and caused by L. infantum[4]. Since non-specific immunity seems to play a major role in leishmaniasis[1], here we will present data on the monocyte function of Leishmania-infected dogs.

MATERIAL AND METHODS

Dogs

Fifteen dogs with generalized leishmaniasis, diagnosed by clinical and serological findings, were employed for this study. Eighteen healthy dogs were used as controls.

Leishmania Isolation and Identification

Parasites were isolated from bone marrow of infected dogs. Briefly, 0.2 ml of bone marrow aspirates were cultured on Tobie's medium modified by Evans[5] and incubated at 24°C for 10-30 days. The isolated strains were kindly typed by the Istituto Superiore di Sanità, Rome, using an electrophoretic assay of isoenzymes[6].

Monocyte Isolation

Peripheral blood lymphomonocytes, isolated on Ficoll-Hypaque gradient[7], were incubated for 1 h at 37°C in petri dishes coated with foetal calf serum (FCS). Adherent cells were detached from dishes by incubation at 4°C in phosphate-buffered saline (PBS) containing 0.2% EDTA and 5% FCS[8]. Monocytes were then removed from dishes by vigorous pipetting and identified by esterase technique (80% of esterase positive cells)[9].

Phagocytosis

5×10^6 monocytes were incubated with Leishmania at 3:1 ratio for 1 h at 37°C on a rocking platform in 0.5 ml of RPMI 1640 (Eurobio, Paris, France) containing 100 μl of autologous and respectively homologous heat-inactivated serum from dogs and 2 drops of heparin[10]. The same procedure was used for the phagocytosis of Candida albicans (monocyte/Candida: 5:1 ratio). Phagocytosis was microscopically evaluated by staining cytocentrifuge preparations with Giemsa. A total of 300 cells was counted in each slide.

Immune Complex (IC) Assay

IC determination was performed by ^{125}I-C1q binding test[11,12].

Statistical Analysis

Analysis was performed by means of paired t-test.

RESULTS

Parasites isolated from bone marrow of infected dogs and typed as L. infantum species were used in the phagocytic assay. Table 1 shows that monocyte phagocytosis from healthy dogs was significantly higher ($0.01 > p > 0.001$) than that observed in infected dogs. Moreover, when monocyte activity in sick dogs was assayed in the presence of serum from healthy dogs, a recovery of phagocytic capacity was observed. By contrast, serum from

Table 1. Monocyte-Mediated Phagocytosis of Leishmania Promastigotes

Donor	Source of serum	Phagocytosis
Healthy Dogs	autologous	43.6+14.2*
"	homologous	29.8+15.3
Infected Dogs	autologous	21.6+8.9
"	homologous	39.4+11.3

*Phagocytosis is expressed as mean+SD.

Leishmania-infected dogs led to a significant ($0.05 > p > 0.02$) inhibition of phagocytosis in healthy dogs. Similar results in terms of either sick serum-induced depression or healthy serum-mediated recovery were observed when phagocytosis was assayed in the presence of Candida albicans (data not illustrated). These findings provide evidence that sera from Leishmania-infected dogs exert a suppressive activity on monocyte-mediated phagocytic response.

To further investigate the suppressive mechanisms, studies have been undertaken to evaluate the presence of soluble circulating IC which may impair the phagocytic function. IC were detected in 83.3% of infected dogs. In fact, the mean value of IC in sick dogs (25.8+10.8 % Clq BA) was significantly ($p < 0.001$) higher than that observed in controls (5.5+2.6 % Clq BA). Since these IC might account for the reduced function, IC-rich sera from infected dogs were treated with polyethylen glycol (PEG)[13] and supernatants were supplemented to the phagocytic system. Table 2 illustrates that, in infected dogs, PEG-treated autologous serum gave rise to a recovery of phagocytosis, this supporting the role for IC in the modulation of immune response.

Table 2. Monocyte Phagocytosis of Leishmania-infected dogs with different sera

Serum	Phagocytosis
Untreated autologous serum	21.6+9.5*
PEG-treated autologous serum	43.8+12.5§

*For legend, see Table 1
§$p < 0.001$

DISCUSSION

There is evidence that phagocytic cells play an important role in animal and human leishmaniasis, and in particular in the lysis of promastigotes[14]. Our data emphasize the importance of monocytes in the defence against Leishmania infection. In fact, in infected dogs, phagocytosis is significantly reduced in comparison with normal dogs. This can represent a mechanism of invasiveness of promastigotes which in normal conditions are well phagocytosed by monocytes and then killed by intracellular oxidative processes[15,16]. The reduction in parasite phagocytosis was also observed in an experimental model using C57Bl/6 mice[17]. Macrophages from infected mice exhibited a reduced ability to ingest L. tropica amastigotes in vitro. Moreover, the phagocytic defect, in our dogs, has been further investigated since it could be also extended to other microorganisms. In this context, we have observed a reduced phagocytosis when monocytes were incubated with Candida albicans. Therefore, the monocyte defect of these animals seems to be a generalized phenomenon. Additionally, the fact that sera from Leishmania-infected dogs decreased the phagocytic capacity of monocytes from healthy dogs indicates that the observed impairment of phagocytosis depends on serum factor(s). This is confirmed by the evidence that healthy sera reverse the reduced monocyte phagocytosis in sick dogs.

In our studies, the recovery of immune functions by using PEG-treated sera from Leishmania-infected dogs, in which IC have been detected, suggests a possible role for IC in determining the phagocytic defect. In this regard, IC have been detected in patients with human leishmaniasis[13,18]. At the same time, IC can inhibit phagocytic capacity of monocytes by interfering with Fc receptors[19]. Additionally, phagocytic and killing defects have also been observed during the acute phase of human visceral leishmaniasis which is characterized by high levels of circulating IC[20]. Moreover, in previous studies we have demonstrated typical renal lesions represented by fibrillar and hyaline thickening of the glomerular mesangium, which may be due to deposits of circulating IC, during the course of chronic canine leishmaniasis[21].

CONCLUSIONS

Our results indicate that IC may play an important role in the monocyte phagocytic process during leishmaniasis. Therefore, these findings emphasize that the study of canine leishmaniasis can represent a suitable model for investigating immunity in the human counterpart.

ACKNOWLEDGEMENTS

Paper supported, in part, by a grant from Ministero Pubblica Istruzione (1986), Rome, Italy.

We thank Dr. Marina Gramiccia (Istituto Superiore Sanità) for typing Leishmania strains.

REFERENCES

1. R.D. Pearson, D.A. Wheeler, L.M. Harrison, and M.D. Kay, The immunobiology of leishmaniasis, Rev. Infect. Dis. 5:907 (1983).
2. D.H. Molyneux and R.W. Ashford, Introduction to leishmaniases, in: "The Biology of Trypanosoma and Leishmania Parasites of Man and Domestic Animals", D.H. Molyneux and R.W. Ashford, eds., Taylor and Francis, London (1983).
3. L. Ceci, F. Petazzi, G. Guidi, and M. Corazza, Modificazioni immunoelettroforetiche in cani affetti da Leishmaniosi, Clin. Vet. 108:268 (1985).
4. M. Gramiccia, L. Gradoni, and E. Pozio, Il genere Leishmania in Italia, Parassitologia 27:187 (1985).
5. D.A. Evans, Kinetoplastidia, in: "Methods of Cultivating Parasites In Vitro", A.E.R. Taylor and J.R. Baker, eds., Academic Press, New York (1978).
6. R. Mazoun, G. Lanotte, N. Pasteur, J.A. Rioux, M.F. Kennou, and F. Pratlong, Ecologie des leishmanioses dans le sud de la France. 16 contribution à l'analyse chimiotaxonomique des parasites de la leishmaniose viscérale méditerranénne. A propos de 55 sauches isolée en Cévenne-Côte d'Azur, Corse et Tunisie, Ann. Parasitol. Hum. Comp. 56:131 (1981).
7. A. Böyum, Isolation of mononuclear cells and granulocytes from human blood, Scand. J. Clin. Lab. Invest. 21 (suppl. 97):77 (1968).
8. K. Kumagai, K. Itoh, S. Hinuma, and M. Tada, Pretreatment of plastic petri dishes with foetal calf serum. A simple method for macrophage isolation, J. Immunol. Methods 29:17 (1979).
9. L.T. Yam, C.Y. Li, and M.H. Crosby, Cytochemical identification of monocytes and granulocytes, Am. J. Clin. Path. 55:283 (1971).
10. L.G. Mandell and W.E. Hook, Leukocyte function in chronic granulomatous disease of childhood, Am. J. Med. 47:473 (1969).
11. R.H. Zubler, G. Lange, P.H. Lambert, and P.A. Miescher, Detection of immune complexes in unheated sera by a modified ^{125}I-Clq binding test, J. Immunol. 116:232 (1976).

12. J.E. Volanakis and R.M. Stroud, Rabbit Clq: purification, functional and structural studies, J. Immunol. Methods 2:25 (1972).
13. S. Sehgal, B.K. Aikat, and A.G. Pathania, Immune complexes in Indian Kala-azar, Bull. WHO 60:945 (1982).
14. K.A. Chang, Antibody-mediated inhibition of phagocytosis in Leishmania donovani human phagocyte interactions in vitro, Am. J. Trop. Med. Hyg. 30:334 (1981).
15. K.A. Chang, Leishmania donovani: promastigote-macrophage interactions in vitro, Exp. Parasitol. 48:175 (1979).
16. R.D. Pearson, J.L. Marcus, D. Roberts, and J.R. Donowitz, Differential survival of Leishmania donovani amastigotes in human monocytes, J. Immunol. 131:1994 (1983).
17. C.B. Panosian and D.J. Wyler, Acquired macrophage resistance to in vitro infection with Leishmania, J. Infect. Dis. 148:1049 (1983).
18. R.D. Pearson, J.E. Alencar, R. Romito, T.G. Naidu, A.C. Young, and J.S. Davis, Circulating immune complexes and rheumatoid factor in visceral leishmaniasis, J. Infect. Dis. 147:1102 (1983).
19. B. Svensson, Serum factor causing impaired macrophage function in systemic lupus erythematosus, Scand. J. Immunol. 4:145 (1975).
20. A. Lazzarin, G. Orlando, M. Galli, and R. Esposito, Defect of leukocyte function and circulating immune complexes in visceral leishmaniasis, Boll. Ist. sieroter. milan. 64: 146 (1985).
21. O. Brandonisio, L. Ceci, P. Bufo, S. Antonaci, and E. Jirillo, Immunological profile of Leishmania infection. Spontaneous canine leishmaniasis: a useful model for studying the immune response in human leishmaniasis, EOS Riv. Immunol. Immunofarmacol. 5:176 (1985).

VARIATION IN LEISHMANIA SPECIES EXPRESSED BY ANTIGENIC GLYCOCONJUGATES AND

EXCRETED FACTOR

R. L. Jacobson, L. F. Schnur and C. L. Greenblatt

Kuvin Center for the Study of Infectious and
Tropical Diseases
Hadassah - Hebrew University
Jerusalem, Israel

INTRODUCTION

Cultured leishmanial promastigotes have glycoconjugates on their surfaces that confer specificity. They also release similar compounds into their growth media. This released material has been variously termed excreted factor (EF), exo-metabolites and shed membrane antigen and has been partially characterized (Schnur et. al., 1972; Decker-Jackson and Honigberg, 1978; Semprevivo and Honigberg, 1980; Slutzky and Greenblatt, 1977, 1979; El-On et. al., 1979; Kameshiro et. al., 1982; Handman et. al., 1984; Turco et. al., 1984). Their use in the serological classification of Leishmania has been described (Schnur, 1982), whereby strains fall into three serotypic categories; A, B and AB, comprizing several subcategories. The same serological determinants have been shown to exist on the surfaces of promastigotes (Jacobson et. al., 1982). These antigens have been shown to be part of a polymorphic family of carbohydrate-rich molecules present in all Leishmania. The major component is a negatively charged glycoconjugate, possibly containing protein (Hernandez, 1983; Turco et. al., 1984), and the A and B types have different electrophoretic mobilities (Slutzky et. al., 1984).

Lectin probes have been used to determine the presence of carbohydrate receptors on Leishmania. Agglutination techniques and fluorescent-labelled lectins have revealed that galactose and mannose and other sugar residues are on both the parasite surface and in the excreted glycoconjugate. Differences have been found in both the quantity and configuration of the sugar moieties among strains of different serotypes (Dwyer, 1981; Jacobson et. al. 1981). Antibodies and lectins appear to compete for reactive sites on the parasite surface, since specific antibody was shown to inhibit lectin-binding to promastigotes (Jacobson, unpublished). The role of these carbohydrate receptors in the host parasite and vector parasite interaction has yet to be elucidated. A multifarious approach has been adopted to determine and compare the biochemical and antigenic nature of leishmanial promastigotes of many strains.

MATERIALS AND METHODS

Twenty strains representing different serotypes were examined (Figure 1 and Table 1). Counter-immunoelectrophoresis was done according to the method described by Closs et. al. (1975). Glycoconjugates were electro-

Table 1. The strains of *Leishmania*

LRC-L	WHO CODE	EF SEROTYPE	SPECIES
137	MHOM/IL/67/Jericho II	A1	L. major
306	MPSA/IL/80/Psammomys 1	A1	L. major
464	IPAP/IL/84/8A1	A1	L. major
505	MHOM/IL/84/ROA	A8	L. major
23	MHOM/IL/60/Ein Gedi-II	A4	L. major
38	MHOM/SU/59/P	A4	L. major
"P"	MHOM/SU/59/P	A4	L. major
448	MMAS/KE/82/NLB-100	A4B2	L. major
31	MHOM/IL/65/Dead Sea	A1B2	L. major
22	MHOM/IL/59/Gabai 159	A2	L. tropica
32	MHOM/IQ/65/Sinai I	A2	L. tropica
36	MHOM/IQ/66/L75	A2	L. tropica
39	MHOM/SU/58/Strain-OD	A2	L. tropica
156	MHOM/IN/77/L113	A2	L. tropica
160	MHOM/IN/77/L117	A2	L. tropica
JISH	MPSM/SA/83/JISH 220	A1	L. arabica
52	MHOM/IN/54/SC23	B2	L. donovani
147	MHOM/ET/71/L100	B1	L. aethiopica
144	MCAV/BR/45/L88	B3	L. enriettii
259	MHOM/BR/77/M2269	Bx	L. m. amazonensis

phoresed against monoclonal antibodies and rabbit polyclonal antisera. Radioimmunoassay inhibition testing (RIA) was done as described by Greenblatt et. al. (1985). Standard purified EFs from L. major (LRC-L137) and L. tropica (LRC-L32), were coated onto microplate wells for two hours at room temperature; plates were washed x3 with PBS-Tween; homologous immune sera were incubated with various concentrations of EFs from different strains; resulting mixtures were applied to the coated wells; after further incubation, wells were washed x3; ^{125}I-labelled protein A was then applied for one hour, washed and adhering radioactivity measured;

$$\% \text{ inhibition} = 100 - \left(\frac{\text{cpm of absorbed sera}}{\text{cpm of unabsorbed sera}} \times 100\right)$$

Flow cytometric analysis (FACS) of formaldehyde - fixed promastigotes incubated with monoclonal antibody WIC 79.3, labelled with fluorescent isothiocyanate (FITC-MAB) was done, as described by Greenblatt et. al. (1985). FITC-lectin labelling for Concanavalin A (Con A), Ricinus 120 (RCA), Peanut (PNA), Soya bean (SBA). and Wheat germ (WGA), (Sigma) was done at a concentration of 5 ug/ml of lectin and 100 - 250 mM of the appropriate inhibiting sugar.

RESULTS

CIE confirmed the main serotypes A, B and AB seen by double diffusion (Fig I) and the uniqueness of their sub-serotypes (Fig II).

RIA showed that quantitative antigenic differences exist among different strains of the same species (Fig III).

FACS analysis of two strains of L. major compared with an L. arabica strain demonstrated inter- and intra- specific differences in PNA and MAB binding over seven days (Fig IV).

FACS analysis of promastigotes of six L. major strains labelled with FITC - lectins and FITC - MAB 79.3 showed considerable quantitative diversity (Fig Va) and even of clones derived from the same parental strain (Fig Vb).

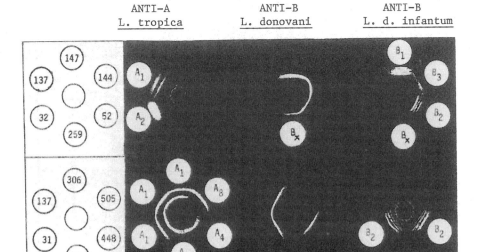

Fig. I Excreted factor (EF) serotypes and sub-serotypes of leishmania strains

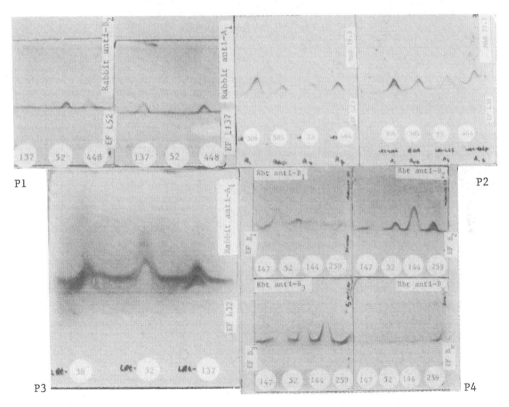

Fig. II Crossed-immunoelectophoresis (CIE) of EFs, comparing their reactions with polyclonal rabbit anti-sera and mouse monoclonal antibodies: plate 1 (P1) confirms the three main leishmanial serotypes A (LRC-L137), B (LRC-L52) and AB (LRC-L448); plate 2 (P2) demonstrates that MAB 79.3 binds to a common component shared by A strains of different sub-types, as defined by rabbit anti-sera; plate 3 (P3) shows components shared by three sub-types A_1, A_2 and A_4 and other components expressing their uniqueness; plate 4 (P4) shows distinct variation among serotype B strains.

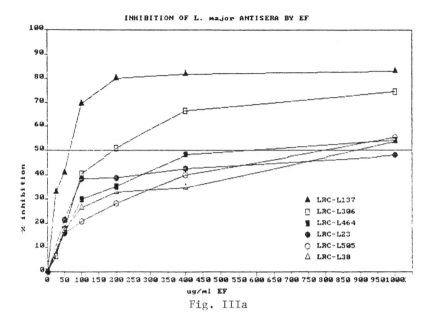

Fig. IIIa

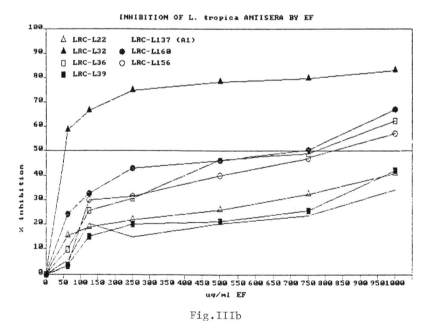

Fig.IIIb

Fig. III Quantitation of antigenicity of excreted factors from the different strains of L. major (a) and L. tropica (b). A radioimmunoassay inhibition test was used.

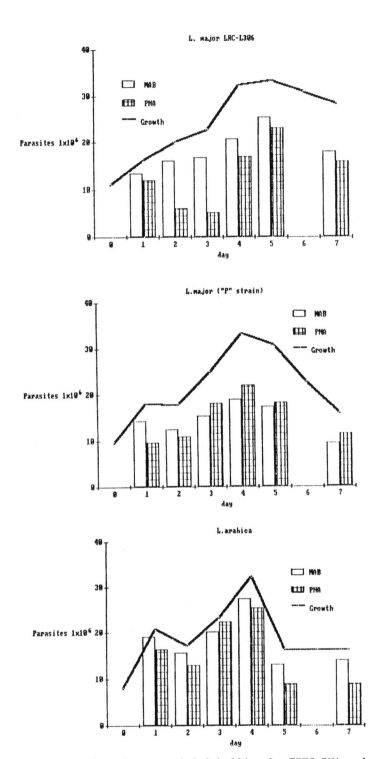

Fig. IV Growth and sequential labelling by FITC-PNA and FITC-MAB 79.3 of L. major (LCR-L306), L. major (P strain) and L. arabica (Jish 220) promastigotes, monitored by flow cytometric analysis (FACS).

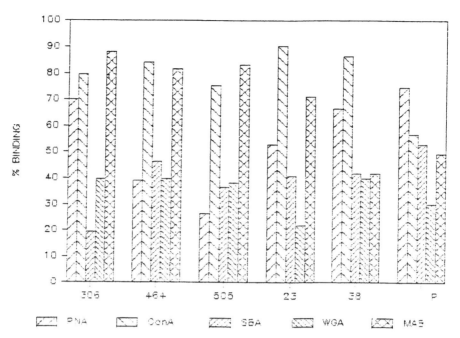

Fig. Va Flow cytometric analysis of the promastigotes of six *L. major* strains labelled with four fluorescent lectins and fluorescent MAB 79.3

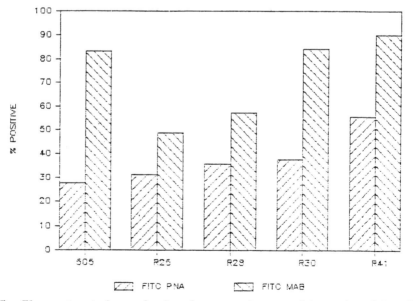

Fig. Vb Flow cytometric analysis of promastigotes of *L. major* (LRC-L505) and four of its clones (R25, R28, R30, and R41) labelled with FITC-PNA and FITC MAB 79.3.

DISCUSSION AND CONCLUSION

The results obtained with these techniques endorsed EF serotypes as useful taxonomic characters, but demonstrate marked antigenic micro-heterogeneity among closely related strains and clones of Leishmania. Among the various strains examined, this variation was seen in both the surface and released glycoconjugates. CIE distinguished qualitative and quantitative differences among glycoconjugates, showing that homologous strains vary in the rates of production and release of these compounds. The RIA inhibition test was particularly useful in measuring the quantitative differences of L. major and L. tropica glycoconjugate antigens to species specific rabbit polyclonal antisera. In the homologous system, 50 ug/ml of EF inhibited binding by 50%, while 750 - 1000 ug/ml of EF was required to obtain the same level of inhibition in most of the other strains of the same species (Fig. III).

The total number of FITC-PNA and FITC-MAB 79.3 labelled promastigotes and the distribution of binding, monitored by FACS, varied considerably among the three strains tested over the seven day period (Fig. IV). Particularly noticeable was the decrease in PNA binding of strain LRC-L306 during early log phase and its subsequent increase at stationary phase. Examination of the promastigote surface glycoconjugates of L. major strains with a panel of different FITC lectins and FITC-MAB 79.3 exposed considerable variations of surface determinants (Fig. Va). The presence of N-acetylglucosamine (WGA binding) on the surface of the promastigotes, detected by FACS, was of interest as the presence of this sugar is not discerned by either direct agglutination or fluorescent microscopy. The comparison of FITC-PNA and FITC-MAB binding to surface glycoconjugates of four clones and their parental strain showed these to be in proportion to one another and were reflected by the amounts released (Fig. Vb); but varied from clone to clone. All these clones were infective to mice.

These antigenic variations described here are probably significant in producing infections, causing pathogenesis, inducing self-cure and establishing protection.

ACKNOWLEDGEMENTS

This study was supported by contract N. NOI-AI-22668-NIH-NIAID and UNDP/World Bank/WHO Special Program TDR. MAB 79.3 was generously donated by Dr. D. Snary, Wellcome Laboratories, London.

REFERENCES

Closs, O., Harboe, M., and Wassum, A. M., 1975, Cross-reaction between mycobacteria. I. Crossed immunoelectrophoresis of soluble antigens of Mycobacterium lepraemurium and comparison with BCG. Scand. J. Immunol. 4, Suppl. 2:173.

Decker-Jackson, J. E., and Honigberg, B. M., 1978, Glycoproteins released by Leishmania donovani. Immunological relationships with host and bacterial antigens and biochemical analysis. J. Protozool. 25:515.

Dwyer, D. M., 1981, Structural, chemical and antigenic properties of surface membranes isolated from Leishmania donovani, in: "The Biochemistry of Parasites", G. M. Slutzky, ed., Pergamon Press, Oxford.

El-On, J., Zehavi, U., Avraham, M., and Greenblatt, C. L., 1983, Leishmania tropica and Leishmania donovani: Solid phase radioimmunoassay using leishmanial excreted factor, Exp. Parasit., 55:270.

Greenblatt, C. L., Handman, E., Mitchell, G. F., Battye, F. L., Schnur, L. F., and Snary, D., 1985, Phenotypic diversity of cloned lines of Leishmania major promastigotes, Z. Parasitenkd. 71:141.

Handman, E., Greenblatt, C. L., and Goding, J. W., 1984, An amphipathic sulphated glycoconjugate of Leishmania: characterization with monoclonal antibodies, EMBO J. 3:2301.

Hernandez, A. G., 1983, in: "Cytopathology of Parasitic Disease", CIBA Foundation Symposium, Pitman, London, 99:138.

Jacobson, R. L., Slutzky, G. M., Greenblatt, C. L., and Schnur, L. F., 1982, Surface reactions of Leishmania I. Lectin mediated agglutination. Ann. Trop. Med. Parasit., 76:45.

Jacobson, R. L., Schnur, L. F., Slutzky, G. M., Greenblatt, C. L., and Doyle, J. J., 1982, Surface reactions of Leishmania II. Correlation between surface antigens and mixed serotypes, Ann. Trop. Med. Parasit., 76:521.

Kaneshiro, E. S., Gottlieb, M., and Dwyer, D. M., 1982, Cell surface origins of antigens shed by Leishmania donovani during growth in axenic culture. Infect. Immun., 37:558.

Schnur, L. F., 1982, in: "Biochemical characterization of Leishmania", Chance, M. L. and Walton, B. C. eds UNDP/ World Bank/WHO, Geneva.

Semprevivo, L. M. and Honigberg, B. M., 1980, Exometabolites of Leishmania donovani promastigotes II. Spontaneous changes of exometabolites after isolation. Z. Parasitenkd., 62:201.

Slutzky, G. M., Yarus, S., Krasner, R. I., Schnur, L. F., and Greenblatt, C. L., 1984, Leishmanial excreted factors (EF) are distinguished by characteristic electrophoretic mobilities, Z. Parasitenkd., 70:549.

Turco, S. J., Wilkerson, M. A., and Clawson, D., 1984, Expression of an unusual acidic glycoconjugate in Leishmania donovani, J. Biol. Chem., 259:3883.

PRELIMINARY STUDIES ON THE DETECTION OF

CIRCULATING ANTIGEN IN VISCERAL LEISHMANIASIS

M.L. Chance, S. Heath, J.M. Crampton and M. Hommel

Liverpool School of Tropical Medicine
Liverpool. L3 5QA, U.K.

INTRODUCTION

Visceral leishmaniasis is endemic in several parts of Africa, the Indian subcontinent and Latin America. The disease also occurs sporadically in China, the Mediterranean basin, South West Asia and southern parts of the USSR. Once overt symptoms have developed the disease is usually considered to be fatal if left untreated. No reliable figures are available for the incidence of infection though the public health importance of the disease can be judged by the severity of the epidemic in Bihar State, India, when 100,000 cases were reported in 1977, followed the next year by a conservatively estimated 40,000 cases.

Definitive diagnosis depends on the isolation and identification of the parasite from biopsy material. This is a serious problem in visceral disease since biopsies of bone marrow or spleen are required which need to be examined by a competent microscopist. The invasive techniques necessary to obtain this material are not without risk particularly in remote rural areas. Although serodiagnostic methods are available they are seriously compromised by their lack of specificity and many cross reactions have been reported including diseases for which the differential diagnosis from visceral leishmaniasis on clinical grounds is difficult. A sure diagnosis based on serology amongst a background of potentially false positive reactions is difficult to achieve.

In addition antibody detection serodiagnostic systems have the potential to generate false positive results due to the persistance of antibody following cure. The use of a system detecting circulating antigen would overcome this difficulty. Circulating immune complexes have been shown in mucocutaneous (Desjeux et al., 1980) and visceral leishmaniasis (Galvao-Castro et al., 1984) but one report indicates that the complexes isolated from a case of visceral leishmaniasis contained only a small amount of parasite antigen (Casali and Lambert, 1979). Our approach to the problem involved isolating immune complexes from cotton rats experimentally infected with L. donovani. These laboratory hosts are capable of maintaining huge parasite loads for long periods of time, in the order of twelve months, and would be expected to contain high concentrations of circulating complexes. Isolated complexes were used to raise a polyclonal rabbit antiserum which was used as a specific reagent to detect leishmanial antigen.

MATERIALS AND METHODS

Two strains of L. donovani were used: an isolate from Ethiopia MHOM/ET/67/HU3;LV9 and an Indian isolate MHOM/IN/39/LV23. Parasites were maintained as promastigotes in HO-MEM culture medium with the addition of 10% foetal calf serum or were passaged as amastigotes in cotton rats (Sigmodon hispidus).

Kala azar serum was a pool from 15 parasitologically confirmed cases from a survey of the Tana river region of Kenya. This serum was a generous gift of Dr. D.H. Smith.

Cotton rat serum was collected from cotton rats with approximately 20 week infections by bleeding by axilar section. Immune complexes were isolated using the polyethylene glycol precipitation method of Maidment et al., (1980).

Rabbits were immunised with 200µg of immune complex protein emulsified in Freund's incomplete adjuvant by multiple subcutaneous injections. After two weeks 50µg of antigen homogenised in PBS was administered intravenously and serum collected one week later.

Anti cotton rat Ig activity was removed from the rabbit serum by passing it repeatedly through a CNBr-sepharose column to which cotton rat immunoglobulin had been bound.

The immunoassay for detecting circulating parasite specific antigens was based at a standard indirect enzyme linked immunosorbant assay (ELISA) as described by Voller (1976). Depending on the species of primary antibody used either peroxidase conjugated anti rabbit or dog IgG or streptavidin biotinylated species specific whole antibody was used. 5-amino salicylic acid was used as the chrogenic reagent. The method described by Laemmli (1970) for sodium dodecyl sulphate - polyacrylamide gel electrophoresis (SDS-PAGE) was used. Electroblotting from polyacrylamide gels was performed by the method of Towbin and Gordon (1984) using a Biorad Transblot cell. Antibody binding was detected using a second antibody conjugated to horseradish peroxidase. 4-chloro-1-napthol was used as the chromogenic agent.

RESULTS

The rabbit anti-circulating immune complex (CIC) serum was characterised in the assay shown in Fig. 1. The optimum concentration of the antigens bound to the microtitre plate was previously determined as 50mg ml^{-1}. The rabbit anti-CIC serum strongly recognised cotton rat immune complexes remaining positive down to a titre of 1:12,800. The antiserum reacted against the homologous CIC antigen and whole amastigote antigen. Antigen derived from promastigotes was negative as was normal cotton rat serum showing that unwanted rabbit anti-rat Ig activity had been removed by the affinity purification proceedure. A further control was performed using hydatid serum which had previously been shown to contain high levels of immune complexes (Craig, 1986). No significant reaction was seen between the rabbit anti-CIC serum and the hydatid serum bound to the plate indicating that non specific reactions involving immune complexes were not occurring in the assay.

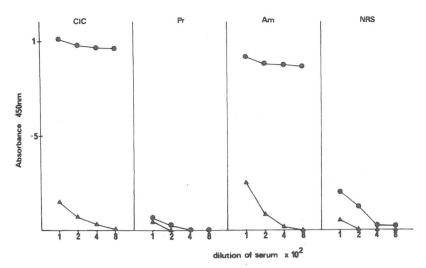

Fig. 1. Titration of rabbit anti CIC serum ● or normal rabbit serum ▲ against: CIC, cotton rat circulating immune complexes; Pr, promastigote antigen; Am, amastigote antigen; NRS, normal cotton rat serum.

The rabbit anti-CIC serum was further characterised in a dot-immunobinding assay in which decreasing amounts of amastigote antigen were adsorbed to nitrocellulose and then probed with a 1:800 dilution of anti-ClC serum. Fig. 2 shows that a strong response was seen with 30ng of amastigote antigen and at 0.3ng a signal was just detected.

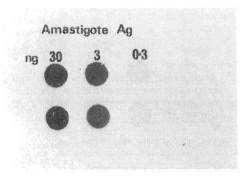

Fig. 2. Immunoblot of duplicate 10-fold dilutions of total amastigote antigen probed with a 1:800 dilution of rabbit anti-CIC serum and detected with anti-rabbit peroxidase conjugate.

The use of the rabbit anti-CIC serum to detect circulating antigen in sera from visceral leishmaniasis patients is shown in Fig. 3. Dilutions of rabbit anti-CIC were bound to a microtitre plate and reacted with 1:200 dilutions of test sera. Only Kala azar serum gave a positive reaction, normal human serum, leprosy serum and rheumatoid arthritis serum gave no reaction.

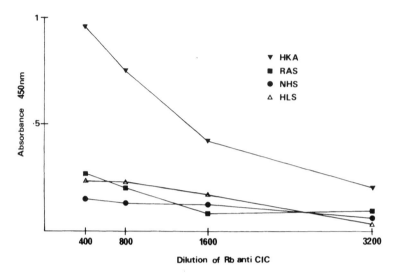

Fig. 3. Titration of immobilised rabbit anti-CIC serum against: HKA, human Kala-azar serum; RAS, rheumatoid arthritis serum; HLS, human leprosy serum; NHS, normal human serum.

We have also tested sera from dogs parasitologically proven to be infected with leishmaniasis and have demonstrated the presence of circulating antigen. Preliminary studies of the characterization of the leishmanial antigen present in the circulating complexes was carried out by separating a total amastigote lysate by SDS-PAGE followed by electroblotting and probing with rabbit anti-CIC serum (Fig. 4).

Two amastigote peptides of 20 and 52kDa were recognised in two different strains of L. donovani. These two peptides were also shown to be present in the circulating immune complexes but not in antigen derived from promastigotes. The component of approximately 77kDa present in the complex may represent undissociated complex. The heavy smearing of the bands in the 20 and 52kDa regions of the complexes may represent some partial recognition of the heavy and light chains (55/25kDa). In order to determine if human Kala azar sera contained antibodies to the two amastigote antigens of 20 and 52kDa and also to confirm that amastigotes did not have associated host (cotton rat) components, whole amastigote peptides were separated by SDS-PAGE and immunoblotted using various sera.

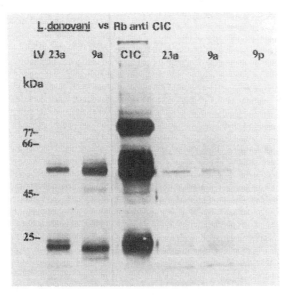

Fig. 4. Immunoblot of L. donovani LV23 and LV9 amastigote antigen (23a, 9a), LV9 promastigote antigen (9p), and cotton rat immune complexes (CIC) probed with either a 1:800 or 1:3200 dilution of rabbit anti CIC serum.

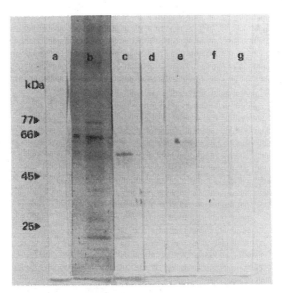

Fig. 5. Immunoblot of L. donovani LV9 amastigote antigen probed with 1:800 dilution of : a) normal human serum, b) human Kala azar serum, c) rabbit anti-CIC serum, d) normal rabbit serum, e) rabbit anti-cotton rat IgG

The results shown in Fig. 5 demonstrate that antibodies to the amastigote 20kDa molecule occur in human Kala azar serum; there does not appear to be a similarly strong response to the 52kDa molecule. The 20 and 52kDa molecules were not recognised by rabbit anti-rat IgG (heavy and light chain specific) confirming that they were not absorbed host components. This serum did however weakly recognise a peptide at 60kDa. No amastigote peptides were shown to bind non specifically to either normal human or rabbit serum.

DISCUSSION

In contrast to the sensitivity of some helminth antigen detection assays, the results obtained in attempts to detect protozoan antigens have been marked by low sensitivities. This study clearly indicates that a sensitive method for detecting circulating L. donovani antigen as a method of diagnosis is feasible. However, there are potential limitations to the assay described here. For example, only immune complexes with free antigen valencies (antigen excess) would be reactive thus circulating antigen would be underestimated. In addition free antigen in sera might compete for binding sites on the immobilised antibody again leading to an underestimation of circulating antigen.

Our experiments showed that the affinity purification of the anti-CIC reagent reduced the anti-Ig antibodies to insignificant levels and that therefore the results obtained with Kala azar serum was due to specific reactions with parasite antigen. Eliminating anti-Ig activity is important in view of the observations of Desjeux et al., (1980) who found anti-IgG antibodies in sera of patients with mucocutaneous leishmaniasis and Carvalho et al., (1983) who found "rheumatoid factor" like antibodies in sera from cases of visceral leishmaniasis.

Although other studies have demonstrated the presense of circulating immune complexes in cases of leishmaniasis no information on the nature of the antigen components of the complexes has been available. This study has provided evidence for two stage specific peptides of 20 and 52kDa. However, apart from the apparent molecular weights nothing else is known of those antigens. They may arise by parasite destruction and breakdown or alternatively they may be exoantigens continuously produced by intracellular amastigotes. Secreted antigens are well known from promastigotes but are also produced by amastigotes. Substantial amounts of amastigote derived exoantigens have been demonstrated, using immunohistochemical techniques, associated with plasma cells (Sells and Burton, 1981).

Further studies are in progress designed to characterise the antigens present in the circulation and to further refine the detecting reagent.

REFERENCES

Carvalho, E.M., Andrews, B.S., Martinelli, R., Dutra, M. & Rocha, H. 1983, Circulating immune complexes and rheumatoid factor in visceral leishmaniasis and schistosomiasis. Am. J. trop. Med. Hyg., 32: 61-68.

Casali, p. & Lambert, p.H. 1979, Purification of soluble immune complexes from serum using polymethylmetacrilate beads coated with conglutinin of Clq. Clin. Exp. Immunol., 37: 295-309

Craig, P.S. 1986, Detection of specific circulating antigen: immune complexes and antibodies in human hydatidosis from Turkana (Kenya) and Great Britain, by enzyme-immunoassay. Parasit. Immunol., 8: 171-188

Desjeux, P., Santoro, F., Afchain, D., Loyens, M. & Capron, A. 1980, Circulating immune complexes and anti IgG antibodies in mucocutaneous leishmaniasis. Am. J. trop. Med. Hyg., 29: 195-198

Galvao-Castro, B., S'a Ferreira, J.A., Marzochi, K.F., Marzochi, M.C., Coutinho, S.G. & Lambert, P.H. 1984, Polyclonal B-cell activation, circulating immune complexes and autoimmunity in human american visceral leishmaniasis. Clin. Exp. Immunol., 56: 58-66

Laemmli, U.K. 1970, Clevage of structural proteins during assembly of the head of bacteriophage T4. Nature (Lond.), 227: 680-685

Maidment, B.W., Papsidero, L.D. & Chu, T.M. 1980, Isoelectric focusing - A new approach to the study of immune complexes. J. Immunol. Methods, 35: 297-306

Sells, P.G. & Burton, M. 1980, Identification of Leishmania amastigotes and their antigens in formalin fixed tissue by immunoperoxidase staining. Trans. R. Soc. trop. Med. Hyg., 75: 461-468

Towbin, H. & Gordon, J. 1984, Immunoblotting and dot immunobinding: current status and outlook. J. Immunol. Methods, 72: 313-340

Voller, A. 1976, Serodiagnosis of malaria. In: Immunology of Parasitic Infections, (Eds. Cohen, S. & Sadun, E.), pp. 107-119, Blackwell Sci. Publ, Oxford.

THE 63kDa PROMASTIGOTE PROTEASE OF LESIHMANIA: ASSESSMENT OF HOST-PROTECTION IN BALB/c MICE USING LIPOSOMES AS ADJUVANT

L. P. Kahl, K-P. Chang* and F. Y. Liew

Department of Experimental Immunobiology, The Wellcome Research Laboratories, Langley Court, Beckenham, Kent BR3 3BS U.K.
*Department of Microbiology and Immunology, University of Health Sciences, The Chicago Medical School, North Chicago, IL 60064 U.S.A.

INTRODUCTION

The 63kDa membrane glycoprotein designated gp63 is a dominant surface antigen of Leishmania constituting 0.5 - 1.0% of total promastigote protein[1-3]. Structural features and the proteolytic function of gp63 were conservatively expressed across seven species of Leishmania (reviewed in ref. 4). The protein was implicated in attachment of L. mexicana mexicana and L. m. amazonensis promastigotes to macrophages[2,5]. A correlation between increased levels of both gp63 expression and its degree of N-glycosylation with the heightened virulence of tunicamycin-resistant L. m. amazonensis variants was observed[6].

The abundance and antigenic dominance of the protein together with its biological roles have posed gp63 as a candidate host-protective antigen of Leishmania. Here we report an evaluation of the efficacy of L. m. amazonensis derived gp63 in conferring protection against experimental murine cutaneous leishmaniasis. In this study, gp63 was administered either free or entraped within liposomes and the various immunised mice were challenged with either the homologous L. m. amazonesis or the heterologous L. major promastigotes.

MATERIALS AND METHODS

Leishmania Stocks and Maintenance

Leishmania mexicana amazonensis (LV78) and L. major (LV39) were obtained from Dr. D. Evans and Dr. R. Neal at the WHO Reference Centre cryobank maintained by the London School of Hygiene and Tropical Medicine. Promastigotes were maintained as described previously[2,7].

Purification of GP63

The 63kDa glycoprotein was purified from NP-40 extracts of L. m. amazonensis promastigotes by monoclonal antibody affinity chromatography (6H12-IgG-coupled Affi-Gel) as described previously[2]. The purified protein was stored either lyophilized or as aliquots of a 1 mg/ml suspension at -70°C for up to twelve weeks prior to immunisation of mice.

Preparation of GP63 Entraped within Liposomes

Liposomes were prepared as dehydration-rehydration vesicles (DRV) according to procedures described by Kirby and Gregoriadis[8,9]. DRV were composed of equimolar phosphatidylcholine distearoyl (DSPC) and cholesterol. Initial experiments involving preparation of DRV using phosphatidylcholine (PC) and its two derivatives DSPC and phosphatidylcholine dipalmitol (DPPC) and a crude extract of soluble L. major antigens revealed that DSPC liposomes were optimal for entrapment of L. major antigens, stability of the DRV preparation and for in vivo T cell priming. This was assessed by prepatency of lesion onset and the size of lesions developing following L. major challenge of immunised mice and by the magnitude of the secondary in vitro proliferative response of primed spleen cells to soluble L. major antigens.

DRV are mainly oligo- and multilamelar although their morphology may be influenced by experimental conditions. The vesicle size of DRV composed of equimolar PC and cholesterol was estimated to be 0.30 ± 0.28 [9]. Entrapment of gp63 into DRV was quantitated by the addition of an ^{125}I-labeled tracer to each DRV preparation[10]. Radioiodination was performed using iodogen[25] and all preparations of ^{125}I-gp63 tracer were 90-98% trichloracetic acid precipitable. Gamma counting of washed hydrated DRV facilitated calculation of entrapment which was 47% and 31% of the material added in experiments 1 and 2 respectively. In inital optimisation experiments, stability of the various DRV preparations was assessed by incorporating 50μl of 0.24M 6-carboxyfluorescein (CF) into the DRV mixture (500μl) followed by fluorimetric analysis. Latency of CF entraped within DSPC liposomes was determined to be 75%. Liposomes with latency values of 70-90% are considered to be stable[9].

Immunisation of Mice and Challenge Infection

All mice used in this study were BALB/c females, eight weeks of age. Mice were obtained from the inbred mouse colonies maintained at The Wellcome Research Laboratories, Beckenham. Two vaccination experiments involving five to seven mice per group were performed. The first involved intravenous (i.v.) immunisation with the following: gp63 in phosphate buffered saline (PBS, 4μg protein); gp63 (4μg) entraped within DSPC liposomes (2.15mg DSPC, lipid:protein = 539:1); empty DSPC liposomes (2.15mg DSPC) and 2×10^7 γ-irradiated (150KRD) L. major. Two injections were given eight days apart and together with controls, immunised mice were challenged with 2×10^5 stationary phase L. major promastigotes thirteen days after the booster immunisation. The parasites were injected subcutaneously on the shaved rump.

In the second experiment, groups of five to seven mice were immunised either four times i.v. or four times subcutaneously (s.c.) with the following: gp63 in PBS (3.5μg protein); gp63 (3.5μg) entraped within DSPC liposomes (1.80mg DSPC, lipid:protein = 507:1); empty DSPC liposomes (1.80mg DSPC) and 2×10^7 irradiated (150 KRD) L. m. amazonensis. The secondary and the two booster immunisations were administered at 7-10 day intervals. Immunised mice, together with naive controls, were challenged with 2×10^6 stationary phase L. m. amazonensis promastigotes seven days after the last injection. In a parallel experiment groups of five naive mice were infected with 2×10^6, 2×10^5, 2×10^4 or 2×10^3 L. m. amazonensis promastigotes harvested from the same stationary phase culture used to prepare the challenge inoculum for the gp63 immunised mice. For all experiments, lesion development in each infected mouse was monitored by measurement of the maximum and minimum lesion diameter. The average lesion diameter for each mouse provided the mean average diameter ± standard error for each group.

RESULTS AND DISCUSSION

The size of lesions developing following L. major infection of mice twice i.v.

immunised with 4 μg of gp63 either free or entraped within liposomes, or with empty liposomes was not significantly retarded compared with that of non-immunised controls throughout a 94 day period of observation. Prepatent periods of lesion onset were similar for all groups with the exception of mice receiving gp63 in PBS. Two of the five mice in this group exhibited a fourteen day acceleration of lesion onset. Although by day 72 and 94 post infection the mean lesion diameter of this group together with those of liposome (+/- gp63) immunised mice did not significantly differ from that of non-immunised controls (data not shown). The lack of protection observed in this experiment may have been due to inadequate antigenic stimulus by two injections of 4 μg of gp63 or, as the gp63 used was purified from L. m. amazonensis, due to the heterologous nature of the challenge. Cross-species reactivity of gp63 for the humoral response had been documented[4]. However, the cross-species reactivity of T cell determinants expressed by gp63 was not known. L. major and L. m. amazonensis derived gp63 may well express both common and species specific T cell stimulatory determinants with recognition of both sets being a prerequisite for curative cell mediated responses. This may be of particular importance in the murine model system studied as the high susceptibility of the BALB/c mice would constitute a stringent test system for any candidate host-protective antigen. Nevertheless, the effectiveness of the γ-irradiated promastigote vaccine in this system has been well documented[11-13] and a defined antigen vaccine would require a similar efficacy. Therefore, a second experiment involving four i.v. injections of gp63 +/- liposomes and homologous L. m. amazonensis challenge was performed.

Purified gp63 conferred only a weak partial protection against the homologous challenge when administered either i.v. or s.c. in PBS without adjuvant. Prepatent periods of lesion onset were similar for both gp63 immunised and control mice but the size of lesions developing in gp63 immunised mice was generally smaller than that observed for controls during the first thirty days of lesion development (days 46-75 post infection; Figure 1a) thereafter lesion size did not differ significantly between the two groups. This weak protection was enhanced by i.v. but not by s.c. administration of gp63 entraped within liposomes (Figure 1a and 1b). Lesion development was delayed by fourteen days and maintained at a size significantly smaller than that of the control group throughout the course of the experiment. Similarly at day 60, 88 and 100, post infection lesions developing in gp63/liposome i.v. immunised mice were significantly smaller than those developing in gp63/PBS i.v. immunised mice (Figure 1a). Although complete protection was not achieved, the data are consistent with an adjuvant effect of DSPC liposomes in T cell priming for a secondary in vivo response to gp63. This i.v. priming was specific for gp63 as i.v. administration of an equal dose of lipid as empty liposomes had no effect (Figure 1a). However, s.c. administration of the same dose of empty liposomes effected a seven day delay in lesion onset and maintenance of lesion size at a level significantly smaller than controls over the first eighty days of infection. Indeed, during this period, the size of lesions developing in gp63/liposome i.v. immunised mice and in empty liposome s.c. immunised mice were very similar (Figure 1b). This indicated that s.c. but not i.v. injection of DSPC liposomes produced a local non-specific activation of effector cells for a leishmanicidal response. In an earlier report liposomes composed of PC/Phosphatidylserine (PS) were found to completely and selectively abrogate lymphokine-induced macrophage microbicidal activity against amastigotes of L. major however, PC liposomes were not suppressive[14]. To our knowledge, there has been no other report of an enhancement of macrophage leishmanicidal activity by s.c. administration of DSPC liposomes. Entrapment of gp63 within liposomes prior to s.c. immunisation eliminated this effect (Figure 1b) suggesting the presence of non-protective determinants of gp63 which preferentially prime T cells when administered in conjnction with DSPC by the s.c. route.

Lesion development in mice immunised i.v. with gp63/liposomes or s.c. with liposomes alone was similar to that obtained following infection of naive mice with 2×10^5 promastigotes (Figure 1b and 1c) suggesting that these procedures primed the BALB/c mouse for cellular responses which effected approximately a tenfold

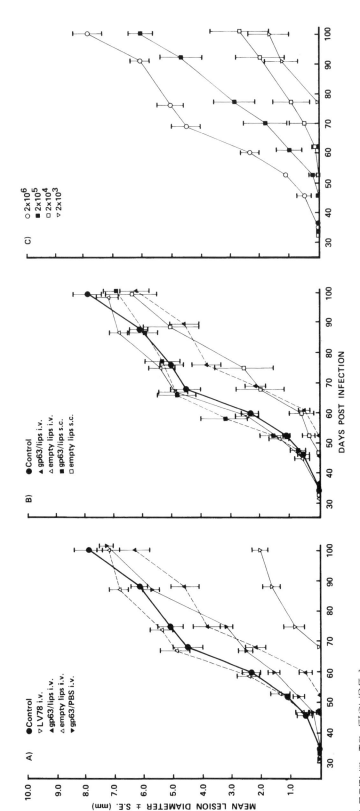

LEGEND TO FIGURE 1

Lesion development in BALB/c mice infected with L. mexicana amazonensis (LV78)

(a) Following four intravenous immunisations with: gp63 (3.5 g) entraped within DSPC liposomes; empty DSPC liposomes; 2×10^7 γ-irradiated LV78 promastigotes, or no immunisation and infection with 2×10^6 LV78 promastigotes.

(b) Following four intravenous or four subcutaneous immunisations with gp63 (3.5 g) entraped within DSPC liposomes or no immunisation and infection with 2×10^6 LV78 promastigotes.

(c) Following infection of naive mice with 2×10^6, 2×10^5, 2×10^4 or 2×10^3 LV78 promastigotes. All promastigotes used for the challenge were harvested from the same stationary phase in vitro culture.

reduction in infectivity of the challenge inoculum. Together the data suggest two independant mechanisms: (i) antigen specific priming of splenic T lymphocytes; and (ii) local s.c. activation of macrophages for leishmanicidal action. Whether or not this is the case and a possible synergy of the two remains to be established.

The protection induced by i.v. immunisation with γ-irradiated promastigotes was stronger than that produced by the various injections with gp63. The characteristics of lesion development in this group were similar to those observed following infection of naive mice with 2×10^3 promastigotes (Figure 1a and 1c) suggesting that the i.v. immunisation with γ-irradiated promastigotes effectively primed the highly susceptible BALB/c mouse for cellular responses which conferred a 700-1,000-fold decrease in infectivity of the challenge inoculum.

CONCLUSIONS

The data described in this report suggest that the 63kDa promastigote glycoprotein is of relevance in immunity against experimental cutaneous leishmaniasis. Both host-protective and non-protective determinants may be expressed on the glycoprotein. Further work is required to confirm this and to identify such determinants. The utility of s.c. administration of DSPC liposomes in promoting leishmanicidal macrophage activity warrants further examination. Nevertheless, the salient point from this study is that purified gp63 (+/- liposomes) was not able to confer a level of protection against challenge infection which approached that achieved using irradiated promastigotes as immunogen. We suggest that gp63 (or carefully identified fragments of the glycoprotein) should be present in, though not as the sole component of, a defined antigen preparation for vaccination against cutaneous leishmaniasis.

ACKNOWLEDGEMENTS

We thank Professor G. Gregoriadis and members of his laboratory at the Academic Department of Medicine, Royal Free Hospital School of Medicine, University of London, Pond Street, London NW3 2QG, for procedures and advice concerning preparation of liposomes. This investigation received financial support from the UNDP/World Bank/WHO Special Programme for Research and Training in Tropical Diseases.

REFERENCES

1. Etges, R. J., Bouvier, J., Hoffman, R. and Bordier, C. Evidence that the major surface proteins of three Leishmania species are structurally related. Mol. Biochem. Parasitol. 14:141 (1985).
2. Chang, C. S. and Chang, K-P. Monoclonal antibody affinity purification of a Leishmania membrane glycoprotein and its inhibition of Leishmania-macrophage binding. Proc. Natnl. Acad. Sci. USA 83:100 (1986).
3. Bouvier, J., Etges, R. and Bordier, C. Identification and purification of membrane and soluble forms of the major surface protein of Leishmania promastigotes. J. Biol. Chem. 260:15504 (1985).
4. Bordier, C. The promastigote surface protease of Leishmania. Parasitol. Today 3:151 (1987).
5. Russell, D. G. and Wilhelm, H. The involvement of the major surface glycoprotein (gp63) of Leishmania promastigotes in attachment to macrophages. J. Immunol. 136:2613 (1986).
6. Kink, J. A. and Chang, K-P. Biological and biochemical characterisation of tunicamycin-resistant Leishmania mexicana: mechanism of drug resistance and virulence. Infect. Immun. 55:1692 (1987).
7. Kahl, L. P. and McMahon-Pratt, D. Structural and antigenic characterisation of a species- and promastigote-specific Leishmania mexicana amazonensis membrane protein. J. Immunol. 138:1587 (1987).
8. Kirby, C. J. and Gregoriadis, G. A simple procedure for preparing liposomes

capable of high encapsulation efficiency under mild conditions. In: Liposome Technology, Vol. I., G. Gregoriadis, Ed., CRC Press, Inc., Boca Raton, FL. (1984).

9. Kirby, C. and Gregoriadis, G. Dehydration-rehydration vesicles: a simple method for high yield drug entrapment in liposomes. Bio. Technol. p.979, Nov. (1984).

10. Fraker, P. J. and Speck, J. C. Protein and cell membrane iodination with a sparingly soluble chloroamide, 1, 3, 4, 6 -tetrachloro-3α, 6 α-diphenylglycoluril. Biochem. Biophys. Res. Commun. 80:849 (1978).

11. Howard, J. G., Nicklin, S., Hale, C. and Liew, F. Y. Prophylactic immunisation against experimental leishmaniasis. I. Protection induced in mice genetically vulnerable to fatal Leishmania tropica infection. J. Immunol. 129:2206 (1982).

12. Liew, F. Y., Howard, J. G. and Hale, C. Prophylactic immunisation against experimental leishmaniasis. III. Protection against fatal Leishmania tropica infection induced by irradiated promastigotes involves $Lyt-1^+2^-$ T cells that do not mediate cutaneous DTH. J. Immunol. 132:456 (1984).

13. Liew, F.Y. Immunological regulation of cutaneous Leishmaniasis. In: Host Resistance Mechanisms. (eds. R. M. Steinman and R. North) Rockefeller Press, New York. pp. 305 (1986).

14. Gilbreath, M. J., Hoover, D. L., Alving, C. R., Swartz, G. M. Jr. and Meltzer, M. S. Inhibition of lymphokine-induced macrophage microbial activity against Leishmania major by liposomes: characterisation of the physicochemical requirements for liposome inhibition. J. Immunol. 137:1681 (1986).

STUDIES ON ANTIGENICITY OF AMPHIPHILIC AND HYDROPHILIC FORMS OF LEISH-

MANIA MAJOR PROMASTIGOTE SURFACE PROTEASE IN THE MOUSE

Denis Rivier, Serge Didisheim, Robert Etges, Clément Bordier, and Jacques Mauël

Institut de Biochimie, Université de Lausanne
CH-1066 Epalinges (Switzerland)

INTRODUCTION

Immunity which develops in CBA mice recovering from Leishmania major infections is, at least partly, T-cell mediated (1). The nature of the parasite antigens that elicit such protective immunity remains however to be determined.

Among the surface molecules of Leishmania promastigotes, an active protease (2) has been described in all species examined so far (3). This promastigote surface protease (PSP) appears to be expressed in higher amounts in the infective form of Leishmania (4) and to be involved in attachment of Leishmania to macrophages, triggering phagocytosis in vitro (5). This molecule can also be used to induce protection against Leishmania infections in mice (Russel et al., personal communication).

In addition, PSP belongs to the growing family of phospholipid-anchored membrane proteins and the hydrophilic form (H-PSP) can be generated from the natural amphiphilic protein (A-PSP) by treatment with inositol specific phospholipase C (6).

In the work presented here, the proliferative assay developed by Corradin et al. (7) was used to study the T-cell response of mice to PSP. We show that proliferation of lymph node cells derived from CBA mice immunized with the amphiphilic or hydrophilic molecule could be induced in vitro by either form of this important Leishmania antigen.

MATERIALS AND METHODS

1 Animals

CBA/T6 mice were obtained from the Swiss Institute for Experimental Cancer Research, Epalinges, Switzerland. Two to three month old mice of either sex were used throughout the experiments

2 Materials

Ovalbumin was purchased from Sigma (St Louis, MO, USA) and Concanavalin A (Con A) was obtained from Pharmacia (Uppsala, Sweden). Complete Freund's adjuvant (CFA) was purchased from Difco Laboratories (Detroit,

MI, USA). Lauryldodecylamine N-oxyde (LDAO) used in the course of purification of PSP was purchased from Fluka (Switzerland).
Phospholipase C (EC 3.1.4.3) preparation Type III from B. Cereus was obtained from Sigma.

3 Parasites

Leishmania major (LV39) isolated from the foot-pads of infected mice were maintained in vitro at 26°C in liquid overlay (Dulbecco's medium) on blood agar (8). Washed promastigotes (50×10^6/ml) in Dulbecco's medium, frozen and thawed three to five times were used as a "total antigen" in the study of lymphocyte proliferation in vitro. Bulk cultures of promastigotes of Leishmania major (LEM 513) were grown at room temperature (ca 25°C) in modified Schaefer's medium (9) in which the erythrocyte lysate was replaced by hemin (6.25 mg/l) and folic acid (12.5 mg/l). Gentamycin sulfate (Sigma, 50 mg/ml) was used as a source of antibiotics. The medium was supplemented with 5% decomplemented foetal or new born calf serum.

4 Purification of promastigote surface protease (PSP)

Washed late log-phase LEM 513 promastigotes were solublilized in 2% Triton X-114 in Tris-HCl buffer, and submitted to phase separation (10,11). PSP contained in the detergent phase was isolated by fast protein liquid chromatography (FPLC) as described by Etges (12). In brief, the detergent phase was diluted approximately 5-fold in 10 mM Tris-HCl, 2.2 mM LDAO, pH 7.5 (DEAE buffer) and then loaded on a column of Fractogel TSK DEAE-650 (S) (Merck, Darmstadt, FRG). Bound proteins were eluted with a gradient of 0-500 mM NaCl in DEAE buffer. Fractions containing PSP were detected by their protease activity. For this determination, the test used was based on the property of PSP to clarify or clot milk powder solutions, by hydrolysis of casein (Bordier et al., unpublished). Pooled DEAE fractions containing protease activity were adjusted to pH 8.0 and diluted 3-fold with 10 mM Tris-HCl, 2.2 mM LDAO, pH 8.0 (Mono Q buffer I) before being applied to a column of Mono Q (Pharmacia, Uppsala, Sweden). Bound proteins were eluted with a gradient of NaCl in Mono Q buffer I. Fractions containing A-PSP were rerun on Mono Q under the same conditions and the resulting A-PSP preparation (in 10 mM Tris-HCl buffer containing 2.2 mM LDAO) was used to immunize mice.

5 Isolation of the amphilic form of PSP (A-PSP) in detergent-free buffer

The preceding preparation of A-PSP was submitted to a final run on Mono Q preequilibrated by extensive washings with 10 mM Hepes, pH 8.0 (Mono Q buffer II containing no detergent). Bound PSP was eluted with a gradient of 0-500 mM NaCl in Mono Q buffer II. This preparation was used throughout the experiments as an antigen for inducing the proliferation in vitro of primed lymph node cells.

6 Conversion of A-PSP by phospholipase C treatment

Phospholipase C was used to generate H-PSP from A-PSP isolated in 10 mM Tris-HCl buffer containing 2.2 mM LDAO (see Materials and Methods, section 4). The pH was adjusted to 6.8 and the final NaCl concentration was 175 mM. The concentration of phospholipase C (3 U/ml) and the duration of the assay (40 min at 30°C) were selected on the basis of previous experiments by Etges et al. (13). Under such conditions, we found that the digestion of 50 to 500 µg of A-PSP per ml of reaction mixture resulted in the transformation of approximately 60% of the protein into its hydrophilic form (H-PSP), as measured by Triton X-114 phase separation methodology (13).

7 Purification of H-PSP

H-PSP generated as described above was isolated from A-PSP by FPLC. The reaction mixture containing both forms of PSP diluted 4-fold in Mono Q buffer I was loaded on a mono Q column. Elution was performed with a gradient of NaCl in Mono Q buffer I, such that bound H-PSP was eluted at approximately 170 mM, while the undigested protein was eluted at higher salt concentration (ca 200 mM) allowing separation of the two molecules. After appropriate dilution in Mono Q buffer II, the H-PSP fractions were submitted to another run on the same Mono Q column as before, but preequilibrated with detergent-free Mono Q buffer II. A final run was performed under the same buffer conditions on a Mono Q column reserved for purification of samples in the absence of detergent. The preparation of H-PSP obtained by this procedure was used for stimulation of lymphocytes in culture as well as for immunization of mice.

8 Sodium dodecyl sulfate-polyacrylamide gel electrophoresis (SDS-PAGE)

SDS-PAGE (7,5 - 15% polyacrylamide linear gradient) was used to analyse the preparations of PSP obtained by the methods described in the previous sections. Prior to SDS-PAGE analysis, part of the samples were heated (100°C for 5 min) and reduced with 1% 2-mercaptoethanol. Under these conditions, amphiphilic and hydrophilic preparations displayed the characteristic migration patterns reported by Bouvier et al. (14). No contaminating protein could be detected after Coomassie Blue staining.

9 Immunization of mice

Purified antigens (A-PSP in 2.2 mM LDAO, purified H-PSP or ovalbumin, OVA) were emulsified in an equal volume of complete Freund's adjuvant (CFA). A total volume of approximately 50 µl was injected subcutaneously at the base of the tail of CBA/T6 mice. Each mouse received a single injection containing 4.5 µg of PSP or 100 µg of OVA.

10 Induction of lymphocyte proliferation in vitro

Ten to thirteen days after immunization, the mice were sacrificed and their inguinal and periaortic lymph node cells were cultured essentially as described by Louis et al. (15). Normal mouse serum (NMS) was used at a concentration of 0.5% to supplement the enriched Dulbecco's modified Eagle's medium (D-MEM). T-cell activation by antigens added to the culture was quantified by the measurement of ^{3}H-methylthymidine (^{3}H-TdR) uptake (7).

RESULTS

1 Proliferative responses of primed lymph node cells induced by A-PSP

Inguinal and periaortic lymph node cells (LNC) prepared from mice immunized with a single injection of 4.5 µg of A-PSP in CFA were exposed in vitro to various dilutions of purified A-PSP. Although this preparation was eluted from a Mono Q column in a buffer without detergent (see Materials and Methods, section 5), it was found to inhibit strongly the Con A (1 µg/ml)-induced proliferation of LNC up to 1/100 dilution (corresponding to an antigen concentration of 18 µg/ml). We observed the same effect with Mono Q fractions from the same run containing no PSP. We concluded that the toxic effect was not due to PSP but to solutes (probably detergent) released in the antigen-containing samples during the Mono Q chromatography purification step.

By further diluting the preparation of A-PSP used as antigen in vitro, a strong proliferative response of A-PSP-primed LNC could be observed (figure 1). The maximum response (5 to 20-fold increase over values obtained when no antigen was added to the cultures) was induced at a concentration of PSP of around 0.3 µg/ml. Interestingly, a suspension of "total L.major antigens", obtained by freeze-and-thawing of whole parasite was also able to induce proliferation in vitro of LNC primed in vivo with purified PSP (figure 1, table 1). Knowing the amount of PSP contained in L.major (0.01 to 0.1 µg/10^6 promastigotes), it was possible to determine that stimulation by both purified A-PSP and total antigen occured in cultures containing PSP in the same range of concentrations.

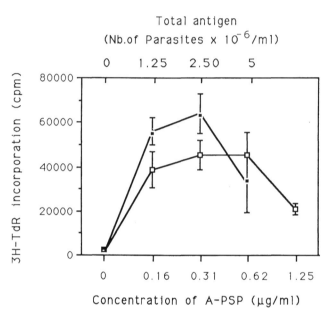

Figure 1. Proliferative response of A-PSP-primed lymph node cells (LNC) from CBA/T6 mice as a function of L.major antigen concentration in culture. LNC were tested in vitro with purified A-PSP (□——□) or "total antigen" from L.major (■——■). Stimulation was assessed after 3 days of culture by the measurement of ^{3}H-thymidine (^{3}H-TdR) uptake. Vertical bars represent the limits of one standard deviation for triplicate culture determinations.

LNC from CBA mice immunized 12 days earlier with purified A-PSP were used for a kinetic study of lymphocyte proliferation in vitro. The maximal response to A-PSP (at an optimal concentration of 0.3 µg/ml) was obtained after 3 to 4 days of culture, not taking into account the 16-h pulse of thymidine. After 5 days of culture, it was observed that the amount of thymidine incorporated by the stimulated cells tarted to decrease (figure 2).

2 Comparison of the proliferative responses of PSP-primed LNC induced by both A-PSP and H-PSP

Preliminary experiments demonstrated that H-PSP obtained as described in Materials and Methods, section 7, did not display the toxic effects observed previously with the A-PSP preparation (see Results, section 1). We attributed this to the fact that a new, detergent-free Mono Q column was used for the final purification step. Under such conditions, the hydrophilic form of PSP could be tested in culture at concentrations as high as 50 µg/ml (corresponding to a 1:10 dilution of the original antigen solution). H-PSP was much less effective than A-PSP at inducing a proliferative response in LNC from A-PSP immunized animals, i.e. the concentration of H-PSP necessary to achieve maximal proliferation was approximately

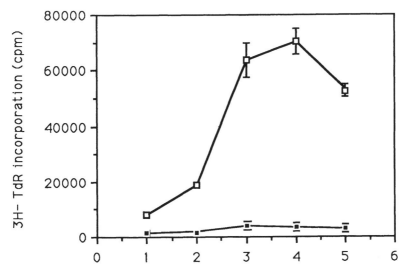

Figure 2. Kinetics of the proliferative response to A-PSP of L.major. CBA/T6 mice were immunized with A-PSP in CFA. Twelve days later their LNC were tested for antigen-induced proliferation. Stimulation with an optimal dose (0.3 µg/ml) of A-PSP (□——□) or no antigen added to the cultures (■——■) was assessed after various times by the measurement of ^{3}H-TdR incorporation using a 16-h pulse.

100-fold higher than when using A-PSP as antigen (data not shown). In order to test whether this could be due to loss of antigenicity of PSP upon phospholipase C treatment, CBA mice were immunized with H-PSP instead of A-PSP and the proliferative responses of their LNC to both forms of antigen tested in vitro. Vigourous responses to H-PSP and also to A-PSP were recorded, with incorporation of thymidine increasing up to 6-fold (H-PSP) or 11-fold (A-PSP) over background values (Table 1). However, the optimal concentrations of H-PSP for in vitro stimulation were high, ranging from 3 to 12 µg/ml. In contrast, A-PSP was inducing maximum response at a concentration as low as 0.3 µg/ml of culture medium. LNC from mice immunized with H-PSP could also respond to the "total antigen" preparation of L.major (Table 1).

Table 1

Specificity of the in vitro PSP-induced proliferation of in vivo primed lymph node cells[a]

Antigen in culture	^{3}H-thymidine incorporation (CPM x 10^{-3})		
	Immunogen[a]		
	A-PSP	H-PSP	OVA
No antigen added	5.2 ± 0.2	3.0 ± 0.2	14.4 ± 7.4
A-PSP (0.3 µg/ml)	61.2 ± 7.6	44.6 ± 7.4	8.5 ± 1.9
H-PSP (6 µg/ml)	13.3*	26.3*	6.5*
"Total antigen" preparation from L.major (0.5 x 10^6 parasites/well)	62.3 ± 4.5	37.4 ± 4.2	6.4 ± 1.8
OVA (500 µg/ml)	5.4 ± 1.2	NT	67.1 ± 20.4

[a] Groups of three CBA/T6 mice each were immunized at the base of the tail either with 4.5 µg of Leishmania promastigote surface protease, amphiphilic (A-PSP) or hydrophilic (H-PSP) or with ovalbumin (OVA) in CFA. Lymph node cells (LNC), derived from these mice 12 (A-PSP, OVA) or 13 (H-PSP) days later, were tested for antigen-induced proliferation. After 3 days of stimulation of LNC in vitro with various antigenic preparations, incorporation of ^{3}H-thymidine was measured using a 16-h pulse. Each value represents the average ± standard deviation of triplicate cultures) or the average (*) of duplicate cultures (variations less than 20%).

In order to study the specificity of the proliferative responses elicited by both the hydrophilic and amphiphilic forms of PSP, LNC from mice immunized with either PSP, or ovalbumin (OVA) were exposed in vitro to homologous or heterologous antigens.
Results reported in Table 1 indicate that LNC primed in vivo with PSP responded to PSP and not to OVA, while LNC primed with OVA responded only to OVA. The proliferative response of LNC from mice immunized against either of these molecules was thus strictly antigen-specific.

DISCUSSION

This report shows that mice primed by injection of the promastigote surface protease (emuslsified in CFA) develop a strong cellular immune response against this molecule, as tested in a lymphoproliferative assay in vitro. Interestingly, a preparation of L.major "total parasite antigen", obtained by freeze-and-thawing whole promastigotes, stimulated the proliferation of PSP-primed lymph node cells to the same extent as the purified molecule. Although the T-cell response of infected animals to PSP remains to be evaluated, PSP can already be regarded as a potent immunogen. Moreover, the observation that PSP-primed mice respond well to whole parasite antigen opens the way to further investigations of the possible immunoprophylactic potential of this material.

Both the hydrophilic and amphiphilic forms of PSP were able to stimulate the proliferation of primed LNC, although the amphiphilic PSP was active at much lower concentration than the phospholipase-digested molecule deprived of its phospholipid anchor. Conceivably, the phospholipid moiety of A-PSP might promote the incorporation of the molecule in the membrane of antigen-presenting cells in such a way that presentation to T-lymphocytes would be improved. The recent results of Carbone et al. (1987) argue in favor of this possibility. These authors have shown that addition of a leader sequence to a cytochrome c-derived peptide led to a 1000-fold increase in the capacity of the molecule to induce the proliferation of a cytochrome c-specific T-cell clone. Concomitantly, a 10-fold increase in binding to liposomes was noted.

In contrast, the hydrophilic PSP would be processed by macrophages like other water-soluble antigens. For such antigens (e.g. human gammaglobulin or cytochrome c), the concentrations required for inducing maximal proliferation of primed LNC *in vitro* may be quite high, ranging from 100 to 500 µg/ml (7). High concentrations of hydrophilic antigens might be necessary to achieve an epitope density sufficient for inducing proliferation, because of losses occuring during antigen processing by macrophages.

ACKNOWLEDGEMENTS

We would like to thank Ms T. Van Pham for advices and help in the establishment of the cell proliferative assay, and Ms A. Ransijn for occasional technical help. The work was supported by grant No. 3.172-0.85 from the Swiss National Science Foundation.

REFERENCES

1. F.Y. Liew, C. Hale, and J.G. Howard, Immunologic regulation of experimental cutaneous leishmaniasis, V. Characterization of effector and specific suppressor T cells, J. Immunol. 128:1917 (1982).

2. R. Etges, J. Bouvier, and C. Bordier, The major surface protein of *Leishmania* promastigotes is a protease, J. Biol. Chem. 261:9098 (1986).

3. J. Bouvier, R. Etges, and C. Bordier, Identification of the promastigote surface protease in seven species of *Leishmania,* Mol. Biochem. Parasitol. 24:73 (1987).

4. M. Kweider, J.L. Lemesre, F. Darcy, J.-P. Kusnierz, A. Capron, and F. Santoro, Infectivity of *Leishmania braziliensis* promastigotes is dependent on the increasing expression of a 65,000-dalton surface antigen, J. Immunol. 138:299 (1987).

5. D.G. Russell and H. Wilhelm, The involvement of the major surface protein (gp63) of *Leishmania* promastigotes in attachment to macrophages, J. Immunol. 136:2613 (1986).

6. C. Bordier, R. Etges, J. Ward, M.J. Turner, and M.L. Cardoso de Almeida, *Leishmania* and *Trypanosoma* surface glycoproteins have a common glycophospholipid membrane anchor, Proc. Natl. Acad. Sci. USA 83:5988 (1986).

7. G. Corradin, H.M. Etlinger, and J.M. Chiller, Lymphocyte specificity to protein antigens I. Characterization of the antigen-induced in vitro T-cell dependent proliferative response with lymph node cells from primed mice, J. Immunol. 119:1048 (1977).

8. R. Behin, J. Mauël, and B. Sordat, Leishmania tropica: pathogenicity and in-vitro macrophage function in strains of inbred mice, Experimental Parasitology 48:81 (1979).

9. F.W.III Schaefer, E.J. Bell, and E.J. Etges, Leishmania tropica: chemostatic cultivation, Exp. parasitol. 28:465 (1970).

10. R. Etges, J. Bouvier, R. Hoffman, and C. Bordier, Evidence that the major surface proteins of three Leishmania species are structurally related, Mol. Biochem. Parasitol. 14:141 (1985).

11. C. Bordier, Phase separation of integral membrane proteins in Triton X-114 solution, J. Biol. Chem. 256:1604 (1981).

12. R. Etges, Identification and partial characterization of the surface protease of Leishmania promastigotes, Ph.D. thesis (1987).

13. R. Etges, J. Bouvier, and C. Bordier, The major surface protein of Leishmania promastigotes is anchored in the membrane by a myristic acid-labeled phospholipid, EMBO J. 5:597 (1986).

14. J. Bouvier, R. Etges, and C. Bordier, Identification and purification of membrane and soluble forms of the major surface protein of Leishmania promastigotes, J. Biol. Chem. 260:15504 (1985).

15. J. Louis, E. Moedder, R. Behin, and H. Engers, Recognition of protozoan parasite antigens by murine T lymphocytes I. Induction of specific T lymphocyte-dependent proliferative response to Leishmania tropica, Eur. J. Immunol. 9:841 (1979).

16. F.R. Carbone, B.S. Fox, R.H. Schwartz, and Y. Paterson, The use of hydrophobic, -helix-defined peptides in delineating the T cell determinant for pigeon cytochrome c, J. Immunol. 138:1838 (1987).

HISTOPATHOGENIC MECHANISMS IN AMERICAN CUTANEOUS LEISHMANIASIS OF MICE

Amalia Monroy-Ostria, Eva Velez-Castro
and Teresa Monroy-Ostria

Departamento de Inmunologia
Escuela Nacional de Ciencias Biologicas, IPN
Mexico City
Mexico

INTRODUCTION

The appearance of specific clinical types of American cutaneous leishmaniasis depends on host genetic factors and the virulence of the parasite. Bradley et al (1979), showed, in mice, that resistance to *Leishmania donovani* is controlled by autosomic gene localized on chromosome 1, designed at Lsh gene. This gene also controls resistance to *Salmonella typhimurium*, *Mycobacteirum bovis* and *Mycobacterium lepraemurium* in mice. It seems that this gene does not have any effect in *Leishmani major* and *Leishmania mexicana* infections. Susceptibility to *Leishmania major* is controlled by the Scl gene which is found on chromosome 8. It also influences infection by *Leishmania mexicana*.

We do not know how these genes act whether directly on the macrophage or possibly eosiniphils, which are involved in host immunological responses mainly in helminthiasis. A few protozoan infectins have been shown to induce an eosinophilic reaction. Grimali et al (1980), demonstrated that histological alterations of cutaneous lesion caused by *Leishmania mexicana mexicana* in C3H mice were characterized by a diffuse mononuclear inflammation with neutrophils and eosinophils. We have performed histological studies of *Leishmania mexicana mexicana* in BALB/c and C57Bl/6 mice performed and found difference in susceptibility.

MATERIALS AND METHODS

Parasites

A strain of *Leishmania mexicana mexicana*, kindly supplied by Dr. Roderigo Zeledon was used (Zeledon et al, 1982). The parasite was maintained by intradermal injection of 3×10^6 amstigotes in phosphate buffered saline (PBS) into the foot pad of golden hamsters. The promastigotes were maintained in RPMI with 13% fetal calf serum.

Antigens

Antigen preparation was as described by Monroy (1983) Briefly: promastigotes at 7 days of culture were washed 3 times with PBS pH 7.2, resuspended in the same solution, frozen and thawed several times until they disintegrated and spun down at 105 000 g for 1 h at 4oC. The supernatant was called soluble antigen (SA) and the pellet insoluble antigen (IA). The promastigotes were washed as above and sonicated 3 times for 1 min periods and spun down as above. Seven day promastigotes were washed 3 times with PBS pH 7.3, smeared on glass slides, allowed to dry, fixed with methanol for 15 min and washed with PBS, pH 7.2

Experimental infection

Female BALB/c, C57Bl/6 and (C57Bl/6 X BALB/c) Fl mice weighing about 20 g, were infected introdermally in the foot pad with 3.5×10^6 or 7.4×10^6 amstigotes in 0.05 ml PBS pH 7.3. The infection was followed by measuring the thickness of the inoculation site every 7 days for 13 weeks. Skin samples were taken from 4 animals of each strain. Half of each sample was fixed with buffered formalin and prepared by conventional techniques for histologicals studies, the other half for electron microscopy studies (Monroy *et al*, 1980).

Skin test

Skin tests were done by intradermal injection of 50 ug of SA (Perez et al, 1978), in the foot pad of infected and uninfected mice, every 15 days for 10 weeks. Skin reactions measured with calipers at 4, 24 and 48 h.

Serum antibodies

Serum antibodies were detected by an indirect immunofluorescent antibody technique as described by Monroy (1983).

RESULTS

With an infection of 3.5×10^6 amastigotes, a nodule developed at the inoculation site in the foot pad after 2 weeks of infection. It grew faster in BALB/c mice than C57BL/6. At 7 weeks the overlaying skin became keratotic, the lesion in the BALB/c ulcerated (small ulcers from 1 to 2 mm in diameter). At 6 weeks the lesion reached its maximum size and the BALB/c mice showed metastasic lesions in the tail and other extremities.

Histology of the lesion 2 weeks after infection in both strains of mice showed an intact epidermis. In the centre of the dermis there were abundant polymorphonuclear cells (PMN) and mononuclear cells (MN) and abundant mature macrophages

Table 1. Histology of skin lesion produced by Leishmania mexicana mexicana in BALB/c and C57Bl/6 mice infected with 3.5 x 10^6 amastigotes.

Time of infection (weeks)	Fibrosis	Necrosis	Parasites	Macrophages	Epithelioid cells	Plasma cells	Lympho-cytes	Giant cells	PMN	Eosinophils
BALB/c										
2	+	+	++	+++	++	+	+	-	+++	
4	-	+	+++	+++	++	+	+	+	++	
6	++	+	+++	+++	++	+	+	+	-	+++
8	++	+	+++	+++	+++	++	+	+	-	++
10	+++	+	+++	+++	+++	++	++	++	-	++
13	+++	+	+++	+++	+++	+++	++	++	-	++
C57Bl/6										
2	+	++	++	+++	++	+	+	-	+++	+++
4	+	+++	++	+++	++	+	+	+	+	+++
6	+	+++	+++	+++	+++	+	++	+	-	+++
8	++	++	+++	+++	+++	+	++	+	-	+++
10	+++	+	+++	+++	+++	++	++	++	-	+++
13	+++	+	+++	+++	+++	+++	+	+	-	+++

The cells were scored as follow: (+)=scanty; (++)=moderate (+++)=abundant.
The necrosis as: (+)=small area; (++)=moderate area; (+++)= extensive
The fibrosis as: (+)=scanty; (++)=moderate ; (+++)=abundant
Parasites as: (+)= 5 to 10 per parasitophorous vacuole (++)= 10 to 20 and (+++)= more than 20

Table 2.- Histology of the skin lesion produced by Leishmania mexicana mexicana in BALB/c, C57Bl/6 and F1 mice infected intradermally with 7.3×10^6 amastigotes.

Time of infection (weeks)	Fibrosis	Necrosis	Parasites	Macrophages	Epithelioid cells	Plasma cells	Lympo-cytes	Giant cells	PMN	Eosinophils
BALB/c										
2	-	+	+++	+++	+++	+	+	-	+++	+++
6	+	+	+++	+++	++	+	+	+	-	++
8	++	+	+++	+++	+++	++	++	++	-	++
10	+++	+	+++	+++	+	++	+	++	-	++
C57Bl/6										
2	+	+	+++	+++	+	+	+	-	+++	+++
6	+	+	+++	+++	++	+	+	+	-	++
8	+	+	+++	+++	++	+	+	++	-	++
10	++	+	+++	+++	+	+	+++	+	-	++
F1										
3	++	++	++	+++	++	+	+	-	+++	+++
6	++	++	++	+++	++	+	++	+	-	++
9	+	+++	+++	+++	+++	++	+	++	-	++
16	+++	+	+++	+++	+	+	+	+	-	++

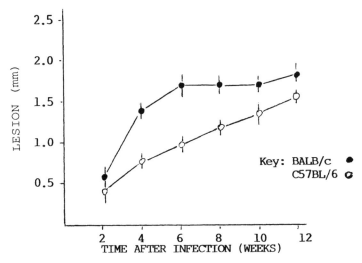

FIGURE 1   CHANGES IN SKIN LESIONS IN BALB/C AND C57BL/6 MICE INFECTED WITH 3.5×10^6 AMASTIGOTES

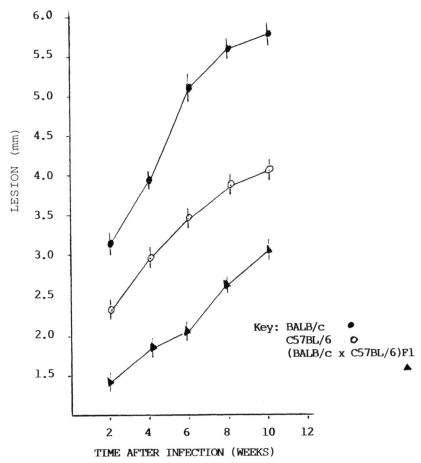

FIGURE 2   CHANGES IN LESIONS IN BALB/C, C57BL/6 AND (BALB/C X C57BL6) FL MICE INFECTED WITH 7.3×10^6 AMASTIGOTES.

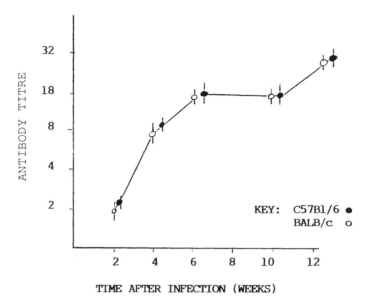

FIGURE 3   ANTIBODY LEVELS IN MICE INFECTED WITH *L.m.mexicana*.

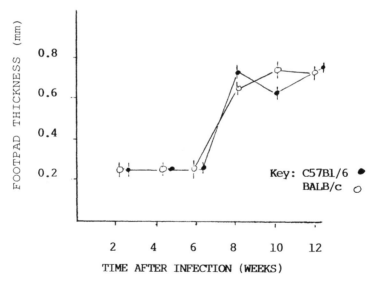

FIGURE 4   DELAYED HYPERSENSITIVITY TO SOLUBLE ANTIGEN IN MICE INFECTED WITH *L.m. mexicana*. THE REACTION WAS READ AT 24 AND 48 Hr. IN BOTH STRAINS OF MICE THE REACTION WAS POSITIVE AT 24 Hr. BECAME NEGATIVE AT 48 Hr. IN ALL THE INFECTION TIME.

and epitheliod cells heavily parasitized in the BALB/c and scanty in the C57Bl/6 mice. Just peripheral to this were some lymphocytes and plasma cells. The necrosis was more scanty in BALB/c than C57Bl/6 mice. Some fibrosis was found at the edge of the lesion.

At 4 weeks, macrophages in the dermis contained more parasites. The parasitophorous vacuoles grew until they coalesced, some of them broke and sometimes necrosis was present. Eosinophils (E) were more abundant in C57Bl/6 mice and were found in most parts of the dermis and accumulated near to the destroyed macrophages.

At 6 weeks in both strains of mice a small crust was observed, the vacuoles were bigger and coalesced, some of them were empty or with parasites grouped in the centre. Many macrophages were heavily infected and many extracellular parasites were seen. In BALB/c mice eosinophils were fewer and were disseminated, but in C57Bl/6 mice they were still abundant and in groups.

At 13 weeks in the BALB/c mice fibrosis occurred from the edge to the centre of the lesion. There were no parasites under the epidermis, but they were still abundant in the centre of the lesion among destroyed macrophages. Plasma cells were more abundant and necrosis was more evident. In the C57Bl/6 mice there were many macrophages and epithelioid cells heavily infected. Fibrosis was evident in the extremes of the lesion. Eosinophils were still abundant and in groups very close to the macrophages with big vacuoles. About 60% of male C57Bl/6 mice recovered spontaneously at this time of infection. The results are summarized in Table 1 and Figure 1. With a dose of 7.3×10^6 amastigotes, the lesions developed more quickly and the infection was more severe than with 3.5×10^6 amastigotes. The C57Bl/6 were not able to control the infection. The F1 mice showed the same behaviour as the C57Bl/6. The results are summarized in Table 2. and Figure 2.

Serum antibodies

Levels of serum antibodies were measured by an indirect immunofluorescent-antibody technique 2, 4, 6, 8, and 13 weeks after infection in BALB/c and C57Bl/6 mice. The sera from uninfected mice were positive without dilution but negative at 1:2. Both strains had the same pattern of antibody production (Figure 3).

Delayed hypersensitivity

Delayed hypersensitivity was measured by introdermal inoculation of *Leishmania mexicana mexicana* AS into C57Bl/6 and BALB/c mice 2, 4, 6, 8 and 10 weeks after infection. The reaction was read 24 and 48 h. In both strains the reaction was positive at 24 h and negative at 48 h. (Figure 4).

DISCUSSION

With 3.5×10^6 amastigotes there was a difference in the time of development of the lesion between strains of mice, from 16 days after infection until 6 weeks. After that the growth was similar until the lesions reached the same size.

In C57Bl/6 a severe necrosis was observed 2 weeks after infection and the parasites were fewer than in BALB/c. Eosinophils were more abundant in C57Bl/6 mice. At 4 weeks, pararsites were more numerous, the BALB/c macrophages looked more vacuolated with more parasites than C57Bl/6. Eosinophils were abundant near the macrophages with empty vacuoles and areas with extracellular parasites. At 8 weeks, parasites were fewer than at 6 in c57Bl/6 but more in BALB/c. Groups of eosinophils were abundant in C57Bl/6 near the damaged macrophages.

Necrosis and eosinophils could play a role in the control of the parasite in the acute phase of the disease. Necrosis has been postulated as an important factor in the elimination of *Leishmania enriettii* in guinea pigs (Monroy et al 1980). Pearson et al (1981), working with *Leishmania donovani*, observed that amastigotes are susceptible to ingestion and killing by PMN and eosinophils. After 10 weeks of infection there was no difference between strains. Fibrosis became important as well as the number of plasma cells but parasites were still growing suggesting that they were avoiding the factors involved in their elimination. Serum antibodies production was similar in both strains, the maximum level was coincident with the peak of plasma cells in the lesion. There was no significative difference in delayed hypersensitivity between strains.

Despite the fact that the delayed hypersensitivity and the serum, antibodies were positive, they did not influence the control of the infection.

CONCLUSIONS

Infection doses influence the outcome of the infection in both strains of mice. With high doses, the infection is similar and uncontrollable. At lower doses the BALB/c mice were initially more susceptible but later the infections were similar.

Necrosis and eosinophils could play an important role in the elimination of the parasite, because in the C57Bl/6 the necrosis was more marked from the beginning of the infection and eosinophils were more abundant all the time and always close to the damaged macrophages.

The infection in the Fl was similar to that in the C57Bl/6. The immune responses measured by antibodies and delayed hypersensitivity do not seem to correlate with the control of the infection.

REFERENCES

Bradley, D.J., Taylor, B.B., Blackwell, J.M. and Freeman, E.P., 1979, Regulation of *Leishmania* population within the host. II mapping of locus controlling susceptibility to visceral leishmaniasis in the mouse. Clin. Exp. Immunol., 37:7

Grimaldi, G. Jr., Moriarty, P.L. and Hoff, R., 1980, *Leishmania mexicana:* immunology and histopathology in C3H mice. Exp. Parasitol., 50:45

Grimaldi, G. Jr., Soares, M.J and Moriarty, P.L , 1984, Tissue eosinophilia and *Leishmania mexicana mexicana* eosinophil interaction in murine cutaneous leishmaniasis., Parasite Immunol., 6: 397

Monroy, O., Ridley, D.S., Heather, C.J. and Ridley, M.J., 1980, Histological studies of the elimination of *Leishmania enriettii* from skin lesions in the guinea pig. Br. J. Exp. Path., 61: 601

Monroy, O.A. 1983, Aspectos histopatologicos relacionados con la respuesta inmun en dos tipos de leishmaniasis., cutanea americana. Tesis Doctoral. Escuela Nacional de Ciencias Biologicas, IPN. Mexico.

Pearson, N.D..and Steigbigel, R.T., 1981, Phagocytosis and killing of the protozoon *Leishmania donovani* by human polymorpho-nuclear leukoctes., J. Immunol., 127: 1438

Perez, H., Arredondo, B. and Gonzalez, M. 1977, Comparative study of American cutaneous leishmaniasis in two strains of inbred mice., Infec. Imm., 22: 301

Perez, H., Labrador, F. and Torrealba, J.W.., 1978, Variations in the response of five strains of mice to *Leishmania mexicana*., Int. J. Parasitol., 9: 27

Zeledon, R., Macoya, G., Ponce, Chaves, F., Murillo, J. and Bonilla, J.A., 1980, Cutaneous leishmaniasis in Honduras Central America.,
Trans Roy. Soc. Trop. Med. Hyg., 70: 276

THE ROLE OF MEMBRANE-STABILIZING DRUGS ON UPTAKE OF LEISHMANIA PARASITES
BY HUMAN MACROPHAGES

A. Kharazmi, A.L. Sørensen, and
H. Nielsen

State Serum Institute, Department of
Clinical Microbiology
Rigshospitalet, 7806, Copenhagen
Denmark

Introduction

More than 12 million people are infected with different species of Leishmania and the annual death toll due to leishmaniasis is over 5000. Treatment of the patients with different forms of leishmaniasis is still a serious problem. Pentavalent antimonials in conventional doses are ineffective against visceral leishmaniasis and at higher doses toxic. The usual second line drugs such as pentamidine and amphotericin B are also toxic and difficult to administer. There is therefore a great need to search for drugs that are safe and can effectively control the disease.

Leishmania promastigotes and amastigotes bind to receptors on the surface of monocytes and macrophages, the host cells for the parasite. Following binding the parasites either actively penetrate into or are phagocytized by the host cells. The interaction of the molecules on the host cell surface with those on the parasite surface are important in the infection of the monocytes/macrophages by the parasite (Blackwell 1985; Chang & Chang 1986; Handman & Goding 1985). Apart from the precise molecular identity of the receptor-ligand interactions involving the known receptors on the macrophage and the ligands on the parasite surface, the cell membrane as a whole plays an important role in host-parasite interactions. Integrity and fluidity of cell membrane is essential in recycling and expression of receptors on the cell surface, and in internalization of the parasite during the ingestion process. Pharmacological alterations of the cell membrane by drugs which can change membrane fluidity may help in inhibition of either receptor-ligand binding or uptake and ingestion of the parasite by the monocytes/macrophages.

Lysosomotropic agents such as chloroquine, methylamine, and a-mantadine interfere with the flow of cell membrane during endocytosis in cultured rat fibroblasts. These drugs inhibit the transfer of extracellular material bound to the plasma membrane from the phagosomal membrane to the lysosomes (Trouet, Tulkens & Schneider 1980). The binding of opiates to their receptors on mouse brain cell membrane can be modulated by lipid fluidity (Heron et al., 1980). Based on the involvement of cell membrane in leishmania-macrophage interactions, and the very important role that cell membrane plays in these interactions, the long range prospect for development of more effective drugs against Leishmania would be to look for drugs which can interfer with parasite interactions at the cell surface.

Membrane-stabiling drugs with lipophilic property could prove to have potential value against Leishmania. The phenothiazine and thioxanthene neuroleptics, and particularly analogs of these drugs with litle or no neuroleptic activity are amongst the important candidates. Chlorpromazine, clopenthixol, and chlorprothixene are the protypes which are used for their antipsychotic, antianxiety, and antiemetic effects. These compounds modify membrane and membrane constituents (Ogiso, Iwaki & Mari, 1981; Suda et al., 1981), alter cyclic nucleotide metabolism (Palmer & Manian, 1979), inhibit actin polymerization (Elias & Boyer, 1979), and exhibit bactericidal activity (Kristiansen & Gaarslev, 1985). Recently there have been several reports on the antiprotozoal activity of some of these compounds. Chlorpromazine exhibits inhibitory effects in vitro against Trypanosoma brucei brucei (Seebeck & Gehr, 1983), and Plasmodium falciparum (Kristiansen & Jepsen, 1985).

The role of membrane-stabilizing drugs on leishmania-macrophage interactions has not been previously studied. The objective of this study was therefore to examine the effect of these drugs on binding and uptake of L. major promastigotes by human monocytes and monocyte-derived macrophages. The rationale is to identify a drug or drugs that can inhibit binding to or ingestion of the parasite by monocyte-macrophages with the idea that the parasite in the extracellular environment will no longer be able to multiply and can easily be controlled by other components of the immune system. One of the advantages of such an approach is to test drugs that are already in clinical use for other diseases and that they are nontoxic.

Experimental design

L. major strain MHOM/SU/73/5-ASKH was obtained from Dr. David Evans, WHO Reference Center for Leishmania, London School of Hygiene and Tropical Medicine. The parasites were grown and maintained in conventional media. The role of several membrane- stabilizing drugs including chlorpromazine, clopenthixol, chlorprothixen, flupentixol, and chloroquine on binding and uptake of parasites by human peripheral blood monocytes and monocyte-derived macrophages (MDM) were studied. The monocytes were isolated from peripheral blood obtained from healthy individuals by Lymphoprep density centrifugation. The mononuclear cells were incubated in Labtek tissue culture chambers for two hours, non-adhering cells were removed and the chambers were further incubated overnight in order to obtain monolayers of MDM. The uptake of parasite by monocytes or MDM was determined by both a radioactive labelling method and by microscopic counting. Monocytes in suspension or MDM as monolayer were incubated with various concentrations of each drug for various time periods. The parasites were then incubated with the monocytes or MDM at ratio of 10:1 for 60 minutes at 37° C. The free parasites were removed by decanting and washing the chambers with monolayers or differential centrifugation of the monocyte suspension. The monocyte or macrophage associated parasites were determined by either counting radioactivity or microscopically.

Results

The data are presented in Tables 1, 2, 3, and 4.

Table 1. Effect of membrane-stabilizing drugs on L.major promastigotes binding/uptake by human macrophages. Monolayers were incubated with various concentrations of each drug for 60 min. after which ^{3}H uracil and ^{3}H thymidine labelled promastigotes were added to each well, incubated at 37° C for another 60 min. Cells washed, removed by Triton- x-100 and radioactivity was counted.

Drug concentrations (uM)	% radioactivity of control (non-treated cells)
Chlorpromazine:	
100	0
50	10
10	76
1	94
Cis(z)-Clopenthixol:	
50	1
10	43
1	52
Trans(E)-Clopenthixol:	
50	0
10	51
1	75
Trans(E)-Flupentixol:	
50	3
10	46
1	86
Trans(E)-Chlorprothixene:	
50	47
10	81
1	107
Chloroquine:	
200	6
40	31
20	52
2	86

Table 2. Effect of membrane-stabilizing drugs on the multiplication of L. major promastigotes. The promastigotes were incubated with various concentrations of each drug and ^{3}H uracil and ^{3}H thymidine overnight. The promastigotes were washed 3 times and radioactivity counted.

Drug concentrations (uM)	% of control counts
Chlorpromazine:	
100	8
50	29
10	64
1	68
Cis(Z)-Clopenthixol:	
100	16
50	37
10	106
1	70
Trans(E)-Clopenthixol:	
100	1
50	14
10	54
1	112
Trans(E)-Flupentixol:	
100	71
50	87
10	50
1	58
Trans(E)-Chlorprothixene:	
100	12
50	66
10	51
1	98

Table 3. Binding of L. major promastigotes preincubated with various concentrations of each drug and ^{3}H uracil and ^{3}H thymidine overnight, washed and added to monolayers. Further incubated for 60 min., washed, and radioactivity was counted.

Drug concentrations (uM)	% of control promastigotes	% of control macrophage
Chlorpromazine:		
10	81	24
1	68	37
Cis(E)-Clopenthixol:		
10	82	67
1	70	33
Trans(E)-Clopenthixol:		
10	61	40
1	112	31
Trans(E)-Flupentixol:		
10	50	37
1	58	26
Trans(E)-Chlorprothixene:		
10	51	34
1	98	45

Table 4. Effect of drugs on L. major promastigotes binding/uptake by human macrophages. Monolayers were incubated with various concentrations of each drug for 60 min. and then washed. The rest of the assay the same as in Table 1.

Drug concentrationes (uM)	% radioactivity of control (non-treated cells)
Chlorpromazine:	
50	80
10	108
Cis(Z)-Clopenthixol:	
50	11
10	121
Trans(E)-Clopenthixol:	
50	2
10	96
Trans(E)-Flupentixol:	
50	28
10	42
Trans(E)-Chlorprothixene:	
50	16
10	76

Discussion

The data presented here indicate that a number of tricyclic phenothiazine and thioxanthene compounds such as chlorpromazine, Cis(Z)- and trans(E)-clopenthixol, Trans(E)-flupentixol, and trans(E)-chlorprothixene at concentrations of 50 uM were able to kill L. major promastigotes in vitro. Furthermore these compounds at lower concentrations inhibited the binding/uptake of L. major promastigotes by human monocyte-derived macrophages. The trans(E)-isomers were as active as the cis(Z)-isomers at comparable concentrations. The trans(E) form of these compounds have no neuroleptic activity (Petersen et al. 1977) therefore their use even at concentrations higher than 50 uM will not cause any neuroleptic side effects.

Anti-leishmanial activity of phenotiazines has been the focus of recent attention. Chlorpromazine was found to kill L. donovani promastigotes, extracellular amastigotes and amastigotes in macrophages (Pearson et al., 1982; Pearson et al., 1984). Zilberstein and Dwyer (1984) showed that clomipramine a compound almost identical to chlorpromazine showed similar effect. The thioxanthenes, another group of neuroleptic drugs with membrane-stabilizing effect are structurally similar to phenothiazines. In general the cis (Z)-isomers of these compounds have dopamine antagonist and neuroleptic effects, whereas the trans (E)-isomers do not (Petersen et al., 1977). Both cis (Z)- and trans (E)-isomers of chlorprothixene has been shown to kill promastigotes and amastigotes of L. donovani (Pearson et al., 1987). Another interesting aspect of some of these drugs such as chlorpromazine, trifluoperazine, and clopenthixol is that they are capable of modulationg the function of phagocytic cells (Lohr, Feix & Kurth, 1984; Rechnitzer, Kristiansen & Kharazmi, 1985; Smith, Bowmann & Iden, 1981).

These compounds appear to affect both the promastigotes and the macrophages. There are several reports on the anti-parasitic activity of some of these compounds(Kristiansen & Jepsen, 1985; Pearson et al, 1984), however, there are no studies on the effect of these drugs on parasite-macrophage interactions. The data presented in Table 3 show that promastigotes which were incubated at very low concentrations (10 uM and 1 uM) of all 5 compounds tested were able to grow in vitro and incorporate radioactivity but their ability to bind the macrophages was markedly reduced.

The mechanism of action of these compounds on the promastigotes and macrophages is not known. These drugs are lipophilic, can stabilize and modulate functions associated with cell membrane such as transport and receptor recycling and inhibit metabolism of certain enzymes (Zilberstein & Dwyer, 1984). They can also interfere with cyclic nucleotide metabolism (Palmer & Manian, 1979). Pearson et al (1982) have shown that exposure of L. donovani promastigotes to 50 ug/ml (150 uM) Chlorpromazine resulted in irreversible loss of motility, loss of nuclear and cytoplasmic detail and disruption of the plasma membrane. The fact that the Cis(Z)- and trans(E)-forms exhibit similar inhibitory effect on macrophages and promastigotes indicate that these inhibitory functions are different from those of neuroleptic and antipsychotic effects.

The potential clinical relevance of these findings needs to be examined. It will be important to search for other membrane-stabilizing drugs which can control the parasite multiplication.

Conclusions

Because of inefficiency and toxicity of available antileishmanial drugs there is a great need to search for more effective and nontoxic drugs. Since cell membrane plays an important role in binding and entrance of Leishmania parasite into its host cell, pharmacological alterations of the membrane to inhibit parasite entry into its target cell appears to be a reasonable approach for control of the disease caused by this parasite. A number of tricyclic phenothiazine and thioxanthene compounds such as chlorpromazine, clopenthixol, flupenthixol, and chlorprothixene at fairly low concentrations appear to inhibit the binding/uptake of L. major promastigote by human macrophages. These compounds affect both the parasite and the macrophage. They exhibit antileishmanial activity and influence the macrophage as well. It is of special interest that the trans(E)-form of these compounds with no neuroleptic activity exhibit similar inhibitory effect on parasite-macrophage interaction. Therefore, the use of trans(E) isomers of these compounds is promising. The potential clinical relevance of these findings needs to be examined in the future.

Acknowledgements

This investigation received financial support from the United Nations Development Programme/World Bank/World Health Organization Special Programme for Research and Training in Tropical Diseases.

References

Blackwell JM (1985) Receptors and recognition mechanisms of Leishmania species. Trans. Roy. Soc. Trop. Med. Hyg. 79: 606-612.

Chang CS, Chang KP (1986) Monoclonal affinity purification of a leishmania membrane glycoprotein and its inhibition of leishmania-macrophage binding. Proc. Nat. Acad. Sci. 83: 100-104.

Elias E, Boyer JL (1979) Chlorpromazine and its metabolites alter polymerization and gelation of actin. Science. 206: 1404-1406.

Handman E, Goding JW (1985) The Leishmania receptor for macrophages is a lipid-containing glycoconjugate. EMBO J. 4: 329-336.

Heron DS, Shinitzky M, Hershkowitz M, Samuel D (1980) Lipid fluidity markedly modulates the binding of serotonin to mouse brain membranes. Proc. Nat. Acad. Sci. 77: 7463-7467.

Kristiansen JE, Gaarslev K (1985) The antibacterial effect of selected neuroleptics on Vibrio cholerae. Acta Path. Microbiol. Immunol. Scand. Sect. B. 93: 49-51.

Kristiansen JE, Jepsen S (1985) The susceptibility of Plasmodium falciparum in vitro to chlorpromazine and the stereo-isomeric compounds cis(Z)-and trans(E)-clopenthixol. Acta Path. Microbiol. Immunol. Scand. Sect. B. 93: 249-251.

Lohr KM, Feix JB, Kurth C (1984) Chlorpromazine inhibits neutrophil chemotaxis beyond the chemotactic receptor-ligand interaction. J. Infect. Dis. 150: 643-652.

Ogiso T, Iwaki M, Mori K (1981) Fluidity of human erythrocyte membrane and effect of chlorpromazine on fluidity and phase seperation of membrane. Biochem. Biophys. Acat. 649: 325-335.

Pearson RD, Manian AA, Harcus Jl, Hall D, Hewlett EL (1982) Lethal effects of phenothiazene neuroleptics on the pathogenic protozoan Leishmania donovani. Science 217: 369-371.

Pearson RD, Manian AA, Hall D, Harcus JL, Hewlett EL (1984) Antileishmanial activity of chlorpromazine. Antimicrob. Agents Chemoth. 25: 571-574.

Pearson RD, Brand JJ, Roberts D, Hewlett EL (1987) Antiprotozoal effects of thioxanthenes against the human pathogen Leishmania donovani. Experientia. In press.

Petersen PV, Nielsen IM, Pedersen V, Jørgensen A, Lassen N (1977) Thioxanthenes in: Psychotherapeutic drugs. ed. E. Udsin & I. Forrest. Marcel Dekker. New York. P. 827-867.

Rechnitzer C, Kristiansen JE, Kharazmi A (1985) In vitro modulation of human neutrophil chemotaxis by cis(Z) - and trans (E)-clopenthixol and chlorpromazine. Acta Pathol. Microbiol. Immunol. Sec. C. 93: 199-203.

Seebeck T, Gehr P (1983). Trypanocidal action of neuroleptic phenothiazenes in Trypanosoma brucei. Mol. Biochem. Parasitol. 9: 197-208.

Smith RJ, Bowmann BJ, Iden SI (1981). Effects of trifluoperazine on human neutrophil function. Immunol. 44: 677-684.

Suda T, Shimizu D, Maeda N, Shiga T (1981). Decreased viscosity of human erythrocyte suspension induced by chlorpromazine and isoxsusprine. Biochem. Pharmacol. 30: 2057-2064.

Trouet A, Tulkens P, Schneider YJ (1980). Subcellular localization of infectious agents: Pharmacological and pharmacokinetic implications. In: The Host Invader Interplay. ed. Van den Bossche, North Hollan H. p. 31-44.

Zilberstein D, Dwyer DM (1984). Antidepressants cause lethal disruption of membrane function in the human protozoan parasite Leishmania. Science 226: 977-979.

GENERATION OF MEGASOMES DURING THE PROMASTIGOTE - AMASTIGOTE
TRANSFORMATION OF LEISHMANIA MEXICANA MEXICANA IN VITRO

L. Tetley, C.A. Hunter, G.H. Coombs and K. Vickerman

Department of Zoology, University of Glasgow
Glasgow G12 8QQ, U.K.

INTRODUCTION

The amastigotes of the Leishmania mexicana complex differ from those of other Leishmania species in possessing unusual large lysosomes, termed "megasomes", which may comprise 15% of the total cell volume. These organelles have a thick (10nm) bounding membrane and markedly heterogeneous contents with electron-dense spherules, vesicles and occasionally elongate crystalloids in a matrix of moderate electron density as seen in transmission electron micrographs (Coombs et al., 1986). They contain acid phosphatase and aryl sulphatase as shown by cytochemistry and a cysteine proteinase demonstrable by immuno-gold staining at the E.M. level (Pupkis et al., 1986). Megasomes are absent from the promastigote stage. The origin of megasomes during amastigote development is unknown. This preliminary investigation describes the mode of formation of megasomes during promastigote-amastigote transformation in vitro, as seen by transmission electron microscopy of sectioned material.

MATERIALS AND METHODS

Parasites

Promastigotes of Leishmania mexicana mexicana (MNYC/B2/62/M379) were grown in HOMEM medium at 25°C as described previously (Pupkis et al., 1986) and harvested during stationary phase (7 days or more after sub inoculation of cultures).

Mouse peritoneal exudate cells (PECs) were obtained from BALB/c mice and the populations pooled and dispensed into Falcon tissue culture flasks at a density of $10^5/cm^2$ and incubated to allow adherence at 34°C for 12 h. Non-adherent cells were then removed by vigorous washing in HBSS and then exposed to the leishmanias.

Promastigotes were introduced to PECs in RPMI 1640 in a ratio of 5/1 for 4 h at 34°C. Infected PEC cultures were harvested at 4, 23, 47, and 73 h and processed for electron microscopy

Electron Microscopy

Infected PECs were released from the bottom of tissue culture flasks by gentle scraping with a rubber pasteur pipette bulb after removal of the medium, and fixed by irrigation with 10 ml of 2.5% glutaraldehyde in 0.1 M phosphate buffer, pH 7.4, 33°C. During 40 mins fixation, the temperature was allowed to drop to 20°C after which the fixed suspension of released, infected PECs was spun at 1500 g for 15 mins, washed twice in 0.1 M phosphate buffer containing 2% sucrose and post-fixed in 1% buffered osmium tetroxide for 1 h. Following removal of osmium with three changes of distilled water, the cells were encapsulated in 1% Seaplaque agarose at 40°C and further processed as small (<1.0 cu mm) blocks through 0.5% aqueous uranyl acetate for 30 mins, alcohol dehydrated and finally Araldite embedded via propylene oxide.

After 2 days polymerization at 60°C, 350 nm or 60 nm sections were mounted on 300 mesh grids and stained with either 2% methanolic uranyl acetate for 5 mins or this stain followed by lead citrate for 5 mins. Exposures were recorded on 70 mm Kodak MP11 roll film using a Zeiss TEM 902 incorporating an electron energy spectrometer for contrast enhancement and thick section imaging. Stereo pair images were recorded with 10° tilt between exposures and are intended for viewing by pocket stereoscope.

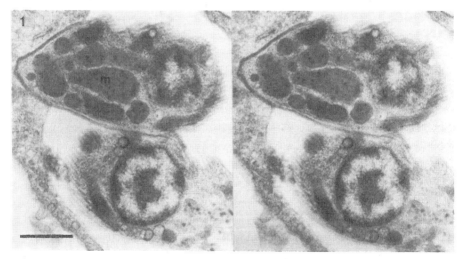

Fig. 1. Stereoscopy of a thick (350 nm) section of amastigotes in the parasitophorous vacuole (electron energy-filtered images). The posterior end of one amastigote is closely applied to the indented vacuole membrane; megasomes fill this region of the parasite. Scale bar = 500 nm.

Key to labelling of figures

er - subtending endoplasmic reticulum; fl - flagellum; fp - flagellar pocket; gly - glycosome; gol - golgi apparatus; kp - kinetoplast; l - lipid droplet; m - megasome; mit - mitochondrion; mvb - multivesicular body; pp - polyphosphate body; ss - swollen saccule; tgn - trans-golgi network.

RESULTS

In sections of the amastigote, megasomes fill the posterior part of the body (Fig. 1); they have a characteristically thick (golgi-processed) bounding membrane, 10 nm across, which distinguishes them from most other cytoplasmic organelles (e.g. glycosomes with a bounding membrane 7 nm across), the exception being the prominent polyphosphate vacuoles which also have a thick membrane (Fig. 2).

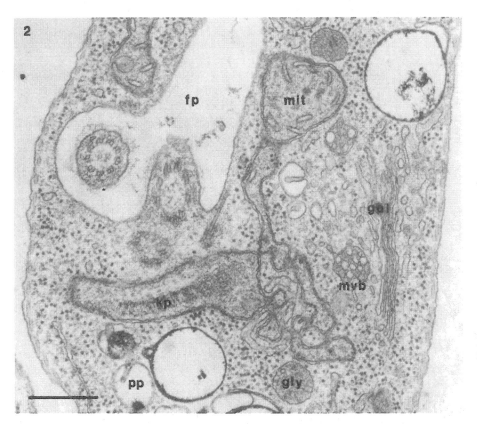

Fig. 2. Promastigote. Longitudinal section of kinetoplast-flagellar pocket-golgi region. Note: multivesicular bodies in trans-golgi region; megasomes are absent. Scale bar = 500 nm.

In the flagellated promastigote stage the golgi apparatus lies alongside the parasite's flagellar pocket. Its cis-region (forming face) is subtended by granular endoplasmic reticulum; its trans-region abuts on small multivesicular bodies (~ 250 nm across). No megasomes are visible in the cytoplasm (Fig. 2), though other cytoplasmic organelles are common to the two stages.

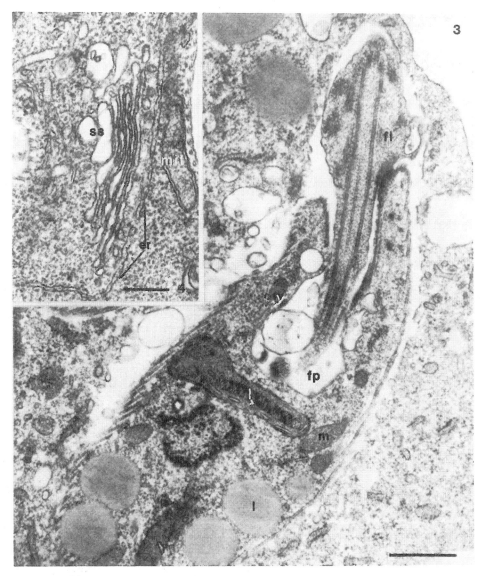

Fig. 3-7 are of transforming parasites 23 h after infection of host macrophages in vitro.

Fig. 3. The extracellular flagellum is being resorbed; the posterior end of the flagellate contains abundant lipid globules; an elongate megasome is visible alongside the kinetoplast. Scale bar = 500 nm.

Fig. 4. Detail of golgi apparatus with subtending ER at cis-face and swollen clear saccules at the trans-face. Scale bar = 500 nm.

By 23 h megasomes have appeared in the trans-golgi region, while the parasites still retain an extracellular flagellum (Fig. 3). The trans-golgi region contains swollen, empty looking sacs and a network of smooth-membraned tubules (Fig. 4). The megasomes appear to arise among the latter as irregular bloated tubule segments (Fig. 5) and to extend from the prenuclear golgi region into the posterior part of the cell where they assume their more characteristic shape (Fig. 6). At times subsequent to 23 h, the transforming parasites have megasomes resembling those of fully transformed amastigotes.

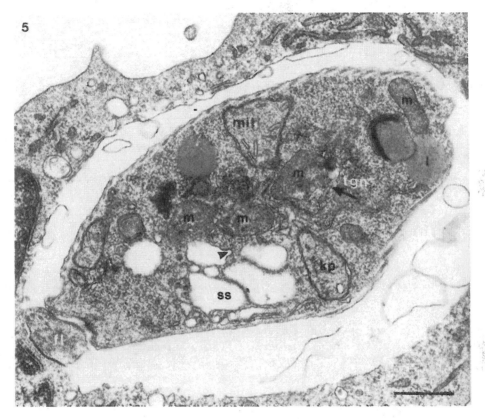

Fig. 5. Megasomes and swollen clear saccules lie alongside one another in the trans-golgi region. Megasomes are continuous within the TGN (at arrow); clathrin-coated vesicles (arrowhead) are associated with the clear saccules but not the megasomes. Note persistent flagellum. Scale bar = 500 nm.

DISCUSSION

Megasomes are clearly lysosomal in nature. They appear to have a role in autophagy (Alexander and Vickerman, 1975), but evidence that their enzymes are released into the parasitophorous vacuole is lacking to date, and their relationship to the swollen parasite-containing vacuoles characteristic of L. mexicana sspp. is obscure.

The finding that megasomes arise from the trans-golgi network (TGN, previously known as GERL - golgi-endoplasmic reticulum-lysosome complex) is in agreement with the proposals of Griffiths and Simons (1986) on the packaging of lysosomal enzymes. We have not observed the TGN-associated clathrin-coated vesicles believed by these workers to be responsible for transport of enzymes to the mature lysosome. The TGN of leishmania amastigotes may participate in other packaging or secretory activities; the function of the swollen golgi saccules with clear contents remains to be determined and may be nothing to do with the generation of megasomes.

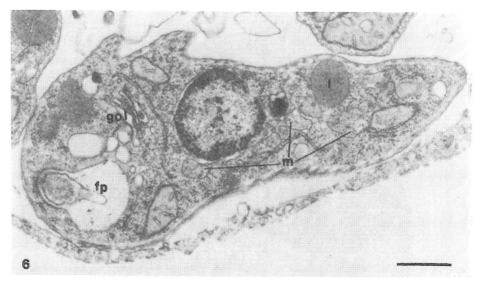

Fig. 6. A chain of megasomes extends from the golgi apparatus to the posterior end of the cell. Lipid droplets are also present in the posterior region. Smooth clear vesicles of the trans golgi-region abut on the flagellar pocket. Scale bar = 500 nm.

As megasomes arise early in the transformation of the promastigote, before loss of the flagellum, they would appear to be important in the survival of Leishmania mexicana in its mammalian host. One possibility is that megasomal proteases are responsible for the production of amines which antagonise the leishmanicidal action of the macrophage hydrolases. In this connexion it is interesting to note that the acquisition of sensitivity by transforming intracellular leishmanias to certain methyl esters of amino acids parallels the production of megasomes (Hunter & Coombs, this meeting). Amastigotes are killed by leucine methyl ester as a result of ester hydrolysis by enzymes in an acidified compartment of the parasite (Rabinovitch et al., this meeting) - presumably the megasome. Infection of macrophages with L. m. mexicana promastigotes and immediate treatment with L-leucine methyl ester results in a substantial reduction in parasite load.

CONCLUSIONS

During the transformation of Leishmania mexicana mexicana promastigotes to amastigotes in vitro, the large lysosomes known as megasomes appear in the trans-golgi region of the parasite's cytoplasm within 24 h of ingestion of the leishmanias by the macrophage host cell, and before the parasite has adopted the amastigote form. Their presence appears to be linked to the survival of the parasite within the parasitophorous vacuole.

ACKNOWLEDGEMENTS

Grants from the Wellcome Trust and from the European Community Sub-Programme on Medicine, Health and Nutrition in the Tropics are gratefully acknowledged.

REFERENCES

Alexander, J. and Vickerman, K. 1975. Fusion of host secondary lysosomes with the parasitophorous vacuoles of Leishmania mexicana-infected macrophages. J. Protozool., 22:502.

Coombs, G.H. 1982. Proteinases of Leishmania mexicana and other flagellate protozoa. Parasitology 84:149.

Coombs, G.H., Tetley, L., Moss, V.A. and Vickerman, K. 1986. Three dimensional structure of the leishmania amastigote as revealed by computer-aided reconstruction from serial sections. Parasitology 92:13.

Griffiths, G. and Simons, K. 1986. The trans golgi network: sorting at the exit site of the golgi complex. Science 234:438.

Pupkis, M.F., Tetley, L. and Coombs, G.H. 1986. Leishmania mexicana: the occurrence of amastigote hydrolases in unusual organelles. Exp. Parasitol., 62:29.

TREATMENT OF EXPERIMENTAL CUTANEOUS AND VISCERAL MURINE LEISHMANIASIS WITH RECOMBINANT GAMMA-INTERFERON

Albrecht F. Kiderlen and Marie-Luise Lohmann-Matthes

Fraunhofer-Institute for Toxicology
Department of Immunology
D-3000 Hannover 61
F.R.G.

INTRODUCTION

Being obligate intracellular parasites in cells of the monocyte/macrophage system leishmanial organisms are, once the infection is established, in essence dependent only on the host qualities of their residence cell and on sufficient recruitment of future host cells. As has been extensively shown, macrophages (Mφ) may be rendered into an activated state of cytotoxicity for a variety of target cells by lymphokine, excreted from adequately stimulated T-cells: The macrophage-activating-factor (MAF) Gamma-interferon (IFN-γ) is a lymphokine that is available as highly pure recombinant material (r-IFN-γ) with high MAF-activity in most test systems. Macrophages that are treated *in vitro* with crude MAF or with r-IFN turn cytotoxic also for intracellular parasites such as invading leishmanial promastigotes or amstigotes [1], as well as for those parasites that have already established intracellular residence [2]. The Mφ-systems should therefore have a dual function, on one hand as a host and on the other as a potent effector system against this intracellular parasite.

The immune response to *Leishmania*-infections is almost exclusively cell-mediated. High titers of specific and non-specific antibodies, characteristic of certain forms of leishmaniasis, and injection of immune sera have no curative effect. In Leishmaniasis, deficiencies in the cell-mediated immune reaction caused for instance by suppressive Mo and T-cell activity have been reported by many authors. It seems therefore plausible that the persistence of infection might be due to inadequate production of MAF/IFN-γ, thus keeping the Mφ in their non-activated "host"-state.

The object of this study was as to extend the data gained in a rapidly developing bacterial infection model [3] to slowly developing infections with chronic aspects as exhibited in the leishmaniases. We chose a cutaneous infection model with *Leishmania major* as causative agent and a systemic infection model caused by *Leishmania donovani*. It was hoped to circumvent the problems of immunosuppression in the infected host as well as problems of drug resistance and endangering side effects of chemotherapy by supporting the bodies own defense mechanism using a natural substance that directly turns the obligate host cell into a leishmanicidal effector cell.

MATERIALS AND METHODS

Animals Six to ten-weeks-old female Balb/c or C57BL/6 mice from Charles River Wiga GmgH, Sulzfeld, FRG.

Recombinant murine interferon-gamma Murine IFN-γ, expressed in *E.coli* was produced by Genentech, San Francisco, USA, and kindly supplied by Boehringer Ingelheim, Ingelheim, FRG.

Leishmania The *Leishmania major* isolate LRC-L38 from a case of cutaneous leishmaniasis in Turkestan, USSR, 1960, was received from F. Ebert, Bernhard-Nocht-Institute fur Schiffs- und Tropenkrankheiten, Hamburg, FRG, and has since been passaged in Balb/c mice. Promastigotes were grown as suspension cultures in RPMI 1640 medium supplemented with 10% fetal calf serum (FCS) at 25°C/6% CO_2.

The *Leishmania donovani* isolate LRCLD51 from a case of Kala-Azar in India, 1954, was also received from F. Ebert and has since been passaged in Cotton Rats (Sigmodon hispidus). Promastigotes were grown as suspension cultures in a 1:1 mixture of RPMI 1640 and Hosmem II medium [4] supplemented with 5% FCS at 25°C/6% CO_2.

In vivo assays

(A) *In vivo* assay; for protection from local (s.c.) infection with *Leishmania major*. Approximately 1 x 10^7 promastigote *Leishmania major* organisms in stationary culture phase were injected s.c. into the hind footpad (day 0). Gamma-interferon was either added to this inoculum or injected separately s.c. into the same footpad or i.v. into a lateral tail vein. Footpad-swelling was measured with a microcaliper (Oditest 20 T/T, Kroeplin GmbH, Schluchtern, FRG). The relative amount of viable *Leishmania major* organisms/foot was determined radiometrically. The mice were sacrificed and the infected foot removed and thoroughly rinsed in 70% ethanol. The foot was then homogenised in 5 ml PBS with a tissue grinder (Ultra Turrax, Janke & Kunkel, Staufen, FRG), the homogenate washed twice (10 min, 3,200 RPM) and resuspended in culture medium (25°C). When viable leishmanial organisms from control mice had transformed and begun to multiply (3-5 days of culture), aliquots were removed from the cultures and cultivated in microtiter plates for 18 h with 1.0 µCi ^{3}H-thymidine. Under these conditions *Leishmania major* organisms were the only cells to significantly incorporate radioactivity. The cells were then harvested and read in a

ß-counter. The relative amount of viable parasites in liver or spleen was determined similarly using a teflon homogeniser (Schutt Labortechnik, Gottingen, FRG).
(B) *In vivo* assay for protection from systemic (i.v.) infection with *Leishmania donovani*. Approximately 2×10^7 promastigote or 5×10^6 amastigote *Leishmania donovani* organisms were injected into a lateral tail vein (day 0). R-IFN-γ was also given i.v. and the relative number of viable *Leishmania donovani* organisms in spleen or liver determined according to the radiometric method described above.

RESULTS

Treatment of subcutaneous Leishmania major-infection in Balb/c mice with recombinant gamma-interferon

Parasite load in infected feet *Leishmania major* susceptible, non-cure Balb/c mice were infected with viable *Leishmania major* organisms into the left hind footpad. Treatment with r-IFN-γ was performed at the times indicated either prophylactically, with the onset of footpad swelling, or with the first signs of ulceration. In Table 1 data from two representative experiments are shown. Experiment 1 demonstrates the dose-dependence of prophylactic application into the infection site. Experiment 2 demonstrates the lower effect of treatment with progression of disease and also the efficiency of systemic treatment of a local infection. In all cases we waited for at least 10 days after termination of treatment, thereby excluding short-term effects.

Table 1. Effects of IFN-γ on local <u>L.major</u>-infection in Balb/c mice

Exp.	Infection (L.major organisms / mouse)	Treatment R-IFN-γ (U/mouse)	Site	Time (days p.i.)	(^{3}H)dThd-incorporation (mean %)	Evaluation date (days p.i.)
1	5×10^6 am+pm	10^3	s.c.	-1,0	105	28
	"	10^4	s.c.	-1,0	21	28
	"	10^5	s.c.	-1,0	3	28
2	1×10^7 am	10^5	s.c.	20,22,24 a)	12	35
	1×10^7 am	10^5	s.c.	28,30,32 b)	39	42
	1×10^7 am	10^5	i.v.	-1,1,3	3	24
	1×10^7 am	10^5	i.v.	17,20,22	25	35
	1×10^7 am	10^5	i.v.	22,24,26 a)	40	35

Groups of 5 mice a) Apparent footpad swelling b) First ulcerations
c) Amount of viable <u>L. major</u> organisms determined radiometrically as described in Materials and Methods and calculated as % related to controls.

Footpad swelling and ulceration In Balb/c mice *Leishmania major* causes progressive swelling and later ulceration of the infected foot. Both parameters are widely used for determining the state of infection. The experiment shown in Figure 1 documents the protective effect of early r-IFN-γ injections either s.c. or i.v. in reduced swelling and ulceration was determined 35 days p.i. A combination of s.c.

and i.v.-treatment was most beneficial at later stage of disease. Again, r-IFN-γ could not completely halt disease progression according to these protocols.

Visceralisation of *Leishmania major* infections
Visceralisation in a typical event following a local infection of Balb/c mice with a high dose of virulent *Leishmania major* organisms. By comparing the amount of viable parasites/spleen with untreated control groups

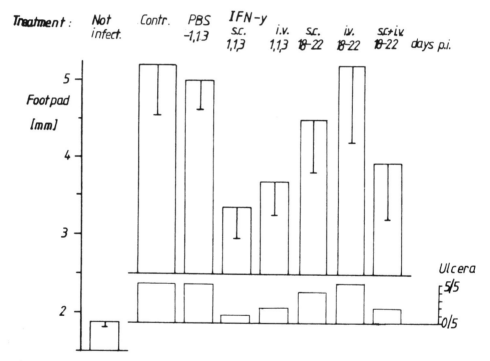

Figure 1   Treatment with r-IFN-γ slows down footpad-swelling and ulcerationin *Leishmania major*-susceptible, non-cure Balb/c mice as determined 35 days post infection (p.i.). Groups of 5 mice + standard deviation.

radiometrically (see Materials and Methods) we show in Figure 2 that r-IFN-γ treatment also substantially lowers visceralisation, especially when mice were treated early during infection.

460

Parasite load in the spleen *Leishmania donovani* susceptible C57BL/6 mice with an inate capacity for keeping the disease under control were treated systemically with r-IFN-γ at early stage of infection according to various protocols. The effect of few doses of r-IFN-γ was similar to the data presented with *Leishmania major* but less significant (data not shown). We therefore attempted a continuous

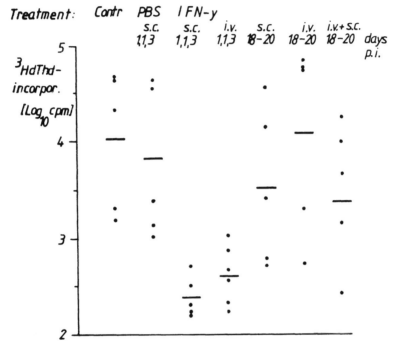

Figure 2   Treatment with r-IFN-γ reduces visceralisation of a sub-cutaneous *Leishmania major*-infection in Balb/c mice as determined radiometrically in spleen homogenates 35 days p.i. Data from the same experiment as Figure 1.

treatment with a relatively low dost of r-IFN-γ (10^3 U/injection) over 9 consecutive days. The results shown in Table 2 indicate a substantial effect of this treatment visualised as a lower parasite load/spleen and reduced splenomegalie. As most mice showed pronounced ulcers (free of parasites!) on the tail coinciding with r-IFN-γ injection into a tail vein, this treatment protocol was abandoned.

Table 2. Effect of long-term, low-dose treatment with r-IFN-γ on systemic infections with Leishmania donovani in C57BL/6 mice.

Treatment (i.v.)	[^{3}H]dThd-incorporation[b] [cpm ± SD]	[%]	Spleen[b] weight [g ± SD]	Spleens positive for L.donovani
Not infected	182 ± 40	0	0.082 ± 0.023	0/5
Infected:				
---	1237 ± 229	100	0.222 ± 0.019	5/5
PBS[a]	1560 ± 350	134	0.237 ± 0.021	5/5
r-IFN-γ	406 ± 187	13	0.190 ± 0.012	3/5

(a) Treatment began 4 hours pre infection with 200 µl PBS/mouse with or without 10^3 U r-IFN-γ given i.v. and was continued for the next 9 consecutive days.
(b) Spleen weights and relative parasite load were determined 33 days post infection as described in Materials and Methods. Means of 5 C57BL/6 mice + standard deviation.

DISCUSSION

In the vertebrate host *Leishmania* organisms are obligate intracellular parasites in cells of the monocyte/macrophage system. With the exception of the infection process as promastigotes and the invasion of new host cells as amastigotes, these parasites can therefore not be reached by factors of the humoral immune response. Instead it has been repeatedly shown that the cellular immune response mechanisms are critical for spontaneous healing from leishmaniasis and, on the other hand, that malfunction of these mechanisms, largely due to suppressive activity of Mφ and T-lymphocytes of helper subset by interactions with parasitised, antigen-presenting Mφ, clonal expansion of these cells and secretion of lymphokines such as MAF/IFN and finally activation of Mφ at the site of infection to enhanced cytotoxicity leading to destruction of the intracellular parasites. *In vitro* data showing the production of MAF/IFN-γ by *Leishmania*-antigen stimulated T-cells and the leishmanicidal activity of MAF/IFN-γ treated Mφ support this theory. It has also been shown by others and ourselves that inteferon-gamma, available as highly pure recombinant material (r-IFN-γ) activates peritoneal and, to a lesser extent, live Mφ *in situ*, as subsequently tested *in vitro*. As this holds true also for sublethally irradiated mice, the injected r-IFN-γ should act directly on Mφ.

With this background we wanted to see if treatment of mice with r-IFN-γ would help resolve or protect from infections with introcellular pathogens involved in exclusively cellular immune reactions. It was our hope to thereby circumvent problems of inadequate immune response caused by suppressor cell activity or clinical immunosuppression as well as problems of host resistance to, and side effects of conventional chemotherapy. In murine listeriosis, an acute, rapidly developing infection model with the facultative intracellular bacterial pathogen *Listeria monocytogenes* the importance of endogeneous IFN-γ production for resolution of the disease and the beneficial effect of treatment with r-IFN-γ has been demonstrated in detail: (i) following sublethal infection, the appearance of IFN in the serum coincides with the beginning of specific T-cell activation and spontaneous healing [5], (ii) treatment of these mice with monoclonal anti r-IFN-γ antibodies hinders the spontaneous resolution [6], (iii) local treatment of mice at the site of s.c. infection or systemic treatment of introvenously infected mice, rIFN-γ significantly reduces the amount of viable bacteria in the respective organ [3], (iv) prophylactic and, to a limited extent, therapeutic treatment of mice that have been infected with an otherwise lethal dose of *Listeria* organisms with r-IFN-γ offers full and dependable protection [7], and (v) a r-IFN-γ treatment that protects mice from lethal listeriosis does not interfere with the development of long-lasting immunity [8].

It must be stressed that murine listeriosis is an acute infection in which spontaneous healing or death are decided within 5-6 days. In the murine leishmaniases spontaneous healing is also possible depending on the infection dose and more so on the genetic background of mice and parasites, but here the development of disease is a matter of months. We report here on the local and systemic treatment of mice with r-IFN-γ before or after infection with Leishmania major (s.c. into a footpad) or with *Leishmania donovani* (i.v.). The results show that:

(i). Treatment of local leishmaniasis by injection of r-IFN-γ at the site of infection is dose and time dependent. The highest relative reduction of parasites is achieved when r-IFN-γ is injected immediately before or early after infection but the effect is still appreciable when treatment begins after footpad swelling. The same effect can be documented as reduced swelling of the foot compared to untreated controls.

(ii) A typical feature of local infection of Balb/c mice with *Leishmania major* is its visceralisation. Local r-IFN-γ-treatment reduces the relative number of parasites invading the spleen.

(iii) Intravenous application of r-IFN-γ has beneficial effects on local parasite burden and visceralisation of cutaneous leishmaniasis. Combined s.c. + i.v.-treatment is beneficial also at late stages of infection.

(iv) With the exception of individual mice treated before or at the very beginning of infection r-IFN-γ provided no sterile cure of cutaneous leishmaniasis.

(v) In visceral leishmaniasis single or few injections of r-IFN-γ showed less effect in parasite reduction as compared to the *Leishmania major* model. Good protection was achieved by 9 repeats of 10^3 U i.v./day whereas the release of the same amount of r-IFN-γ over 7 days into the peritoneum using an implanted osmotic mini-pump (data not shown) was less effective.

(vi) Continuous treatment with r-IFN-γ i.v. or i.p. caused histotoxic side-effects (necrosis) at the site of injection resp. at the site of the r-IFN-γ secreting pump. When treatment was terminated, the tissue healed. We therefore abandoned this method of therapy.

A typical symptom of viceral leishmaniasis (Kala Azar) in hepatosplenomegaly. We found that a large part of the expanded cell populations causing these symptoms in both organs are early differentiation stages of the Mφ-system: Mφ-precursor cells that are not yet phagocytic or adherent, that exhibit typical Mφ-surface markers, that are spontaneously cytotoxic for YAC-1 tumor cells, the yeast phase of *Candida albicans* and promastigote *Leishmania* organisms and that will mature to typical Mφ under adequate culture conditions [9]. These cells represent a pool for future hosts, as well as for leishmanicidal effector cells. The role of this cell population in the course of visceral leishmaniasis and especially the effect of r-IFN-γ treatment at a later stage of infection when these cells are abundant is under current investigation.

Treatment of Leishmaniases with r-IFN-γ is best in the early stage of infection. The reduced effect in later stages might be due to changes in the Mφ population under the inflammatory recruitment conditions leading to an increase in young "inflammatory" Mφ with better host and poorer effector cell properties than the resident cells that dominate in the beginning. Others, using a different test system, have reported a reduction of parasite multiplication in the liver of Leishmania donovani infected mice treated with r-IFN-γ [10]. A sterile protection from leishmaniasis by IFN-γ-treatment can so far not be expected. The incorporation of r-IFN-γ in liposomes has achieved higher levels of in vivo activation of liver and splenic Mφ (Hockertz, et al., in preparation), the effect of this application form on visceral leishmaniasis is currently under investigation. According to our results, a therapy with r-IFN-γ, complementary to chemotherapy, thereby reducing the necessary dose (and the side effects!) seems to be a sensible perspective.

CONCLUSIONS

The aim of the experiments summarised here was to test the efficiency of immunotherapy with recombinant gamma-interferon in intracelular infection models.involving almost exclusively T-cell mediated immune reactions. We have reported previously that r-IFN-γ treatment was very successful in murine listeriosis, an acute, very rapidly developing infection by the bacterium Listeria monocytogenes. Leishmania infections, in contrast, develop slowly thereby evoking a multitude of phenomena that suppress an effective immune response. In in vitro tests we found no macrophage population that would not be activated by r-IFN-γ to cytotoxicity for Leishmania organisms. Furthermore, r-IFN-γ was shown to activate macrophages also under in vivo conditions. Treatment of Balb/c mice, infected locally with Leishmania major, with r-IFN-γ according to different protocols caused a marked reduction of viable parasites when tested 35 days post infection. The effect was best at an early stage of infection, but still appreciable up to ulceration of the infection site. Visceralization of the parasite was also reduced. An absence of parasites was only very rarely documented. Treatment of C57BL/6 mice, infected with Leishmania.donovani was also effective at the beginning of infection, but needed repeated injections. Treatment at a later stage is still under investigation, as visceral leishmaniasis involves complex cellular reactions, some of which are discussed.

According to our present state of knowledge, the treatment of Leishmaniasis with r-IFN-γ should be beneficial especially in speeding up resolution in self-cure cases. Treatment of non-selfcure cases with r-IFN-γ alone, even when employing better application procedures (e.g. liposomal delivery), will probably be confronted with relapses as soon as the treatment is stopped. Also, additional information on the in vivo effect of r-IFN-γ on cells other than mature macrophage during Leishmania donovani-infection is needed.

REFERENCES

1. Nacy, C.A. Fortier, A.F. Meltzer, Buchmeier, N.A and Schreiber,R.D.(1985)
   J. Immunol. 135:3505 .

2. Mauel, J. and Buchmuller, Y. (1987)
   Eur. J. Immunol. 17:203

3. Behrens R.L. and Marr,J.J.(1978)
   J. Parasitol 64:160

4. Kiderlen, A.F. Kaufmann, S.H.E. and Lohmann-Matthes,M-L.
   Eur. J. Immunol. 14:964 (1984).

5. Nakane A.and Minagawa,T. (1984)
   Cell Immunol. 88:29

6. Buchmeier N.A. and Schreiber, R.D. (1985)
   Proc. Natl. Acad. Sci. USA 82:7404

7. Kiderlen, A.F. and Lohmann-Matthes, M-L (1987)
   submitted

8. Kiderlen, A.F. and Lohmann-Matthes, M-L (1987)
   in: "Proceedings of 18th International Leucocyte Culture Conference", Academic Press, New York

9. Baccarini, M. Kiderlen, A.F. Decker, T. and Lohmann-Matthes M-L. (1986)
   Cell. Immunol. 101:339

10. Murray, H.W. Stern, J.J. Welte, K. Rubin, B.Y. Carriero,S-M. and Nathan, C.F.(1987).
    J. Immunol. 138-2290

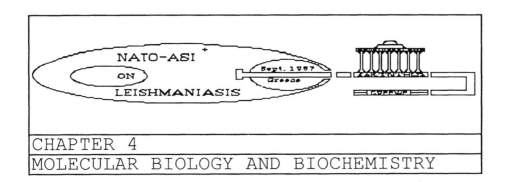

CHAPTER 4
MOLECULAR BIOLOGY AND BIOCHEMISTRY

MOLECULAR BIOLOGY AND BIOCHEMISTRY: AN OVERVIEW

Graham H. Coombs

Department of Zoology
University of Glasgow
Glasgow G12 8QQ, Scotland, U.K.

Many of the more exciting recent discoveries in the field of leishmaniasis have resulted from the application of the techniques of biochemistry and molecular biology, so it was perhaps not surprising that this session contained more contributions than any other at the meeting. Several of the papers highlighted areas of current controversy. Most notable, perhaps, was the issue of the surface-located proteinase(s); its identity, characteristics and functional significance, and even what it should be called. The occurrence of large amounts of a glycoprotein of molecular weight approximately 63 kDa on the surface of cultured promastigotes of several species of Leishmania has been recognised for some years, and several groups have been investigating it with a view to use in a vaccine or diagnosis. These studies have revealed a good deal of information on the protein including, most intriguingly, that it possesses proteolytic activity. Initial findings indicated that it is an unusual enzyme, perhaps most akin to a metalloproteinase optimally active at alkaline pH (see Bordier et al.). Subsequent studies have produced different results, however, and at this meeting evidence was presented (Olafson et al.) showing different substrate specificity and an acid pH optimum. The two sets of data seem incompatable and the only reasonable conclusion at present is that different enzymes were being studied. Which, if either, is the major surface protein may be revealed from gene-cloning and sequencing studies. The sequence revealed at the meeting (Button et al.) appears to have little homology with the known sequences of other proteinases. Clearly further studies are required to clarify the situation, and in particular to elucidate the functional significance of the protein(s) and assess their potential for use in diagnosis, vaccines and as drug targets. These studies may also provide us with a more acceptable name for the protein than the much used gp63 (Gp63, p63). This suffers not only from its anonymity but also from the differences in molecular weight of the glycoprotein found by various groups for a variety of species and strains - the figures range from 58-72 kDa! I prefer the name "promastigote surface proteinase", but this falls if there is more than one enzyme and it is (they are) also present on amastigotes; current evidence suggests that it or a closely related molecule probably is. Clearly a more specific name is required. Yet despite the offer of a reward, and discussions late into the night, an acceptable name was not forthcoming at this meeting; I imagine, however, that this issue will have been resolved before the next one.

Another area of dispute concerned the cytosolic pH of leishmania cells, with evidence being presented by Zilberstein suggesting that it is surprisingly low (approximately pH 6.2). Using different methodology, Mukkada and coworkers found it to be pH 6.8 or above. It seems likely that the differences resulted from the use of alternative analytic techniques; in particular, the contribution from various organelles is uncertain at present. It may be that a method that allows quantitation of the pH in individual organelles will resolve the issue. Both groups, however, agree that the internal pH can be maintained over a wide range of external pH, and particularly intriguing is the finding that amastigotes of L. donovani can withstand lower external pH than can promastigotes - more evidence that they are adapted for living in an acid environment.

Possibly related to pH homeostasis or modification of the parasitophorous vacuole is the production of D-lactate by leishmanias. So far this has been shown only for L. braziliensis panamensis promastigotes, but nevertheless it is a most surprising and exciting discovery. It raises again the question of the selective advantage to cells of this apparently valueless pathway. The greater production of D-lactate under anaerobiosis also poses the question as to whether such conditions are encountered in vivo; one of the major difficulties we face continually is our lack of detailed knowledge of the environment in which the amastigotes reside.

In the past, research on leishmanias has tended to follow the exciting leads that came out of studies on trypanosomes and other trypanosomatids. Trypanothione metabolism will clearly be another example of this. It is becoming increasingly clear, however, that leishmanias and the leishmaniases provide excellent systems for studying a variety of fundamental biological phenomena - notably cell differentation and survival and growth intracellularly. Our understanding of these processes is increasing slowly, although the availability of leishmania metacyclics should advance studies immensely. Already it is clear that these infective promastigotes differ at the molecular level in many ways from multiplicative promastigotes, although the trigger for transformation is yet to be discovered. The observed phenotypic differences between the two promastigote populations have consequences for the use of isoenzyme analysis as a method of identification; care must be given to ensure that similar promastigote populations are used in all experiments and results should be interpreted with some caution. There is now evidence from isoenzyme and chromosome analysis of natural isolates for the occurrence of genetic exchange between leishmanias, although this has yet to be confirmed experimentally. It suggests, however, that in this respect leishmanias are similar to salivarian trypanosomes.

The session included many interesting papers demonstrating how the application of modern techniques has provided new information on the genotypic and phenotypic characteristics of leishmanias and ways in which they can be used to identify the parasites. It should be noted, however, that several areas of great current interest, which are being extensively studied by various groups, were mentioned only fleetingly in the formal part of the meeting. Purine and pyrimidine metabolism being one major example. There was also surprisingly little new information on the glycosomes of leishmanias, although it was suggested that they may be the site of action of the antileishmanial antimonials. This could explain their specificity towards leishmanias rather than mammalian cells, but not the drugs' lack of toxicity towards promastigotes and other trypanosomatids. It is good that more workers are taking an interest in elucidating the mode of action of these compounds, which are, after all, the most important antileishmanial drugs currently available, and more information on their action is becoming available. The meeting seemed to provide an ideal opportunity for discussing in some detail the current evidence and ideas, but unfortunately this did not occur. Indeed it seems that many people are becoming increasingly wary of revealing new findings at scientific meetings and prefer simply to reiterate published work or, at best, disclose findings about to be published. Perhaps this is an inevitable consequence of the need to compete and the possibly great rewards, financial and otherwise, awaiting the successful. A consequence, however, is that despite the amazing advances made in information technology new findings often are disseminated more slowly now than they would have been in the past. Sometimes it appears that the scientific community does not so much work together towards the greater goal, but instead competes for individual glory. We must wait to see whether this approach will have the desired effect and lead to more rapid progress.

BIOCHEMICAL MECHANISMS OF PENTOSTAM

Jonathan D. Berman and
Max Grogl

Division of Experimental Therapeutics
Walter Reed Army Institute of Research
Washington, DC 20307-5100   USA

INTRODUCTION

Although treatment with antimonials may have been used by the ancient Greeks, and pentavalent antimonials such as sodium stibogluconate (Pentostam) have been the drugs of choice since the 1940s, in early 1985 Mottram and Coombs still could write that "there are no reports on the mechanism of antileishmanial antimonials".[1]

Our recent investigations have provided some knowledge into the biochemical mechanisms of Pentostam and are summarized in this communication.

CHEMICAL PROPERTIES OF PENTOSTAM

The generally assumed structure for sodium stibogluconate consists of two Sb atoms bound to two gluconate molecules, with three sodium atoms as counterions.

For this structure, the molecular weight is 746 and an elemental analysis of % carbon = 19.3, % hydrogen = 2.3, % sodium = 9.3, and % Sb = 32.6 can be calculated. A 100 mg Sb/ml water solution, the formulation in clinical use, would contain 307 mg Pentostam/ml (411 mM Pentostam). If all the sodium atoms dissociated from the Sb-carbohydrate moeities, the osmolarity of the 100 mg Sb/ml solution would be 1644 mosm.

We investigated the actual osmolarity, molecular weight, elemental analysis and NMR spectrum of Pentostam.

Osmolarity

The osmolarity of several lots of Pentostam, ^{125}Sb-Pentostam, and Glucantime were determined. The mean osmolarity of three Pentostam lots tested was 789 mosm. A clinically ineffective lot had an osmolarity >1000 mosm. A clinically effective lot of Glucantime had an osmolarity of 842 mosm, whereas an ineffective lot had a much higher osmolarity of 1241 mosm.

Gel Chromatography P₂ gel chromatography of ^{125}Sb-Pentostam revealed label spread between the solvent front and one column volume. Chromatography of Vitamin B₁₂ (MW=1355 daltons) and glucose (MW=180 daltons) standards indicates that entities of MW=100-4000 would elute between the solvent front and one column volume. Thus, ^{125}Sb-Pentostam appears to be a mixture of a large number of species of MW=100-4000 daltons.

Elemental Analysis One lot of unlabeled Pentostam had an elemental analysis of % carbon = 19.7, % hydrogen = 3.0, % sodium = 5.3, and % Sb = 27.8.

NMR Analysis This lot of unlabeled Pentostam was also found to have at least 20 peaks on ^{13}C NMR analysis, in contrast to the 6 carbon peaks expected from gluconic acid.

The chromatographic, elemental analysis, ^{13}CNMR, and osmometric data each indicate that Pentostam does not have the simple structure normally postulated. The components of Pentostam must be much more closely associated than the figure implies, resulting in a molecular weight greater than that expected and an osmolarity 1/2 that anticipated. Pentostam may be accurately described as an unknown number of complexes of Sb and carbohydrates derived from gluconic acid.

BIOCHEMICAL PROPERTIES OF PENTOSTAM

Chromatography When ^{125}Sb-Pentostam was incubated with L. mexicana amastigotes, organism sonicates that did not contain reducing agents or SDS demonstrated two peaks of radioactivity (MW = 45,000 and >300,000 daltons) on Sephadex G-200 chromatography. SDS-PAGE under reducing conditions was performed to more precisely determine the molecular weights of the components to which ^{125}Sb bound. SDS-PAGE of amastigotes revealed 9 subunits of molecular weight 14,000-68,000 daltons, as well as material that did not penetrate the 5% stacking gel (lines A in Fig. 1). Thus, the molecular weights of labeled species determined by the two techniques are very similar. Since amastigote extracts treated with proteases showed no radioactivity between 14,000 and 68,000 daltons on either Sephadex G-200 or SDS-PAGE chromatography (lines B in Fig. 1), these bands represent ^{125}Sb bound to protein.

Uptake of ^{125}Sb-Pentostam by Leishmania

Both Croft et al. and Berman et al. have shown that radiolabeled Pentostam is concentrated by amastigotes. After 24 hours the stibogluconate space was approximately 24 times greater than the water space.[2] The concentration of Pentostam in amastigotes exposed to 1.6 mM drug for 1 hour is 48 mM (concentration factor of 30).[3] The most likely explanation for concentration of Sb by amastigotes is binding to amastigote proteins.

Inhibition of Amastigote Biochemical Reactions

Intermediary Metabolism To investigate the effect of Pentostam on amastigote metabolism, it was necessary to first determine in vitro effective Pentostam concentrations. When L. mexicana amastigotes were exposed to 150, 300, and 500 μg Sb/ml for 4 hours and the number of promastigotes derived from the amastigotes were determined 2 days later, the numbers were 75%, 62%, and 39% of control, non-Sb exposed organisms.[4]

In control L. mexicana amastigotes (organisms not exposed to Sb), the rate of CO_2 formation from the 1-carbon of glucose was 2-4 times the rate of CO_2 formation from the 6-carbon (Table 1).[5] Since the 1-carbon is oxidized

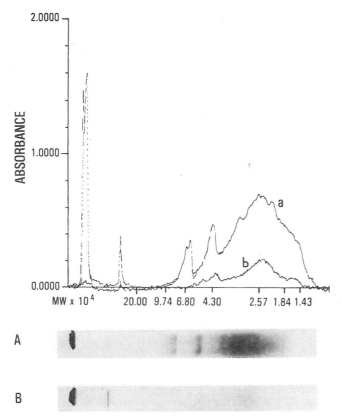

Figure 1. Components of L. mexicana (WR 227) tissue derived amastigotes reactive with ^{125}Sb-Pentostam. Extracts of ^{125}Sb-treated L. mexicana amastigotes were made by sonication and Chapso treatment and applied to SDS-polyacrylamide gels. Bottom: Panel (a): fluorogram of amastigote extract; 80 µg protein. Panel (b): fluorogram of amastigote extract treated with proteinase K; 80 µg. Top: Spectrophotometric measurements of fluorograms were done utilizing white light. The densitometric tracings of panels a and b are superimposed.

Table 1. Rates of metabolism of precursors to CO_2 in stibogluconate-treated L. mexicana amastigotes at pH 7.4

Precursor	Precursor conc (mM)	Precursor metabolized to CO_2 at [Sb] (μg/ml)			
		0	150	300	500
[1-^{14}C]Glucose	0.21	2.7 ± 1.1*	97 ± 10†	87 ± 13†	86 ± 14†
[6-^{14}C]Glucose	0.21	0.90 ± 0.15	89 ± 11	52 ± 13	31 ± 8
[U-^{14}C]Glucose	0.21	0.85 ± 0.28	90 ± 6	90 ± 12	76 ± 13
[1-^{14}C]Palmitate	0.21	1.3 ± 0.27	74 ± 11	40 ± 11	33 ± 10
[U-^{14}C]Palmitate	0.21	0.60 ± 0.07	49 ± 12	15 ± 6	12 ± 2
[2-^{14}C]Acetate	0.41	11 ± 2.7	98 ± 5.5	93 ± 7	94 ± 6

Amastigotes that had been pretreated for 4 hr with the indicated concentration of antimony in the form of stibogluconate were exposed to ^{14}C-labeled precursor (labeled at the indicated carbon), and the formation of $^{14}CO_2$ was determined.

* Nmoles precursor metabolized to $CO_2/10^8$ cells/hr (mean ± SE: N=4-7).

† Percent control metabolism (mean ± SE: N = 4-7).

Table 2. Inhibition of Leishmania amastigote purine trinucleotide formation by stibogluconate[a]

Sb treatment (μg/ml)	% Control cpm in:			TP/DP
	MP	DP	TP	
150	99(92-106)	115(105-126)	105(96-114)	6.4(5.5-7.2)
300	150(148-151)	148(129-167)	100(84-115)	5.3(3.9-6.7)
500	160(107-213)	144(142-146)	44(36-52)	2.0(1.9-2.1)
0 (control)	117	273	1,960	7.2

[a] One milliliter of amastigotes (30×10^6) exposed to 0 to 500 μg of Sb and to [^{14}C]hypoxanthine for 4 h were trichloracetate acid (TCA) treated, and 2.5 μl of the trioctylamine-Freon extract of the TCA supernatant was chromatographed on thin-layer plates. Spots corresponding to nucleoside monophosphates (MP), diphosphates (DP), and triphosphates (TP) were cut out and counted. Data represent counts perminute in Sb-exposed organisms expressed as a percentage of control counts (mean of two experiments [range]). Mean control values (counts per minute) are also listed.

before carbons 2-6 in the hexose monophosphate shunt, but is equivalent to the 6-carbon in glycolysis, the increased rate of 1-carbon over 6-carbon metabolism to CO_2 has been taken as an approximation of the rate of activity of the hexosemonophosphate shunt. On this basis, the hexosemonophosphate shunt was found to be 1.5-3.0 times faster than glycolysis in amastigotes.

As Hart and Coombs reported,[6] oxidation of the first carbon of fatty acids (here, palmitic acid) was approximately twice as fast as oxodation of the rest of the molecule. This comparison suggests that half of 1-carbon catabolism to CO_2 occurs in a pathway that removes only that carbon and, therefore, will not generate acetate. The rate of utilization of [U-^{14}C]palmitate to CO_2 may better reflect catabolic processes that generate 2-carbon moieties suitable for entry into the citric acid cycle. In this case, the rate of utilization of fatty acids for processes that are likely to generate NADH was slightly less than the rate of glucose metabolism via glycolytic enzymes.

Exposure of amastigotes to 150-500 µg Sb/ml resulted in a dose-dependent decrease in formation of CO_2 from [6-^{14}C]glucose via glycolytic enzymes and from [^{14}C]palmitate via fatty acid β-oxidation. The lack of stibogluconate inhibition of the acetate-to-CO_2 pathway (Table 1) indicates that stibogluconate treatment did not inhibit utilization of acetate generated by glycolytic enzymes or β-oxidation. Thus, inhibition of CO_2 formation from glucose and fatty acid resulted from inhibition of a process between the uptake of the precursors and the generation of acetate.

Utilization of glucose in the hexosemonophosphate shunt was relatively unaffected by stibogluconate; this indicates that stibogluconate did not inhibit glucose transport into the cell or phosphorylation of glucose to glucose-6-phosphate. Inhibition of formation of CO_2 from [6-^{14}C] glucose may be due to inhibition of the generation of acetate from glucose-6-phosphate, that is, due to inhibition of glycolytic enzymes such as phosphofructokinase themselves. Alternatively, the fact that Leishmania promastigotes and, presumably, amastigotes segregate their glycolytic enzymes into organelles (glycosomes) suggests that inhibition of glycosome structure or function by stibogluconate may result in inhibition of glycolytic enzymes.

The manner in which fatty acids are presented to β-oxidative enzymes has not been clarified for Leishmania, but the fact that oxidation of 1-carbon of palmitate was inhibited to approximately the same extent as oxidation of the rest of palmitate suggests that some basic aspect of fatty acid transport, rather than β-oxidation per se, may be inhibited by stibogluconate.

Purine Nucleotide Formation   Control amastigotes exposed to [^{14}C]hypoxanthine for 4 h demonstrated a nucleoside triphosphate-to-diphosphate (TP/DP) ratio of 7.2 (Table 2).[4] The incorporation of label into amastigotes exposed to 500 µg of Sb per ml demonstrated a 56% decrease in nucleoside triphosphate and a 44 to 60% increase in nucleoside monophosphates and diphosphates. The TP/DP ratio decreased by a factor of 3.6, from 7.2 in controls to 2.0 (Table 2). The specific block in formation of ATP from ADP in Pentostam-exposed amastigotes suggests that inhibition of bioenergetics may lead to inhibited ATP synthesis.

SUMMARY

Pentostam, an uncharacterized complex of Sb^V and carbohydrate derived from gluconic acid, is concentrated by Leishmania amastigotes via protein binding. Biochemical consequences of the interaction of amastigotes with Pentostam are inhibition of parasite bioenergetics and inhibition of ATP synthesis.

REFERENCES

1. J.C. Mottram and G.H. Coombs. Enzyme activities of amastigotes and promastigotes and their inhibition by antimonials and arsenicals. Exper. Parasitol. 59:151 (1985).
2. S.L. Croft, K.D. Neame and C.A. Homewood. Accumulation of [^{125}Sb] sodium stibogluconate by Leishmania mexicana amazonensis and Leishmania donovani in vitro. Comp. Biochem. Physiol. 68C:95 (1981).
3. J.D. Berman, J.V. Gallalee, and B.D. Hansen. Leishmania mexicana: uptake of sodium stibogluconate (Pentostam) and pentamidine by parasite and macrophages. Exper. Parasitol. 64:127 (1987).
4. J.D. Berman, D. Waddell and B.D. Hanson. Biochemical mechanisms of the antileishmanial activity of sodium stibogluconate. Antimicrobial Agents Chemotherapy. 27:916 (1985).
5. J.D. Berman, J.V. Gallalee, and J.M. Best. Sodium stibogluconate (Pentostam) inhibition of glucose catabolism via the glycolytic pathway, and fatty acid β-oxidation in Leishmania mexicana amastigotes. Biochem. Pharmacol. 36:197 (1987).
6. D.T. Hart and G.H. Coombs. Leishmania mexicana: Energy metabolism of amastigotes and promastigotes. Exper. Parasitol. 54:397 (1982).

EFFECTS OF SINEFUNGIN ON CELLULAR AND BIOCHEMICAL

EVENTS IN PROMASTIGOTES OF LEISHMANIA d. donovani

Françoise Lawrence, and Malka Robert-Géro

Institut de Chimie des Substances Naturelles
C.N.R.S.
91190 Gif-sur-Yvette (France)

INTRODUCTION

Sinefungin is a nucleoside antibiotic produced by Streptomyces griseolus and Streptomyces incarnatus. This molecule is composed of an adenosine moiety in which the 5'end is linked by a carbon-carbon bond to an ornithine residue. Sinefungin is an antifungal and antiparasitic agent in vivo and in vitro (for ref. see: M. Robert-Géro "et al.", this issue). In order to understand the mechanism of action of sinefungin, we studied the effects of this nucleoside on cellular and biochemical events in Leishmania d. donovani promastigotes.

MATERIALS AND METHODS

Leishmania d. donovani (strain LRC L32) originated from the World Health Organisation's International Reference Center for leishmaniasis. Mouse peritoneal macrophages, cell line P388D, were provided by Dr. A. Adam (Orsay, France). Cells were grown in a semi-defined medium as described previously[1] in presence or absence of sinefungin for various lengths of time. Cells were then labelled with appropriate radioactive precursor. After 1 h. the cells were sedimented and rinsed twice with cold phosphate buffered saline. The uptake into soluble pool and the incorporation into macromolecules were obtained from cold-TCA soluble, hot-TCA soluble and insoluble materials.[2] Protein concentration was determined by the Lowry procedure.[3]

The phosphorylation of nucleosides was carried out on a 0.5M cold perchloric acid extract which had been neutralized and chromatographed on cellulose thin layer plate.[4]

DNA was extracted as described by Blin and Stafford[5] and analyzed on CsCl gradients.

DNA polymerase activity was measured with partially purified enzyme using two assays : the PPi assay[6] and incorporation of thymidine.[7]

S-adenosylmethionine (AdoMet) synthesis was measured by incorporation of [^{35}S]-L-methionine into AdoMet which was isolated by cellulose thin layer chromatography.

Protein synthesis pattern was assayed on SDS-polyacrylamide gel electrophoresis as described by Laemmli.[8]

RESULTS

Growth, Morphology, Motility and Macromolecular Syntheses

The growth of L. d. donovani promastigotes was inhibited by low concentration of sinefungin.[1] With 0.026 µM sinefungin the increase in cell number was 30% that of control culture after the first 24 hours treatment and 2% for the next 24 hours. With 0.130 µM the growth was completely and irreversibly inhibited.

Sinefungin induced modifications in the shape and motility of promastigotes. The long slender flagellated promastigotes became progressively more rounded and their motility decreased and then ceased. The proportion of round-shaped and immobile forms was time and concentration dependant. With 2.6 µM sinefungin the changes were observable after 3 to 6 hours contact : the percentage of these round immobile forms represented 20±7, 45±5 and 83±5 of the cell population after 6, 16 and 24 hours treatment respectively.

Studies of macromolecular biosyntheses showed that sinefungin drastically inhibited the incorporation of thymidine into the DNA of promastigotes.[4] After 6 hours in the presence of 0.026 µM and 0.26 µM sinefungin, the incorporation of thymidine was inhibited by 70% and 91% respectively, despite an increase in the amount of radioactivity in the acid soluble pool. Under similar conditions uridine incorporation and uptake were both moderately decreased; however the uptake of uridine into the acid-soluble fraction was inhibited to a lesser degree (21 and 41%) than the incorporation into the acid-insoluble material (36 and 61%) suggesting a slight effect on RNA synthesis. Leucine incorporation into proteins was weakly inhibited by the drug (3 and 19%).

DNA Synthesis

The inhibition of thymidine incorporation into DNA was concentration dependant (as shown by the values cited previously) and time dependant : sinefungin treatment (0.26 µM) for 1, 2, 4 and 6 hours inhibited the incorporation of thymidine by 48±5, 78±9, 82±8 and 91±3 percent respectively.

This inhibition seemed specific for parasites since in macrophages (host cells) no such effect could be observed, even treatments with 10 to 100 times higher concentrations and incubations up to 24 hours did not alter thymidine incorporation into the macrophages.[4]

Analysis of the DNA on CsCl gradient showed that the incorporation of thymidine was less inhibited in kinetoplastic DNA (kDNA : 43±18% inhibition) than in nuclear DNA (nDNA : 77±4% inhibition) after 6 hours treatment with 0.26 µM sinefungin. The buoyant densities for kDNA and nDNA were respectively similar in control and treated cells.[4]

The inhibition of DNA synthesis in promastigotes by sinefungin can be antagonized by AdoMet : although AdoMet addition alone did not cause an increase in thymidine incorporation of a control culture, cultures with this compound in the medium were not as sensitive to sinefungin inhibition as parallel cultures grown without AdoMet. Thus with 0.26 µM sinefungin, the presence of 2 to 20 µM AdoMet elicit the doubling of thymidine incorporation compared to sinefungin alone (Fig. 1); S-adenosyl-homocysteine (AdoHcy) was significantly less efficient in antagonizing the effect of sinefungin since to obtain similar effect, concentrations 50 fold higher than those of AdoMet were needed.

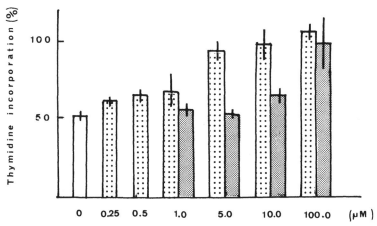

Fig. 1. Antagonism between AdoMet and Sinefungin for Thymidine Incorporation

Promastigotes (5.10^6 cells/ml) were cultured in a medium containing 0.26 µM sinefungin either alone ☐ or with various concentrations of AdoMet ▨ or AdoHcy ▧ for 4 hours; then the cultures were labelled with thymidine for 30 minutes. Incorporation into DNA was measured in TCA insoluble material. The 100% value was obtained from parallel cultures carried out without any addition.

Attempts to explain the mechanism of action of sinefungin have shown that the decline in the labelling of DNA did not result from an inhibition of the transport of thymidine into the cells (since the amount of label found in the acid-soluble pool increased upon sinefungin treatment) nor from an inhibition of nucleoside phosphorylation (either ribo- or deoxyribo-).[4]

Preliminary results on the effect of sinefungin on <u>in vitro</u> DNA polymerase activity were not very reproducible. The inhibitory effect was poor (23%±15 at 10 µM sinefungin) and seemed to increase upon preincubation of the partially purified enzyme with the drug.

Table 1. Synthesis of S-Adenosyl Methionine in Control and
Sinefungin-treated Cells

	% Radioactivity in AdoMet		
	1 h	4 h	20 h
Control	7.25	3.38 ± 0.44	7.54 ± 0.81
Sinefungin 2.6 µM	6.85	3.85 ± 0.82	7.31 ± 0.09
Treated/control	0.94	1.14	0.97

Leishmania promastigotes (5.10^6 cells/ml) were cultured with or without 2.6 µM sinefungin for various lenghts of time, and then labelled for 30 min with 200 µci/ml [^{35}S]-L-methionine. Cells were then sedimented, rinsed twice with PBS and extracted 2 min with cold 1M perchloric acid. The perchloric extract was neutralized with KOH on ice, using phenol red as internal indicator. After centrifugation to remove the perchlorate salts, 10 and 20 µl were chromatographed along with unlabelled carriers on thin layer cellulose plates, using n-Butanol/acetic Acid/H_2O (60/15/25, vol/vol) as solvent.
The radioactivity accompanying the carriers was determined by liquid scintillation counting. Results are expressed as the percentage of radioactivity found in AdoMet.

S-Adenosyl-Methionine Synthesis

Since AdoMet is structurally related to sinefungin and since AdoMet antagonized the effect of the drug on thymidine incorporation we studied the effect of sinefungin on AdoMet synthesis (Table 1) : Treatment of the promastigotes with 2.6µM sinefungin up to 24 hours did not affect significantly the percentage of radioactivity found in AdoMet. This indicates that sinefungin did not inhibit the synthesis of AdoMet within these cells.

Protein Synthesis

Although amino acid incorporation into proteins was not affected by treatment with 2.6 µM sinefungin for 1 hour[4] the electrophoretical pattern of the labelled proteins was modified : in sinefungin treated promastigotes some proteins became overlabelled (Fig. 2). The apparent molecular weight of the three main inducible proteins (estimated on the bases of their mobilities on SDS-polyacrylamide gels) were 90 000, 80 000 and 70 000. Additional bands were observed after longer period of treatment. Their molecular weight being 110 000, 54-56 000, 35-38 000, 32 000, 18 000 and 16 000 d.

Comparison of Electrophoretical Patterns
of Proteins Synthesized in Presence or
Absence of Sinefungin.

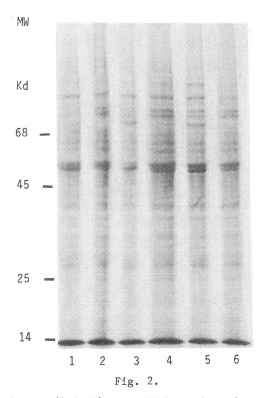

Fig. 2.

Sinefungin (2.6 µM) was added to the cultures of
L. d. donovani promastigotes (5.6 10^6 cells/ml).
The cells were then labelled with [^{35}S]-L-methionine (200 µCi/ml) for 30 min. Lanes 1,3,5 :
sinefungin treated cells for 24 hrs, 3 hrs and 1
hr respectively; lanes 2,4,6 : control cells at
similar timing.

The synthesis of the sinefungin-induced proteins followed different kinetics. They appeared more or less rapidly following the sinefungin stimulus and their synthesis lasted for a limited period. The maximal intensity of 70 000 and 90 000 proteins appeared faster than that of the 80 000 protein. The 90 000 protein decreased rapidly after 3 hours treatment while the 80 000 protein decreased slowly after 6-16 hours and the 70 000 protein after 24 hours. The response towards sinefungin treatment was found to decrease gradually in magnitude as the age of the culture advanced except for the 70 000 protein. The synthesis of these sinefungin induced proteins depended on the translation of newly transcribed mRNA, the presence of actinomycin impairing the overexpression of these proteins.

Protein methylase I (arg) and III (lys) activities in a crude extract were competitively inhibited by sinefungin, however the apparent Ki values were higher than those observed in avian and mammalian cells.[9] Furthermore aminoacid analysis of proteins from a 12 000 g supernatent showed that the N-methylations of the aminoacid residues were not significantly inhibited in treated cells.[9]

DISCUSSION

Sinefungin has been reported to inhibit the growth of various Leishmania species.[1,10,11] Until now the most spectacular effect of sinefungin on the promastigotes of L. donovani is the inhibition of DNA synthesis. The effect is species specific since it occurred in various Leishmania promastigotes[4,10] and Plasmodiun falciparum but not in host cells (macrophages).[4] The unresponsiveness of the macrophages is not due to a lack of uptake of sinefungin within the cells nor to a metabolic inactivation since the drug is able to inhibit amastigote multiplication within the macrophages.[11,12] The explanation of such a specificity might be in differences in DNA synthesis processes between parasites and macrophages.[13] The replication of DNA is an enzymatically complex processes and it requires many activities and various factors in addition to the DNA polymerase.[14,15] It has been reported that DNA polymerase from the trypanosomatidae was biochemically and immunologically distinct from its mammalian counterpart.[16,17]

The fact that kDNA synthesis is less sensitive to sinefungin inhibition than nDNA could reflect either a lower penetration of the drug into the kinetoplast or a different sensitivity of the target. Another possibility is that the ionization of sinefungin is different in these two cellular compartments, leading to a modified efficiency of the drug.

Our results on the effect of sinefungin on DNA polymerase activity conflict those of Nolan et al.[10] reporting inhibition of DNA polymerase of L. mexicana in vitro by sinefungin (Ki = 15 nM), the drug being a competitive inhibitor of dATP. However our data fit well with the observation by Bachrach's group who found that in P.falciparum the synthesis of the only DNA polymerase of the parasite (DNA polymerase alpha) is triggered by high levels of spermine and spermidine.[18] In this case sinefungin lowered the level of these polyamines[19] and thus the DNA polymerase of the parasite is no more induced and DNA synthesis could not occur.

CONCLUSION

The precise mechanism of inhibition of thymidine incorporation by sinefungin is not yet completely elucidated. The fact that the inhibition by sinefungin can be antagonized by AdoMet suggests that the cellular target(s) in promastigote might be a specific methylase related to DNA replication. In this respect it is interesting to consider the data of Noguchi et al.[20] describing an enzymatic complex named "replitase" containing DNA polymerase and DNA methylase activities fully associated with newly synthesized DNA. The other approach under study is the possibility that as in P.falciparum the polyamine level is lowered in the presence of sinefungin and that prevents the induction of the DNA polymerase of the parasite.

ACKNOWLEDGEMENTS

This work was supported by Grants from the World Health Organisation UNDP/World Bank/Who Special Programme for Research and Training in Tropical Diseases.

REFERENCES

1. P. Paolantonacci, F. Lawrence and M. Robert-Gero, Differential effect of Sinefungin and Its Analogs on the Multiplication of Three Leishmania Species, Antimicrob. Agents Chemother., 28:528 (1985).
2. W.C. Schneider, Phosphorous Compounds in Animal Tissues. Extraction and Estimation of Desoxypentose Nucleic Acid and of Pentose Nucleic Acid, J. Biol. Chem., 161:293 (1945).
3. O.H. Lowry, N.J. Rosebrough, A.L. Farr and R.J. Randall, Protein Measurement with the Folin Phenol Reagent, J. Biol. Chem., 193:265 (1951).
4. P. Paolantonacci, F. Lawrence, L. Nolan and M. Robert-Gero, Inhibition of Leishmanial DNA Synthesis by Sinefungin, Biochem. Pharmacol., 36:2813 (1987).
5. N. Blin and D.W. Stafford, A General Method for Isolation of High Molecular Weight DNA from Eukaryotes, Nucleic Ac. Res., 3:2303 (1976).
6. Sigma Technical Bulletin, New DNA Polymerase Assay, n°.8014 (1984).
7. G.P. Noy and A. Weissbach, HeLa Cell DNA Polymerases : The Effect of Cycloheximide in vivo and Detection of a New Form of DNA Polymerase α, Biochim. Biophys. Acta, 477:70 (1977).
8. U.K. Laemmli, Cleavage of Structural Proteins during the Assembly of the Head of Bacteriophage T4, Nature, 227:680 (1970).
9. P. Paolantonacci, F. Lawrence, F. Lederer and M. Robert-Gero, Protein Methylation and Protein Methylases in Leishmania donovani and Leishmania tropica Promastigotes, Mol. Biochem. Parasitol., 21:47 (1986).
10. L.L. Nolan, W. Hanson and V. Waits, Molecular Target of Antileishmanial Action of Sinefungin. (in Preparation).
11. U. Bachrach, L.F. Schnur, J. El-On, C.L. Greenblatt, E. Pearlman, M. Robert-Gero and E. Lederer, Inhibitory Activity of Sinefungin and SIBA (5'deoxy-5'-S-isobutylthioadenosine) on the Growth of Promastigotes and Amastigotes of Different Species of Leishmania, FEBS Letters, 121:287 (1980).
12. R.A. Neal and S.L. Croft, An in vitro System for Determining the Activity of Compounds against the Intracellular Amastigote Form of Leishmania donovani, J. Antimicrob. Chemother., 14:463 (1984).

13. T.W. North and D.J. Wyler, DNA Synthesis in Promastigotes of Leishmania major and L. donovani, Mol. Biochem. Parasitol., 22:215 (1987).
14. J.L. Campbell, Eukaryotic DNA Replication in "Ann. Rev. Biochem.", C.C. Richardson, P.D. Boyer, I.B. Dawid, A. Meister Eds, Annual Review Inc., Palo Alto, U.S.A. (1986).
15. J.W. Chase, K.R. Williams, Single-stranded DNA Binding Proteins Required for DNA Replication, in "Ann. Rev. Biochem.", C.C. Richardson, P.D. Boyer, I.B. Dawid, A. Meister Eds, Annual Reviews Inc., Palo Alto, U.S.A. (1986).
16. A.M. Holmes, E. Cheriathundam, A. Kalinski and L.M.S. Chang, Isolation and Partial Characterisation of DNA Polymerase from Crithidia fasciculata, Mol. Biochem. Parasitol., 10:195 (1984).
17. A.D. Solari, Tharaud D., Y. Repetto J., Aldunate, A. Morello and S. Litvak, In vitro and in vivo Studies of Trypanosoma cruzi DNA Polymerase. Biochem. Int., 7:147 (1983).
18. Y.G. Assaraf, L. Abu-Elheiga, D.T. Spira, H. Desser and U. Bachrach, Effect of Polyamine Depletion on Macromolecular Synthesis of the Malarial Parasite, Plasmodium falciparum, Cultured in Human Erythrocytes, Biochem. J., 242:221 (1987).
19. E. Messika, J. Golenser, M. Robert-Gero, E. Lederer and U. Bachrach, Effect of Sinefungin on the Development and Polyamine Metabolism of Plasmodium falciparum, 3rd Congress on Parasites in Jerusalem, p. 22 (1987).
20. H. Noguchi, G. Prem Veer Reddy and A.B. Pardee, Rapid Incorporation of Label from Ribonucleoside Diphosphates into DNA by a Cell-Free High Molecular Weight Fraction from Animal Cell Nuclei, Cell, 32:443 (1983).

METABOLISM AND FUNCTIONS OF TRYPANOTHIONE

WITH SPECIAL REFERENCE TO LEISHMANIASIS

Alan H. Fairlamb

Department of Medical Protozoology
London School of Hygiene and Tropical Medicine
London, U.K.

INTRODUCTION

Over a century has passed since the causative organism of cutaneous leishmaniasis was discovered. The history of trypanothione is considerably shorter than that, and, following the initial observations in 1982, our knowledge of trypanothione has increased rapidly. Thus, reviews of this unusual spermidine-containing peptide need to be frequently updated. The purpose of this article is two-fold: to revise an earlier review in the NATO-ASI series (Fairlamb and Henderson, 1987); and to highlight specific areas of the biochemistry of trypanothione that may be exploited for chemotherapeutic intervention against leishmaniasis. Most of our present knowledge has been obtained from studies on other trypanosomatids, but preliminary studies on leishmania suggests that these findings are also applicable to this group of organisms.

TRYPANOTHIONE AND CONTROL OF CELLULAR REDOX

Trypanothione was discovered during studies on glutathione reductase activity in <u>Trypanosoma brucei</u>. A low-molecular weight thiol-containing co-factor was found to be essential for the enzymatic reduction of glutathione disulphide (GSSG) by NADPH (Fairlamb and Cerami, 1985). This co-factor was present in extracts of all trypanosomatids, including leishmania, but absent in a variety of mammalian, bacterial and plant extracts. The compound was purified as its disulphide and the structure determined to be N^1,N^8-bis(glutathionyl)spermidine (Fairlamb et al., 1985). As it is unique to trypanosomatids, we have chosen trypanothione as an appropriate trivial name.

The structure and the terminology of the biochemically important oxidation states of this molecule are given in Figure 1. Note that the two molecules of glutathione are attached in covalent linkage from the glycine carboxyls to the terminal amino groups of spermidine. In the cell, essentially all of the trypanothione is present as the dithiol, dihydro- trypanothione, due to the action of the NADPH-dependent enzyme trypanothione reductase. This enzyme is incapable of reducing GSSG directly. However, GSSG and other intracellular disulphides are reduced indirectly by means of non-enzymatic thiol-disulphide exchange with dihydrotrypanothione. The net result of these reactions is NADPH-dependent disulphide reduction as found in most other organisms.

Control of intracellular redox is regarded as essential for many cellular functions, including the synthesis or degradation of proteins, regulation of enzyme activity and protection against reactive oxygen compounds or free radicals (see review by Meister and Anderson, 1983). Thus, compounds that either reduce the levels of the substrate, trypanothione, or inhibit trypanothione reductase itself, might be expected to damage these parasites.

TRYPANOTHIONE AND DEFENCE AGAINST OXIDATIVE DAMAGE

All organisms living in aerobic environments appear to have evolved defence mechanisms against toxic oxygen metabolites which are produced internally as an inevitable consequence of their metabolism. In addition, parasites need to defend themselves from reactive oxygen species, generated externally by the host immune-defence system in an attempt to destroy the invading parasites.

In the scheme outlined in Figure 2, most of the oxygen consumed during oxidative metabolism proceeds via a direct 4-electron reduction of dioxygen to form H_2O without the formation of partially reduced oxygen species as free intermediates. The enzyme par excellence catalyzing this reaction is of course cytochrome oxidase. However, a small proportion of the oxygen used also undergoes either a 1-electron reduction to form superoxide anion $[O_2^-]$ (by reduced flavins, quinones, etc) or a 2-electron reduction to form hydrogen peroxide $[H_2O_2]$ (by amino acid oxidase, urate oxidase, etc). If O_2^- and H_2O_2 are allowed to accumulate, then formation of the highly reactive hydroxyl radical $[OH\cdot]$ will be favoured through the Haber-Weiss reaction, catalyzed by transition metal ions. Hydroxyl radicals (or related radical species) can then lead to damage to DNA, membrane lipids and other essential components with disastrous consequences to the cell.

No enzymatic defence mechanism is available to remove $OH\cdot$ once it is formed. Thus, most organisms have developed a strategy of minimising the formation of $OH\cdot$ by maintaining the precursors O_2^- and H_2O_2 at vanishingly small concentrations. This is achieved by the concerted action

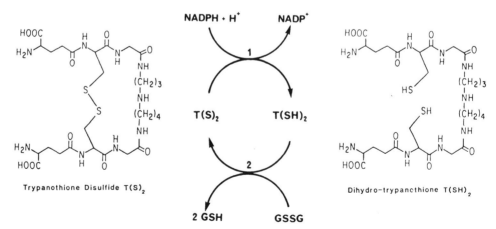

Fig. 1. Reduction of glutathione disulphide (GSSG) in trypanosomatids. Reaction 1 is catalyzed by trypanothione reductase and reaction 2 occurs non-enzymatically.

of: i) superoxide dismutase and ii) peroxidases such as glutathione peroxidase or catalase.

The first line of defence, superoxide dismutase [SOD], is present in both trypanosomes (T.brucei and T.cruzi) and leishmanias (Leishmania tropica) and appears to be similar to the iron-containing SOD from Crithidia fasciculata (Le Trang et al., 1983). Crithidial Fe-SOD is closely related to bacterial Fe-SOD, but only distantly related to the human Mn- and Cu-,Zn-containing enzymes. It can be estimated that the intracellular concentration of Fe-SOD in Crithidia is approximately 10^{-6} M, which is about 10 times lower than that calculated for mammalian tissues (Fridovich, 1978). Thus, leishmania and other trypanosomatids can prevent accumulation of O_2^- within the cell, but they do so at the expense of promoting the formation of H_2O_2.

Many anti-trypanosomal compounds, including nitroheterocyclics and quinones, are thought to selectively kill parasites by promoting the formation of toxic oxygen species through redox cycling (Docampo and Moreno, 1986). This involves an enzymatic 1-electron reduction of the drug and its spontaneous reoxidation by molecular oxygen forming O_2^-. Since trypanothione plays a central role in defence against oxidative damage, a potent synergism might be predicted between these compounds and inhibitors of trypanothione metabolism. Further work is necessary to test this hypothesis.

Until recently, it was thought that trypanosomatids were deficient in the enzymes that form the second line of defence: the removal of hydrogen peroxide (see review by Docampo and Moreno, 1986). However, Penketh and Klein (1986) have shown that appreciable amounts of exogenously added H_2O_2 can be metabolized by bloodstream T.brucei-- despite the fact that these organisms contain essentially no catalase or glutathione peroxidase. We subsequently demonstrated that reduction of H_2O_2 by extracts of T.brucei requires NADPH and dihydrotrypanothione, proceeding via the cyclical activity of a trypanothione-dependent peroxidase and reductase (Henderson, et al., 1987a). This mechanism parallels the glutathione peroxidase and reductase of mammalian cells. A similar trypanothione peroxidase activity has been identified in C.fasciculata, but it is not yet known whether a similar enzyme activity is present in Leishmania spp.

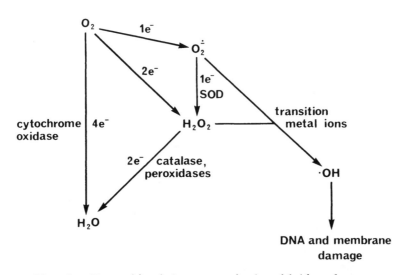

Fig. 2. Enzymatic defences against oxidative damage.

Table 1. A comparison of the properties of trypanothione reductase [TR] and glutathione reductase [GR].

Parameter	TR		GR
	C.fasciculata	T.cruzi	human
Subunit mass	53.8 kDa	50 kDa	52.5 kDa
Oligomeric structure	dimer	dimer	dimer
Cofactor	FAD	FAD	FAD
Catalytic disulphide	yes (Cys-Cys)	yes (?)	yes (Cys-Cys)
Turnover number (min^{-1})	31,000	12,600	14,200
Substrate specificity (K_m)			
NADPH	7 µM	5 µM	8.5 µM
Trypanothione disulphide	51 µM	45 µM	none
Glutathionylspermidine disulphide	149 µM	275 µM	none
Glutathione disulphide	none	none	65 µM

Data are from Shames et al. (1986), Henderson et al. (1987b), and Krauth-Siegel et al. (1987).

TRYPANOTHIONE REDUCTASE AS A TARGET FOR CHEMOTHERAPY

At present, trypanothione reductase is a principal target for the rational design of new trypanocidal drugs. Leishmania are similar to trypanosomes in that they contain trypanothione reductase. Despite the size difference, both promastigotes and purified amastigotes of L.mexicana amazonensis contain comparable amounts of activity (400 and 414 nmol min^{-1} mg^{-1}, respectively) (Chang and Fairlamb, unpublished). After correction for differences in assay conditions, these levels are in the same range as those for C.fasciculata and T.cruzi. Unfortunately, the leishmanial enzyme has not been fully characterised as yet. However, purification has been achieved from C.fasciculata (Shames et al., 1986) and T.cruzi (Krauth-Siegel et al., 1987). Both have similar physical and chemical properties to mammalian glutathione reductase (Table 1). In C.fasciculata, the amino acid sequence of the active site shows strong homology with glutathione reductase. However, these enzyme classes show significant differences in their substrate specificity: GSSG is not a substrate for trypanothione reductase; neither is trypanothione disulphide a substrate for glutathione reductase.

The molecular basis for this specificity has been examined using chemically synthesized analogues of trypanothione (Henderson et al., 1987b). These studies show that the spermidine moiety of trypanothione can be replaced by a variety of functional groups, suggesting that the substrate binding domain of trypanothione reductase is much less specific than glutathione reductase. Indeed, by attaching such functional groups to nitrofurans, nitroimidazoles or quinones, trypanothione reductase can be tricked into reducing compounds that bear virtually no resemblance to trypanothione disulphide (Henderson, Ulrich, Fairlamb and Cerami, unpublished). As described above, these compounds undergo redox-active cycling to form O_2^- and H_2O_2 and thus might be exploited as a means of inducing parasite-specific oxidative damage.

In summary, two potential approaches to chemotherapy present themselves. First, to inhibit the enzyme trypanothione reductase and consequently interfere with the normal functions of trypanothione (maintenance of intracellular redox and removal of peroxides). Second, to subvert the enzyme into generating toxic oxygen metabolites within the target cell, thereby swamping its oxidative defences. Such work will be greatly aided by knowledge of the three dimensional structure of the enzyme. Trypanothione reductase from T.cruzi is now available in crystalline form (Krauth-Siegel et al., 1987) and sequence data from this and other species will be available soon.

BIOSYNTHESIS OF TRYPANOTHIONE AND THE EFFECT OF DFMO

In Leishmania, both promastigotes and amastigotes are capable of synthesizing putrescine, spermidine and spermine from ornithine (reviewed by Bacchi, 1981 and Bacchi and McCann, 1987). The first enzyme in the polyamine biosynthetic pathway, ornithine decarboxylase [ODC], is sensitive to inhibition by difluoromethylornithine [DFMO], a drug currently undergoing clinical trials for the treatment of African sleeping sickness (reviewed by Schecter et al., 1987). Recently, Kaur et al. (1986) have reported that growth of L.donovani promastigotes in culture can be completely blocked by DFMO. After exposure to DFMO for 70 h, cells were completely depleted of putrescine and contained about 50% less spermidine than controls. The cytosatic effects of DFMO on Leishmania braziliensis guanensis and Leishmania donovani both in vivo and in vitro are described in a separate article (see Keithly and Fairlamb, this volume). These initially promising results suggest that inhibition of polyamine metabolism by DFMO or other compounds could form the basis for the development of new therapeutic agents.

Metabolic labelling studies with intact or cell-free lysates of C.fasciculata are consistant with the biosynthetic route to trypanothione shown in Figure 3 (Fairlamb et al., 1986). Synthesis from the precursors spermidine and glutathione proceeds via a series of ATP-dependent enzyme-catalyzed reactions with glutathionylspermidine as intermediate. Since leishmania also contain glutathionylspermidine, it can be inferred that a similar pathway exists in these organisms. Purification and characterization of these enzymes is underway. Information on the biochemical mechanisms of these proteins is of prime importance for drug development, since these enzymes are unique to the parasites, unlike those catalysing the preceding biochemical steps.

In view of the initial results obtained with DFMO against Leishmania, some new findings on the effects of DFMO on the biochemistry of African trypanosomes should be mentioned. Treatment of T.brucei infections in vivo causes profound metabolic, biochemical and morphological changes, associated with cytostasis and subsequent elimination of the parasite by the host immune system (reviewed by Bacchi and McCann, 1987). Depletion of the polyamines putrescine and spermidine is associated with a significant reduction in the cells content of glutathionylspermidine and trypanothione (Fairlamb et al., 1987). In the light of these findings and the previous discussion, we have proposed that the pronounced synergism found between DFMO and certain other drugs may be due to depletion of these important metabolites (see Figure 3). Similar considerations should be applied to Leishmania. It should also be noted that DFMO-resistant mutants of T.brucei procyclic trypomastigotes have been produced under laboratory conditions (Phillips and Wang, 1987; Bellofatto et al., 1987). Although the precise mechanism of how resistance is achieved remains unclear (both groups have failed to find amplification of the ODC gene), it is significant that mutants grow normally in the presence of drug with markedly depleted polyamine levels, while maintaining glutathionylspermidine and dihydrotrypanothione at normal levels. This finding supports the contention that these metabolites are essential for survival of the parasites.

Glutathionylspermidine was originally discovered in Escherichia coli, where it is formed solely in the stationary phase of growth (Tabor and Tabor, 1975). In contrast, this metabolite is present as a minor component in logarithmically growing bloodstream (Fairlamb et al., 1987) and procyclic T.brucei (Bellofatto et al., 1987), C.fasciculata (Fairlamb et al., 1986) and Leishmania (Keithly and Fairlamb, unpublished). As noted in Table 1, glutathionylspermidine disulphide is a substrate for trypanothione reductase, albeit less efficient than trypanothione disulphide, and could thus play a minor role in control of cellular redox. Curiously, in stationary phase C.fasciculata, dihydrotrypanothione is replaced by N^1-glutathionylspermidine as the most abundant intracellular thiol (Shim and Fairlamb, 1987). Whether these changes in metabolite levels actually induce or merely reflect stationary phase growth conditions is not known. Accumulation of glutathionylspermidine in stationary phase would appear to function as a means of regulating the levels of free unconjugated spermidine. On restoration of growth conditions, glutathionylspermidine [GSH-SPD] is rapidly converted to free spermidine [SPD] and dihydrotrypanothione [T(SH)$_2$] as follows:

$$2 \text{ GSH-SPD} \longrightarrow \text{T[SH]}_2 + \text{SPD}$$

As might be expected from this equation, the level of unconjugated GSH does not change during this 'metabolic shuffle'. This process is essentially

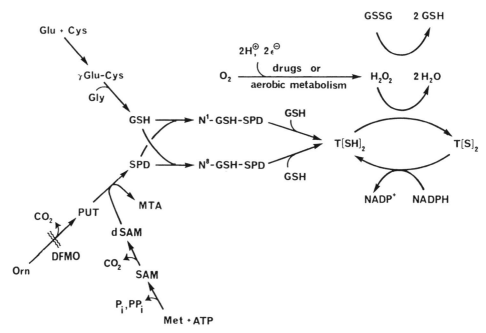

Fig. 3. Biosynthetic pathway to trypanothione. The abbreviations used are: Orn, ornithine; put, putrescine; spd, spermidine; PP$_i$, inorganic pyrophosphate; SAM, S-adenosylmethionine; dSAM, decarboxylated S-adenosylmethionine; MTA, methylthioadenosine; GSH-SPD, glutathionylspermidine; T[SH]$_2$, dihydrotrypanothione.

complete within 15 min and precedes de novo synthesis of polyamines. This mechanism may be advantageous to the cell for rapidly releasing free spermidine required for macromolecular biosynthesis. It would be interesting to determine whether leishmania promastigotes in stationary phase show similar properties as this could be advantageous to the organism during the invasion and transformation process on entering the mammalian host. If glutathionylspermidine does indeed regulate the intracellular levels of spermidine, then inhibition of this process could interfere with normal cell growth and development.

CONCLUSION

Although studies on trypanothione are still in their infancy, our current knowledge points to a pivotal role for this peptide in several essential metabolic functions of these parasites. Thus, the trypanothione system represents a particularly important target for the development of new and better drugs.

ACKNOWLEDGEMENTS

The author would like to thank Ms C. Strobos for assistance in preparing the manuscript. The work reviewed here was supported by grants from the National Institutes of Health, UNDP/World Bank/WHO Special Programme for Research and Training in Tropical Diseases, The Rockefeller Foundation and the Wellcome Trust.

REFERENCES

Bacchi, C. J., 1981, Content, synthesis, and function of polyamines in trypanosomatids: Relationship to chemotherapy, J. Protozool., 28:20-27

Bacchi, C. J., and McCann, P. P., 1987, Parasitic protozoa and polyamines, in: "Inhibition of Polyamine Metabolism," P. P. McCann, A. E. Pegg, and A. Sjoerdsma, eds., Academic Press, San Diego.

Bellofatto, V., Fairlamb, A. H., Henderson, G. B., and Cross, C. A. M., 1987, Biochemical changes associated with alpha-difluoromethylornithine uptake and resistance in Trypanosoma brucei, Mol. Biochem. Parasitol., in press.

Docampo, R., and Moreno, S. N. J., 1986, Free radical metabolism of antiparasitic agents, Fed. Proc., 45:2471-2476.

Fairlamb, A. H., and Cerami, A., 1985, Identification of a novel, thiol-containing co-factor essential for glutathione reductase enzyme activity in trypanosomtids, Mol. Biochem. Parasitol., 14:187-198.

Fairlamb, A. H., and Henderson, G. B., 1987, Metabolism of trypanothione and glutathionylspermidine in trypanosomatids, in: "Host-Parasite Molecular Recognition and Interaction in Protozoal Infections," K.-P. Chang and D. Snary, eds., NATO-ASI Series, Heidelberg.

Fairlamb, A. H., Blackburn, P., Ulrich, P., Chait, B. T., and Cerami, A., 1985, Trypanothione: A novel bis(glutathionyl)spermidine cofactor for glutathione reductase in trypanosomatids, Science, 227:1485-1487.

Fairlamb, A. H., Henderson, G. B., and Cerami, A., 1986, The biosynthesis of trypanothione and N^1-glutathionylspermidine in Crithidia fasciculata, Mol. Biochem. Parasitol., 21:247-257.

Fairlamb, A. H., Henderson, G. B., Bacchi, C. J., and Cerami, A., 1987, In vivo effects of difluoromethylornithine on trypanothione and polyamine levels in bloodstream forms of Trypanosoma brucei, Mol. Biochem. Parasitol., 24:185-191.

Fridovich, I., 1978, The biology of oxygen radicals, Science, 201:875-880.
Henderson, G. B., Ulrich, P., Fairlamb, A. H., and Cerami, A., 1986, Synthesis of the trypanosomatid metabolites trypanothione, and N^1-mono- and N^8-mono-glutathionylspermidine, J. Chem. Soc. Chem. Commun., 593-594.
Henderson, G. B., Fairlamb, A. H., and Cerami, A., 1987a, Trypanothione dependent peroxide metabolism in Crithidia fasciculata and Trypanosoma brucei, Mol. Biochem. Parasitol., 24:39-45.
Henderson, G. B., Fairlamb, A. H., Ulrich, P., and Cerami, A., 1987b, Substrate specificity of the flavoprotein trypanothione disulphide reductase from Crithidia fasciculata, Biochemistry, 26:3023-3027.
Kaur, K., Emmett, K., McCann, P. P., Sjoerdsma, A., and Ullman, B., 1986, Effects of DL-alpha-difluoromethylornithine on Leishmania donovani promastigotes, J. Protozool., 33:518-521.
Krauth-Siegel, R. L., Enders, B., Henderson, G. B., Fairlamb, A. H., and Schirmer, R. H., 1987, Trypanothione reductase from Trypanosoma cruzi: Purification and characterization of the crystalline enzyme, Eur. J. Biochem., 164:123-128.
Le Trang, N., Meshnick, S. R., Kitchener, K., Eaton, J. W., and Cerami, A., 1983, Iron-containing superoxide dismutase from Crithidia fasciculata, J. Biol. Chem., 258:125-130.
Meister, A., and Anderson, M. E., 1983, Glutathione, Annu. Rev. Biochem., 52:711-760.
Penketh, P. G., and Klein, R. A., 1986, Hydrogen peroxide metabolism in Trypanosoma brucei, Mol. Biochem. Parasitol., 20:111-112.
Phillips, M. A., and Wang, C. C., 1987, A Trypanosoma brucei mutant resistant to alpha-difluoromethylornithine, Mol. Biochem. Parasitol., 22:9-17.
Schecter, P. J., Barlow, J. L. R., and Sjoerdsma, A., 1987, Clinical aspects of inhibition of ornithine decarboxylase with emphasis on therapeutic trials of eflornithine (DFMO) in cancer and protozoan diseases, in: "Inhibition of Polyamine Metabolism," P. P. McCann, A. E. Pegg, and A. Sjoerdsma, eds., Academic Press, San Diego.
Shames, S. L., Fairlamb, A. H., Cerami, A., and Walsh, C. T., 1986, Purification and characterization of trypanothione reductase from Crithidia fasciculata, a newly discovered member of the family of disulfide-containing flavoprotein reductases, Biochemistry, 25:3519-3526.
Shim, H., and Fairlamb, A. H., 1987, Levels of polyamines, glutathione and glutathione-spermidine conjugates during growth of the insect trypanosomatid Crithidia fasciculata, J. Gen. Microbiol., in press.
Tabor, H., and Tabor, C. E., 1975, Isolation, characterization, and turnover of glutathionylspermidine from Escherichia coli, J. Biol. Chem., 250:2648-2654.

THE STEROLS OF LEISHMANIA PROMASTIGOTES AND AMASTIGOTES: POSSIBLE IMPLICATIONS FOR CHEMOTHERAPY

L.J. Goad[1], J.S. Keithly[2], J.D. Berman[3], D.H. Beach[4] and G.G. Holz[4]

[1]Department of Biochemistry, University of Liverpool, P.O. Box 147, Liverpool L69 3BX U.K.; [2]Department of Microbiology Cornell University Medical College, 1300 York Avenue, New York, N.Y. 10021 U.S.A. [3]Division of Experimental Therapeutics Walter Reed Army Institute of Research, Washington, DC 20307-5100, U.S.A.; [4]Department of Microbiology and Immunology S.U.N.Y., Health Science Center at Syracuse, Syracuse, N.Y. 13210, U.S.A.

INTRODUCTION

The major sterol identified [1] in the promastigotes of several Leishmania species is ergosta-5,7,24(28)-trien-3β-ol (11, Fig 1) and this is often accompanied by variable amounts of ergosta-5,7,22E-trien-3β-ol (ergosterol, 12). The presence of lanosterol (1) and a range of other trace sterols (2-10) in Leishmania [1,2], together with the results of labelling studies with [2-^{14}C]mevalonic acid [2-4], indicate that the major promastigote C_{28}-sterols are produced by the routes shown in Fig. 1. Similar metabolic routes are operative in many fungi which elaborate ergosterol (12) as the major sterol. When Leishmania promastigotes are cultured on a medium containing serum the cells contain considerable amounts of cholest-5-en-3β-ol (cholesterol) [1,2]. This cholesterol is derived from the serum lipoproteins and it does not appear to be metabolised by the promastigotes to C_{28}-sterols such as 11 or 12 [2].

A range of imidazole and triazole antifungal drugs have been designed which block the cytochrome P-450 dependent C-14 demethylation step in fungal ergosterol synthesis [5-7]. This causes the accummulation of 14α-methyl compounds such as lanosterol (1) and obtusifoliol (3) with a concomittant decline in ergosterol (12). It is believed that this change in sterol composition results in a disruption of membrane function with consequential effects upon membrane enzymes and that this is the basis, at least in part, of the fungistatic and fungitoxic effects of these antifungal compounds [7].

The imidazole, ketoconazole, has been tested for activity against Leishmania species and shown to inhibit growth of L. mexicana mexicana promastigotes [4] and the propogation of amastigotes of three species of Leishmania in human and mouse macrophages [8-10]. Ketoconazole has also proved effective against visceral leishmaniasis in the golden hamster [11] and cutaneous and mucocutaneous lesions in man [12-16].

The similarity of sterol patterns between Leishmania and fungi prompted us to test the effect of the antifungal drug ketoconazole against L. mexicana

mexicana. Growth of both the promastigotes [2, 4] and amastigotes [3] was inhibited and 14α-methylsterols, particularly 4α,14α-dimethylcholesta-8,24-dien-3β-ol (2), accumulated and there was a decrease in the amount of C_{28}-sterols (9 and 11). It thus appears that the inhibitory effects of ketoconazole on Leishmania are probably the result of impaired sterol synthesis as in the case of fungi.

In the host animal, the Leishmania amastigotes reside in macrophage cells which have the capacity to synthesise cholesterol. Therefore we considered it important to determine the sterol composition of the amastigotes to ascertain if any sterols are present that possibly could be derived from the macrophages (or plasma lipoproteins). The uptake and utilisation of host sterols by the amastigote could have important implications for the successful use of imidazole drugs, or other sterol synthesis inhibiting drugs, against leishmaniasis.

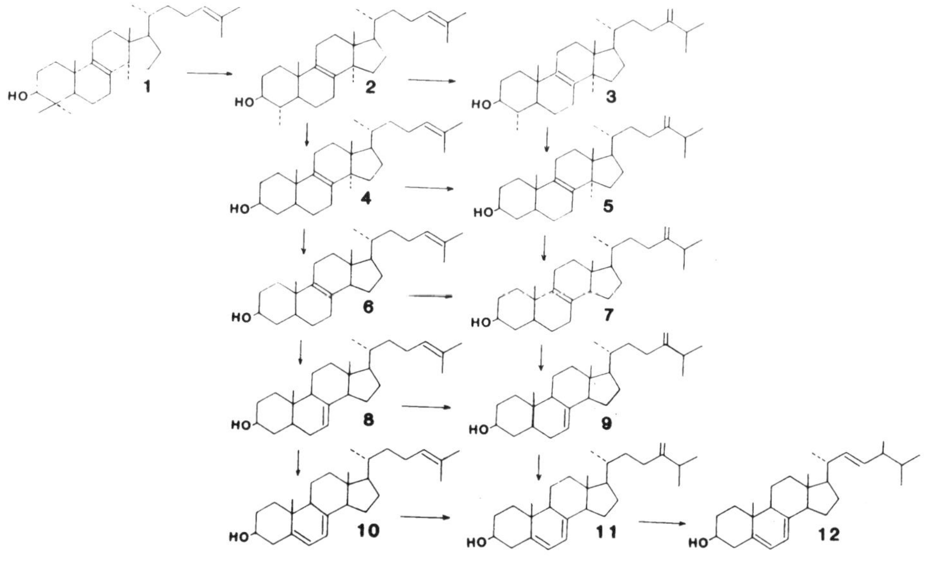

Fig. 1. Sterols of Leishmania species.

MATERIALS AND METHODS

Amastigotes of L. braziliensis guyanensis (wild type, clones 1-A, 7-D, 8-2 and 8-3) and L. mexicana mexicana (WR227) were propagated in murine macrophage cells (J774.1) for 3-4 days [3]. The macrophages were lysed by two passages through a 30-gauge needle and the freed amastigotes were purified by differential centrifugation employing a Percoll gradient by the methods described previously [3].

Promastigotes of L. braziliensis guyanensis and L. mexicana mexicana were cultured as described elsewhere in Schneider's Drosophila medium or the RE III medium of Steiger and Steiger, respectively [2].

Samples of lyophilised cells were extracted twice with chloroform-methanol (2:1) and the volume of solvent reduced. The extract was then partitioned with petroleum ether to provide the sterol containing fraction [2, 7].

The sterols were analysed by GC-MS on a VG 70-70H mass spectrometer (source 220ºC, 70ev, 4kV, 200μA) with a Finnigan Incos 2300 Data System and employing a fused silica bonded phase capillary column (BP-1, 25m x 0.25mm, on column injection at 50ºC, then rapid heating to 250ºC, then 4ºC/min to 280ºC). A few samples were analysed on a Hewlett-Packard 59085B GC-MS system fitted with a DB-1N (15m x 0.25mm) capillary column, initial temperature 70ºC, then raised to 250°C at 20°C/min, then to 260°C at 4°C/min. Sterol identifications were based upon comparisons of mass spectra and GC retention times with those of authentic compounds.

RESULTS AND DISCUSSION

(a) Promastigotes

The promastigote forms of both L. braziliensis guyanensis and L. mexicana mexicana contained appreciable amounts of cholesterol (50-60% of total sterol). This will have been obtained from the serum in the growth media. The major C_{28}-sterol in L. mexicana mexicana was ergosta-5,7,24(28)-trien-3β-ol (11, about 30% of total sterol) and this was accompanied by ergosta-7,24(28)-dien-3β-ol (9, 7%). Small amounts of lanosterol (1, 4%) and 4α,14α-dimethylcholesta-8,24-dien-3β-ol (2, 2%) were also detected.

L. braziliensis guyanensis (clone 1-A) by contrast contained ergosta-5,7,22-trien-3β-ol (12, ergosterol, 30%) as the principal C_{28}-sterol. Also present was ergosta-7,24(28)-dien-3β-ol (9, 10%). The wild type and other clones had similar compositions, some with traces of 1 and 2, but in no case was more than a minor amount of ergosta-5,7,24(28)-trien-3β-ol (11) observed. L. braziliensis guyanensis differs from other species of Leishmania so far analysed [1] which although in several cases produce ergosterol (12) still have the 24-methylene compound 11 as the major of these two components. Sterol 11 is a probable precursor to ergosterol (12) (see Fig. 1) and it thus appears that L. braziliensis guyanensis has a more evolved biosynthetic pathway leading to ergosterol as the predominant sterol. By contrast the L. mexicana mexicana promastigotes display little or no ability to introduce the Δ^{22}-bond required to produce ergosterol (12).

(b) Macrophage cells

As a prelude to determining the sterol composition of amastigotes it was first considered desirable to identify the sterols of the host macrophage cells. The two major components were readily identified from their characteristic GC retention times and mass spectra as cholesterol (90%, m/z 386, 321, 368, 313, 301, 275, 255, 213) and cholesta-5,24-dien-3β-ol (13, desmosterol, 10%, m/z 384, 369, 366, 351, 300, 271, 253, 213, 69). Cholesterol is the predominant sterol of mammalian tissues while demosterol (13) is an immediate precursor of cholesterol.

(c) Amastigotes

The recovered amastigotes of L. braziliensis guyanensis (Clone 1-A) gave a GC profile (Fig. 2) revealing a large amount of cholesterol (peak 251) and desmosterol (peak 268) but in addition other peaks (288 and 311) had the retention times of C_{28}-sterols. The identities of the cholesterol and desmosterol were confirmed by their mass spectra. However, the mass spectrum of peak 268 revealed a second co-chromatographing minor component with a molecular ion at m/z 398 and this, coupled with the retention time, allowed the probable identification of the compound as ergosta-5,22-dien-3β-ol (14).

The GC peak 288 had a mass spectrum displaying three molecular ions at m/z 400, 398 and 396 and a range of diagnostically valuable fragmentation ions. The library search by the data system provided an identification of the m/z 400 component as ergost-5-en-3β-ol (15, m/z 400, 382, 367, 315, 213) which was in accord with its retention time when compared to that of an authentic sample.

A second data system library search was then performed for the difference spectrum obtained by subtraction of the mass spectrum of 15 from the original mixture mass spectrum. The m/z 398 compound was easily identified as ergosta-5,24(28)-dien-3β-ol (16) because of the large fragment ion at m/z 314, This ion

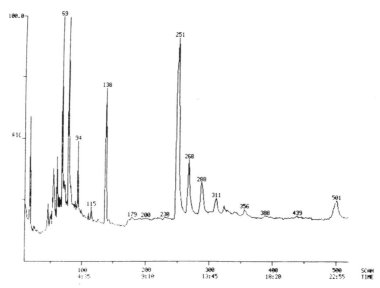

Fig. 2. GC-MS analysis of the sterols from amastigotes of L. braziliensis guyanensis.

arises by a characteristic loss of part of the side chain (84 a.m.u.) due to the McLafferty rearrangement which occurs in sterols with a 24-methylene group in the side chain [17]. Also a large ion at m/z 271 was observed in the mass spectrum which is consistent with the presence of sterol 16.

A third library search was finally made for the difference spectrum remaining after subtraction of the spectra of both 15 and 16 from the original mixture mass spectrum. A remarkably good fit was obtained for the identification of the m/z 396 sterol as ergosterol (12, m/z 396, 363, 253, 211, 159, 147, 145) which was again consistent with its GC retention time.

Peak 311 in the GC analysis (Fig. 2) gave a mass spectrum revealing two compounds which were readily identified as ergost-7-en-3β-ol (m/z 400, 385, 273, 255, 229, 213) and ergosta-7,24(28)-dien-3β-ol (9, m/z 398, 383, 365, 314, 271, 255, 229, 227, 213). GC peak number 356, although a minor component, gave a good mass spectrum revealing it to be stigmasta-7,24(28)-dien-3β-ol (17, m/z 396, 314, 271, 253, 213) which was identified in larger amounts in the amastigotes of L. mexicana mexicana (see below). Amastigotes of the other clones of L. braziliensis guyanensis gave similar sterol profiles.

GC-MS analysis of the sterols obtained from L. mexicana mexicana amastigotes showed again cholesterol (40% of total sterol) but rather less desmosterol (1%) while ergosta-7,24(28)-dien-3β-ol (9) was the main C_{28}-sterol A most significant observation was that ergosta-5,24(28)-dien-3β-ol (16) comprised 7% of the mixture. The location of the ring system double bond at the C-5/C-6 position in 16 was confirmed by GC-MS analysis of the trimethylsilyl ether derivatives of the sterol mixture. The TMS-derivative of 16 gave a base peak at m/z 129 and an ion (rel. int. 14%) at m/z 341 $[M-129]^+$ which are typical fragment ions of a Δ^5-sterol TMS-ether [18]. In contrast to the sterols of L.

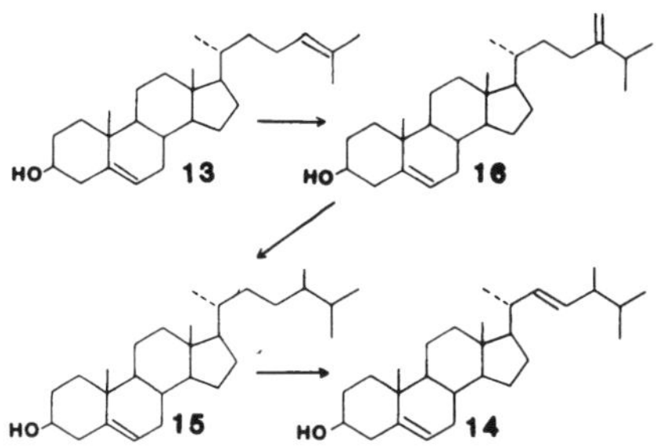

Fig. 3. Suggested route for production of Δ^5 24-methylsterols from desmosterol (13) in Leishmania amastigotes.

braziliensis guyanensis there was no evidence for the presence of ergosta-5,22-dien-3β-ol (14) or ergost-5-en-3β-ol (15) in the amastigotes of L. mexicana mexicana. However, appreciable amounts of two C_{29}-sterols were found and identified as stigmasta-7,24(28)-dien-3β-ol (17, 9% of total sterols, m/z 412, 392, 314, 299, 271, 255, 213) and stigmasta-5,7,24(28)-trien-3β-ol (18, 10%, m/z 410, 395, 377, 351, 211, 159, 157, 145, 143). The mass spectra of the trimethylsilyl ether derivatives of the two C_{29}-sterols were consistent with these identifications.

The C_{29}-sterols have previously been observed in only small amounts in the sterol mixtures obtained from the promastigotes of most Leishmania species [1] although promastigotes of L. major contain an appreciable (5-8%) amount (unpublished observation). Sterols with the stigmastane skeleton are typically found in algae and higher plants and evidence is now emerging that 24-ethylsterols may play some essential role in plant cell growth [20]. The appearance of significant amounts of sterols 17 and 18 in the amastigote form of Leishmania thus presents an intrigueing problem regarding their function. There must also be some signal which triggers increased C_{29}-sterol formation when the promastigote form develops into the amastigote in the host macrophage cell.

Equally significant is the presence of Δ^5-sterols alkylated at C-24 (14, 15, 16) in the amastigotes. This type of Δ^5-sterol has not been reported in the promastigotes which produce Δ^7- and $\Delta^{5,7}$-sterols, and like most fungi, Leishmania species may lack the ability to reduce the Δ^7-bond of $\Delta^{5,7}$-sterols to yield Δ^5-sterols [21]. We postulate that the Δ^5-sterols (14, 15, 16) are produced (Fig. 3) in the amastigote from desmosterol (14) that is a product of the host macrophage cell and which has been absorbed, together with cholesterol, by the amastigote. It is noteable that L. braziliensis guyanensis promastigotes produce ergosterol (12) with the 24-methyl Δ^{22}-side chain and the amastigotes can also apparently convert desmosterol to ergosta-5,22-dien-3β-ol (14) requiring the same side chain modifications. By contrast L. mexicana mexicana, which produces predominantly the 24-methylene sterol 11 in the promastigotes, must have little or no $\Delta^{24(28)}$-reductase or Δ^{22}-desaturase activities. Moreover, the amastigotes of this species can only apparently produce the 24-methylene derivative 16 from desmosterol and not the 24-methyl or Δ^{22}-compounds 14 or 15.

It has recently been shown that trace amounts of 24-methylsterols are essential for growth of yeast cells [22-24] and other fungi [25] while C_{27}-sterols (cholesterol, 5α-cholestanol) can satisfy a bulk requirement for membrane structures [26]. It is possible that C_{28}-sterols may play a similar essential role for cell division and growth in Leishmania amastigotes and this can be fulfilled by sterols 14-16 produced from host desmosterol. If this situation indeed pertains it has significant implications for the chemotherapy of leishmaniasis when employing drugs such as imidazole or allylamine antifungals [27] which block de novo sterol synthesis at an early stage in the sequence. The amastigotes may be able to survive the inhibition of endogenous de novo sterol synthesis by utilising absorbed host cholesterol for membrane functions and 24-alkyl sterols synthesised from absorbed desmosterol, for some other vital function where the C-24 substituted side chain structure is a critical requirement. Perhaps significantly, there have been a few reports of the ineffective use of imidazole drugs against cutaneous leishmaniasis in mice and man [28-30]. These possibilities are now being actively explored in our laboratories.

CONCLUSIONS

The promastigotes of L. braziliensis guyanensis and L. mexicana mexicana contain cholesterol, derived from the medium, and synthesise $\Delta^{5,7}$ C_{28}-sterols. Ergosta-5,7,22-trien-3β-ol is the major product of L. braziliensis guyanensis but in L. mexicana mexicana ergosta-5,7,24(28)-trien-3β-ol predominates. There is no evidence of Δ^5-C_{28}-sterols in promastigotes.

The amastigote forms of these Leishmania species contain cholesterol and desmosterol which are products of the host macrophage cell. The amounts of $\Delta^{5,7}$-C_{28}-sterols are diminished but the C_{29}-sterols stigmasta-7,24(28)-dien-3β-ol and stigmasta-5,7,24(28)-trien-3β-ol appear and account for about 20% of the sterol in the case of the L. mexicana mexicana amastigotes. Δ^5-C_{28} sterols are also found in the amastigotes. L. mexicana mexicana contains ergosta-5,24(28)-dien-3β-ol but L. braziliensis guyanensis contains in addition ergost-5-en-3β-ol and ergosta-5,22-dien-3β-ol. We suggest that these sterols are synthesised in the amastigote by transmethylation of desmosterol which has been taken up from the host macrophage cell.

The possibilty that the C_{28}-sterols are essential for Leishmania growth and cell division is discussed. The implications of utilisation of host sterol for membranes and for Δ^5-C_{28} sterol production are considered in relation to the use of chemotherapeutic drugs which are effective through inhibition of de novo sterol synthesis.

REFERENCES

1. L. J. Goad, G. G. Holz and D. H. Beach, Sterols of Leishmania species. Implications for biosynthesis. Mol. Biochem. Parasitol. 10: 161-170 (1984).
2. L. J. Goad, G. G. Holz and D. H. Beach, Sterols of ketoconazole-inhibited Leishmania mexicana mexicana promastigotes. Mol. Biochem. Parasitol. 15: 257-279 (1985).
3. J. D. Berman, L. J. Goad, D. H. Beach and G. G. Holz, Effects of ketoconazole on sterol biosynthesis by Leishmania mexicana mexicana amastigotes in murine macrophage tumor cells. Mol. Biochem. Parasitol. 20: 85-92 (1986).
4. J. D. Berman, G. G. Holz and D. H. Beach, Effects of ketoconazole on growth and sterol biosynthesis of Leishmania promastigotes in culture. Mol. Biochem. Parasitol. 12: 1-13 (1984).
5. H. B. Levine, Ketoconazole in the management of fungal disease. ADIS Press, Balgowlah, Australia (1982).
6. H. Van den Bossche, W. Lauwers, G. Willemsens, P. Marichal, F. Cornelissen and W. Cools, Molecular basis for the antimycotic and antibacterial activity of N-substituted imidazoles and triazoles: the inhibition of isoprenoid biosynthesis. Pestic. Sci. 15: 188-198 (1984).
7. H. Van den Bossche, Biochemical targets for antifungal azole derivatives: Hypothesis on the mode of action. Curr. Topics in Med. Mycol. (M.R. McGinnis ed.) Vol.1, pp 313-351, Springer-Verlag, New York (1985).
8. J. D. Berman, Activity of imidazoles against Leishmania tropica in human macrophage cultures. Am. J. Trop. Med. Hyg. 30: 566-569 (1981).
9. J. D. Berman, In vitro susceptibility of antimony resistant Leishmania to alternative drugs. J. Infect. Dis. 145: 279 (1982).

10. J. D. Berman and L. S. Lee, Activity of anti-leishmanial agents against amastigotes in human monocyte-derived macrophages and in mouse peritoneal macrophages. J. Parasitol. 70: 220-225 (1984).
11. W. Raether and H. Seidenath, Ketoconazole and other potent anti-mycotic azoles exhibit pronounced activity against Trypanosoma cruzi, Plasmodium berghei and Entamoeba histolytica in vivo. Z. Parasiteuk. 70: 135-138 (1984).
12. F. G. Urcuyo and N. Zaias, Oral ketoconazole in treatment of leishmaniasis. Int. J. Dermatol. 21: 414-416 (1982).
13. L. Weinrauch, R. Livshin and J. El-On, Cutaneous leishmaniasis treatment with ketoconazole. Cutis 32: 288-294 (1983).
14. L. Weinrauch, R. Livshin, Z. Evan-Paz and J. El-On, Efficacy of ketoconazole in cutaneous leishmaniasis. Arch. Dermatol. Res. 275, 353-354 (1983).
15. J. Viallet, J. D., MacLean and H. Robson, Response to ketoconazole in two cases of longstanding cutaneous leishmaniasis. Am. J. Trop Med. Hyg. 35: 491-495 (1986).
16. D. Borelli, A clinical trail of itraconazole in the treatment of deep mycoses and leishmaniasis. Rev. Infect. Dis. 9: (Suppl. 1) S57-S63 (1987).
17. I. J. Massey and C. Djerassi, Structure and stereochemical applications of mass spectrometry in the marine field. J. Org. Chem. 44: 2448-2456 (1979).
18. C. J. W. Brooks, E. C. Horning and J. S. Young, Characterisation of sterols by gas chromatography-mass spectrometry of the trimethylsilyl ethers. Lipids 3: 391-402 (1968).
19. C. J. W. Brooks, B. A. Knights, W. Sucrow and B. Raduchel, The characterisation of 24-ethylidene sterols. Steroids 20: 487-497 (1972).
20. P. A. Haughan, J. R. Lenton and L. J. Goad, Paclobutrazol inhibition of sterol biosynthesis in a cell suspension culture and evidence of an essential role of 24-ethylsterol in plant cell division. Biochem. Biophys. Res. Commun. 146: 510-516 (1987).
21. E. I. Mercer, The biosynthesis of ergosterol. Pestic Sci. 15: 133-155 (1984).
22. R. J. Rodriguez, C. Low, C. D. K. Botema and L. W. Parks, Multiple functions for sterols in Saccharomyces cerevisiae. Biochim. Biophys. Acta 837: 336-343 (1985).
23. W. J. Pinto and W. R. Nes, Stereochemical specificity for sterols in Saccharomyces cerevisiae. J. biol. Chem. 258: 4472-4476 (1983).
24. C. Dahl, H-P. Biemann and S. Dahl, A protein kinase antigenically related to pp60 possibly involved in yeast cell cycle control: Positive in vivo regulation by sterol. Proc. Natl. Acad. Sci. USA., 84: 4012-4016 (1987).
25. W. D. Nes and R. C. Heupel, Physiological requirement for biosynthesis of multiple 24β-methylsterols in Gibberella fujikuroi. Arch. Biochem. Biophys. 244: 211-217 (1986).
26. R. J. Rodriguez and L. W. Parks, Structural and physiological features of sterols necessary to satisfy bulk membrane and sparking requirements in yeast sterol auxotrophs. Arch. Biochem. Biophys. 225: 861-871 (1983).
27. L. J. Goad, G. G. Holz and D. H. Beach, Effect of the allylamine antifungal drug SF 86-327 on the growth and sterol synthesis of Leishmania mexicana mexicana promastigotes. Biochem. Pharmacol. 34: 3785-3788 (1985).
28. L. Weinrauch and J. El-On, The effect of ketoconazole and a combination of rifampicin/amphoterin B on cutaneous leishmaniasis in laboratory mice. Trans R. Soc. Trop. Med. Hyg. 78: 389-390 (1984).
29. L. Weinrauch, R. Livshin, G. P. Jacobs and J. El-On, Cutaneous leishmaniasis: failure of topical treatment with imidazole derivatives on laboratory animals and man. Arch. Dermatol Res. 276: 133-134 (1984).
30. J. S. Keithly and S. G. Langreth, Inefficacy of metronidazole in experimental infections of Leishmania donovani, L. mexicana and Trypanosoma brucei brucei. Am. J. Trop. Med. Hyg. 32: 485-496 (1983).

Acknowledgments: We thank Mark Prescott, Department of Biochemistry, Liverpool University, for the excellent GC-MS analyses.

ASSESSMENT OF THE USE IN THE DIAGNOSIS OF LEISHMANIASIS OF BIOTINYLATED KINETOPLAST DERIVED DNA SEQUENCES

Douglas C Barker

MRC Outstation of NIMR, Molteno Laboratory
Department of Pathology, University of Cambridge
CAMBRIDGE CB2 3EE

INTRODUCTION

Any of the 15 subspecies of Leishmania at present identified as infective to man can cause the single cutaneous lesion which is the commonest clinical sign of the disease. The wide spectrum of symptoms which may result from the progression of the disease can, at least partially, be related to the subspecies of Leishmania. However the well known problems [1] of genuine or apparent self healing, metastisizing complications of cutaneous manifestations of visceral or secondary infections and immunopathology make clinical diagnosis difficult. The epidemiologists have the time consuming tasks of dissection of sandflies and patient culturing of organisms from the infected tissue of reservoir hosts to incriminate vectors and hosts in transmission. Both the clinical diagnosis and the epidemiologists' problems could be alleviated by a rapid, cheap and accurate method of identification.

At the beginning of this decade (1980) the WHO/TDR programme focussed attention on the diagnostic problems of the biochemical characterisation of Leishmania in a PAHO workshop [2]. The use of kinetoplast DNA hybridisation was advocated by Barker et al. [in 2] and sufficient sequence divergence in minicircular DNA demonstrated to make DNA probes feasible. Endonuclease digestion of kDNA and Southern filter hybridisation was initially used to identify an unknown organism [3]. Wirth and McMahon Pratt [4] developed the rapid and accurate dot blot method which enabled identification of whole organisms lysed on nitrocellulose. This was a major advance because the method eliminated the need to culture unknown Leishmania isolates. 'In situ' hybridisation diagnostic methods using microscopy [9, 12, 14, 17, 18] have similar advantages.

Since these early studies, progress in research in many laboratories over the last seven years has been outstanding in establishing DNA hybridisation as a useful additional tool in the diagnosis of Leishmania [5-12]. All minicircles so far DNA sequenced in both Trypanosoma and Leishmania have a 13 bp conserved sequence [Reviewed in 12] at the origin of replication [13]. Despite this fact, the sequence divergence, even in the 120 bps spanning the origin of replication, is sufficient to prevent significant cross hybridisation between members of different complexes [5-12]. Kennedy [14], Lopes and Wirth [7], Jackson et al. [8], Barker et al. [9] and Lawrie et al. [15] have all used recombinant DNA methods to select cloned sequences of kDNA from Old and New World Leishmania which, when used as probes, have complex, species, strain and isolate specificity. Recently, Rogers and Wirth [16] have demonstrated that, even within one single cloned minicircle of L. m. amazonensis, DNA sequences can be selected with different taxonomic specificities.

One major disadvantage of these methods for field use has been that the most sensitive detection systems normally make use of radioactively labelled DNA probes. Our own limited field experience and that of many other field workers indicates that, for field use, simpler and safer detections systems are necessary. Recently, we have compared the efficiency of biotinylation of kDNA by ultraviolet light photoactivation and by nick translation. This communication reports both the encouraging and discouraging results we have had in the evaluation, by filter and microscopy 'in situ' hybridisation, of these biotinylated probes. The use of minicircle derived complex, species and subspecies kinetoplast DNA and specific sequence recombinant DNA probes for non-radioactive detection of sequence homology for field identification is assessed.

MATERIALS AND METHODS

Detailed instructions for most of our methods of DNA preparation, endonuclease digestion, electrophoresis, blotting, filter and 'in situ' hybridisation, making radioactive or biotinylated probes and general procedures are contained in a laboratory manual of simplified methods for the DNA characterisation of Leishmania [17] which is available at the NATO/ASI, and free of charge from the Director, WHO/TDR Programme, Geneva, Switzerland.

Photobiotinylation

An expanded protocol for this method is given in a second paper by the same author which can be found in the Workshop on Characterisation and Taxonomy of Leishmania.

Dot blots and Southern Filter and 'In situ' Hybridisations

Dot blots containing serial dilutions of leishmania were made according to the method of Wirth and McMahon Pratt [4] as modified by Spithill and Grumont [6]. Endonuclease digestions, Southern filter transfers and 'in situ' preparations, prehybridisation, hybridisation, stringency wash, radioactive and non-radioactive probe DNA labelling and detection were all as given previously [3, 5, 9, 12, 17].

RESULTS

'In situ' Hybridisation by Light Microscopy

Bio-11-dUTP labelled kDNA probes. Figure 1 illustrates the quality of results which can now be achieved. Promastigotes of a Leishmania braziliensis guyanensis MHOM/BR/75/M4147 and L. mexicana mexicana NYC/BZ/62/M379 were smeared on microscope slides. Hybridisation was with a probe made by the nick translation labelling of kDNA, isolated from a L. b. braziliensis MHOM/BR/75/M2903, with the biotinylated nucleotide Bio-11-dUTP. To detect the hybridised sequence, the slides were incubated with streptavidin followed by incubation with a biotin-labelled polymer of alkaline phosphatase. The steptavidin bound to both the Bio-11-dUTP, which had hybridised to the kinetoplast DNA of the organism, and to the biotin-labelled alkaline phosphatase. This resulted in the localization of the enzyme at the site of L. b. braziliensis kDNA hybridisation. The application of the chromogenic substrate gave a purple-blue deposit where hybridisation had occurred (Figure 1b). The localisation of the colour deposit was much better than we had previously achieved. Careful analysis of the stages given in the methods, indicated that the crucial step was adequate denaturation of both the probe and organism DNAs simultaneously by the steam treatment at 85°C. The

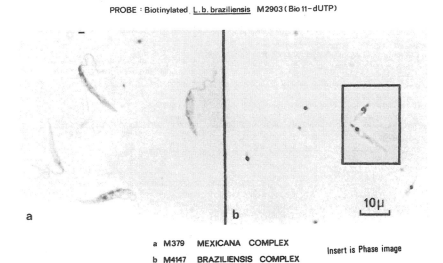

Fig. 1. Promastigotes of (a) L. m. mexicana and (b) L. b. guyanensis hybridised 'in situ' with biotinylated kDNA from L. b. braziliensis. Sequential application of streptavidin, biotinylated alkaline phosphate and a chromogenic substrate results in the localisation of stain on the kinetoplast of the L. b. guyanensis indicating sequence homology with L. b. braziliensis. A phase contrast insert has been included to highlight the preserved morphology of the promastigotes. No stain is visible on the kinetoplasts of L. m. mexicana indicating lack of sequence homology between L. m. mexicana and L. b. braziliensis.

morphology of the much larger organism L. m. mexicana (Figure 1a) indicated that little, if any, disruption of these cells had occurred. The lack of staining of the kinetoplast confirmed the total lack of sequence homology between members of the mexicana and braziliensis complexes. The kinetoplast, under bright field illumination, was very darkly stained in the L. b. guyanensis cells (Figure 1b); however, it was difficult to see the whole cells. Figure 1b insert is a phase contrast image of the two leishmania promastigotes immediately to the left of the insert showing adequate, if not ideal, morphology of these smaller cells.

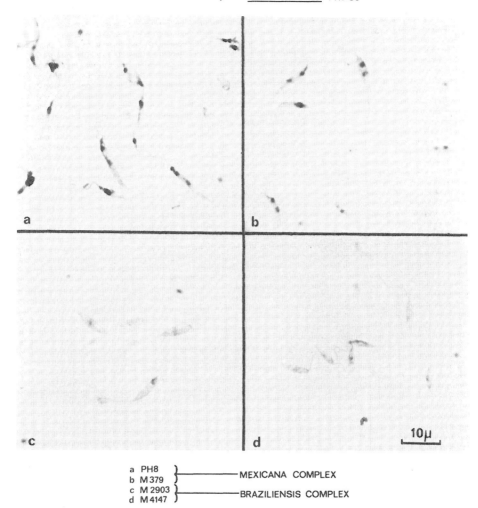

Fig. 2. Promastigotes of (a) L. m. amazonensis, (b) L. m. mexicana, (c) L. b. braziliensis, and (d) L. b. guyanensis hybridised 'in situ' with photobiotinylated kDNA from L. m. amazonensis. After application of the detection system, intense staining can be seen in the kinetoplast of L. m amazonensis (a) indicating total sequence homology; less intense staining of the kinetoplast of L. m. mexicana (b) indicating a degree of partial homology. No staining of the kinetoplast of L. b. braziliensis (c) or L. b. guyanensis (d) was observed indicating a lack of sequence homology between the braziliensis strains and L. m. amazonenesis.

Photobiotinylated kDNA Probes

Figure 2 illustrates the excellent result which can be achieved using the photobiotinylation protocol given in the methods section of this author's paper in "Characterisation and Taxonomy of Leishmania" Workshop.

Promastigotes of four reference strains of Leishmania:IFLA/BR/67/PH8 L. m. amazonensis and NYC/BZ/62/M379 L. m. mexicana representing the mexicana complex; MHOM/BR/75/M2903 L. b. braziliensis and MHOM/BR/75/M4147 L. b. guyanensis representing the braziliensis complex were smeared on microscope slides. Hybridisation was with a probe made by photobiotinylating kDNA from L. m. amazonensis PH8C5 which is a clone of organisms derived from one single individual promastigote (David Evans, personal communication and gift). Detection of the hybridised sequences was as given in the text for Figure 1. This resulted in localisation of the colour deposit whereever the L. m. amazonensis biotinylated kDNA probe had hybridised. Figure 2a showed very intense staining of the kinetoplast of L. m. amazonensis PH8. It is also quite noticeable that there is a lesser, but significant, accumulation of stain on the nucleus. Figure 2b showed that the kinetoplast of L. m. mexicana M379 was stained to a lesser extent than the kinetoplast of L. m. amazonensis but enough for us to assert that the kinetoplast of L. m. mexicana has DNA sequences within it which hybridise to L. m. amazonensis kDNA from a cloned strain.

Figure 2c and d showed no staining of the kinetoplast of either of the braziliensis complex strains L. b. braziliensis M2903 and L. b. guyanensis M4147. Interestingly, there was a small amount of colour recorded from the nucleus of both strains but particularly of L. b. guyanensis.

These results confirm the lack of sequence homology between minicircle sequences of the mexicana and braziliensis complexes.

Dot Blot Hybridisation

The Wirth and McMahon Pratt [4] dot blot method has attractions for field use. It eliminates the need for elaborate kDNA extraction from unknown isolates. Organisms can be transferred directly from lesions or from culture on to nitrocellulose paper and lysed 'in situ'. The nitrocellulose paper with immobilised DNA can then be probed with kDNA, nuclear DNA or recombinant DNA probes. This method has been used by Wirth et al. [11] successfully to diagnose leishmaniases in patients from Manaus where DNA probes clearly detected infections in more patients than either histopathology or culturing. The major disadvantage of this methodology is the requirement for a radio-isotope, therefore, alternative methods for labelling DNA should be used in field situations [11].

In the following experiments we have made a direct comparison between the use of radioactive and biotin labelled probe hybridised to dot blots. Replicate filters were prepared, each containing serial dilutions (10^7-10^4) of promastigotes, from four reference strains of Leishmania: L. m. amazonensis IFLA/BR/67/PH8 clone 5; L. b. guyanensis MHOM/BR/75/M4147; L. m. mexicana NYC/BZ/62/M379 and L. b. braziliensis MHOM/BR/75/M2903.

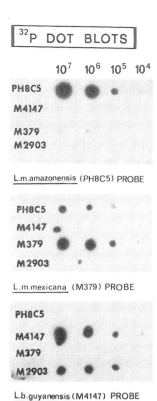

Fig. 3. Promastigotes of four strains of Leishmania, L. m. amazonensis PH8C5, L. b. guyanensis M4147, L. m. mexicana M379 and L. b. braziliensis M2903 were dotted on to nitrocellulose membrane filters to give dots containing 10 million, 1 million, 100 thousand and 10 thousand organisms. Each replicate filter was hybridised with radioactively labelled kDNA as indicated under each autoradiograph above. The autoradiographs show which dots contain DNA sequences homologous to the probes used.

Radioactive Probes

In the first series of experiments, DNA probes were made by nick translation of kDNA in the presence of radioactively labelled nucleotide. Figure 3 illustrates the results. The top autoradiograph is of a filter hybridised with radioactively labelled kDNA of L. m. amazonensis. The hybridisation signal can be seen to progressively decrease with number of organisms but can still be observed in the dot containing 10000 L. m. amazonensis promastigotes. The L. m. amazonensis kDNA has also hybridised to a very limited extent with the dots containing 10 million and 1 million promastigotes of L. m. mexicana. No hybridisation occurred to any dot of L. b. braziliensis or L. b. guyanensis.

The middle autoradiograph is of a replicate filter hybridised with radioactively labelled kDNA of L. m. mexicana. There are two artifact black areas which do not correspond to any dot. The kDNA of L. m. mexicana has hybridised strongly to its homologous DNA and a signal can be seen above the dot blot containing 10000 organisms. L. m. amazonensis must contain many more copies of a kDNA sequence which is homologous to a sequence present in L. m. mexicana in low copy number. This is evident from the observation that in the top autoradiograph, L. m. amazonensis kDNA hybridises only weakly to L. m. mexicana but, in the middle autoradiograph L. m. mexicana kDNA has hybridised fairly strongly to L. m. amazonensis in the dot containing 10000 organisms. No hybridisation to L. b. guyanensis or L. b. braziliensis can be detected. The bottom autoradiograph is of a replicate filter hybridised with L. b. guyanensis kDNA radioactively labelled. No hybridisation can be detected with any dot of L. m. amazonensis or L. m. mexicana. The progressive decrease in hybridisation signal can be observed with the homologous dots down to the dot containing 10000 L. b. guyanensis promastigotes. Almost equally strong hybridisation of the L. b. guyanensis probe is observed to promastigotes of L. b. braziliensis as a very faint signal can detected over the dot containing 10000 promastigotes. The results from all three filters probed with radioactive kDNA is that the method can discriminate well between the two mexicana complex strains and between them and braziliensis strains which show almost identical hybridisation and, therefore, sequence homology.

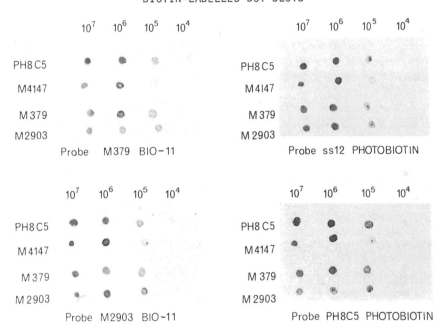

Fig. 4.   Promastigotes of four strains of Leishmania L. m. amazonensis PH8C5, L. b. guyanensis M4147, L. m. mexicana M379 and L. b. braziliensis M2903 were dotted onto nitrocellulose membrane filters to give dots containing 10 million, 1 million, 100 thousand and 10 thousand organisms. Each replicate filter was hybridised with a biotin-11-dUTP or photobiotin kDNA probe or a single stranded recombinant DNA probe as indicated under each photograph. The detection system has reacted with every dot indicating that no discrimination can be accomplished by this method.

509

Replicate filters of those used in the experiments described above were used for hybridisation with biotin-labelled kDNA from L. m. mexicana, L. b. braziliensis, L. m. amazonensis and a biotin-labelled single stranded recombinant DNA probe which hybridises with kDNA from braziliensis complex isolates. It is evident even from a cursory examination of the photographs of all four filters in Figure 4, that no discrimination can be made between the braziliensis and mexicana strains. There is a progressive decrease in staining related to the number of organisms. But, at any one dilution, all four dots show an equal amount of staining regardless of whether the probe DNA was biotin-11-dUTP or photobiotin labelled.

Southern Filter Hybridisation

Southern filter hybridisation. A number of experiments have been performed by this method using both biotin-11-dUTP and photobiotinylated

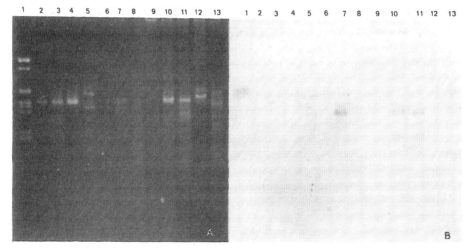

Fig. 5. (a) Photograph taken under ultraviolet light of ethidium bromide stained fragments of kDNA which had previously been digested with the endonuclease Hae III and electrophoresed in a 2% agarose gel. 1 Bacteriophage PM2 molecular weightmarker DNA. 2 L. b. braziliensis M2903. 3 L. b. guyanensis M4147. 4 L. b. panamensis LS94. 5 L. m. mexicana M379. 6 Blank. 7 L. m. amazonenesis PH8. 8 L. d. infantum LEM78. 9 L. b. M7649. 10 L. sp MTB581/583. 11 L. sp. R163. 12 L. braziliensis R300. 13 L. d. donovani DD8. (b) Nitrocellulose filter containing fragments seen in (a) hybridised with biotin-11-dUTP labelled kDNA of L. m. amazonensis. The probe has hybridised strongly to the homologous DNA in track 7 and to the mexicana complex minicircle fragments in tracks 10 and 11 containing the Leishmania species MTB581/583 and R163.

probes [9, 12, 17]. Kinetoplast DNA from L. b. braziliensis MHOM/BR/75/M2903, L. b. guyanensis MHOM/BR/75/M4147, L. b. panamensis MHOM/PA/71/LS94, L. m. mexicana NYC/BZ/62/M379, L. m. amazonensis IFLA/BR/67/PH8, L. d. infantum CAN/TN/78/LEM78 and L. d. donovani MHOM/IN/80/DD8 standard bacteriophage PM2 DNA and from two braziliensis complex isolates from Brazil L. b. braziliensis MHOM/BR83/M7649 and L. braziliensis MHOM/BR/XX/R300 and to two mexicana complex isolates PRO/BR/XX/MTB/581/583 and MHOM/BR/XX/R163, both Leishmania species probably L. m. amazonensis were digested with the endonuclease Hae III and the fragments electrophoretically separated on a 2% agarose gel (Figure 5a). The gel was treated and the DNA fragments Southern transferred using standard methods [17]. The filter was hybridised with Bio-11-dUTP labelled kDNA of L. m. amazonen sis. After application of the streptavidin/alkaline phosphatase detection system, staining of the minicircle fragments was observed (Figure 5b) in the track containing the homologous L. m. amazonensis DNA and staining to the minicircle DNA of two Leishmania species MTB581/583 and R163. No hybridisation has occurred to the minicircle DNA of any other isolate or strain nor to the bacteriophage DNA fragments.

DISCUSSION

We have tried to establish why biotinylated DNA probes can distinguish between species when used in microscopy 'in situ' or Southern filter kDNA hybridisations but show no discrimination with the dot blot method. When substrate alone is applied to replicate filters of those used in Figures 3 and 4, no colour reaction can be seen. It, therefore, seems unlikely that native alkaline phosphatase is present on the surface of, or is released from, Leishmania. However, if no probe is hybridised to the filters, application of the detection system results in all dots showing colour. Similar results with all dots showing colour can be obtained by not hybridising and not using streptavidin or using a streptavidin/alkaline phosphatase conjugate or using avidin and biotin blocking reagents. Our present working hypothesis is that lysing whole leishmania on nitrocellulose releases from the organism some substance which binds biotin, attached or unattached, to alkaline phosphatase or streptavidin.

CONCLUSIONS

Biotinlyated kDNA can be used for 'in situ' or Southern filter hybridisation to discriminate between Leishmania species. By microscopy 'in situ' techniques the hybridised biotinylated probe kDNA can be detected in the 10^{-13} g of kDNA in a single kinetoplast. Some amastigotes must be observed in tissue (or promastigotes in sandfly guts) before the technique can be applied. At the present time, dot blot hybridisation can discriminate between two or more species with 1000 organisms containing 10^{-10} g of kDNA using radioactive probes. No discrimination can be achieved with biotin labeled probes on dot blots.

Future research must aim towards the use of non-radioactive probes with dot blot hybridisation. Increasing the sensitivity of non-radioactive detection, possibly by enzyme amplification methods using a microtitre tray assay, is a priority. The final aim is to totally eliminate the need for radioactive isotopes, expensive X-ray film, and costly enzymes so that DNA diagnosis can become a cheap alternative method in hospital laboratories.

REFERENCES

1. Peters, W. (1986) "Leishmaniases in Biology and Medicine" Peters, W. and Killick-Kendrick, R., eds, Academic Press, London
2. Chance, M.L. and Walton, B.C. (1982) Biochemical Characterization of Leishmania WHO, Geneva. 263-276
3. Arnot, D.E. and Barker, D.CEE. (1981) Biochemical identification of cutaneous leishmania by analysis of kinetoplast DNA II. Sequence homologies in leishmania kDNA, Mol. Biochem. Parasitol. 3:47-56
4. Wirth, D.F. and McMahon-Pratt, D. (1982) Rapid identification of Leishmania species by specific hybridisation of kinetoplast DNA in cutaneous lesions. Proc. Nat. Acad. Sci. USA 79:6999-7003
5. Barker, D.C. and Butcher, J. (1983) The use of DNA probes in the identification of leishmaniasis: discrimination between isolates of the Leishmania mexicana and L. braziliensis complexes. Trans. R. Soc. Trop. Med. Hyg. 77:285-297
6. Spithill, T.W. and Grumont, R.J. (1984) Identification of species, strains and clones of Leishmania by characterization of kinetoplast DNA mini-circles. Mol. Biochem. Parasitol. 12:217-236
7. Lopes, U.G. and Wirth, D.F. (1986) Identification of visceral Leishmania species with cloned sequenceS of kinetoplast DNA. Mol. Biochem. Parasitol. 20:77-84
8. Jackson, P.R., Lawrie, J.M., Stiteler, J.M., Hawkins, D.N., Wohlhieter, J.A. and Rowton, E.D. (1986) Detection and characterization of Leishmania species and strains from mammals and vectors by hybridisation and restriction endonuclease digestion of kinetoplast DNA. Vet. Parasitol. 20:195-215
9. Barker, D.C., Gibson, L.J., Kennedy, W.P.K., Nasser, A.A.A. and Williams, R.H. (1986) The potential of using recombinant DNA species-specific probes for the identification of tropical Leishmania. Parasitology 91:S139-S174
10. Wirth, D.F. and Rogers, W.O. (1985) "Rapid identification of infectious agents" Kingsburg, D.T. and Falbow, S., eds 127-137, Academic Press, New York
11. Wirth, D.F., Rogers, W.O, Barker, R., Dourado, H., Suesebang, L. and Albuquerque, B. (1986) Leishmaniasis and Malaria: New tools for epidemiologic analysis. Science 234:975-979
12. Barker, D.C. (1987) DNA diagnosis of human leishmaniasis. Parasitol. Today. 3:177-184
13. Ntambi, J.M. and Englund, P.T. (1985) J. Bio. Chem. 260:5574-5579
14. Kennedy, W.P.K. (1984) Novel identification of differences in the kinetoplast DNA of Leishmania isolated by recombinant DNA techniques and'in situ' hybridisation. Mol. Biochem. Parasitol. 12:313-325
15. Lawrie, J.M., Jackson, P.R., Stiteler, J.M. and Hockmeyer, W.T. (1985) Identification of pathogenic Leishmania promastigotes by DNA:DNA hybridization with kinetoplast DNA cloned to E. coli plasmids. Am. J. Trop. Med. Hyg. 34:257-265
16. Rogers, W.O. and Wirth, D.F (1987) Kinetoplast DNA minicircles: Regions of extensive sequence divergence. Proc. Natl. Acad. Sci. USA 84:565-569
17. Barker, D.C. (1986) in: "Characterisation of Leishmania sp. by DNA hybridization probes" pp 57, WHO, Geneva
18. van Eys, G.J.J.M., Schoone, G.J., Lighart, G.S., Laarman, J.J. and Terpstra, W.J. (1987) Detection of Leishmania parasites by DNA in situ hybridization with non-radioactive probes. Parasitol. Res. 73:199-202

ACKNOWLEDGEMENTS

I am grateful that the investigations received the financial support of the Medical Research Council (UK) and the UNDP/WORLD BANK/WHO/TRD programme ID 840412. I would like to thank Lorna Gibson and Roger Williams for their active participation in this work and for their sometimes sceptical and always critical evaluation of our results. My thanks is also due to Miss Tracy Askin for typing the manuscript.

APPLICATION OF TOTAL AND RECOMBINANT DNA PROBES IN THE DIAGNOSIS OF

LEISHMANIA INFECTIONS

> G.J.J.M. Van Eys, G.J. Schoone, G.S. Ligthart, J.A. Schalken*
> and W.J. Terpstra
> Laboratory of Tropical Hygiene
> Royal Tropical Institute, Amsterdam, The Netherlands
> Laboratory of Biochemistry*
> University of Nijmegen, Nijmegen, The Netherlands

INTRODUCTION

Detection and classification of Leishmania parasites is still laborious and time-consuming. Detection of Leishmania infections depends largely on microscopic screening of smears and tissue sections, whereas classification relies on geographical area, pathology of the infection and more recently immunological and biochemical properties of the parasite. At this moment isoenzyme analysis is the most satisfactory method for the determination of Leishmania parasites. The main disadvantage of this method is that one has to culture the parasites.
The developments in the field of molecular biology have induced the application of new techniques for the detection and characterization of Leishmania. Investigators tried to take advantage of a peculiarity that the Leishmania shares with the trypanosome parasites: the presence of a kinetoplast. The kinetoplast has properties that seemed to make it a promising tool for the diagnosis of Leishmania infections. The presence of several thousands of mostly homologous minicircles, the high variability of the minicircles between isolates and the relatively simple procedures to obtain pure kinetoplast DNA seemed to qualify this organelle for further study. Restriction enzyme analyses provided not only evidence of considerable differences between Leishmania of different strains but also between isolates of the same strain (Arnot and Barker , 1981; Jackson et al.,1984; Kennedy, 1984; Lawrie et al.,1985). Hybridization of Southern blots of kDNA with total kDNA or recombinant probes showed that kinetoplast minicircles contain conserved sequences and variable sequences. However, from the data presented so far, no strain specific probes or hybridization patterns have been documented (Barker and Butcher, 1982; Spithill and Grumont, 1984; Kennedy, 1984; Lawrie et al., 1985; Lopez and Wirth, 1986). So, recently attention has been focussed on the more complex nuclear DNA. Genomic and cDNA libraries have been constructed and clones coding for tubulin (Comeau et al, 1986; Bishop and Miles, 1987; Spithill and Samaras, 1987), ribosomal spacers (Ramirez and Guevara, 1987), and surface antigens (Sheppard and Dwyer, 1986) have been isolated. Data published in

the papers mentioned above indicate that such clones can be used for the classification of isolates and for the synthesis of specific Leishmania antigens. However, the value of such recombinant DNA probes for the diagnosis of leishmaniasis will depend largely on the techniques in which they will be applied.

At this moment three DNA techniques are under investigation for the detection and classification of Leishmania parasites: Southern blotting, dot blot and in situ hybridization. Southern blotting is the method of choice for the classification of Leishmania strains, whether kDNA or nuclear DNA derived recombinant probes are used. The combination of specific probes with reproducible hybridization patterns has the potential of detailed characterization of Leishmania parasites (Kennedy, 1984; Lopez and Wirth, 1986; Ramirez and Guevarra, 1987). To achieve this the development of strain specific probes will be necessary. The method is not a serious candidate for routine diagnosis of Leishmania infections since it needs culturing of the parasites and can only be performed in well equipped laboratories. Dot blot and in situ hybridization do not have the disadvantages of the Southern blot technique. Several investigators have applied dot blot analyses with different types of probes (Wirth and McMahon Pratt, 1982; Spithill and Grumont, 1984; Lawrie et al., 1985; Lopez and Wirth, 1986). They concluded that dot blot assays need a relatively small number of parasites, are easy to perform and rather inexpensive, and therefore might be a useful technique under field conditions. However, studies on other parasites have shown the need for proper controls and the replacement of radio-isotopes by non-radioactive labels to make this technique applicable in the clinical setting (McGlauglin et al.,1986, 1987). In situ hybridization is a rather new technique. It has been performed on Leishmania with radioactive-labelled probes (Kennedy, 1984) and with biotin-labelled probes (Van Eys et al., 1987). In these studies total DNA and kDNA probes were used. The method has the advantage of combining a hybridization signal with the visualization of the parasites morphology. Such a specific staining will improve detection, but for characterization of the parasite specific recombinant probes will be needed. In this paper we describe the use of recombinant probes in the different assay systems. The use of kDNA, cDNA and genomic DNA probes on different types of clinical samples was investigated and the potential of the different assay techniques and their fields of application will be discussed.

MATERIALS AND METHODS

Parasites: Leishmania promastigotes were cultured in Dwyer's medium (Dwyer, 1972) or in RPMI 1640, both media supplied with 15% FCS. The strains used were kindly provided by Dr.D. Evans (London), Dr. J. Alvar (Madrid), Dr. J. Schottelius (Hamburg), Dr. P. Jackson (Washington) and Dr. A. Harith (Amsterdam). Strains are referred to by the code, mentioned by the donors, or has been described previously (Van Eys et al., 1987). Parasites were grown to a density of approximately 10^7 per ml. They were collected by centrifugation (350g, 30 min, 10°C) and washed twice with PBS.

Sample preparation for in situ hybridization: Promastigotes were layered on microscopic slides, air dried and fixed by immersion in methanol (10 min, 20°C). Infections of mice and preparation of impression smears have been described previously (Van Eys et al., 1987). Tissues were fixed in a 2% buffered formaldehyde solution for 16 h at 4°C. Embedding and sectioning of the tissues were done according to standard histological procedures.The in situ hybridization procedure itself has recently extensively been described (Van Eys et al.,1987). In addition, the DAB precipitate signal was enhanced by siver amplification treatment (Amersham). Preparation of genomic DNA, poly A-RNA, and biotin- and 32P-labelled DNA probes, as well as procedures for Southern blotting and dot blotting, construction of genomic and cDNA libraries and selection of recombinant clones have been described elsewhere (Southern, 1976; Maniatis et al., 1982; Van Eys et al., 1987). All fragments were ligated in the vector pUC19 (Yanisch-Perron et al., 1985).

RESULTS

From the three types of DNA libraries that were constructed (genomic, kDNA and cDNA), clones were selected on the basis of their reactivity and specificity. Clones selected from the kDNA library varied in size from about 100 bp up to 1 kbp. Clones from the cDNA library were up to 4 kbp in length. If the genomic library was made with total parasite DNA almost all selected clones turned out to be kDNA minicircle clones, and even after gradient centrifugation most of the clones were kinetoplast derived. This is due to the selection of clones with total DNA probes. Therefore we isolated nuclear DNA fragments by gel electrophoresis and used these for the construction of genomic libraries. After a first screening by preferential, and a second sceening by dot blot hybridization, 8 kinetoplast and 8 nuclear DNA clones were selected for further experiments. In addition, we had four rib somal clones from a Trypanosoma brucei library (a generous gift from Dr. T. White, Amsterdam).

Southern blotting of the selected clones showed that most clones can be used for characterization of Leishmania strains. A number of the cDNA clones showed cross-hybridization between different strains but are useful on the basis of differences in the blotting pattern (Fig. 1a). Clone 7-118, for instance, shows the same pattern for visceral Leishmania, a different pattern for old world cutaneous Leishmania and no reaction for new world cutaneous Leishmania. On the other hand, clone 7-131 shows differences in reactivity and pattern to the different visceral Leishmanias, and very little reaction to other strains (Fig.2a). A few cDNA clones are almost strain specific (Fig. 2b). Of the kDNA probes most of them are isolate specific, in the sense that different isolates of the same strain showed no or limited cross-hybridization (Fig. 2b,c). Differences in blotting patterns were not observed, due to the restriction enzymes used and the method of electrophoresis applied. The ribosomal probes showed no marked differences in hybridization intensity, but showed variations in the patterns (Fig. 1b).

Dot blot assays showed the increased specificity of recombinant probes over total DNA probes, with the exception of the ribosomal probes (Fig. 3).However, the cDNA probes as well as the kDNA probes have to be tested on greater panels of well characterized isolates. The former for reasons of strain specificity, the latter to find out the variability of the minicircle within a particular strain.

When in situ hybridization is performed with biotin-labelled total DNA probes, nuclei as well as kinetoplast hybridize clearly. This has been observed in preparations of promastigote cultures, impression smears and in tissue sections of infected animals (Fig. 4a,d,f,g,i). Hybridization with bacterial DNA or

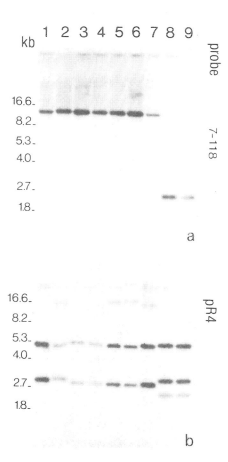

fig.1

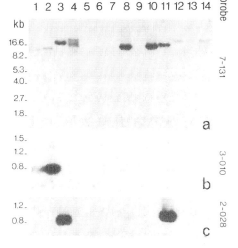

fig.2

Fig. 1a: Southern blot of a 0.7% agarose gel with Hind III digested DNA of 9 Leishmania strains. The blot is hybridized to probe 7-118, selected from a L.donovani cDNA library. The strains are (from 1 to 9): L.infantum (Angeles); L.infantum (LV140); L.infantum (Itmap); L.donovani 1s; L.donovani WR352; L.chagasi (PP75); L.chagasi (IMP); L.major (Githure); L.major (AMC9836). Note that the visceral Leishmania give the same pattern whereas the two L.major isolates give another pattern.

Fig. 1b: The same blot hybridized to a probe derived from the Trypanosoma brucei ribosomal gene (White et al., 1987). With this probe it is also possible to differentiate between certain groups of strains.

Fig. 2a: DNA of 14 Leishmania strains was digested by Eco RI and fragmented on a 0.7% agarose gel. The blot was hybridized to probe 7-131, derived from a L.donovani cDNA library. The DNA had been isolated from (1-14): L.major AMC9836; L.major (Githure); L.donovani 1s; L.infantum Angeles; human; mouse; leptospira; L.chagasi PP75; L.chagasi IMP; L.donovani WR352; L.donovani 1s; L.br. braziliensis; L.m. amazonica WR669; L.m. mexicana WR544. Note the differences between the two L.chagasi and the two L.donovani isolates.

Fig. 2b: Hybridization of the same blot with probe 3-010, from a L.major kDNA library, shows no cross-hybridization with other strains. except AMC9836. However the hybridization with this isolate is only 10% of that with L.major (Githure) for the same quantity of DNA.

Fig. 2c: Hybridization of the same blot with probe 2-028, from a L.donovani 1s kDNA library. Only very weak cross-hybridization is found for PP75, whereas no hybridization is found for WR352.

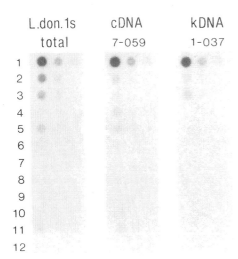

Fig. 3: DNA of different Leishmania strains was spotted on nitrocellulose and and hybridized to different L.donovani probes. The DNA was spotted in quantities of 100, 20 and 4 ng. The different isolates are (from 1-12): L.donovani 1s; L.donovani WR352; L.chagasi PP75; L.chagasi IMP; L.don.donovani; L.major AMC9836; L.br.braziliensis; L.br. guanensis; L.mex.mexicana WR544; L.mex.amazonensis WR669; L.infantum LV140; human DNA.

DNA of Giardia lambia showed no such hybridization (results not shown). Application of biotin labeled recombinant DNA probes showed specific hybridization of the nucleus, when a cDNA probe is used, and specific staining of the kinetoplast, when a kDNA probe is used (fig. 4b,e,h). Strain specificity is not complete. cDNA probes from Leishmania donovani cross-hybridize somewhat with other old-world Leishmania strains. Concentrations of probe and assay conditions influence the level of cross-hybridization. Similar cross-hybridizations have been observed for cDNA probes from Leishmania major and for kDNA probes at various levels. Further study of the hybridization conditions and generation of more specific probes will be necessary.

DISCUSSION

Detection and classification of Leishmania is still troublesome. The methods used for the detection either have a low sensitivity, like microscopic screening of clinical samples, or are time consuming, such as the culturing of parasites. The most prominent method of characterization today is iso-enzyme analysis, which is also time-consuming. In addition, these methods need a laboratory setting and a trained and experienced staff. Development of new methods for the detection and characterization of Leishmania should aim for procedures that can be routinely performed by unspecialized personel working in laboratories with limited facilities. We think that DNA based techniques might be helpful to achieve these goals.

The results of the three different hybridization techniques show that these techniques have different fields of application and different limitations. Southern blotting can only be used with recombinant DNA probes, is a complicated and time-consuming technique, and needs culturing. Hence, the technique might prove to be useful for characterization of Leishmania parasites but will be of very limited value for the diagnosis. Probes derived from kDNA show weak hybridization with DNA from isolates of supposedly the same strain of Leishmania. This indicates that these probes are more isolate specific than strain specific. A study on large groups of isolates within one strain but

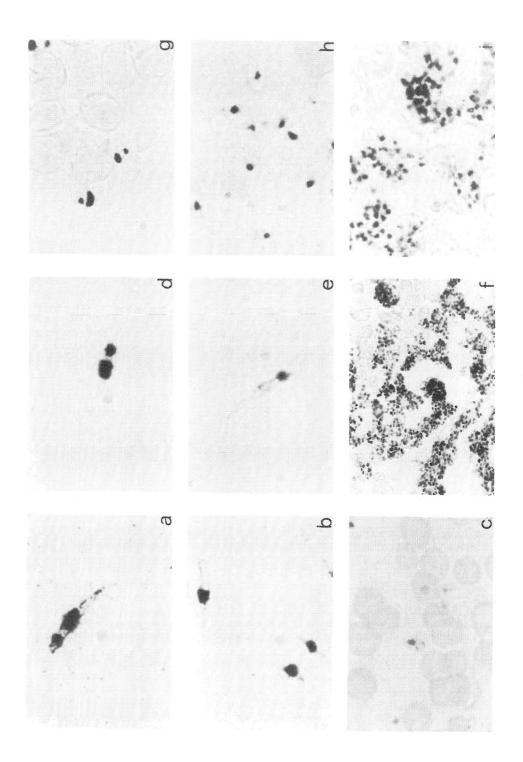

originating from different geographical areas will be needed to estimate the value of this approach. To some extend this is also true for the cDNA probes. We have probed a relatively small number of isolates or reference strains with these probes. For a number of our cDNA probes we have found strain specificity, but since we did not screen greater number of isolates within and without the strains involved, Leishmania donovani and Leishmania major, a final evaluation of these probes and the potential of this method has to wait for the outcome of those experiments.

As a diagnostic tool the dot blot hybridization assay has a number of advantages over Southern blotting. For a dot blot a relatively small number of parasites will be sufficient (Wirth and McMahon Pratt, 1982). Also, the processing of clinical samples is rather simple and the assay can be performed in a short period of time without sophisticated equipment. For the detection of Leishmania infections total DNA probes will work. However, as can be deduced from our results, strain specific probes are a necessity, if one wants to detect and classify in one assay. For the classification of Leishmania parasites this technique depends on the development of strain specific recombinant probes, or on combinations of such probes. We have presented data on 32P-labelled probes. The use of highly sensitive radioactive probes will be useful for well-equipped laboratories. However, the clinical situation will ask for non-radioactive labelling of the probes. In our hands this results in a tenfold decrease of sensitivity when using commercially available staining kits. The recent gains in sensitivity and the increasing simplicity of operation of these kits may soon overcome the present drawbacks of non-radioactive probes, and turn the dot blot assay into a clinically relevant diagnostic tool.

The availability of non-radioactive labels is also essential for the applicability of the in situ hybridization assay. In situ hybridization with radioactive probes is a difficult, slow and cumbersome technique, certainly not useful for routine diagnosis. Our results demonstrate that this technique can be performed with biotin-labeled total DNA as well as specific recombinant DNA probes. Total DNA probes have the advantage of providing a strong signal for the kinetoplast as well as for the nucleus. The stable configuration of kinetoplast and nucleus facilitates recognition of the Leishmania parasites. Besides, use of total DNA probes will not demand a high signal amplification, and this will diminish background problems. The considerable degree of cross-hybridization of total DNA probes with isolates of different

Fig. 4: In situ hybridization with biotin labelled probes. Diaminobenzidine was used as substrate and the signal of the formed precipitate was enhanced by silver. Promastigotes (a,b,d,e) are hybridized with total DNA probes of L.donovani (a) or L.major (d), and with recombinant probes 7-059 from a L.donovani cDNA library (b) or 3-010 from a L.major kDNA library (e). Amastigotes in impression smears of a L.major infected mouse as observed after Giemsa staining (c) and after hybridization to a total DNA probe of L.major (g) or recombinant probe 3-010 (h). Amastigotes were demonstrated in sections of paraffin embedded tissue of hind limb of a L.major infected mouse, using a total DNA probe (f,i). Note the visualisation of both nucleus and kinetoplast when total DNA probes are applied, whereas only one of them can be seen when recombinant probes are applied. Magnification was 1000x, except for (f) 400x.

strains and the impossibility to quantitate the signal indicate that this approach cannot be used for the characterization of the parasites. Still, in situ hybridization with total DNA probes migth be a worthwhile asset for the detection of Leishmania infections. The availability of recombinant DNA probes increases the diagnostic value of this technique considerably. This will enable the investigator to characterize the parasite with one or a few strain specific probes. Combination of a few recombinant clones, especially nuclear and kinetoplast, might turn out to be superior in terms of sensitivity and specificity. With such probes it is possible to detect and identify the Leishmania parasite simultaneously. Our results show that biotin-labelled recombinant probes work in this hybridization system. The generation of sufficient numbers of specific clones and the screening of those clones will be the tedious job for the years to come. An additional advantage of the in situ hybridization, either with total or recombinant DNA probes, is that it can be applied on routinely taken clinical samples. This is not only of clinical importance but also presents opportunities for retrospective and epidemiological investigations.

Although the practical use of hybridization assays still has to be proven, we think that these assays have great potential. The Southern blotting technique might serve as a worthwhile addition to other classification systems like iso-enzyme analysis. It has the advantage that DNA, unlike proteins, is relatively stable and its structure and sequence is not changed by conditions inside or outside the parasite. The dot blot and in situ hybridization assays might be of diagnostic value. The best opportunities for the latter two assays will, in our opinion, be in the field of (muco)cutaneous leishmaniasis, where smears of ulcers or tissue samples offer good material for these assays.

The presented data cover one particular area of DNA techniques that might be applied: DNA hybridization assays. We want to mention two other techniques. Firstly, restriction enzyme analysis of kinetoplast minicircle DNA has been investigated by several groups, for Leishmania as well as for Trypanosoma. Under natural conditions the mutation frequency of the kDNA is apparently of such a degree that different restriction patterns are found within one strain (Lawrie et al., 1985; Jackson et al., 1984; Kennedy, 1984). This may reflect the lack of evolutionary selection, since no convincing data have been presented for transcription of minicircle DNA, and therefore no properties of the parasite will depend on this DNA (Hoeimakers and Borst, 1978; Fouts and Wolestenholmes, 1979). The degree of kDNA divergence and the fact that culturing is needed to perform restriction enzyme analysis, makes this technique, in our opinion, unfit for routine diagnosis. Secondly, the generation of fusion-proteins from cDNA expression libraries of Leishmania parasites. Such proteins can be applied in immuno-assays like ELISA and agglutination tests, or for the production of antisera and monoclonals. The integration of DNA and immuno-techniques will combine the highly pure recombinant antigens with proven and established assay systems. A serious disadvantage is that such assay will tell little about the stage of the infection, unless stage specific antigens can be found. We think that this approach has great potential for the diagnosis of visceral leishmaniasis, whereas hybridization assay will perform better in cases of (muco)cutaneous leishmaniasis.

CONCLUSIONS

   Diagnosis of leishmaniasis may be improved by recently developed DNA based techniques. Hybridization techniques have been shown to be able to detect as well as characterize Leishmania parasites. Three techniques are discussed within the scope of this paper. Southern hybridization has been found to be too complicated for routine diagnosis of leishmaniasis, but probably very helpful in the classification of these parasites. Dot blot and in situ hybridization have been shown to offer opportunities for improved detection of Leishmania parasites. Development of strain specific recombinant probes provided these techniques with the possibility for characterization of the parasites. Although the generation of such strain specific recombinant probes will ask for a great effort, the techniques themselves are rather simple, sensitive, specific and relatively fast.

REFERENCES

Arnot, D. E., Barker, D. C., 1981, Biochemical identification of cutaneous leishmanias by analysis of kinetoplast DNA. II. Sequence homologies in Leishmania kDNA. Mol. Biochem. Parasitol. 3: 47-56.

Barker, D. C., Butcher, J., 1983, The use of DNA probes in the identification of leishmanias: discrimination between isolates of the Leishmania mexicana and L.braziliensis complexes. Trans. Roy. Soc. Trop. Med. Hyg. 77: 285-279.

Bishop, R. P., Miles, M. A., 1987, Chromosome size polymorphisms of Leishmania donovani. Mol. Biochem. Parasitol. 24: 263-272.

Comeau, A. M., Miller, S. I., Wirth, D. F., 1986, Chromosome location of four genes in Leishmania. Mol. Biochem. Parasitol. 21: 161-169.

Dwyer, D. M., 1972, A monophasic medium for cultivating Leishmania donovani in large numbers. J. Parasitol. 58: 847-848.

Jackson, P. R., Wohlhieter, J. A., Jackson, J. E., Sayles, P., Diggs, C. L., Hockmeyer, W.T., 1984, Restriction endonuclease analysis of Leishmania kinetoplast DNA characterizes parasites responsible for visceral and cutaneous disease. Am. J. Trop. Med. Hyg. 33: 808-819.

Kennedy, W. P. K., 1984, Novel identification of differences in the kinetoplast DNA of Leishmania isolates by recombinant DNA techniques and in situ hybridization. Mol. Biochem. Parasitol. 12: 313-325.

Lawrie, J. M., Jackson, P. R., Stiteler, J. M., Hockmeyer, W. T., 1985, Identification of pathogenic Leishmania promastigotes by DNA: DNA hybridization with kinetoplast DNA cloned into E.coli plasmids. Am. J. Trop. Med. Hyg. 34: 257-265.

Lopes, U. G., Wirth, D. F., 1986, Identification of viseral Leishmania species with cloned sequences of kinetoplast DNA. Mol. Biochem. Parasitol. 20: 77-84.

Maniatis, T., Fritsch, E. F., Sambrook, J., 1982, Molecular cloning: A laboratory manual. Cold Spring Harbor Laboratories, Cold Spring Harbor, NY.

McLaughlin, G. L., Ruth, J. L., Jablonski, E., Steketee, R., Cambell, G. H., 1987, Use of enzyme- linked synthetic DNA in diagnosis of falciparum malaria. Lancet, March 28, 714-715.

Ramirez, J. L., Guevarra, P., 1987, The ribosomal gene spacer as a tool for taxonomy of Leishmania. Mol. Biochem. Parasitol. 22: 177-183.

Sheppard, H. W., Dwyer, D. M., 1986, Cloning of Leishmania donovani genes encoding antigens recognized during human visceral leishmaniasis. Mol. Biochem. Parasitol. 19: 35-43.

Southern, E. M., 1975, Detection of specific sequences among DNA fragments separated by gel electrophoresis. J. Mol. Biol. 98: 503-517.

Spithill, T. W., Grumont, R. J., 1984, Identification of species, strains and clones of Leishmania by characterization of kinetoplast DNA minicircles. Mol. Biochem. Parasitol. 12: 217-236.

Spithill, T. W., Samaras, N., 1987, Genomic organization, chromosomal location and transcription of dispersed and repeated tubulin genes in Leishmania major. Mol. Biochem. Parasitol. 24: 23-37.

Van Eys, G. J. J. M., Schoone, G. J., Ligthart, G. S., Laarman, J. J., Terpstra, W. J., 1987, Detection of Leishmania parasites by DNA in situ hybridization with non-radioactive probes. Parasitol. Res. 73: 199-202.

White, T. C., Rudenko, G., Borst, P., Three small RNAs within the 10 kb trypanosome rRNA transcription unit are analogous to Domain VII of other eukaryotic 28S rRNAs. Nuc. Acids Res. 14: 9471-9489.

Wirth, D. F., McMahon Pratt, D., 1982, Rapid identification of Leishmania species by specific hybridization of kinetoplast DNA in cutaneous lesions. Proc. Natl. Acad. Sci. USA 79: 6999-7003.

Yanisch-Perron, C., Vieira, J., Messing, J., 1985, Improved M13 phage cloning vectors and host strain: nucleotide sequences of M13mp18 and pUC19 vectors. Gene 33: 103-119.

ACKNOWLEDGEMENTS

We gratefully acknowledge Nel Kroon and Jelle Zaal for their cooperation and Ariane Heibloem for secretarial assistance.

BIOTINYLATED kDNA FROM Leishmania braziliensis

Martin Lopez, Ysabel Montoya, Alejandro Llanos Cuentas and
Jorge Arevalo

Instituto de Medicina Tropical "Alexander von Humboldt"
Universidad Peruana Cayetano Heredia
P.O. Box 5045, Lima 100, PERU

INTRODUCTION

The lesions caused by the Leishmania braziliensis complex begin as a cutaneous lesion. In some cases, as those produced by L. braziliensis braziliensis, the lesion very often progresses towards destruction of mucouse tissues. In the Amazonian jungle, an area endemic for mucocutaneous Leishmaniasis it is common that people, specially new settlers, develop ulcerative lesions that are often diagnosed incorrectly as Leishmaniasis. Differential diagnosis between Leishmania and other etiological agents causing skin diseases is thus required. A potential diagnostic method would be the direct demonstration of parasites in lesions by DNA hybridization with DNA probes from Leishmania.

Another use for DNA probes will be in epidemiological studies to determine the percentage of infected Lutzomyias. At present for that type of studies microscopic examination of freshly disected guts from sandflies is required. This method implies highly trained personnel and is very time consuming. Furthermore it could give false positives since other flagellates could be found in the vector. We have reported the characterization of a Leishmania-like flagellate, HS-55, isolated from an Andean insect vector. Its isoenzymatic pattern did not match with those obtained with standard reference strains recommended by the World Health Organization (WHO), neither reacted with monoclonal antibodies nor with kDNA probes specific for L. braziliensis and L. mexicana.[1] This isolate also did not infect peritoneal macrophages from Balb/c mice, which are highly susceptible to Leishmania infection (unpublished results).

The kinetoplast DNA (kDNA) minicircles of trypanosomatids, due its large number of copies are suitable for use as probes. Wirth and Pratt[2] described the use of kDNA probes for the characterization of Leishmanias. Several studies using this approach has been carried out succesfully.[3-7] In all of these studies DNA was labelled with ^{32}P. The relative short half life of the radioisotope, the laboratory facilities required for autorradiography, the need for trained personnel to handle radioactive material and the availability of adequate systems to dispose radioactive waste limits the application of radiolabelled DNA probes to properly equipped laboratories, usually not found in countries were tropical diseases are endemic.

A few years ago Leary et al.[9] described a nonradioactive detection system that could replace the use of ^{32}P. It takes advantage of the extremely high binding affinity of Avidin for molecules containing Biotin. Thus, incorporation of the analogue Bio-dUTP in the DNA can be detected enzymatically after reacting the modified DNA with a biotinylated alkaline phosphatase-Avidin complex which gives a color reaction with a specific substrate.

Recently there was a report on the use of radiolabelled DNA probes to detect Leishmania parasites using crude biopsies blotted on Nitrocellulose (NC) paper.[7] The authors were able to detect as few as 50 parasites. Attempts to use biotinylated DNA probes for hybridization with crude samples blotted on NC paper were not successful.[10] A high background developes at the place where the sample is applied. This difficulty is the reason why biotinylated DNA probes are used to detect either purified DNA or parasites fixed on slides by in situ hybridization.[10-13] These approaches would not be practical for use as routine diagnostic methods. Here we present studies of hybridization with biotinylated kDNA from Leishmania under experimental conditions that allow the levels of sensitivity attained with radiolabelled probes and discuss its potential use for diagnosis.

MATERIALS AND METHODS

Parasites

Leishmania parasites were isolated from biopsies or aspirates of patient lesions and grown in a cell free biphasic medium as described elsewhere.[1]

MHOM/BR/75/M2903 (L. braziliensis braziliensis), MHOM/BR/75/M4147 (L. brazilienis guyanensis), IFLA/BR/67/PH8 (L. mexicana amazonensis), and MNYC/BZ/62/M379 (L. mexicana mexicana) were used as reference strains.[14]

Preparation of Blotted Parasites

Different numbers of washed prasites in 2 µl of 0.9% saline solution were blotted on NC paper. Leishmania DNA was denatured and fixed by floating the filter on 0.5 N NaOH for 5 min. After neutralization by two incubations of 5 min each with 1 M Tris pH 7.5, the filter was washed twice in 0.5 M Tris pH 7.5, 0.5 M NaCl.

In order to lower the background we incubated the blotted parasites with Proteinase K (100 µg/ml) in 0.1 M Tris pH 7.5 at 37°C for 30 min before hybridization. Filters were air dried and then baked at 80°C for two hours.

Crude Biopsy Blotting Procedure

Biopsies were taken from lesions with disposable 4 mm biopsy punches. The tissue was processed in three different ways. Firstly, it was smashed directly on the NC paper, then air dried and stored at room temperature until used. Secondly, the tissue was grinded with a glass homogenizer in 800 µl of saline solution. The homogenate was then passed through NC paper with the aid of a 96 wells minifold filtering apparatus and washed twice with 2X SSC. The blotted samples were then air dried and stored at room temperature until their use. Thirdly, samples were processed as in the second procedure with the only difference that 800 µl of 5% citric acid (about pH 2) were used during the homogenization. The homogenates were rapidly neutralized with a 1 M Tris pH 8 solution.

DNA Hybridization

The procedures for Leishmania kDNA purification and its labelling by nick translation with either ³²P or Bio-dUTP have been described in detail elsewhere.[1,15]

For the nonradioactive DNA hybridization method we have adapted the conditions described by Leary et al.[8] to detect small number of parasites. Leishmania parasites blotted on NC paper were prehybridized with 10 ml of a solution containing 50 mM phosphate buffer pH 6.5, 50% deionized formamide, 5X SSC, 5X Denhardt's solution and 100 ug/ml salmon sperm DNA for 2 hours at 42°C in a siliconized plastic container. The prehybridization solution was then replaced by a similar one containing 10% Dextran sulfate (Sigma) and 500 ng/ml of heat denatured specific kDNA probe (0.15-0.40 ml of DNA probe solution/cm² NC paper). After an overnight incubation at 42°C with gentle rocking the filters were washed as follows: Twice with 250 ml of 2X SSC-0.5% SDS, Once with 250 ml of 1X SSC-0.5% SDS and finally once with 250 ml of 0.1X SSC-0.5% SDS. Washes were made at 55°C for 30 min each. The filters were afterwards air dried at room temperature.

Enzymatic development

Dried blotted hybridized samples were hydrated in AP 7.5 buffer solution (0.1 M Tris pH 7.5, 0.1 M NaCl, 2 mM $MgCl_2$, 0.05% Triton X-100) containing 3% BSA (Sigma) and 2% dehydrated milk for 30 min at 37°C. After baking the samples at 80°C for half an hour the filters were rehydrated under the same conditions mentioned above. The filters were dripped of excess liquid, transferred to a glass petri dish and exposed to Streptavidin and alkaline phosphatase at room temperature in a two step reaction. Firstly, 1 - 2 ml of Streptavidin (Calbiochem) in AP 7.5 solution (3.6 µg/ml) were added to the filter for 10 min. After removing the excess of Streptavidin by two washes with 50 ml each of AP 7.5 solution, the filters were incubated 10 min with 1-2 ml of biotinylated alkaline phosphatase (0.9 µg/ml in AP 7.5 solution). All further procedures were as described by Leary et al.[8] except that we used a glass petri dish instead of a plastic bag for the enzymatic degradation of substrate to colored product.

Characterization of Plasmid Recombinant DNA

We have inserted MboI restriction fragments of kDNA from different New World Leishmania isolates into the BamHI site of the pBR322. Crude plasmid DNA from Ampicillin resistant and Tetracycline sensitive bacterial colonies was obtained by the alkaline extraction procedure.[16] Two microliters of each extract were blotted on NC paper followed by a Proteinase K treatment. Those clones which were positive by dot blot were further characterized by Southern blot hybridization using our biotinylated kDNA probes. In this case Proteinase K treatment was unnecessary.

RESULTS

Optimal conditions for biotinylating 4 µg of Leishmania kDNA were the following: incubation with 400 pg of DNAse and 20 units of DNA polymerase I for 30 min at 16°C. Using these labelling conditions we were able to detect down to one thousand parasites. Below this number the background made it difficult to discriminate between a positive with small number of parasites and a false positive. To detect less than 1000 parasites per dot blot with this nonradioactive method we attempted to improve the contrast between control and positive samples.

Two steps where important to improve the detection level of parasites. First, an incubation of the samples with Proteinase K (100 µg/ml) at 37°C for 30 min before the hybridization step reduced the background at the place where the parasites were blotted. Second, an incubation of blotted samples with 2% milk powder solution in 0.1 M Tris pH 7.5 buffer after the hybridization step avoided any nonspecific adsorption of the colorimetric product to the NC paper after the enzymatic development. These treatments abolished the background almost completely. With these treatments we were able to detect as few as 100 whole parasites dot blotted on NC paper using biotinylated kDNA probes after an overnight period of enzymatic development (Figure 1). With ^{32}P labelled DNA probes, five days of autorradiography using intensifier screens were necessary to detect the same number of parasites.

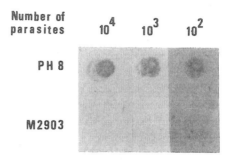

Fig. 1. Detection of whole parasites blotted on NC paper. Different numbers of parasites where blotted as described in Materials and Methods. PH8 and M2903 are reference strains of L. mexicana amazonensis and L. braziliensis braziliensis respectively. Filters were hybridized with a biotinylated kDNA probe from PH8 as described in Materials and Methods. Filters with 10^4 parasites blotted were color developed after 3 min. Filters with 10^3 parasites were developed for 20 min. Filters with 100 parasites required overnight developement.

Biotinylated kDNA probes were able to discriminate between L. braziliensis and L. mexicana complexes (Figure 2). Furthermore as we reported previously[1] all peruvian isolates where undistinguishable from the L. braziliensis reference strains. Unfortunately total kDNA as probe was not able to detect differences at the subspecies level.

To discriminate between Uta and Espundia, the two clinical forms of Leishmaniasis in Peru, by the use of DNA probes, it is necessary to clone subspecies specific DNA fragments. In order to search for plasmid recombinant DNAs containing these specific kDNA sequences, we used the nonradioactive detection system here described. For example kDNA fragments from Leishmania LC39 (isolated from a typical Uta lesion) were inserted into the BamHI site of the plasmid pBR322. Crude plasmid extracts from Ampicillin resistant, Tetracycline sensitive bacteria were blotted on NC paper and treated with Proteinase K. After hybridization with homologous biotinylated kDNA, only clone Uta 2 seemed to carry a kDNA fragment (Figure 3). This was further confirmed by Southern blot Hybridization (Figure 4). This clone did not hybridize with the L. mexicana kDNA probe. Unfortunately this clone used as target DNA hybridized with biotinylated probes from the L. braziliensis complex (M2903 and M4147) and the Espundia LC03 isolate (data not shown).

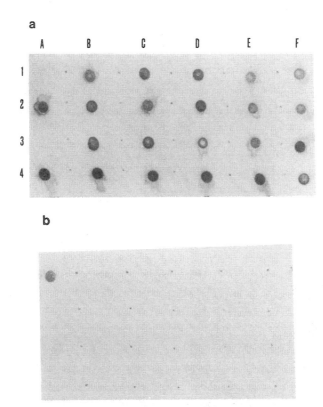

Fig. 2. Characterization of Leishmania isolates from different regions of Peru with biotinylated kDNA probes. Column A corresponds to standard reference strains recommended by the WHO. Coordinates 1A and 1C are PH8 and M379 respectively. Coordinates 1B and 1D are M2903 and M4147 respectively (see Materials and Methods). The other coordinates correspond to peruvian isolates from Andean and Selvatic regions. Figure 2(a) corresponds to a filter hibridized with biotinylated L. braziliensis kDNA probe. Figure 2(b) corresponds to biotinilated L. mexicana kDNA probe.

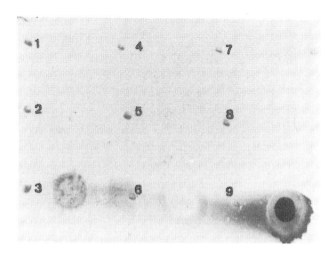

Fig. 3. Dot blot of bacteria containing recombinant DNA hybridized with biotinylated kDNA probes from L. braziliensis. kDNA from Leishmania LC39 was cloned in pBR322. Bacterial colonies with plasmid containing insert were blotted on NC paper and hybridized as described in Material and Methods. Sample 9 was a positive control, M2903 (L. braziliensis). Sample 3, Uta 2 gave a strong positive reaction.

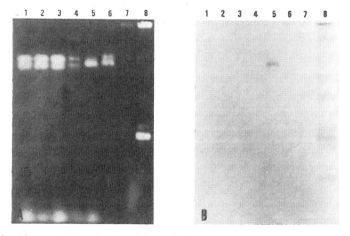

Fig. 4. Southern blot of recombinant plasmids prepared from Ampicillin resistant, Tetracycline sensitive colonies after transformation with pBR322 and Leishmania LC39 kDNA potential recombinants. Lane 8 is an Eco RI digestion of kDNA from L. braziliensis (M2903) and constitutes a positive control. Lanes 6 is an Eco RI digest of a L. mexicana (PH8). Lanes 1 to 6 correspond to potential recombinant plasmids. Figure 4A shows the ethidium bromide staining of the 1.2 % agarose gel electrophoresis. Figure 4B shows the corresponding Southern blot hybridized with biotinylated kDNA from M2903. Lane 5 corresponds to Uta 2 clone.

The use of biotinylated DNA probes to detect Leishmania from biopsies obtained from lesions was tested with three different methods of biopsy preparation as described in Materials and Methods. When biopsies were touch blotted on NC paper we were able to detect positive hybridization. The intensity of the color reaction was however very small (data not shown), which makes this method of preparation inadequate at present. Results of biopsies previously homogenized were more encouraging. Figure 5 shows homogenates from lesions obtained from experimentally infected hamsters. Biopsies homogenated in citrate (Fig. 5A) appear to give stronger positive reactions than those homogenated in saline (Fig. 5B). With citrate homogenates (Fig. 5A) 4 out of 6 samples gave positive reaction. The control sample, normal hamster tissue gave a much lighter color reaction. It should be noted that the percentage of positivity obtained in these preliminary studies is higher than that obtained by conventional detection techniques (direct microscopical observation of smears and *in vitro* culture).

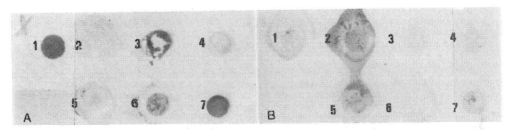

Fig. 5   Hybridization of biopsies from experimentally infected hamsters with kDNA probe specific for L. braziliensis labelled with Biotin dUTP. A) Samples homogenized with 5% citric acid and rapidly neutralized with 1M Tris pH 8. B) Samples homogenized with 0.9% saline solution Sample 5 in Fig. 5A is tissue from non-infected hamster (control).

Figure 6 shows the use of biotinylated kDNA from L. braziliensis when tested on biopsies from human patients. The samples where homogenized with citrate. Two out of six samples are clearly positive. Control of normal human tissue gave only a light reaction.

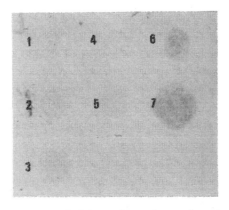

Fig. 6   Hybridization of biopsies from human patients with biotinylated kDNA probes specific for L. braziliensis isolates. Sample 3 was obtained fro a non-infected human biopsy (control).

DISCUSSION

The results presented here and elsewhere[1] demonstrate that nonradioactive kDNA probes are as specific and sensitive as radiolabelled ones. The use of nonradioactive detection systems should be important for research on tropical diseases to be carried out in Third World countries where these diseases constitute public health problems. In these countries access to facilities for work with radioactive material is usually difficult.

We have used biotinylated kDNA probes to characterize Leishmania isolates from different geographical areas of Peru. So far we have characterized more than two hundred isolates and shown that all of them belong to the L. braziliensis complex.

Currently we are using this nonradioactive kDNA probes in three related research lines. Firstly, in the development of subspecies specific DNA probes to discriminate between parasites causing Andean cutaneous Leishmaniasis (Uta) and Selvatic Leishmaniasis. In this regard we used this probes to identify clones containing Leishmania sequences. Secondly, we will apply the biotinylated kDNA probes for the direct demonstration of the presence of Leishmania in insect vectors. Vectors captured in endemic areas will be directly smashed on NC paper and subjected to hybridization and detection procedures such as those described in the present report. Thirdly, we are working towards the development of a rapid diagnostic test for the presence of Leishmania parasites in crude biopsies obtained from lesions. The preliminary results reported here show that such a diagnostic test is feasible. Further studies are being carried out in order to confirm this possibility and further improve sensitivity.

CONCLUSIONS

Experimental conditions have been adapted for the use of non-radioactive kDNA probes from Leishmania for detection of parasites in crude samples blotted on NC paper. The probes are as sensitive and specific as ^{32}P radiolabelled ones. The potential of biotinylated DNA probes for diagnosis is envisaged.

ACKNOWLEDGEMENTS

We wish to thank Dr. J. Bellatin and Dr. M. Arana for help in preparing this manuscript. Dr. Humberto Guerra and Dr. Juan Carlos Palomino for critically reviewing it. This work was supported by the UNDP/World Bank/WHO Special Programme for Research and Training in Tropical Diseases (Director's Initiative Fund Grant number 840169) and the United States Agency for International Development (Project 936-5542, Obligation 5361463).

KARYOTYPE ANALYSIS OF LEISHMANIA DONOVANI

Richard P. Bishop and Michael A. Miles

Wolfson Unit/Department of Medical Protozoology
London School of Hygiene and Tropical Medicine
Keppel Street
London   WC1E 7HT

INTRODUCTION

Kinetoplastid protozoa of the genus Leishmania are the causative agents of leishmaniasis which has recently been estimated to affect 20 million people, mainly in developing countries (Barker, 1987). A number of biochemical techniques have been applied to differentiate the organisms causing the various clinical forms of the disease, the most successful being the use of isoenzymes (Peters, 1986) and schizodeme analysis of DNA (Morel and Simpson, 1980).

The recent development of pulsed field gradient gel electrophoresis (PFGGE) (Schwarz and Cantor, 1984) and orthogonal field alternation gel electrophoresis (DFAGE) (Carle and Olsen, 1984) has for the first time allowed the chromosomes of Leishmania, which do not condense at any phase of the mitotic cycle, to be visualised. These techniques, in which large DNA prepared in an agarose matrix is size-fractionated through an agarose gel by the alternate application of two mutually perpendicular electrical fields, represent an exciting new development in the molecular characterization of Leishmania and other parasitic protozoa.

We have applied OFAGE to the karyotpye analysis of the L. donovani complex of organisms which are responsible for human visceral leishmaniasis. The analysis included stocks representing the recognised subspecies of L. donovani, Indian L. donovani donovani, Mediterranean L. donovani infantum, and South American L. donovani chagasi as well as several African stocks L. donovani (sensu lato).

MATERIALS AND METHODS

For details of methods and table of L. donovani stocks used see Bishop and Miles (1987).

RESULTS

The results section summarises work which is presented in detail in Bishop and Miles (1987).

Existence of chromosome size polymorphisms between L. donovani stocks

Pulse switching times between 40 and 200 seconds were used to analyse the karyotypes of L. donovani stocks. Using an 80 second switching time 15 chromosome sized bands were observed whereas using a 200 second switching time a further 7 chromosomes could be seen suggesting a minimum chromosome complement of 22 for L. donovani. The accuracy of this estimate is affected by non-stoichiometry of bands, perhaps caused by clonal heterogeneity of parasite populations, and the possible failure of some chromosomes to enter the gel. Clear differences were apparent between the 11 L. donovani stocks tested both in the size of specific chromosomes and in the overall pattern of ethidium bromide staining. Size polymorphisms were most apparent between the six smallest chromosomes when a 40 second pulse switching time was employed.

Three L. d. chagasi stocks and three L. d. infantum stocks were more similar karyotypically to one another than they were to two L. donovani donovani stocks.

The Ethiopian L. donovani (sensu lato) stock HU3 exhibited the most distinct karyotype of those examined and possessed the smallest chromosome seen in any stock (approximately 240kb in size).

Homologies of L. donovani chromosomes

To investigate the homology relationships of L. donovani chromosomes within and between stocks, DNA from specific chromosomes was isolated from OFAGE gels by electroelution, radiolabelled with $\alpha^{32}P$, and hybridised to Southern blots of other OFAGE gels.

An Indian L. donovani donovani chromosome 1 probe was found to hybridise both to itself and to chromosomes 4 and 13/15 in all stocks thus demonstrating the presence of homologous repetitive elements on these three chromosomes. The small 240kb chromosome of HU3 exhibited hybridisation both to itself and to a large chromosome present in all stocks but when washed at high stringency did not exhibit significant hybridisation to the small chromosomes of other L. donovani stocks with the exception of the Sudanese stock Khartoum.

Mechanisms of chromosome size polymorphisms

A chromosome equivalent to chromosome 3 of Indian L. d. donovani appeared to be absent from several L. d. chagasi and L. d. infantum stocks.

To investigate this apparent absence on L. donovani donovani chromosome 3 probe was hybridised to a blot onto which DNA from the chromosomes of L. d. chagasi and L. d. infantum stocks had been transferred after fractionation by OFAGE. The L. d. donovani chromosome 3 probe was found to hybridise predominantly to itself and to chromosome 2 of L. d. chagasi and L. d. infantum (hybridisation also occurred to a large chromosome present in all stocks). Hybridisation of an L. d. donovani chromosome 2 probe to the same blot (after stripping off the chromosome 3 probe) also resulted in hybridisation to chromosome 2 of L. d. infantum and L. d. chagasi.

The existence of sequences on L. d. chagasi and L. d. infantum chromosome 2 homologous to both chromosomes 2 and 3 of Indian L. donovani suggests that interchromosomal transposition may be involved in generating the observed chromosome size polymorphisms.

Chromosomal location of α and β tubulin genes

Trypanosoma brucei α and β tubulin gene probes were used to map the corresponding L. donovani genes to specific chromosomes. β tubulin was situated on three chromosomes 21/22, 13 and 7 with hybridisation being strongest to the large chromosome 21/22, suggesting that the main tandem repeat of the β tubulin genes (Spithill and Samaras, 1985) is situated on this chromosome. By contrast α tubulin was found to hybridise only to chromosome 9. In both α and β tubulin the gene arrangement was highly conserved between different L. donovani stocks.

DISCUSSION

OFAGE fractionation has revealed the existence of chromosome size polymorphisms between L. donovani stocks, similar size polymorphisms have also been observed in L. major (Spithill and Samaras, 1986) and Plasmodium falciparum (Van der Ploeg et al., 1985; Corcoran et al., 1986). These polymorphisms appear useful for stock identification, of the 11 stocks examined only the two Indian stocks examined, Patna II and DD8, possessed indistinguishable karyotypes. Karyotype analysis appears more sensitive than isoenzyme analysis in that the L. donovani subspecies Indian L. d. donovani, Mediterranean L. d. infantum, South American L. d. chagasi and African L. donovani (sensu lato) are all karyotypically distinct whereas they are not so clearly differentiated by isoenzymes (Lainson et al., 1981; Schnur, et al., 1981; Le Blancq and Peters, 1986). The fact that L. d. chagasi and L. d. infantum stocks tested exhibit karyotypic similarities not shared with L. d. donovani provides support for the hypothesis of Killick-Kendrick et al. (1980) that visceral leishmaniasis is not native to South America but was introduced from the Mediterranean. A recent study of Leishmania nuclear DNA evolution (Beverley et al., 1987) also concluded that L. d. chagasi and L. d. infantum were more closely related to one another than to other L. donovani stocks analysed.

The discovery of small chromosomes in HU3 and Khartoum with no apparent equivalent in other L. donovani stocks but exhibiting homology to a single large chromosome in all stocks suggests that these chromosomes may be derived from the large chromosome and are perhaps analogous to two Plasmodium chromosomes' one of which is an incomplete copy of the other (Van der Ploeg et al., 1985). A process of "chromosome duplication" might also explain the hybridisation of the L. donovani chromosome 1 to two larger chromosomes 4 and 13/15 although it is not yet known whether the cross hybridisation of these chromosomes is due purely to the existence of shared repetitive sequences or is indicative of more general homology. The discovery that a single chromosome in L. d. chagasi and L. d. infantum exhibits homology to chromosomes 2 and 3 of L. d. donovani implies either that an inter-chromosomal transposition has occurred or that variant forms of the two chromosomes are co-migrating in the gel. A similar experiment in L. major (Spithill and Samaras, 1986) in which two seperate chromosome probes were observed to hybridise to a single polymorphic chromosome band also suggested translocation of DNA between chromosomes as a likely mechanism for the generation of chromosome size polymorphisms in Leishmania.

It can be concluded that the genome of Leishmania is unstable and that chromosomal evolution is rapid as evinced by the existence of karyotypic differences between closely related L. donovani subspecies and even individual stocks. By contrast on the evidence of the tubulin genes the chromosomal location of protein coding genes is relatively conserved.

ACKNOWLEDGEMENTS

We thank the Wolfson Foundation, the Medical Research Council and the Nuffield Foundation for financial support. MAM is a Wellcome Trust Senior Lecturer.

REFERENCES

Barker, D.S. 1987, DNA diagnosis of human leishmaniasis, Parasitology Today 3, 177-184.

Beverley, S.M., Ismach, R.P. and McMahon-Pratt, D. 1987, Evolution of the genus Leishmania as revealed by comparisons of nuclear DNA restriction fragment patterns. Proc.Natl.Acad.Sci. USA, 84, 484-488.

Bishop, R.P. and Miles, M.A. 1987, Chromosome size polymorphisms of Leishmania donovani, Molecular and Biochemical Parasitology, 24, 262-272.

Carle, G.F. and Olson, M.V. 1984, Separation of chromosomal DNA molecules from yeast by orthogonal-field alternation gel electrophoresis. Nucleic Acids res. 12, 5647-5664.

Corcoran, L.M., Forsyth, K.P., Bianco, A.E., Brown, G.V. and Kemp, D.J. 1986, Chromosome size polymorphisms in Plasmodium falciparum can involve deletions and are frequent in natural parasite populations. Cell 44, 87-95.

Killick-Kendrick, R., Molyneux, D.H., Rioux, J.A. and Leaney, A.J. 1980, Possible origins of Leishmania chagasi. Ann.Trop.Med.Parasitol. 74, 563-565.

Lainson, R., Miles, M.A. and Shaw, J.J. 1981, On the identification of viscerotropic Leishmaniasis. Ann.Trop.Med.Parasitol. 75, 251-253.

Le Blancq, S.M. and Peters, W. 1986, Leishmania inthe Old World: 4. The distribution of L. donovani (sensu lato) zymodemes. Trans.R.Soc.Trop.Med.Hyg. 80, 367-377.

Morel, C.M. and Simpson, L. 1980, Characterisation of pathogenic trypanosomatidae by restriction endonuclease fingerprinting of kinetoplast DNA minicircles. Am.J.Trop.Med.Hyg. 29, 1070-1074.

Peters, W. and Killick-Kendrick, R. 1986, "Leishmaniases in Biology and Medicine", Academic Press, London.

Schnur, L.F., Chance, M.L., Ebert, F., Thomas, S.C. and Peters, W. 1981, The biochemical and serological taxonomy of visceralizing Leishmania. Ann.Trop.Med.Parasitol. 75, 131-144.

Schwarz, D.C. and Cantor, C.R. 1984, Separation of yeast chromosome sized DNAs by pulsed field gradient gel electrophoresis. Cell 37, 67-75.

Spithill, T.W. and Samaras, N. 1985, The molecular karyotype of Leishmania major and mapping of α- and β-tubulin gene families to multiple unlinked chromosomal loci. Nucleic Acids Res. 13, 4155-4161.

Spithill, T.W. and Samaras, N. 1986, Chromosome size polymorphisms and mapping of tubulin gene loci in Leishmania. UCLA Symp.Mol.Cell.Biol. 42, 1-11.

Van der Ploeg, L.H.T., Smits, M., Ponnudruai, T., Vermeulen, A., Meuwissen, J.H. and Langsley, G. 1985, Chromosome sized DNA molecules of Plasmodium falciparum. Science 229, 658-661.

ABNORMALLY MIGRATING CHROMOSOME IDENTIFIES LEISHMANIA

DONOVANI POPULATIONS

N.Gajendran, J.-Cl.Dujardin *, D.Le Ray *,
G.Matthyssens, S.Muyldermans, and R. Hammers

Vrije Universiteit Brussel, Instituut voor
Moleculaire Biologie, Paardenstraat 65,
1640 Sint-Genesius-Rode, Belgium
* Institute of Tropical Medicine,
Nationalestraat 155, Antwerp, Belgium

INTRODUCTION

In recent years karyotyping of protozoan parasites by separation of chromosome sized DNA molecules has been made possible by relaxation migration gel electrophoresis using alternating electric fields and adequate electrode geometry (Carle & Olson, 1984). Several different electrode configurations have allowed the separation of DNA molecules up to two megabases in size (Chu et al., 1986). These methods have allowed distinction between different strains of malaria parasites (Kemp et al., 1985; Van Der Ploeg et al., 1985), chromosome assignment of genes in Trypanosoma (Van Der Ploeg et al. 1984; Gibson et al., 1986) and recently species identification in Trypanosoma (Majiwa et al., 1985) and Leishmania (Scholler et al., 1986).

When different stocks of Leishmania were submitted to karyotyping by OFAGE, a chromosome of L.donovani showed an abnormal migratory pattern. We have made an attempt to analyse this chromosome and discuss here the results of our findings.

MATERIALS AND METHODS

Chromosomal DNA from Leishmania promastigotes was prepared as described for trypanosomes (Van Der Ploeg et al., 1984). The OFAGE apparatus used was as described by Carle and Olson, 1984. Gels were made of 1.5 % agarose and run for 20 hours at 15 C, 300 V, 260 mA and then stained with ethidium bromide. For the gel seen in Fig.1B, the time of electrophoresis was 12 hours and run at 7 C. Isolation of Kinetoplast DNA was as previously described (Simpson and Berliner, 1974).

Isolation of L.donovani nuclei: promastigotes were lysed in 20mM Pipes pH 7.5, 15 mM NaCl, 60 mM KCl, 14 mM beta mercapto-ethanol, 0.5 mM EGTA, 4 mM EDTA, and 15 mM spermine and 0.1 % NP_{40} and 1 mM PMSF (freshly solubilised in ethanol). The nuclei were purified by sedimentation through a 1.5 M sucrose cushion in a SW 27 rotor for 45 min at 25000 rpm. The pellet was washed twice in buffer A (0.3 M sucrose, 20 mM NaCl, 10 mM Tris pH 7.5, and 4 mM $MgCl_2$).

Micrococcal nuclease digestion: The nuclear preparation (1.5 mg DNA/ml) was made in 1 mM $CaCl_2$ and digested with 150 U/ml micrococcal nuclease at 37 C. Aliquots were taken out at 30 sec, 1 min, 2 min, 4 min, 8 min, and 15 min, and the digestion stopped with 10 mM EDTA (final concentration). All samples were dialysed against TE buffer (10 mM Tris-HCl pH 7.5, 10 mM EDTA), and then centrifuged. Part of the supernatant was loaded on a nucleoprotein gel. This is a normal agarose gel but the buffer is made up of 20 mM Tris pH 8.0, 2 mM EDTA and the gel is run in a cold room. The rest of the supernatant was deproteinised with proteinase K in 0.1 % SDS and then phenol/chloroform extracted and applied on a gel.

Exonuclease III digestion in agarose blocks was performed as described previously (Bernards et al., 1982). The blocks were then washed with TE buffer and subject to OFAGE. Isolation of L.donovani total RNA (Guanidinium/Cesium Chloride method), Southern transfer and nick-translation were performed as described by Maniatis et al., 1982. The pre-hybridization, hybridization (overnight) and washing (high stringency) was performed as described in the instruction booklet for the Hybond N-filters entitled "membrane transfer and detection methods" from Amersham.

RESULTS

When different species of Leishmania were submitted to karyotyping by OFAGE, L.donovani (ITMAP 263) showed a chromosome which jumped out of line and migrated along a different track with respect to the other chromosomes (fig.1A). It had an anomolous migration and its position relative to the other chromosomes was dependent upon field geometry and conditions of OFAGE (fig.1B).

The isolated DNA of the chromosome did not hybridize to the kinetoplast DNA but hybridized to the nuclear DNA. Micrococcal nuclease digestion gave a typical nucleosome repeat ladder and southern blot hybridization with the labelled DNA of the chromosome showed hybridization to the nucleosome repeat ladder (fig.2). Lanes 2 and 10 contain the 15 min and 30 sec digestions. Lanes 3,5,6,7,8 and 9 contain

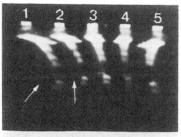

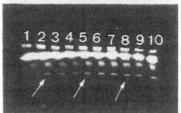

Fig.1. (A) An OFAGE gel of L.donovani with CD 1 (arrows). (B) CD 1 (arrows) migrating first.

the DNA extracted from the chromatin as obtained after 30 sec, 1 min, 2 min, 4 min, 8 min and 15 min digestions. Lane 1 contains total DNA from L.mexicana. Lane 4 is a PM2-Hae III digested DNA used as a size marker. Lengths are from top to bottom 1900, 1485, 915, 860, 695, 614, 531, 352, 317, 282, 167 bp.

Southern hybridization to karyotype blots of L.donovani stocks with the labelled DNA of CD 1 showed no significant hybridization to the other chromosomes (fig.3B). CD 1 is seen as a doublet here (fig.3A). Lanes 1, 2, and 3 are L.donovani stocks (ITMAP 263, ITMAP 263 clone 10 and Tunis respectively) with CD 1 showing hybridization (arrows). Lane 4 contains L.tropica (Bokhara), lane 5 contains L.mex.amazonensis (LV 98) and lane 6 contains L.b.braziliensis (LV 65). EXO III digestion in the agarose block before performing the electrophoresis left CD 1 intact while digesting all the other hromosomes as observed after OFAGE (not shown).

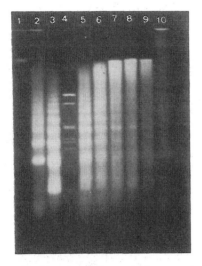 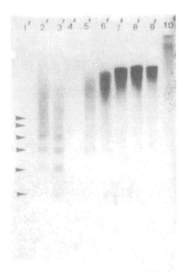

Fig.2A. A nucleosomal repeat ladder as seen after a micrococcal nuclease digestion of nuclear DNA.

Fig.2B. Southern hybridization with the labelled DNA of CD 1 to the nucleosomes.

CD 1 was found in 6 of the stocks previously identified as L.donovani and was absent in the other species of Leishmania when examined by OFAGE. When Karyotype blots of 24 other stocks of Leishmania were hybridized with the labelled DNA of CD 1, hybridization was found in those L.donovani stocks having CD 1. In the L.donovani stocks without CD 1, hybridization was found on another chromosome band (table 1), the size of which differs depending on the stock (fig.4). The intensity of the hybridizing signal also differed in the latter case. Lanes 1, 3, 5, 6, and 7 are all L.donovani stocks (CRC L64, Khartoum LV 711, ITMAP 263, and LRC-L133 respectively). Lane 2 contains Leishmania sp. (M35), Lanes 4 and 8 contain L.tropica (Syria and LV 305 respectively). One exception to this was the WHO reference strain L.b.braziliensis M2903, which also showed hybridization on another chromosome band (Table I).

Adding up the DNA lengths of the bands seen after electrophoresis of a Pst I digest of the isolated CD 1 comes to 30 Kb. Some of the smaller fragments were of a higher intensity on ethidium bromide staining and on hybridization than some of the larger fragments.

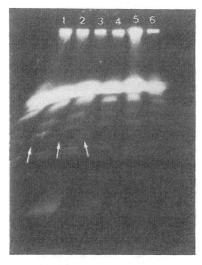

Fig.3A. An OFAGE gel with CD 1 seen as two bands (arrows).

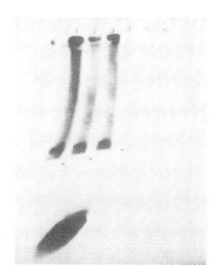

Fig.3B. Southern hybridization to the OFAGE gel (3A) with the labelled CD 1.

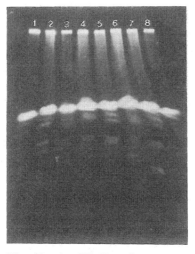

Fig.4A. An OFAGE gel containing Leishmania stocks.

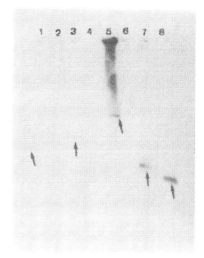

Fig.4B. The gel (4A) hybridized with the labelled DNA of CD 1.

Hybridization with the labelled DNA of CD 1 to the Northern blot containing the total RNA (lane 1) L.donovani (ITMAP 263) promastigotes, and total (lane 2) and poly A+ RNA of Trypanosoma b. rhodesiense (lane 3: resistant form, lane 4 sensitive form) (Rifkin, 1984) showed hybridization to bands of about 1 Kb and 1.3 Kb (fig.5B) in the L.donovani total RNA.

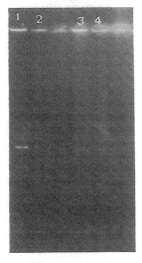

Fig.5A. An agarose gel containing total RNA of L.donovani (lane 1).

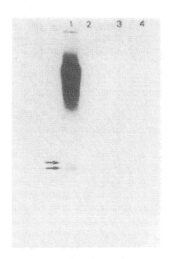

Fig.5B. Hybridization to the Northern blot (5A) with the labelled DNA of CD 1.

Table 1. PFG gels of Leishmania stocks probed with CD 1.

Stocks	Code	No Hybridization	Hybridization
L.d.donovani	MHOM/IN/80/DD8	−	+
L.donovani	K 42	+	+
L.donovani	1-S	+	+
L.donovani	LRC-L51	+	+
L.donovani	VP74,LRC-L61	+	+
L.donovani	Tunis	+	+
L.d.infantum	ITMAP263	+	+
L.donovani	L13	−	+
L.donovani	LRC-L133/ITMAP1899	−	+
L.donovani	CRCL64	−	+
L.donovani	KhartoumLV711	−	+
L.donovani	L28	−	+
L.d.chagasi	MHOM/BR/74/PP75	−	+
L.tropica	Syria	−	−
L.tropica	LV305	−	−
L.tropica	Bokhara	−	−
L.tropica	Kenya	−	−
L.tropica	DM	−	−
L.tropica	Pakistan,ITMAP1929	−	−
L.mex.amazonensis	LV78	−	−
L.b.braziliensis	LV65	−	−
L.b.braziliensis	MHOM/BR/75/M2903	−	+
L.tarentolae	LV108	−	−
L.tarentolae	Senegalensis	−	−
L.adleri		−	−
Leishmania.sp.	M35		

+ : Hybridization to a chromosome and/or presence of CD 1.
− : No hybridization and/or absence of CD 1.

Discussion

When different species of Leishmania were submitted to karyotyping by OFAGE, L.donovani (ITMAP 263) showed a chromosome (designated CD 1) which jumped out of line, and migrated along a different track with respect to the other chromosomes (fig.1A). This is more evident when there is a skewed field in the OFAGE apparatus. This CD 1 has an anomolous migration and its position relative to the other chromosomes is dependent upon field geometry and conditions of OFAGE (fig.1B). Its migration would suggest that the chromosome is circular as there have been a number of reports(Chu et al., 1986; Maurer et al., 1987) that circular molecules have a different migration in field-alternation gel electrophoresis. On some occasions CD 1 is resolved into a doublet (fig.3A). The resolution into a doublet in only some positions in the gel is most likely due to the inhomogeneous electric field while the doublet itself could be due to the different levels of supercoiling of the DNA.

Since the isolated DNA of CD 1 did not hybridize to the kinetoplast DNA but hybridized to the nuclear DNA, it points to the fact that it is of nuclear origin (not shown). Moreover the typical nucleosomal repeat ladder obtained from the microccocal nuclease digestion showed that it was compacted in regularly spaced nucleosomes (fig.2A). Indeed this is as expected since microccocal nuclease will cut between the nucleosomes and hence yield bands of 1 nucleosome, 2 nucleosomes, etc., on a gel after a limited digest. Hybridization to the Southern blot of this digest with the labelled DNA of CD 1 (fig.2B) confirms this and the fact that the L.mexicana DNA does not hybridize with the probe indicates that the signal seen in the lanes is specific for CD 1.

When karyotype blots of L.donovani stocks were hybridized with the labelled DNA of CD 1, there was no significant hybridization to the other chromosomes (fig.3B). This shows that the chromosome does not share sequences with the other chromosomes and hence does not have the common telomeric sequences and this is suggestive of its circular conformation. The enzyme exonuclease III (EXO III) will digest accessible 3' hydroxyl ended DNA but not closed-circular DNA molecules. EXO III digestion of the chromosomes in the agarose block, before performing the electrophoresis, leaves CD 1 intact while digesting all the other chromosomes (not shown). This confirms that it is of a closed-circular topology.

The size of CD 1 is, because of its anomolous migration in OFAGE, difficult to determine. The position of migration in a gel, after an ECOR I digest of the DNA of the chromosome, indicates that it is more than 20 Kb. Furthermore, adding up the sizes of the bands after a Pst I digestion of the isolated CD 1 comes to 30 Kb. This is only an approximate estimate of the size as the intensities ,after ethidium bromide staining and after hybridization of some of the smaller bands was higher than some of the larger bands. This indicates that some of the bands could be present in a higher copy number than the other bands within the chromosome or there could be heterogeneity in the copy number of the whole chromosome as two bands were sometimes observed in OFAGE. Hybridization with cloned fragments (of a Pst I digest) showed hybridization only to a fragment of the same size as the ^{32}P labelled cloned fragment (i.e. to itself) and not to the other fragments of the digest. These results indicate that the chromosome does not consist of extensively repeated small sequences.

When other stocks of Leishmania were examined by OFAGE, CD 1 was only present in some of the stocks previously identified as L.donovani and was absent in the other species of Leishmania. Hybridization with the labelled DNA of the chromosome to karyotype blots of 29 other stocks of

Leishmania also indicated CD 1 to be specific to the
L.donovani/L.infantum-complex (table I). L.donovani stocks having CD 1
will light up with the probe. In the L.donovani stocks that did not have
CD 1, hybridization is found on another chromosome band, the size of
which differs depending on the stock (fig.4B). The intensity of the
signal also differs implying that the amount of sequence homology with CD
1 varies. In contrast the non-L.donovani stocks do not show any
significant hybridization. One exception to this concerned Leishmania
braziliensis braziliensis. Out of six L.braziliensis stocks tested, one
(MHOM/BR/75/M2903) showed hybridizing material located on one of the
chromosomes. Checking by isoenzyme typing confirmed the identity of the
WHO reference strain M2903.

A chromosome with an altered migration in OFAGE has already been
described as characterizing a particular drug (methotrexate) resistant
species of Leishmania major (Garvey et al., 1986; Beverly et al., 1984;
Coderre et al., 1983). Gene amplification due to methotrexate has also
been shown to occur in certain resistant variants of human cell lines
(Maurer et al., 1987). However, in our case, CD 1 is found in six of the
L.donovani stocks that were cultured without exposure to methotrexate and
hence cannot have arisen through drug (methotrexate) driven gene
amplification as shown for the L.major extrachromosomal circular DNA
molecule. Furthermore our results with the hybridization with cloned
fragments of CD 1 indicates that the hybridization seen in the L.donovani
stocks (that do not have CD 1) is not to a complete CD 1 sequence in all
the stocks.

In Leishmania hertigi virus like particles were reported to have
been found (Molyneux, 1974), distributed throughout the cytoplasm of the
promastigotes. We cannot exclude the possibility of CD 1 being a virus,
however it is of nuclear origin and not cytoplasmic. Furthermore electron
microscopy of L.donovani (ITMAP 263) did not reveal any virus like
particles in the cytoplasm.

The observation of the hybridizing material in the L.b.braziliensis
strain (M2903) raises the interesting question of the possibility of
genetic exchange between sympatric Leishmania classified as belonging to
different species, as opposed to phylogenetic relationships. So far
genetic exchange in Leishmania has not been shown to occur although
recent evidence indicates its possibility (Evans et al., 1987). Genetic
exchange has been shown to occur in Trypanosoma, both in the fly and in
the host (Jenni et al., 1986; Paindavoine et al., 1986; Zampetti-Bosseler
et al., 1986; Tait, 1983).

Another interesting question raised is whether CD 1 carries any
genes involved in the biology of the parasite. The Northern blot (Fig.5B)
indicates the presence of transcripts. Since CD 1 does not appear to
share sequences with the other chromosomes, the observed transcripts are
most likely due to the expression of genes that are present on the
chromosome. A plasmid has been introduced into Crithidia (Hughes et al.,
1986) and recently a chromosome has been introduced into a trypanosome by
the technique of electroporation (Gibson et al., 1987). These
developments may now facilitate the investigation towards understanding
the biology of Leishmania experimentally.

Conclusion

The DNA molecule in L.donovani that has a different migration in
OFAGE, is compacted into nucleosomes and is of nuclear origin. Our
results are consistent with the hypothesis that this chromosome is
circular. We have designated this chromosome CD 1 (circular DNA 1).

Hybridization to other species of Old World Leishmania indicates that CD 1 is specific to some isolates of the L.donovani/L.infantum-complex. Related sequences were found in members of the L.donovani/L.infantum-complex and in a single L.b.braziliensis strain. Hybridization to L.donovani total RNA shows the existence of transcripts.

ACKNOWLEDGEMENTS

We thank Dr.P.Desjeux, Dr.El Amin El Rouffaie and Dr.D.Evans for the gift of some of the Leishmania stocks. This work was supported by an EEC Science and Technology for Development Programme and by the Belgian Medical Research Council (FGWO) grants to D.Le Ray. This work was also supported by an FGWO contract (No. 3.0027.85) to G.Mathyssens/S.Muyldermans.

REFERENCES

Beverly, S.M., Coderre, J.A., Santi, D.V., Schimke, R.T.: Unstable DNA amplifications in methotrexate-resistant Leishmania consist of extrachromosomal circles which relocalize during stabilization. Cell, **38**, 431-439 (1984).

Carle, G.F., Olson, M.V.: Separation of chromosomal DNA molecules from yeast by orthogonal-field-alternation gel electrophoresis. Nucleic Acids Res., **12** (14), 5646-5664 (1984).

Chu, G.F., Vollrath, D., Davis, R.W.: Separation of large DNA molecules by contour-clamped homogeneous electric fields. Science, **234**, 1582-1585 (1986).

Coderre, J.A., Beverly, S.M., Schimke, R.T., Santi, D.V. Overproduction of a bifunctional thymidylate synthetase dihydrofolate reductase and DNA amplification in methotrexate-resistant Leishmania tropica. Proc. Natl. Acad. Sci. USA, 80, 2132-2136 (1983).

Evans, D.A., Kennedy, W.P., Chapman, C.J., Smith, V.: Evidence for the occurence of genetic exchange in the genus Leishmania. "LEISHMANIASIS: THE FIRST CENTENARY (1885-1985) NEW STRATEGIES FOR CONTROL, "Plenum Press, New York.

Garvey, E.P., Santi, D.V.: Stable amplified DNA in drug-resistant Leishmania exists as extrachromosomal circles. Science, **233**, 535-540 (1986).

Gibson, W.C., Borst, P.: Size-fractionation of the small chromosomes of Trypanozoon and Nannomonas trypanosomes by pulsed field gradient gel electrophoresis. Mol. Biochem. Paras. **18**, 127-140 (1986).

Gibson, W.C., Miles, M.A.: The karyotype and ploidy of Trypanosoma cruzi. EMBO, **5** (6), 1299-1305 (1986).

Gibson, W.C., White, T.C., Laird, P.W., Borst, P.: Stable introduction of exogenous DNA into Trypanosoma brucei. EMBO, **6** (8), 2457-2461 (1987).

Hughes, D.E., Simpson, L.: Introduction of plasmid DNA into the trypanosomatid protozoan Crithidia fasciculata. Proc. Natl. Acad. Sci. USA, **83**, 6058-6062 (1986).

Jenni, L;, Marti, S., Schweizer, J., Betschart, B., Le Page, R.W.F., Wells, J.M., Tait, A., Paindavoine, P., Pays, E., Steinert, M.: Hybrid formation between African Trypanosomes during cyclical transmission. Nature, **322**, 173-175 (1986).

Kemp, D.J., Corcaran, L.M., Coppel, R.L., Stahl, H.D., Bianco, A.E., Brown, G.V., Anders R.F.: Size variation in chromosomes from independent cultured isolates of Plasmodium falciparum. Nature, **315**, 347-350 (1985).

Majiwa, P.A.O., Masake, R.A., Nantulya, V.M., Hamers, R., Matthyssens,G.: Trypanosoma (Nannomonas) congolense: Identification of two karyotypic groups.'EMBO, **4** (12), 3307-3313 (1985).

Maniatis, T., Fritsch, E.F., Sombrook, J., Molecular cloning, A laboratory manual, Cold Spring Harbour Laboratory, N.Y. (1982).

Maurer, B.J., Lai, E., Hamkalo, B.A., Hood, L., Attardi, G. Novel submicroscopic extrachromosomal elements containing amplified genes in human cells. Nature, **327**, 434-437 (1987).

Molyneux, D.H.: Virus-like particles in Leishmania parasites. Nature, **249**, 588-589 (1974).

Paindavoine, P., Zampetti-Bosseler, F., Pays, E., Schweizer, J., Guyaux, M., Jenni, L., Steinert, M.: Trypanosome hybrids generated in tsetse flies by nuclear fusion. EMBO, **5** (13), 3631-3636 (1986).

Rifkin, M.R.: Trypanosoma brucei: Biochemical and morphological studies of cytotoxicity caused by normal human serum. Exper. Paras., **58**, 81-93 (1984).

Scholler, J.K., Reed, S.G., Stuart, K.: Molecular karyotype of species and subspecies of Leishmania. Mol. Biochem. Paras., **20**, 279-293 (1986).

Simpson, L., Berliner, J.: Isolation of the Kinetoplast DNA of Leishmania tarentolae in the form of a network. J.Protozool. **21** (2), 382-393 (1974).

Tait, A.: Sexual processes in the kinetoplastida. Parasitology, **86**, 29-57 (1983).

Van Der Ploeg, L.H.T., Shwartz, D.C., Cantor, C.R., Borst, P.: Antigenic variation in Trypanosoma brucei analyzed by electrophoretic separation of chromosome-sized DNA molecules. Cell, **37**, 77-84 (1984).

Van Der Ploeg, L.H.T., Smits, M., Ponnudurai, T., Vermeulen, A., Meuwissen, J.H.E.TH., Langsley, G.: Chromosome-sized DNA molecules of Plasmodium falciparum. Science, **229**, 658-660 (1985).

Zampetti-Bosseler, F., Schweizer, J., Pays, E., Jenni, L., Steinert, M.: Evidence for haploidy in metacyclic forms of Trypanosoma brucei. Proc. Natl. Acad. Sci., USA, **83**, 6063-6064 (1986).

KINETOPLAST DNA PROBES FOR THE IDENTIFICATION OF THE OLD WORLD CUTANEOUS LEISHMANIASES

C.J. Chapman, W.P.K. Kennedy, and D.A. Evans

Department of Medical Protozoology/Wolfson Unit
London School of Hygiene and Tropical Medicine
Keppel Street, London, WC1E 7HT

INTRODUCTION

The cutaneous leishmaniases of the Old World are socially and medically important conditions caused by species of the genus Leishmania transmitted by sandflies of the family Phlebotominae. They can be highly disfiguring diseases, and rapid initial diagnosis and identification of the causative organism are extremely important to the subsequent treatment and follow-up of infected individuals. Likewise in any leishmaniasis control programme the rapid and accurate identification of organisms is of paramount importance, especially as most of the leishmaniases are zoonoses (Lainson and Shaw, 1979). Often, species of Leishmania causing different forms of the disease, are endemic to the same geographical region, for example those from a country such as Saudi Arabia where L. major, L. arabica, L. tropica and L. donovani are all found (Peters et al., 1985, 1986).

In addition, the epidemiologies of the cutaneous leishmaniases are not always fully understood, and sensitive and specific detection methods of identification of the parasite from vector and reservoir hosts, and patients are needed. This is particularly appropriate in the case of Leishmania arabica where the vector and infectivity to man have yet to be proven (Peters et al., 1986).

At present the classical method for the identification of the parasite is that of isoenzyme electrophoresis, which is time consuming, and difficult to apply in the field, requiring initial isolation and extensive cultivation of the organism from sandfly or animal. Other methods are presently being sought to improve identification of these organisms - the most promising being the use of species specific monoclonal antibodies (McMahon-Pratt and David, 1981; Delbarra et al., 1982) and DNA probes, the potential of which has been discussed by Barker (1987) and Kennedy (1983). These methods can detect a small number of organisms with minimal, if any, culturing of the organism required.

Leishmanial kinetoplast DNA (kDNA) is made up of a large network of catenated minicircles and maxicircles. The minicircle fraction evolves rapidly and the sequences differ not only between species but also within individual species and subspecies (Borst and Hoeijmakers, 1979).

Whole kDNA has previously been used for the detection of some species of Leishmania (Wirth and Pratt, 1982; Barker et al., 1982; Barker and Butcher, 1983). However, kDNA cross hybridisation is observed between certain cutaneous and visceral organisms (Lawrie et al., 1985). Cloned sequences of kDNA have been used to isolate L. donovani-specific probes (Lawrie et al., 1985; Lopez and Wirth, 1986).

Here we report the use of cloned sequences of kDNA to isolate diagnostically useful parasite-specific probes for the detection of Leishmania arabica, L. major and L. tropica in the field.

MATERIAL AND METHODS

Parasite cultivation

Leishmania were initially isolated into Evans modified TMB medium, and once sufficiently dense in number were transferred into MEM:FCS:EBLB medium for mass cultivation where they were maintained by weekly passage (Evans et al., 1984).

Isolation of kDNA

kDNA was extracted from approximately 10^{10} Leishmania of the species L. arabica (MPSM/SA/83/JISH220) zymodeme LON 64, L. major (MPSM/SA/74/JISH252) LON 4, and L. tropica (MHOM/SU/74/K27) LON 7. The method used was essentially that of Kennedy (1984) with the following modifications. The cell pellet was washed twice in NET 100 (100 mM NaCl, 100 mM EDTA, 10 mM Tris-Hcl, pH 8.0). The washed pellet was resuspended in a solution of 3% sodium sarcosine and 1 mg ml^{-1} proteinase K (Sigma) in NET 100 at a cell concentration of 10^9ml^{-1}. This was then passed through a 23G needle and incubated at 37°C overnight. The DNA was centrifuged and purified as described previously (Kennedy, 1984).

Blots of promastigotes

Leishmania were grown as described above. The cell number was determined using a haemocytometer and aliquots adjusted in phosphate buffered saline so that 10^7, 10^6, 10^5, 10^4, 10^3, 10^2, 10 and 1 parasites were applied per dot. The parasites were dotted onto Hybond-N (Amersham) filters in a Hybri-dot manifold (BRL). The filters were floated on a solution of 10% SDS for 3 minutes followed by a solution containing 0.5 M NaOH/1.0 M NaCl for 10 minutes, they were then neutralised in 1.0 M Tris-HCl pH 8.0 for 2 x 10 minutes and finally treated in a solution of 2 x SSC (1 x SSC: 150 mM NaCl, 15 mM Na$_3$ citrate, pH 7.0) for 5 minutes. These were then air dried and baked under U-V light for 10 minutes.

Blots of kDNA

Appropriate dilutions of kDNA were applied to Hybond-N filters in a Hybri-slot manifold (BRL). These were then washed with 1 x TE buffer (10 mM Tris-HCl, 0.1 mM EDTA, pH 8.0), air dried and baked under U-V light for 10 minutes.

Restriction enzyme digests

All digests were performed according to manufacturers instructions. Hae III. Taq Y1, Acc I and Sma I were purchased from Anglian Laboratories.

Radioactive labelling of kDNA

Total kDNA was labelled with {^{32}P} dCTP (Amersham) by nick translation with Esherichia coli DNA polymerase I (Boehringer) (Rigby et al., 1977). The labelled DNA was separated from unincorporated label using a Sephadex G-50 column. This was washed with 2 x SSC.

Electrophoresis

1.5% agarose gels (Sigma Type II) containing 1 µg ml^{-1} ethidium bromide were run in Tris-borate/EDTA (TBE Buffer (90 mM Tris, 2.5 mM EDTA, 80 mM Boric acid, pH 8.3)) also containing 1 µg ml^{-1} ethidium bromide. Electrophoresis was carried out on a BRL H4 horizontal gel electrophoresis apparatus, at 40 V overnight. Gels were visualised under long wave U-V light and photographed.

Gel blotting and transfer to Hybond-N paper

Pre-treatment of the gel and blotting conditions were as described by Wahl et al. (1979). Transfer was performed at room temperature overnight in 10 x SSC buffer.

Southern hybridization and autoradiography

Southern hybridizations were performed according to Wahl et al. (1979) and Southern (1975), the filters were air dried, baked under U-V light for 10 minutes and soaked for a minimum of 4 hours at 42°C in prehybridization solution (5 x SSC, 5 x Denhardt's solution, 50% formamide, 100 µg ml^{-1} denatured salmon sperm DNA). The prehybridization solution was then removed and replaced with hybridization solution (5 x SSC, 1 x Denhardt's solution, 50% formamide, 100 µg ml^{-1} denatured salmon sperm DNA, 0.1% SDS). Labelled DNA was added and the filter incubated overnight at 42°C. Filters were washed in 2 x SSC/0.1% SDS at 65°C for 4 x 30 minutes. Filters were then sealed in a polythene bag and exposed to XAR-5 film at -70°C with intensifying screens. This procedure was also applied for hybridization with blotted promastigotes and kDNA.

Cloning experiments

The plasmic pUC 13 was digested with either Acc I or Sma I. The ends were then treated at 37°C for 1 hour with calf intestinal alkaline phosphatase (Sigma) at 2 units µg^{-1} of DNA in CIAP buffer (1 mM MgCl$_2$, 0.1 mM ZnCl$_2$, 1mM Spermidine, 50 mM Tris-HCl, pH 8.0). The plasmic was then phenol: chlorofom (1:1) extracted and ethanol precipitated. L. major (JISH 252, LON 4 and NIH173, LON 1) and L. tropica (K27, LON 7) kDNAs were digested with Hae III and L. arabica (JISH 220, LON 64) kDNA digested with Taq YI to completion. These were also extracted and precipitated as above.

Ligation reaction. The digested kDNA was mixed with the plasmid vector pUC 13 to give a molar ratio of 4:1 (fragment:plasmid) and incubated overnight in the presence of T$_4$ DNA ligase (Boehringer) at 14°C. Hexamine cobalt chloride was added at a concentration of 10 mM to the blunt ended ligations. Competent TG1 cells were transformed with the recombinant DNA, and plated out onto L-broth plates containing 100 µg ml^{-1} ampicillin in the presence of 10 mM IPTG and 2% XGal (Maniatis et al., 1982).

Screening and selection of recombinant plasmids

Ampicillin resistant colonies containing insert were isolated and

propagated overnight in microtiter plates containing 0.2 ml YT-broth
(1% {w/v} tryptone, 0.5% {w/v} yeast extract, 0.5% {w/v} NaCl) and 100 μg
ml^{-1} ampicillin. The recombinant plasmids were screened with {^{32}P}-
radiolabelled kDNAs by the colony hybridization technique (Maniatis et al.,
1982). Species specific colonies were isolated, cloned and the plasmid
DNA purified by the alkaline lysis method (Birnboin and Doly, 1979). This
DNA was radiolabelled and used to probe known and unknown Leishmania
isolates, including the Leishmania WHO reference strains (Evans, 1985) and
a range of L. major strains of different zymodemes (LeBlanq et al., 1986)
and L. arabica (Peters et al., 1986), to determine their specificity and
sensitivity.

RESULTS

Taq YI digestion of Leishmania arabica and Hae III digestion of
L. major and L. tropica kDNA, followed by cloning into pUC13 resulted
in the production of species-specific probes. The L. arabica-specific
clone, C5, was seen to hybridise only to this species and to the putative
L. major/L. arabica hybrid MD26, LON 62 (Evans et al., submitted). No
cross-hybridisation can be seen with any of the L. major strains tested.
At least 0.1 ng kDNA could be detected and 10^4 organisms clearly distinguished on nylon membranes, with this probe.

The L. major probe, T, hybridises only to the L. major and the
L. arabica complexes, having particular affinity for L. major LON 1
(except Russian strains belonging to this zymodeme), and for LON 4,
LON 65, LON 70 and the putative hybrid LON 62. This probe is the least
sensitive of the three, but can still detect 10^5 of the above Leishmanias.

The L. tropica probe, 87B, also hybridises only to the L. tropica
complex, being more sensitive for some strains than others. 0.01 ng K27
kDNA was identifiable, and as few as 10^3 K27 whole parasites, whilst a
larger number of other L. tropica parasites were needed before an
identification could be made. At 10^6-10^7 organisms all L. tropica
isolates can be distinguished from other Leishmania.

When these probes were used to identify unknown isolates of
Leishmania, in particular from Sudan and Saudi Arabia, they were found
to correctly identify the Old World cutaneous leishmanial samples involved
when 10^6-10^7 parasites were used. No false positive results were obtained,
however, a few isolates were not identified due to insufficient parasite
number being applied to the membranes.

A fuller account of these results will be published elsewhere
(Chapman et al. in preparation).

DISCUSSION

Kinetoplast DNA of Leishmania has been used to distinguish isolates
for both taxonomic and clinical purposes. The use of cloned sequences
of kDNA to produce diagnostic tools has been discussed by Barker et al.
(1986), and a diagnostic probe for L. donovani has been produced
previously using similar methods (Lawrie et al., 1985; Lopez and Wirth,
1986). As can be seen here, probes for 3 species of Old World cutaneous
leishmaniases, L. arabica, L. major and L. tropica have been produced
by using cloned sequences of kDNA. The clones described are species-
specific and can identify 10^4-10^7 leishmanial organisms dotted onto nylon
membrane, the number of organisms that can be identified being dependant
on the strain involved.

One of the obvious advantages of this technique over classical identification methods, such as isoenzyme electrophoresis, is the minimal need for parasite culture. The application of these probes to the identification of leishmanial organisms isolated directly from human and animal lesions, and from the sandfly vector, without in vitro cultivation, is presently being investigated. In situ hybridisation, and biotinylated probes are also being evaluated as diagnostic tools for the field.

CONCLUSIONS

Here we have showed that specific kDNA probes can be developed to identify the causal agents of Old World cutaneous leishmaniasis, L. arabica, L. major and L. tropica using cloned fragments of minicircle kDNA. These can then be used to provide a rapid alternative method for diagnosis of cutaneous leishmaniasis.

ACKNOWLEDGEMENTS

We would like to thank Mrs V Smith for help with parasite culture. This work was partially funded by an MRC research studentship, the Wolfson Foundation, the University of London and a UNDP/World Bank/WHO Special Programme for Research and Training in Tropical Diseases grant to Professor W. Peters.

REFERENCES

Barker, D.C., 1987, DNA diagnosis of Human Leishmaniasis, Parasitol. Today, 3, 177-184.

Barker, D.C., Arnot, D.E. and Butcher, J., 1982, DNA characterization as a taxonomic tool for identification of kinetoplastic flagellate protozoans, in: Proceedings of the Workshop of the Pan Characterization of Leishmania, Washington D.C., 1980, ed. M.L. Chance and B.C. Walton, pp.139-180. Geneva: UNDP/World Bank/WHO.

Barker, D.C. and Butcher, J., 1983, The use of DNA probes in the identification of leishmaniasis: discrimination between isolates of the Leishmania mexicana and L. braziliensis complexes, Trans. Roy. Soc. Trop.Med.Hyg. 77, 285-297.

Barker, D.C., Gibson, L.J., Kennedy, W.P.K., Nasser, A.A.A. and Williams, R.H., 1986, The potential of using recombinant DNA species-specific probes for the identification of tropical Leishmania. Parasitol. 91, S139-S174.

Birnbain, H.C. and Daly, J., 1979, A rapid extraction procedure for screening recombinant plasmid DNA. Nuc.Acid.Res. 7, 1513-1523.

Borst, P. and Hoeijmakers, J.H.J, 1979, Kinetoplast DNA, Plasmid 2, 20-40.

Delbarra, A.A.L., Howard, J.G. and Snary, D., 1982, Monoclonal antibodies to Leishmania tropica major. Specificities and antigen location. Parasitology, 85, 523-532.

Evans, D.A., 1985, Leishmania reference strains, Parasitology Today, 1, 172-173.

Evans, D.A., Lanham, S.M., Baldwin, C.I. and Peters, W., 1984, The isolation and isoenzyme characterization of Leishmania braziliensis subsp. from patients with cutaneous leishmaniasis acquired in Belize, Trans.Roy.Soc.Trop.Med.Hyg. 78, 35-42.

Kennedy, W.P.K., 1984, Novel identification of differences in the kinetoplast DNA of Leishmania isolates by recombinant DNA techniques and 'in situ' hybridization, Mol.Biochem.Parasitol., 12, 313-323.

Lainson, R. and Shaw, J.J., 1979, The role of animals in the epidemiology of South American leishmaniasis, in: "Biology of the Kinetoplastida" ed. W.H.R. Lumsden and D.A. Evans (Academic, London), Vol. 2, pp.1-116.

Lawrie, J.M., Jackson, P.R., Stiteler, J.M. and Hockmeyer, W.T., 1985, Identification of pathogenic Leishmania promastigotes by DNA; DNA hybridisation with kinetoplast DNA cloned into E. coli plasmics, Am.J.Trop.Med.Hyg. 34, 257-265.

Leblanq, S.M., Schnur, L.F. and Peters, W., 1986, Leishmania in the old world: 1. The geographical and hostal distribution of L. major zymodenes, Trans.Roy.Soc.Trop.Med.Hyg. 80, 99-112.

Lopez, U.G. and Wirth, D.F., 1986, Identification of visceral Leishmania species with cloned sequences of Kinetoplast DNA, Mol.Biochem.Parasitol. 20, 77-84.

Maniatis, T., Fritsch, E.F. and Sambrook, J., 1982, Molecular cloning, a laboratory manual. Cold Spring Harbor Laboratory Publications.

McMahon-Pratt, D.M. and David, J.R., 1981, Monoclonal antibodies that distinguish between 'New World' species of Leishmania. Nature, London, 291, 581-583.

Peters, W., Elbihari, S. and Evans, D.A., 1986, Leishmania infecting man and wild animals in Saudi Arabia. 2. Leishmania arabica n.sp. Trans.Roy.Soc.Trop.Med.Hyg. 80, 497-502.

Peters, W., Elbhari, S., Lui, C., LeBlanq, S.M., Evans, D.A., Killick-Kendrick, R., Smith, V. and Baldwin, C.I., 1985, Leishmania infecting man and wild animals in Saudi Arabia. 1. General Survey. Trans. Roy.Soc.Trop.Med.Hyg. 79, 831-839.

Rigby, P.W.J., Diekman, R.C. and Berg, P., 1977, Labelling deoxyribonucleic acid to high specific activity in vitro by nick translation with DNA polymerase. Int.J.Mol.Biol. 113, 237-251.

Southern, E., 1975, Detection of specific sequences among DNA fragments separated by gel electrophoresis. J.Mol.Biol. 98, 503.

Wahl, G.M., Stern, M. and Stark, G.R., 1979, Efficient transfer of large fragments from agarose gels to diazobenzylmethyl paper and rapid hybridization by using dextron sulphate. Proc.Natl.Acad.Sci. USA, 76, 3683-3687.

Wirth, D.F. and Pratt, D. McMahon, 1982, Rapid identification of Leishmania species by specific hybridization of kinetoplast DNA in cutaneous lesions. Proc.Natl.Acad.Sci. USA, 6999-7003.

SMALL NUCLEIC ACIDS IN LEISHMANIA

K. Stuart, P. Tarr, R. Aline Jr., B. Smiley,
J. Scholler, and J. Keithly

Seattle Biomedical Research Institute
4 Nickerson St.
Seattle, WA 98109-1651 USA

INTRODUCTION

The detection of autonomously replicating genetic elements such as viruses or plasmids in Leishmania may be significant to disease processes and useful for molecular biological studies. Virus-like particles have been detected by electron microscopy in Leishmania hertigi (Molyneux, 1974), Endotrypanum (Croft et al., 1986), and also in Entamoeba, Plasmodia, and Naegleria fowleri (Diamond and Mattern, 1976). In addition, double stranded RNAs which appear to be viral in origin have been observed in Trichomonas vaginalis and Giardia lamblia (Wang and Wang 1986; 1986b). We report here the detection of a 250 kb DNA (LD1) and a 6 kb RNA (LR1) both of which may be autonomously replicating genetic elements.

METHODS

Leishmania stocks were grown as promastigotes and examined by pulse field gel electrophoresis (PFGE) as described previously (Scholler et al., 1986). Total cell RNA was isolated according to Feagin et al., (1985) which entailed sedimentation through cesium chloride; total cell nucleic acids were isolated by treatment with 1% SDS and 1 mg/ml proteinase K in 25 mM EDTA for 1 hr at 50° C followed by phenol/chloroform extraction and ethanol precipitation. LD1 was isolated by preparative PFGE and LR1 was isolated by preparative conventional agarose gel electrophoresis of SDS/proteinase K treated cell lysates from which the bulk of chromosomal DNA had been removed by potassium acetate precipitation (Maniatis et al., 1982).

Nuclei were isolated by centrifuging Triton X-100 lysates of live cells at 2,000 xg for 10 min (Shapiro and Young, 1981). The postnuclear supernatant was further fractionated on a linear-log sucrose density gradient centrifuged at 40,000 rpm in an SW 40 rotor for 2 hrs. cDNA was prepared from isolated LR1 by random priming (Persons and Finn, 1986) and cloned into bluescribe vector. Clones containing LR1 sequence were identified by colony hybridization using the first strand synthesis material as a probe.

RESULTS

LD1 was found in <u>Leishmania braziliensis braziliensis</u> MHOM/BR/75/M2903 while LR1 was found in <u>Leishmania braziliensis guyanensis</u> MHOM/SR/81/CUMC1 (Fig. 1) but not in 10 other stocks of <u>Leishmania</u> (see Scholler et al., 1986). The intense ethidium bromide staining relative to

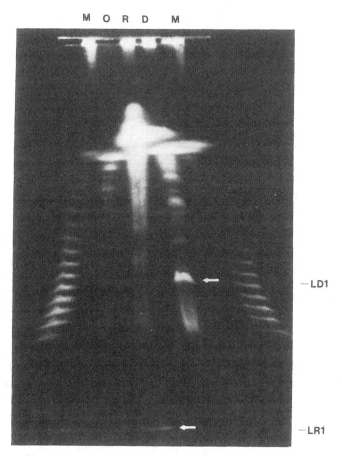

Fig. 1. Two types of small nucleic acids. Ethidium bromide stained PFG electrophoretogram of Leishmania chromosomal DNAs. M, lambda ladder size markers; O, <u>L. braziliensis guyanensis</u> M4147; R, <u>L. braziliensis guyanensis</u> CUMC1 clone 1-A; D, <u>L. braziliensis braziliensis</u> M2903. The 250 kb LD1 and 6 kb LR1 are indicated by arrows.

the size of LD1 and LR1 indicates that both of these nucleic acids are multicopy relative to the chromosomal DNAs. LD1 stained green-yellow with acridine orange implying that it is DNA while LR1 stained red-orange suggesting it is RNA.

The DNA nature of LD1 was confirmed by its susceptibility to DNAse but not RNAse (Fig. 2). Its mobility under different conditions of PFGE and its susceptibility to Bal 31 exonuclease (data not shown) indicate that it is linear. LD1 is also a double stranded DNA based upon its susceptibility to restriction endonucleases and its ability to be nick translated (Fig. 3). When nick translated LD1 was hybridized to restriction endonuclease digested isolated LD1 or total cell DNA, the same DNA fragments were detected indicating that LD1 sequences are not highly reiterated on the

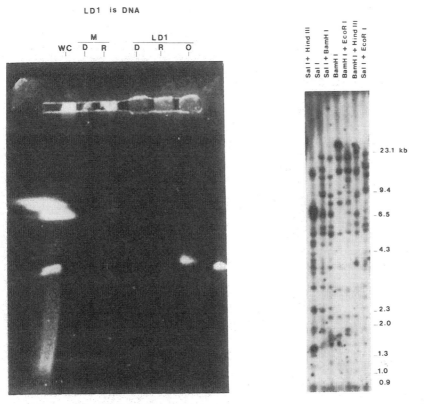

Fig. 2. LD1 is DNA. Ethidium bromide stained PFG electrophoretogram of isolated LD1 after DNase or RNase treatment. WC, L.b.b. M2903 total cellular DNA; M, lambda ladder; LDI, isolated LD1; D, incubated with 1 ug/ml RNase-free DNase; R, incubated with 1 ug/ml RNase A; O, untreated LD1. Incubations were for 30 min at 37°C.

Fig. 3. LD1 is double stranded DNA. Autoradiogram of L.b.b. M2903 genomic DNA digested with various restriction endonucleases, electrophoresed on a 0.7% agarose gel, transferred to nitrocellulose and probed with isolated LD1 that had been radiolabelled by nick translation as described in Myler et al. (1984). Marker sizes are shown to the right.

(other) chromosomal DNAs. This experiment preferentially detects repeated sequences and thus we cannot exclude the possibility that some unique LD1 sequences are present on other chromosomes. The restriction fragments detected a total of 115 kb while intact LD1 is about 250 kb. While it is possible that LD1 is a twofold repeat it is more likely that many restriction fragments co-migrated or ran off the gel. Interestingly, as reported elsewhere (Gajendran et al., 1987a; 1987b), a circular DNA (CD1) from L. donovani hybridized to LD1 as discussed below.

The RNA nature of LR1 is confirmed by its susceptibility to RNAse and alkali but not to DNAse (Fig. 4). Its susceptibility to RNAse was not altered by the addition of NaCl to 200 mM (not shown) showing that the RNA is single stranded. LR1 is largely, if not exclusively, restricted to the cytoplasm; the 6 kb RNA is detected in the cytoplasmic but not the nuclear fraction (Fig. 5). In addition, LR1 exists in a complexed form, presumably

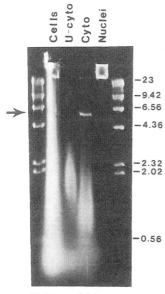

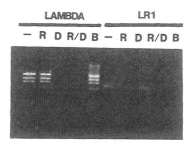

Fig. 4. LR1 is RNA. Ethidium bromide stain of Hind III digested lambda DNA and isolated LR1 treated with 1 ug/ml RNase A (R), 1 ug/ml RNase-free DNase (D), RNase A and RNase-free DNase (R/D), or 50 mM NaOH (B). Samples were incubated for 10 min at 37°C and electrophoresed on a 0.8% agarose gel. For the NaOH treated samples, HCl was added to pH 7.5 prior to electrophoresis.

Fig. 5. LR1 is predominantly in the cytoplasm. Ethidium bromide stain of an 0.8% agarose gel of 10^9 L.b.g. CUMC1 clone 1-A cells treated with 1% SDS and 20 ug/ml proteinase K for 1 hr at 65°C (CELLS); cytoplasm from 10^8 cells without SDS/proteinase K treatment (U-CYTO); cytoplasm from 10^8 cells treated with SDS and proteinase K (CYTO); nuclei from 2×10^8 cells treated with SDS and proteinase K (NUCLEI). Marker sizes (in kb) are shown to the right. LR1 is indicated by the arrow.

with proteins, since the cytoplasmic 6 kb RNA band is not detected in the absence of proteinase K and SDS treatments. Sucrose density gradient analysis of the cytoplasmic fraction reveals that the 6 kb RNA is present in a fraction with a sedimentation coefficient of about 140 S (Fig. 6). This confirms that the majority of the LR1 is not a free RNA but is present in a particulate form. Electron microscopy of the negatively stained material from the sucrose gradient fraction containing LR1 reveals particles that are about 40 nm in diameter (Fig. 7).

A 497 nucleotide sequence of one region was determined from two cDNAs that contained overlapping sequence (Fig. 8). This sequence contains a 143 codon open reading frame but neither the nucleotide sequence nor the derived amino acid sequence has convincing homology to any sequences in available data bases. The greatest homology was to the L protein of vesicular stomatitis virus (VSV). The FASTP initial and optimized scores (Lipman and Person, 1985) were 54 and 66, respectively, at 6 standard deviations above the mean, a value which approaches significance.

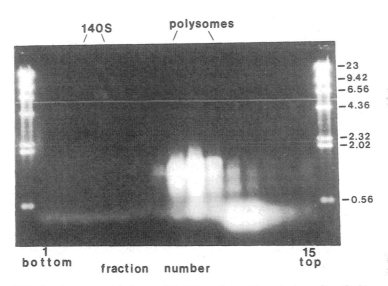

Fig. 6. LR1 is in a particle. Ethidium bromide stain of a 0.8% agarose gel of 20 ul aliquots of sucrose gradient fractions treated with 1% SDS and 20 ug/ml proteinase K for 1 hr at 65°. Cytoplasm from 10^{10} cells (0.5 ml) was centrifuged through a linear-log sucrose gradient and 1 ml fractions collected. Marker sizes (in kb) are shown to the right.

DISCUSSION

The properties of the multicopy DNA and RNA that we have detected in some stocks of Leishmania are consistent with them being autonomously replicating genetic elements. It appears likely that LD1 contains integrated sequences homologous to the circular DNA (CD1) observed by Gajendran et al. (1987a; 1987b). Further characterization of the properties of LD1 is required to determine if it has the characteristics of a plasmid, virus, or other self replicating genetic element. LD1/CD1 appears to be a transmissable DNA based on its presence in a circular or (integrated) linear form in some but not all stocks and a variety of species of

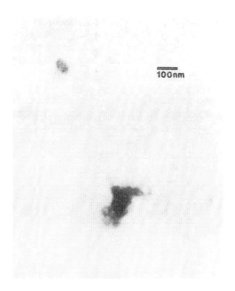

Fig. 7. EM of LR1 particle. An electron micrograph of negatively stained sucrose gradient fraction containing LR1. Diameter of the spherical particles is 40-50 nm.

Leishmania. This transmissibility further implies that some or all of the CD1 sequence has an exogenous origin. Additionally, it is likely that the non-CD1 sequences of LD1 and the other chromosomes within which CD1 is integrated are endogenous in origin. The multicopy nature of LD1 but not other chromosomes within which CD1 is integrated implies that LD1 copy number control differs from that of other chromosomes and perhaps is under the control of the CD1 replication origin. LD1 does not contain the H sequence or dihydrofolate reductase/thymidylate synthetase, rRNA, or tubulin genes (Scholler et al., 1986) and the parasites were not exposed to inhibitors such as methotrexate. Thus, the multicopy nature of LD1 is probably not the result of drug resistance.

```
           10        20        30        40        50        60        70        80        90
CCCAGGATGTTCAACGTTCGCGCTATGGAGTTACATACACTGTCCCATCCCAACGGTCCATTGGGTTGTGCTGCCACTGTTCCATCACGGTTTTCTGTAT 100
  P  G  C  S  T  F  A  L  W  S  Y  I  H  C  P  I  P  T  V  H  W  V  V  L  P  L  F  H  H  G  F  L  Y

GCTTGTCCTTCTTTCCTTGTTGCAAGTTCAGGATGGGCATGTTCTAATGCTCGTGAATGTGACCATTTGCAGCCCACAGCCAACGAGAAGACCAAAAATC 200
  A  C  P  S  F  L  V  A  S  S  G  W  A  C  S  N  A  R  E  C  D  H  L  Q  P  T  A  N  E  K  T  K  N

ACAAATTACCCCATATGTCACCGGCCGTCGTCGCAATTCTTGTGAATAGATCATCGGACGGCAGCACGCAATTCATCTCGTCGAGCCTCTGCATGCTTAG 300
  H  K  L  P  H  M  S  P  A  V  V  A  I  L  V  N  R  S  S  D  G  S  T  Q  F  I  S  S  S  L  C  M  L  R

ACTGCCGACATCTAGCCTTCTTCTTGCTTCAGTCTCAAGATCGATCTCATTGACACCACGCCCCAGCAAACACTTCATCTCAACCAACTGCGGTAGCAAG 400
  L  P  T  S  S  L  L  L  A  S  V  S  R  S  I  S  L  T  P  R  P  S  K  H  F  I  S  T  N  C  G  S  K

CAGACATCCCTCTATGCTTTATGTATATGTTGATGTCATCAGCGAAGCGAGGCTATCCGACAACACACATTAAAGCCCACAACACACAAAACC          500
  Q  T  S  L  Y  A  L  C  I  C  *
```

Fig. 8. LR1 open reading frame. The amino acid translation of the longest open reading frame derived from two overlapping cDNA clones.

LR1 is probably a single stranded RNA virus. It resembles the virus-like particles described in <u>Leishmania hertigi</u> (Molyneux, 1974) and <u>Endotrypanum</u> (Croft et al., 1986) in size and cytoplasmic location. The true relationship will await hybridization or serological analyses. Although, the possible homology of the LR1 sequence to VSV may be fortuitous, VSV is a single stranded RNA virus with general characteristics similar to LR1. In addition, it is intriguing that the sandfly is the vector of LR1 as well as VSV, possibly indicating an interesting biological relationship.

Both LD1 and LR1 were detected in stocks of <u>Leishmania</u> isolated from human cutaneous lesions. At this time there is no obvious correlation between the presence of LD1 (CD1) or LR1 and specific disease characteristics. It is unlikely, however, that the presence of self replicating genetic elements would be without effect on the parasite and thus there may be a consequence to the disease or to vector susceptibility. These questions require further investigation.

CONCLUSIONS

<u>Leishmania</u> contain small nucleic acids that have the properties expected for self replicating acquired genetic elements. One of these (LD1/CD1) is a DNA that appears to exist either integrated into chromosomal DNA or in a circular form. This is reminiscent of plasmids or viruses. The other (LR1) is a cytoplasmic single stranded RNA that occurs in a particle. This is similar to RNA viruses, some of which are found in the sandfly. Further experimentation is required to determine the precise character of these elements, in particular transmission experiments and studies on the effects of these elements on the parasites and the course of the disease.

ACKNOWLEDGEMENTS

We thank R.A. Sutherland for excellent technical assistance. This study received support from NIH grant AI24771 and the Rockefeller Foundation. KS is a recipient of a Special Fellowship from the Burroughs Wellcome Fund.

REFERENCES

Croft, S.L., Chance, M.L., and Gardener, P.J., 1986, Ultrastructural and biochemical characterization of stocks of <u>Endotrypanum</u>, Ann. Trop. Med. Parasitol., 74:586.
Diamond, L., and Mattern, C., 1976, Protozoal viruses, Adv. Virus Res., 20:87.
Feagin, J.E., Jasmer, D.P., and Stuart, K., 1985, Apocytochrome b and other mitochondrial DNA sequences are differentially expressed during the life cycle of <u>Trypanosoma brucei</u>, Nucl. Acids Res., 13:4577.
Gajendran, N., Dujardin, J.P., LeRay, D., Matthyssens, G., and Hamers, R. 1987a, Abnormally migrating chromosomes identify <u>Leishmania donovani</u> strains, <u>in</u>: "Leishmaniasis: the first Centenary (1885-1985) new strategies for control," D.T. Hart, ed., Plenum, New York.
Gajendran, N., Dujardin, J.P., Stuart, K., and Hamers, R. 1987b, Circular and linear forms of small nucleic acids in <u>Leishmania</u>, <u>in</u>: "Leishmaniasis: the first Centenary (1885-1985) new strategies for control," D.T. Hart, ed., Plenum, New York.

Lipman,, D.J. and Pearson, W.R., 1985, Rapid and sensitive protein similarity searches, Science, 27:1435.

Maniatis, T., Fritsch, E.F., and Sambrook, J., 1982, "Molecular Cloning, a Laboratory Manual", Cold Spring Harbor Laboratory, Cold Spring Harbor, New York.

Molyneux, D.H., 1974, Virus-like particles in Leishmania parasites, Nature, 249:588.

Myler, P.J., Allison,J., Agabian, N., and Stuart, K., 1984, Antigenic variation in African trypanosomes by gene replacement or activation of alternate telomeres, Cell, 39:203.

Persons, D.A., and Finn, O.J., 1986, A rapid and efficient method for preparing cDNA from RNA in agarose gel slices, BioTech., 4: 398.

Shapiro, S. Z., and Young, J.R., 1981, An immunochemical method for mRNA purification. Application to messenger RNA encoding trypanosome variable surface antigen, J. Biol. Chem., 256:1495.

Scholler, J.K., Reed, S.G., and Stuart, K., 1986, Molecular karyotype of species and subspecies of Leishmania, Mol. Biochem. Parasitol., 20:279.

Wang, A.L., and Wang, C.C., 1986a, The double-stranded RNA in Trichomonas vaginalis may originate from virus-like particles, Proc. Natl. Acad. Sci. USA, 83:7956.

Wang, A.L., and Wang, C.C.,1986b, Discovery of a specific double-stranded RNA virus in Giardia lamblia, Molec. Biochem. Parasitol., 21:269.

GENE EXPRESSION IN THE INFECTIVE PROMASTIGOTES OF

LEISHMANIA MAJOR

Deborah F. Smith, Paul D. Ready*, Richard M.R. Coulson, Susan Searle and Antonio J.R. Campos

Department of Biochemistry and *Department of Pure and Applied Biology, Imperial College of Science and Technology, London SW7 2AZ

INTRODUCTION

We are studying the molecular events which accompany the differentiation of Leishmania major promastigotes in vitro, an understanding of which could be important in developing prophylactics against infective-stage promastigotes inoculated by sandfly vectors.

The changes in parasite morphology which occur during development of Leishmania in the sandfly vector have been extensively studied (Killick-Kendrick, 1979). In particular, a characteristic promastigote form has been observed, in the midgut and in the head, which is highly motile and of short body length (Sacks and Perkins, 1984, 1985). This form is abundant only as population growth slows and is believed to be the form inoculated by the fly into its mammmalian host. The molecular characterisation of the infective form requires quantities of messenger RNAs and proteins that can only be provided by a simple in vitro promastigote differentiation system; there are relatively small numbers of promastigotes in a sandfly's gut.

It has been shown that L. major promastigotes, growing in monophasic culture media, undergo a sequential development (or differentiation) from non-infective to infective forms, associated with a change from log.-phase to stationary-phase of growth (Sacks and Perkins, 1984,1985). The highly virulent infective forms are morphologically similar to the sandfly proboscis forms and are further characterised by strain-variable resistance to complement (Franke et al., 1985) and an absence of receptor sites for peanut agglutinin (PNA); this plant lectin effectively agglutinates all log. phase, complement-sensitive, non-infective forms (Sacks et al., 1985).

We have further characterised this in vitro culture system and are using it to study the changes in gene expression that occur during promastigote differentiation, with the aim of identifying those genes which are expressed in the parasite form inoculated by the sandfly vector.

MATERIALS AND METHODS

Parasites. The Friedlin strain of L. major (London zymodeme 1) used in all experiments was maintained on slopes of biphasic NNN medium at 23° C. Parasites were subcultured into Schneider's Drosophila medium (Gibco) containing 10% heat-inactivated fetal calf serum (FCS, Gibco) and 100ug/ml gentamycin and incubated at 23° or 26° C. In all RNA isolation experiments, log. phase cultures = 3 day cultures, 0% infective forms;

stationary phase cultures = 10 day cultures, 60 - 80 % infective forms. The concentration of glucose in culture media was determined by standard methods.

   Peanut lectin agglutination. In our hands, the agglutination procedures of Sacks et al. (1985) yielded supernatants of infective forms contaminated with many small rafts of agglutinated non-infective forms. We found that a higher purity could be obtained by sucrose gradient centrifugation of the agglutination mix (Ready and Smith, unpublished).

   RNA extraction and analysis. Pelleted washed parasites were lysed in 5M guanidinium isothiocyanate and the RNA isolated by density gradient centrifugation (Maniatis et al., 1982). Poly-adenylated RNA was selected by chromatography through oligo (dT) cellulose. RNA was analysed on neutral agarose gels, after denaturation with glyoxal and dimethylsulphoxide as described (Maniatis et al., 1982), followed by transfer to nylon membranes (Hybond N, Amersham). DNA probes were radio-labelled by nick translation (Rigby et al., 1977) or by oligo-labelling (Feinberg and Vogelstein, 1984). Post-hybridisational washes were either at low stringency (2 x SSC, 0.5% SDS, 65° C) or at high stringency (0.2 x SSC, 0.5% SDS, 65° C).

   DNA probes. The human hsp probe used was a cDNA clone, comprising 75% of the coding region (Hunt and Morimoto,1985). The T. brucei β-tubulin probe was also derived from a cDNA clone, encoding 60% of the coding region (Thomashow et al., 1983). The L. major actin probe was a Eco R1/Sal 1 fragment encoding the whole gene, derived from a lambda genomic clone (Smith and Searle, unpublished).

   cDNA cloning and screening. cDNA was synthesised from poly A+ RNA extracted from late stationary phase organisms containing 70% infective forms, using the method of Watson and Jackson (1983). 25,000 plaques were replica-plated onto Hybond N discs and initially screened with log. phase specific RNA, radiolabelled using $^{32}P\gamma$ ATP and T_4 polynucleotide kinase (Maniatis et al., 1982). After probe removal, the same plaques were then rescreened with radiolabelled RNA from stationary phase organisms. Plaques that showed increased hybridisation or which only hybridised with the latter probe were picked, purified and their DNA isolated.

   Genomic cloning and screening. Total L. major DNA was isolated by the method of Cowman et al., 1984. A genomic library was constructed by the insertion of partial Sau 3A fragments into the Bam Hl sites of bacteriophage lambda EMBL 4 and screened by standard methods (Kaiser and Murray, 1985).

RESULTS

   Growth characteristics of in vitro cultures. Promastigotes of L. major, Friedlin (F) strain, were cultured at 26° C and growth and differentiation monitored by counting the organisms, by observing their morphological forms and by agglutinating samples with peanut lectin(PNA). Typically, logarithmic growth ceased after 4-5 days at this temperature, when the cells entered the stationary phase. Morphologically, promastigotes which were actively dividing had a characteristic cigar-shaped body and a flagellum 1-1.5 x as long. In stationary phase, 60 - 80% of these log. phase organisms differentiated into promastigotes which were highly motile and had a shorter body and longer flagellum as described by Sacks and Perkins (1984). These forms may correspond to the head forms seen in the sandfly. We also observed a population of varying size of "round-bodied" forms in stationary phase cultures (see below). The ability of stationary phase organisms to differentiate is strain-specific: P strain (MRHO/SU/59) transforms at a lower frequency (10 - 20%) under our conditions.

   Agglutination with peanut lectin (PNA) was used to monitor the extent of differentiation in these cultures. We confirmed the findings of Sacks et al.(1985) that the highly motile, stationary phase forms (infective organisms) were not agglutinated by this lectin while the log. phase forms (non-infective organisms) were. The round-bodied forms were also resistant to PNA agglutination. The % increase in infective forms closely correlated with the transition from log. phase but continued to increase in stationary phase, reaching a plateau after 7 days in culture. At this stage in the growth cycle, it is possible to use PNA to agglutinate all non-infective organisms from a large-scale culture and to recover the infective organisms by centrifugation.

Days in culture		3	5	7	10
Glucose concentration (mM)	+GS	54	40	36	38
	-GS	4.0	3.8	2.0	0.2
Parasites/ml of culture	+GS	5×10^4	7×10^5	5×10^6	4×10^6
	-GS	2×10^4	7×10^5	3×10^6	1.5×10^6

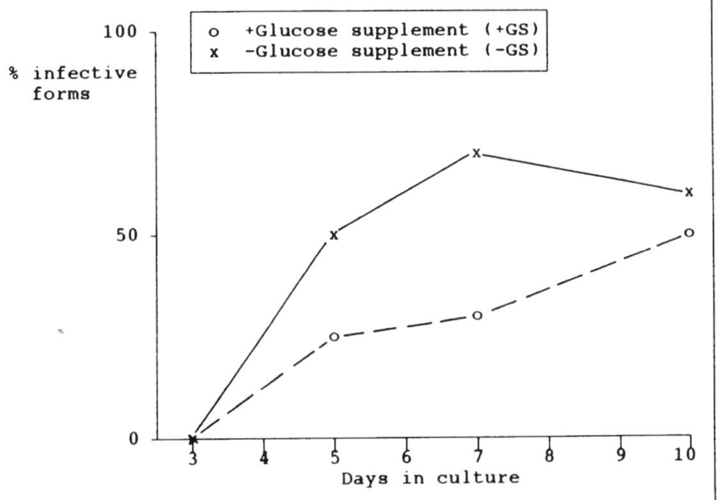

Figure 1. Growth of L. Major F strain +/- glucose. Cultured promastigotes were counted, agglutinated with peanut lectin and the medium glucose concentration determined. %infective forms = % non-agglutinated parasites. (One of 5 reproducible experiments).

Effect of sugars on transformation rate. Sugars can affect the development of Leishmania in sandflies (Warburg and Sclein, 1986). To test the effects of excess extracellular sugars on promastigotes growing in culture, we conducted a number of experiments in which the culture media were supplemented with various sugars on the day of parasite inoculation. We observed that the addition of sucrose, fructose or trehalose (all added to 1% (w/v) final concentration) had no effect on the growth rate or transformation frequency of F strain organisms. Conversely, the addition of 1% glucose reproducibly caused a decrease in the rate at which the promastigotes differentiated into infective forms (Figure 1). The difference was approximately 50% after 7 days in culture, although the number of parasites was unaltered. The same effect was also seen if the glucose supplement was made 1, 2 or 3 days into the culture period. From the glucose concentrations recorded during the growth cycle, it is evident that the glucose supplemented organisms are in an environment which is not being depleted of sugar, but they still transform albeit at a slower rate. If such organisms are kept for longer periods (up to 21 days), they still do not reach the same level of differentiation as do the untreated controls. We can only speculate as to the importance of this observation in the development of the parasite and its relevance in vivo (see later).

Molecular differences between infective and non-infective organisms. In vivo protein labelling experiments and in vitro translation of promastigote mRNA show some differences in protein profiles between log. and stationary phase organisms (data not shown) but such methods will not allow the detection of small changes in molecules which may be crucial to the transforming parasite. One way to study these molecular events is to look for changes in gene expression, by an analysis of RNA populations and the proteins they encode.

Analysis of RNA from log. and stationary phase cultures: the use of heterologous gene probes To look for changes in gene expression which accompany promastigote differentiation, we used a number of cloned genes (which encode proteins that are evolutionarily highly conserved) to probe L. major RNA from different developmental stages. Of a number of such genes used, 2 showed specific increases in the levels of transcript detected. These were the β-tubulin gene of T. brucei (Thomashow et al., 1983) and the human gene encoding the heat shock protein 70 (hsp 70) (Hunt and Morimoto, 1985).

The β-tubulin gene hybridised to transcripts in all developmental stages of L. major. In log. phase organisms, one major transcript of 2.2 Kb and one minor transcript of 2.8 Kb were found (Figure 2A, lane 1), both of which were polyadenylated. Stationary phase poly A+ RNA showed these 2 bands plus an additional transcript of 3.4 Kb (Figure 2A, lane 2). In total amastigote RNA (lane 3), the largest transcript was absent, while the 2.8 Kb band showed an abundance equivalent to the 2.2 Kb band. Taking into account the approximately 50-fold difference in the amounts of poly A+ RNA found in lanes 1 and 2 compared to lane 3, these results demonstrate both quantitative and qualitative differences in the amounts of β-tubulin transcript found in different stages:

Size of transcript (Kb)	Abundance (relative to Log.*)		
	Log.	Stationary	Amastigote
3.4	-	10 +	-
2.8	1+ *	5+	200+
2.2	100+	50+	200+

It is known that there are at least 3 non-allelic β-tubulin loci in L. major, one of which encodes the 2.2Kb transcript (Spithill and Samaras, 1987). We suggest that the 3 developmentally-regulated transcripts shown in Figure 3 could arise from dispersed genes which encode proteins of different function in the Leishmania life cycle.

Figure 2B shows the pattern of transcripts found after probing total RNA from infective organisms with the β-tubulin probe. RNA isolated from stationary phase infective organisms (lane 3) shows the same number of transcripts as seen with total stationary phase RNA (Figure 2A, lane 2). This result confirms our prediction that infective promastigotes can have abundant RNAs although we can not say that the pattern of β-tubulin transcription shown is specific for these forms alone, because the "non-infective" sample was contaminated with "infective" forms (lane 2).

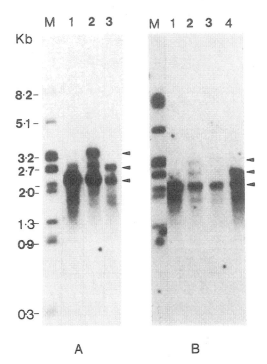

Figure 2. Autoradiogram of L. major transcripts with homology to β-tubulin. Size-separated RNAs from different promastigote stages were transferred and hybridised with a T. brucei β-tubulin probe.
A: 1 ug poly A+ RNA from log.(1) and stationary(2) phase, 1 ug total RNA from amastigotes(3). B: 1 ug of total RNA from log.
(1), stationary:infective + non-infective forms(2), stationary:infective forms(3) and amastigotes(4). M: DNA markers.

The human hsp70 gene hybridised to a 3.2 Kb transcript in L. major (Figure 3A), which was shown to be a polyadenylated RNA (data not shown). This transcript was present in non-infective organisms, at a level approximately equivalent to that of actin mRNA (which represents <5% of total mRNA). As the parasites differentiated to 70% infective forms, the level of this transcript increased by >2-fold (after 10 days in culture). Hybridisation of the same filter with a ribosomal gene probe showed that the amounts of RNA loaded in each lane were equivalent. When the same RNA samples were probed for actin mRNA (Figure 3B), little variation in the amount of this mRNA was observed over the same time course. In an independent experiment, it was shown that the level of the L. major hsp 70 RNA only increased during promastigote differentiation but did not increase following the transformation to amastigotes (Figure 4). (The small decrease in transcript level seen between lanes 10 and A is an artefact of loading.)

The observed increase in the L. major hsp 70 mRNA level may be due to an increase in transcription, but it might also be due to storage or decreased translation of this molecule.

cDNA cloning. Although the use of heterologous probes described above has yielded 2 genes which may be developmentally-regulated in L. major, this approach cannot be used to detect the subtle and potentially most interesting changes in gene expression between the non-infective and infective parasite forms. It was therefore decided to construct a complementary (c) DNA library from stationary phase RNA and to

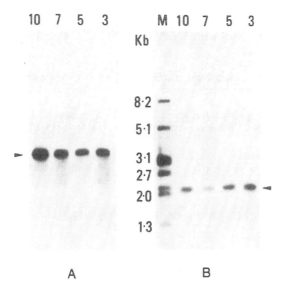

Figure 3. Autoradiogram of L. major transcripts with homology to actin/hsp 70. RNAs, treated as in Figure 2, were hybridised with A: human hsp 70 probe (low stringency); B: actin probe (high stringency). 10 ug total RNA per lane from 3,5,7,10 day cultures (as in Figure 1). M: DNA markers.

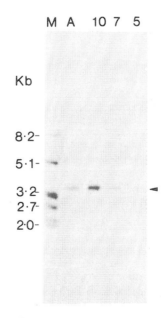

Figure 4. Autoradiogram of L. major transcripts with homology to hsp 70. RNAs, treated as in Figure 2, were hybridised with the human hsp 70 probe. 5 ug total RNA per lane from 5,7,10 day cultures and amastigotes. M: DNA markers.

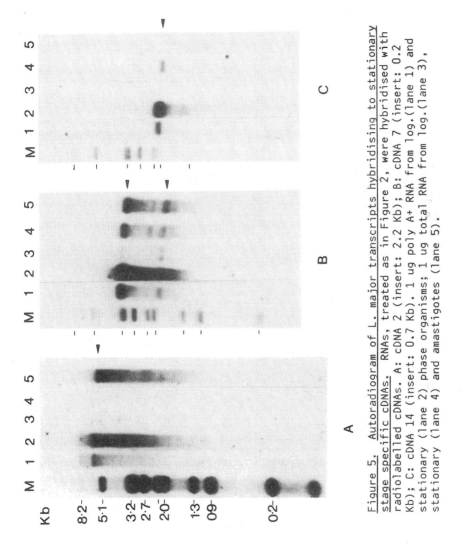

Figure 5. Autoradiogram of L. major transcripts hybridising to stationary stage specific cDNAs. RNAs, treated as in Figure 2, were hybridised with radiolabelled cDNAs. A: cDNA 2 (insert: 2.2 Kb); B: cDNA 7 (insert: 0.2 Kb); C: cDNA 14 (insert: 0.7 Kb). 1 ug poly A+ RNA from log.(lane 1) and stationary (lane 2) phase organisms; 1 ug total RNA from log.(lane 3), stationary (lane 4) and amastigotes (lane 5).

differentially screen the cloned sequences with RNA from log. and stationary phase parasites. This approach should allow the detection of genes whose expression is increased in stationary phase infective organisms.

The first screen of this cDNA library yielded 18 positive phage plaques which hybridised strongly with stationary phase RNA but weakly with log. phase RNA. After subsequent screens, 6 individual cDNA clones, all different from one another, were hybridised to size-separated denatured RNA transferred to nylon membranes. The results from some of these experiments (Figure 5) show a number of different patterns of expression of the genes from which these sequences derive. In Figure 5A, cDNA 2 hybridised to a 6 Kb poly A+ RNA which increased in amount between log. and stationary phase (A, lanes 1 and 2). However, when total RNA was probed with the same cDNA, a hugh increase in the amount of this transcript between promastigotes and amastigotes was also detected (Figure 5A, lanes 3-5).

cDNA 7 hybridised to 2 poly A+ transcripts (3.2 Kb and 1.8 Kb) in log. phase organisms (Figure 5B, lane 1), both of which increased in stationary phase RNA (lane 2). In total RNA, this pattern was also seen, but no further increase was observed in amastigote RNA (Figure 5B, lanes 3-5). 2 additional faint transcripts were seen, however, at 2.2 and 2.4 Kb, and the smaller of these was present in stationary phase RNA (lane 4). We believe that this cDNA may encode the hsp 70 gene identified by Van der Ploeg et al.,(1985).

cDNA 14 hybridised to a 2.1 Kb poly A+ transcript which increased from log. to stationary phase (Figure 5C, lanes 1 and 2). An additional faint transcript of 1.5 Kb was seen in both RNAs. This transcript disappears on the transformation from promastigote to amastigote: it is undetectable in total amastigote RNA (Figure 5C, lane 5) although may be transcribed at a low level.

These cDNA clones therefore show different developmental patterns of hybridisation as follows:

cDNA clone	Transcript Size (Kb)	Abundance (relative to Log.)		
		Log.	Stationary	Amastigote
2	6.0	1+	3+	100+
7	3.2	1+	10+	10+
	2.4	-	-	1+
	2.2	-	2+	1+
	1.8	1+	2+	3+
14	2.1	1+	20+	-
	1.5	(+)	1+	(-)

We are at present further characterising these cDNAs and others in order to identify their gene products. We know that none encode either of the tubulin proteins but that all are transcribed at a relatively high level (>0.1% of total mRNA). The differential RNA screen of the cDNA library which produced these clones would not be sensitive enough to detect genes transcribed at very low levels; we intend to rescreen a larger number of recombinants with a more sensitive, "subtractive probe" in order to identify genes of this type.

Further characterisation of the L. major hsp 70 genes. In view of the increased abundance of a L. major RNA showing homology to the human hsp 70 gene during promastigote differentiation, we decided to clone the gene as a preliminary to a more rigorous study of its transcriptional regulation and function. A previous report has demonstrated the presence of a similar gene in L. major, showing homology to the heat-inducible hsp 70 gene of D. melanogaster (Van der Ploeg et al.,1985). A genomic library, constructed in bacteriophage lambda EMBL was screened using the human hsp 70 gene probe and a number of clones isolated and characterised (Campos, Searle and Smith, unpublished). Preliminary work indicates that there are a number of different L. major genes which share homology with the human hsp 70 gene. The gene mapped in Figure 6, λLm hsp 70.1, is situated on a 4.3 Kb Eco R1/ Bam H1 fragment within the genome and shows homology to the human probe only at its 5' end. When the human hsp 70 gene is used to probe size-fractionated L. major genomic DNA (Figure 7), however, 3 additional Eco R1/ Bam H1 genomic fragments are recognised (Figure 7, lane 2). One of these, of > 12 Kb, hybridises very strongly, suggesting a number of repeated homologous genes on this fragment. A similar result is suggested by the Eco R1/Hind III digest (lane 3), which shows 4 hybridising bands, only one of which can be attributed to the gene cloned in λLm hsp 70.1.

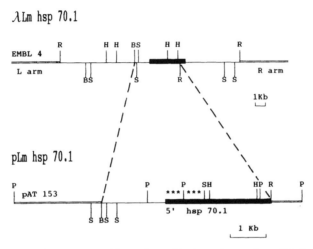

Figure 6. Restriction maps of λLm hsp 70.1 and pLm hsp 70.1.
λLm hsp 70.1 is a genomic clone in the vector EMBL4. The central 4.4 Kb Eco R1/ Bam H1 fragment containing most of the coding region (solid block) is sub-cloned into the vector pAT 153 to give pLm hsp 70.1. The 5' end of the gene has been determined by S1 nuclease mapping. ***:region of homology with the human hsp 70 probe. R: Eco R1; B: Bam H1; S: Sal 1; H: Hind III; P: Pst 1.

These results show the presence of at least 3 genes related to the human hsp 70 gene in L. major. A small family of hsp 70 related genes has been described in T. brucei (Glass et al., 1986), but these are clustered in a close tandem array. The gene described in Figure 6 cannot form part of a similar array as it has >5 Kb of untranscribed DNA on either side of it.

λLm hsp 70.1 hybridises to a number of transcripts in total L. major RNA, in addition to the 3.2 Kb transcript which is recognised by the human hsp 70 probe (Figure 3). If a 5' specific probe is hybridised to size-fractionated parasite RNAs (Figure 8, 0.98 Pst), 3 transcripts, of 3.2, 4.5 and 5.5 Kb, are found in stationary phase organisms. Each is found in increased amounts in amastigotes, although the 3.2 Kb RNA increases by a greater proportion. If the same RNA filter is then rehybridised with a more 3' probe (Figure 8, 1.1 Hind), the same 3 fragments are seen but that at 3.2 Kb is by far the most abundant and is again up-regulated after the

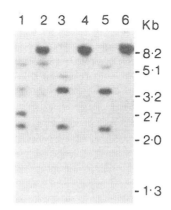

Figure 7. Autoradiogram of L. major genomic DNA with homology to hsp 70. Genomic DNA was digested, Southern blotted (using standard techniques) and hybridised with the human hsp 70 probe at low stringency. Lane 1: Bam H1/Hind III: Eco R1/ Bam H1; 3: Eco R1/ Bam H1; 5: Hind III; 6: Eco R1.

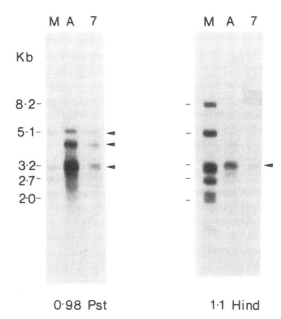

Figure 8. Autoradiogram of L. major hsp 70 transcripts. RNAs, treated as in Figure 2, were hybridised with the 5' specific 0.98 Kb Pst 1 fragment or with the internal 1.1 Kb Hind III fragment from the gene encoded in pLm hsp 70.1 (Figure 6). 5 ug total RNA from 7 day (stationary) or amastigotes (A). M: DNA markers.

transformation to amastigotes (Figure 8, 1.1 Hind, lane A). This transcript is specific for the cloned gene, λ Lm hsp 70.1. We have not yet determined the identity of the larger transcripts but believe that they share homology to λLm hsp 70.1, at its 5' end.

These results suggest that the L. major hsp genes show different patterns of expression during development, and therefore, that they may be induced by different stimuli. It has been proposed that the transformation from promastigote to amastigote in vivo, which is accompanied by a change in temperature from that of the insect vector (25 - 29 $^\circ$C) to that of the mammalian host (37°C), might constitute a heat shock to the organisms and result in a change in transcription in the hsp genes. While the mRNA encoded by one of our cloned genes does increase from promastigote to amastigote, that encoded by another does not, but instead increases as the promastigote becomes infective. This pattern of gene expression is similar to that shown by the human hsp 70 gene (Figure 5). Both genes are constituitively-expressed.

DISCUSSION

The general aims of the work described here are, firstly, to identify molecules that could be useful in vaccination and/or as a target for chemotherapy and would have the advantage of being specific for the forms which are inoculated into the human host. Secondly, we would wish to be able positively to identify infective promastigotes in sandflies, by detection of specific surface or intracellular molecules.

To achieve these general aims, several approaches could be made. A number of workers have concentrated on the search for stage-specific surface antigens, using either human sera from diagnosed cases of leishmaniasis to identify iodinated surface proteins (Heath et al., 1987) or specific monoclonal antibodies to bind surface carbohydrates (Handman et al., 1984). Another approach, described in this paper, is to identify stage-specific proteins by searching for increased expression of their genes. This approach has the potential to identify both surface and intracellular molecules. In addition, it provides the opportunity to further our understanding of the novel mechanisms controlling gene expression in the trypanosomatids (Borst, 1986).

The ability to reproduce promastigote differentiation in vitro has been crucial to this work. Confirming previously reported work (Sacks and Perkins, 1984), our experiments show that in vitro differentiation is dependent on the length of time that the organisms spend in culture and on the strain used. It has not yet been proven that the infective forms which differentiate in vitro are those forms which are normally inoculated by sandflies in nature.

We have developed a method of separating infective promastigotes from stationary cultures which gives preparations of 80 - 100 % purity. This work has allowed us to confirm that these infective forms do contain elevated amounts of specific messenger RNAs, although we have routinely used whole stationary cultures of the high transforming F strain to provide large amounts of nucleic acids.

Analysis of total and poly A+ RNA from both infective and non-infective promastigotes identified 2 genes whose transcription may be increased during differentiation: L. major genes encoding β-tubulin and an hsp 70 protein. The differential screening of the cDNA library identified other genes which may be up-regulated in infective stage promastigotes. The identity of these genes and their products will be determined using a number of strategies. DNA sequence analysis of the cDNA clones will allow the identification of open reading frames for protein synthesis and may yield information as to the proteins themselves. Antibodies raised to fusion proteins expressed from the cloned genes will be used to locate, to isolate and to characterise the function of the native proteins.

The observation that a L. major gene with homology to a human hsp 70 gene undergoes increased expression in infective promastigotes is intriguing, given the different functions which have been proposed for the hsp 70 proteins in other organisms. They are believed to have multiple functions concerned with the assembly and dis-assembly of protein aggregates in eukaryotic cells. Of particular interest are the glucose-regulated hsp 70 proteins (grps) which are found in high amounts in secretory cells, and are regulated by extracellular glucose concentration (Pelham, 1986).

The identification of a family of hsp 70-related genes in L. major must therefore give rise to speculation as to the number of hsp-like proteins and their function in this organism. Our results indicate that at least one of the genes may be heat-inducible and that this is encoded by the cloned gene, λ Lm hsp 70.1. Another of the genes may show increased expression during promastigote differentiation, and we speculate that extra-cellular glucose concentration could be important in its regulation, given our observed inhibition of promastigote differentiation in the presence of high glucose levels. A role for glucose regulation in the production of infective promastigotes in vivo can be postulated from the observation that engorged female sandflies stop taking sugars from plant saps until the bloodmeal is completely digested (Killick-Kendrick and Killick-Kendrick, 1987). As it is at the end of blood meal digestion that infective parasites are found in the mid-gut and head of the fly, these organisms must presumably differentiate in an environment of decreasing (blood) sugar concentration.

The roles of the hsp-related proteins in L. major are therefore, a subject of some interest. The isolation of related proteins, all of which are dominant immunogens, from a wide range of other parasites is intriguing, given the intracellular location of these proteins in all the organisms so far tested (Ardeshir et al, 1987; Hedstrom et al., 1987).

Acknowledgements. This work is supported by a grant from the Wellcome Trust to D.F.S.

References

Ardeshir, F., Flint, J.E., Richman, S.J. and Reese, R.T., 1987, A 75 kd merozoite surface protein of Plasmodium falciparum which is related to the 70 kd heat-shock proteins, EMBO.J., 6:493.
Borst, P., 1986, Antigenic variation in Trypanosomes, Ann. Rev. Biochem., 55:701.
Cowman, A.F., Bernard, O., Stewart, N. and Kemp, D.J., 1984, Genes of the protozoan parasite Babesia bovis that rearrange to produce RNA species with different sequences, Cell, 37: 653.
Feinberg, A.P. and Vogelstein, B., 1984, A technique for radiolabelling DNA restriction endonuclease fragments to high specific activity, Analytical Biochemistry, 137: 266.
Franke, E.D., McGreevy, P.B., Katz, S.P. and Sacks, D.L., 1985, Growth cycle dependent generation of complement resistant Leishmania promastigotes, J. Immunol, 134:2713.
Glass, D.J., Polvere, R.I. and Van der Ploeg, L.H.T., 1986, Conserved sequenc and transcription of the hsp70 gene family in Trypanosoma brucei, Mol. and Cell. Biol., 6: 4657.
Handman, E., Greenblatt, C.L. and Goding, J.W., 1984, An amphipathic sulphated glycoconjugate of Leishmania: characterisation with monoclonal antibodies, EMBO J., 3:2301.
Heath, S., Chance, M.L., Hommel, M. and Crampton, J.M., 1987, Cloning of a gene encoding the immunodominant surface antigen of L. donovani promastigotes, Mol. Biochem. Parasitol., 23:211.
Hedstrom, R., Culpepper, J., Harrison, R.A., Agabian, N. and Newport, G., 1987, A major immunogen in Schistosoma mansoni infections is homologous to the heat-shock protein Hsp70, J. Exp. Med., 165: 1430.

IN VITRO AND IN VIVO DIFFERENTIATION OF L.MEXICANA-Hsp70 GENE EXPRESSION

Michal Shapira[1], Juan G. McEwen[1] and Charles L. Jaffe[2]

Department of Chemical Immunology[1] and Biophysics[2]

The Weizmann Institute of Science, Rehovot 76100, Israel

INTRODUCTION

Expression of heat shock proteins (Hsp's) is a universal response to exposure of cells to stress of various kinds. It is believed to play an important role in protecting the organism against unphysiological growth conditions, and in acquisition of thermotolerance, through mechanisms which are still not uniquely agreed upon. For review see references[1-3]. Most abundant are proteins of Mr 70 and 83-90 Kd, which are both highly conserved throughout evolution. Proteins of the Hsp70 family all share the characteristic of binding to ATP[4-6], and are believed to be involved in prevention or disruption of hydrophobic aggregates through an ATP-dependent mechanism[7]. Recently it has also been shown that RNA splicing is interrupted by heat shock and rescued by Hsp70 expression[8]. Most organisms also produce one or more small heat shock proteins, with Mr of 18-30 Kd. These small Hsp's show a lower degree of structural conservation among species. In some organisms, heat shock genes are expressed independently of environmental stress at specific stages of development[9].

Parasites with a biphasic life cycle are an interesting system for studying the heat shock response, since they are adapted for survival in a wide range of temperatures. Indeed proteins which are highly homologous to members of the Hsp70 family have been detected in schistosomiasis[10], in the trypanosomatid family[11,12] and in malaria. Interestingly, in malarial merozoite a 75 Kd protein which bears high homology to drosophila Hsp70 is distributed on the cell surface, and therefore may be involved in processes which allow invasion and survival within the host cells[13]. In this report we follow the expression of heat shock genes in both life stages of leishmania, along with studying their mode of regulation.

MATERIALS AND METHODS

Parasites

Leishmania mexicana amazonensis, isolate LTB 0016 was subcloned by the limiting dilution technique, and propagated in vitro in Schneider's drosophila medium at 26°C as promastigotes. Amastigotes were obtained from foot lesions of Balb/c mice, and purified over Percoll gradients[14]. In addition, amastigotes were also obtained by infecting peritoneal macrophages with promastigotes at 35°C, after which excess promastigotes were washed out. The infection rate and proliferation of the amastigotes within the macrophage phagolysosome, was monitored by Giemsa staining of the infected macrophages.

Metabolic Labeling Experiments

10^8 cells/ml of parasites from late log to stationary phase promastigotes culture grown in DMEM were labeled metabolically with 40μci/ml of ^{35}S-methionine, in methionine depleted DMEM, supplemented with 2% FCS. Promastigotes were labeled for 30-60 minutes either at 26°C or at 35°C, after 1 hour of heat shock at 35°C. Lesion amastigotes were labeled over night immediately post isolation under similar labeling conditions at 35°C. Amastigotes grown in vitro within peritoneal macrophages were labeled over night seven days post infection. All labeled cells were washed x3 with cold PBS, dissolved in sample buffer and analyzed by fluorographs of SDS PAGE.

Immunoblotting

SDS gels of cell extracts were blotted to nitrocellulose, and reacted with the specific antibodies. For detection of Hsp70, monoclonal antibody B.10 was used, generously donated by Dr. S. Lindquist. Tubulin was detected by a polyclonal serum raised in rabbits against chicken tubulin. The total protein content is demonstrated by amido black staining of the blot.

RESULTS

Temperature Elevation Induces Morphological Changes as in Stage Differentiation

Transfer of the promastigote culture of L.mexicana from 26°C to 35°C resulted in morphological changes similar to those which occur during promastigote-amastigote stage transformation. Within several hours the flagellum shortened extensively, causing loss of motility, and the cell shape rounded up. These changes were shown in a Giemsa staining of promastigotes cultured at 26°C and promastigotes exposed to a 48 hrs heat shock at 35°C in Fig. 1. Parallel to the temperature shift, proliferation rate was reduced several fold. These changes were reversible, and a transfer back to 26°C resulted in the transformation back to a promastigote culture.

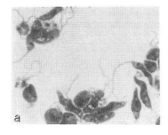 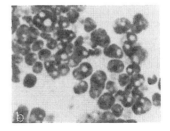

Fig. 1. Light microscopy (x1000) of Giemsa stained L. mexicana amazonensis promastigotes at (a) 26°C and (b) 35°C, after 48 hours.

Heat Shock Proteins are Constitutively Expressed in Amastigotes, as well as in Heat Shocked Promastigotes

Promastigotes cultured at 26°C and heat shocked at 35°C, as well as amastigotes isolated from foot lesions, or grown within peritoneal macrophages, were metabolically labeled by ^{35}S-Methionine. As depicted in Fig. 2, a protein of 70 Kd was constitutively expressed in the amastigote stage. The amastigotes were labeled at 35°C. Promastigotes transferred to 35°C also produced a major heat shock response, and expressed proteins of 70 and 84 Kd. The appearance of major heat shock proteins was accompanied by a severe reduction in the synthesis of tubulin, at both life stages. Hsp 84 was also constitutively expressed in amastigotes of L.donovani and L. major, but not in L.mexicana amazonensis although extensively synthesized in heat shock promastigotes of that strain. It is possible that Hsp84 was not detected in gels of L.mexicana amastigotes due to protein degradation in the samples, and the final conclusion with respect to Hsp84 is yet to come.

Characterization of Hsp70 with Monoclonal Antibodies

In order to specifically characterize the protein detected at Mr 70,000 d as a member of the Hsp70 family of proteins described in the literature, gel blots of extracts from heat shocked promastigotes, were reacted with specific antibodies. Monoclonal antibody B.10 which is directed against Drosophila Hsp70, gave a strong cross reaction with proteins of Mr 68,000 and 70,000 d (Fig. 3). This monoclonal antibody recognizes proteins of the Hsp70 family from various species and is probably directed against a conserved epitope. Since our study relates to tubulin expression as well, this protein was also immunologically characterized. Fig. 3, demonstrates recognition of tubulin by polyclonal serum raised against chicken tubulin, at Mr 55 Kd.

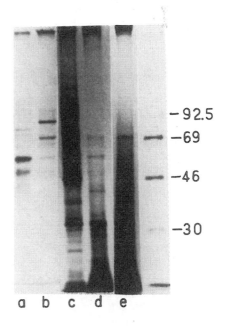

Fig. 2. Metabolic labeling of L. mexicana promastigotes and amastigotes with ^{35}S-methionine (a) Cultured promastigotes at 26°C, (b) cultured promastigotes after 1 hr at 35°C, (c) non infected peritoneal macrophages, (d) infected macrophages with amastigotes, 7 days post infection, (e) lesion amastigotes.

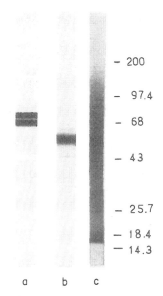

Fig. 3. Immunoblotting of heat shocked L. mexicana promastigotes. (a) Binding of monoclonal antibody B.10. specific for drosophila Hsp70, (b) binding of polyclonal sera raised in rabbit against chicken tubulin, (c) amido black staining of the total amount of proteins on the blot.

DISCUSSION

In this report we follow the synthesis and regulation of the major heat shock proteins in both life stages of Leishmania mexicana promastigotes and amastigotes. Using metabolic labeling of cells, we show that an Hsp70 like protein is constitutively expressed in amastigotes of Leishmania mexicana. This has been shown both for lesion amastigotes and amastigotes grown in vitro within peritoneal macrophages. Hsp70 is also expressed in heat shocked promastigotes, immediately after transfer from 26°C to 35°C, as also shown by other groups[11,12]. Expression of Hsp70 is accompanied by a severe reduction in tubulin synthesis. Tubulin expression has been shown to be stage specific, and its down regulation may be a result of either temperature elevation, or the appearance of Hsp70. The unavailability of a reproducible transformation system in Leishmania and other protozoal organisms, leaves that question still open. Nevertheless, the constitutive expression of Hsp70 in the amastigote stage suggests that this protein is essential for acquisition of thermotolerance and survival within the mammalian host, and most probably is involved in processes that lead to stage differentiation.

The 70 Kd protein that is extensively expressed at 35°C is homologous to the drosophila Hsp70, as shown by cross-reactivity at the immunological level and at the nucleic acid level as well. The role of this protein in leishmania is still unknown. Studies in other systems have shown that Hsp70 is involved in ATP-dependent disruption of protein hydrophobic aggregates[4-6], and it is acceptable that the intracellular survival of the parasite within the mammalian host, at 35°C forms constant stress conditions. Proteins which bear high homology to the drosophila Hsp70 are common in other parasites with biphasic life cycle such as schistosomiasis[10] and malaria[13].

CONCLUSIONS

Expression of the Hsp70 gene in leishmania has been studied in promastigotes of both 26°C and 35°C, and in lesion amastigotes. Hsp70 is constitutively expressed in the amastigote stage as well as in heat shocked promastigotes. Expression of Hsp70 parallels a reduction in tubulin synthesis, both in amastigotes and promastigotes transferred to 35°C. Hsp70 may be essential for acquisition of thermotolerance and for leishmanial stage differentiation.

REFERENCES

1. E.A Craig. The heat shock response in: CRC Critical Reviews in Biochemistry. pp. 239-280 (1985).
2. S. Lindquist. The heat shock response. Ann. Rev. Biochem. 55:1151-1191 (1986).
3. M.J. Schlesinger. Heat shock proteins: The search for functions. J. Cell Biol. 103:321-325 (1986).
4. T.G. Chappel, W.J. Welch, D.M. Schlossman, K.B. Palter, M.J. Schlesinger and J.E. Rothman Uncoating ATPase is a member of the 70 Kd family of stress proteins. Cell 45:3-13 (1986).
5. W.J. Welch, J.R. Feramisco. Rapid purification of mammalian 70,000-Dalton stress proteins: Affinity of the proteins for nucleotides. Mol. Cell Biol. 5:1229-1237 (1985).
6. H.R.B. Pelham and M.J. Lewis. Involvement of ATP in the nuclear and nucleolar functions of the 70 Kd heat shock protein. EMBO J. 4:3137-3143 (1985).
7. H.R.B. Pelham. Speculations of the functions of the major heat shock and glucose regulated proteins. Cell 46: 959-961 (1986).
8. J.Yost and S. Lindquist. RNA splicing is interrupted by heat shock and is rescued by heat shock protein synthesis. Cell 45: 185-193 (1986).
9. C. Schuldt and P.M. Kloetzel. Analysis of cytoplasmic 19S Ring-type particles in Drosophila which contain Hsp23 at normal growth temperatures. Develop. Biol. 110:65-74 (1985).
10. R. Hedstrom, J. Culpepper, R.A. Harrison, N. Agabian and G. Newport. A major immunogen in Schistosoma mansoni infection is homologous to the heat shock protein Hsp70. J. Exp. Med. 165:1430-1435 (1987).
11. E. Lawrence and M. Robert-Gero. Induction of heat shock and stress proteins in promastigotes of three Leishmania species. Proc. Natl. Acad. Sci. USA. 82:4414-4417 (1985)..
12. K.W. Hunter, C.L. Cook and E.G. Hayunga. Leishmania differentiation in vitro: Induction of heat shock proteins. Biochem. Biophys. Res. Commun. 125:755-760 (1984)..
13. F. Ardeshir, J.E. Flint, S.J. Richman and R.T. Reese. A 75 Kd merozoite surface protein of Plasmodium falciparum which is related to the 70 Kd heat-shock proteins. EMBO J. 6:493-499 (1987).
14. K.P. Chang. Human outaneous leishmania in a mouse macrophage line: Propagation and isolation of intracellular parasites. Science. 209:1240 (1980).
15. T. Maniatis, E.F. Fritch, J. Sambrook. Molecular cloning - laboratory manual. (1982).
16. H.R.B. Pelham and R.J. Jackson. An efficient mRNA dependent translation system from reticulocyte lysates. Eur. J. Biochem. 67:247 (1976).

Funding was provided by the John and Catherine T. MacArthur Foundation.

THERMOREGULATED ANTIGEN EXPRESSION BY LEISHMANIA PROMASTIGOTES

Thomas E. Fehniger*, Genene Mengistu, Amare Gessesse,
Hiwot H/Mariam, and Yohannes Negesse

Armauer Hansen Research Institute
P.O. 1005
Addis Ababa, Ethiopia

INTRODUCTION

The biochemical characterization of antigens expressed by Leishmania ssp have often been limited to the promastigote form of the organism because it is difficult to obtain adequate quantities of amastigotes for extended studies. To this date the direct analysis of amastigote antigens has not been possible for some species (ie. L. aethiopica) due to the lack of experimental animal or in vitro infection models. However the development of protective or immunotherapeutic anti-leishmanial vaccines will require the deliniation of T-cell and antibody effector activities against both promastigote and amastigote expressed antigenic determinants.

Amongst the species in which models of experimental infection exist, it has been possible to directly compare promastigotes and purified amastigotes at the molecular level. These studies have shown that the bilateral differentiation of organisms between the two forms is accompanied by significant changes in metabolic and energy utilization pathways[1,2], levels of specific mRNA transcription[3,4], and antigen expression[5,6]. The underlying factors and mechanisms which control the differentiation process are not currently understood however recent evidence suggests that temperature may provide a regulating influence. While the standard conditions for growing promastigotes is normally 22-28°C., the average ambient temperature within the insect vector, recent studies have demonstrated a close homology between promastigotes cultured at higher temperatures (ie. 37°C) and amastigotes, in cell morphology and gene expression[7,8]. Detailed studies of the thermo-induced gene products have identified particular molecules that are related to the family of heat shock proteins (HSP) whose expression is conserved throughout nature, in promastigotes cultured at 37-40°. When directly compared to amastigotes the high temperature cultured promastigotes show similar patterns of synthesis for the HSP of 22-28, 50-54, 69-74, and 80-90 kilodaltons (kd) in molecular weight not observed in organisms grown at standard temperature conditions[8,9,10]. Although the biological role of these thermo-induced molecules in Leishmania differentiation has not been established, these studies have demonstrated that changes in protein synthesis occur which can be associated with the temperature of growth. These studies further show that the patterns of protein expression which occur in organisms cultured at low and high temperature appear to approximate the specific protein profiles of the two morphological forms of the organism.

---

* address correspondence: Karolinska Institute, Department of Infectious Diseases, Roslagstulls Hospital, P.O. 5651, 114 89 Stockholm, Sweden.

The differences in antigen expression, observed between the infective promastigote and intracellular amastigote forms, may play a critical role in influencing host immune reactivity and subsequent disease limitation or progression. The factors which control these variations in antigen expression have not as yet been determined. Since amastigote to promastigote, and promastigote to amastigote conversion can occur simultaneously, the potential for expressing either shared or form specific gene products exists during both stages of differentiation. Hence, we can postulate that the regulation of expression for particular gene products most probably occurs at the level of either RNA transcription of "active" genes or at post transcriptional RNA processing and/or translational pathways[3,4]. The existence of thermal induced genetic elements and regulatory proteins which control specific gene expression have been well documented in both prokaryotic and eukaryotic systems[11]. Thus, it is possible that the temperature at which Leishmania organisms are grown may play a significant role in controlling the expression of particular gene products and the subsequent antigenic profile of the organism.

We have investigated whether changes in antigen expression occur when $25°$ grown promastigotes are cultured at $37°$. Our results show that temperature shifts can promote significant changes in the antigenic profile of Leishmania organisms. Following $37°$ incubation, the induced synthesis of molecules which are antigenically related to amastigote stage expressed determinants, can be demonstrated using antibodies present in infected patient serum. These changes in antigen expression may provide Leishmania parasites with a mechanism for evading host immunity during the initial phases of infection and thus contribute to the organisms' pathogenicity.

MATERIALS AND METHODS

Parasite Stocks. WHO Reference Bank isolates of L. tropica (MHOM/SU/74/K27), L. major (MHOM/SU/73/SASKH) and L. donovani strain LV-9 were obtained as generous gifts from Prof. W. Peters and Dr. J. Blackwell respectively, London School of Hygiene and Tropical Medicine (LSHTM), London, England. L. aethiopica isolates were obtained from biopsies of patients presenting at the All Africa Leprosy Rehabilitation and Training Hospital (ALERT), Addis Ababa, Ethiopia, and were confirmed for species identification by isozyme analysis by Dr. D. Evans, LSHTM.

Organism Propagation. Promastigotes cultured at $25°C$ were grown using standard conditions in RPMI 1640 medium supplemented with 20% heat inactivated fetal calf serum (FLOW), 100 u/ml. penicilin, and 100 ug/ml. streptomycin[12]. This temperature represented the ambient room temperature of the laboratory in Addis Ababa, located at an elevation of 2,200 meters. Parasites were allowed to grow to stationary phase growth cycle before analysis or high temperature incubation. Organisms were cultured at $37°C$ in a Flow Incubator 220, in an atmosphere of 5% carbon dioxide and air, under conditions of free gas exchange, in 100 ml. aliquots in 250 ml. flasks, for a period of 1-5 days. Following culture all organisms were harvested by washing extensively 5 times in 50 ml. volumes of tris-buffered saline ((TSB), 50 mM tris, 150 mM NaCl, pH 7.4), containing 1.2 mM phenyl methyl sulfonyl fluoride (Sigma) and 200 U/ml. Trasylol (Bayer), resuspended in the same buffer and stored at $-70°C$ until use. Amastigotes were purified from spleens and livers of adult Balb/c mice following 10-14 weeks after intra-peritoneal infection as previously described[13].

Serum Samples. Sera from patients clinically and histopathologically diagnosed with either a): localized or diffuse cutaneous leishmaniasis, were obtained under approved guidelines and protocol of the Research Committee of the ALERT Hospital; or b): visceral leishmaniasis, were obtained under approval of the Armed Forces Hospital, Addis Ababa, Ethiopia.

Analysis of Parasite Antigens. Whole cell lysates of organisms were obtained by mixing washed cells from above with a SDS-PAGE sample buffer (pH 6.8) containing 2% SDS, and 5% B-2-mercaptoethanol, final concentration. Samples were placed in a boiling water bath for 5 minutes, and then centrifuged at 14K RPM for 5 minutes to pellet insoluble material. Samples (50 ug protein/0.5 cm gel surface) were separated by the SDS-PAGE electrophoresis system of Laemlli[14], using preparative 10% polyacrylamide resolving slab gels crosslinked 2.6% with bis-acrylamide, of 0.7 mm thickness. Determinations of relative molecular weight were extrapolated using commercial standards (Pharmacia) and beta-galactosidase (Sigma). Following separation the gels were either stained with Coomassie Brilliant Blue, for glyco-conjugates using the periodate silver stain of Tsai and Frasch[15], or Western Blotted onto nitrocellulose (Sartorius, 0.2 micron) using high concentration glycine buffer, as previously described[16].

Serum antibody reactivity with nitrocellulose bound antigen strips was determined using the following previously unpublished procedure. Individual strips were pre-treated to block non-specific binding by rocking in a bath of 0.05% Brij 58 detergent (Sigma) in TSB for one hour, and then incubated overnight by gentle rocking at room temperature with human serum samples diluted 1/40 in the Brij-TSB buffer. Strips were then washed in the same buffer, 4 x 15 minutes, and then incubated with peroxidase conjugated rabbit anti-human IgG, IgM, IgA (heavy and light chain specific (Dako)), for two hours as above. Strips were washed for one hour and then incubated for one hour with 1/100 diluted peroxidase conjugated swine anti-rabbit IgG (Dako). Strips were washed with Brij-TSB 4 x 15 minutes and then with distilled deionized water for 5 minutes. Color development was achieved by reacting with the substrate solution (final concentration: 0.01% 4-chloro-1-naphthol (Sigma) dissolved in DMSO, and 0.003% hydrogen peroxide, in TSB, pH 7.4), using vigorous shaking (150 rpm), for 10 minutes.

RESULTS

Effect of Temperature on L. donovani Promastigote Antigen Expression

When L. donovani (LV-9) promastigotes were cultured at 37°C, changes in the antigenic proile of the organisms occurred within the first day of culture, and were maintained over 3 days of culture. In figure 1A the reactivity of antibodies from a L. donovani infected patient serum are shown with antigens expressed by promastigotes grown at 25°C (lane A), at 37°C for 1 day (lane B), and at 37°C for 3 days (lane C).

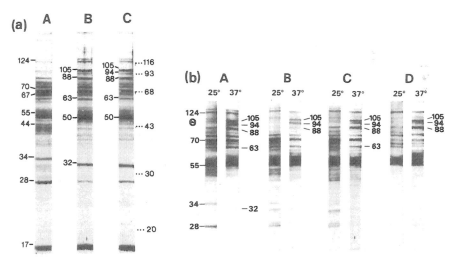

Fig. 1. Differences in antigen expression between L. donovani promastigotes cultured 25°C and 37°C detected with patient serum antibodies. (a) Kinetics of change. Promastigotes were grown at 25° (lane A), 37° for 1 day (lane B) or 37° for 3 days (lane C). Whole cell lysates were seperated by SDS-PAGE, immuno-blotted, and reacted with serum from a patient with visceral leishmaniasis. (b). Crossreactivity of 37° induced antigens with antibodies present in infected patients. Four individual sera (lanes A-C) were reacted with promastigotes grown at 25° or 37° for 3 days.

While many of the major antigenic determinants such as the 55 kd tubulin protein (also 17, 28, and 70 kd antigens) expressed by 25°C grown cells were maintained throughout 37°C culture, significant changes in the profile were observed. The 37°C grown organisms expressed prominent antigenic bands of 32, 50, 63, 88, 94, and 105 kd which were either not detected or equivalently expressed by 25°C grown organisms. Conversely, some antigens expressed by 25°C grown organisms were not expressed equally at 37°C, notably molecules of 34, 40-44, and 67 kd. The relatively strong reactivity of this serum sample from a patient with established disease suggested that the induced determinants most probably are antigenically related to molecules which are expressed by amastigotes during infection. To determine whether the observed antibody reactivity was limited to particular patients we tested four other serum samples from patients diagnosed with visceral leishmaniasis. The antibody reactivities of these sera with promastigotes cultured at 25°C, and at 37°C for 3 days, is shown in figure 1B. While some differences in individual patient seroreactivity was seen, all of the samples tested contained antibodies which recognized the higher molecular weight antigens of 63, 88, 94, and 105 kd particularly expressed by the 37°C grown L. donovani cells.

A comparison of the total protein profiles of the L. donovani organisms cultured at 25°C, or at 37°C for 1 or 3 days (Fig. 2A) showed a correlative increase in the relative amounts of molecules with molecular weights analogous to those of the antigens induced in the 37°C grown organisms. The increased expression of the 50, 63, 88, and 105 kd proteins was detectable following the first day of 37°C culture. In addition to the differences in total protein profiles in organisms cultured under the two temperature conditions, a change in glycoconjugate expression was also observed (Fig. 2B). Several molecules (32, 39, 41, 48, 60, 63, 80, and 94 kd) which stained with the periodate silver technique were expressed following 37°C culture, which were not similarly seen at 25°C. Three of the induced antigens (70, 88, and 105 kd) were negatively stained and thus most probably are not glyco-proteins in composition.

Antigen Expression by L. donovani Amastigotes

To determine if molecules similar to those seen in 37°C grown promastigotes are expressed by amastigotes, we analyzed organisms purified from infected animals following separation on SDS-PAGE and immunoblotting as above. In figure 3, the serum antibody

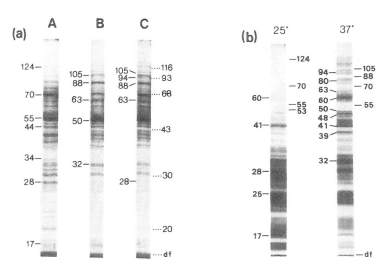

Fig. 2 Differences in protein and glycoconjugate profiles of L. donovani promastigotes cultured at 25°C and 37°C. (a) Coomassie Blue stained gel of promastigotes cultured at 25° (lane A), 37° for 1 day (lane B), or 37° for 3 days (lane C). (b) Periodate silver stained gel of glyco-conjugates expressed by promastigotes at 25° and after 3 days of 37° culture. Note negative staining of 55, 70, 88, and 105 kd molecules.

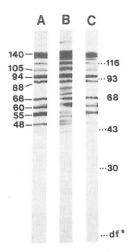

Fig. 3. Antigens of L. donovani amastigotes reactive with patient antibodies. Purified amastigotes were separated by SDS-PAGE, immunoblotted, and reacted with three individual sera (lanes A-C) from patients with visceral leishmaniasis.

binding reactivities of three patients (lanes A, B, C) with visceral leishmaniasis are shown. A general trend in the recognition of higher molecular weight molecules was observed. Major antigenic determinants recognized commonly by the patients included molecules of 48, 55, 60, 68, 88, 94, 105, and 140 kd. Therefore amastigotes do appear to express molecules of similar molecular weight to the 88, 94, and 105 kd antigens induced in 37° grown promastigotes. However further studies on the immunological and biochemical relationships of the amastigote and thermo-induced molecules will be required to confirm their identities.

Thermo-Regulated Antigen Expression in Other Leishmania Species

The expression of thermo-regulated antigens is not restricted to the LV-9 isolate of L. donovani tested but appears to be a common property of several different Leishmania ssp. In figure 4A, the Western blots of three isolates of L. aethiopica, 190/85 (lanes A), 1773/85 (lanes B), and 1471/85 (lanes C), cultured at 25°C and 37°C, are shown following incubation with a L. aethiopica infected patient serum sample. While some micro-heterogeneity in antigen expression was observed between the individual isolates, enhanced expression of 38, 57, 64, 67, and 94 kd antigens occurred in all three of the samples, following 37°C incubation.

The antigens induced at 37°C appear to possess crossreactive epitopes which are conserved on a variety of molecules expressed by several different Leishmania ssp. Figure 4B shows that antigens expressed at 37°C by L. major (lanes A) of 28, 42, 45, 67, 70, and 80 kd, L. tropica (lanes B) of 35, 46, 66, 70, 80, and 94 kd, and L. aethiopica (lanes C) of 94 kd, are recognized by antibodies which develop in patients infected with L. donovani. Again, these determinants did not appear to be equivalently expressed by these same isolates at 25°C. The induced antigens detected in the different species differed in molecular weight, and thus are not identical, however, their crossreactivity with patient antibodies indicates that at least a subset of the epitopes expressed on these molecules are antigenically if not structurally related.

DISCUSSION

The two dimorphic stages of Leishmania parasite differentiation are associated with growth within either the insect vector or the mammalian host. The environments which organisms occupy as infective promastigotes residing in the insect midgut or as amastigotes within phagocytic macrophages are sufficiently different to suggest that

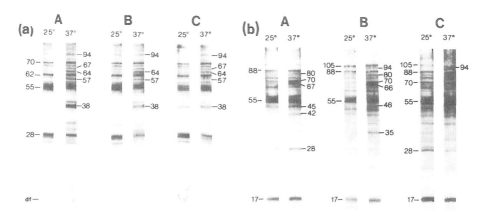

Fig. 4. Thermo-regulated antigen expression by different Leishmania ssp. Promastigotes grown at 25°C, and 37°C for 3 days were separated by SDS-PAGE and immuno-blotted. (a) L. aethiopica isolates (lanes A-C) reacted with serum from L. aethiopica infected patient. (b) Crossreactivity of thermo-regulated antigens. Isolates of L. major (lanes A), L. tropica (lanes B), and L. aethiopica (lanes C), reacted with serum from patient with visceral leishmaniasis infected with L. donovani.

specialized mechanisms for growth maintainance have evolved which are differentially utilized in response to particular changes in the conditions encountered. One of the environmentally determined conditions which changes between promastigote and amastigote form development is the ambient temperature maintained by the host. Promastigotes are readily grown in vitro at 22-28°C., the temperature which corresponds to growth in the insect vector, however several previous studies have documented the similarities which relate promastigotes cultured at higher temperature with amastigotes. These include changes in morphology (cylidrical flagellates to non-motile spherical bodies), and in the expression of specific gene products [7-10]. The results presented in this study suggest that antigen expression by promastigotes changes shortly after encountering the temperature which occurs within the mammalian host following infection.

We have examined the influence of temperature on antigen expression in four species of Leishmania which cause either cutaneous (L. aethiopica, L. major, and L. tropica) or disseminating visceral disease (L. donovani). Promastigotes from each of these species cultured in vitro in the same medium, under two temperature conditions (25° and 37°), were found to change their pattern of antigen expression. The promastigotes cultured at 37° expressed several antigenic molecules that were not equivalently expressed during 25° culture. These high temperature induced determinants are "amastigote-like", as defined by their crossreactivity with serum antibodies from infected patients with established disease. In addition, when the patterns of antigen expression of 25° grown promastigotes, 37° grown promastigotes, and amastigotes are directly compared on immuno-blots, the 37° grown organisms show striking similarity to the tissue derived amastigotes.

The antigenic profile of each of the different species tested in this study varied following 37° culture. These differences may be due to evolutionary divergence between particular species. However, the specific thermo-induced molecules expressed by the different species are antigenically related to one another. This is evidenced by the serological crossreactivity of antibodies in L. donovani infected patient serum with 37° expressed antigens of L. major, L. tropica, and L. aethiopica. Therefore at least some epitopes on these determinants are conserved between different species of Leishmania. The possible benefits of using thermal manipulation for experimental purposes can be best exemplified in studies of L. aethiopica. Since amastigotes of L. aethiopica are difficult to obtain due to the lack of experimental models, culture temperature manipulation may provide a useful means of acquiring sufficient quantities of amastigote related determinants for characterization and immuno-biological study.

We have used L. donovani as a model system to analyze the kinetics, and establish preliminary biochemical characterizations, of the antigens in which temperature influenced regulation of expression is observable. Changes in the antigenic profile of molecules reactive with patient serum antibodies occurred within 24 hours following culture at 37°. Both qualitative and quantitative modulations in the antigenic profile of 25° grown promastigotes were observable. Promastigotes grown at 37° selectively expressed immunogenic determinants with molecular weights of 32, 50, 63, 88, 94, and 105 kd. The expression of these antigens was stable over 5 days of 37° culture (data not shown). The relative high molecular weights of these molecules argues against their origin as simple breakdown products of previously expressed promastigote antigens. A corresponding increase in the relative amounts of the antigenic molecules seen on immuno-blots of 37° cultured organisms was seen on gels stained for total protein. Since patterns of glyco-conjugate expression also differed between 25° and 37° culture conditions, we conclude that whole pathways of post-transcriptional protein processing are probably affected by the temperature change. Moreover, the changes in glyco-conjugate expression may be related to the reported differences in glycosylation which seperate infective and non-infective promastigotes [17].

The biological significance and activities of the molecules in which thermo-regulated expression occurs in Leishmania ssp has not as yet been determined. It is possible that these induced molecules are related to heat shock proteins, as suggested previously[8-10]. However, since their expression occurs at temperatures which the organism has adapted for its stages of growth, the functions of these proteins probably differ from the activities of protective adaptation ascribed to HSPs during periods of stress[11]. We have found that in L. donovani cells cultured at 37°, a glyco-protein antigen of 63 kd is induced, which is similar in size to the conserved surface protein which has been previously descibed as the attachment ligand to host macrophages[18-19]. It is concievable that the expression of molecules which are particularily necessary for establishing infection in the mammallian host are regulated by environmental influences such as temperature.

The role which thermo-regulated molecules play in the interactions between the pathogen and the host deserve particular attention. One possible consequence of the thermo-regulated expression of particular molecules by Leishmania promastigotes is that the infective form of the parasite has the capacity, through differential gene expression, to partially shield its antigenic identity during the initial phase of infection. This could allow the organism to establish intra-cellular residence before significant immune reactivity to key determinants develops. The possibility that the induced antigens could function as immuno-regulatory determinants, effecting specific suppression or promoting antibody mediated masking which hinders effector cell function once infection is established, might also be addressed in further studies.

CONCLUSIONS

The results of this study demonstrate that thermo-modulated changes in antigen expression occur in Leishmania species. These changes were detectable at the level of differences in the specific patterns of antigen recognition by serum antibody from patients with established disease, and protein and glyco-conjugate staining of cell lysates separated on SDS-PAGE gels. The temperature induced changes in antigen expression were observed in parasites causing cutaneous (L. aethiopica, L. major, and L. tropica) and visceralizing (L. donovani) disease. Promastigotes cultured at 37^oC expressed "amastigote-like" antigenic determinants which were not equivalently expressed by promastigotes cultured at 25^oC. The results of this study suggest that the changes in antigen expression which occur between the promastigote and amastigote form of the parasite can at least in part be regulated by the temperature in which organisms are grown. The antigenic variation which differentiates the insect vector and mammalian host stages of Leishmania may play an important role in the disease process. The use of this model system may provide access to biologically important molecules which are not available for study using conventionally cultured promastigotes and may contribute to our understanding of the molecular basis of pathogenicity of this organism.

REFERENCES

1. D. T. Hart, and G.H. Coombs, Leishmania mexicana. Energy metabolism of amastigotes and promastigotes, Exp. Parasitol., 54:397, (1982).
2. J. C. Meade, T.A. Glaser, P.F. Boneventure, and A.J. Mukkada, Enzymes of carbohydrate metabolism in Leishmania donovani amastigotes, J. Protozool., 31:156, (1984).
3. M. Wallach, D. Fong, and K-P. Chang, Post-transcriptional control of tubulin biosynthesis during Leishmania differentiation, Nature, 299:656, (1982).
4. S. M. Landfear, and D.F. Wirth, Control of tubulin gene expression in the parasitic protozoan Leishmania enrietti, Nature, 309:716, (1982).
5. E. Handman, and J.M. Curtis, Leishmania tropica: Surface antigens of intracellular and flagellate forms, Exp. Parasitol., 54:243, (1982).
6. E. Handman, H.M. Jarvis, and G.F. Mitchell, Leishmania major: Identification of stage specific antigens and antigens shared by promastigotes and amastigotes, Parasit. Immunol., 6:233, (1984).
7. K. W. Hunter, C.L. Cook, and S.A. Hensen, Temperature induced in vitro transformation of Leishmania mexicana, 1. Ultrastructural comparison of culture transformed and intracellular amastigotes, Acta Tropica, 39:143, (1982).
8. K. W. Hunter, C.L. Cook, and E.G. Hayunga, Leishmania differentiation in vitro: Induction of heat shock proteins, Biochem. and Biophys. Res. Commun., 125:755 (1984).
9. L. H. van der Ploeg, S.H. Giannini, and C.S. Cantor, Heat shock genes: Regulatory role for differentiation in parasitic protozoa, Science, 228:1443, (1985).
10. F. Lawrence, and M. Robert-Gero, Induction of heat shock and stress proteins in promastigotes of three Leishmania species, Proc. Nat. Acad. Sci. U.S.A., 82:4414, (1985).
11. R. H. Burdon, Heat shock and heat shock proteins, Biochem. J., 240:313, (1986).
12. L. D. Hendricks, D.E. Wood, and M.E. Hajduk, Hemoflagelates: commercially available liquid media for rapid cultivation, Parasitol. 76:209, (1978).
13. D. T. Hart, K. Vickerman, and G.H. Coombs, A quick simple method for purifying Leishmania mexicana amastigotes in large numbers, Parasitol., 82:345, (1981).
14. U. K.Laemlli, Cleavage of structural proteins during the assembly of the head of bacteriophage T4, Nature, 227:680, (1970).
15. C. M. Tsai, and C.F. Frasch, A sensitive silver stain for detecting lipopolysacharides in polyacrylamide gels, Anal. Biochem., 119:115, (1982)
16. T. E. Fehniger, A.M. Walfield, T.M. Cunningham, J.D. Radolf, J.N. Miller, and M.A. Lovett, Purification and characterization of a cloned protease resistant Treponema pallidum specific antigen, Infect. Immun., 46:598, (1984).
17. D. L. Sacks, S. Hieny, and A. Sher, Identification of cell surface carbohydrate and antigenic changes between non-infective and infective developmental stages of Leishmania major promastigotes, J. Immunol., 135:564, (1985).
18. R. J. Etges, J. Bouvier, R. Hoffman, and C. Bordier, Evidence that the major surface proteins of three Leishmania species are structurally related, Mol. and Biochem. Parasitol., 14:141, (1985).
19. D. G. Russell, and H. Wilhelm, The involvement of the major surface glycoproteins (gp 63) of Leishmania promastigotes in attachment to macrophages, J. Immunol., 136:2613, (1986).

A SIMPLE, HIGHLY REPETITIVE SEQUENCE IN THE LEISHMANIA GENOME

John Ellis and Julian Crampton

Wolfson Unit of Molecular Genetics
Liverpool School of Tropical Medicine
Liverpool L3 5QA

INTRODUCTION

Leishmania are simple unicellular protozoa which are tramsitted by the bite of an infected sandfly, producing a spectrum of clinical diseases in man[1]. Since their discovery in 1903, the organisation of the genome of this clinically important protozoan has received little attention. We have used DNA hybridisation studies to identify many of the repetitive DNA sequences in the Leishamania genome. Here we report the characterisation of the most highly repetitive DNA sequence that we have been able to isolate. Differences in copy number and organisation of this sequence within the Leishmania genome may well contribute to the chromosome size variations previously reported by other investigators.

The commercial exploitation of hypervariable DNA sequences have recently been highlighted by the elegant work of Jeffreys et al[2] who used a simple repetitive DNA sequnce for the fingerprinting of human DNA. DNA fingerprints have proven a powerful method for individual identification, establishing family relationships and in forensic science. We report here that the simple repetitive sequence described above may also be used for the DNA fingerprinting of Leishamania strains and species.

Repetitive DNA seqeunces with their high copy number are particularly amenable for use as DNA probes in the detection of parasites in clinical material. The simple, highly repetitive sequence described in this report has been used to derive a synthetic, oligonucleotide probe which may be used as a sensitive means for the detection of this parasite.

MATERIALS AND METHODS

Cultivation of Parasites and Preparation of DNA

Leishamania were grown in HOMEM medium supplemented with 10% heat-inactivated fetal calf serum at 26°C. Cells were used immediately for DNA preparation or stored at -70°C for use later.

Genomic DNA was extracted the by procedure of Van der Ploeg[3] and essentially involved the use of Sarkosyl and proteinase K followed by two successive rounds of ethidium bromide/cesium chloride centrifugation.

Cot Analysis of L.donovani Genomic DNA

Renaturation of LV9 genomic DNA was followed using S1 nuclease analysis coupled with TCA precipitation[4]. Driver DNA was sheared by sonication to a mean size of 700bp and tracer DNA was prepared by nick translation of genomic DNA to activities greater than 5×10^7 cpm/ug.

Preparation of a sheared genomic DNA library

Genomic DNA was sonicated to a mean size of 700bp and blunt-ended using T4 polymerase. This DNA was then ligated into the EcoRV site of pAT153 and transformed into E.coli strain MC1060. Recombinants were screened at high density using the method of Hanahan and Meselsohn[5], washed and autoradiographed at -70°C with an intensifying screen.

Oligonucleotide synthesis

The oligonucleotide 3'-CCCAATCCCAATCCCAAT-5' was synthesised using the B-cyanoethylamidite chemistry adapted for use with controlled-pore glass supports[6]. Deprotection and cleavage of the synthesised oligonucleotide was accomplished using concentrated ammonia solution.

Radiolabelling and hybridisation of DNA probes

Double-stranded DNA was radiolabelled by the procedure of nick-translation[7]. The probes were boiled before use and hybrisations were performed overnight in 5 x SSC, 50% formamide, 1mM EDTA and 100ug/ml denatured, sonicated herring sperm DNA at 43°C.

Oligonucleotides were kinased at the 5' position using γ-ATP (Amersham, 5000Ci/mMol) and T4 polynucleotide kinase as described by Maniatis, Fritsch and Sambrook[8], followed by desalting on Sephadex G-25. Hybridisation of the oligo-probes was performed at 37°C for two hours in 6 x SSC, 10 x Denhardt's, 10ug/ml yeast tRNA and 100ug/ml denatured, sonicated herring sperm DNA.

Dot blots

Total parasite DNA was denatured for 10 minutes in 0.5M NaOH, 5 x SSC at room temperature. The solution was then neutralised and dotted onto nitrocellulose using a dot blot manifold (S & S) connected to a suction pump. The nitrocellulose was rinsed in 6 x SSC and the filter baked at 80°C for two hours.

Cultured promastigotes were lysed directly on nitrocellulose according to the procedure of Massamba and Williams[9].

RESULTS

Cot Analysis of L.donovani Genomic DNA

Non-linear regression analysis of the renaturation of LV9 DNA allows the separation of genomic DNA into 3 components and Table 1 shows the proportions of these fractions in the genome of LV9, along with the calculated complexities of each of component. About 10% of the DNA failed to reassociate and was probably considerably degraded. By a summation of the total number of bases present in each of the 3 components, it can be calculated that the haploid genome size of LV9 is of the order of 3.3×10^7 bp. No allowance has been made in this calculation for the possible effect of GC content on the rate of reassociation.

Table 1. Renaturation data for L.donovani strain LV9

Component	Fraction of Genome	Cot $_{1/2}$	Sequence Complexity	Reiteration Frequency
1	0.1387	$3-7 \times 10^{-6}$	6-12	$3-7 \times 10^5$
2	0.186	0.324	9.7×10^4	73
3	0.6212	23.6	2.4×10^7	1

Peparation and Screening of a Sheared Genomic Library

With a view to the cloning and subsequent identification of repetitive DNA sequences from the L.donovani genome, genomic DNA was sheared and cloned as detailed in the methods. Between 5-10 clones were obtained/ng of genomic DNA used in the ligation reaction. Screening of this library with a total genomic DNA probe should allow the identification of highly repeated DNA sequences in the genome. 22,500 clones of an amplified stock were screened with ^{32}P-labelled nick-translated, genomic DNA. Overnight autoradiography of the washed filters revealed approximately 0.17% of the clones showing a strong hybridisation signal. These clones were assumed to be homologous to sequences present at high copy number in the LV9 genomic DNA. No hybridisation was detected with a kinetoplast DNA probe.

Preliminary Characterisation of Genomic Repetitive Clones

8 clones (called pRs) showing the strongest hybridisation to LV9 genomic DNA in our colony screen were grown in L-broth and plasmid DNA purified. This DNA was nick-translated and used as a probe onto Southern blots of HaeIII digested genomic DNA from LV9 and LV710 and the result is shown in Figure 1A. Numerous bands of hybridisation were evident in many size ranges. This result was interpreted as representing a high level of dispersion of this repetitive sequence throughout the Leishmania genome. This experiment also revealed slight differences in the organisation of these sequences within the genomes of these 2 Leishmania donovani strains (indicated by the arrow heads). All the pRs series of clones showed exactly the same hybridisation pattern implying that they represent members of the same class of repetitive sequences.

PRs2A was subsequently hybridised to HindIII digests of genomic DNA from a variety of Leishmania species (Figure 1B). The patterns of hybridisation seen in these blots indicated significant differences in the genomic distribution of this repetitive sequence. Strong hybridisation was present to several large DNA fragments in the strains DD8 and LEM235. The single representative of L.donovani chagasi had a more dispersed pattern of hybridisation to the pRs2A probe. This is also true of a second L. donovani chagasi (LV474) strain that we have studied.

Subcloning and DNA sequence Analysis

Insert DNAs from 2 of the pRs clones were gel purified and subcloned into M13 and sequenced by the dideoxy method[11]. Sequence analysis of pRs2A and 11A revealed in addition to flanking, apparently non-repetitive sequences, large blocks of the simple hexanucleotide sequence 5' CCCTAA 3' repeated in tandem. These constituted approximately 50% of the inserted DNA sequences; clone 2A contained 27 repeats of this sequence and 11A contained two runs of the basic repeat with 4 and 13 copies.

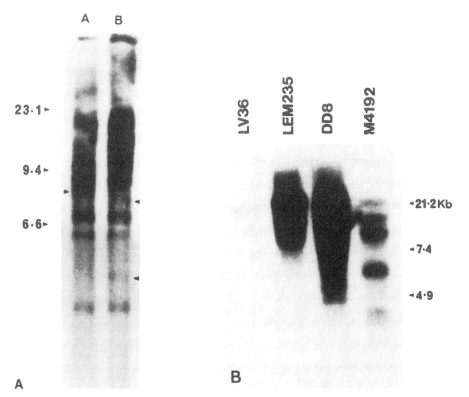

Figure 1   Southern Blot Analysis of Leishmania DNAs probed with the CCCTAA repeat. A: HaeIII digests of LV710 (Lane A) and LV9 (Lane B) genomic DNA. B:HindIII digested genomic DNA from 4 different Leishmania species.

Copy Number Determination

DNA sequence analysis indicated that the repeat sequence CCCTAA constituted 2.7% of the total mass of the recombinant plasmid pRs11A. Consequently, it was possible to determine the copy number of this sequence within the Leishmania genome by a comparative DNA hybridisation methodology as described in the Methods.

The copy number of the CCCTAA repeat was determined for LV9 and other Leishmania isolates and the results are summarised in Table 2.

Table 2   Variation in copy number of the CCCTAA repeat in different Leishmania isolates.

Organism	Origin	Copy Number/ Haploid Genome
L.donovani		
LV9	Ethiopia	5.8×10^5
DD8	India	1.5×10^5
L.donovnai chagasi		
M4192	Brazil	2.3×10^5
L.donovani infantum		
LEM235	Tunisia	3.3×10^4
L.major		
LV561	Jordan	3.3×10^4

Variation of this sequence not only occurs between different Leishmania species, but also appears to vary between isolates of the same species. The L. donovani isolates LV9 and DD8 contain very different numbers of the sequence under study.

Organisation of the CCCTAA repeat within the genome of L.donovani

In order to determine the distribution the CCCTAA repeat within the genome of L.donovani, intact chromosomal DNA from LV9 promastigotes was prepared and separated by Pulse Field Gradient Electrophesis (PFGE) using the method of Carle and Olson[11]. After staining with Ethidium Bromide the DNA was denatured and Southern blotted and hybridised to the ^{32}P-labelled oligonucleotide probe containing the CCCTAA repeat unit. A switching time of 85 seconds was used. Figure 2A shows the ethidium stained gel and Figure 2B the Southern transfer hybridised to the CCCTAA repeat sequence.

Hybridisation at very low intensity was apparent to all of the chromosomal DNA molecules seen on these gels. This is to be expected if these sequences were either located randomly throughout the genome or if they were exclusively located at the telomeric sites on all chromosomes as in the Trypanosoma[12]. However, the data of Blackburn and Challoner [13] does support the latter notion that these sequences are confirmed to telomeric locations in the Leishmania.

Fingerprinting of Leishmania DNAs using the CCCTAA repeat

Genomic DNA from a variety of Leishmania isolates were digested with a number of different restriction enzymes and subsequently electrophoresed through a 1% agarose gel. Southern blots were then hybridised to a ^{32}P-labelled probe containing the CCCTAA repeat sequence, the filters washed at high stringency and autoradiographed. The result obtained for just two Leishmania isolates is shown in Figure 3A (L.donovani chagasi, M4192) and 3B (L.major, LV561). This experiment confirmed the initial observations (see above) that hybridisation was present to a large number of restriction fragments of many different sizes. It is clear from these and similar experiments that is should be possible to use the CCCTAA repeat probe as a means of fingerprinting different Leishmania isolates.

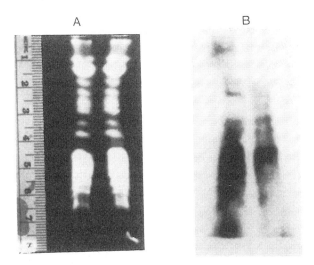

Figure 2. Chromosomal distribution of the CCCTAA repeat. Pulsed field electrophoresis of L.donovani strain LV9 using 85 second switch time. A: Ethidium bromide stained gel and B: Southern transfer hybridised to CCCTAA.

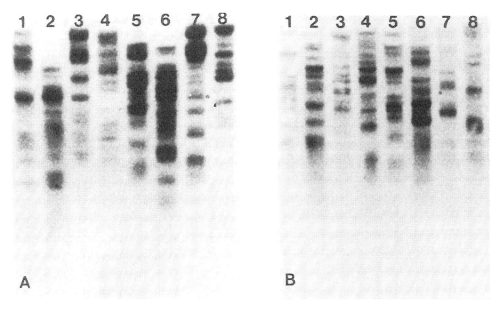

Figure 3. Fingerprinting of Leishmania DNAs. Southern hybridisation of L.donovani chagasi (A) and L.major (B) DNAs digested with 1:HindIII, 2:PvuII, 3:SmaI, 4:BamHI, 5:EcoRV, 6:XhoI, 7:XbaI, 8:DraI

Sensitivity of the CCCTAA oligo probe for the detection of L.donovani

The sensitivity of the kinased 18 mer oligonucleotide as a DNA probe for the detection of LV9 was determined by hybridisation to doubling dilutions of genomic DNA dotted onto nitrocellulose filters (Figure 4A). After hybridisation at 37°C for two hours with a probe concentration of 8ng/ml the filter was washed in 2 x SSC at room temperature. The filter was then autoradiographed at -70°C with a preflashed film and screen. Densitometric scanning of the film exposed for 18 hours revealed that 0.1pg of genomic DNA or 244 parasites could just be detected (Fig.4B). This level of sensitivity was at the limit of radioisotope detection, since even with longer exposures there was no further differentiation from background.

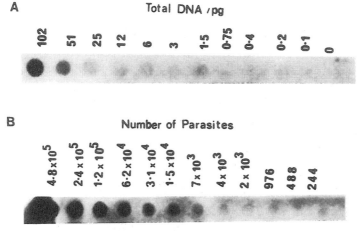

Figure 4. Sensitivity of the CCCTAA repeat for detecting L.donovani
The ^{32}P-labelled 18 mer oligonucleotide was hybridised to A: doubling dilutions of LV9 genomic DNA and B: LV9 parasites lysed in-situ on nitrocellulose.

DISCUSSION

We report here evidence for the presence of a highly repetitive DNA sequence in the genome of L.donovani and other related species of Leishmania. Analysis of the cloned DNA sequences has indicated that this repetitive sequence consists of a simple hexanucleotide, 5' CCCTAA 3'. This sequence is identical to the telomeric repeats found in Trypanosoma brucei and other species[12]. Our results of hybridisation of the repeat to Southern blots of PFGE gels indicates that the sequence is widely distributed in the genome and may occur at the telomeres of chromosomes of L.donovani[13].

There is considerable heterogeneity observed in the distribution and copy number of this repeat and associated hybridising sequences throughout the genomes of different Leishmania species. Results reported here support the notion that use of this simple repetitive sequence may have value as a means of fingerprinting the DNA of different Leishmania isolates. Indeed, we have yet to witness the same pattern of hybridisation of this repeat to any 2 Leishmania isolates. However, using restriction enzymes that are considered to be 'infrequent cutters', many of the Old World isolates considered to be L.donovani are truely similar. Two isolates previously typed and described as L.donovani chagasi showed a pattern of hybridisation which is very different from that of the Old World Leishmania. This supports the karyotype profiles of Giannini et al[14] in suggesting that L. donovani chagasi is probably an indigenous parasite of South America.

Finally, the use of an oligonucleotide probe derived from a number of copies of the hexanucleotide repeat can provide a rapid and sensitive means of detecting target DNA sequences. Hybridisation of a specific 18 mer to Leishmania genomic DNA occurs at extremely low probe concentrations and is complete within 2 hours. The realisation that simple telomeric sequences are not conserved between genera[13] implies that a good level of specificity may be obtained in that this sequence may be viewed as being specific for Leishmania and Trypanosoma species.

REFERENCES

1. P.E.C. Manson-Bahr and F.I.C Apted, "Manson's Tropical diseases", Bailliere Tindall (1983)
2. A.J. Jeffreys, V. Wilson and S.L. Thein, Individual-specific 'fingerprinting' of human DNA, Nature, 316:176 (1985)
3. L.H.T. Van der Ploeg, M. Smits, T. Ponnudurai, A. Vermeulen, J.Meuwissen and G. Langley, Chromosome-sized DNA molecules of Plasmodium falciparum, Science 229:658 (1984)
4. R.J. Britten, D.E. Graham, F.C. Eden, D.M. Painchaud and E.N. Davidson, J. Mol. Evol., 9:1 (1976)
5. D. Hanahan and M. Meselsohn, Plasmid screening at high colony density, Gene, 10:62 (1980)
6. M.J. Gait, "Oligonucleotide Synthesis - a Practical Approach" IRL Press, Oxford (1984)
7. P.W.J Rigby, M. Deckmann, C. Rhodes and P. Berg, Labelling DNA to high specific activity in vitro by nick-translation with DNA polymerase I. J.Mol. Biol. 113:1237 (1977)
8. T. Maniatis, E.F. Fritsch and J. Sambrook "Molecular Cloning. A laboratory Manual" Cold Spring Harbor, USA. (1982)
9. N.N. Massamba and R.O. Williams, Parasitology 88:55 (1984)
10. F. Sanger, S. Nicklen and A.R. Coulsen, DNA sequencing with chain termination inhibitors. Proc. Nat. Acad. Sci. 74:5463 (1977)
11. G.F. Carle and M.V. Olson, Nucl. Acids Res. 12:5647 (1984)
12. L.H.T. Van der Ploeg, A.Y.C. Liu and P. Borst, Structure of the growing telomeres of Trypanosomes. Cell 36:459 (1984)
13. E.H. Balckburn and P.B. Challoner Cell 36:447 (1984)
14. S.H. Giannini, M. Schittini, J.S. Keithly, P.W. Warburton, C.R. Cantor and L.H.T. Van der Ploeg, Karyotype analysis of Leishmania species and its use in classification and clinical diagnosis. Science 232:762 (1986)

CLONING AND CHARACTERISATION OF LEISHMANIA DONOVANI GENES CODING FOR IMMUNODOMINANT ANTIGENS

John M. Kelly, Mark L. Blaxter, Elaine Kellet, and Michael A. Miles
Wolfson Unit/Department of Medical Protozoology
London School of Hygiene and Tropical Medicine
Keppel Street
London   WC1E 7HT   UK

INTRODUCTION

Organisms of the <u>Leishmania donovani</u> complex are the causative agents of human visceral leishmaniasis. The genetics of <u>L. donovani</u> are not well understood, no prophylatic immunisation is available and medical and epidemiological studies of the disease and its transmission are greatly inhibited by lack of a reliable, specific and rapid means of diagnosis.

<u>Leishmania</u> express a range of antigens on their surface and it is of interest to examine the roles of these antigens in the infection process, in survival within the macrophage lysosomes and in interaction with the host immune system. Purified antigens which elicit a species-specific immunological response could form the basis of a rapid means of diagnosis.

In an attempt to define candidate diagnostic reagents or vaccines and to gain more understanding of <u>Leishmania</u> genetics we have isolated several cDNA clones which correspond to immunodominant antigens of <u>L. donovani</u> from a λgt11 expression library. The characteristics and properties of two of these cDNA clones are described.

METHODS

Construction and screening of λgt11 expression library

Blunt-ended double stranded cDNA was made from 2µg of polyA$^+$ RNA isolated from <u>L. donovani</u> promastigotes (MHOM/ET/67/HU3) using the RNase H method (1). The cDNA was tailed with E.CORI linkers and ligated with 1µg of ECORI cut, phosphorylated λgt11 arms (2). The products of ligation were packaged into infective phage particles using a Gigapack kit (Stratagene).

A single high titre (>1:2000) visceral leishmaniasis serum (codename TF1) was chosen to screen the library. The patient from whom the serum was taken had become infected in Sudan, and was successfully treated in the Hospital for Tropical Diseases, London. This serum was strongly reactive with <u>L. donovani</u> antigen on Western blots. Screening was performed on 10^5 phage plaques by the method of Hyunh et al. (2) using radioiodinated protein A (Amersham) as the secondary screening reagent. Positive plaques were detected after overnight autoradiography at -70°C. These plaques were rescreened at lower density until single clones could be picked. They were stored as amplified phage stocks, and lysogenised into E. Coli Y1089 (2).

Identification of native antigen by western blotting

The serum used to screen the library reacted to many Leishmania antigens. In order to identify the native antigens which corresponded to selected cDNA clones, the serum was first affinity purified against the expression fusion protein immobilised on nitrocellulose filters (3). Leishmania antigen was prepared for SDS-polyacrylamide gel electrophoresis (PAGE) from both promastergotes and amastergoted. The cells were extensively washed in PBS before lysis to remove media contamination. Whole membrane preparations were made from freeze-thawed lysed promastigotes by the method of Dwyer (4). Fusion proteins were prepared from lysogens as described (2). 7-20% gradient SDS-PAGE of the above antigens (40mg per track) were run and transferred onto nitrocellulose by western blotting (5). Antibody diluted 1 in 100 was added and the filters incubated with gentle shaking for 1 hour. Excess unbound antibody was washed off with PBS and the secondary antibody (1 in 1000dilutions of mouse anti-human immunoglobulin heavy and light chains conjugated to horseradish peroxidase) added and incubated for a further hour. The bound peroxidase was visualised by reaction with H_2O_2 and chloronapthol.

Specificity of human leishmaniasis sera in recognising fusion proteins

Lysogen lysates were fractionated on 8% preparative SDS-PAGE gels and the proteins transferred onto a nitrocellulose filter by western blotting. The filter was cut into 5mm wide longitudinal strips and probed (as above) with 1 in 100 dilutions of sera from patients with leishmaniasis and other infections. Reaction with the fusion proteins was scored on a +/- basis. As a control, strips containing λgt11 wild type lysogen lysate were also probed. These gave negative results in all cases.

Analysis of RNA and DNA

High molecular weight genomic DNA was isolated from Leishmania cells by the proteinase K method (6). The DNA was phenol extracted and dialysed prior to restriction digestion and southern hybridisation. RNA was extracted from cells after lysis with 4M guanidinium thiocyanate and pelleted by centrifugation through a 5.7m Caesium Chloride gradient (7). Northern analysis was performed under standard conditions (6). Orthogonal field alteration gel electrophoresis (OFAGE) was carried out as described previously (8).

RESULTS

A λgt11 expression library was constructed with mRNA from the promastigote form of L. donovani (African isolate HU3).$6x10^5$ clones were obtained, of which >80% were recombinants (Methods). Aliquots from this library were screened with serum TF1 which had been obtained from a patient infected with visceral leishmaniasis in Sudan. Several cDNA clones that expressed β.galactosidase/L. donovani antigen fusion proteins were detected (Methods). These clones were purified to homogeneity and two were studied in more detail.

Clone BT4. This cDNA clone contained a 1.9kb DNA insert and expressed a 140-150kd fusion protein. Antibodies against the fusion protein were selected from total TFI serum by plaque affinity purification (3). The purified antibodies reacted with a 60/64kd doublet band on western blots of whole L. donovani promastigote antigen and with a 60kd band on western blots of L. donovani membrane antigen. One interpretation of these data is that the 60kd membrane-associated molecule is the processed form of a cystolic 64kd precursor. The antigen was not expressed in freshly isolated amastigotes. Bands of a similar size were detected on western blots of whole promastigote antigen from a series of other Leishmania species. Anti-BT4 antibodies were found universally in the sera of visceral leishmaniasis patients (20/20+ve) irrespective of geographical location. They were not detected in sera from patients with cutaneous leishmaniasis or with T. cruzi infection (50/50-ve).

On northern blots, the BT4 cDNA hybridised to a large promastigote-specific RNA transcript of 20kb. Data from southern analysis of genomic DNA suggested that the BT4 gene was present as a single copy. Orthogonal field alteration gel (OFAG) electrophoresis indicated that the chromosomal location was conserved in all Leishmania species investigated. Homologous sequences were not detected outside the genus Leishmania.

M13 sequencing of the 1.9kb cDNA insert revealed a 1.2kb open reading frame and 0.7kb of untranslated 3'-end sequence. It can be inferred from this that the insert contains sufficient genetic information to code for up to 2/3rds of the amino acid sequence including the -COOH terminus. The insert was also used to probe an EMBL-3 genomic library of L. donovani (HU3)DNA. Overlapping clones corresponding to one gene were isolated.

Clone CT1. Antibodies against the CT1 fusion protein were isolated from visceral leishmaniasis serum TF1 by plaque affinity purification. These antibodies identified a 68kd band on western blots containing antigen isolated from whole L. donovani promastigotes and antigens obtained by treating promastigotes with 0.1% NP40. At this concentration NP40 detergent will extract surface membrane proteins from intact cells. The antibodies were non-reactive with antigen prepared from freshly prepared amastigotes. CT1 native antigen thus appears to be a promastigote-specific peripheral membrane protein. Bands homologous to the CT1 antigen were identified on western blots of promastigote antigen from a series of other Leishmania species. Anti-CT1 fusion protein antibodies were detected in some but not all visceral leishmaniasis sera (11/20+ves) (Methods). Positive reactivity was not related to geographical origin of patients with cutaneous leishmaniasis or T. cruzi infections (50/50-ve).

The CTI cDNA clone, which contains a 600bp insert, hybridised on northern blots to an abundant promastigote specific mRNA of 3.5kb. The genes coding for this mRNA were located on a single chromosome and were organised as a series of 3.6kb tandem repeats. The sequence and structure of these genes were highly conserved within the kinetoplastids.

DISCUSSION

This report describes the preliminary characterisation of two cDNA clones which correspond to promastigote specific antigens that are expressed early in the differentiation of amastigotes to promastigotes before morphological changes are apparent. The mechanisms governing such stage specific gene expression in Leishmania and other kinetoplastids are not understood. It is not clear how promoters and other transcription regulating sequences function. Isolation and analysis of genomic clones corresponding to these stage specific genes is therefore a preliminary step towards such an understanding.

As the prognosis of visceral leishmaniasis patients is poor in the absence of medical intervention it is important to provide a reliable diagnosis as soon as possible after infection has occurred and to provide diagnostic reagents for epidemiological studies. The ability to clone Leishmania antigens such as those described is a step in this direction. The assay system used here to characterise the serum specificity of these antigens (western blot analysis) was chosen because of the widespread anti-E.Coli activity in human sera: the fusion proteins migrate clear of most other proteins and thus preabsorption of the sera with E.Coli antigen was not necessary. Also fusion proteins need not be purified from the lysogen lysate. For practical purposes with a view to a rapid and accurate means of diagnosis this assay could be refined by purification of the fusion protein in bulk and adaptation to the ELISA system.

The BT4 antigen which is described here has obvious diagnostic potential. The generation of an antibody response to the antigen was limited to visceral leishmaniasis patients despite the presence of homologous genes and immunologically cross-reactive antigens in parasites causing cutaneous leishmaniasis. This could be due to different location of parasite infection in visceral leishmaniasis patients, different processing of the antigen by the immune system or different antigenic presentation compared to other Leishmania. It is now our intention to test this and other cloned antigens for their ability to stimulate specific T-cell responses using a modification of the T-cell blotting technique ((9) in collaboration with P. Kaye LSHTM). On the basis of detailed analysis including both T-cell and B-cell mapping of epitopes, synthetic peptides will be made and their ability to elicit immunity in experimental animals will be assessed.

CONCLUSIONS

cDNA clones corresponding to two L. donovani antigens have been isolated and characterised. The cDNAs were used to identify the native antigens, examine genomic structure and chromosomal location and expression of the antigen gene. One of the clones (BT4) corresponded to a 60kd membrane-associated antigen, the other (CT1) to a 68kdal peripheral membrane antigen. Antibodies against the BT4 fusion protein were detected universally in the sera of visceral leishmaniasis patients. This report demonstrates the feasibility of expression cloning as a means of defining specific visceral leishmaniasis reagents, of providing insight into Leishmania genetics and gene expression and ultimately as a means of providing antigens as candidates for a synthetic vaccine.

ACKNOWLEDGEMENT

We thank the Wolfson Foundation and Wellcome Trust for financing the research: MAM is a Wellcome Trust Senior Lecturer.

REFERENCES

(1) U. Gubler and B.J. Hoffman, Gene, 25, 263-269 (1983).
    A simple and very efficient method for generating cDNA libraries.

(2) T.V. Hyunh, R.A. Young and R.W. Davis, pp.49-78. "DNA Cloning, A practical approach" Vol. I, Glover D. (ed.) IRL Press, Oxford (1985).

(3) L.S. Ozaki, D. Mathei, M. Jendoubi, P. Druihle, T. Blisnick, M. Guillotle, O. Puijalon, and L.P. Da Silva. J. Immunol. Methods 89, 213-219 (1986).
Plaque antibody selection: Rapid immunological analysis of a large number of recombinant phages clones positive to sera raised against Plasmodium falciparum antigens.

(4) D.M. Dwyer, pp.9-28. "The Biochemistry of Parasites" Slutzky, G.M. (ed.), Pergamon Press, Oxford, UK (1981).

(5) H. Towbin, T. Staehlin and J. Gordon. Proc. Nat. Acad. Sci. USA 76, 4350-4354 (1977).
Electrophoretic transfer of proteins from polyacrylamide gels to nitrocellulose sheets: Procedure and some applications.

(6) T. Maniatis, E.M. Frisch and J. Sambrook, "Molecular Cloning: A laboratory manual". Cold Spring Harbour Laboratory, Cold Spring Harbour, USA (1982).

(7) J.M. Kelly, A.C.G. Porter, Y. Chernajovsky, S.G. Gilbert, G.R. Stark and I.M. Kerr EMBO.J. 5, 1601-1606 (1986).
Characterisation of a human gene inducible by α- and β-interferons and its expression in mouse cells.

(8) R.P. Bishop and M.A. Miles. Molec. and Biochem. Parasit. 24, 263-272 (1987).
Chromosome size polymorphisons of Leishmania donovani.

(9) J.L. Lamb and D.B. Young. Immunol., 60, 1-5 (1987).
A novel approach to the identification of T-cell epitopes in Mycobacterium tuberculosis using human T-lymphocyte clones.

SURFACE ANTIGENS OF LEISHMANIA INFANTUM IDENTIFIED BY MONOCLONAL
ANTIBODIES: ISOLATION OF A MONOMERIC AND AN OLIGOMERIC FORM OF A MAJOR
L.INFANTUM ANTIGEN

Ketty Ph. Soteriadou*, Athina K. Tzinia*, Maria
G. Hadziantoniou+ and Socrates J. Tzartos*

Laboratories of *Biochemistry and +Parasitology
Hellenic Pasteur Institute, 127 Vassilissis Sofias
Avenue, Athens 11521, Greece

INTRODUCTION

Leishmania, species-specific [1-5], stage-specific [2,4,6] and cross-reactive antigens [7,8], have been identified using as tools monoclonal antibodies (mAbs). However, little is known about the pathophysiological importance of these molecules.

A major Leishmania surface glycoprotein of approximately 63.000 mol.wt. termed p63, has been identified using kala-azar sera and human cutaneous leishmaniasis sera [7]. The p63 appears to be common among a great number of Leishmania species and is recognized by rabbit anti-L. donovani immune sera [8-10]. A p63 has been purified from Leishmania mexicana amazonensis (L.m.amazonensis) by mAb affinity binding and this glycoprotein inhibits Leishmania-macrophage binding [11]. The involvement of the L.m.mexicana p63 in the attachment of Leishmania promastigotes to macrophages has also been reported [12]. p63 was characterized as an integral membrane protein [13]. A hydrophilic form was identified during its purification [14]. It has also been demonstrated that p63 is a protease [15], designated as promastigote surface protease (PSP) [16], and has a common membrane anchor with Trypanosoma VSG (variant surface glycoprotein) [17].

In this report we describe the identification and partial purification of the monomeric and oligomeric form of a predominant L.infantum protein of 58.000 mol.wt. which posses proteolytic activity. The observed in vitro inhibition of L.infantum promastigote-macrophage interaction caused by the mAbs recognizing the above proteins, implies that the 58kDa monomer and oligomer might be involved in the binding of promastigotes to macrophages and could subsequently be used for immunoprophylaxis. Current information on p63 combined with our results suggest that the 58kDa protein identified in this study is the major surface Leishmania protein, p63.

MATERIALS AND METHODS

Leishmania

The L.infantum strain (HOM-Gr-78-L4) used was isolated in Greece from human visceral leishmaniasis [18]. Promastigotes were cultured at 27°C in a monophasic medium consisting of hemoglobin (1g/L), neopeptone (5g/L), brain-heart infusion (5g/L), lactalbumin hydrolysate (3g/L), 14mM glucose and 1% human hemolysed blood (M.Hadziantoniou, PhD Thesis).

Preparation of Leishmania membranes

Membrane preparations of L.infantum promastigotes were obtained according to Dwyer [19].

Production of mAbs

Balb/c mice were immunized with intact or detergent solubilized promastigote membranes in incomplete Freund's adjuvant. Fusions were carried out according to the "direct cloning" method of Tzartos et al.[20] a modification of the classical cell fusion technique of Kohler and Milstein [21]. The modification is based on the introduction of agar immediately after fusion of the cells.

Solid-phase radioimmuoassay

A solid phase radioimmunoassay (RIA) was used to identify hybrids secreting mAbs to L.infantum [22].

Electrophoresis

Sodium dodecyl sulfate-polyacrylamide gel electrophoresis (SDS-PAGE) was performed on 7.5% or 10% gels according to Laemmli [23].

Western blotting

Isolated L.infantum membranes were electrophoretically transferred from SDS-polyacrylamide gels to nitrocellulose paper according to the procedure first described by Towbin et al. [24]. The nitrocellulose strips were incubated with hybridoma supernatants, rabbit anti-mouse immunoglobulins and ^{125}I-protein A in the order given.

Limited digestion

L.infantum membranes were incubated at room temperature for 1 hr in the presence of 0.1ug/well Staphylococcus aureus V8 protease [8]. The resulting digests were first analyzed by SDS-PAGE and then by Western blotting using the anti-L.infantum mAbs as probes.

Iodination

Lactoperoxidase-catalyzed iodination was used [25].

Gel filtration

Hydrophilic forms of the studied antigens in PBS were loaded on a Superose 12 TM-column and analyzed by FPLC (Pharmacia). The column was equilibrated with PBS pH 7.4. Fractions (0.5 ml) were collected and subjected to SDS-PAGE followed by protein staining and/or analyzed by Western blotting. In some experiments where a small amount of ^{125}I-labelled material was added to the sample, the eluants were counted to detect any radioactivity present.

L.infantum infection of mouse macrophages

Mouse macrophage cell line J774G8 was cultured on cover slips placed in Petri dishes. The cells (10^6/ml) were allowed to adhere at 37°C in an atmosphere of 10% CO_2, for a minimum of 1 hr. The cover slips were then washed to remove non-adherent cells, and L.infantum promastigotes, either non-treated or treated with mAbs, were added at a ratio of 10 parasites per cell. After 1 hr incubation cover slips were washed vigorously with medium, fixed in methanol and stained with Giemsa [26]. The number of cells infected was determined by counting 500 cells in a Giemsa-stained culture.

RESULTS

Ten stable hybridomas, producing mAbs to promastigote membrane antigens, were produced according to the "direct cloning" method [20] and detected by a solid-phase RIA, using intact, isolated membranes. All ten mAbs produced were IgM molecules.

Identification and characterization of membrane antigens recognized by anti-L.infantum mAbs

The identification of membrane antigens by the ten mAbs was carried out by Western Blotting followed by autoradiography. Blots of SDS-solubilized L.infantum membranes, heated at 100°C (with or without 2-ME) before analysis by SDS-PAGE, showed that all 10 L.infantum mAbs recognized a band at 58kDa. However, when non heat-treated solubilized membranes (in the presence or absence of 2-ME) were used, the above mAbs gave two distinct recognition patterns: Eight of the mAbs still recognized the 58kDa band (e.g LD16 and LD23) whereas two (mAbs LD20 and LD24) recognized, in addition to the 58kDa, bands of higher mol.wt. (approximately 200kDa, Fig.1). Occasionally, when membranes were not heated before analysis by SDS-PAGE, multiple intermediate mol.wt. bands were detected which may represent proteolytic breakdown products of the 200kDa band. The presence of 2-ME in the sample buffer did not affect the migration of the high mol.wt. bands.

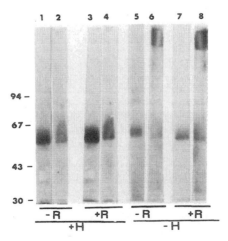

Figure 1. Autoradiographs of L.infantum membranes identified by Western blotting using mAbs to L.infantum as probes. SDS-PAGE (7.5%) was performed under reducing (+R), or non- reducing conditions (-R). Membranes were either heated at 100°C (+H), or non-heated (-H). mAb LD16 recognized only a 58kDa band under all conditions (lanes 1,3,5,7). LD20 recognized a 58kDa when membranes were heated (lanes 2,4), and in addition to the 58kDa, a band of approximately 200kDa when membranes were not heated (lanes 6,8).

Autoradiographs of ^{125}I-labelled isolated membranes, subjected to SDS-PAGE, showed that a 58kDa polypeptide was mainly labelled. The ^{125}I-labelled polypeptide co-migrated with the 58kDa polypeptide detected on blots by the mAbs (data not shown).

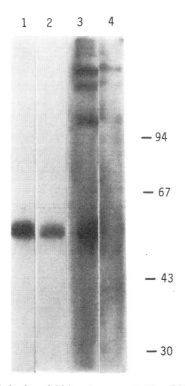

Figure 2. Generation of hydrophilic forms of the 58kDa monomer and oligomer. L.infantum membranes were dialyzed against PBS for 4hr and then centrifuged. Both the pellet and the supernatant were analyzed by Western blotting. The antigens recognized by mAbs LD16 and LD20 were detected both in the supernatant (lanes 1,3 respectively) and the pellet (lanes 2,4 respectively).

The possibility that the 58kDa polypeptide detected by both groups of mAbs (i.e. binding or not to the high molecular weight bands) is identical was investigated by peptide mapping. It was showed that all four mAbs tested (two of each group) recognized the same digests (data not shown). Thus, they recognized the same 58kDa polypeptide. The above results strongly suggest the existence of a monomeric and an oligomeric form of the 58kDa polypeptide.

Identification, partial purification and proteolytic activity of hydrophylic forms of the 58kDa monomer and oligomer

Hydrophylic forms of the 58kDa monomer and oligomer were obtained as indicated in Fig.2 and were isolated by gel filtration by FPLC. Absorbance at 280nm revealed four major peaks (Fig.3). The contents of each peak were analyzed by SDS-PAGE. Gels were either stained for protein or analyzed by Western blotting. Oligomeric forms of the 58kDa protein were detected, by the mAbs, in the second peak (~200kDa). The 58kDa protein was detected in the third peak (~60kDa) (Fig. 4a). Staining for protein gave the same results (Fig. 4b). The presence of the 58kDa protein in the third peak was confirmed by the analysis of ^{125}I- labeled supernatant (whose major labelled antigen is the 58kDa band) which showed that the major peak co-migrated with the third peak of the unlabeled supernatant (Fig.4).

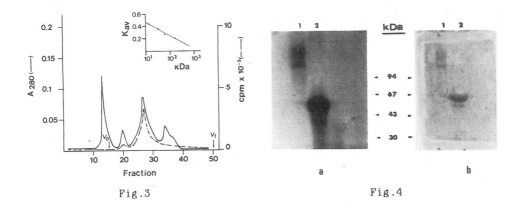

Fig.3 Fig.4

Figure 3. Partial purification of the hydrophilic 58kDa monomer and oligomer by gel filtration. A Superose-TM column (FPLC, Pharmacia) was equilibrated with PBS pH 7.4 and calibrated with a IgG mAb (150kDa), BSA (67kDa), ovalbumin (43kDa), and ribonuclease A (13.7kDa). The column then was loaded with hydrophilic forms of the studied antigens (supernatant). When the column was loaded with a small amount of iodinated supernatant and fractions measured for radioactivity, a major radioactive peak was detected coinciding with the peak of 60kDa (dotted line).

Figure 4. Detection of the 58kDa monomer and oligomer partially isolated by gel filtration as described in Fig.4. Fractions of the second and third peak (lanes 1,2 respectively) were pooled, concentrated by ultrafiltration and analyzed by SDS-PAGE (7.5%). Samples were neither heated nor reduced. a) Western blotting analysis. The blots were probed with a mixture of mAbs (LD16 and LD20). b) Staining for protein.

The partially purified by gel filtration hydrophylic forms of the 58kDa monomer and oligomer were found to possess proteolytic activity (data not shown).

Inhibition of parasite attachment to macrophages caused by the anti-L.infantum mAbs

We have also investigated mAbs interference with parasite penetration into mouse macrophages (Fig.5). mAbs LD16, LD23 (capable of monomeric antigen recognition) inhibited about 30% parasite attachment to mouse macrophages and mAbs LD20, LD24 (capable of monomeric and oligomeric antigen recognition) exhibited about 50% inhibition. Anti-tubulin mAb and anti-acetylcholine receptor mAbs [20] did not affect promastigote binding to macrophages (Fig.5). Therefore, the surface antigens recognized by these mAbs may play an important role in parasite-macrophage interaction.

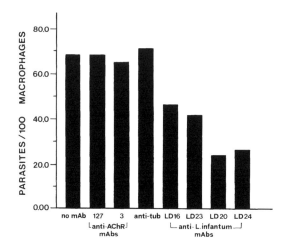

Figure 5. Effect of anti-L.infantum mAbs on the attachment of promastigotes to mouse macrophage cell line J774G8. The anti-L.infantum mAbs LD16, LD23 and LD20, LD24 inhibited about 30% and 50% parasite attachment respectively. Anti-AChR (acetylcholine receptor) mAbs and the anti-tubulin mAb (anti-tub) used as negative controls had no effect on the binding of L.infantum to cells.

DISCUSSION

In this study we identifed a monomeric and oligomeric form of a 58kDa L.infantum antigen. Hydrophylic forms of the 58kDa monomer and oligomer, possessing proteolytic activity, were detected and partially purified. The characteristics of the studied antigens are the following:

a) The 58kDa oligomer appears to be a heat modifiable Leishmania membrane antigen. Heating of oligomers in SDS may result in their dissociation and when analyzed by SDS-PAGE they migrate as monomers [27].

b) The 58kDa oligomer comprises non-covalently associated subunits.

c) The oligomeric conformations favour binding of mAbs LD20 and LD24 to the corresponding epitopes whereas the epitopes of the other eight mAbs (i.e. LD16 and LD23) seem to be on the sites of attachment of the 58kDa subunits.

d) The 58kDa is recognized by all our mAbs implying that this protein is very immunogenic.

e) Predominant ^{125}I labelling of the 58kDa.

f) The 58kDa monomer and oligomer play an important role in parasite-macrophage binding as observed by the 30% and 50% inhibition of parasite attachment to mouse macrophages when using the corresponding mAbs.

The experimental evidence presented above in addition to the recognition by the two groups of our mAbs of the p63 or PSP from L.major

LEM 513 (kindly provited by Dr. C. Bordier) support the identity of the 58kDa antigen as the PSP.

ACKNOWLEDGEMENTS

We are grateful to Profs. Ch. Serie and G. Cohen for their valuable suggestions and encouragement during the course of this work and Dr C. Bordier (Universite de Lausanne) for supplying p63 from L.major LEM 513 and for valuable discussions.

LITERATURE CITED

1. D. McMahon-Pratt, and J. R David, Monoclonal antibodies that distinguish between New World species of Leishmania, Nature 291:581 (1981).
2. C. L. Jaffe, and D. McMahon-Pratt, Monoclonal antibodies specific for Leishmania tropica. I. Characterization of antigens associated with stage and species-specific determinants, J. Immunol. 131:1987 (1983).
3. C. L. Jaffe, E. Bennett, G. Jr. Grimaldi, and D. McMahon- Pratt, Production and characterization of species-specific monoclonal antibodies against Leishmania donovani for immunodiagnosis, J.Immunol. 133:440 (1984).
4. E. Handman, and R. E. Hocking, Stage specific, strain-specific and cross reactive antigens of Leishmania species identified by monoclonal antibodies, Infect.Immun. 37:28 (1982).
5. C. L. Greenblatt, G. M Slutzky, L. de Ibarra, and D. Snary, Monoclonal antibodies for serotyping Leishmania strains, J. Clin.Microbiol. 18:191 (1983).
6. D. Fong, and K. P. Chang, Surface antigenic change during differentiation of a parasitic protozoan, Leishmania mexicana:Identification by monoclonal antibodies, Proc. Natl.Acad. Sci. USA 79:7366 (1982).
7. D. A. Lepay, N. Nogueira, and Z. Cohn, Surface antigens of Leishmania donovani promastigotes, J. Exp. Med. 157:1562 (1983).
8. V. Colomer-Gould, L. G. Quintao, J. Keithly, and N. Nogueira, A common major antigen on amastigotes and promastigotes of Leishmania species, J. Exp. Med. 162:902 (1985).
9. R. J. Etges, J. Bouvier, R. Hoffman, and C. Bordier, Evidence that the major surface proteins of three Leishmania species are structurally related, Mol. Biochem. Parasitol. 14:141 (1985).
10. P. R. Gardiner, C. L. Jaffe, and D. M. Dwyer, Identification of cross-reactive promastigote cell surface antigens of some leishmanial stocks by ^{125}I-labeling and immunoprecipitation. Infect. Immun. 43:637 (1984).
11. C. S. Chang, and K. P. Chang, Monoclonal antibody affinity purification of a Leishmania membrane glycoprotein and its inhibition of Leishmania- macrophage binding, Proc. Natl. Acad. Sci. USA 83:100 (1986).
12. D. G. Russell, and H. Wilhelm, The involment of the major surface glycoprotein (gp63) of Leishmania promastigotes in attachment to macrophage, J. Immunol. 136:2613 (1986).
13. R. Etges, J. Bouvier, and C. Bordier, The major surface protein of Leishmania promastigotes is anchored in the membrane by a myristic acid-labeled phospholipid, EMBO J. 5:597 (1985).
14. J. Bouvier, R. J. Etges, and C. Bordier, Identification and purification of membrane and soluble forms of the major surface protein of Leishmania promastigotes, J. Biol. Chem. 260:15504 (1985).

15. R. Etges, J. Bouvier, and C. Bordier, The major surface protein of Leishmania promastigotes is a protease, J. Biol. Chem. 261:9098 (1986).
16. C. Bordier, The promastigote surface protease of Leishmania, Parasit. Today 3:151 (1987).
17. C. Bordier, R. J. Etges, J. Ward, M. J. Turner, and M.L.Cardoso de Almeida, Leishmania and Trypanosoma surface glycoproteins have a common glycophospholipid membrane anchor, Proc. Natl. Acad. Sci. USA 83:5988 (1986).
18. N. Tzamouranis, L. F. Schnur, A. Garifallou, E. Pateraki, and C. Serie, Leishmaniasis in Greece. I. Isolation and identification of the parasite causing human and canine visceral leishmaniasis, Ann. Trop. Med. Parasitol. 78:363 (1984).
19. D. M. Dwyer, Isolation and characterization of surface from Leishmania donovani promastigotes, J. Protozool. 27:176 (1980).
20. S. J. Tzartos, Monoclonal antibodies as probes of the acetylcholine receptor and myasthenia gravis, Trends Biochem. Sci. 9:63 (1984).
21. G. Kohler, and C. Milstein, Continuous cultures of fused cells secreting antibody of predefined specificity, Nature 256:495 (1975).
22. J. W. Stocker, and C. H. Heusser, Methods for binding cells to plastic: application to a solid-phase radioimmunoassay for cell-surface antigens, J. Immunol. Methods 26:87 (1979).
23. U. K. Laemmli, Cleavage of structural proteins during the assembly of the head of bacteriophage T4, Nature 227:680 (1970).
24. H. Towbin, T. Staehelin, and J. Gordon, Electrophoretic transfer of proteins from polyacrylamide gels to nitrocellulose sheets: procedure and some applications, Proc. Natl. Acad. Sci. USA 76:4350 (1979).
25. C. Dissous, C. Dissous, and A. Capron, Isolation and characterization of surface antigen from Schistosoma mansoni schistosomula, Mol. Biochem. Parasitol. 3:215(1981).
26. K. P. Chang, and D. Fong, Cytopathology of parasitic disease, Pitman Books, London (Ciba Foundation symposium 99) p. 113 (1983).
27. S. K. Armstrong, and C. D. Parker, Heat-modifiable envelope proteins of Bordetella pertussis, Infect. Immun. 54:109 (1986).

This work was supported by the Greek General Secretariat of Research and Technology, and the French Delegation Generale a la Recherche Scientifique et Technique.

SEQUENCE ANALYSIS OF THE MAJOR SURFACE GLYCOPROTEIN

OF *LEISHMANIA MAJOR**

Linda L. Button, Robert W. Olafson[+] and W. Robert McMaster

Department of Medical Genetics
University of British Columbia
Vancouver, B.C. Canada V6T 1W5

INTRODUCTION

During the initial stages of infection by *Leishmania*, the interaction between parasites and macrophages in the mammalian host is mediated by macrophage receptors and cell surface molecules on *Leishmania* . Parasites are engulfed by phagocytosis, then differentiate from extracellular promastigotes to intracellular amastigotes which reside within the lysosomal compartment of the macrophage. The following experimental evidence suggests the importance of the major surface glycoprotein of *Leishmania* promastigotes, gp63, for the establishment of parasitism resulting in Leishmaniasis in humans (for recent review, see Bordier, 1987). The structure of gp63 and the protease activity associated with gp63 is conserved among several diverse species of *Leishmania* (Bouvier et al. 1987, Colomer-Gould et al. 1985, Etges et al. 1985, Gardiner et al. 1984, Lepay et al. 1983). Pretreatment of macrophages with either purified gp63 (Chang & Chang 1986) or anti-gp63 antibody (Russell & Wilhelm 1986) results in the inhibition of promastigote binding to macrophages. The level of gp63 expression on the surface of promastigotes is directly related to the infectivity of *Leishmania* for the host macrophages (Kweider et al. 1987). Although macrophage receptors which bind *Leishmania* have been described, such as the complement receptor type 3 (Blackwell et al. 1985, Mosser & Edelson 1985) and the mannose-fucose receptor (Wilson & Pearson 1986), the specific recognition between these receptors and gp63 has not yet been demonstrated.

In this report, we describe the analysis of the protein structure of gp63, predicted from the DNA sequence of a cloned gp63 gene from *Leishmania major* (Button, Olafson & McMaster, 1987). This represents a step toward using recombinant gp63 for studying the function of gp63 on *Leishmania* as well as the interaction between gp63 and specific macrophage receptors, and potentially for developing a synthetic vaccine against Leishmaniasis.

---

[*] Supported by grants from the MRC (Canada) to WRM and the UND/World bank/WHO Special Programme for Research Training in Tropical Diseases to WRM and RWO.

[+] Department of Biochemistry and Microbiology, University of Victoria, Victoria B.C., Canada V8W 2Y2

METHODS

Amino Terminal protein sequence of gp63

L. major gp63 was purified by Triton X-114 phase separation (Bouvier et al. 1985). Promastigotes of the L. major S strain (Neva et al. 1979, provided by Dr. Neil Reiner) were grown in large scale cultures of Medium 199 plus 10% fetal calf serum to a density of 2×10^7 cells per ml. Cells (1×10^{11}) were harvested by centrifugation at 10,000 x g for 10 min., washed in TBS [10 mM Tris-HCl, 0.15 M NaCl (pH 7.5)], resuspended in 50 ml TBS, and solubilized by the addition of Triton X-114 to 1%. After homogenizing the cells and removing the nuclei by centrifugation at 10,000 x g for 10 min., the extract was heated to 30°C. The condensed detergent phase was separated by underlaying a cushion of 6% (w/v) sucrose in TBS and centrifuging at 1600 x g for 30 min. The detergent phase was dialysed against 0.1% SDS, the protein was then concentrated by ultrafiltration and ethanol precipitated. The protein was solubilized in 10% SDS and gp63, the major constituent, was isolated by preparative sodium dodecyl sulphate polyacrylamide gel electrophoresis (SDS-PAGE). Following electrophoresis, gp63 was eluted and dialysed against 0.1% SDS. Purified gp63 was subjected to amino acid sequence analysis on an Applied Biosystems 470A gas-phase sequencer which gave a provisional 23 residue sequence for the N-terminus of gp63.

Oligonucleotide probe for gp63

A 50 base oligonucleotide (50-mer) with a unique DNA sequence which encodes residues 3-19 at the N-terminus of gp63 was designed based on the limited data available for codon usage with Leishmania genes (Grumont et al. 1986, WRM unpublished data), The 50-mer probe and a 15-mer primer, complementary to the 3' end of the 50-mer, were synthesized using an Applied Biosystems DNA synthesizer. The 50-mer was labelled to a high specific activity (10^8 cpm/μg) by extending the 15-mer primer with DNA Polymerase I, Klenow fragment (Hellman & Pettersson 1987).

Isolation and characterization of genomic DNA clones which encode gp63

A genomic DNA library prepared for the L. major S strain was screened by colony hybridization with the 50-mer probe (Button, Olafson & McMaster, 1987). Gp63 clones were characterized by restriction enzyme mapping, Southern hybridization and DNA sequence analysis of the 50-mer binding site region. The purified clones cross-hybridized and contained the same DNA sequence for the 50-mer binding site region, hence the clone with the longest 3' region was selected for DNA analysis of the gp63 gene. A 2.2 kilobasepair (kbp) EcoRI fragment was subcloned in the bacteriophage vector M13mp19 for DNA sequence analysis of both DNA strands (Button, Olafson & McMaster, 1987). The single 1.8-kbp open reading frame was translated to give the predicted protein structure of gp63. Computer analysis (Seqnce, Delaney Software Ltd.) of the sequence provided the codon usage, amino acid composition, secondary structure prediction (Garnier et al. 1978), and hydropathy profile (Kyte & Doolittle, 1982) of gp63.

RESULTS and DISCUSSION

Design of a Unique Oligodeoxynucleotide Probe which Encodes the N-terminal Amino acid Sequence of L. major gp63.

The predominant protein component in the Triton X-114 phase separation method used to purify gp63 had a relative molecular mass (M_r) of 63 kDa under reducing conditions of SDS-PAGE. The mobility of the protein increased to Mr 50 kDa with nonreducing conditions of SDS-PAGE, and the purified protein bound the lectin

Concanavalin A (data not shown). By these criteria, previously shown for gp63 (Bouvier, Etges, & Bordier 1985), the purified protein in our preparation was identified as gp63. Shown in Figure 1 is the N-terminal amino acid sequence of gp63 purified from *L. major* promastigotes. The predicted DNA sequence, including codon redundancies, that encodes the N-terminus is shown below the protein sequence and underlined are the bases chosen for the synthesis of the 50 base oligonucleotide probe (50-mer). Either G or C was selected for the wobble position of each codon, as this strong G/C bias was shown for other genes in *Leishmania* (Grumont et al. 1986, WRM unpublished results). The DNA sequence of this region in the isolated gp63 clones revealed the close agreement between the predicted codons in the synthetic oligonucleotide and those used in the gp63 gene. There was only 5 mismatches over 50 nucleotides, and 4 of the 5 mismatches were the result of a G versus C choice for the wobble positions in the 50-mer. The predicted protein sequence agreed with 21 of the 23 residues determined for the N-terminus of gp63. The two mismatches at positions 18 and 19 were actually Thr and Asp for the translated DNA sequence but were assigned as Lys and Thr for the provisional amino acid sequence.

```
                     1                                    18 19
     i    v  r  d  v  n  w  g  a  l  r  i  a  v  s  t  e  d  l  k  t  p  a  y
     ii   GTGCGGGACGTGAACTGGGGCGCGCTGCGCATCGCGGTGTCCACGGAGGACCTGAAGACGCCGGCGTAC
               CA C  T  C  T        G  C  C  G  A  C  C  G  C  A  T  C  A  C  C  C  T
               A  A     A           A  A  A  A  T  A  A  A  A        A        A  A  A
               T  T     T           T  T  T  T     T  T  T  T        T        T  T  T
     iii  GTGCGCGACGTGAACTGGGGCGCGCTGCGCATCGCCGTCTCCACCGAGGACCTCACCGACCCCGCCTAC
     iv   v  r  d  v  n  w  g  a  l  r  i  a  v  s  t  e  d  l  t  d  p  a  y
```

i   N-terminal amino acid sequence of *L. major* gp63
ii   Predicted DNA sequence including redundancies and sequence of DNA probe (underlined)
iii   Actual DNA sequence of gp63 gene (differences to oligonucleotide probe are underlined)
iv   Translated amino acid from gp63 gene (differences to protein sequence are underlined)

Figure 1   50 base oligonucleotide probe encoding the N-terminus of gp63 based on codon usage in *Leishmania*.

Codon Usage in *Leishmania*

The DNA sequence of the *L. major* gp63 gene together with the predicted protein sequence, was analyzed for codon usage and the results are summarized in Table I. The base composition and codon usage for the gp63 gene corresponds to the high G plus C content of the *Leishmania* genome and the strong preference for G or C in the wobble position of codons for the relatively few *Leishmania* genes that have been characterized. The average G/C content for both the coding region and the untranslated regions was about 68%. There was a strong bias (84%) for either G or C in the third or wobble positions of the codons, whereas the G/C content of the first and second positions of the codons (67% and 52%, respectively) reflected the average G/C content in the *Leishmania* genome (60%). This base preference for G/C versus A/T in the third position of codons is apparently confined to the coding region since it is not obvious in the untranslated regions for the gp63 gene. Presumably, this analysis of base distribution for the gp63 gene is applicable in predicting the coding regions and reading frames for other *Leishmania* genes.

Table I   Codon Usage in the *L. major* gene encoding unprocessed gp63

0-TTT-Phe-0.000	3-TCT-Ser-0.005	1-TAT-Tyr-0.002	2-TGT-Cys-0.003
16-TTC-Phe-0.027	6-TCC-Ser-0.010	14-TAC-Tyr-0.023	21-TGC-Cys-0.035
0-TTA-Leu-0.000	1-TCA-Ser-0.002	0-TAA-Stop .000	0-TGA-Stop .000
2-TTG-Leu-0.003	5-TCG-Ser-0.008	0-TAG-Stop .000	6-TGG-Trp-0.010
4-CTT-Leu-0.007	3-CCT-Pro-0.005	6-CAT-His-0.010	6-CGT-Arg-0.010
13-CTC-Leu-0.022	8-CCC-Pro-0.013	17-CAC-His-0.028	21-CGC-Arg-0.035
2-CTA-Leu-0.003	5-CCA-Pro-0.008	2-CAA-Gln-0.003	3-CGA-Arg-0.005
16-CTG-Leu-0.027	18-CCG-Pro-0.030	23-CAG-Gln-0.038	6-CGG-Arg-0.010
1-ATT-Ile-0.002	2-ACT-Thr-0.003	1-AAT-Asn-0.002	4-AGT-Ser-0.007
14-ATC-Ile-0.023	17-ACC-Thr-0.028	17-AAC-Asn-0.028	17-AGC-Ser-0.028
1-ATA-Ile-0.002	2-ACA-Thr-0.003	1-AAA-Lys-0.002	3-AGA-Arg-0.005
8-ATG-Met-0.013	17-ACG-Thr-0.028	13-AAG-Lys-0.022	1-AGG-Arg-0.002
7-GTT-Val-0.012	8-GCT-Ala-0.013	6-GAT-Asp-0.010	11-GGT-Gly-0.018
21-GTC-Val-0.035	35-GCC-Ala-0.058	27-GAC-Asp-0.045	34-GGC-Gly-0.057
1-GTA-Val-0.002	8-GCA-Ala-0.013	1-GAA-Glu-0.002	3-GGA-Gly-0.005
33-GTG-Val-0.055	34-GCG-Ala-0.057	20-GAG-Glu-0.033	3-GGG-Gly-0.005

Predicted Primary and Secondary Structures of L.major prepro-gp63

The primary protein structure of gp63 translated from a *L. major* gene is shown in Figure 2 together with the predicted secondary structure. The protein contains 601 amino acids and the N-terminal sequence determined for purified gp63 from *L. major* promastigotes is located at position 101 to 123. The 100 residue extension at the N-terminus of gp63 on the cell surface of promastigotes indicates that gp63 is synthesized as a precursor protein with a calculated molecular weight of 64,121 excluding any glycosylation. The removal of the N-terminal peptide in processing of the precursor protein yields a mature protein of 501 amino acids with a calculated molecular weight of 53,949 excluding any glycosylation. This is consistent with asparagine-linked glycosylation accounting for 10 - 15% of the molecular mass for gp63 as shown by tunicamycin or endoglycosidase-H treatment (Chang & Chang 1986, Chang et al. 1986). The hydropathy profile of the entire gp63 protein is shown in Figure 3 and indicates that gp63 contains regions of hydrophobic and hydrophilic amino acid sequence. The predicted secondary structure (Figure 2) indicates that gp63 may not have a predominant structural form as all four folding patterns are represented. A putative hydrophobic leader sequence, also referred to as a signal peptide or pre sequence, is evident at position 21 to 39 followed by a potential cleavage site, Ala-Xxx-Ala (Von Hienje 1983). The pre sequence is then followed by a 61 residue region prior to the mature N-terminus. This region may constitute a "pro" region that is common in many proteases and may regulate the protease activity of gp63. Since Val-101 is the N-terminal residue for mature gp63, the propeptide is removed by proteolytic cleavage between His-100 and Val-101. Studies have shown that gp63 is anchored in the promastigote membrane by a glycoinositol phospholipid covalently attached to the carboxy terminus (C-terminus), (Etges, Bouvier, Bordier, EMBO 1986). The hydropathy profile depicts a hydrophobic C-terminal tail of 12 residues for the predicted protein sequence of gp63. This hydrophobic region may be involved in post-translational modification of gp63 and may be proteolytically removed prior to the addition of the lipid tail in a similar manner as that seen in the modification of the variant surface glycoprotein of *Trypanosoma brucei* (Cross, G.A.M. 1987). The calculated hydropathic values for gp63, -0.17 and -0.24 with and without the C-terminal protein tail respectively, are consistent with the hydrophilic properties of gp63 in the absence of the phospholipid tail.

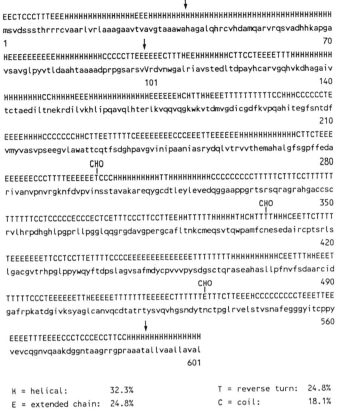

Figure 2 Translated Amino Acid Sequence and Predicted Secondary Structure of gp63

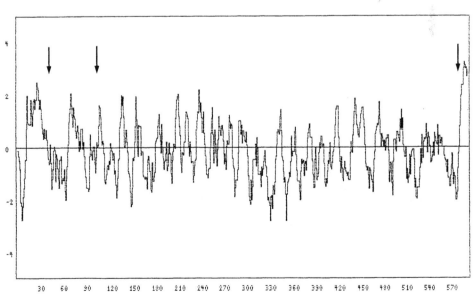

Figure 3   Hydropathy Profile of prepro-gp63 (arrows indicate potential cleavage sites)

Consistent with the N-linked glycosylation described previously for gp63, the primary structure of gp63 has three potential N-linked glycosylation sites, Asn-Xxx-Ser/Thr, located in the mature gp63. Studies are currently in progress to determine the location and structure of these N-linked carbohydrate units. An interesting tripeptide recognition sequence, Arg-Gly-Asp, or R-G-D, occurs at residue 375 in the primary structure of gp63. The R-G-D sequences in some binding proteins are involved in the recognition by specific receptors (Ruoslahti & Pierschbacher 1986) and this may also hold true for gp63 interactions with macrophage receptors.

The amino acid composition of the mature form of gp63,ie.the pre-pro peptide is removed, is shown in Table II. Relevant to the protein structure of gp63 is the high cysteine content and the potential for several disulfide bonds in the primary structure of gp63. Since the protease activity associated with gp63 is inhibited by iodoacetamide (Etges, Bouvier, Bordier 1986), at least one unpaired cysteine may be required in the active site of gp63.

Table II   Amino Acid Composition of *L. major* Promastigote Cell Surface gp63:

Alanine	58 -- 0.1158	Arginine	30 -- 0.0599
Asparagine	18 -- 0.0359	Aspartate	28 -- 0.0559
Cysteine	21 -- 0.0419	Glutamine	22 -- 0.0439
Glutamate	21 -- 0.0419	Glycine	45 -- 0.0898
Histidine	16 -- 0.0319	Isoleucine	16 -- 0.0319
Leucine	32 -- 0.0639	Lysine	13 -- 0.0259
Methionine	6 -- 0.0120	Phenylalanine	16 -- 0.0319
Proline	30 -- 0.0599	Serine	28 -- 0.0559
Threonine	33 -- 0.0659	Tryptophan	5 -- 0.0100
Tyrosine	14 -- 0.0279	Valine	49 -- 0.0978

CONCLUSION

The use of oligonucleotide probes with a unique sequence that is based on codon usage is a valid approach for isolating genes in *Leishmania* as shown for the gp63 gene. The protein structure, predicted from the DNA sequence of a cloned gp63 gene, revealed several characteristics of the promastigote major surface glycoprotein. Primarily, the gene is expressed as prepro-gp63, with both an N-terminal signal peptide region and and adjacent propeptide region. Although the mature gp63 protein has a relative molecular mass of 63 kDa, the calculated molecular weight is 54 kDa in the absence of glycosylation. N-linked glycosylation at the three potential sites in the primary structure can account for this discrepancy.

REFERENCES

Blackwell, J. M., R. A. B. Ezekowitz, M. B. Roberts, J. Y. Channon, R. B. Sim, and S. Gordon. 1985. Macrophage complement and lectin-like receptors bind Leishmania in the absence of serum. J. Exp. Med. 162:324.

Bordier, C. 1987. The promastigote surface protease of Leishmania. Parasitol. Today 3: 151-153.

Bouvier, J., R.J. Etges, and C. Bordier. 1985. Identification and purification of membrane and soluble forms of the major surface protein of Leishmania promastigotes. J. Biol. Chem. 260:15504-15509.

Bouvier, J., R. Etges, and C. Bordier. 1987. Identification of the promasitigote surface protease in seven species of Leishmania. Mol. Biochem. Parasitol. 24: 73-79.

Button, L.L., Olafson, R.W., and McMaster, W.R. 1987. Molecular cloning of the major surface antigen of Leishmania. Nature (submitted).

Chang, C. S., and K. -P. Chang. 1986. Monoclonal antibody affinity purification of a Leishmania membrane glycoprotein and its inhibition of Leishmania-macrophage binding. Proc. Natl. Acad. Sci. USA 83:100-104.

Chang, C.S., T.J. Inserra, J.A. Kink, D. Fong, and K.-P. Chang. 1986. Expression and size heterogeneity of a 63 kilodalton membrane glycoprotein during growth and transformation of Leishmania mexicana amazonensis. Mol. Biochem. Parasitol. 18:197-210.

Colomer-Gould, V., L. Galvao Quintao, J. Keithly, and N. Nogueira. 1985. A common major surface antigen on amastigotes and promastigotes of Leishmania species. J. Exp. Med. 162:902-916.

Cross, G.A.M. 1987. Eukaryotic protein modification and membrane attachment via phosphatidylinositol. Cell 48:179-181.

Etges, R., J. Bouvier, and C. Bordier. 1986. The major surface protein of Leishmania promastigotes is anchored in the membrane by a myristic acid-labeled phospholipid. EMBO J. 5:597-601.

Etges, R., J. Bouvier, and C. Bordier. 1986. The major surface protein of Leishmania promastigotes is a protease. J. Biol. Chem. 261:9098-9101.

Etges, R.J., J. Bouvier, R. Hoffman, and C. Bordier. 1985. Evidence that the major surface proteins of three Leishmania species are structurally related. Mol. Biochem. Parasitol. 14:141-149.

Gardiner, P. R., C. L. Jaffe, and D. M. Dwyer. 1984. Identification of cross-reactive promastigote cell surface antigens of some Leishmanial stocks by 125I labelling and immunoprecipitation. Infect. Immun. 43:637-643.

Gardnier, J., Osguthorpe, D.J. and Robson B. 1978. Analysis of the accuracy and implications of simple methods for predicting the secondary structure of globular proteins. J. Mol. Biol. 120:97-120.

Grumont, R., W. L. Washtien, D. Caput, and D. V. Santi. 1986. Bifunctional thymidylate synthase-dihydrofolate reductase from Leishmania tropica: Sequence homology with the corresponding monofunctional proteins. Proc. Natl. Acad. Sci. U.S.A. 83:5387-5391.

Hellman, L. and U. Pettersson. 1987. Analysis of closely related genes by the use of synthetic oligonucleotide probes labeled to a high specific activity. Gene Anal. Techn. 4:9-13.

Kweider, M., J.-L. Lemesre, F. Darcy, J.-P. Kusnierz, A. Capron, and F. Santoro. 1987. Infectivity of Leismania Braziliensis promastigotes is dependent on the increasing expression of a 65,000-dalton surface antigen. J. Immunol. 138:299-305.

Kyte, J. and R.F. Doolittle. 1982. A simple method for displaying the hydropathic character of a protein. J. Mol. Biol. 157:105-132.

Lepay, D. A., N. Nogueira, and Z. A. Cohn. 1983. Surface antigens of Leishmania donovani promastigotes. J. Exp. Med. 157:1562-1572.

Mosser, D. M., and P. J. Edelson. 1985. The mouse macrophage receptor for C3bi (CR3) is a major mechanism in the phagocytosis of Leishmania promastigotes. J. Immunol. 135:2785.

Neva, F. A., D. Wyler, and T. Nash. 1979. Cutaneous Leishmaniasis- a case with persistent organisms after treatment in presence of normal immune response. Am. J. Trop. Med. Hyg. 28:467-471.

Ruoslahti, E. and M. D. Pierschbacher. 1986. Arg-Gly-Asp: A versatile cell recognition signal. Cell 44:517-518.

Russell, D.G. and H. Wilhelm. 1986. The involvement of gp63, the major surface glycoprotein, in the attachment of Leishmania promastigotes to macrophages. J. Immunol. 136: 2613-2620.

Von Heijne, G. 1983. Patterns of amino acids near signal sequence cleavage sites. Eur. J. Biochem. 133:17-21.

Wilson, M.E. and R.D. Pearson. 1986. Evidence that Leishmania donovani utilizes a mannose receptor on human mononuclear phagocytes to establish intracellular parasitism. J. Immun. 136:4681-4688.

STRUCTURE FUNCTION STUDIES ON LEISHMANIA SURFACE MEMBRANE PROTEINS

Robert W. Olafson[1], Raymond A. Dwek[2], Thomas W. Rademacher[2], Kwang-Poo Chang[3], and Michael A. J. Ferguson[2]

Department of Biochemistry and Microbiology, University of Victoria, Victoria, B.C., Canada[1], Department of Biochemistry Oligosaccharides Group, University of Oxford, Oxford, England[2] and Department of Microbiology/Immunology, University of Health Sciences, Chicago Medical School, North Chicago, Il., USA[3]

INTRODUCTION

Elucidation of the molecular features of parasite cell surfaces is crucial to our understanding of parasite-host cell recognition as well as parasite survival in phagolysosomes. Recent studies have implicated a membrane glycoprotein and lipophosphoglycan in both of these phenomena[1,2,3]. Indeed, cell surface carbohydrates now appear to be critical to immunity[4,5], macrophage binding and internalization[6,2], as well as definition of infective and non-infective developmental stages[7,8]. This report emphasizes on-going structure and function studies of Leishmania glycoproteins as part of our general interest in parasite cell surface molecules.

MATERIALS AND METHODS

Affinity chromatography and preparative electrophoresis was performed as previously described [2,9]. Ion exchange HPLC was carried out on a MonoQ (Pharmacia) column using a pH 8.5 NH_4HCO_3 buffer with a linear NaCl gradient of 0-1M developed in 120 minutes. Reverse phase HPLC was performed on a Beckman ODS column using a 0.1% TFA mobile phase with a linear gradient of 60% acetonitrile developed in 30 min. Enzyme digests were performed on performic acid oxidized bovine insulin (250 µg/ml) in 200 mM sodium formate buffer, pH 4.0 at 37°. The detergent Mulgofen BC720 was a GAF product, New York, NY, while all other reagents were obtained from Sigma Chemical Co. Exoglycosidases were purified from the given sources by standard procedures[10].

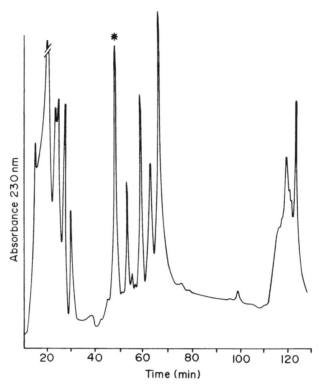

Fig. 1. Ion-exchange HPLC of detergent solubilized L. major pellicular membranes developed with a NaCl gradient as described in the Methods section. The asterisk indicates the elution position of the 63KD acid protease.
Detection sensitivity was 0.3 AUFS.

RESULTS AND DISCUSSION

A combination of affinity chromatography, HPLC and automated preparative SDS-PAGE electrophoresis procedures has made possible the isolation of the L. major gp63 and L. donovani acid phosphatase glycoproteins. As a result the N-terminal sequences have recently been determined for oligonucleotide probe synthesis, in collaboration with Dr. R. McMaster and Drs. D. Dwyer and P. Bates (unpublished results). Major interest in our laboratory has been focussed on the 63,000 M_r acid protease from L. donovani and L. major. Enzyme activity has been followed during isolation of this glycoprotein using ion-exchange HPLC of detergent solubilized (Mulgofen BC720) and concanavalin A concentrated material (Fig. 1). Since the enzyme activity had previously been shown to be maximum near pH 4.0 for L. mexicana[11], pH-stat activity determinations were obviated and replaced with analytical reverse phase HPLC separation of hydrolyzed peptides (Fig. 2). We were initially interested to ascertain the number of discrete enzyme activities associated with the solubilized membrane preparation. Subsequently we have shown that digests of performic acid oxidized insulin with detergent solubilized membrane preparations are less active at all pH values away from pH 4.0. At pHs above 5.5 no activity was found after incubation for 48 hours at 37°. With the possible exception of a protease with an

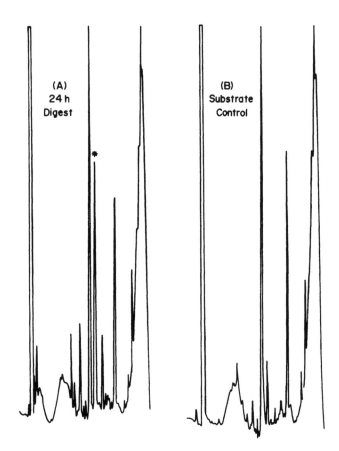

Fig. 2. Reverse phase HPLC separation of performic acid oxidized insulin peptides arising from a 24 hour digest with acid protease (A). Panel (B) shows the elution profile for the oxidized insulin substrate control. Hydrolysis conditions were as described in the Methods section.

unusual and absolute micronutrient requirement or sensitivity to detergent, it can be concluded that the L. major and L. donovani membranes do not have a basic protease activity against denatured protein. Moreover, on separation of the membrane components by ion-exchange HPLC, only one major peak was found to have acid protease activity. Oxidized insulin peptides arising from proteolysis with the latter enzyme were isolated and subjected to amino acid and amino terminal analysis. Results of this study indicated that the acid protease was a broad specificity protease not unlike mammalian pepsin. Cleavage sites at the carboxyl terminal side of Leu, Ala, Phe, Gly and Tyr were observed. If this enzyme is truly analogous to pepsin, then the specificities could be very broad indeed, with many residues of secondary preference. To characterize further the L. donovani acid protease, we also investigated the relative sensitivity to a number of serine and sulfhydryl directed protease inhibitors. Figure 3 shows the time course study of proteolysis of oxidized insulin as a function of the appearance of a specific peptide (asterisked in figure 2). Surprisingly, at 300 micromolar inhibitor concentrations, leupeptin and the sulfhydryl directed inhibitor E64 were not measurably inhibitory - nor was the trypsin inhibitor TLCK. A suggestion of inhibition was seen with TPCK, the chymotrypsin inhibitor, but not at a statistically significant level. On the other hand alkylation with iodoacetate at pH 8.5 completely destroyed enzyme activity suggesting the presence of a sulfhydryl group in the active site. It was of interest that the soluble cytoplasmic fraction of L. donovani was observed to have both acidic (pH 4.0) and basic (pH 8.0) protease activity towards oxidized insulin and that this activity was not inhibited by 300 micromolar TPCK, TLCK or Leupeptin.

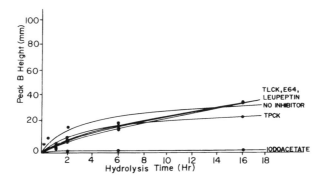

Fig. 3. Time course study of the effect of leupeptin, E64, tosylphenylchloromethyl ketone (TPCK), tosyllysylchoromethyl ketone (TLCK), and iodoacetic acid on acid protease activity. Inhibitor concentrations were 300 mM and exposure was made 30 min. prior to introduction of substrate.

A preliminary experiment has also been conducted on L. donovani amastigote membranes to ascertain whether they have acid protease activity. Very high levels of activity were found at pH 4.0. In order to distinguish this activity from possible host membrane contamination, the acid protease activity will be compared with spleen cell enzyme activity by amino acid and N-terminal analysis of isolated peptide products. This work is on-going.

Since gp63 has been shown to provide a macrophage lectin binding site[1,2], we have recently undertaken a chemical characterization of the oligosaccharides on the surface of the L. mexicana glycoprotein. The objective is to carry out a comparative study of gp63 carbohydrate structures on several species of Leishmania. The molecule was isolated by immunoaffinity chromatography using a Sepharose-linked monoclonal antibody, as described earlier[1]. Oligosaccharides from the glycoprotein were released quantitatively and intact by hydrazinolysis as described by Ashford et al[12]. The reducing termini of the pooled oligosaccharides were radioactively labelled by reduction with tritiated sodium borohydride and charged material was separated by high voltage paper electrophoresis. The neutral sugars were chromatographed on a BioGel P4 gel permeation column as previously described[12]. Figure 4 shows the presence of four major oligosaccharides equivalent in hydrodynamic mass to dextran polymers of 8.0, 9.0, 10.0 and 11.0 glucose units (g.u.). A smaller set of radioactive peaks, eluting between 3.6 and 2.4 g.u., was subsequently

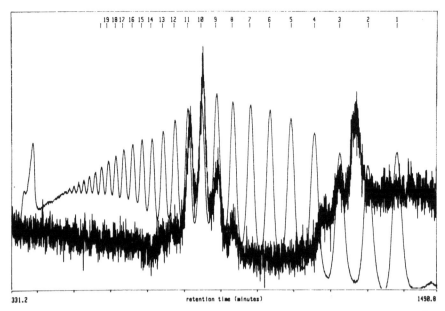

Fig. 4. Bio-Gel P-4 gel permeation chromatography of L. mexicana gp63 oligosaccharides reductively labelled with tritium. Elution position is indicated relative to a hydrolyzed dextran standard detected by refractive index monitoring and indicated in the figure by the oscillating profile.

shown by hydrolysis and reducing end terminal analysis on borate high voltage electrophoresis, to be glucose - presumably originating from the previous affinity chromatography isolation procedure. There is thus no evidence of O-linked sugars at this early stage of analysis but unequivocal determination will require further investigation. In a biosynthetic study, the Asn-linked oligosaccharides of L. mexicana had been proposed to be of the oligomannose type, with possible transient non-reducing end glucosylations[13]. However, on exposure to Jack Bean α-mannosidase only the g.u. 8.0 and 9.0 structures were lost from the high molecular weight group, with simultaneous appearance of a new peak at g.u. 5.6 (equivalent to the elution position of $ManGlcNAc_2$) and g.u. 4.7. The structural identity of the latter species has yet to be determined. Two major peaks remained at elution positions g.u. 10.1 and 9.3, indicating the presence of terminal sugars other than α-linked mannose (Fig. 5). Since Russell had provided evidence for terminal GlcNAc residues on gp63 of L. mexicana[4], the former pair of oligosaccharides were treated with Jack Bean β-hexosaminidase and rechromatographed. However, the peaks at g.u. 10.1 and 9.3 occupied the same elution position, indicating that the terminal saccharide is not a simple GlcNAc or GalNAc-Mannose linkage susceptible to β-hexosaminidase cleavage. The possibility that the end terminal sugars are glucose residues remains plausible and is presently under investigation.

CONCLUSION

From these studies it appears that a single sulfhydryl dependent, pepsin-like acid protease is present on the membrane of L. donovani with no evidence for the presence of basic proteases. The nature of the

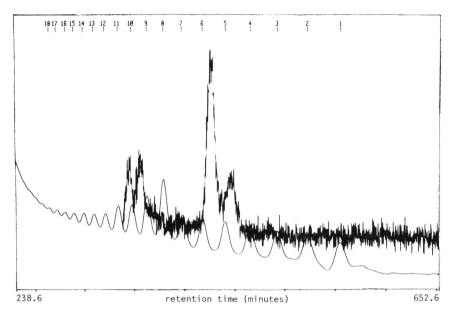

Fig. 5. Bio-Gel P-4 gel permeation chromatography of Jack Bean α-mannosidase digested, L. mexicana gp63 oligosaccharides isolated from g.u. positions 8.0, 9.0, 10.0 and 11.0 as shown in figure 4. New oligosaccharide elution positions were observed at g.u. 4.7, 5.6, 9.3 and 10.1.

oligosaccharide structures on gp63 are being actively pursued in our laboratory at this time. Preliminary investigations of the N-linked oligosaccharides of L. mexicana gp63 have indicated that they are of the high mannose type but more complicated than previously speculated. It is hoped that comparative structural studies of this glycoprotein across species and between life cycle stage may help elucidate the functional basis of the acid protease in the pathology of the Leishmaniases.

REFERENCES

1. C.S. Chang and K.-P. Chang, Monoclonal antibody affinity purification of a Leishmania membrane glycoprotein and its inhibition of Leishmania-macrophage binding, Proc. Natl. Acad. Sci. USA, 83:100 (1986).
2. D.G. Russell and H. Wilhelm, The involvement of the major surface glycoprotein (gp63) of Leishmania promastigotes in attachment to macrophages, J. Immunol. 136:2613 (1986).
3. E. Handman and J.W. Goding, The Leishmania receptor for macrophages is a lipid-containing glycoconjugate, EMBO J. 4:329 (1985).
4. R.M. Gorczynski, Do sugar residues contribute to the antigenic determinants responsible for protection and/or abolition of protection Leishmania-infected BALB/C mice?, J. Immunol. 137:1010 (1986).
5. K.M. Williams, J.B. Sacci and R.L. Anthony, Identification and recovery of Leishmania antigen displayed on the surface membrane of mouse peritoneal macrophages infected in vitro, J. Immunol. 136:1853 (1986).
6. J.M. Blackwell, Roll of macrophage complement and lectin-like receptors in binding Leishmania parasites to host macrophages, Immunol. Lett. 11:227 (1985).

7. D.L. Sacks, S. Hieny and A. Sher, Identification of cell surface carbohydrates and antigenic changes between noninfective and infective developmental stages of Leishmania major promastigotes, J. Immunol. 135:564 (1985).
8. E.M.B. Saraiva, A.F.B. Andrade and M.E.A. Pereira, Cell surface carbohydrate of Leishmania mexicana amazonensis: difference between infective and non-infective forms, Eur. J. Cell Biol. 40:219 (1986).
9. R.W. Olafson, A. Wallace and R. McMaster, Isolation and characterization of Leishmania membrane proteins, NATO ASI Series (Chang, K.-P. ed.) in press.
10. A. Kobata, Use of endo- and exoglycoidases for structural studies of glycoconjugates, Anal. Biochem. 100:1 (1979).
11. G. Chaudhuri and K.-P. Chang, Acid protease activity of gp63: possible role in virulence, NATO ASI Series (Chang, K.-P. ed.) in press.
12. D. Ashford, R.A. Dwek, J.K. Welply, S. Amatayakul, S.W. Homans, H. Lis, G.N. Taylor, N. Sharon and T.W. Rademacher, The β1-2D-xylose and α1-3L-fucose substituted N-linked oligosaccharides from Erythrina cristagalli lectin, Eur. J. Biochem. 166:311 (1987).
13. A.J. Parodi, J. Martin-Barrientos and J.C. Engel, Glycoprotein assembly in Leishmania mexicana, Biochem. Biophys. Res. Commun. 118:1 (1984).

THE PROMASTIGOTE SURFACE PROTEASE OF LEISHMANIA:

pH OPTIMUM AND EFFECTS OF PROTEASE INHIBITORS

Robert Etges, Jacques Bouvier, and Clement Bordier

Institut de Biochimie
Universite de Lausanne
CH-1066 Epalinges
Switzerland

INTRODUCTION

Surface glycoproteins of *Leishmania* promastigotes are readily identified by radioiodination. Commonly, a large proportion of the label is incorporated into a single component, a glycoprotein of 59 to 72 kDa, termed gp63 [1-7]. In the case of *Leishmania major* (LEM 513), promastigotes have been shown to contain 5×10^5 copies of gp63 [8], corresponding to 10,000 monomers per μm^2 [9]. In all the species examined, gp63 is anchored in the pellicular membrane of the promastigote by a glycophospholipid [10] which is structurally similar to the anchor of the variant surface glycoprotein (VSG) of another flagellated kinetoplastic protozoan, *Trypanosoma brucei* [11].

Protease activities have been detected in several species of *Leishmania*. Fong and Chang [12] briefly described two major enzymatic activities with molecular masses of 43 and 68 kDa in *Leishmania Mexicana amazonensis* promastigotes which were active on gelatin and fibrinogen after SDS-PAGE separation. Coombs [13] and Pupkis and Coombes [14] found a particulate protease in promastigotes and suggested that a soluble 67 kDa protease was common to both promastigotes and amastigotes of this species. Soluble acidic protease activities, probably of lysosomal origin, were superficially examined in extracts of *Leishmania donovani* and *Leishmania braziliensis* promastigotes [15,16]. However, in none of these cases was the enzyme examined in great detail.

During the purification of gp63, we found that the major surface glycoprotein of *Leishmania major* possess a endopeptidase activity [17,18]. Although the identity of this protease and the activities described by others has not been established, it is now known that homologous surface proteases occur on cultured promastigotes of most, if not all, isolates of *Leishmania* that have been examined [7,18]. During the life cycle of the parasite, the protease is found on promastigotes of *Leishmania infantum* in the midgut of *Phlebotomus perniciosus* [19]. Herein we describe the pH optimum and inhibitors sensitivity of the promastigote surface protease (PSP) with azocasein and fibrinogen as substrates.

RESULTS

THE pH OPTIMUM OF *Leishmania major* PSP

The pH optimum of *Leishmania major* (LEM 513) PSP was determined in a mixed-buffer system on two different polypeptide substrates. In the first method azocasein (4 mg/ml) was digested with 1 µg of the hydrophilic enzyme (H-PSP) in 0.5 ml of 50 mM each of HEPES, citric acid, boric acid, Na_2HPO_4 adjusted to 0.5 pH unit intervals with 1 M NaOH or 1 M HCL (azocasein precipitates below pH 4.0, and releases acid-soluble material that absorbs at 366 nm above pH 11). After a 30 min incubation at 37°C, an equal volume of 5% TCA was added on ice, and the absorbance of the TCA soluble material was determined after centrifugation at 366 nm. As shown in Figure 1a (closed symbols), PSP digests azocasein in solution in the absence of detergent. The pH optimum of the reaction is 8 to 10 [17].

In the second assay, using a rapid zymographic method with bovine fibrinogen (Mr 340,000) as a substrate copolymerized in a polyacrylamide gel containing 0.1% SDS [20], purified PSP was resolved on a single-sample gel (1 µg cm-1) containing 240 µg ml-1 fibrinogen. After electrophoresis, the gel was washed extensively in distilled H_2O and cut into 11 slices. Each gel slice was equilibrated at one pH unit intervals between pH 4 and 12 in the buffer mixture described above, incubated overnight at 42°C, then stained with Coomassie blue and destained (Figure 1b).

The protease activity is detected as a transparent band on a Coomassie blue-stained fibrinogen background. The degree of fibrinogenolytic activity in each gel piece was determined by semi-quantitative densitometry (Figure 1a, open symbols). On the fibrinogen substate, PSP demonstrates a broader range of optimum activity from pH 7 to 10. Similar results are obtained with the PSP of *Leishmania mexicana amazonensis* (LV 79) and *Leishmania donovani* (1S 2D) (data not shown).

Fibrinogen-SDS-PAGE analysis was used to investigate the effects of several substances known to inhibit other proteases on the activity of *Leishmania* PSP (Figure 2a & b). In this case, amphiphilic PSP was purified from surface-radioiodinated promastigotes and resolves as a single-sample on a fibrinogen containing gel.

After extensive washing in 10 mM Tris-HCl at pH 8.5 containing 140 mM NaCl (TBS), the gel was cut into 1 cm slices and incubated as above in the presence of the designated substance in TBS. Following the incubation, the gel pieces were stained in Coomassie blue (Figure 2a), then dried and fluographed to demonstrate the presence of PSP (Figure 2b)

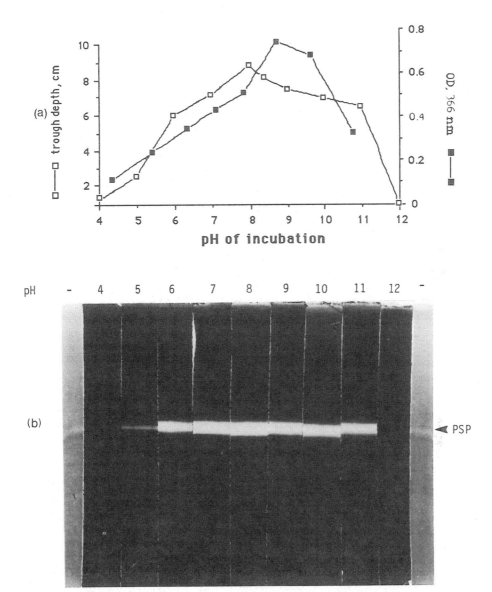

Figure 1a & b Activity of *Leishmania major* PSP as a function of pH

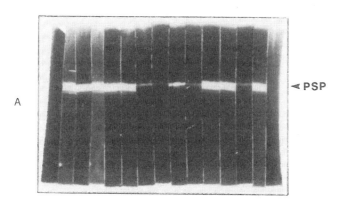

```
       2   4   6   8   10  12   14
     1   3   5   7   9   11  13   15
```

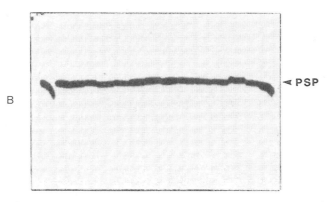

Figure 2a & b Effects of several inhibitors on the activity of *Leishmania major* PSP analysed by fibrinogen-SDS-PAGE.

Table 1. Substances tested for their effect on the activity of *Leishmania major* PSP with azocasein and fibrinogen-SDS-PAGE.

No detectable inhibition:

    1 mN diisopropylfuorophosphate (DFP)
    1mM phenylmethane-sulfonylfluoride (PMSF)
    1 mM N-p-tosyl-L-lysine chloromethylketone (TLCK)
    20 µg ml^{-1} (29.5 µM) antipain
    20 µg ml^{-1} (44 µM) leupeptin
    20 µg ml^{-1} (29 µM) pepstatin
    8000 U ml^{-1} aprotinin
    10 ug ml^{-1} (49 nM) soybean trypsin inhibitor
    0.5 µM L-trans-epoxysuccinylleucylamido-(4-guanidino)-butane (E-64)
    6 & 30 nM N-(alpha-rhamnopyranosyl-oxyhydroxyphosphinyl)-L-leucyl-L-tryptophan (phosphoramidon)
    10 mM Na_2 EDTA
    10 mM Na_2 EGTA
    ·1 - 10 mM $CaCl_2$
    1 - 10 mM $MgCl_2$
    10 mM iodoacetamide
    0.1 mM dithiothreitol

Weak inhibition (less than 10%):

    1 mM dithiothreitol
    1 mM 2-mercaptoethanol
    10 mM p-chloromercuriphenylsulfonic acid (PCMPSA)*
    1 mM AgCl

Strong inhibition (more than 90%):

    10 mM 1,10-phenanthroline
    10 mM dithiothreitol
    1 mM $HgCl_2$
    1 mM $ZnCl_2$
    1 mM $FeCl_2$
    1 mM $CoCl_2$
    1 mM $CuSO_4$

  *Inhibition detected only with azocasein as substrate

Gel slices were treated as follows:
1 and 15 were fixed and stained immediately after electrophoresis (negative control).
2 was incubated in buffer alone (positive control).
3 was incubated with 20 μg ml^{-1} (29.5 uM) antipain, 20 μg ml^{-1} (44 μM) leupeptin, 20 μg ml^{-1} (29 μM) pepstatin.
4: 6 nM phosphoramidon.
5: 30 nM phosphoramidon.
6: 1 mM N-ptosyn-Ll lysine chloromethylketone (TLCK).
7: 0.1 mM $ZnCl_2$.
8: 1 mM $ZnCl_2$;
9: 0.1 mM $CoCl_2$.
10: 1 mM $CoCl_2$.
11: 50 mM Na_2EDTA.
12: 50 mM Na_2EGTA.
13: 1 mM 1, 10-phenanthroline.
14: 10 mM p-chloromercuri-phenylsulfonic acid (pCMPSA).

Only Zn Cl_2, orthophenanthroline, and to a lesser extent $CoCl_2$, inhibit the activity of PSP. Similar results are obtained using azocasein as substrate (data not shown). A more extensive list of inhibitors, tested on both substrates, is shown in Table 1.

The results obtained with inhibitors, and the uniformly negative results with synthetic chromogenic peptide substrates (not shown), preclude the precise characterization of the substrate specificity, or the identification of a specific reactive amino acid of the promastigote surface protease. However, the incapacity of diisopropylfluorophosphate (DFP) and phenylmethylsulfonyl-fluoride to inhibit the activity of PSP suggests only that the *Leishmania* protease is not likely to be a serine esterase.

CONCLUSION

The elucidation of the substrate specificity and enzymatic mechanism of *Leishmania* PSP could lead to the rational design of a substrate analogue that would inactivate specifically the parasite's enzyme. Should the activity of PSP prove to be necessary for the establishment of infection and survival for the amastigote form of the parasite in the mammalian host, such a compound could be modified to a pharmacologically active drug for the treatment of Old and New World leishmaniases.

REFERENCES

1   Lepay, D.A.; N. Nogueira, and Z. Cohn 1983.
     J. Exp. Med. 157, 1562-1572.
2   Gardiner, P.R.; C.L. Jaffe, and D.M. Dwyer 1984.
     Infect. Immun. 143, 637-643.
3   Etges, R.; J. Bouvier, R. Hoffman, and C. Bordier 1985.
     Mol. Biochem. Parasitol. 14, 141-149.
4   Misle, J.A., M.E. Marquez, and A.G. Fernandez 1985.
     Z. Parasitenkd. 71, 419-428.

5   Russell, D.G.; and H. Wilhelm 1986.
       J. Immunol. 136, 2613-2620.
6   Legrand, D.; P. Desjeux, E. Prina, F. Le Pont, and S.F.
       Breniere 1986. C.R,Acad.Sci. Paris 303,607-612
7   Bouvier, J.; R. Etges, and C. Bordier 1985.
       Mol Biochem. Parasitol. 24, 73-79.
8   Bouvier, J.; R. Etges, and C. Bordier 1985.
       J. Biol. Chem. 260, 15504-15509.
9   Bordier, C. 1987
       Parasitol Today 3, 151-153.
10 Etges, R., J. Bouvier, and C. Bordier 1986.
       EMBO J. 5, 587-601.
11 Bordier, C.; R. Etges, J. Ward, M.J. Turner, and M.L.
       Cardoso de Almeida 1986. P.N.A.S. 83,5988-5991
12 Fong, D. and K.-P Chang 1982.
       J. Cell Biol. 91, 43A.
13 Coombes, G.H.   1982.
       Parasitol. 84, 149-155.
14 Pupkis, M.F. and G.H. Coombs 1984.
       J. Gen. Micobiol. 130, 2375-2383.
15 Camargo, E.P.; S. Itow, and S.C. Alfieri 1978.
       J. Parasitol. 64, 1120-1121.
16. Steiger, R.F.; F. van Hoof, J. Bontemps, M. Myssens-
       Jadin, and J.-E. Druetz 1979.
       Acta Tropica 36,335-341
17 Etges, R.; J. Bouvier, adn C. Bordier 1986.
       J. Biol. Chem. 261, 9098-9101.
18 Etges, R.; J. Bouvier, and C. Bordier 1987.
       NATO-ASI Series "Host-Parasite Cellular and
       Molecular Interactions in Protozoal Infections",
       K.-P Chang and D. Snary (eds). Springer Verlag
       Heidelberg. pp. 165-168.
19 Grimm, F.; Jenni, L., Bouvier, J., Etges, R.
       and Bordier C. 1987. Acta Tropica, in press.
20 Lonsdale-Eccles, J.D.; and G.W.N. Mpimbaza 1986.
       Eur. J. Biochem. 155, 469-473

PROTEOLYSIS IN LEISHMANIA: SPECIES DIFFERENCES AND DEVELOPMENTAL CHANGES IN

PROTEINASE ACTIVITY

Michael J. North[1], Barbara C. Lockwood[2], David J. Mallinson[2] and Graham H. Coombs[2]

[1]Department of Biological Science, University of Stirling Stirling, FK9 4LA, U.K. and [2]Department of Zoology, University of Glasgow, Glasgow G12 8QQ, U.K.

INTRODUCTION

Proteolysis probably plays an important part in the life cycle of many parasitic protozoa (North, 1982). A complete understanding of proteolysis in any organism is dependent on a knowledge of the enzymes involved and of their properties. It is now apparent that in most cells proteolytic enzymes are present in multiple forms and the task of identifying individual enzymes can be difficult. Two methods have been used to distinguish the different proteinases present in species of Leishmania. The first involved gel electrophoresis and represents a development of an approach which was used initially to demonstrate qualitative differences between the enzymes of the promastigote and amastigote stages of L. mexicana mexicana (North and Coombs, 1981). A quantitative difference in activity between the two stages was demonstrated in proteinase assays based on protein substrates (Coombs, 1982), and subsequent work allowed substrate specificities to be differentiated through the use of chromogenic and fluorogenic peptides as substrates (Pupkis and Coombs, 1984). The second method used in the present study involved chromogenic peptides. In this paper data are presented on the proteinase activities present in three species of Leishmania, L. m. mexicana, L. donovani and L. major, at different stages of the life cycle. In particular, we have compared the activities in mid-log phase promastigotes (thought to be equivalent to those in the midgut of the sandfly) and stationary-phase populations of promastigotes (thought to contain high numbers of metacyclic promastigotes) or the purified metacyclic promastigotes where possible. We have also investigated amastigotes, the form that grows in mammals. In this way we have been able to determine whether metacyclic promastigotes synthesise proteinases as a preadaptation for survival in mammals. These results together with those of previous investigations demonstrate the importance of developmental regulation among the proteinases, and reveal enzymes whose presence at particular stages of the life cycle suggests specific roles in the host-parasite relationship.

MATERIALS AND METHODS

Samples of L. mexicana mexicana, MNYC/BZ/62/M379, L. major, MHOM/SA/83/RKK2, and L. donovani, MHOM/ET/67/L82, were obtained as described by Mallinson and Coombs (1986) and stored as cell pellets at -70°C until required. Parasite lysates were prepared by addition of 0.25% (v/v) Triton X-100 in 0.25 M sucrose unless otherwise indicated.

The method used for the analysis of proteinases by electrophoresis on polyacrylamide gels has been described in detail elswhere (Lockwood et al., 1987a,b). Briefly the procedure involves subjecting parasite lysates to electrophoresis on gels containing 0·2% gelatin and then incubating the gels successively in 2·5% (v/v) Triton X-100, buffer (normally 0·1 M sodium acetate/acetic acid, pH 5·5), staining solution and destaining solution. Proteinase activity is observed as clear bands against a stained background.

Proteinase assays were carried out using nitroaniline-derivatives as substrates as described by North et al. (1983). The assays were conducted at 37°C and pH 6·0 in the presence of 1 mM dithiothreitol unless otherwise indicated. Activity was measured as an increase in absorbance at 405 nm due to the release of 4-nitroaniline. Specific activities were determined assuming a molar extinction coefficient of 9500 and are given in units of nmol product released per minute per mg protein. Protein was determined by the method of Sedmak and Grossberg (1977) using bovine albumin as standard.

The substrates were obtained from the following sources: Bz-Arg-Nan (Bz, N-benzoyl; Nan, 4-nitroaniline), Bz-Val-Gly-Arg-Nan, Bz-Pro-Phe-Arg-Nan, Bz-Phe-Val-Arg-Nan (Sigma, Poole, England); Cbz-Arg-Arg-Nan (Cbz, N-carbobenzoxy), Ac-Phe-Gly-Nan (Ac, acetyl), Suc-Val-Pro-Phe-Nan (Suc, succinyl), Suc-Phe-Pro-Phe-Nan (Novabiochem, Läufelfingen, Switzerland) and Cbz-Tyr-Lys-Arg-Nan, Suc-Ala-Ala-Pro-Phe-Nan and Suc-Ala-Ala-Pro-Leu-Nan (Bachem, Bubendorf, Switzerland).

RESULTS AND DISCUSSION

Two methods have been used to distinguish the proteinases in unfractionated lysates of Leishmania species, gel electrophoresis and assays based on chromogenic peptides. Separation and detection of proteinases can be achieved by electrophoresis on polyacrylamide gels containing gelatin (gelatin-PAGE), and some of the details of the enzymes detected in different cell types of L. mexicana mexicana, L. donovani and L. major have been reported elsewhere (Lockwood et al., 1987b). In L. mexicana mexicana there appeared to be two distinct groups of proteinases. One group consists of enzymes which have apparent molecular weights in the range from 60000 to 130000 and are found at all stages of the life cycle. It has not yet been possible to determine whether there are developmental changes in individual enzyme activities, although increased activity is apparent in amastigotes. The second group of proteinases consists of enzymes of low apparent molecular weight (16000 to 36000) which are subject to developmental regulation. At the promastigote stage they are absent during the mid-log phase but are apparent, albeit at low levels, in populations of stationary phase cells. They are, however, abundant in amastigotes. Significantly there are qualitative differences between the promastigote and amastigote enzymes.

Leishmania donovani differs from L. m. mexicana in that it lacks the low molecular weight proteinases. A number of high molecular enzymes with properties similar to those of L. m. mexicana are present and some interesting developmental changes are apparent. For example, a 130000-M_r proteinase is present at a low level in mid-log phase promastigotes, in increased amounts in stationary phase promastigotes and is most abundant in amastigotes. Leishmania donovani has a 90000-M_r enzyme which is apparently specific to stationary phase promastigotes. A 63000-68000-M_r enzyme can be detected at all stages.

In common with L. donovani and L. m. mexicana, L. major has high molecular weight proteinases. We have now shown that these enzymes are present not only at the promastigote and metacyclic stages but also in amastigotes (Fig. 1). One of the higher molecular weight proteinases, which has an apparent molecular weight of 120000, resembles the 130000-M_r enzyme of L. donovani in its regulation. It is barely detectable in mid-log phase promastigotes but is present at an increased level at the metacyclic stage, while the highest activity is found in amastigotes. As in the other two

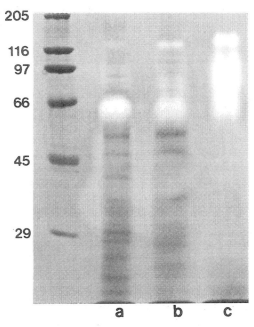

Fig. 1. Developmental changes in the proteinases of Leishmania major revealed by gelatin-PAGE. Samples of (a) mid-log phase promastigotes, (b) metacyclics promastigotes or (c) amastigotes were subjected to electrophoresis on gelatin gels. Proteinase bands were developed by incubation at pH 5·5 in the presence of 1 mM dithiothreitol

species a 63000-68000-$\underline{Mr}$ proteinase is present throughout. There are no lower molecular weight proteinases detectable in amastigotes, in which respect L. major resembles L. donovani rather than L. mexicana mexicana,.

The two groups of proteinases, the larger enzymes found in all stages of all three species and the smaller enzymes unique to L. m. mexicana, can be distinguished from one another by their sensitivity to proteinase inhibitors. A range of putative inhibitors have been tested, but only one agent, 1,10-phenanthrolene, has been found to inactivate the higher $\underline{Mr}$ enzymes. In contrast, a number of reagents, including antipain and leupeptin, inhibit the L. m. mexicana low $\underline{Mr}$ enzymes, indicating that these proteinases are of the cysteine type (EC 3.4.22.-). The size, inhibitor sensitivities and developmental changes of the proteinases revealed by gelatin-PAGE analyses indicate that they include the enzymes previously purified from L. m. mexicana (Pupkis and Coombs, 1984). These were a 67000-$\underline{Mr}$ proteinase found in amastigotes and promastigotes, which must be a representative of the high molecular weight group, and an amastigote-specific enzyme of 31000 molecular weight, which must be one of the low molecular weight cysteine proteinases.

The properties of the high molecular weight proteinases also reveal a marked similarity to the proteinase activity associated with gp63, the major surface antigen of Leishmania species. The enzyme activity of this glycoprotein was first demonstrated for L. major (Etges et al., 1986) and it has now been shown to be present on all of the Leishmania species examined (Bouvier et al., 1987), including the three considered here. The shared properties include inhibition by phenanthrolene and binding to conconavalin A (Lockwood et al., 1987b). Since it is present at all stages of all species and is of a similar size, it seems likely that this 63000-68000-$\underline{Mr}$ proteinase observed on gelatin gels is the same as gp63.

Table 1. Hydrolysis of arginine containing peptide-nitroanilides by promastigotes[a].

Substrate[b]	Specific Activity[c]		
	L. major	L. donovani	L. m. mexicana
Bz-R	6·0	12·5	8·5
Cbz-RR	9·2	20·3	8·4
Bz-FVR	2·1	10·1	6·0
Cbz-YKR	2·4	12·1	3·0
Bz-VGR	6·6	18·6	7·8
Bz-PFR	7·2	14·9	7·7

[a]Lysates were prepared from mid-log phase promastigotes.
[b]The substrates used were Bz-Arg-Nan (Bz-R), Cbz-Arg-Arg-Nan (Cbz-RR), Bz-Phe-Val-Arg (Bz-FVR), Cbz-Tyr-Lys-Arg-Nan (Cbz-YKR), Bz-Val-Gly-Arg-Nan (Bz-VGR) and Bz-Pro-Phe-Arg-Nan (Bz-PFR).
[c]Specific activities are in units of nmol min^{-1} (mg protein)$^{-1}$.

The analysis of the purified proteinases of L. m. mexicana showed that two groups of enzyme can also be distinguished by their specificity towards chromogenic and fluorogenic peptide substrates (Pupkis & Coombs, 1984). The 67000-Mr enzyme hydrolysed a number of derivatives containing arginine at the P_1 position (as defined by Schechter & Berger, 1967). The activity was non-specific since the derivatives were hydrolysed at similar rates irrespective of which amino acid residues were present at the P_2 and P_3 positions. In contrast, the 31000-Mr enzyme showed a preference for particular amino acids in the P_2 and P_3 positions and hydrolyzed the substrate Bz-Pro-Phe-Arg-Nan at significantly faster rates than any other nitroanilide tested. Amastigote lysates hydrolysed the latter substrate considerably more rapidly than did promastigote lysates. When the Bz-Pro-Phe-Arg-Nan hydrolysing activity of L. m. mexicana was compared with the same activity in three other species, with only one of these, L. m. amazonensis, was the substrate hydrolysed rapidly (Pupkis et al., 1986). As with L. m. mexicana, high activity was specific to amastigotes. Amastigotes of L. major and L. donovani contained low activity. These results indicated that Bz-Pro-Phe-Arg-Nan represents a relatively specific substrate for the low molecular weight enzymes, although it must be emphasised that there is some hydrolysis, albeit at a much reduced rate, with promastigote lysates.

We have now extended the range of peptide derivatives tested with Leishmania lysates to establish, in particular, whether there is a preferred substrate for promastigote activity. None of the following were hydrolysed at a significant rate (specific activity of less than 0·2 nmol min^{-1} (mg protein)$^{-1}$) by lysates prepared from promastigotes of L. major, L. donovani or L. mexicana mexicana: Suc-Ala-Ala-Pro-Phe-Nan, Suc-Ala-Ala-Pro-Leu-Nan, Suc-Phe-Pro-Phe-Nan, Suc-Val-Pro-Phe-Nan and Ac-Phe-Gly-Nan. When arginine-containing peptide derivatives were tested, these were all hydrolysed by promastigote lysates at rates similar to those for substrates tested previously (Table 1). No obvious substrate preference was apparent, confirming the broad specificity of the promastigote enzymes for this type of substrate.

Three arginine-containing nitroanilides were selected for a comparison between the three species at different cell stages (Table 2). The unique nature of the Bz-Pro-Phe-Arg-Nan-hydrolysing activity of L. mexicana mexicana amastigotes is confirmed by the data. The small but significant difference between the Bz-Pro-Phe-Arg-Nan-hydrolysing activity of mid-log phase and stationary phase promastigotes of L. m. mexicana correlates with the appearance

Table 2. Hydrolysis of peptide-nitroanilides by lysates of Leishmania at different stages of the life cycle

Species - stage	Specific Activity on Substrates[a]		
	Bz-R	Cbz-RR	Bz-PFR
L. major			
- mid-log phase promastigotes	7.4	11.3	8.9
- metacyclic promastigotes	13.4	11.1	15.3
L. donovani			
- mid-log phase promastigotes	12.5	20.3	14.9
- stationary phase promastigotes	16.4	17.6	12.7
- amastigotes	17.3	26.6	35.2
L. m. mexicana			
- mid-log phase promastigotes	10.3	8.6	7.1
- stationary phase promastigotes	12.3	9.6	15.4
- amastigotes	38.2	35.8	105.1

[a]The substrates used were Bz-Arg-Nan (Bz-R), Cbz-Arg-Arg-Nan (Cbz-RR) and Bz-Pro-Phe-Arg-Nan (Bz-PFR). The values are from replicate assays and are in units of nmol min^{-1} (mg protein)$^{-1}$.

of low molecular weight proteinase bands in stationary phase promastigotes (Lockwood et al., 1987b).

Use of the specific cysteine proteinase inhibitor E64 provided confirmation that the Bz-Pro-Phe-Arg-Nan-hydrolysing activity in mid-log phase promastigotes differed from that in amastigotes. The former activity was not inhibited by 10 μg E64 ml^{-1} whereas the amastigote activity was reduced by 85%. Interestingly, there was some inhibition (~30%) of the activity in stationary phase promastigotes, probably because some low molecular weight proteinases were present. With amastigotes, the activity towards Bz-Arg-Nan and Cbz-Arg-Arg-Nan was also inhibited by E64, suggesting that the low molecular weight cysteine proteinases do have some activity towards these substrates. Omission of dithiothreitol from the assay had no affect on the promastigote activity towards Bz-Pro-Phe-Arg-Nan but reduced the amastigote activity by over 80%. These results are consistent with the activity in amastigotes, but not that in promastigotes, being due to cysteine proteinases.

A comparison of the activities with different substrates may provide clues as to the relationship between the amastigote proteinases and analogous mammalian enzymes. Mammalian cells possess a number of cysteine proteinases, the best characterised being cathepsin B, cathepsin H and cathepsin L. Since the specific activities for the hydrolysis of Bz-Arg-Nan and Bz-Arg-Arg-Nan by L. m. mexicana amastigotes were similar, the proteinases involved differ from cathepsin B, an enzyme with a preference for the latter substrate (Kirschke and Barrett, 1985). The high activity observed with Bz-Pro-Phe-Arg-Nan suggests that the enzymes are more like cathepsin L, which hydrolyses substrates containing Phe-Arg but has low activity towards those containing Arg-Arg. An important characteristic of mammalian cathepsin L is its high activity towards protein substrates.

The relationship between the higher molecular weight Leishmania proteinases and well-characterised enzymes in other organisms remains to be established. The data obtained to date do not readily suggest to which of the four well-defined proteinase classes they belong. The leishmania enzymes do not appear to be cysteine proteinases since they are not activated by DTT and are not inhibited by agents such as antipain, leupeptin or E64. Lack of inhibition with pepstatin or phenylmethylsulphonyl fluoride (PMSF) suggests that they are not aspartic or serine proteinases, although their non-specific activity towards a range of arginine derivatives is a trypsin-like characteristic. Phenanthroline is the only substance which has been found to have an effect on the activity. This agent is, however, of limited use for establishing the proteinase class. It is a chelating agent which is usually considered to be an inhibitor of metalloproteinases, but there are a number of instances, especially among protozoan enzymes, in which inhibition of cysteine proteinases by phenanthrolene has been noted (North, 1982). It seems possible that the high molecular weight Leishmania proteinases represent a unique class of proteinases which have no well-characterised counterparts in other systems.

The cell stage-dependent changes in the peptide nitroanilide-hydrolysing activity of L. m. mexicana are reminiscent of the situation observed in African trypanosomes (North et al., 1983). With Trypanosoma brucei it was possible to differentiate two types of activity, a DTT-dependent activity specific for Bz-Pro-Phe-Arg-Nan and a DTT-independent activity of broader specificity. Significantly, the former was detected only in the bloodstream forms. Thus with both Leishmania and Trypanosoma species cysteine proteinase activity detected with Bz-Pro-Phe-Arg-Nan is characteristic of the stages of the life cycle in the mammalian host.

All of the results obtained to date are consistent with the view that the high cysteine proteinase activity of Leishmania species is associated with the megasome (Pupkis et al., 1986). Only those species which possess megasomes have cysteine proteinase activity, megasomes and high cysteine proteinase activity are both specific features of the amastigote stage, and the presence of cysteine proteinase in megasomes has been demonstrated by immunocytochemistry (Pupkis et al., 1986). The acquisition of cysteine proteinase by L. m. mexicana probably represents a necessary preparation for the intracellular stage of the life cycle. The importance of cysteine proteinase to the organism is indicated by the fact that inhibitors of the enzymes, notably antipain, have antileishmanial activity and inhibit the growth of L. m. mexicana amastigotes (Coombs et al., 1982, Coombs and Baxter, 1984).

Developmental changes in proteinase activities are not, however, confined to the cysteine proteinases, and regulation can also be seen among the high molecular weight group of enzymes. For example, there is one enzyme specific to the stationary phase promastigotes of L. donovani, and there are enzymes found in both L. major and L. donovani which are much more abundant in amastigotes than in promastigote forms. Whether these fulfil a function equivalent to the developmentally-regulated cysteine proteinases of L. mexicana mexicana has still to be investigated. With the exception of the gp63 proteinase activity the precise localisation of the high molecular weight proteinases has not been established.

The finding that the gp63 glycoprotein possesses proteinase activity has stimulated interest in the proteinases of Leishmania. Nevertheless it should be emphasised that further study of other proteolytic enzymes are likely to prove to be equally important since they include proteins whose activities undergo significant changes during the life cycle. This suggests an involvement of the proteinases in the adaptation of the parasite to life in its different hosts.

CONCLUSIONS

1. Two distinct groups of proteinases are apparent in Leishmania species, one group of higher molecular weight enzymes, representatives of which are present in all of the species examined, and a group of low molecular weight proteinases which were detected only in L. m. mexicana.

2. The low molecular weight proteinases were detected at low activity in stationary phase, but not in mid-log phase populations of promastigotes. They were abundant in amastigotes.
3. The presence of low molecular weight proteinases correlates with a specific dithiothreitol-dependent hydrolytic activity towards the chromogenic peptide Bz-Pro-Phe-Arg-Nan. This activity is E64-sensitive.
4. High molecular weight enzymes were found in all stages in all species investigated. Some developmental changes were apparent. A 63000-68000-M_r enzyme is common to all stages and all species and may be the cell surface proteinase gp63.
5. The high molecular weight enzymes have broad specificity towards arginine-containing chromogenic peptides. No specific substrate has yet been demonstrated. Phenanthrolene is the only effective inhibitor found to date.
6. Overall the results highlight the difference between L. m. mexicana and the other species with respect to proteinase content, a difference which correlates with the presence of megasomes.

ACKNOWLEDGEMENTS

We wish to thank the Medical Research Council and The Wellcome Trust for financial support.

REFERENCES

Bouvier, J., Etges, R. and Bordier, C., 1987, Identification of the promastigote surface protease in seven species of Leishmania, Mol. Biochem. Parasitol. 24, 73-79.

Coombs, G. H., 1982, Proteinases of Leishmania mexicana and other flagellate protozoa, Parasitology 84, 149-155.

Coombs, G. H. and Baxter, J, 1984, Inhibition of Leishmania amastigote growth by antipain and leupeptin, Ann. Trop. Med. Parasitol. 78. 21-24.

Coombs, G. H., Hart, D. T. and Capaldo, J., 1982, Proteinase inhibitors as antileishmanial agents, Trans. Roy. Soc. Trop. Med. Hyg. 76, 660-663.

Etges, R., Bouvier, J. and Bordier, C., 1986, The major surface protein of Leishmania promastigotes is a protease, J. Biol. Chem. 261, 9098-9101.

Kirschke, H. and Barrett, A. J, 1985, Cathepsin L - a lysosomal cysteine proteinase., in: "Intracellular Protein Catabolism," E. A. Khairallah, J. S. Bond and J. W. C. Bird, eds., pp. 61-69, Alan R. Liss, New York.

Lockwood, B. C., North, M. J., Scott, K. I., Bremner, A. F. and Coombs, G. H., 1987a, Comparative analysis of trichomonad proteinases using a highly sensitive electrophoretic method, Mol. Biochem. Parasitol, 24, 89-95.

Lockwood, B. C., North, M. J., Mallinson, D. J. and Coombs, G. H., 1987b, Analysis of Leishmania proteinases reveals developmental changes in species-specific forms and a common 68-kDa activity, FEMS Microbiol. Lett., in press.

Mallinson, D. J. and Coombs, G. H., 1986, Molecular characterisation of the metacyclic forms of Leishmania, IRCS Med. Sci. 14, 557-558.

North, M.J., 1982, Comparative biochemistry of the proteinases of eucaryotic microorganisms, Microbiol. Rev. 46, 308-340.

North, M. J. and Coombs, G. H., 1981, Proteinases of Leishmania mexicana amastigotes and promastigotes: analysis by gel electrophoresis, Mol. Biochem. Parasitol, 3, 293-300.

North, M. J., Coombs, G. H. and Barry, J. D., 1983, A comparative study of the proteolytic enzymes of Trypanosoma brucei, T. equiperdum, T. evansi, T. vivax, Leishmania tarentolae and Crithidia fasciculata, Mol. Biochem. Parasitol. 9, 161-180.

Pupkis, M. F. and Coombs, G. H., 1984, Purification and characterization of proteolytic enzymes of Leishmania mexicana mexicana amastigotes and promastigotes, J. Gen. Microbiol. 130, 2375-2383.

Pupkis, M. F., Tetley, L. and Coombs, G. H., 1986, Leishmania mexicana: amastigote hydrolases in unusual lysosomes, Exp. Parasitol. 62, 29-39.

Schechter, I. and Berger, A., 1967, On the size of the active site in proteases. I. Papain, Biochem. Biophys. Res. Commun. 27, 157-162.

Sedmak, J. J. and Grossberg, S. E., 1977, A rapid, sensitive and versatile assay for protein using Coomassie Brilliant Blue G250, Anal. Biochem. 79, 544-552.

THE LEISHMANIA DONOVANI LIPOPHOSPHOGLYCAN:

STRUCTURE AND FUNCTION

Salvatore J. Turco

Department of Biochemistry
University of Kentucky College of Medicine
Lexington, KY 40536 U.S.A.

INTRODUCTION

The protozoan parasite Leishmania donovani is able to live in two harsh hydrolytic environments in its digenetic life cycle: as an extracellular promastigote in the alimentary tract of its sandfly vector and as an intracellular amastigote in lysosomes of macrophages of its mammalian host. That L. donovani has adapted to survive in such hostile environments is most likely due to protection conferred by specialized molecules on the parasite's cell surface. We have discovered that L. donovani synthesizes and expresses a unique, cell surface glycoconjugate called lipophosphoglycan (1-4). Our long-term objective is to provide insight into the biochemistry of this major glycoconjugate of L. donovani. In this report, the structure and possible biological role of lipophosphoglycan are proposed.

MATERIALS AND METHODS

Cells

Promastigotes of Leishmania donovani were obtained and passaged as described elsewhere (1). Starter cultures were grown at 25°C to an average density of 3×10^7 cells/ml in Dulbecco's modified Eagle medium supplemented with 0.3% bovine serum albumin, adenosine (0.05 mM), xanthine (0.05 mM), biotin (1 mg/l), Tween 80 (40 mg/l), hemin (5 mg/l), and triethanolamine (0.5 ml/l). For isolation and purification of large amounts of LPG, one liter cultures of Brain-Heart Infusion supplemented with ethanolamine (1 ml/l), hemin (5 mg/l), and xanthine (0.01 mM) were seeded with 50-100 ml of starter cultures. Cells were grown at 25°C in a controlled environment incubator shaker to a density of $4-5 \times 10^7$ cells/ml.

Extraction and Purification of LPG

Ten liters of exponentially-growing L. donovani promastigotes (approximately 10^{11} cells) were extracted as described previously (1). Briefly, the cells were separated from the culture medium by centrifugation and washed with 250 ml of phosphate-buffered saline (1). The cells were then extracted sequentially (with 15 ml of each solvent at 4°C) as follows: twice with chloroform/methanol/water (3:2:1), 1-4 times with 4 mM $MgCl_2$, and three times with chloroform/methanol/water (1:1:0.3). LPG was then extracted from the resulting delipidated residue fraction by four extractions at 4°C with 15 ml of water/ethanol/diethylether/pyridine/NH_4OH (15:15:5:1:0.017) (solvent E). The extract was dried by evaporation under reduced pressure, resuspended in 5 ml of 40 mM NH_4OH and 1 mM EDTA, and applied to a column (4.6 cm x 30 cm) of Sephadex G150 equilibrated in 40 mM NH_4OH and 1 mM EDTA. The fractions containing LPG were pooled, dried by lyophilization, and desalted by elution through a column (1 cm x 5 cm) of Sephadex G25 equilibrated in 40 mM NH_4OH. The dried LPG was resuspended in 4 ml of solvent E and was precipitated from the pooled fractions by adding an equal volume of methanol and chilling the sample at -20°C for 16 h. Purified LPG can then be resuspended in solvent E.

RESULTS

L. donovani promastigotes synthesize and express on their cell surface a novel glycoconjugate called lipophosphoglycan (LPG). This complex carbohydrate is a major glycoconjugate since it contains over half of the total carbohydrate bound to macromolecules in L. donovani. Based on the results summarized below and described in detail elsewhere (1-4), we propose the structure of LPG as shown in Figure 1. LPG is a heterogeneous glycoconjugate (average molecular weight ~ 9 Kd) containing as its salient feature a repeating phosphorylated disaccharide unit of [PO_4→6Gal(β1→4)Manα1]. The repeating unit is attached to an unusual lyso-alkylphosphatidylinositol lipid anchor via a phosphoheptasaccharide carbohydrate core containing 3 galactose, 2 mannose, 1 glucose, and 1 unacetylated glucosamine residue.

Purification of LPG

We developed a rapid and simple method for purifying the L. donovani LPG to homogeneity. LPG can be extracted from the parasites with solvent E after removal of lipids and metabolites as described elsewhere (1,3). LPG can then be precipitated from contaminating proteins by adding an equal volume of methanol and chilling the sample at -20°C for 16 h. After resuspending the precipitate in solvent E, LPG prepared in this manner was judged to be homogeneous by analysis on SDS polyacrylamide gels and thin layer chromatography (3).

Characterization of the repeating disaccharide unit

In an early observation (1), LPG was found to be extremely labile to mild acid hydrolysis (0.02 N HCl, 15 min, 60°C) yielding one major carbohydrate fragment and several minor fragments. We have completed the characterization of the main carbohydrate fragment as the phosphorylated disaccharide PO_4→6Gal(β1→4)Man (Fig. 2). The presence of 4-substituted mannose in LPG was determined by methylation linkage analysis (GLC-mass spectrometric analysis of the partially methylated alditol acetates). This was an especially significant discovery considering that

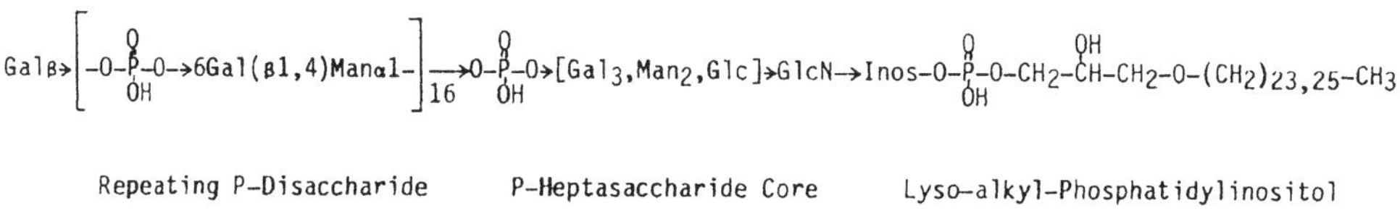

Galβ→[-O-P(O)(OH)-O→6Gal(β1,4)Manα1-]$_{16}$ →O-P(O)(OH)-O→[Gal$_3$,Man$_2$,Glc]→GlcN→Inos-O-P(O)(OH)-O-CH_2-CH(OH)-CH_2-O-$(CH_2)_{23,25}$-CH_3

Repeating P-Disaccharide   P-Heptasaccharide Core   Lyso-alkyl-Phosphatidylinositol

Fig. 1. Structure of Lipophosphoglycan

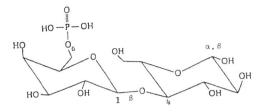

Fig. 2. Structure of the Repeating Unit of LPG

4-substituted mannose is highly unusual in glycoconjugates from eukaryotic cells. Thus, LPG may prove to be highly antigenic due to an epitope possessing this unusual carbohydrate linkage. Repeating units of $PO_4 \rightarrow 6Gal(\beta 1 \rightarrow 4)Man\alpha 1$ linked together by α-glycosidic linkages are also unique in a eukaryotic glycoconjugate. The location of the phosphate group on the 6-hydroxyl group of the galactose residue and the anomeric configuration of the phosphate group attached to the anomeric carbon of the mannose residue were determined by ^{1}H-NMR in collaboration with Dr. Steven W. Homans and coworkers, Department of Biochemistry, University of Oxford, England. We determined that there are an average of sixteen phosphorylated disaccharide units in the overall glycoconjugate structure.

Characterization of the lipid moiety of LPG

The lipid region of LPG, which is believed to be the anchoring unit for this cell surface macromolecule, has been characterized according to the experimental protocol in Figure 3. We performed a series of hydrolytic degradations on LPG and in each case, the lipid products were characterized by gas-liquid chromatography-mass spectrometry (3). Analysis has shown the glycan portion of LPG to be covalently linked to a novel lyso-phosphatidylinositol lipid in which the glycerol backbone is in ether linkage with a alkyl side chain. Support for this conclusion is based on results obtained following treatment of LPG with a

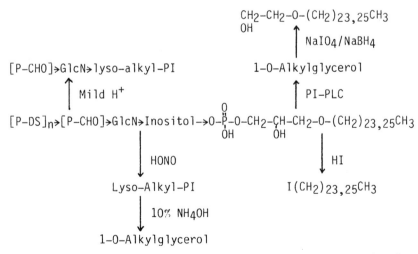

Fig. 3. Structure of the LPG Lipid Region and its Reaction Products. P-DS = Phosphorylated disaccharide units; P-CHO = Phosphocarbohydrate core.

phosphatidylinositol-specific phospholipase C (PI-PLC) isolated from Staphylococcus aureus or 10% NH4OH; both treatments released the same lipid species. Structural characterization of the PI-PLC-released lipid via GC-MS indicated the presence of two saturated, unbranched hydrocarbons: one with a C_{24} alkyl chain comprising approximately 78% of the lipid with the remaining 22% as a C_{26} alkyl chain. Periodate sensitivity demonstrated that the alkyl chain is linked to the C-1 position of the glycerol backbone. Ammonolysis of intact LPG and subsequent carbohydrate analysis also revealed the presence of a heptasaccharide structure linked to the inositol of the lipid moiety. Information obtained from further digestion with nitrous acid showed an unacetylated glucosamine attached to the lyso-PI lipid. Thus, these results indicate that L. donovani anchors its LPG with a unique lipid component.

Partial characterization of the carbohydrate core

The repeating phosphorylated disaccharide units are attached to the lyso-alkyl-PI anchor via a phosphocarbohydrate core containing three galactose, two mannose, one glucose, and one unacetylated glucosamine residue bound to the inositol residue. This sugar composition is comparable to the composition of the carbohydrate core of the VSGs of African trypanosomes (5). Experiments are in progress to determine the complete structure of this phosphoheptasacccharide core.

Comparison of the glycolipid anchors of LPG and protein

Interestingly, the phosphoheptasaccharide-lipid domain of LPG is similar to the carbohydrate-containing phosphatidylinositol anchor that has been reported for a growing number of eukaryotic membrane proteins (see ref. 6 for a review). LPG is the first reported occurrence of an analogous lipid anchoring a polysaccharide. The main structural difference in the two lipid anchors is a conventional diacylated PI for proteins and a lyso-alkyl PI for LPG (Fig. 4).

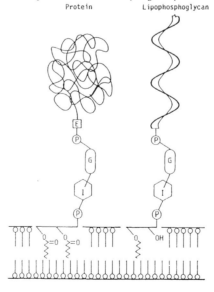

Fig. 4. Schematic Representation of Proteins, such as the Trypanosomal VSGs (5), and LPG Anchored in Membranes. Abbreviations: I, inositol; G, glycan core; P, phosphate; and E, ethanolamine. In this schematic representation, all sixteen phosphorylated disaccharide units are illustrated as a ribbon-like, consecutive sequence.

Cell surface localization of LPG

We established the important fact that LPG is located on the cell surface of the parasite (2). This conclusion was confirmed using a galactose oxidase/NaB[^{3}H]$_4$ technique of radiolabeling cell surface macromolecules. Incorporated radioactivity was analyzed by gel filtration on Sephadex G-100, chromatography on ricin agglutinin-coupled agarose, and lability to mild acid hydrolysis. The rationale for the use of this technique was based on prior information that the LPG possesses a terminal galactose residue. With the knowledge of the molar ratio of phosphate/LPG provided through the quantitative analysis of LPG (3), the cellular copy number for LPG was estimated. The extraction of 1 liter of cells (4×10^{10}) yields approximately 1.5 µmol of total phosphate contained in LPG, resulting in a cellular copy number of 1.25×10^6 molecules of LPG/cell. From estimates of the total cell surface area of the parasite and the percentage occupied by the polar head group of an individual phosphatidylinositol, the cell surface copy number of LPG could account for at least 25% of the total cell surface area. Depending on the conformation of LPG on the parasite's surface, the percentage may even be higher.

Release of LPG from the cells into the culture medium

Importantly, metabolically-labeled LPG is found in the culture medium following incubation of promastigotes with carbohydrate precursors (2). This "medium" LPG occurs in two structurally distinct forms. One form very tightly binds to bovine serum albumin in the medium and structural analysis revealed no obvious difference relative to the cellular LPG. A likely interpretation is that the lipid moiety of LPG interacts with a hydrophobic binding pocket of albumin facilitating LPG's release from the parasite's surface. However, the other form of medium LPG is structurally quite different from cellular LPG. This form of LPG appears to be similar in size as determined by gel filtration, but unlike cellular LPG, it does not bind to phenyl-Sepharose suggesting it lacks the hydrophobic region of LPG. A detailed characterization of this hydrophilic LPG found in the medium is required to determine the identity of the modification in the structure that releases it from the cell surface. It is possible that a lipid cleavage reaction enables the material to be released from cells. This is analogous to the phenomenom with the related trypanosomatid Trypanosoma brucei in which an endogenous PI-specific phospholipase C liberates the variable surface glycoprotein from the cell surface into the culture medium (7,8). Thus, similarities in the carbohydrate core and of the phosphatidylinositol lipid anchors of the leishmanial LPG and the trypanosomal VSGs (Fig. 4) suggest a possible phospholipase cleavage of LPG to release it from the parasite. It is also possible that the enzyme that releases LPG from the parasite might be an endoglycosidase.

Relationship of growth phase to the expression of LPG

We have found that while LPG is present throughout the various phases of growth of L. donovani, it is preferentially expressed during the latter part of logarithmic phase and in the stationary phase. This conclusion is based on the results of three experiments using parasites at various phases of growth: 1) incorporation of [^{3}H]mannose into LPG during 1 h of metabolic labeling of the cells; 2) cell surface labeling of LPG by the galactose oxidase/NaB[^{3}H]$_4$ method; and 3) total carbohydrate determination of LPG. It should be noted that Sacks and coworkers (9,10) have shown that L. major promastigotes maintained in stationary phase are much more infectious than parasites growing logarithmically. These investigators propose that a LPG-like molecule undergoes a structural modification of a terminal galactose residue as the parasite enters the stationary phase.

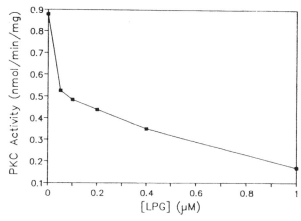

Fig. 5. Inhibition of Protein Kinase C Activity by LPG. Rat brain protein kinase C was assayed using [γ-^{32}P]ATP and histones as substrates and diacyl glycerol, phosphatidylserine, and calcium as cofactors. LPG in the designated concentration was added in the phosphatidylserine vesicles. After 3 min of incubation at 30°C, the reaction mixture was stopped by the addition of 5% trichloroacetic acid and the mixture was applied to an ascending paper chromatographic system using 5% trichloroacetic acid as the solvent. Radioactivity remaining at the origin of the chromatogram was quantitated and plotted.

Inhibition of protein kinase C activity by LPG

In order for L. donovani to survive in phagolysosomes of host cells, the parasite must circumvent the macrophage's potent oxidative burst. We hypothesize that this is accomplished by inhibition of the activation of the macrophage's protein kinase C by LPG. In a preliminary set of experiments, protein kinase C was isolated from rat brain (11) and its activity was shown to be inhibited by submicromolar concentrations of LPG (Fig. 5). In addition, LPG was found to be a competitive inhibitor with respect to diolein, a noncompetitive inhibitor with respect to phosphatidylserine, and had no significant effect on protein kinase A.

DISCUSSION

Cell surface components most likely play a key role in the survival of the Leishmanial parasites in the hostile environments and in confrontation with host-immune responses. However, in spite of their virtually certain relevance to the disease processes, only a limited amount of information is available regarding the biochemistry of complex carbohydrate-containing macromolecules of Leishmania. In early studies, several groups of investigators working with various human leishmanial species reported that promastigotes release antigenically active glycoconjugates into the culture medium (12-14). Using monoclonal antibodies, Handman and coworkers (15-19) have isolated and characterized a lipid-containing glycoconjugate from L. major. They have ascribed certain striking properties to this glycoconjugate. First, it is involved in attachment of the parasites to macrophages. During the movement of the parasite into the phagolysosome, the leishmanial glycoconjugate appears on the surface of the infected macrophage where it should be available to the immune system. Secondly, they further showed that immunization with the glycoconjugate protects mice against cutaneous leishmaniasis. Thirdly, the glycoconjugate isolated from a virulent clone of L. major could be passively incorporated into avirulent promastigotes of L. major which lost the capacity to synthesize this macromolecule. Such passive transfer of the lipid-containing glycoconjugate had conferred on the avirulent strain the ability to survive in macrophages in vitro. The L. donovani LPG appears to be structurally similar to the glycoconjugate of L. major.

It is not known how L. donovani survives in obviously hostile environments throughout its life cycle. To survive and proliferate, L. donovani must evade the action of degradative enzymes and the products of the oxidative burst in phagolysosomes of host macrophages. Toxic oxygen molecules, such as hydrogen peroxide, superoxide anion, and hydroxy radicals, are normally generated during the oxidative burst by activated phagocytic cells for the killing of microbes. Both the promastigote and amastigote forms of L. donovani are extremely sensitive to these toxic oxidative metabolites and are rapidly killed in vitro (20,21). Thus, in order to escape destruction, the parasite must somehow circumvent the induction of the oxidative burst. It is noteworthy that the presence of intracellular leishmanial parasites strongly inhibits the oxidative burst in lymphokine-activated or lipopolysaccharide-stimulated mouse peritoneal macrophages, as measured by chemiluminescence, reduction of cytochrome c and nitro blue tetrazolium, and hexose monophosphate shunt levels (22).

An important enzyme in macrophages that is believed to be responsible for initiating the oxidative burst is the phospholipid, Ca^{++}, and sn-diacylglycerol-dependent protein kinase (protein kinase C) (23-25). One of the proteins that is reported to be phosphorylated by protein kinase C following its induction is the NADPH oxidase which directly produces superoxide ions (25,26). Among a number of reported inhibitors of protein kinase C in cultured leukemic cells is a lyso-alkylphospholipid (27), a molecule analogous to the lipid portion of LPG. Our preliminary results suggest that the molecular basis of the previously described inhibition of the oxidative burst by L. donovani may be due to the inhibitory effect of its LPG on protein kinase C of the host macrophages.

In another aspect of the oxidative burst, Glew and coworkers (28,29) have shown that a tartrate-resistant acid phosphatase from L. donovani plays an important role in suppressing toxic metabolite production. Their observations suggest that the phosphatase causes inhibition by dephosphorylating critical substrates that enable the cell to become activated, rather than by directly affecting the oxidative pathway involved in generating superoxide and H_2O_2.

A potentially important finding of our structural work on the L. donovani LPG is the presence of a heptasaccharide core containing 3 galactose, 2 mannose, one glucose and one glucosamine residue. This composition is similar to the composition of the carbohydrate core of the variable surface glycoproteins (VSGs) of African trypanosomes (7). The carbohydrate core of the latter is believed to be the cross-reacting determinant for all VSGs. Thus, similarities in the carbohydrate core and of the phosphatidylinositol anchors of the leishmanial LPG and the trypanosomal VSGs warrant further investigation and possibly may lead to similar treatments for both classes of parasites.

CONCLUSIONS

The major, cell surface glycoconjugate of Leishmania donovani promastigotes is lipophosphoglycan. The structure of this unique macromolecule has been elucidated as a polymer of repeating phosphorylated disaccharide units linked via a phosphoheptasaccharide core to a novel lyso-alkylphosphatidylinositol lipid anchor. A possible, important physiological role of lipophosphoglycan as a negative effector of protein kinase C in host macrophages is proposed.

ACKNOWLEDGEMENTS

This investigation received financial support from UNDP/WORLD BANK/WHO Special Programme for Research and Training in Tropical Diseases, NIH Grant AI20941, and an NIH Research Career Development Award AM01087

REFERENCES

1. Turco, S. J., Wilkerson, M. A., and Clawson, D. R. (1984) J. Biol. Chem. 259, 3883-3889.
2. King, D. L., Chang, Y. D., and Turco, S. J. (1987) Mol. Biochem. Parasitol. 24, 47-54.
3. Orlandi, P. A., and Turco, S. J. (1987) J. Biol. Chem. 262, 10384-10391.
4. Turco, S. J., Hull, S. R., Orlandi, P. A., Shepherd, S. D., Homans, S. W., Dwek, R. A., and Rademacher, T. W., Biochemistry, in press.
5. Ferguson, M. J. A., Low, M. G., and Cross, G. A. M. (1985) J. Biol. Chem. 260, 14547-14555.
6. Low, M. G. (1987) Biochem. J. 244, 1-13.
7. Cardosa de Almeida, M. L., Allan, L. M., Turner, M. J. (1984) J. Protozool. 31, 53-60.
8. Fox., J. A., Duszenko, M., Ferguson, M. A. J., Low, M. G., and Cross, G. A. M. (1986) J. Biol. Chem. 261, 15767-15777.
9. Sacks, D. L., and Perkins, P. V. (1984) Science 223, 1417-1419.
10. Sacks, D. L., Heiny, S., Sher, A., (1985) J. Immunol. 135, 564-569.
11. Walton, G. M., Bertics, P. J., Hudson, L. G., Vedvick, T. S., and Gill, G. N., (1987) Anal. Biochem. 161, 425-437.
12. Decker-Jackson, J. E., and Honigberg, B. M. (1978) J. Protozool. 19. 514-525.
13. Semprevivo, L. H. (1978) Proc. Soc. Exp. Biol. Med. 159, 105-110.
14. El-On, J., Schnur, L. F., and Greenblatt, C. L. (1979) Exp. Parasitol. 47, 254-269.
15. Dwyer, D. M. (1980) J. Protozool. 27, 176-182.
16. Handman, E., Greenblatt, C. L., and Goding, J. W. (1984) EMBO J. 3, 2301-2306.
17. Handman, E., and Goding, J. W. (1985) EMBO J. 4, 329-336.
18. Handman, E., Schnur, L. F., Spithill, T. W., and Mitchell, G. F. (1986) J. Immunol. 137, 3608-3613.
19. Handman, E., and Mitchell, G. F. (1985) PNAS 82, 5910-5914.
20. Murray, H. W. (1981) J. Exp. Med. 153, 1302-1315.
21. Pearson, R. D., and Steigbigel, R. T. (1981) J. Immunol. 127, 1438-1443.
22. Buchmuller-Rouiller, Y., and Mauel, J. (1987) Infect. and Immun. 55, 587-593.
23. Wilson, E., Olcott, M. C., Bell, R. M., Merrill, A. H., and Lambeth, J. D., (1986) J. Biol. Chem. 261, 12616-12623.
24. Pontremoli, S., Melloni, E., Salamino, F., Sparatore, B., Michetti, M., Sacco, O., and Horecker, B. L. (1986) BBRC 140, 1121-1126.
25. Gennaro, R., Florio, C., and Romeo, D. (1985) FEBS Lett. 180, 185-190.
26. Cross, A. R., and Jones, O. T. G. (1986) Biochem. J. 237, 111-116.
27. Helfman, D. M., Barnes, K. C., Kinkade, J. M., Vogler, W. R., Shoji, M., and Kuo, J. F. (1983) Cancer Res. 43, 2955-2961.
28. Remaley, A. T., Kuhns, D. B., Basford, R. E., Glew, R. H., and Kaplan, S. S. (1984) J. Biol. Chem. 259, 11173-11175.
29. Das, S., Saha, A. K., Remaley, A. T., Glew, R. H., Dowling, J. N., Kajiyoshi, M., and Gottlieb, M. (1986) Mol. Biochem. Parasitol. 20, 143-153.

IMMUNOCHEMICAL CHARACTERIZATION OF THE LEISHMANIA DONOVANI 3'-NUCLEOTIDASE

Katie B. Pastakia and Dennis M. Dwyer

Cell Biology and Immunology Section
Laboratory of Parasitic Diseases
National Institute of Allergy and Infectious Diseases
National Institutes of Health
Bethesda, Maryland 20892 USA

INTRODUCTION

3'-nucleotidase (3'NT) is an externally oriented surface membrane enzyme of Leishmania donovani.[1,2] The enzyme is a glycoprotein of apparent $M_r=43,000$, capable of hydrolyzing 3'-nucleotides and also exhibits exonuclease activity.[1-3] As Leishmania have an absolute requirement for preformed purines, it has been suggested that the 3'NT might function in the acquisition of these essential nutrients from the growth medium.[1,2] It was recently shown, in a related trypanosomatid, Crithidia fasciculata, that 3'NT activity was regulated by the levels of exogenously supplied purines.[4] Similar regulation of 3'NT activity was observed with L. donovani in the current study. To facilitate the further characterization of this enzyme, a rabbit antiserum was rasied against the 3'NT isolated from L. donovani promastigotes. Results of immunochemical studies with this antiserum are presented in this report.

MATERIALS AND METHODS

1. Culture conditions. L. donovani (WHO designation: MHOM/SD/00/1S-2D) promastigotes were grown in medium 199 with 10% (v/v) fetal bovine serum.[1] For purine depletion studies, cells were grown in a chemically defined medium (RE-III minus BSA)[4] with various concentrations of adenosine.

2. Assay of 3'NT activity. Protein and enzyme determinations with intact cells and subcellular fractions were done as previously described.[1] Enzyme activity is expressed as nmol P_i released from 3'-AMP per min at 30°C.

3. Staining of 3'NT activity in gels. Samples of isolated 3'NT or immuno-precipitates (below) were separated by SDS-PAGE using 10% gels. Following SDS removal and incubation with 3'-AMP, the product of enzyme activity was visualized in gels using the malachite green-molybdate reagent.[3]

4. Immunochemical methods. 3'NT was isolated from promastigote surface membranes as previously described.[3] An antiserum against the isolated enzyme was raised in a rabbit by multiple, subcutaneous injections. Immunoprecipitations with this serum were done at 4°C for 4-18 hr. Immune complexes were recovered on Protein A-Sepharose CL-4B (Pharmacia), washed 3 times in 10 mM Tris-HCl/150 mM

NaCl/0.1% (v/v) Triton X-100, pH 7.5 buffer and eluted from the beads with SDS-sample buffer by boiling for 3 min. Supernatants from these were analyzed by SDS-PAGE.

RESULTS AND DISCUSSION

The effect of various concentrations of exogenously added adenosine as the sole purine source on the 3'NT activity of L. donovani promastigotes was examined. As shown in Table 1, the specific activity of 3'NT was significantly enhanced when the organisms were deprived of adenosine. The cells showed ≈10-fold increase in enzyme specific activity under purine starvation conditions suggesting that the 3'NT is regulated by purine levels in the growth medium. Similar observations have been reported with the related trypanosomatid, Crithidia fasciculata.[4] These results suggest that the 3'NT is an inducible enzyme system.

Table 1. Effect of adenosine concentration in the growth medium on the 3'NT activity of L. donovani promastigotes.

[Adenosine] in Medium μM	3'NT Specific Activity (nmol/mg protein/min)
25	290
10	520
5	1686
1	1350
0	2496

Promastigotes were grown in complete, defined medium (RE-III minus BSA) to a density of 1.4×10^7 cells/ml, harvested, washed, and resuspended in the same medium lacking adenosine. These cells were inoculated at a density of 1.8×10^6/ml into fresh medium containing 0 to 25 μM adenosine. After 55 hr of growth, the cultures were harvested, washed and assayed for 3'NT activity and protein.

The 3'NT was isolated from promastigote surface membranes and analyzed by SDS-PAGE. Subsequent to removal of SDS, the enzyme was renatured and its activity visualized in the gel (Fig. 1). In such gels, two major and one minor band of 3'NT activity (apparent M_r = 43,000, 37,000 and 90,000, respectively) were detected. Under similar conditions, spent growth medium showed a single activity stained band of M_r=37,000. Surface membrane preparations treated under these conditions have been reported to contain a single band of 3'NT activity at M_r=43,000.[5] The band of M_r=37,000 observed in both the isolated 3'NT preparations and the spent growth medium presumably represents a degradation product of the native enzyme.

A rabbit antiserum was raised against isolated 3'NT and used in a variety of immunochemical studies. The anti-3'NT serum readily agglutinated intact promastigotes. Further, this antibody was shown to inhibit the activity of the isolated 3'NT by ≈30% (Fig. 2A). This result suggests that the anti-3'NT serum contains some antibodies which affect the active site configuration of the enzyme. The antiserum also precipitated 3'NT activity in a concentration-dependent manner (Fig. 2B).

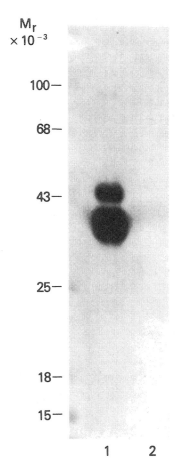

Fig. 1. Activity staining of renatured 3'NT after SDS-PAGE. Staining of 3'NT activity in gels was done as in Materials and Methods. Lane 1, isolated 3'NT, 20 µg protein, activity 0.055 µmol/min; lane 2, 50 µl of 100-fold concentrated spent growth medium (RE-III minus BSA).

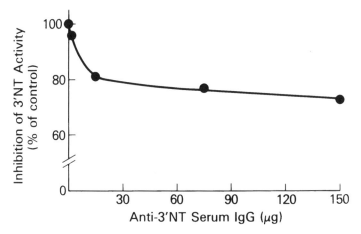

Fig. 2A. Inhibition of 3'NT activity by anti-3'NT serum. Isolated 3'NT was incubated with purified IgG from anti-3'NT serum and controls contained equivalent amounts of IgG from normal (preimmune) rabbit serum. 3'NT activity was measured as indicated in Materials and Methods.

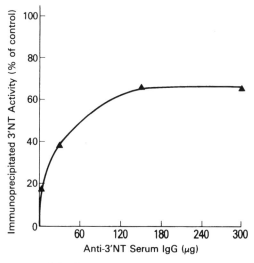

Fig. 2B. Immunoprecipitation of 3'NT activity by anti-3'NT serum. Immune complexes formed after incubation of the enzyme and IgG were adsorbed onto Protein A-Sepharose beads, washed and assayed for enzyme activity.

Immunoprecipitates of 3'NT were separated by SDS-PAGE, the enzyme activity renatured and stained in the gel. In such gels, two bands of 3'NT activity were observed of apparent M_r=43,000 and 37,000, respectively (Fig. 3). These results further substantiate the apparent M_r of the 3'NT (cf. Fig. 1).

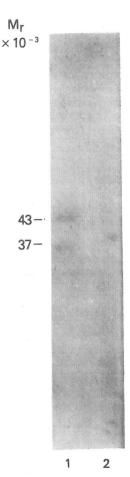

Fig. 3. Immunoprecipitated 3'NT stained for activity after SDS-PAGE. Immunocomplexes on Protein A-Sepharose beads were washed, eluted in SDS sample buffer, boiled for 3 min and the supernatants separated on 10% gels by SDS-PAGE. Subsequently, the gel was processed for activity staining. Immunoprecipitation with: Lane 1, anti-3'NT serum; lane 2, normal preimmune rabbit serum.

To analyze further the properties of this enzyme, the isolated 3'NT was iodinated with $Na^{125}I$ and Iodogen. Immunoprecipitates of the radiolabeled enzyme with anti-3'NT serum were analyzed by SDS-PAGE and autoradiography. As shown in Fig. 4, two polypeptides of M_r=43,000 and 37,000 were immunoprecipitated by the antiserum. These corresponded to the two major activity- stained bands observed in gels with both the isolated enzyme and immunoprecipitates, above (cf. Figs. 1,3). Immunoprecipitates of the radiolabeled enzyme contained three additional polypeptides of M_r=63,000, 26,000 and 18,000. The band of M_r=63,000 was recognized by anti-p63 serum (kindly provided by J. Bouvier and C. Bordier) indicating that p63 (promastigote surface protease)[6] copurified with the 3'NT. The other two bands present in the radio-immunoprecipitates may represent subunits of the enzyme, degradation products or polypeptides which copurify with the 3'NT.

To characterize the polypeptides recognized by the anti-3'NT serum, poly(A$^+$)mRNA from L. donovani was translated in an in vitro rabbit reticulocyte lysate system. The radiolabeled translation products were reacted with either preimmune serum or antiserum and the immunoprecipitates processed for SDS-PAGE/autoradiography. The anti-3'NT serum specifically precipitated two

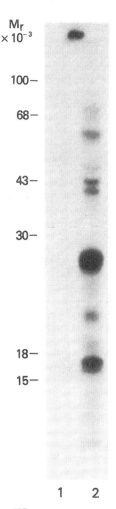

Fig. 4. Autoradiograph of ^{125}I-3'NT immunoprecipitates. ^{125}I-labeled 3'NT was reacted with anti-3'NT serum or with normal (preimmune) rabbit serum. Immune complexes were recovered as in Fig. 3 and analyzed by autoradiography. Immunoprecipitation with: Lane 1, normal (preimmune) rabbit serum; Lane 2, anti-3'NT serum.

polypeptides of M_r=70,000 and 40,000 (Fig. 5). Further, these two polypeptides were competed out by the addition of 3'NT to the immunoprecipitation reaction. These results demonstrate that the anti-3'NT serum recognized translated, nascent polypeptides. From their M_r, these polypeptides presumably correspond to the nascent enzyme prior to its secondary modification (e.g. glycosylation).

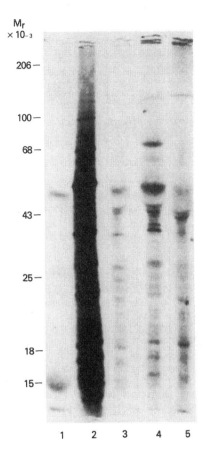

Fig. 5. SDS-PAGE/autoradiograph of immunoprecipitated in vitro translation products. [^{35}S]methionine-labeled in vitro translation products were reacted with normal or immune rabbit serum. Immune complexes were processed for SDS-PAGE as mentioned in Materials and Methods and analyzed by fluorography. Lane 1, minus RNA control; Lane 2, total in vitro translated products; Lanes 3-5, immunoprecipitates with preimmune serum, anti-3'NT serum and anti-3'NT serum in the presence of added 3'NT, respectively.

CONCLUSIONS

1. The 3'NT of L. donovani promastigotes is regulated by extracellular purine levels. Depletion of adenosine as the sole purine source leads to increased 3'NT activity.

2. The 3'NT was isolated from promastigote surface membranes. This glycoprotein was renatured in SDS-PAGE gels. Two major bands of apparent $M_r=43,000$, and 37,000, and a minor band of $M_r=90,000$ were stained for enzyme activity.

3. A rabbit anti-3'NT serum was raised which both inhibited and immunoprecipitated the enzyme. Immunoprecipitates, renatured after SDS-PAGE, showed enzyme activity at apparent $M_r=43,000$ and 37,000.

4. From in vitro translated products of L. donovani poly(A$^+$)mRNA, the anti-3'NT serum immunoprecipitated two specific polypeptides of apparent $M_r=70,000$ and 40,000. These presumably correspond to the nascent 3'NT polypeptides prior to their glycosylation/secondary modification.

REFERENCES

1. M. Gottlieb, and D. M. Dwyer, Evidence for distinct 5'- and 3'-nucleotidase activities in the surface membrane fraction of Leishmania donovani promastigotes, Mol. Biochem. Parasitol. 7: 303-317 (1983).
2. D. M. Dwyer and M. Gottlieb, Surface membrane localization of 3'- and 5'-nucleotidase activities in Leishmania donovani promastigotes, Mol. Biochem. Parasitol. 10:139-150 (1984).
3. M. Gottlieb and G. W. Zlotnick, 3'-nucleotidase of Leishmania donovani -- evidence for exonuclease activity, in "Molecular Strategies for Parasitic Invasion," N. Agabian, H. Goodman and N. Noguiera, eds., UCLA Symposium on Molecular and Cellular Biology, New Series, Vol. 42, Alan R. Liss, Inc., New York (1986).
4. M. Gottlieb, Enzyme regulation in a trypanosomatid: effect of purine starvation on levels of 3'-nucleotidase activity, Science 227:72-74 (1985).
5. G. W. Zlotnick, M. C. Mackow and M. Gottlieb, Renaturation of Leishmania donovani 3'-nucleotidase following sodium dodecyl sulfate-polyacrylamide gel electrophoresis, Comp. Biochem. Physiol. 87B:629-635 (1987).
6. R. Etges, J. Bouvier, and C. Bordier, The major surface protein of Leishmania promastigotes is a protease, J. Biol. Chem. 261:9098-9101 (1986).

INTERRELATIONS BETWEEN GLUCOSE AND ALANINE CATABOLISM, AMMONIA

PRODUCTION, AND THE D-LACTATE PATHWAY IN LEISHMANIA BRAZILIENSIS

J.J. Blum[1], D.G. Davis[2], T.N. Darling[1], and R.E. London[2]

[1]Department of Physiology, Duke University Medical Center Durham, NC 27710 and [2]National Institute of Environmental Health Sciences, Research Triangle Park, NC 27709

INTRODUCTION

L. braziliensis promastigotes catabolize glucose to CO_2 and release several incompletely oxidized products. These products, identified by NMR spectroscopy, include succinate, alanine, pyruvate, acetate, and lactate (Darling et al, 1987). Under anaerobic conditions, glycerol becomes a major product and lactate production increases, but glucose consumption decreases ("reverse" Pasteur effect). Enzymatic assays showed that the lactate formed is the D-stereoisomer, and that it is formed via methylglyoxal synthase and glyoxalases I and II (Darling and Blum, submitted for publication). D-lactate dehydrogenase does not appear to be present. The regulation and function of the methylglyoxal pathway in Leishmania are not yet known.

The formation of alanine from glucose implies proteolytic degradation of cellular proteins and extensive transamination of the amino acids so formed. Further support for the occurrence of proteolysis during incubation is production of ammonia (Darling et al, 1987). L. tropica also degrade intracellular protein, even in the presence of glucose (Simon and Mukkada, 1983). These observations suggest that glucose alone cannot meet all the metabolic requirements of the cell and that amino acids play a vital role in Leishmania metabolism. Furthermore, the presence of a large intracellular pool of alanine (Simon et al, 1983; Darling et al, 1987) and its utilization during starvation (Simon et al, 1983) suggests that alanine plays a central role in the intermediary metabolism of this parasite. Therefore, using NMR spectroscopy, we have identified the products formed from [3-^{13}C]alanine and from [2-^{13}C]glucose, and have studied the interaction between alanine and glucose. To gain insight into the control of proteolysis in Leishmania, we also examined ammonia and alanine production in the presence and absence of substrate or of proteolytic inhibitors.

METHODS

Leishmania braziliensis panamensis promastigotes (MHOM/PA/82/WR470) were grown as described (Darling and Blum, 1987). Cells in early stationary phase were harvested by centrifugation, washed, and resuspended in Hanks' balanced salt solution, and used for NMR spectroscopy or for assay of metabolites, as described (Darling et al, 1987). [3-^{13}C]Alanine and [2-^{13}C]glucose were obtained from Merck, Sharpe and Dohme Isotopes, Montreal, Canada.

RESULTS AND DISCUSSION

Metabolism of [2-^{13}C]glucose in the presence and absence of alanine

Promastigotes incubated with [2-^{13}C]glucose as sole exogenous carbon source released labeled succinate, acetate, alanine, lactate, and pyruvate (Fig. 1A), as expected from a comparable study with [1-^{13}C]glucose (Darling

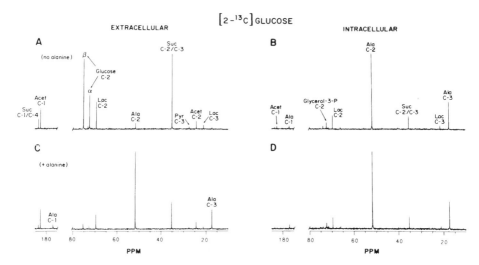

Fig. 1. Promastigotes were washed and resuspended with [2-^{13}C]glucose (5.55 mM initially plus 2.77 mM added at 30 min) in the absence (panels A and B) or presence (panels C and D) of L-alanine (2 mM added at t=0, 15, 30, and 45 min), and incubated aerobically for 60 min at 26°C. ^{13}C-labeled metabolites released into the medium (panels A and C) or obtained by perchloric-acid extraction of the cells (panels B and D, see Darling et al, 1987, for details) are shown. In addition to the signals shown, a small pyruvate C-2 signal at 206.0 PPM was observed in both extracellular samples. NMR shifts not listed in Darling et al (1987) include: acetate C-1, 182.5 PPM; succinate C-1/C-4, 183.4 PPM; alanine C-1, 176.9 PPM. Lac, lactate; suc, succinate; acet, acetate; ala, alanine; pyr, pyruvate.

et al, 1987). The label positions in these products were consistent with catabolism via the glycolytic pathway and formation of D-lactate by the methylglyoxal pathway. In addition, [3-^{13}C]lactate, [3-^{13}C]pyruvate, [2-^{13}C]acetate, and [3-^{13}C]alanine were released, indicating some label redistribution via the Krebs cycle, CO_2 fixation, and/or the pentose phosphate pathway. The succinate C-2 and/or C-3 peak was large relative to the succinate C-1/C-4 peak even considering the attenuation of the carboxyl signal. Since [2-^{13}C]glucose forms predominantly [1-^{13}C]acetyl CoA which would form succinate C-1/C-4, the large succinate C-2/C-3 peak suggests that most of the succinate is formed by CO_2 fixation onto P-enolpyruvate or pyruvate C-2 and then reversal of the Krebs cycle to succinate. Other evidence, reviewed by Marr (1980) supports formation of succinate by reverse flow in the Krebs cycle and suggests pyruvate carboxylase as the primary pathway of CO_2 fixation. It should be noted that although the signal for lactate C-1 (183.5 ppm) is very near to that for succinate C-1/C-4 (183.4 ppm), we assign the observed signal to succinate because it is unlikely that there would be more lactate C-1 than lactate C-3.

The intracellular pool contained alanine, succinate, acetate, and lactate, and also showed a spectral line corresponding to [2-^{13}C]glycerol-3-phosphate (Fig. 1B). A small amount of glycerol C-2 (73.3 ppm) was observed in the extracellular sample, in agreement with our observation that promastigotes produce only a small amount of glycerol under aerobic conditions (Darling et al, 1987). The absence of [2-^{13}C]glucose inside the cell (Fig. 1B) indicates that its rate of entry into the cell does not exceed the cell's capacity to metabolize it.

The same cells were also incubated with [2-^{13}C]glucose in the presence of unlabeled alanine (Figs. 1C, 1D). The spectrum of the labeled products (Fig. 1C) was closely similar to that of the labeled products released in the absence of alanine (Fig. 1A). The ability to resolve the [1-^{13}C]alanine peak probably reflects the greater production of labeled alanine. Neither did the presence of alanine affect the rate of glucose utilization. The ∼ 8 mM glucose added decreased to 0.25 and 0.5 mM in the presence and absence of added alanine, respectively. A separate experiment confirmed that alanine had no effect on glucose utilization. The labeling pattern of the intracellular pools was almost identical in the presence (Fig. 1D) as in the absence (Fig. 1B) of unlabeled alanine. Thus the addition of alanine had little effect on the pattern of label flow from [2-^{13}C]glucose, despite the fact that it is metabolized at a rapid rate (Keegan et al, 1987).

Metabolism of [3-^{13}C]alanine in the presence and absence of glucose

A complementary experiment was performed in which promastigotes were incubated with [3-^{13}C]alanine in the presence and absence of unlabeled glucose. When [3-^{13}C]alanine was the sole carbon source, [2-^{13}C]acetate was the only product besides CO_2 (Fig. 2A). When unlabeled glucose was also present, however, [2,3-^{13}C]succinate, [3-^{13}C]lactate and [2-^{13}C]alanine were released into the medium, as well as [3-^{13}C]pyruvate and [2-^{13}C]acetate (Fig. 2C). In addition, a small peak at 58.7 ppm was present. We tentatively identify this as [1-^{13}C]ethanol although the expected labeling of ethanol would be primarily of C-2 with, perhaps, a smaller peak of [1-^{13}C]ethanol, as observed in C. fasciculata catabolizing [1-^{13}C]glucose (de los Santos et al, 1985). Ethanol production has also been reported for T. lewisi and Strigomonas oncopelti (Ryley, 1958), but it has not to our knowledge been reported as a product of Leishmania metabolism. Further studies are required to be certain that this product is indeed ethanol and to establish the pathway for its synthesis.

While the presence of glucose clearly facilitated the flow of label from [3-^{13}C]alanine into products other than acetate, net utilization of alanine appeared to be reduced (cf. Figs. 2A and 2C). This was confirmed by enzymatic assay, which showed that alanine consumption decreased from about 600 to 150 nmol/mg protein·hr upon addition of 5 mM glucose. Thus whereas alanine had little effect on glucose utilization, glucose markedly reduced alanine utilization.

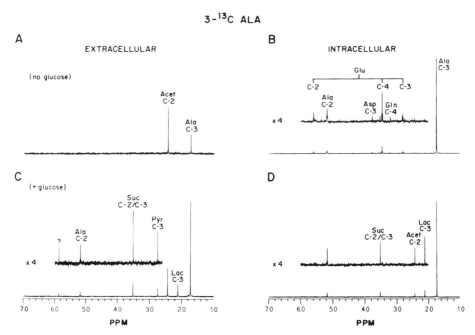

Fig. 2. Promastigotes were washed and resuspended with [3-^{13}C]L-alanine (2 mM added at t=0, 15, 30, and 45 min) in the absence (panels A and B) or presence (panels C and D) of glucose (5.55 mM, plus 2.77 mM at t=30 min). For further details, see legend to Fig. 1. Insets are at 4-fold gain. Signals not listed in Fig. 1 are: glutamate C-2, C-4, and C-3, 55.8, 34.5, and 28.1 PPM, respectively; aspartate C-3, 37.8 PPM; glutamine C-4, 31.9 PPM. Glu, glutamate; asp, aspartate, gln, glutamine.

In the intracellular pools, peaks corresponding to [2-^{13}C]-, [3-^{13}C]-, and [4-^{13}C]glutamate, [3-^{13}C]aspartate, and [4-^{13}C]glutamine were present in addition to [3-^{13}C]alanine itself and [2-^{13}C]alanine (Fig. 2B). The condensation of [2-^{13}C]acetyl CoA with unlabeled oxaloacetate (derived, presumably, from proteolysis) would form [4-^{13}C]α-ketoglutarate, which would yield [4-^{13}C]glutamate upon transamination and [4-^{13}C]glutamine by the action of glutamine synthetase. Label incorporation into [2-^{13}C]- and [3-^{13}C]glutamate can be accounted for by two pathways. Label from [4-^{13}C]α-ketoglutarate would appear in positions 2 and 3 after multiple turns of the Krebs cycle and randomization of label at fumarate. Alternatively, fixation of CO_2 into [3-^{13}C]pyruvate followed by randomization could also yield [2-^{13}C]- and [3-^{13}C]α-ketoglutarate and thus [2-^{13}C]- and

[3-^{13}C]glutamate. These reactions would also account for the [3-^{13}C] aspartate peak. The splitting of the glutamate peaks and of the alanine C-2 peak (Fig. 2B) indicates small amounts of the doubly labeled compounds.

When glucose was added in addition to the [3-^{13}C]alanine, the ^{13}C-labeled aspartate, glutamate, and glutamine were not visible (Fig. 2D). Instead ^{13}C-labeled acetate, lactate, and succinate (i.e., the products released into the medium) were present (Fig. 2C). Thus when alanine is sole carbon source it appears to be metabolized largely by transamination to pyruvate followed by decarboxylation to acetyl CoA and, by an as yet unknown mechanism, release of acetate. Some of the acetyl CoA enters the Krebs cycle as shown by the presence of succinate, which is not released from the cells. The transamination of alanine is with oxaloacetate and α-ketoglutarate, forming the aspartate and glutamate peaks observed intracellularly. Glutamate dehydrogenase probably serves to release most of the amino groups derived from the alanine as ammonia. In the presence of glucose the rate of alanine consumption is greatly reduced and the intracellular levels of ^{13}C-labeled glutamine, glutamate, and aspartate remain too small to be observed in the NMR spectrum.

Proteolysis by washed promastigotes

Although the degradation of intracellular proteins by L. tropica promastigotes began almost immediately after suspending the cells in nutrient-free buffer, glucose had no noticeable effect on the rate of ^{3}H-leucine release until after 1 hr of incubation (Simon and Mukkada, 1983). L. braziliensis incubated for 30 min in the absence of exogenous substrates produced ammonia and consumed alanine at about equal rates (Table 1). Since the cells were washed only once, it is possible that some of the alanine consumed was exogenous, but most was the large intracellular pool of alanine (Simon et al, 1983; Darling et al, 1987). The addition of glucose - but not, however, of acetate - reduced ammonia formation by over 70% and caused a net production of alanine as well as of ammonia. Further evidence for degradation of cellular protein was obtained from cells that were suspended in buffer for 1 hr before glucose or acetate were added (Table 1). The rate of alanine production was then negligible but appreciable amounts of ammonia were released. These rates were not significantly changed if acetate was added, but glucose markedly decreased the rate of ammonia release while increasing that of alanine. Since [2-^{14}C]acetate is oxidized to ^{14}CO$_2$ at about one-third the rate of [1-^{14}C]glucose (data not shown), these observations suggest the rate of oxidation of these substrates is not a major factor in determining the rate of proteolysis. Contrary to our previous suggestions that glucose inhibited proteolysis, which was based on measurement of ammonia production only (Darling et al, 1987), the present data show that the primary effect of glucose is not to inhibit proteolysis (see also Simon and Mukkada, 1983) but rather to markedly change the ratio of alanine to ammonia released, presumably by providing pyruvate for transamination.

Simon and Mukkada (1983) found that the proteolytic inhibitor TLCK did not inhibit proteolysis until about 1 hr after its addition, whereas phenylmethylsulfonyl fluoride inhibited ^{3}H-leucine release within minutes after its addition. We have found that neither chymostatin, leupeptin, nor antipain (100 µg/ml) altered the rate of ammonia formation during a 1 hr incubation in buffer. Much more work is required to establish the nature of this protease and the factors that regulate its activity. In particular, it would be interesting to ascertain whether a ubiquitin or a calcium-activated neutral protease is present.

Table 1. Effects of Glucose and Acetate on Ammonia and Alanine Production

	Ammonia	Alanine
	(nmol/min·mg protein)	

Additions

I. Added immediately after cells were resuspended in buffer

—	4.07 ± 1.16 (4)	-3.51 ± 0.62 (4)
Acetate	4.29 ± 0.94 (4)	-2.90 ± 0.96 (4)
Glucose	1.15 ± 0.21 (4)	1.31 ± 0.42 (4)

II. Added 1 hr after cells were resuspended in buffer

—	2.80 ± 0.81 (4)	0.31 ± 0.24 (5)
Acetate	3.00 ± 0.72 (3)	0.17 ± 0.23 (4)
Glucose	0.85 ± 0.14 (3)	3.10 ± 0.73 (4)

Promastigotes were washed and resuspended in Hanks' balanced salt solution (without glucose) as described in METHODS. Immediately after resuspension (Expt. 1) or after 1 hr incubation at 26°C (Expt. II), 1.3 mM acetate or 7.3 mM glucose were added as indicated and the cells incubated for 30 min. Samples were then taken for assay of alanine and ammonia. The means ± standard errors are shown, with the number of experiments in parentheses. A minus sign indicates utilization.

D-lactate production by ellipsoidal forms

Heating L. braziliensis promastigotes at 34°C for 72 hr transforms them to amastigote-like forms, and for shorter durations reversibly converts them into a morphologically and metabolically intermediate ellipsoidal (E) form (Darling and Blum, 1987). The rate of glucose utilization by the 6-hr heated E-forms is less than that of promastigotes, but the NMR spectra are similar (Darling et al, 1987). In one experiment promastigotes consumed 453 nmol glucose/mg protein·hr and produced 171 of D-lactate, while 6-hr heated E-forms consumed 219 nmol glucose/mg protein·hr and produced 114 of D-lactate. Thus the rate of D-lactate production relative to glucose utilization does not change dramatically upon transformation to the E-form. We have not yet examined amastigotes or other species of Leishmania, but culture forms of Trypanosoma brucei gambiense did not release D-lactate when incubated anaerobically with glucose (Balber, Darling, and Blum, unpublished). At present we have no information on the rates of proteolysis or its control during the heat-induced shape transformation of L. braziliensis, but this clearly deserves attention.

CONCLUSIONS

L. braziliensis promastigotes contain a large intracellular pool of alanine which is consumed during nutrient deprivation. Ammonia is produced even after the alanine pool is exhausted, indicating continuing and highly regulated proteolysis. Adding glucose to starving cells causes a shift to the release of alanine instead of ammonia but does not decrease proteolysis for at least 30 min. Exogenous alanine is transaminated with α-ketoglutarate and, to a lesser extent, oxaloacetate, forming glutamate and aspartate, respectively. The pyruvate so formed is catabolized to acetate and CO_2, but is not used by the methylglyoxal pathway. Adding glucose decreases exogenous [3-^{13}C]alanine utilization and causes a marked redistribution of label into other products. Alanine, however, has no effect on [2-^{13}C]glucose utilization and causes little change in the pattern of label incorporation except for the amount incorporated into alanine. Identification of the major products of glucose and of alanine metabolism has provided new insight into the organization of intermediary metabolism in L. braziliensis promastigotes and the role of proteolytic degradation during brief starvation, but much more remains to be learned.

ACKNOWLEDGEMENTS

T.N. Darling was supported by the Medical Scientist Training Program (NIH grant 5-T32-GM07171). We are grateful to Alvernon Hayes for his excellent technical assistance.

REFERENCES

Darling, T. N., and Blum, J. J., 1987, In vitro reversible transformation of Leishmania braziliensis panamensis between promastigotes and ellipsoidal forms, J. Protozool., 34:166-168.

Darling, T. N., Davis, D. G., London, R. E., and Blum, J. J., 1987, Products of Leishmania braziliensis catabolism: Release of D-lactate and, under anaerobic conditions, glycerol, Proc. Natl. Acad. Sci. USA, In press.

de los Santos, C., Buldain, G., Frydman, B., Cannata, J. J. B., and Cazzulo, J. J., 1985, Carbon-13-nuclear magnetic resonance analysis of [1-^{13}C]glucose metabolism in Crithidia fasciculata. Evidence of CO_2 fixation by phosphoenolpyruvate carboxykinase, Eur. J. Biochem., 149:421-429.

Keegan, F. P., Sansone, L., and Blum, J. J., 1987, Oxidation of glucose, ribose, alanine, and glutamate by Leishmania braziliensis panamensis, J. Protozool., 34:174-179.

Marr, J. J., 1980, Carbohydrate metabolism in Leishmania, in: "Biochemistry and Physiology of Protozoa", 2nd edition, Vol. 3, Academic Press, NY.

Pupkis, M. F., and Coombs, G. H., 1984, Purification and characterization of proteolytic enzymes of Leishmania mexicana mexicana amastigotes and promastigotes, J. Gen. Microbiol., 130:2375-2383.

Ryley, J. F., 1956, Studies on the metabolism of the protozoa. 7. Comparative carbohydrate metabolism of eleven species of trypanosome, Biochem. J., 62:215-222.

Simon, M. W., and Mukkada, A. J., 1983, Intracellular protein degradation in Leishmania tropica amastigotes, Molec. Biochem. Parasitol., 7:19-26.

Simon, M. W., Jayashimhulu, K., and Mukkada, A. J., 1983, The free amino acid pool in Leishmania tropica promastigotes, Molec. Biochem. Parasitol., 9:47-57.

LEISHMANIA AMASTIGOTES: ADAPTATIONS FOR GROWTH

IN AN ACIDIC IN VIVO ENVIRONMENT

Antony J. Mukkada, Theresa A. Glaser, Steven A. Anderson and Steven K. Wells

Department of Biological Sciences, University of Cincinnati, Cincinnati, Ohio 45221, USA

INTRODUCTION

The amastigote stage of Leishmania is an obligate intracellular parasite proliferating within the phagolysosomes of macrophages in vertebrate hosts (1,12). The macrophage represents a hostile environment for most microbes since it is endowed with mechanisms designed to destroy conventional organisms after phagocytosis. A limited number of parasites such as the agents of trypanosomiasis, toxoplasmosis, tuberculosis, leprosy, legionnaires' disease and epidemic typhus can resist killing by macrophages. These agents escape destruction by developing adaptive devices which generally prevent or minimize contact between them and the microbicidal substances within the lysosomes (2,6,9,17,19). Leishmania species are unique in that they allow fusion of the phagosome with lysosomes but survive and multiply in the resulting phagolysosomes. The phagolysosomal environment in murine, and human phagocytes is distinctly acidic with a pH between 4.0 and 5.0 (4,7,8). Amastigote survival in vivo must involve strategies affecting several levels of host parasite interactions. However, this discussion will be restricted to some of the adaptations which enable the parasite to cope with an acidic environment.

MATERIALS AND METHODS

Leishmania donovani (Sudan 1S) amastigotes were isolated from infected hamster spleens by a method we developed (13). Promastigotes were maintained in medium 199 (Gibco) supplemented with 15% heat inactivated fetal calf serum. Transport of labeled substrates was followed by a filtration technique described before (15). ATPase activity was assayed by following the release of inorganic phosphate by the method of Lanzetta et al (11).

RESULTS AND DISCUSSION

Activation of Amastigote Metabolism by Acid pH

We postulated that the extraordinary resistance of amastigotes to the acidic environment is at least in part due to the ability of the parasites to use the protons (H$^+$) plentifully available in the environment, to their own advantage. Recently we reported that several important physiological activities in L. donovani amastigotes show an acidic pH optimum which coincides with the pH of the intraphagolysosomal environment in which they reside (16). It was found that incorporation of nucleic acid precursors thymidine and uridine, the metabolism of glucose and proline as well as respiration occur optimally at pH 4.5-5.5 in amastigotes while these same activities occur optimally at around pH 7.0 in promastigotes (Fig. 1). It appears that amastigote metabolism is activated by the high hydrogen ion concentrations in their natural acidic habitat.

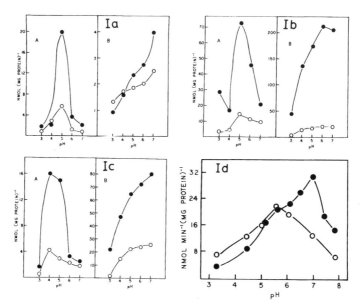

Fig. 1. Effect of pH on physiological activities in L. donovani amastigotes and promastigotes. 1a. Incorporation of [^{3}H] thymidine (0-0) and uridine (●-●). A. amastigotes, B. promastigotes. 1b. [^{14}C] proline metabolism. ●-●, CO$_2$ evolution; 0-0, incorporation into trichloroacetic acid insoluble material A. amastigotes, B. promastigotes. 1c. [^{14}C] glucose metabolism. ●-●, CO$_2$ evolution; 0-0, incorporation into trichloroacetic acid precipitable material. A. amastigotes, B. promastigotes. 1d. Respiration in amastigotes (0-0) and promastigotes (0-0). Reprinted from reference 16.

Acid pH Dependence of Substrate Transport

An interesting coincidence is that transport of substrates such as proline also occurs optimally at pH 5.5 in amastigotes (Fig. 2). Lowering the pH of the suspending medium from 7.0 to

5.5 resulted in a stimulation of the rate of transport as predicted while raising the pH from 5.5 to 7.0 had the opposite effect (Fig. 3). Thus in amastigotes, transport which is the first step in metabolism is dependent on the acid pH characteristic of the phagolysosomal environment. On the other hand, the pH optimum for the uptake of proline and 2-deoxy-D-glucose in promastigotes is around 7.0. Acidification of the medium to pH 5.5 drastically reduced transport in promastigotes.

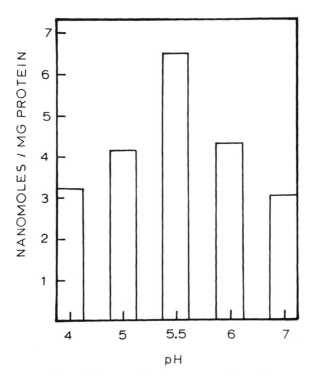

Fig. 2. Effect of pH on proline transport in L. donovani amastigotes.

Utilization of Proton Gradients in Transport

The proton rich phagolysosomal environment contributes to a gradient of protons across the membranes of resident amastigotes. The question is whether the amastigotes exploit this proton gradient to drive active uptake of substrates. Active transport in promastigotes has already been shown to be driven by an electrochemical gradient of protons across the membrane (14,20). To see if the same is true of amastigotes, uptake was followed under conditions that dissipate transmembrane proton gradients. Proline transport in amastigotes was severely inhibited when treated with ionophores such as carbonyl cyanide-m-chlorophenylhydrazone (CCCP), nigericin and valinomycin. Although these agents differ in the specific mechanisms of action, they all share the common feature in impeding the establishment of pH and electrical gradients by translocating protons and ions across the membrane. Uptake inhibition by these ionophores confirms the dependence of amastigotes on transmembrane proton gradients (pH gradients) for uptake. The protons in the in vivo environment could serve as a steady reservoir.

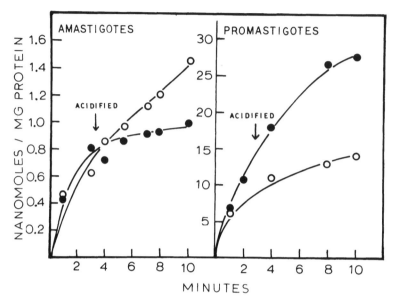

Fig. 3. Effect of acidification on proline transport in L. donovani amastigotes and promastigotes. Uptake was initiated at pH 7.0 and at the arrow enough HCl was added to lower the pH to 5.5. ●-●, control, 0-0, uptake after acidification.

The parasite is able to maintain a transmembrane proton gradient largely through the activity of a proton extruding ATPase (proton pump) located on the plasma membrane. This ATPase is present in both stages but because of the ease of growing promastigotes, much of the data are derived from this stage. Continuous monitoring of unbuffered cell suspensions showed acidification of the medium giving direct evidence for proton extrusion (Fig. 4). Proton extrusion was inhibited upon addition of the ATPase inhibitor, N,N'-dicyclohexyl carbodiimide (DCCD). This ATPase is Mg^{+2} dependent, shows a pH optimum at 6.7, is insensitive to ouabain and oligomycin but is sensitive to DCCD and vanadate. Plasma membranes were purified according to the method of Gottlieb and Dwyer (5) and were solubilized in Zwittergent 3-14 and subjected to nondissociating polyacrylamide gel electrophoresis (10). Activity staining of native gels revealed one or two bands of ATPase activity. When these bands were sliced, solubilized and run on SDS-PAGE gels (10), three protein bands were apparent at Mr 70 Kd, 100 Kd, and 105 Kd. The 70 Kd band was the most prominent. Subsequently, bands from the native gels and 70 Kd denatured proteins were mixed and injected into rabbits to produce a polyclonal antiserum. Immunoblotting showed recognition of a protein band at 70 Kd in lysates of both amastigotes and promastigotes. It also recognized a 105 Kd protein in promastigote lysates. The 70 Kd protein binds with [^{14}C] DCCD. It would seem that the 70 Kd - DCCD binding protein is the proton pump or that it is a breakdown product of the pump which is a 105 Kd protein.

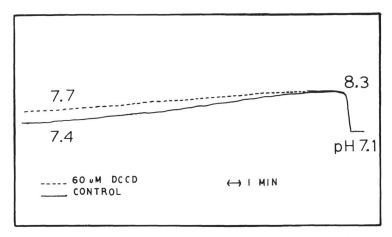

Fig. 4. Effect of DCCD on proton extrusion by L. donovani promastigotes.

Intracellular pH and Ion Regulation

The maintenance of physiological pH is most important for an organism such as Leishmania which cycles between acidophilic and neutrophilic stages. Promastigotes normally live within the gut of the sandfly at a slightly alkaline pH while the amastigotes live at pH 4.0-5.0. It is especially important for an organism which depends on proton motive force to drive transport. Intracellular pH was determined (1) from the distribution of the radiolabelled weak acid 5,5-dimethyl-[2^{14}C] oxazolidine-2-4-dione (DMO) according to the method of Rottenberg (18), and (2) by the [^{31}P] NMR spectra according to den Hollander et al (3). The results from both procedures were in close agreement. As shown in Fig. 5 promastigotes maintained an intracellular pH (pHi) between 6.8-7.4 when suspended at external pH's (pHe) ranging from 5.0-7.4. Below pHe 5.0, they were unable to maintain physiological pH. Amastigotes maintained physiological pH internally at an external pH as low as 4.0.

As would be expected, in both stages the pH gradient (ΔpH) is greatest when the external pH is the lowest. ΔpH makes a greater contribution to proton motive force in amastigotes living at pH 5.0 than in promastigotes living at pH 7.0. Starved cells lose the ability for pH homeostasis but incubation in presence of an energy source such as glucose, preserves it fully. Treatment with ionophores such as nigericin, and CCCP as well as the ATPase inhibitor DCCD, results in significant reduction in the pH gradient.

The proton pumping ATPase undoubtedly plays a major role in intracellular pH regulation. However, exploratory experiments indicate the involvement of other cation exchange systems the principal one being a Na^+/H^+ antiporter. This is a nearly universal system which carries out the electroneutral exchange of external Na^+ for internal H^+ and is fully reversible depending on the direction of the ion gradients. Besides its role in in-

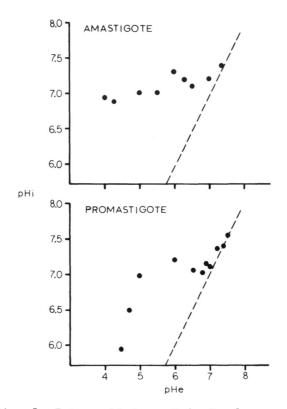

Fig. 5. Intracellular pH in L. donovani amastigotes and promastigotes at varying external pH's

tracellular pH regulation, this antiporter would function to remove toxic Na^+ ions from the cells. As shown in Fig. 6, addition of Na^+ (NaCl) to cells in a Na^+-free medium, triggered a rapid drop in external pH indicating exchange of external Na^+ for internal H^+. As in other systems, Na^+ could be replaced with lithium to produce the same effect. Monensin is an ionophore that mimicks the Na^+/H^+ antiporter. Addition of monensin enhanced the release of H^+ from the cells. Cells treated with amiloride, a known blocker of Na^+/H^+ antiporter, failed to show H^+ efflux upon addition of Na^+.

Potassium is another cation that seems to play a significant role in pH homeostasis in Leishmania. It was observed that the acidification of the medium when the cells were supplied with a readily metabolizable energy source such as glucose was further enhanced in combination with K^+ (Fig. 7). The acidification (proton efflux) of the medium was accompanied by an influx of K^+ which was reflected in a decrease of K^+ in the medium. This acidification and K^+ uptake are both inhibited by DCCD. When the pH of a cell suspension in presence of glucose and K^+ was raised from 6.0 to 7.2 by the addition of tetramethyl ammonium hydroxide (TMAH), there was a rapid influx of K^+ (Fig. 8). This was obliterated in presence of DCCD. These results together with DCCD inhibition of proton pumping, seem to suggest that K^+ is required as a counter ion for the proton extruding plasma membrane ATPase. Whether the exchange of K^+ for H^+ is linked as a K^+/H^+ antiporter or operates separately is not clear at this time. Fig. 9 is a tentative model for pH and ion regulation in amastigotes.

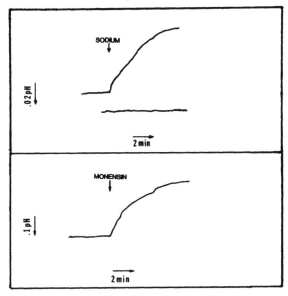

Fig. 6. Effect of sodium (NaCl) (5mM) and monensin (5μM) on H^+ release from L. donovani promastigotes.

CONCLUSIONS

Amastigotes of Leishmania are well adapted for survival and growth within the acidic in vivo environment. Their success depends in part on the development of physiological and biochemical activities which operate optimally at high proton concentrations characteristic of their natural environment. The parasite is fully capable of maintaining a constant intracellular pH in an environment so rich in protons. This is achieved through proton extrusion and the exchange of internal H^+ for external cations such as Na^+ and K^+. The maintenance of constant intracellular pH is crucial since many events in growth and development beginning with DNA replication require a physiological pH.

The DCCD and vanadate sensitive plasma membrane ATPase which is a proton extruding pump, plays a major role in maintaining a constant intracellular pH and a proton gradient across the membrane that is conducive for active transport. This ATPase is thus critically important in the biology of the parasite and could be a potential target for chemotherapy. It will also be interesting to see whether the manipulation of the intraphagolysosomal pH by using lysosomotropic agents such as ammonium chloride, methylamine and chloroquine will inhibit parasite growth.

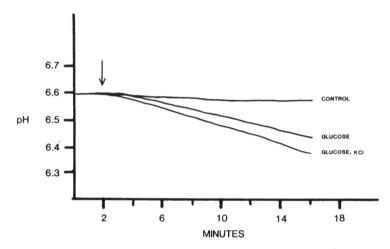

Fig. 7. Stimulation of H^+ release by 5mM K^+ (KCl). Change in pH was followed with a continuously recording pH meter (radiometer).

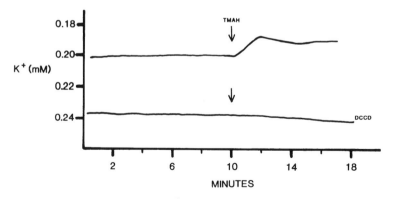

Fig. 8. Influx of K^+ induced by the alkalinization of external medium by tetramethylammonium hydroxide (TMAH) and its inhibition by DCCD (50μM)

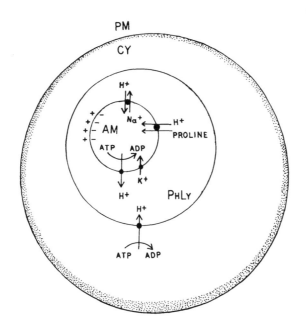

Fig. 9. Hypothetical model for pH and ion regulation in *Leishmania* amastigotes. AM, amastigote; CY, cytoplasm; PHYL, phagolysosome; PM, peritoneal macrophage.

REFERENCES

1. Alexander, J. and Vickerman, K. 1974. J. Protozool. 22:502-508.
2. Armstrong, J.A. and D'Arcy Hart, P. 1971. J. Exp. Med. 134:713-723.
3. den Hollander, J.A., Ugurbil, K., Brown, T.R. and Shulman, R.G. 1981. Biochemistry 20:5871-5880.
4. Geisow, M.J., D'Arcy Hart, P. and Young, M.R. 1981. J. Cell Biol. 89:645-652.
5. Gottlieb, M. and Dwyer, D.M. 1981. Exp. Parasitol. 52:117-128.
6. Horwitz, M.A. 1983. J. Exp. Med. 158:2108-2126.
7. Horwitz, M.A. and Maxfield, F.R. 1984. J. Cell Biol. 99:1936-1943.
8. Jensen, M.S. and Bainton, D.F. 1973. J. Cell Biol. 56:379-390.
9. Jones, T.C. and Hirsch, J.G. 1972. J. Exp. Med. 136:1173-1194.
10. Laemmli, V.K. 1974. Nature 227:680-685.
11. Lanzetta, R.A., Alvarez, L.J., Reinach, P.S. and Candia, O.A. 1979. Anal. Biochem. 100:95-97.
12. Lewis, D.H. and Peters, W. 1977. Ann. Trop. Med. Parasitol. 71:295-312.
13. Meade, J.C., Glaser, T.A., Bonventre, P.F. and Mukkada, A.J. 1984. J. Protozool. 31:156-161.
14. Mukkada, A.J. 1985. in "Transport Processes: Iono-and Osmoregulation," Gilles, R. and Gilles-Baillien, M. ed. Springer-Verlag, Berlin, p. 326-333.

15. Mukkada, A.J., Long, G. and Romano, A.H. 1973. Biochem. J. 132:155-162.
16. Mukkada, A.J., Meade, J.C., Glaser, T.A. and Bonventre, P.F. 1985. Science 229:1099-1101.
17. Nogueira, N. and Cohn, Z.A. 1978. J. Exp. Med. 146:288-297.
18. Rottenberg, H. 1978. Methods Enzymol. 55:547-569.
19. Walker, T.S. and Winkler, H.H. 1978. Infect. Immun. 22:200-208.
20. Zilberstein, D. and Dwyer, D.M. 1985. Proc. Natl. Acad. Sci. USA 82:1716-1720.

ABROGATION OF SKIN LESIONS IN CUTANEOUS LEISHMANIASIS

BY ULTRAVIOLET B IRRADIATION

Suzanne Holmes Giannini

Univ. Md. Sch. Med.
Dept. Med., Ctr. Vac. Devel.
Baltimore MD 21201

Edward C. De Fabo

George Washington Univ.
Dept. Dermatol.
Washington DC 20006

INTRODUCTION

The leishmaniases remain serious public health problems in the tropics and semitropics. These regions receive two to ten times as much solar ultraviolet radiation (UV) as do the temperate or arctic zones.

UV in the sunburn portion of the solar spectrum, between 290 and 320 nm wavelengths (UVB), when applied locally to skin at the site of antigen application, inactivates skin-associated lymphoid tissue functions leading to antigen-specific anergy [1,2], and in some cases, to tolerance [3].

Solar UVB may modulate the immune response to infectious agents of cutaneous disease, especially those like the Leishmania, that are acquired through exposed (unclothed) skin. Leishmania are deposited by their sandfly vectors in the epidermis and upper layer of the dermis, where they will encounter the cells of the skin-associated lymphoid tissues, and also UVB in sunlight.

UVB causes an impressive array of immunological effects, including depression of cell-mediated immune responses such as contact hypersensitivity [4-10] and delayed type hypersensitivity [11-13], altered rates of secretion of lymphokines [14,15; reviewed in 16], alteration in lymphocyte homing patterns [17,18] and the induction of T suppressor cells [19,20]. The effective doses of UVB range from 150 Joules per square meter (J m^{-2}) to damage epidermal antigen-presenting cells (Langerhans cells) [21], to 22,800 J m^{-2} to alter lymphocyte homing patterns [17], to 49,000 J m^{-2} to cause systemic suppression of contact hypersensitivity [22-24] and 86,400 J m^2 to cause immunologic unresponsiveness to UV-induced tumors [25].

It may seem that kilojoule exposures are non-physiological, and that humans would rarely receive such high levels of UVB in sunlight. This is not the case. In the latitudes between +25° North and -25° South, the midday UVB flux at the ground reaches from 2.4 to 4.0 watts per square meter [calculated from ref. 26 and 27; and J. Frederick, personal communication, 1986], so that within a 3 to 5 day period, humans could readily be exposed to even the highest experimental levels of biologically effective UVB. Systemic immunosuppressive effects do not depend on the rate of exposure, but rather depend on the cumulative dose of UVB [25,28]. Thus doses that are fractionated and delivered over several days, are as effective as when they are given all at once. It would be surprising indeed if exposure to kilojoule levels of UVB radiation did not also affect the immune response to infectious agents, and susceptibility to clinical disease.

Sunlight or UVB irradiation of mouse skin causes immunological and fine structural alterations resembling those seen in human skin, such as changes in Langerhans cell morphology [21,29]. Human skin damaged by long-term exposure to sunlight shows a diminished ability to mount cell-mediated immune responses to contact allergens and to commonly encountered antigens [30]. The susceptibility of mice to UVB induced suppression of contact hypersensitivity is strain-specific and is unrelated to pigmentation [2]. It appears that this degree of variability in susceptibility to UVB may also obtain in humans. The immune responses of some individuals are more UVB-sensitive than the immune responses of others [J.W. Streilein, personal communication, 1987]. These similarities between human and murine responses to UVB further support the use of mouse models for UVB studies.

To elucidate the effects of UVB on immunological determinants of resistance to leishmanial disease, we have developed a mouse model, the male B10.129(10M)Sn [31] infected with Leishmania major [32,33]. In earlier studies, we have shown that low doses of UVB irradiation (wavelengths 280 - 320 nm) convert these chronically susceptible male mice into apparently resistant hosts that heal their skin lesions [34,35]. The effective dose (2100 J m^{-2}, delivered in 14 doses of 150 J m^{-2}) is similar to levels of UVB exposure from sunlight in the tropics and semitropics, where leishmaniasis is endemic.

Surprisingly, the L. major-infected, lesion-free UVB irradiated mice have the same numbers of parasites in skin at the injection site and in the draining lymph nodes as do the unirradiated, diseased mice [35]. Furthermore, the experimental levels of UVB do not affect parasite viability or numbers in vitro in a mouse macrophage-like cell line, the J774A.1, even though these exposures kill many host cells [34]. So it seems that the primary targets of UVB in skin are the host cells and not the leishmania. Thus the UVB irradiated mice are heavily infected despite being asymptomatic.

The Leishmania-infected, UVB irradiated mice, unlike their unirradiated counterparts, develop minimal delayed type hypersensitivity responses, and respond to a challenge infection at a distal skin site as if they have never before been exposed to leishmania. UVB affects immunological memory to L. major as early as 2 weeks post infection [35]. From this it is clear that resistance or susceptibility to disease are promoted by early immunological events occurring in the skin and draining lymph nodes, events that are significantly perturbed by UVB irradiation.

What are the active wavelengths for abrogation of primary lesion development in cutaneous leishmaniasis? The answer is important epidemiologically because wavelengths longer than 310 nm or so predominate in the terrestrial solar spectrum at ground level while shorter UVB wavelengths are absorbed more efficiently by the ozone layer [27]. Alternatively, UVB effects could be caused principally by shorter wavelengths, which are more efficient in damaging the antigen-presenting cells of the skin (Langerhans cells) [9], in inducing local [36] and systemic [7] suppression of contact hypersensitivity, and in inducing immunologic unresponsiveness to UV-induced tumors [28].

To address this question, we investigated the effects of narrow band UVB at either end of the UVB spectrum, 290 nm and 320 nm.

MATERIALS AND METHODS

Animals   Male B10.129(10M)Sn [31] mice were obtained from Jackson Laboratories (Bar Harbor, ME, USA) at 4 to 8 weeks of age. In these mice, local irradiation with sub-erythematous doses of broad-band UVB abrogates the induction of contact hypersensitivity to contact allergens applied to irradiated skin. In mice infected with L. major, lesion development is abrogated by broad-band UVB irradiation of the injection site during the first month post infection with L. major [34,35].

Parasites   Leishmania were a cloned line of the WR300 strain of L. major, from Senegal [37]. The parasites were cultivated in vitro, counted, and injected into mice as described [33,38]. Leishmania promastigotes were harvested from stationary phase, when they are most infective [39,40].

UV irradiator   The narrow-band UV source was a unique interference filter monochromator capable of producing narrow-band radiation in the UVB and UVC regions. The system consisted of narrow bandpass UV interference filters of half bandwidth 2-3 nm coupled to a 2.5 kW xenon arc. The filters transmitted 10-20% of the incident energy and blocked transmission of wavelengths outside the main bandpass to <0.01% from X ray to far infrared, thus minimizing heat production. Irradiances ranged from 0.05 to 0.5 W/m^2 depending on wavelength. The field size produced by this arrangement (50-60 cm^2) is large enough to irradiate the dorsal surfaces of three mice simultaneously [7]. Mice were rotated on a carousel to ensure uniform exposure.

UV doses (irradiances):   To control for systemic effects of UVB irradiation, doses of narrow band UVB were used that cause similar levels of systemic suppression, 20 to 40%. At 290 nm, this was 720 J/m^2; and at 320 nm, 1650 J/m^2 [7,9].

The 290 nm UVB was delivered in 5 hour-long exposures of ~145 $J\,m^{-2}$, the 320 nm UVB, in 5 exposures of ~330 J/m^2.

UV irradiation of mice   The skin on the dorsal surface of the trunk was shaved with electric clippers prior to each irradiation as needed. A minimum of 3 to 4 weeks was required for lesions to develop, so that irradiation was completed and shaving terminated well before symptoms occurred. Unirradiated control mice were also shaved.

During exposure to the UV source, mice were confined individually in plastic narrow, open-top cages. To control for possible effects of stress and handling, unirradiated mice were similarly confined for comparable periods.

Irradiation schedule   The schedule was based on studies of UVB induced systemic suppression of contact hypersensitivity [7,9], and was planned to activate the immune suppressor network of mice prior to their exposure to leishmanial antigen. Mice were irradiated twice at -3 to -8 days before infection, and then twice +5 to +8 days post infection. Exposure to UVB in a time window of -3 days to -15 days before application of antigen induces systemic suppression of contact hypersensitivity (CHS). Continued irradiation after infection was necessary to maintain local immunosuppression, because skin cells begin to regain surface markers characteristic of antigen presentation within 96 hours [41] while leishmania persist in both normal and irradiated skin for several months [34].

Infection of mice   Ten µl containing 1×10^6 L. major promastigotes (the infective form in nature) were injected intradermally, resulting in a visible "bleb" at the injection site for each mouse.

Assessment of lesion development At 3 weeks after infection, mice were anaesthetized and lesion diameters were measured in two dimensions with spring-loaded calipers.

Assay for parasite dissemination Mice were necropsied and leishmania were enumerated in skin and lymphoid tissues by a limiting dilution culture technique, which can detect a single L. major planted into a culture well [38]. Serial tenfold dilutions of triturated skin at the primary and challenge injection sites, distal skin sites, regional and distal lymph nodes and spleen were cultured.

Statistical analysis Significance of results was determined by the Wilcoxon Rank Sum test [42].

RESULTS

Determination of active wavelengths of UVB irradiation that affect lesion development following infection with L. major. In two experiments, infected mice whose injection sites were irradiated with 320 nm UVB developed significantly smaller lesions than unirradiated mice ($p<0.01$). UVB of 290 nm wavelength had no discernible effect on skin lesions, when compared with unirradiated mice (Table I).

Determination of active wavelengths affecting parasite dissemination. In both experiments, as with broad band UVB irradiated mice [34], parasites were present in the skin to the same extent in all 3 groups, regardless of gross pathology. In a small series of animals, it appeared as though 290 nm UVB promoted dissemination of parasites, in that parasites were recovered from two or more disseminated sites in the majority of mice irradiated with 290 nm. In contrast, unirradiated mice or mice irradiated with 320 nm UVB all had one or fewer metastases (Table II).

TABLE I. UVB WAVELENGTHS AFFECTING SKIN LESIONS IN MURINE CUTANEOUS LEISHMANIASIS

Treatment[b]	Lesion diameter (x 0.1 mm)[a]	
	Expt. 1	Expt. 2
no UVB	232 ± 53	236 ± 39
290 nm UVB	260 ± 53	233 ± 55
320 nm UVB	156 ± 59[c]	172 ± 20[c]

[a] Mean lesion diameters ± standard deviations for groups of 2 to 6 mice, 3 weeks post infection with 1×10^6 L. major
[b] Infected mice received no UVB, or UVB at 290 nm or at 320 nm calculated to cause ~30% systemic suppression of CHS
[c] Significantly different from unirradiated controls ($p<0.01$)

TABLE II. EFFECTS OF NARROW BAND UVB
RADIATION ON PARASITE DISSEMINATION FROM
THE PRIMARY INJECTION SITE[a]

Groups	Skin at injection site	Disseminated sites[c] (number of sites)			
		0	1	2	>2
Untreated					
mouse 1	+	+			
mouse 2	+		+		
320 nm UVB					
mouse 3	+	+			
mouse 4	+		+		
mouse 5	+		+		
290 nm UVB					
mouse 6	+		+		
mouse 7	+			+	
mouse 8	+				+

[a] see footnotes to Table I; mice shown are from Expt. 2
[b] parasites found in triturates of tissues assayed by limiting dilution culture technique [38]
[c] distal skin, draining and distal lymph nodes, and spleen were assayed

DISCUSSION

Results show that UVB induced abrogation of lesion development is not due solely to systemic immunosuppression, because both 290 nm and 320 nm wavelengths induce similar levels (~30%) of suppression of contact hypersensitivity [7], while only 320 nm UV affects pathogenesis (Table I).

That the active wavelengths affecting pathogenesis in cutaneous leishmaniasis are near 320 nm is particularly significant to natural infections, because the longer wavelengths of solar UVB reach the earth's surface in high fluences. Thus the doses of the active wavelengths in sunlight are likely to be high enough to affect pathogenesis in some humans infected with Leishmania.

It is critical to identify the active wavelengths affecting protective immunity in leishmaniasis, especially since this immunity is depressed by broad band UVB [34,35]. Although it is premature to draw firm conclusions from our limited set of data, these wavelengths might be closer to 290 nm, since irradiation with this wavelength UVB exacerbated parasite dissemination in a small series of animals (Table II). In the tropics near the equator, fluences of wavelengths near 290 nm are of relatively constant high levels, and exposure to them could predispose humans to more severe leishmanial disease. This would hold even more if humans become infected with species of Leishmania capable of dissemination [43].

UVB has profound effects on the outcome of other infectious diseases as well. For example, UVB can reactivate recurrent herpes simplex labialis [44,45] and recurrent genital herpes in humans [46]. In primary herpes simplex virus type I (HSV-I) infections in the mouse, UVB affects viral titers [47], and reactivates HSV-I infections in mice [48] and rabbits [49]. High exposure of immunosuppressed humans to sunlight is associated with increased incidence of viral warts (papillomas) on sun-exposed skin [50,51].

Lesions of herpes zoster [52] and cutaneous leishmaniasis in humans [53] have been ameliorated by treatment with UV. Unfortunately, exposure to UVB during the host's initial encounter with infectious agents can also depress the induction of delayed type hypersensitivity to Leishmania major [34,35] and to herpes simplex types I [12] and II [13] in mice. These observations are consistent with the finding that a first exposure to a contact allergen via UVB irradiated skin not only fails to sensitize the host, but also induces a tolerance to subsequent exposure to the antigen [1-3]. UVB-induced depression of cell-mediated immune responses that are critical to the acquisition of protective immunity may profoundly affect susceptibility to more serious and systemic forms of infectious disease upon re-exposure. More studies are needed to identify the active wavelengths affecting cell-mediated immune responses and the effects of narrow-band UVB irradiation on protective immunity in leishmaniasis.

CONCLUSIONS

UVB irradiation of skin at the injection site, applied around the time of initial infection, abrogated the induction of skin ulcers and also of anti-leishmanial cell-mediated immune responses in a mouse model for cutaneous leishmaniasis. But despite the absence of overt skin lesions, the UVB irradiated mice were as heavily infected as the unirradiated controls with lesions. Thus UVB irradiation during the first contact with Leishmania leaves the host non-immune and heavily parasitized, although free of obvious skin ulcers.

Both the effective doses and active wavelengths of UVB modulating pathogenesis occur naturally in sunlight in the tropics and semitropics, where the leishmaniases are endemic. Solar UVB may affect pathogenesis and immunity in leishmanial infections occurring in nature.

The consequences of chronic UVB exposure are poorly understood, so it is unknown whether people living in the tropics become resistant to UVB with long exposure. Susceptibility to the immunosuppressive effects of UVB is likely to be genetically determined [Streilein, personal communication], so that some individuals may not be affected even by high exposures. Nevertheless, it is likely that acute exposure to UVB radiation, particularly at the time of initial infection, influences the outcome of the infection process and development of clinical disease.

ACKNOWLEDGMENTS

This study was supported by USPHS Grant AI23956 and a grant from the University of Maryland Biotechnology Center. We are grateful to Drs. John E. Frederick and J. Wayne Streilein for permission to cite their unpublished data. We thank Dr. Edmond A. Goidl for a critical review of the manuscript. Drs. Frances P. Noonan and Janice Longstreth provided many helpful discussions. Mrs. Gail Hudson aided in the culture assay for leishmania.

REFERENCES

1. Kripke, M. 1984. Immunolog. Rev. 80: 87.
2. Streilein, J.W. 1983. J. Invest. Dermatol. 80: 12S.
3. Bergstresser, P.R., Elmets, C.A. and Streilein, J.W. 1983. In J.A. Parrish [ed.]. The Effect of Ultraviolet Radiation on the Immune System. Skillman, NJ: Johnson & Johnson Baby Products Co., pp.73-86.
4. Noonan, F.P., DeFabo, E.C., and Kripke, M.L. 1981. Springer Semin. Immunopathol. 4: 293.
5. Noonan, F.P., De Fabo, E.C. and Kripke M.L. 1981. Photochem. Photobiol. 34: 683.
6. Noonan, F.P., Kripke, M.L., Pedersen, G.M., and Green, M.I. 1981. Immunology 43: 524.
7. De Fabo, E.C., and Noonan, F.P. 1983. J. Exp. Med. 158: 84.
8. Toews, G.B., Bergstresser, P.R. and Streilein, J.W. 1980. J. Immunol. 124: 445.
9. Noonan, F.P., Bucana, C., Sauder, D.N. and De Fabo, E.C. 1984. J. Immunol. 132: 2408.
10. Kripke, M.L., and McClendon, E. 1986. J. Immunol. 137: 443.
11. Morison, W.L., Bucana, C., and Kripke, M.L. 1984. Immunology 52: 299.
12. Howie, S., Norval, M. and Maingay, J. 1986. J. Invest. Dermatol. 86: 125.
13. Hayashi, Y., and Aurelian, L. 1986. J. Immunol. 136: 1087.
14. Ansel, J., Luger, T.A., Kock, A., Hochstein, D. and Green, I. 1984. J. Immunol. 133: 1350.
15. Gahring, L., Baltz, M., Pepys, M.B. and Daynes, R. 1984. Proc. Natl. Acad. Sci. USA 81:1198.
16. Luger, T.A. 1986. Photodermatology 3: 123.
17. Spangrude, G.J., Bernhard, E.J., Ajioka, R.S. and Daynes, R.A. 1983. J. Immunol. 130: 2974.
18. Daynes, R.A., Spangrude, G.J., Roberts, L.K. and Krueger, G.G. 1985. J. Invest. Dermatol. 85: 14s.
19. Fisher, M.S. and Kripke, M.L. 1982. Proc. Nat. Acad. Sci. (USA) 74: 1688.
20. Granstein, R.D. 1985. J. Invest. Dermatol. 84: 206.
21. Aberer, W., G. Schuler, G. Stingl, H. Honigsmann and K. Wolff. 1981. J. Invest. Dermatol. 76: 202.
22. Fisher, M.S., and M.L. Kripke. 1982. Science 216: 1133.
23. Funnell, S.G.P. and Keast, D. 1986. Photodermatology 3: 64.
24. Kripke, M.L. and W.L. Morison. 1986. Photodermatology 3: 4.
25. De Fabo, E.C., and M.L. Kripke. 1979. Photochem. Photobiol. 30: 385.
26. Frederick, J.E. 1986. In J.G. Titus [ed.], Effects of Changes in Stratospheric Ozone and Global Climate, Vol.I. Overview. Washington, D.C.: U.S. Environmental Protection Agency, pp. 121-128.
27. Frederick, J.E. and D. Lubin. 1987. Manuscript submitted to J. Geophys. Res.
28. DeFabo E.C., and Kripke, M. 1980. Photochem. Photobiol. 32: 183.
29. Scheibner, A., Hollis, D.E., McCarthy, W.H. and Milton, G.W. 1986. Photodermatology 3: 15.
30. O'Dell, B.L., Jessen, R.T., Becker, L.E., Jackson, R.T. and Smith, E.B. 1980. Arch. Dermatol. 116: 559.
31. Snell, G.D. and Bunker, H.P. 1965. Transplantation 3: 235.
32. Blackwell, J.M. et al. 1985. Immunogenetics 21: 385.
33. Giannini, M.S.H. 1986. Parasite Immunol. 8: 31.
34. Giannini, M.S.H. 1986. Infect. Immun. 51: 838.
35. Giannini, M.S.H. 1986. In J.G. Titus [ed.] Effects of Changes in Stratospheric Ozone and Global Climate, Vol. 2, Stratospheric Ozone.

Proceedings of UNEP/EPA International Conference on Health and Environmental Effects of Ozone Modification and Climate Change. Washington, D.C.: U.S. Environmental Protection Agency, pp. 101-112.
36. Elmets, C.A., LeVine, M.J. and Bickers, D.R. 1985. Photochem. Photobiol. 42: 391.
37. Strobel, M., Ndiaye, G., Renaud-Steens, C., Dedet, C.P. and Marchand, J.P. 1978. Med. Mal. Infect. 8: 98.
38. Giannini, M.S.H. 1985. Trans. Roy. Soc. Trop. Med. Hyg. 79: 458.
39. Giannini, M.S.H. 1974. J. Protozool. 21: 521.
40. Sacks, D.L. and Perkins, P.V. 1984. Science 223: 1417.
41. Bergstresser, P.R., Toews, G.B., and Streilein, J.W. 1980. J. Invest. Dermatol. 75: 73.
42. Wilcoxon, R., and Wilcox, R.A. 1964. In: Some Rapid Approximate Statistical Procedures. Pearl River, N.Y.: Lederle Laboratories, pp. 7-8.
43. Anonymous. 1984. The Leishmaniases. WHO Tech. Rep. Ser. 701.
44. Wheeler, C.E. Jr. 1975. J. Invest. Dermatol. 65: 341.
45. Spruance, S.L. 1985. J. Clin. Microbiol. 22: 366.
46. Klein, K.L., and Linnemann, C.C. Jr. 1986. Lancet 1: 796.
47. Harbour, D.A., Hill, T.J. and Blyth, W.A. 1977. Arch. Virol. 54: 367.
48. Blyth, W.A., Hill, T.J., Field, H.J. and Harbour, D.A. 1976. J. Gen. Virol. 33: 547.
49. Spurney, R.V., and Rosenthal, M.S. Amer. J. Ophthalmol. 73: 609.
50. Boyle, J., MacKie, R.M., Briggs, J.D., Junor, B.J.R. and Aitchison, T.C. 1984. Lancet 1: 702.
51. Dyall-Smith, D., and Varigos, G. 1985. Austral. J. Derm. 26: 102.
52. Szigeti, B., Chapiro, J. and Saint-Girons, J.M. 1976. J. Radiologie 57: 37.
53. Mutinga, M.J. and Mngola, E.N. 1974. East African Med. J. 51: 68.

EVIDENCE FOR HYBRID FORMATION IN THE GENUS LEISHMANIA

D.A. Evans[1], V. Smith[1], R. Killick-Kendrick[2], R.A. Neal[1] and W. Peters[1]

[1] Department of Medical Protozoology, London School of Hygiene and Tropical Medicine, Keppel Street, London WC1
[2] Imperial College Field Station, Silwood Park, Ashurst Lodge, Ascot, Berkshire, U.K.

INTRODUCTION

Until recently it was generally assumed that reproduction in the genus Leishmania was by asexual binary fission, and that a sexual process was denied to these organisms. Studies on Leishmania isolated from man, wild animals and sandflies in the Al-Ahsa oasis of the Eastern Province of Saudi Arabia (Evans et al., 1988), have revealed the presence of organisms which appear to be hybrids.

In this communication we examine the evidence for and against these organisms being hybrids, and describe experimental work designed to produce hybrid leishmanial organisms under laboratory conditions.

MATERIALS AND METHODS

Isolation and passage of leishmanial organisms. Isolates from human patients were obtained by inoculation of material obtained by a variety of different methods (needle aspiration and/or various biopsy techniques) from cutaneous lesions. Those from animal and sandfly sources were obtained by the inoculation of tissues or in the case of sandflies, gut contents, into BALB/c mice, and subsequently from the lesions that developed in these animals into modified Tobie's medium.

Organisms. Details of the provenances of the leishmanial organisms used in this study are given in Table 1.

Amastigotes. These were raised by the intradermal inoculation of organisms (initially promastigotes were the inoculum, thereafter amastigotes were used) into the hind footpads of hamsters.

Infection of sandflies. Laboratory reared female Phlebotomus papatasi from a colony of flies established from individuals captured in the Al-Ahsa area of Saudi Arabia, were fed amastigotes of either L.major, L.arabica or a mixture of L.major and L.arabica purified from BALB/c mouse or hamster lesions. The amastigotes were suspended in in defibrinated hamster blood to a concentration of approximately 2×10^5 amastigotes per ml.,then introduced into a magnetically stirred, water-jacketed feeding chamber maintained at $37°C$, and finally covered with a chick skin membrane. When mixed feeds of L.arabica and L.major were offered to the flies approximately equal numbers of the two parasites were used in the mixture.

Dissection of sandflies. Flies which had fed on bloodmeals containing mixed amastigotes of L.major and L.arabica were killed with ethyl acetate vapour, and surface washed by immersion in sterile proline balanced salts solution (PBSS) containing 100 ug/ml. gentamycin. Each washed fly was then placed in a drop of PBSS on a sterile microscope slide and it's head and wings removed. The gut of the fly was then removed using sterile dissecting needles, and transferred to a small drop of sterile MEM/FCS/EBLB medium which contained 100 ug gentamycin/ml. A sterile coverslip was placed over the drop of culture medium which contained the fly gut, and this examined under a phase contrast microscope for the presence of leishmanial promastigotes. Promastigotes were expelled from infected guts by gentle pressure on the coverslip, which was then removed and the culture medium containing the released promastigotes taken up into a sterile micro-pipette.

Table 1. Strains of Leishmania

International Code	Place of origin	Zymodeme LON-	Species
MPSM/SA/83/JISH220	Jisha (Al-Ahsa)	64	L.arabica
MPSM/SA/83/JISH224	Jisha (Al-Ahsa)	64	L.arabica
MPSM/SA/84/JISH231	Jisha (Al-Ahsa)	64	L.arabica
MPSM/SA/84/JISH238	Jisha (Al-Ahsa)	64	L.arabica
MCAN/SA/84/MD94	Hofuf (Al-Ahsa)	64	L.arabica
MCAN/SA/83/MD26	Omran (Al-Ahsa)	62	hybrid
MPSM/SA/84/JISH249	Jisha (Al-Ahsa)	62	hybrid
MHOM/SA/84/JISH118	Jisha (Al-Ahsa)	4	L.major
MPSM/SA/84/JISH213	Hofuf (Al-Ahsa)	4	L.major
MCAN/SA/84/MD62	Hofuf (Al-Ahsa)	4	L.major
MHOM/SA/84/JISH118	Jisha (Al-Ahsa)	4	L.major
MHOM/SA/83/RKK2	Hofuf (Al-Ahsa)	4	L.major
IPAP/SA/82/PAPATASI-3	Hofuf (Al-Ahsa)	4	L.major

Cloning of promastigotes from infected sandflies. Four different methods were used. 1. Dilutions of suspensions of the promastigotes released from an infected fly gut were made in MEM/FCS/EBLB medium and hanging micro-drop preparations made as described in Evans & Smith (1986). Drops containing single promastigotes were sealed into glass capillaries and incubated at 23°C (Evans & Smith, 1986). 2. The suspension of released promastigotes was diluted with sterile PBSS so that it contained approximately 3×10^3 organisms/ml and spread-plates made on blood agar after the method of Hill et al. (1983). The plates were sealed into plastic bags containing cotton wool soaked in sterile saline and incubated at 23°C. Individual colonies which developed on the plates were picked up on sterile needles and transferred to modified Tobie's medium. 3. The gut contents of infected flies were inoculated into tubes of modified Tobie's medium, incubated at 23°C until growth of promastigotes was observed. Clones of these cultured promastigotes were then made using the method of Evans & Smith (1986).
4. Essentially as 3 except that spread plates were made as in 2.

In vitro cultivation of promastigotes. Promastigotes were retrieved from storage in liquid nitrogen by rapid thawing followed by immediate transfer to modified Tobie's medium (Evans et al., 1984) and incubation at 23°C. Subsequent passages were into MEM/FCS/EBLB medium (Evans et al., 1984) or a modification of this medium in which the foetal calf serum component was replaced with inspissated bovine serum (Evans, 1986).

Cultivation of mixed promastigote populations. Both wild type non-cloned and cloned promastigotes of L.arabica and L.major were grown together, wild type with wild type, and cloned with cloned organisms. Approximately equal numbers (ca. 10^3) of exponentially dividing promastigotes of L.arabica and L.major were inoculated into modified Tobie's medium and incubated at 23°C. Samples were taken from the mixed cultures after 24 h, 72 h and 1 week incubation periods, and clones prepared using the method of Evans & Smith (1986). Second samples taken after 24 h from the mixed cultures were spread thickly on to blood agar plates to enable the mixed population of promastigotes to grow in extremely close association with one another. The spread plates were incubated as described above, and after 10 days samples from areas with confluent lawn type growth of organisms and also some from individual colonies, were inoculated into modified Tobie's medium. Clones were prepared from log phase cultures as described above.

Isoenzyme characterization. Eleven enzymes (ALAT, ASAT, ES, GPI, 6-PGD, PGM, PEP-D, SOD, MPI, MDH and NH) were examined by the methods described in Peters et al. (1985). An initial quick screen for the detection of recombinant organisms was by the examination of GPI and MPI.

RESULTS

Isoenzyme characterization of Leishmania isolated from Al-Ahasa. The isoenzyme profiles of 132 stocks of Leishmania from human, wild animal and sandfly sources have been examined and each stock assigned an appropriate London zymodeme (LON) number. One hundred and twenty four were L.major zymodeme LON4, 1 was L.major LON65 (differing from LON4 in esterase), 5 were L.arabica LON64 and 2 (JISH249 and MD26) had hybrid-like profiles and were assigned to zymodeme LON62 (Fig. 1).

Identification of the products of mixed feeds to Phlebotomus papatasi

Sandflies dissected on days 7 and 9 after a feed containing amastigotes of L.arabica (JISH220) mixed with L.major (JISH118 clone 6) and promastigotes from their guts cloned into culture as described above, yielded a total of 19 cultures. Cultures of promastigotes cloned using the hanging drop and capillary growth system of Evans & Smith (1986) yielded only pure cultures of either L.arabica or L.major. No mixtures or putative hybrids were detected using isoenzyme methods. Cultures derived from individual colonies picked off blood agar spread plates were, however, found to consist of isoenzymically pure L.arabica and L.major plus several cultures which were obvious mixtures of L.arabica and L.major, no organisms with the putative hybrid isoenzyme profiles of MD26 and JISH249 were detected.

Identification of the products of co-cultivation of L.arabica and L.major

(a) Cultivation on Tobie's medium. Cloned cultures derived from mixed L.arabica/L.major promastigotes, whether these were from mixtures of wild type non-cloned starting material, or from cloned material gave similar results. Cloned cultures set up from samples taken after 24 and 72 h, were isoenzymically either L.arabica or L.major; samples taken and cloned after 1 week were all L.arabica.

(b) Cultivation on blood agar plates. Cultures derived from individual colonies after either 1 or 2 weeks growth on blood agar were all isoenzymically L.arabica.

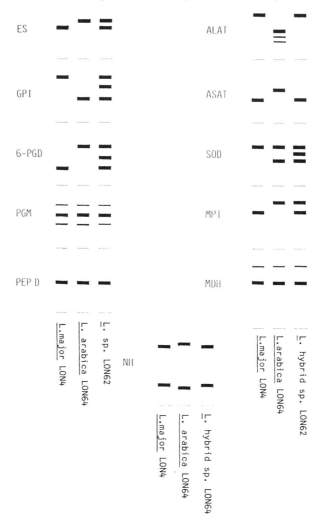

Figure 1.

DISCUSSION

Zoonotic cutaneous leishmaniasis (ZCL) is endemic in the Al-Ahsa area in and around the oasis town of Hofuf which is situated in the Eastern Province of the Kingdom of Saudi Arabia. Leishmania major zymodeme LON4 is the causative organism in the majority of cases of human and animal leishmaniasis in this area (93% in the present study). Only one strain of L.major (LON65) KFUH7352 (Peters et al., 1985) showed an isoenzyme difference in any of the 12 enzymes used to delineate zymodeme LON4 from the other 'LON' zymodemes. The difference was in ES where in the place of the single band of LON4 a triple band was detected. The other leishmanial organisms isolated being L.arabica and the putative hybrid organisms JISH249 and MD26. The isolations of L.major were from man, Psammomys obesus, Meriones libycus, Canis familiaris and Phlebotomus papatasi; while those of L.arabica and of the putative hybrid from P.obesus and C. familiaris.

The evidence that MD26 and JISH249 may be hybrids of L.major and L.arabica is presented in Evans et al. (1988) and is based on isoenzyme analysis where heterozygous banding patterns were seen (see also Fig.1); the use of highly specific kDNA probes which revealed a degree of DNA sequence homology between the L.arabica and the putative hybrids which was not seen between L.major and L.arabica; that after the separation of chromosomes from these organisms by orthogonal field alternation gel electrophoresis (OFAGE), a DNA probe hybridized to chromosome 7 in L.major, chromosome 9 in L.arabica and to both chromosomes 7 and 9 in MD26 and JISH249, something that was not seen in the examination of any other Leishmania of Old World origin, strong evidence that MD26 and JISH249 are indeed hybrids.

As far as is known, Ph.papatasi is the sole vector of leishmaniasis in the Al-Ahasa area (Killick-Kendrick et al., 1985), and although all the leishmanias isolated from Ph.papatasi thus far in these studies have been L.major LON4, we have assumed that this sandfly is also the vector both of L.arabica and the putative hybrid. If this is the case, and work reported here shows that L.arabica will develop in Ph.papatasi, then we have a relatively small geographical area with 2 main leishmanial parasites (L.major and L.arabica) circulating in the wild animal population and sharing a common vector. The chances, therefore, of these 2 different 'species' of Leishmania coming into close contact, either in a sandfly or a wild animal, are increased, and at least one of the conditions assumed necessary for genetic exchange being satisfied.

The experiments reported here in which attempts have been made to produce hybrid leishmanias in the laboratory are very preliminary, and the results presented are from 4 in vitro, and 1 set of sandfly experiments. Our failure to find any evidence of genetic recombination having taken place is hardly surprising at this stage of proceedings. The in vitro experiments in which L.major and L.arabica were mixed in culture used both cloned and non-cloned organisms. Non-cloned organisms were included in case the cloning procedure had selected incompatible or 'non-mating' promastigotes. The experiment in which a mixture of amastigotes from cloned L.major and from non-cloned L.arabica were fed to flies may seem somewhat perverse; it was really a preliminary experiment and organisms were used that were available when a suitable batch of flies had hatched.

REFERENCES

Evans, D.A. (1986) An inexpensive easily available replacement for foetal calf serum in media for the in vitro cultivation of Leishmania spp. Z. Parasitenkd 72: 567-572.

Evans, D.A., Lanham, S.M., Baldwin, C.I. and Peters, W. (1984) The isolation and isoenzyme characterization of Leishmania braziliensis subsp. from patients with cutaneous leishmaniasis acquired in Belize. Trans. Roy. Soc. Trop. Med. Hyg. 78: 35-42.

Evans, D.A. and Smith, V. (1986) A simple method for cloning leishmanial promastigotes. Z.Parasitenkd 72: 573-576.

Evans, D.A., Kennedy, W.P.K., Elbihari, S., Chapman, C.J., Smith, V. and Peters, W. (1988) Hybrid formation within the genus Leishmania? Parassitologia (submitted for publication).

Hill, J.O., North, R.J. and Collins, F.M. (1983) Advantages of measuring changes in the number of viable parasites in murine models of experimental cutaneous leishmaniasis. Infection and Immunity 39: 1087-1094.

Killick-Kendrick, R., Leaney, A.J., Peters, W., Rioux, J-A., and Bray, R.S. (1985) Zoonotic cutaneous leishmaniasis in Saudi Arabia: incrimination of Phlebotomus papatasi as the vector in Al-Hassa oasis. Trans. Roy. Soc. Trop. Med. Hyg. 79: 252-255.

Peters, W., Elibihari, S., Ching Liu, Le Blancq, S.M. Evans, D.A., Killick-Kendrick, R., Smith. V. and Baldwin, C.I. (1985) Leishmania infecting man and wild animals in Saudi Arabia 1. General Survey. Trans. Roy. Soc. Trop. Med. Hyg. 79: 831-839.

ACKNOWLEDGEMENTS

This study is part of the National Leishmaniasis Research Programme based on King Faisal University, Dammam, and was funded in part by the King Abdul Aziz Centre for Science and Technology and by the EPILEISH component of the UNDP/World Bank/WHO Special Programme for Research and Training in Tropical Diseases.

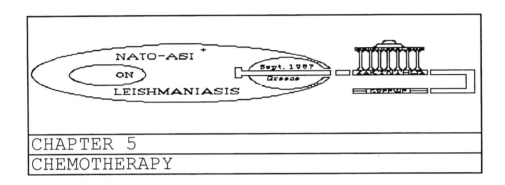

CHAPTER 5
CHEMOTHERAPY

CHEMOTHERAPY - OVERVIEW

L.G.Goodwin

Wellcome Tropical Institute

200 Euston Road, London NW1

It is fifty years since the publication of the important book of reviews on the medicinal use of organic antimony compounds by Schmidt and Peter (1937) and of the first reports of the use of Solustibosan in leishmaniasis (Weese, 1937; Kikuth & Schmidt, 1937). Trivalent tartar emetic had long ago been replaced by the much less toxic phenylstibonic acid derivatives Neostibosan, Neostam and Ureastibamine. The introduction of Solustibosan, an even less toxic pentavalent derivative of the tartar emetic type, with the metal joined to carbon through oxygen, was a further advance by German scientists. During the war years, Pentostam and Glucantime were developed in Britain and France to replace Solustibosan and since then, alas, nothing more active or less toxic has been discovered. Pentostam and Glucantime are still recommended by WHO (1984) as the first line treatment for visceral leishmaniasis.
   A second category of remedies includes Pentamidine, Amphoteracin B, Allopurinol ribnucleoside and Ketoconazole - compounds developed for other purposes that heve been found of some use against various forms of leishmanial infection.
In a third category are substances with activity against leishmania parasites in vitro, too few of which have been tested against infections in laboratory animals and are therefore of as yet unknown potential. And there are extensive, exciting studies of the biochemistry of leishmania parasites and the cells they live in, indicating points of possible interference by antimetabolites and inhibitors that might eventually be developed into useful drugs.
   Dr. Ralph Neal, at the Forum that followed the Lecture Session on Chemotherapy drew the attention of all research workers to the need to define the stage in this series to which their studies referred. Many substances that show activity in vitro or in biochemical systems fail to become useful drugs because of the prolonged time and very high cost of toxicological and formulation studies needed before any clinical trial can take place nowadays.

Pentavalent Antimonials

The standard WHO regimen of Pentostam or Glucantime, given at a dose level of 20 mg/kg antimony daily for 20-30 days was found by Berman and by Tavares et al. in recent assessments to be effective and reasonably free from side effects. If these occurred - cough, nausea, abdominal pain and ECG changes - they disappeared when treatment stopped.

Pentavalent antimonial preparations of this kind are not clearly defined chemical entities, the degree of polymerization depending upon the method of manufacture and Berman, in an attempt to clarify this issue, suggests that the determination of osmolarity would be a suitable method of standardizing sodium stibogluconate solutions. Of great interest has been the development of new methods of drug delivery, in liposomes, niosomes or microparticles, that are picked up by macrophages, the cells in which leishmania parasites are found. Croft et al. and Hunter et al. describe experimental work in vitro and in vivo carried out with these preparations, which can show more than 100 fold enhanced activity. They hold great promise as more effective and less toxic treatments and it is to be hoped that after some 10 years of work, one of these preparations will soon receive a good clinical trial in comparison with the standard regimen.

The cutaneous leishmaniases present a special problem that is in need of careful, controlled clinical trials. Some types of cutaneous lesions heal themselves, often very slowly, and few clinical trials to date have included a parallel control series of patients left untrerated for comparison for long enouogh. Only when this has been done will it be possible to judge whether treatment with any drug has been of advantage, and therefore justified. As Berman points out,treatment should be effective and no worse than the disease itself.There is also a need for more drugs to be tried, in suitable vehicles, by local application.

Failures of treatment with antimony are not uncommon and research shows that there may be several different reasons for this. Allen and Neal, using infected macrophages in vitro, have shown that some species of Leishmania have innate resistance to pentavalent antimony and that it is also possible to induce resistance in a particular strain of parasite. The pharmacodynamics of antimony in different patients varies and, mnoreover, Carter et al., by counting parasites in the organs of infected BALB/c mice, found that although the liver was cleared by preparations of Pentostam, the numbers of parasites in the spleen and bone marrow were unaffected. This suggests that the drug may not reach an effective concentration in all parts of the body, allowing parasites to survive in the more "remote" organs. But the cure of leishmania infections also depends upon the activity of a restored immune response and in BALB/c mice this would not be very effective.

There is a further point concerning the activity of sodium stibogluconate that, in recent work, appears to have been overlooked. After an intravenous or intramuscular dose, most of the antimony is excreted very rapidly by the kidney in the pentavalent state.

Antimony that accumulates in the tissues after a succession of doses is, however, reduced to the trivalent state and living mammalian cells will also reduce pentavalent to trivalent antimony in vitro (Goodwin and Page,1943). Pentostam in a single dose has no detectable trypanocidal activity in infected mice,but shows a small effect if repeated doses are given (Goodwin, 1944) and its trivalent analogue, 'Triostam', once used for the treatment of schistosomiasis, is, like tartar emetic, a potent trypanocide. All this suggests that, like arsenic, antimony in the pentavalent state is likely to be innocuous and needs to be reduced to be effective. Perhaps it is easier to reduce by living cells when presented to them in liposomes or other carriers. Hunter et al. showed how efficiently antimony in the new carrier systems accumulates in the livers of mice, but the method of estimation used (124Sb) took no account of valency. What effect does Triostam have on leishmania-infected macrophages in vitro? And what would be its effect if incorporated into liposomes or niosomes? One would expect liposomes of Triostam to be much more active than Pentostam - but probably also more toxic to host cells as well. There seems to be room for further studies in this area.

Compounds developed for other purposes

A wide range of drugs in clinical use for other diseases has been tried against cutaneous leishmaniasis and as a second treatment for visceral infections that have not been cured by antimony. Amphoteracin B and pentamidine have often been successful when antimony treatment has failed, but have more severe side effects.

Leishmania synthesizes purines by the salvage pathway and this is a target for allopurinol ribonucleoside; this drug has been reported to have a beneficial effect on cutaneous leishmaniasis in Panama.

Ketoconazole and its congeners, developed for the treatment of fungal infections, show activity against leishmania amastigotes in vitro. These compounds inhibit the oxidation and removal of the 14 alpha - methyl group of lanosterol; the metabolic chain is blocked, abnormal steroids accumulate and growth and reproduction are reduced but do not cease. Beach et al. suggest that the metabolic functions of the sterols are affected, and also their role as "spacers" in stabilizing the plasma membrane of the parasite.

Ketoconazole has shown promise in the treatment of patients infected with the L. mexicana complex. It also deserves assessment when applied locally to cutaneous lesions.

Sinefungin, a natural nucleoside produced by Streptomyces spp. is another potent antifungal agent with high activity against Leishmania and a range of other parasitic protozoa, both in vitro and in laboratory animals (Robert-Gero et al.).

It inhibits the incorporation of thymidine into DNA. Unfortunately it also has severe toxic effects in mammals, causing tubular necrosis of the kidney and has therefore not been tried clinically. Attempts are in progress to prepare less toxic derivatives by genetic engineering.

Laboratory work shows that when some of the "second line" drugs are given at the same time as Pentostam, antagonism of action results. Studies are needed of the best associations of drugs to use in human infections, and in which order to give them to achieve the best clinical response.

Candidate remedies in course of developmemnt

Substances that interfere with metabolic processes and that have not yet been through the toxicological screen are further from reaching the stage of clinical trial, but there are some interesting candidates.

Certain 8-aminoquinoline derivatives have activity against leishmania both *in vitro* and *in vivo* (Neal, 1987). One of them, WR6026 is under continuing investigation.

DFMO inhibits ornithine decarboxylase and therefore, polyamine synthesis. Keithly and Fairlamb found it to have high activity against some leishmanias in vitro and in mouse infections. Its action is antagonized by pentavalent antimony.

Amino acid esters are trapped in lysosomes, where they are hydrolysed, release the amino acid and disrupt the organelles. *Leishmania* amastigotes live within acidified, long-lived phagolysosomes in the host's macrophages and Rabinovitch found that L-leucine methyl ester killed some leishmanias in vitro, but was not equally active against all species. Hunter et al. also studied the compound; it was active only against species such as *L. mexicana mexicana*, whose amastigotes possess large lysosome-like organelles (megasomes) of their own. Amino acid esters have no effect on leishmania infections in mice and have no immediate promise as chemotherapeutic agents.

Ribosome inactivating proteins (RIPs) such as abrin and ricin are very toxic plant products that are attracting attention for possible use in viral infections and cancer. Cenini and Stirpe found that some of the Type 1 (single chain) RIPs - saporins and dianthins - inactivated *L. infantum* ribosomes and could be conjugated with anti-leishmania antibodies to form "immunotoxins". Such products have the potential for being targeted to reach the parasite and kill it in its macrophage. A long way off but not, perhaps, a dream?

After more than 70 years of antimony - the first case of cutaneous leishmaniasis was treated with tartar emetic by Vianna in 1913 - we badly need some new drugs. As the complex, interlinked metabolic patterns and immunological responses of parasites and host cells continue to be unravelled, the opportunities for devising elegant, specific inhibitors and blockers increase. But in the meantime, it is always worth while to try a "hunch" and those whose work shows promising results in vitro should always find out at an early stage whether or not their compounds work *in vivo*.

References

Goodwin, L.G. (1944) J. Pharm. exp. Therap., 81:224.
Goodwin, L.G. and Page, J.E. (1943) Biochem. J., 37:198.
Kikuth, W. and Schmidt, H. (1937) Chinese med. J., 52:425.
Neal, R.A. (1987) in "The Leishmaniases in Biology and
    Medicine".Vol.2:793. W. Peters and R.
    Killick-Kendrick eds.,Academic Press, London.
Schmidt, H and Peter, F.M. (1937) Ergebnisse u. Fortschritte
    der Antimontherapie, G.Thieme, Leipzig.
Weese, H. (1937) Chinese med. J., 52:421.
WHO (1984) Tech. Rep. Ser., 701, Geneva.

THE FUTURE FOR ANTILEISHMANIAL CHEMOTHERAPEUTIC AGENTS: A REVIEW

Jonathan D. Berman

Division of Experimental Therapeutics
Walter Reed Army Institute of Research
Washington, DC 20307-5100 USA

KEY WORDS   Pentostam, Glucantime, Antimony, Ketoconazole, allopurinol
ribonucleoside, Leishmania tropica, Leishmania mexicana,
Leishmania braziliensis, Leishmania donovani

Issues in Treating Cutaneous Leishmaniasis

The utility of antileishmanial agents will probably vary with the form of leishmaniasisns being treated. One way to categorize the cutaneous leishmaniases is to divide them into L. tropica and L. mexicana complexes on the one hand, and L. braziliensis complex on the other hand (Table 1) Except in rare cases, cutaneous leishmaniasis due to L. tropica complex in the Old World and to L. mexicana complex in the New World is thought to consist of single ulcerative lesions that do not frequently undergo lymphatic metastasis and that self cure in a few months to a year. It is hoped that the natural history of these syndromes will be carefully studied in the future and that the data will support these generalizations. If so, these diseases constitute relatively uncomplicated outpatient problems. Ironically, the mild nature of these diseases has made it difficult to decide on appropriate therapy. The generally accepted therapy for all forms of leishmaniasis is pentavalent antimony (Sb) in the form of Pentostam or Glucantime, but it could be argued that the reversible T-wave depressions accompanying Sb therapy[1] should be avoided in treatment of an outpatient problem. In addition, the drug is given parenterally, and not all patients view 20 injections as being clearly preferable to the possibility of a few months of a non-debilitating skin ulcer.

To avoid Sb therapy, a very wide variety of orally administered drugs used for other diseases (nifurtimox, metronidazole, cycloguanil, dehydroemetine, isoniazid and rifampin, trimethoprim-sulfamethoxazole, dapsone, ketoconazole) has been utilized to treat cutaneous leishmaniasis. Because these drugs are already in clinical use, they are generally safe and easy to administer. However, therapeutic success with some of these agents (such as metronidazole, isoniazid plus rifampin, trimethoprim-sulfamethoxazole) was later countered by less favorable reports (as in Table 2). There are as yet no contradictory reports for others of these agents. Nevertheless, for cutaneous leishmaniasis which undergoes variable but potentially rapid self-cure, it is prudent to require demonstration of activity in a randomized trial utilizing no-treatment controls before an agent can be considered effective.

Table 1 Postulated Future of Present Antileishmanial Chemotherapeutic Agents

Disease	Organism	Therapy	Comments
Cutaneous	L. tropica and L. mexicana complexes	Sb:20 MKD x 20 day	Initial Regimen
		Sb:10-20 MKD x 10 day	Evaluate in trials
		Sterol inhibitors	Probably effective
		Purine analogs	Probably effective
		Topical measures	Superficially attractive
	L. braziliensis complex	Sb:20 MKD x 20 day	Initial Regimen
		Sb:10-20 MKD x 10 day	Evaluate in trials
		Sterol inhibitors	Possibly effective
		Purine analogs	Possibly effective
Mucosal	L. braziliensis complex	Sb:20 MKD x 30 day	Standard Regimen
Visceral	L. donovani complex	Sb:20 MKD x 30 day	Standard Regimen
		WR 6026	in Phase I
		Liposomal preparation	in Preclinical evaluation

MKD = mg/kg/day

An even wider variety of local therapies (several means of mechanical excision, application of heat and cold, local injections, and topical applications) have also been employed for L. tropica and L. mexicana disease. Although superficially attractive, in reality these therapies are not necessarily without local morbidity, and it requires ingenuity to make these approaches simple to administer. In addition, local therapy is appropriate only after it has been determined that disease in the region of the world under consideration is indeed localized, and each local therapeutic regimen has to be shown to be more effective than no treatment.

Recommendations to Treat Cutaneous Leishmaniasis

In lieu of therapy that is truly appropriate on the basis of ease of administration, lack of toxicity, and demonstrated efficacy, the prudent recommendation for the isolated case of disease due to or in an area endemic for L. tropica or L. mexicana complex is treatment with the regimen that has the best chance of being effective. In my opinion, this regimen is 20 mg Sb/kg/day, with no upper limit on daily dose, for 20 days (Table 1). Physicians who have more clinical material could engage in trials to determine if other regimens are competitive with this long-term, high dose Sb regimen. The trials might be organized in the following manner. First, for each major endemic region, this regimen of Sb (20 MKD x 20 days) should be compared to no treatment in a randomized study. If the time to cure and cure rate in Sb-treated patients is not significantly less than the natural cure time and cure rate, the reason could be use of one pentavalent antimonial (Pentostam or Glucantime) rather than the other, injection by one route (intravenous or intramuscular) rather than the other, or that Sb therapy simply is no better than no treatment at all. There are no reports on the relative efficacy of Pentostam vs. Glucantime or on intravenous vs. intramuscular injection. Whether Sb treatment for cutaneous disease is effective on the basis of statistical significance is an open question. As Table 2 indicates, in Algeria Glucantime (17 mg Sb/kg/day for 15 days) was no better than no treatment.[2] On the other hand, at Walter Reed a high dose of Pentostam has been shown to be more effective than a low dosage. 20 mg Sb (Pentostam)/kg/day, with no upper limit on daily dose for 20 days cured 19/19 patients with Panamanian cutaneous disease, whereas 10 mg/kg/day for 20 days cured 16/21 patients (p=.03). The study was double-blind and randomized.[3]

Table 2   Comparison of two oral agents to no-treatment and to Glucantime treatment for L. major disease in Algeria.

Treatment Regimen	# Patients	# Cured (%) 1 month after treatment
None	108	59 (55%)
Glucantime: 17 mg Sb/kg/d x 15 day	97	47 (48%)
Trimethoprim-Sulfamethoxazole: 160-320 mg trimethoprim per day x 15 day	99	54 (55%)
Metronidazole: 1.5-3.0 g per day x 15 day	80	41 (51%)

Adapted from reference 2.

When and if the efficacy of long-term, high-dose Sb treatment is established, treatment regimens utilizing lower Sb dosages, shorter Sb courses, or oral or local therapies could be compared to the high-dose, long-term Sb cure rate.

There are now oral agents that are based on Leishmania specific biochemical pathways. Leishmania synthesize purines via the salvage pathway. Amastigotes as well as promastigotes have an unusual hypoxanthine phosphoribosyltransferase, nucleoside phosphotransferase, and adenylosuccinate synthetase and lyase.[4] These enzymes convert hypoxanthine and inosine analogs such as allopurinol and allopurinol ribonucleoside into analogs of inosine monophosphate, adenosine monophosphate, adenosine diphosphate, adenosine triphosphate, and RNA. The means by which these purine analogs generate cytotoxicity is very unclear. Amastigote and promastigote sterol biosynthesis is comparable to that of many fungi, and distinct from that of mammalian cells, in having ergostane-series sterols as the major demethylated sterol and in the susceptibility of lanosterol demethylating enzymes to imidazoles such as ketoconazole.[5,6] A practical advantage of the similarity in fungal and leishmanial sterol biosynthesis is that potential antileishmanial agents can be developed for clinical use without having to be financially justified on the basis of their utility for a parasitic disease. Allopurinol ribonucleoside is curing a majority of cases of cutaneous leishmaniasis in Panama (Saenz and Rogers; personal communication). Ketoconazole cured 6 of 6 patients in Nicaragua,[7] 4 of 4 with L. mexicana but only 1 of 4 with L. braziliensis in Belize,[8] at least 11 of 14 with L. braziliensis disease in Panama (Saenz and Berman, unpublished data), 2 of 12 with L. braziliensis disease in French Guiana,[9] two Algerians,[10] one Ethiopian,[11] and one Saudi Arabian.[11] The opinion of this reviewer is that allopurinol ribonucleoside and ketoconazole are modestly active agents that will be effective for modestly aggressive cutaneous disease. Thus, allopurinol ribonucleoside and ketoconazole are likely to be chemotherapeutically useful for the outpatient problems of Old World cutaneous disease, L. mexicana complex disease in the New World, and less aggressive L. braziliensis disease.

Treatment for aggressive L. braziliensis disease, with its frequent lymphatic metastasis, is conceptually simpler because local therapy is inappropriate for disseminated disease. Individual cases should be treated with 20 mg Sb/kg/day, with no upper limit on daily dose, for 20 days. Trials of Sb versus no treatment, shorter Sb courses, and oral agents should be undertaken and may lead to optimal treatment regimens.

Mucosal and Visceral Disease

For established mucosal and visceral disease, 20 mg Sb/kg/day for 20 days or more appears to bring about initial cure in virtually all cases. For example, Anabwani et al. demonstrated initial cures in 20/20 patients with Kenyan childhood kala-azar, although the relapse rate may have been as high as 14%.[12] Thakur initially cured 62/63 patients with Indian kala-azar.[13]

Non-antimonial therapy of visceral leishmaniasis is likely to require development of agents still in preclinical evaluation, such as WR 6026, liposomes, and perhaps new purine analogs or imidazoles. Unfortunately, the oro-nasal mucosa is not part of the visceral reticuloendothelial system and should not benefit from preclinical agents targeted to viscerally infected organs. No present chemotherapeutic agent can reasonably be expected to replace Sb therapy for mucosal disease.

Present recommendations to treat the small but not insignificant number of cases of cutaneous, mucosal, and visceral disease that do not demonstrate complete initial cure with Sb, or that relapse after initial cure, are: more Sb, combinations of Sb and oral agents, pentamidine, or amphotericin B. There is insufficient data on the efficacy and toxicity of these choices to decide which has the most favorable therapeutic index.

SUMMARY

Logical drug development in a biochemical sense involves recognition of parasite-specific biochemical pathways and synthesis of drugs that act on those pathways. Logical clinical drug development involves determining the maximum drug dosage that is safe, investigating the efficacy of such a regimen, and (if that regimen is effective) determining if lesser drug dosages are also effective. The 1980's have seen logic applied to the clinical evaluation of Pentostam regimens in that a regimen of 20 mg Sb/kg/day for 20-30 days has been found to be safe and the efficacy of this and lower dosages is beginning to be determined. Biochemical logic has also been instituted with the emphasis on orally administrable agents acting on parasite purine and steroid biosynthesis. Continuation of these efforts should bring about significant advances in our antileishmanial armamentarium.

REFERENCES

1. J.D. Chulay, H.C. Spencer, and M. Mugambi. Electrocardiographic changes during treatment of leishmaniasis with pentavalent antimony (sodium stibogluconate). Am. J. Trop. Med. Hyg. 34:702 (1985).
2. S. Belazzoug and R.A. Neal. Failure of meglumine antimonate to cure cutaneous lesions due to Leishmania major in Algeria. Trans. Roy. Soc. Trop. Med. Hyg. 80:670 (1986).
3. W.R. Ballou, D.M. Gordon, J. Andujar, J.B. McClain, G.D. Shanks, J.D. Berman, and J.D. Chulay. Safety and efficacy of high-dose sodium stibogluconate therapy of American cutaneous leishmaniasis. Lancet 2:13 (1987).
4. D.L. Looker, R.L. Berens, and J.J. Marr. Purine metabolism in Leishmania donovani amastigotes and promastigotes. Mol. Biochem. Parasitol. 9:15 (1983).
5. L.J. Goad, G.G. Holz, and D.H. Beach. Sterols of Leishmania species: Implications for biosynthesis. Mol. Biochem. Parasitol. 10:161 (1984).
6. J.D. Berman, L.J. Goad, and D.H. Beach, G.G. Holz. Effects of ketoconazole in sterol biosynthesis by Leishmania mexicana mexicana amastigotes in murine macrophage tumor cells. Mol. Biochem. Parasitol. 20:85 (1986).
7. F.G. Urcuyo and N. Zaias. Oral ketoconazole in the treatment of leishmaniasis. Int. J. Derm. 21:414 (1982).
8. D.S. Jolliffe. Cutaneous leishmaniasis from Belize-treatment with ketoconazole. Clin. Exp. Derm. 11:62 (1986).
9. J.P. Dedet, P. Jamet, P. Esterre, P.M. Glipponi, C. Genin, and G. Lalande. Failure to cure Leishmania braziliensis guayanensis cutaneous leishmaniasis with oral ketoconazole. Trans. Roy. Soc. Trop. Med. Hyg. 80:176 (1986).
10. S. Belazzong, A. Ammar-Khodja, M. Belkaid, and O. Tabet-Derraz. La leishmaniose cutanee du Nord de L'Algeria. Bull. Soc. Path. Ex. 78:615 (1985).
11. J. Viallet, J.D. Maclean, and H. Robson. Response to ketoconazole in two cases of longstanding cutaneous leishmaniasis. Am. J. Trop. Med. Hyg. 35:491 (1986).

12. G.M. Anabwani, G. Dimiti, J.A. Ngira, and A.D.M. Bryceson. Comparison of two dosage schedules of sodium stibogluconate in the treatment of visceral leishmaniasis in Kenya. Lancet. 1:210 (1983).
13. C.P. Thakur, M. Kumer, S.K. Singh, D. Sharma, U.S. Prasad, R.S.P. Singh, P.S. Dhawan, and V. Achari. Comparison of regimen of treatment with sodium stibogluconate in kala-azar. Br. Med. J. 288:895 (1984).

CHEMOTHERAPY OF MEDITERRANEAN VISCERAL LEISHMANIASIS WITH MEGLUMINE ANTIMONIATE

Luis Tavares, Celia Carvalho, and Eduardo Monteiro

Department of Infectious Diseases
Hospital Santa Maria
1600 Lisboa
Portugal

INTRODUCTION

Over the last years many trials have been performed to obtain adequate new drug delivery systems which could carry drugs directly to macrophages. In such systems, liposome [1] or cell ghosts [2] could carry smaller amounts of conventional drugs with a high efficacy and obviously lower toxicity. However, they are as yet only experimental systems.

Clinical administration of pentavalent antimonial compounds (ie Glucantime or Pentostam) in a 20 day course of 20 mg Sb^{5+}/kg of body weight/day is the recommended first choice therapy for visceral leishmaniasis [3]. Other drugs like Allopurinol or Pentamidine have been tried but they should be regarded as second choice agents due to their relative lack of efficacy or higher toxicity.

The present study of fourteen adult patients with parasitologically proven visceral leishmaniasis is aimed to evaluate the clinical efficacy and toxicity of the treatment with meglumine antimoniate. We report here the results of clinical and laboratory treatment as well as toxicity data.

PATIENTS AND METHODS

Between 1977 and 1986, fourteen patients with visceral leishmaniasis were treated at the Department of Infectious Diseases, Hospital Santa Maria in Lisbon. The records have been reviewed - the clinical features, methods of diagnosis, the results of physical examinations, treatment regimens and laboratory tests, especially haematological, serological, hepatic and renal function tests and ECG records.

Clinical cure was defined as an improvement in clinical condition and a return to normal in the laboratory investigations. Relapse was defined as the reappearance of parasites after a clinical cure.

RESULTS

All patients were adults with a mean age of 30 ranging from 21 to 68 years. The male/female ratio was 2.5:1. All were previously healthy and had lived in Portugal for several years before admission.

Diagnosis

Every patient had parasitologically confirmed visceral leishmaniasis. Thirteen of the 14 had a positive bone marrow stained preparation, and one had a positive blood culture. In addition 2 out of 4 had positive liver biopsy. No splenic aspiration was performed.

Clinical Picture

Fever was universally present with an irregular pattern. Anorexia and nausea, vomiting or diarrhoea were symptoms rerported by 12/14 patients. Other complaints were: sweating 11, asthenia 10, weight loss 9, and less frequently, epistaxis or hematoemesis 8, and headaches, only 4 patients.

Physical Examination

Enlargement of the spleen and liver were present in 13/14 patients. Other frequent findings were pallor 8, lymphadenopathy 4, and jaundice in one patient.

Laboratory Data

Hypergammaglobulinemia was present in all patients; in 3 it was more than 50 g/l. The leucocyte count was lower than $4.0 \times 10^9/l$ in 11 patients and all patients had an erythrocyte count of less than $4.0 \times 10^{12}/l$.

Treatment

Every patient was initially treated with Glucantime (meglumine antimoniate-Specia); 1 vial = 5 ml with a 28.35% Sb^{5+} content (one vial equivalent to 425 mg of pentavalent antimony). The drug was administered deeply IM in two or three divided doses according to the following schedule:

2 courses of 10 days	(with a 10 day interval)	5 patients
3 courses of 10 days	(with a 10 day interval)	1 "
2 courses of 15 days	(with a 15 day interval)	5 "
1 course of 20 days		2 "

In one patient the treatment was stopped on day 10 because of moderately severe side effects. In this particular patient treatment was followed with rifampin 1200 mg PO, daily for 10 days.

The daily dosage of antimony ranged from 12.5 to 22.7 mg of Sb^{5+}/kg, (mean 16.8) and the maximal total dose/patient was 1271 mg/kg.

Toxicity

No local reaction at the site of injection was reported. Four patients experienced no untoward reaction related to the antimonial compound. Except for the ECG changes (see below) the adverse side effects were:

urine erythrocytes	5	patients
abdominal pain/diarrhoea	3	"
oedema of lower limbs	2	"
depression	1	"
myalgia	1	"
hyperuricemia	1	"

In one patient severe oedema of the lower limbs and intense myalgia occurred and the treatment was discontinued. We noted no change in hepatic and renal function assessed by serological profiles.

The initial ECG pattern was normal in all the patients. Changes were recorded in 9 patients in the ST-T segments. In 6 the ST deviation was more than 2mm and/or T-wave inversion was present. All ECG changes reverted to normal at various times after the end of treatment.

Follow-up
Clinical cure was observed in all patients and no relapses have so far occurred.

DISCUSSION

Various toxic effects of antimonial compounds have been described, including cough, chest or abdominal pain, collapse and sudden death; ECG changes (prolonged QT interval and ST segment/T wave changes) are almost always present. The toxic effects observed in our series of patients were minor; even the patient for which treatment with meglumine antimoniate was interrupted ceased to complain a few days after the last dose.

No hepatic or major renal side-effects were observed and all the patients were clinically cured. Although maglumine antimoniate has been held responsible for major adverse reactions such as agranulocytosis [5], many reports testify to the safety of and tolerance to pentavalent compounds [6,7,8,9]; even in pregnancy [10].

Geographical differences in the susceptibility of leishmanial infections to antimony have been recognized [11], but treatment failure can be due, at least in part, to inadequate dosage or duration of treatment [12, 13]. One of our patients was successfully treated with Rifampin, which raises the interesting question of the effect of antimycobacterial agents on visceral leishmaniasis [14].

In view of the toxicity of Amphotericin B, the relative failure of Metranidazole [15, 16] and that of Allopurinol when used alone [17, 18], pentavalent antimony compounds because of their safety and clinical efficacy should remain the first line chemotherapeutic agents for the treatment of visceral leishmaniasis.

REFERENCES

1. R.R.C. New, M.L. Chance, S.C. Thomas and W. Peters, Antileishmanial Activity of antimonials trapped in liposomes, Nature, 272:55-56 (1978).

2. J.D. Berman, J.B. Gallallee, J.S. Williams and W.D. Hockmeyer, Activity of pentamidine-containing human red cell ghosts against visceral leishmaniasis in the hamster, Am. J.Trop.Med.Hyg., 35:297-302 (1986).

3. Comite d'Experts de l'OMS. Rpports techniques, 701, OMS, Geneve (1984).

4. P.J. Rees, Drugs, in: "Manson's Tropical Diseases", P.E.C. Manson-Bahr, 18th Ed, Bailliere-Tindal, London (1982).

5. F.G. Rodero, I.M. Jeromini V.O.T. Ducasse and A.P. Gonzalez, Agranulocitosis por glucantime durante el tratamiento del Kala-Azar
Med. Clin. (Barc.), 84:840 (1985).

6. B. Costa, F. Vidal, A. Llorente, F. Furquet and C. Richart, Kala-Azar en el area de Tarragona
Rev. Clin. Esp., 177:473-474 (1985).

7. A. Andreoli, M. Cambie, D. Manzoni, G. Bonora, G. Gargantini, G. Giaracuni and L. Perletti, Descrizione di un caso di leishmaniosi viscerale
Minerva Ped., 37:479-484 (1985).

8. C.N. Chunge, G. Gachihi, R. Muigai, K. Wassunna, J.R. Rashid, J.D. Chulay, G. Anabwani, C.N. Oster and A.D.M. Bryceson, Visceral leishmaniasis unresponsive to antimonial drugs III. Successful treatment using a combination of sodium stibogluconate plus allopurinol, Trans. R. Soc. Trop. Med. Hyg., 79:715-718 (1985).

9. C.P. Thakur, M. Kumar, S.K. Singh, D. Sharma, U.S. Prasad, R.S.P. Singh, P.S. Dhawan and V. Achari, Comparison of regimens of treatment with sodium stibogluconate in Kala-Azar,
Brit. Med. J., 288:895-897 (1984).

10. P. Massip, C. Goutner, Y. Dupic and P. Navarrot, Kala-Azar chez la femme enceinte,
Presse Med., 15:933 (1986).

11. L. Yan-jia, A review of kala-azar in China from 1949 to 1959.
Trans. R. Soc. Trop. Med. Hyg., 76:531-537 (1982).

12. A.D.M. Bryceson, J.D. Chulay, M. Ho, M. Mugambii, J.B. Were, R. Muigai, C. Chunge, G. Gachihi, J. Meme, G. Anabwani and S.M. Bhatt, Visceral leishmaniasis unresponsive to antimonial drugs. I. Clinical and immunological studies,
   Trans.Roy.Soc.Med.Hyg., 79:700-704 (1985).

13. A.D.M. Bryceson, J.D. Chulay, M. Mugambi, J.B. Were, G. Gachihi, C.N. Chunge, R. Muigai, S.M. Bhatt, M. Ho, H.C. Spencer, J. Meme and G. Anabwani, Visceral leishmaniasis unresponsive to antimonial drugs. II. Response to high dosage sodium stibogluconate or prolonged treatment with pentamidine,
   Trans,. R. Soc. Trop. Med. Hyg., 79:705-714 (1985).

14. A.S. Neto, E.N. Sousa, H.B. Valente, R. Guimaraes, J.A. Richardo, F.M. Conceicao-Silva, C.D. Silva-Pereira, P. Abranches and S. Rosa, Un cas original de leishmaniose viscerale,
   Presse Med. 15:1286 (1986).

15. M. Mishra, B.D. Thakur and M. Choudhary, Metronidazole and Indian kala-azar: results of a clinical trial,
   Brit. Med. J., 291:1611 (1985).

16. J.S. Keithly and S.G. Langreth, Inefficacy of metronidazole in experimental infections of *Leishmania donovani*, *L. mexicana*, and *Trypanosoma brucei brucei*,
   Am. J. Trop. Med. Hyg., 32:485-496 (1983).

17. P.A. Kager, P.H. Rees, B.T. Wellde, W.T. Hockmeyer and W.H. Lyerly, Allopurinol in the treatment of visceral leishmaniasis,
   Trans. R. Soc. Trop. Med. Hyg., 75:556-559 (1981).

18. T.K. Jha, Evaluation of allopurinol in the treatment of kala-azar occurring in North Bihar, India,
   Trans. R. Soc. Trop. Med. Hyg., 77:204-207 (1983).

THE *IN VITRO* SUSCEPTIBILITY OF MACROPHAGES INFECTED WITH AMASTIGOTES OF *LEISHMANIA* SPP. TO PENTAVALENT ANTIMONIAL DRUGS AND OTHER COMPOUNDS WITH SPECIAL RELEVANCE TO CUTANEOUS ISOLATES

Sarah Allen and R.A. Neal

Department of Medical Protozoology
London School of Hygiene and Tropical Medicine
Winches Farm Laboratories
St. Albans, Herts AL2 3BE

INTRODUCTION

Variation in clinical response to treatment of leishmaniasis with pentavalent antimonial compounds has been reported on many occasions. It has been assumed that the variations arise from the patient or drug potency since there has previously been no way of checking the sensitivity of the parasites. The development of *in vitro* infected macrophage systems has allowed drug sensitivity to be monitored (Berman and Wyler, 1980; Neal and Matthews, 1982).

Preliminary studies with *L.major*, *L.brasiliensis* and *L.panamensis* promastigotes showed that uniform macrophage infections were found on day 2 and 3 after infection, but that after 5 days incubation, no amastigotes were observed in the macrophages. Since it is necessary to incubate the infected macrophages for 5 to 7 days to demonstrate an effect with antimony compounds, the use of promastigotes was abandoned in favour of amastigotes. The use of amastigotes from infected animals makes the procedure more lengthy and cumbersome, but the amastigote technique provides baseline data for future comparison with promastigote infections.

Herein we describes the effect of pentavalent antimonials on mouse peritoneal macrophages infected *in vitro* with different strains of *Leishmania* amastigotes.and the nomenclature used is that proposed by Lainson and Shaw (1987).

MATERIALS AND METHODS

Parasites

Strains of different *Leishmania* were grown in culture (Schneider's medium + 10% foetal calf serum or 4N medium) and inoculated into the hind footpad of hamsters. All cultures were characterised by Dr D.A. Evans (London School of Hygiene and Tropical Medicine) using isoenzyme analysis to confirm the specific status of the strains.

The strains were:

L.donovani	MHOM/ET/67 HU3;
	MHOM/SD/Waits-Hanson Sb resistant*
	(Professor W.L. Hanson, Georgia, USA)
L.panamensis	MHOM/PA/67/Boynton
L.brasiliensis	MHOM/BO/67/Atenzana, MHOM/PE/66/L280
L.guyanensis	MHOM/BR/86/607M, MHOM/BR/86/620M
	(Dr W. Rogers, Manas, Brazil)
L.amazonensis	MOYR/BR/72/M1824,
	MPRO/BR/72/M1845,
	MHOM/BR/85/M10111,
	MHOM/BR/85/M1132
	(Professor R. Lainson, Belem, Brazil)
L.mexicana	MNYC/BZ/62/M379, MHOM/CR/69/O-CR-B
L.major	MHOM/DZ/82/LIPA 60,
	MHOM/DZ/82/LIPA 64,
	MHOM/DZ/82/LIPA 67
	(Dr S. Belazzoug, Algiers, ALgeria),
	MHOM/SA/84/JISH 118,
	MHRO/SU/59/NEAL-P,
	MHOM/SA/85 JISH 1181,
	MHOM/SA/86/J3125
	(Dr R. Kubba, Al-Khobar, Saudi Arabia)
L.tropica	MHOM/AF/82/K001
	MHOM/AF/82/K002,
	MHOM/AF/82/K003

Infected stabilates were cryopreserved. Individual strains were kindly donated by named colleagues.

Amastigote Suspensions

Hamster footpad lesions 1-2 months old were used for isolation of amastigotes. Amastigotes were released from infected tissue by grinding in RPMI 1640 + 10% FCS + gentamicin 50 mg/l medium. The amastigotes were washed twice, then resuspended in about 2 ml of medium. The number of amastigotes was determined by quantitating against 1×10^8 suspension (10^8/ml) of polystyrene beads (Neal and Reeve, unpublished data) and counted after Giemsa staining. The number of amastigotes was adjusted to contain 1×10^6/ml.

Macrophages and Infection with Amastigotes

Washed macrophages (4×10^5/ml) from the peritoneal cavity of soluble starch-induced mice were plated in 8 chamber tissue culture slides (Lab-tel Products, Miles Laboratories) and amastigotes added in the ratio of 2.5 to each macrophage. Infected macrophages were incubated in 5% CO_2 in air at either 37ºC for *L.donovani* or 33ºC for *Leishmania* causing cutaneous leisions *in vivo*.

Susceptibility to Drugs and Compounds Used

The protocol was similar to that described earlier (Neal and Croft, 1984) and involved exposure of the infected macrophages to different concentrations of drugs in RPMI 1640 + 10% FCS medium for 7 days. Sodium stibogluconate was prepared by diluting the "Pentostam" formulation (Wellcome Foundation Ltd, batches B52462 and A56530). Meglumine antimoniate (Rhone-Poulenc, batch 848 (CA 7735400) was prepared as a solution. The concentration of these drugs is given as mg of pentavalent antimony according to the manufacturers' information. Other drugs were formulated as described earlier (Neal and Croft, 1984).

Assessment of Drug Response

After Giemsa staining, the proportion of macrophages free of amastigotes was determined microscopically. The data were analysed by linear regression analysis and 50% suppressive concentrations were calculated. Fiducial limits (P95) gave acceptable limits in each experiment.

No toxicity to macrophages was seen with the antimonials.

RESULTS

Macrophage Infections
About 60-85% of the macrophages contained amastigotes. The mean number of amastigotes per macrophage varied in different experiments but at 24 hr it was about 5, increasing to approximately 10 at 7 days, indicating a 2 fold increase in numbers.

Effect of Temperature
The effectiveness of pentavalent antimonials was studied on macrophages infected with amastigotes of L.amazonensis M 10111. The results showed that incubation of the infected macrophages with drugs at 35ºC or 33ºC did not significantly alter the response. The response of L.amazonensis M 10111 to meglumine antimoniate at the two temperatures gave identical ED_{50} values of 21 $mgSb^V$/litre.

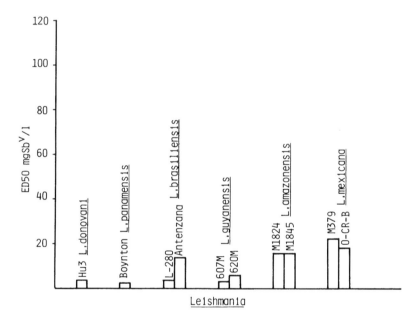

FIGURE 1 *LEISHMANIA* SP SENSITIVE TO PENTAVALENT ANTIMONY

Response to Pentavalent Antimonial Drugs
The response of different strains to sodium stibogluconate is summarized in the histograms shown in Figs 1 to 3. The HU3 strain of L.donovani has been used for other chemotherapy studies and the mean response for the most recent 5 experiments is shown in Figure 1. The New World isolates L.panamensis, L.guyanensis and one strain of L.brasiliensis (L-280) were as sensitive as the reference L.donovani. However, another strain of L.brasiliensis (Atenzana), L.amazonensis and L.mexicana were less susceptible.

The susceptibility of Old World cutaneous *Leishmania* was less than those determined for New World strains (Figure 2). One strain of *L.major* (JOSH 118) from Saudi Arabia and two of *L.tropica* from Afghanistan gave 50% suppressive values of over 40 mgSb^V/litre. All strains were isolated from patients before treatment or from reservoir hosts.

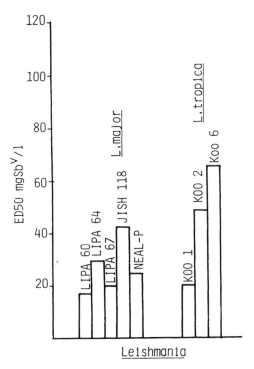

FIGURE 2 *LEISHMANIA* SP LESS SENSITIVE TO PENTAVALENT ANTIMONY

The laboratory developed antimony resistant strain of *L.donovani* showed very little response to sodium stibogluconate at the highest level tested, 81 mgSb^V/litre (Figure 3). This is compared with strains of *L.major* and *L.amazonensis* isolated from patients who had received two or more treatments with sodium stibogluconate. The response of one *L.major* strain (JISH 1181) was similar to that of an untreated patient (JISH 118, Figure 2), while a strain from another treated patient (J 3125) was highly non-responsive to a level similar to that of the laboratory drug resistant *L.donovani*. The two isolates of *L.amazonensis* were from two patients with diffuse cutaneous leishmaniasis who had received many treatments and relapsed after each treatment. The *in vitro* response of the isolates were much less than those of *L.amazonensis* isolated from reservoir hosts (Figure

1) and the resistance of one strain (M 10111) approached that of the laboratory antimony resistant strain of *L.donovani*.

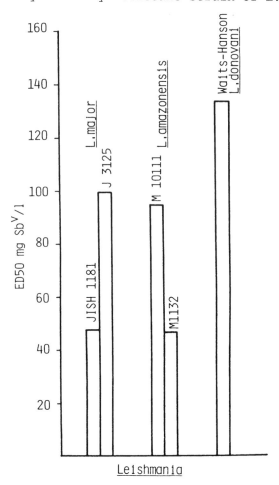

FIGURE 3 *LEISHMANIA* SP HIGHLY RESISTANT TO PENTAVALENT ANTIMONY

The response to meglumine antimoniate parallelled that to sodium stibogluconate. Meglumine antimoniate, however, was generally more active *in vitro*, by a factor of about 4 fold or less. It was less active than sodium stibogluconate against two strains of *L.major* (LIPA 60 and 64) and against *L.tropica* (strain K002) no effect was observed at concentrations up to 81 mgSb^V/litre.

Response to Other Drugs
No systematic studies have been undertaken but limited data of the response to paromomycin and amphotericin B with the non-responsive strains are shown in Table 1. In general the strains remained sensitive to these drugs.

DISCUSSION

There are two possible interpretations of our results. Firstly, that some species of *Leishmania* are innately less susceptible to antimonial compounds than others. Thus *L.panamensis*, *L.guyanensis* and one isolate of *L.brasiliensis* were as sensitive as the reference *L.donovani* HU3 strain while *L.major* and *L.tropica* were less susceptible. *L.amazonensis* and *L.mexicana* were intermediate in susceptibility. Further studies are required with the *L.brasiliensis* group owing to conflicting results with the two isolates tested and with the *L.mexicana* complex to decide whether the results are due to experimental variation.

The low susceptibility of *L. major in vitro* correlates with the difficulty in curing infections in mice. It is not possible to cure a mouse with non-healing *L.major* infections; the beneficial effect is only temporary and the parasites resume development after the drug treatment has stopped (Neal, 1964). It is possible that the drug fails to reach the parasites in the skin. The low susceptibility of *L.major in vitro*, however, does not seem to correlate with the use of antimonial drugs for treatment of the lesions in man. Such clinical evidence is not strong and the publication of a controlled clinical trial of these drugs against *L. ajor* lesions is awaited. A low susceptibility of *L.major in vitro* is also reported by Berman and Lee (1984).

The second interpretation is that acquired antimony resistance is present in certain strains. The very high ED_{50} values for the *L.donovani* Sb^V-resistant strain correlates with the lack of susceptibility *in vivo*. Hamster infections are not affected by a dose level of 500 mgSb/kg/day x 5 days, about 30x the ED_{50} of normal *L.donovani* strains (Hanson and Neal, unpublished data).

The low susceptibility of *L.major* isolates from unresponsive patient J 3125 is of considerable interest. This patient was not cured after receiving 3 courses of sodium stibogluconate treatment (Dr R. Kubba, unpublished data). This correlates with the results of the infected macrophage *in vitro* tests since the J 3125 strain did not respond to a high antimony concentration (81 mg/l) *in vitro*.

Two isolates of *L.amazonensis*, M 10111 and M 1132 were also insensitive to antimony *in vitro*. These strains were isolated from two patients with diffuse cutaneous leishmaniasis (DCL) who had received approximately one course of treatment per year with either sodium stibogluconate or meglumine antimoniate since 1971 and 1968 respectively (Peters et al., 1981; Lainson, 1982 and unpublished data). It is not surprising to find that the 50% suppressive concentrations were extremely high. It seems likely that selection of less susceptible amastigotes had occurred during the many treatments of the two DCL patients in the absence of a protective immune response.

The results with *L.major* indicate that antimony resistance may develop relatively quickly. Antimony resistance is not affected by amastigote/promastigote transformation since parasites from the unresponsive patients and the laboratory drug resistant strain were sent to London as promastigote cultures, then established in hamsters. The results support the need for using an adequate dose schedule for treatment.

Recent studies of the pharmacokintics of sodium stibogluconate have shown that the peak antimony blood level is about 10-15 mgSb^V/l (reviewed by Bryceson, 1987). No information is available on spleen or liver concentration, but assuming that the blood level is equalled in the tissues, it is clear that the 50% suppressive levels of the unresponsive strains and the Old World cutaneous strains are above the achievable blood level. This would suggest that cure rates by direct antiparasite effects would be low.

The presence of acquired drug resistance has been suspected from clinical unresponsiveness by a number of workers. Berman *et al.* (1982) studied the susceptibility of *L.panamensis* strains *in vitro*, but were unable to observe a consistent correlation with clinical response, although some strains were clearly less sensitive than others. Bryceson *et al.* (1985a,b) and Chunge *et al.* (1985) demonstrated the failure of a few kala azar patients to respond to sodium stibogluconate treatment. Earlier studies by Ercoli (1964) in Venezuela with strains of *Leishmania* from DCL patients, showed a difference in response of mouse infections to treastment with meglumine antimoniate according to whether the patients had received no previous treatment or many treatments. The evidence, although clear, was difficult to evaluate because of the failure to cure mouse infections with normal strains of cutaneous *Leishmania*. However, from the *in vitro* evidence with parasites from similar patients given above, it is likely that Ercoli's studies did represent true acquired drug resistance.

Previously reported data (Neal & Croft, 1984) showed that meglumine antimoniate was more active *in vitro* than sodium stibogluconate. In most comparisons this was also true for the present data. However, there was a reversal of relative activity between the two antimonial compounds in individual expeiments with *L.major* Lipa 64 and with the unresponsive *L.amazonensis* M 1132. In addition, against *L.tropica* K002, a concentration related response was not observed with meglumine antimoniate. No rationale for these variations is apparent.

The efficacy of Paromomycin and Amphotericin B on *Leishmania* spp. that were classed as having either inherent or acquired non-responsiveness, showed a response similar to that previously reported for *L.donovani* (Neal and Croft, 1984). Thus it would be expected that patients infected with similar strains of *Leishmania* would respond to treatment with these drugs. The effectiveness of drugs other than antimonials was reported by Berman (1982).

ACKNOWLEDGEMENTS

We would like to thank the following colleagues; Dr S. Belazzoug, Prof. S.L. Hanson, Dr R. Kubba, Prof. R. Lainson, Mr W. Rogers and Prof. W. Peters, for generously donating strains, and to Mr C. Kimber for providing strains cryopreserved in the WHO Reference Bank. We are also grateful to the Wellcome Trust and to UNDP/World Bank/WHO Special Programme for Research and Training in Tropical Diseases for financial support.

REFERENCES

Berman, J.D., 1982, *In vitro* susceptibility of antimony-resistant *Leishmania* to alternative drugs, J. Infectious Dis., 145:279.

Berman, J.D., Chulay, J.D., Hendricks, L.D. and Oster, C.N., 1982, Susceptibility of clinically sensitive and resistant *Leishmania* to pentavalent antimony *in vitro*, Am. J. Trop. Med. Hyg., 31:459.

Berman, J.D. and Lee, L.S., 1984, Activity of antileishmanial agents against amastigotes in human monocyte derived macrophages and in mouse peritoneal macrophages, J. Parasitology, 70:220.

Berman, J.D. and Wyler, D.J., 1980, An *in vitro* model for investigation of chemotherapeutic agents in leiahmaniasis, J. Infectious Dis., 142:83.

Bryceson, A., Therapy in man, in: "The Leishmaniases in Biology and Medicine", W. Peters & R. Killick-Kendrick, eds, Academic Press (1987).

Bryceson, A.D.M., Chulay, J.D., Ho, M., Mugami, M., Were, J.B., Muigai, R., Chunge, C., Gachihi, G., Meme, J.,Anabwani, G. and Bhatt, S.M., 1985a, Visceral leishmaniasis unresponsive to antimonial drugs. I. Clinical and immunological studies, Trans. R. Soc. Trop. Med. Hyg., 79:700.

Bryceson, A.D.M., Chulay, J.D., Mugambi, M., Were, J.B., Gachihi, G., Chunge, C.N., Muigai, R., Bhatt, S.M., Ho, M., Spencer, H.C., Meme, J. and Anabwani, G., 1985b, Visceral leishmaniasis unresponsive to antimonial drugs. II. Response to high dosage sodium stibogluconate or prolonged treatment with pentamidine, Trans. R. Soc. Trop. Med. Hyg., 79:705.

Chunge, C.N., Gachihi, G., Muigai, R., Wasunna, K., Rashid, J.R., Chulay, J.D., Anabwani, G., Oster, C.N. and Bryceson, A.D.M., 1985, Visceral leishmaniasis unresponsive to antimonial drugs. III. Successful treatment using a combination of sodium stibogluconate plus allopurinol, Trans. R. Soc. Trop. Med. Hyg., 79:715.

Ercoli, N., 1964, Studies on the therapeutic resistance of cutaneous *Leishmania* infections, Chemotherapia, 8:3.

Lainson, R., Leishmaniasis, in: "CRC Handbook Series in Zoonoses", Section C Parasitic Zoonoses, Vol. I, L. Jacobs, ed., CRC Press, Florida (1982).

Lainson, R. and Shaw, J.D., Evolution, classification and geographical distribution, in: "The Leishmaniases in Biology and Medicine", W. Peters & R. Killick-Kendrick, eds, Academic Press (1987).

Neal, R.A., 1964, Chemotherapy of cutaneous leishmaniasis: *Leishmania tropica* infections in mice, Ann. Trop. Med. Parasitol., 58:420.

Neal, R.A. and Croft, S.L., 1984, An *in vitro* system for determining the acitvity of compounds against the intracellular amastigote form of *Leishmania donovani*, J. Antimicrobial Chemotherapy, 14:463.

Neal, R.A. and Matthews, P.J., 1982, *In vitro* antileishmanial proportions of pentavalent antimonial comounds, Trans. R. Soc. Trop Med. Hyg., 76:284.

Peters, W., Lainson, R., Shaw, J.J., Robinson, B.L. and Franca, Leao, A., 1981, Potentiating action of Rifampicin and Isoniazid against *Leishmania mexicana amazonensis*, Lancet, 23:1122.

RELAPSE IN KALA AZAR : FAILURE OF SODIUM STIBOGLUCONATE TO CLEAR PARASITES FROM ORGANS OTHER THAN THE LIVER

K.C. Carter,[1,2], J. Alexander,[1], A.J. Baillie,[2] and T.F. Dolan,[2]

Department of Immunology[1] and Pharmacy[2]
University of Strathclyde
George Street
Glasgow G1 1XW, UK.

INTRODUCTION

Relapse in Kala-azar is a common problem, occurring in 5-30% of patients (Chulay et al, 1983, Sanyal and Arora, 1979). Although this could be attributed to re-infection, there is a strong possibility that it may at least partly be due to treatment failure. Two recent studies suggest that removal of parasites from certain tissue sites may be difficult.

Anabwani et al (1983) compared the response of patients to two dosage regimes of sodium stibogluconate. After 9 weeks treatment with 10 mg Sb kg^{-1} body weight, 2 out of 28 patients still had positive spleen counts, suggesting that removal of parasites from this site was difficult. Similarly, removal of parasites from the bone marrow also seems difficult since Wickramsinghe et al (1971) recovered L.donovani amastigotes from bone marrow aspirates of 2 out of 3 patients after two weeks of daily sodium stibogluconate injections.

However, in the majority of chemotherapeutic studies using animal models of L.donovani infection, the efficacy of various treatments has been based purely on liver parasite burdens (Black et al, 1977; Adinolfi et al, 1985; Alving et al, 1986; Baillie et al, 1986). Thus these studies would have failed to discover if stibogluconate treatment removed parasites from the deeper sites. In this study therefore, the effect of stibogluconate therapy on parasite numbers in the spleen, liver and bone marrow has been compared using the experimental protocol described by Baillie et al (1986), which has been shown to clear parasites from the liver.

MATERIALS AND METHODS

Materials

Sodium stibogluconate (Pentostam) equivalent to 0.32

mg Sb mg^{-1} was obtained from the Wellcome Foundation, UK. Synthetic (>99% pure) L-α-phosphatidylcholine (DPPC) and ash free cholesterol (CHOL) were obtained from Sigma. The single chain non-ionic surfactant (Surfactant I, Baillie et al, 1985) was obtained from L'Oreal, France. These materials were used as received and other reagents were of analytical grade. Liposomes and niosomes comprised 70% amphiphile (DPPC or non-ionic surfactant) and 30% CHOL, on a molar basis, and were prepared using procedures already described (Baillie et al, 1986).

Animals

Eight to ten week-old inhouse bred BALB/c mice which originated from breeding pairs from Bantin and Kingman Ltd. colony (The Field Station, Grimston, Aldborough, Hull) were used throughout experiments. Aged matched female B10.D2/n/O1a (B10.D2) mice obtained from OLAC (1976) Ltd. were also used. Golden Syrian hamsters (Mesocricetus auratus) obtained from the Anatomy Department, Glasgow University were used to maintain the parasite.

Parasite

Leishmainia donovani strain MHOM/ET/67/L82 (LV9), obtained from Dr. G. Coombs, Glasgow University was harvested and maintained as described by Carter et al (1987). Mice were injected into the tail vein (without anaesthetic) with 1-2 x 10^7 amastigotes in 0.2ml.

Parasite distribution

Mice were killed by cervical dislocation and impression smears of the spleen and liver taken after weighing the organs. A smear of the bone marrow was obtained by cutting off the end of the right femur, nearest the 'knee' joint, and inserting a 25G needle into the bone. The bone marrow sample was smeared on to a glass slide. Smears were fixed in methanol, stained in 10% Giemsa (Gibco) and the number of amastigotes per 1000 host cell nuclei counted. The number of Leishman-Donovan units (LDU) was calculated per organ for the liver and spleen using the formula : LDU = number of amastigotes per 1000 host cell nuclei x the organ weight (g) (Bradley and Kirkley, 1977).

Experimental design

In a typical experiment mice were treated on 7 days and 8 post-infection and parasite numbers in the liver, spleen and bone marrow assessed 6 days later. Groups of 5 mice were injected into the tail vein (without anaesthetic) with 0.2ml of one of the following preparations; distilled water, free sodium stibogluconate, niosomal or liposomal sodium stibogluconate.

Presentation and statistical analysis of data

Parasite burden of the spleen and liver is expressed as mean LDU/organ ± standard error, whereas the bone marrow counts are expressed as mean number of parasites/1000 host cells ± standard error. Results were analysed using an independent 't' test or a one way analysis of variance on the $\log_{10}$ transformed data.

RESULTS

Treatment with free sodium stibogluconate (equivalent to a total antimony dose of 2 mg) had no significant effect on L.donovani spleen and bone marrow parasite burdens in either BALB/c or B.10D2 mice ($p>0.05$, Table 1). However, it did cause a significant reduction in liver parasite burdens : a 97% suppression in BALB/c mice and a 73% suppression in B10.D2 mice, compared with controls.

The carrier forms of the drug (both niosomal and liposomal) were also unable to reduce parasite numbers in the spleen and bone marrow of BALB/c mice ($p>0.25$, Table 2), although they did cause a significantly greater reduction in the liver parasite burdens compared with free drug treatment ($p<0.01$). Thus the carrier forms of sodium stibogluconate were more active, even though the drug concentration was nearly a tenth of the free drug dose. However there was no difference in the therapeutic effect of the two carriers ($p>0.10$).

DISCUSSION

The results clearly demonstrated that both the free and carrier form of sodium stibogluconate had an organ dependent antileishmanial effect. They were capable of significantly reducing the liver parasite burden but failed to limit parasites numbers in the spleen and bone marrow.

Various methods have been attempted to overcome this problem (Carter et al, 1987) including : (a) increasing the total antimony dose given to animals from 2 to 10 mg but maintaining the same two day treatment regimen; (b) increasing the total antimony dose given from 2 to 5 mg by using a 'multiple dosing' regimen; and (c) using smaller sized liposomes to deliver the drug in an attempt to avoid clearance from the circulation by Kupffer cells. However, none of these therapeutic regimens were able to reduce parasite numbers in the deeper organs.

Assuming that a similar organ dependent antileishmanial effect occurs in man, and the results of Wickramsinghe et al (1987) and Anabwani et al (1983) do support this view, then a failure to eradicate all foci of infection could possibly lead to a generalised recolonization of the body. This would seem to occur in the mouse model as Carter et al (1987) found that organ counts obtained fifty days post-drug treatment (i.e. day 58 post-infection) demonstrated that the liver parasite burden had increased to 37% of the control value, compared to 1.5% normally obtained on day 6 post-treatment (i.e. day 14 post-infection). There is however, also the possibility that the liver parasite population could have originated from the few parasites left in the liver after drug treatment.

TABLE 1

The effect of sodium stibogluconate treatment on L.donovani parasite burdens of different organs of two mouse strains.

BALB/c mice[1]	n	Parasite Burdens		
		Spleen	Liver	Bone Marrow
Controls[a]	7	53±13	3748±379	23±10
2mg Sb[b]	8	99±24	127±31	101±26
B10.D2 mice[2]				
Controls[a]	4	174±23	7074±520	1704±259
2mg Sb[b]	5	121±25	1895±282	1343±263

Mice, infected with 1×10^7 (1) or 2×10^7 (2) L.donovani, were treated on days 7 and 8 post-infection with either water[a] or sodium stibogluconate[b] with the total antimony dose shown. On day 14 post-infection the number of parasites in the spleen, liver and bone marrow was determined. The results are expressed as the mean LDU ± standard error for the spleen and liver, and as the mean number of amastigotes/1000 host cell nuclei for the bone marrow. The number of animals per treatment 'n' is shown.

TABLE 2

The effect of three different sodium stibogluconate preparations on L.donovani spleen, liver and bone marrow burdens.

	n	Parsite Burdens		
		Spleen	Liver	Bone Marrow
Control[a]	5	65±21	4428±268	34±4
free drug[b]	5	61±15	67±30	35±13
niosomal drug[c]	5	57±19	4±4	94±42
liposomal drug[d]	5	53±15	1±1	32±5

BALB/c mice, infected with 2×10^7 L.donovani, were treated on days 7 and 8 post-infection with one of the following : water[a]; Free drug[b] (total antimony dose 2mg); niosome encapsulated drug[c] (total antimony dose 320ug); or liposome encapsulated drug[d] (total antimony dose 320ug). On day 14 post-infection the parasite burdens of the three organs were assessed. Results are expressed as described in Table 1.

However, if incomplete removal of parasites from all foci of infection is a feature of sodium stibogluconate therapy, why does relapse not occur to a greater extent in Kala-azar? Is it possible that the immune status of the host could be important?

Visceral leishmaniasis is associated with a deficient cell-mediated immune response, demonstrated by a number of features. Patients with the active disease fail to respond to parasite antigen in delayed hypersensitivity skin tests (Manson-Bahr, 1959); their lymphocytes are unresponsive in vitro to specific antigen stimulation (Sacks et al, 1987); and the ratio of circulating T helper/inducer to T suppressor/T cytotoxic cells is greatly reduced (Koech, 1987). After successful chemotherapy all of these responses are reversed and the majority of individuals develop an acquired immunity to re-infection (Napier, 1946). Therefore chemotherapy seems to influence the cell-mediated immunity of the host, possibly by reducing the parasite load to a level low enough for the immune response of the host to resolve the infection itself.

The effect of chemotherapy on the immune response of the host is an area which has received little attention. We are currently studying this using inbred mice that are naturally susceptible (Lsh^s) to L.donovani. Such mice can display 3 phenotypic patterns of infection which are H-2 linked : 'early-cure' ($H-2^{s,r}$); 'cure' ($H-2^b$); and 'non-cure', including B10.D22 and BALB/mice ($H-2^{d,q,f}$) (Blackwell et al, 1980). However, the H-2 linked influence can be circumvented by varying the parasite dose given to animals, so that mice which normally would cure become non-curing (Ulczak and Blackwell, 1983). In man, individuals could similarly have a 'curing' phenotype but because of high parasite loads become 'non curing'. These individuals would be anticipated not to relapse after chemotherapy, while 'non-curing' phenotypes would succumb to infection. This is a problem we hope to bypass by designing a drug targetting regimen which would completely eradicate parasites from all sites in the body.

CONCLUSIONS

The possibility that relapse in Kala-azar was due to chemotherapy failure was investigated in the mouse model. Infected mice were treated on days 7 and 8 post-infection with sodium stibogluconate, in the free or carrier form. On day 14 post-infection the number of parasites in the spleen, liver and bone marrow was determined. It was found that both forms of drug treatment caused a significant reduction in parasite liver burdens, but failed to affect parasites residing in the spleen and bone marrow. It is therefore proposed that relapse in visceral leishmaniasis can partly be attributed to the organ dependent antileishmanial effect of sodium stibogluconate.

ACKNOWLEDGEMENTS

This study was supported by the Medical Research Council. J. Alexander holds a Wellcome Trust Lectureship and T.F. Dolan is supported by SERC. The donations of Pentostam and the non-ionic surfactant are gratefully acknowledged.

REFERENCES

Adinolfi, L.E., Bonventre, P.F., Vander Pas, M. and Eppstein, D.A. (1985) Synergistic effect of glucantime and a liposome-encapsulated muramyl dipeptide analog in therapy of experimental visceral leishmaniasis. Infect. and Immun., 48:409.

Alving, C.R. (1986) Liposomes as drug carriers in leishmaniasis and malaria. Parasit. Today, 2:101.

Anabwani, G.M., Ngira, J.A., Dimiti, G. and Bryceson, A.D.M. (1983) Comparison of two dosage schedules of sodium stibogluconate in the treatment of visceral leishmaniasis in Kenya. Lancet, 29 July, 1983, 211.

Baillie, A.J., Florence, A.T., Hume, L.R., Muirhead, G.T. and Rogerson, A. (1985) The preparation and properties of niosomes - non-ionic surfactant vesicles. J.Pharm.Pharmacol., 37:863.

Baillie, A.J., Coombs, G.H., Dolan, T.F. and Laurie, J. (1986) Non-ionic surfactant vesicles, niosomes, as a delivery system for the anti-leishmanial drug, sodium stibogluconate. J.Pharm.Pharmacol., 38:502.

Black, C.D.V., Watson, G.J. and Ward, R.J. (1977) The use of pentostam liposomes in the chemotherapy of experimental leishmaniasis. Trans.Royal Soc.Trop.Med.Hyg., 71:550.

Blackwell, J.M., Freeman, J.C. and Bradley D.J. (1980) Influence of the H-2 complex on acquired resistance to Leishmania donovani infection in mice. Nature, 283:72.

Bradley, D.J. and Kirkley, J. (1977) Regulation of Leishmania populations within the host. 1. The variable course of Leishmania donovani infections in mice. Clin.Exp.Immunol., 30:119.

Carter, K.C., Baillie, A.J., Alexander, J. and Dolan, T.F. (1987) submitted J.Pharm.Pharmacol. The therapeutic effect of sodium stibogluconate in BALB/c mice infected with L.donovani is organ dependent.

Chulay, J.D., Bhatt, S.M., Muigai, R., Ho, M., Gochihi, G., Were, J.B., Chunge, C. and Bryceson, A.D. (1983) A comparison of three dosage regimens of sodium stibogluconate in the treatment of visceral leishmaniasis in Kenya. J.Infect.Dis., 148:148.

Koech, D.K. (1987) Subpopulations of T. lymphocytes in Kenyan patients with visceral leishmaniasis. Am.J.Trop.Med.Hyg., 36:497.

Manson-Bahr, P.E.C. (1959) East African kala-azar with special reference to the pathology, prophylaxis and treatment. Trans.Roy.Soc.Trop.Med.Hyg., 53:123.

Napier, L.E. (1946) in "The Principles and Practice of Tropical Medicine", p.134, Macmillan, New York.

Sacks, D.L., Lal, S.L., Shrivastava, S.N., Blackwell, J. and Neva, F.A. (1987) An analysis of T cell responsiveness in Indian Kala-azar. J.Immunol., 138:908.

Sanyal, R.K. and Arora, R.R. (1979) Assessment of drug therapy of Kala-azar in current epidemic in Bihar.J.Commun.Dis., 11:198.

Ulczak, O.M. and Blackwell, J.M. (1983) Immunoregulation of genetically controlled acquired response to Leishmania donovani. Infection if mice : the effects of parasite dose, cyclophosphamide and sublethal irradiation. Parasite Immunol., 5:449.

Wickramasinghe, S.N., Abdalla, S.H. and Kaisili, E.G. (1987) Ultrastructure of bone marrow in patients with visceral leishmaniasis. J.Clin.Path., 40:267.

FROM LYSOSOMES TO CELLS, FROM CELLS TO LEISHMANIA:

AMINO ACID ESTERS, POTENTIAL CHEMOTHERAPEUTIC AGENTS ?

Michel Rabinovitch

Department of Immunology
Institut Pasteur
Paris, France

INTRODUCTION

Amino acid esters are weak bases, with pKs between 7 and 8, which, in their non-protonated species, easily permeate through cell membranes. Similar to other weak bases such as methylamine or chloroquine, the esters can be trapped by protonation within the acidified milieu of lysosomes (de Duve et al., 1974). However, amino acid esters are not only trapped but also hydrolyzed by as yet uncharacterized lysosomal enzymes. Lysosomal accumulation of the more charged, and thus, less permeant amino acids, may result in osmotic swelling and disruption of the organelles (Goldman and Kaplan, 1973; Reeves, 1979). Possibly related to the lysosomal effects, certain amino acid and dipeptide esters have been shown to be selectively toxic to mammalian cells (Thiele et al., 1983; Thiele and Lipsky, 1985, 1986). This selectivity is highlighted by the prevention of murine graft versus host disease by a short exposure of the donor bone marrow cells to the dipeptide ester L-Leu-L-Leu-OMe (Charley et al., 1986; Thiele et al., 1987).

Leishmania amastigotes lodge within acidified, long lived phagolysosomes of host macrophages (reviewed in Rabinovitch, 1985). We postulated that amino acid esters accumulated in the parasitophorous vacuoles could be further concentrated in the amastigote lysosomes and might damage the parasites. We could show that certain L-amino acid esters and amides kill intracellular and isolated amastigotes of Leishmania mexicana amazonensis (Rabinovitch et al., 1986, 1987) and that several features of the parasite destruction were similar to those described for lysosomal disruption by the compounds.

Lysosomal and Cellular effects of Amino acid Esters

   Amino acid and peptide methyl esters were first shown by Goldman and her collaborators (Goldman and Kaplan, 1973; Goldman and Naider, 1974) to disrupt lysosomes in liver subcellular fractions. Damage to the organelles was assessed by loss of latency of acid phosphatase activity, release of non-sedimentable activity into the medium, and decreased turbidity of lysosomal suspensions. This pioneering report emphasized that ester hydrolysis was required for lysosome disruption and postulated that the organelles were damaged by the rapid accumulation of the relatively impermeant, osmotically active amino acid. However, direct evidence for amino acid accumulation could not be obtained. Disruptive activity was mainly associated with esters of hydrophobic amino acids (Met, Leu, Trp, Ala, Phe).

   Goldman's model received support from the work of Reeves and his collaborators. Tritiated methyl esters were used to examine the kinetics of amino acid accumulation in, and efflux from, lysosome-rich liver fractions (Reeves, 1979). The importance of lysosomal acidification was also demonstrated (Reeves and Reames, 1981). Similar studies, involving lysosome-rich fractions of leukocytes, lymphoblasts, fibroblasts and thyroid epithelial cell lines, not only permitted the discovery of a selective defect of cystine transport in cystinotic human subjects and in I cell disease fibroblasts (Steinherz et al., 1982; Gahl et al., 1982, 1983; Jonas et al.,, 1982; Pisoni et al., 1985, 1986; Tietze et al., 1986), but led to the characterization of several carrier-mediated transport systems in lysosomal membranes (Bernar et al., 1986; Pisoni et al., 1987). It could also be shown that amino acids accumulated in lysosomal fractions prepared from cells preincubated with labeled esters (Gahl et al., 1982; Ransom and Reeves, 1983). As an example, over 70% of the counts taken up by rat polymorphonuclear leukocytes incubated with tritiated Leu-OMe were associated with a granule-rich fraction, and codistributed with the lysosome-like azurophilic granules (Ransom and Reeves, 1983).

   Evidence that amino acid esters can damage lysosomes of living cells was first given by Reeves et al. (1981) in experiments in which rat hearts were perfused with medium containing high (10 mM) concentrations of Leu-OMe. Although the hearts continued to beat normally, they displayed ultrastuctural and biochemical evidence of lysosomal damage.

   Thiele and his associates reported that in vitro exposure of human blood mononuclear cells to certain amino acid esters resulted in selective destruction or functional inactivation of monocytes, NK cells and certain subpopulations of cytotoxic lymphocytes (Thiele et al., 1983; Thiele and Lipsky, 1985 a,b, and 1986; Charley et al., 1986; Tiele et al., 1987). Interestingly, macrophages derived from explanted monocytes were much more resistant to the compound. Sensitivity of NK cells depended upon the generation by monocytes or neutrophils present in the cell population, of low concentrations of a more toxic dipeptide ester, Leu-Leu-OMe (Thiele and Lipsky, 1985 a,b). NK function of lymphocyte populations depleted of monocytes, was only reversibly inhibited by 50 mM Leu-OMe, an inhibition probably due to lysosomal alkalinization. Although the functional assay used for NK cells did not yield precise ED50 values, detailed studies involving a series of dipeptide esters emphasized the requirement of non-polar amino acids such as Leu, Phe, or Val for irreversible inactivation of NK cells (Thiele and Lipsky, 1985 b).

In contrast to irreversible cell damage induced by rather low concentrations of Leu-OMe or dipeptide esters, other cell types, although they accumulated amino acids in lysosomes (as indicated by cytoplasmic vacuolization), survived exposure to distinctly higher concentrations of the compounds. These cells include macrophages, fibroblasts, epithelial cells such as Hela (Rabinovitch and F. Darcy, unpublished), myocytes, endothelial cells and several lymphoid cell lines (Thiele and Lipsky, 1986). It is not known whether the differences in cellular sensitivity to the esters are related to relative abundance of lysosomes, extent of acidification of the organelles, relative abundance and specificity of lysosomal enzymes, numbers and kind of amino acid transporters on lysosomal membranes (Bernar et al., 1986), relative lysosomal fragility or consequences of the leakage of lysosomal contents in the cytosol. One or more of these parameters may account for the sensitivity of _Leishmania_ amastigotes to the amino acid derivatives.

MATERIALS AND METHODS

Amino acid esters and amides were purchased from Sigma Chemical Co., St. Louis, MO and from Bachem Feinchemikalien, Budendorf, Switzerland. _Leishmania mexicana amazonensis_ LV 79 (Chance et al.,, 1974) was given to us by Dr. J.P. Dedet in 1980 and maintained by amastigote transfers in hamsters and Balb/C mice. Isolation of amastigotes from mouse lesions, preparation and infection of murine macrophage cultures, treatment of infected macrophages and of isolated amastigotes by amino acid esters or other compounds, were as previously described (Rabinovitch et al., 1986; Alfieri et al., 1987). In most experiments, 80% or more of the macrophages were infected by one or more amastigotes. Toxicity of the compounds to intracellular parasites was assessed by scoring microscopically the percent of macrophages containing one of more amastigotes. Viability of isolated amastigotes was estimated by the tetrazolium MTT reduction assay (Mosmann, 1983). Recently, solubilization of the formazan with dimethylsulfoxide (Carmichael et al., 1987) was found to increase the sensitivity and speed of the technique. ED50 (concentrations for half maximal killing) were estimated from plots of % optical density against concentration (Rabinovitch et al., 1987). Labeled amino acid esters were prepared by esterification of tritiated amino acids with methanol-acetyl chloride (Reeves and Reames, 1981; Steinherz et al., 1982) and ester purity was assessed by thin layer chromatography. Parasites were incubated with labeled esters and either washed on glass fiber filters on a cell harvester, or rapidly centrifuged through an oil cushion. Total radioactivity as well as radioactivity associated with free amino acid and with the ester form were determined (Ramazeilles and Rabinovitch, in preparation).

RESULTS

Amino acid and Dipeptide ester Specificities of Amastigote Destruction

For both intracellular and isolated amastigotes, the most active of the methyl esters assayed was that of Leu, followed by those of Trp, Met, Glu (dimethyl ester), Phe and Tyr (Rabinovitch et al., 1986, 1987). The ED50 for isolated amastigotes ranged from about 0.6 mM for Leu-OMe to 3.8 mM for Tyr-OMe. A one hour pulse with 1 mM Leu-OMe cured more than 90% of heavily infected macrophages or killed more than 90% of isolated amastigotes. In the experiments with infected macrophages the pulse was followed by a 18 h chase to allow digestion of the damaged parasites ; this made scoring of infected and non-infected cells easier. In both instances, the methyl esters of Ile, Val, Ala, Gly, Ser, His and Pro were inactive at concentrations of 5 or 10 mM. This specificity is compatible with substrate recognition by one or more parasite enzymes. As in previous studies with lysosomes (Goldman and Kaplan, 1973), esters of D-amino acids were not leishmanicidal. Benzyl esters, such as Leu-OBzl (ED50 for isolated amastigotes, 0.07 mM) showed much greater activity than their methyl homologs. Indeed, the benzyl esters of Val, Ile or Gly, were quite active (ED50 of 0.2, 0.22, and 0.9 mM respectively), contrasting with the inactivity of the methyl esters of the same amino acids. As expected from the work of Thiele and collaborators (1985 b), the dipeptide Leu-Leu-OMe was more active than Leu-OMe on infected macrophages and isolated parasites (ED50 = 0.094 mM). In addition, Ile-Ile-OMe (prepared by Odile Siffert, Institut Pasteur) displayed substantial activity (ED50 = 0.23 mM, contrasting with the inactivity of Ile-OMe (Rabinovitch et al., 1986 and unpublished).

Destruction of amastigotes by Amino acid Amides

There is at present no information on the enzymes involved in the toxicity of amino acid esters for the amastigotes. Because several proteinases can cleave both amino acid esters and amides (Knight, 1977), we compared the leishmanicidal activity of a series of amino acid amides with that of the methyl esters (Rabinovitch and Zilberfarb, submitted). The amides were generally less active than the esters and several were more toxic to macrophages, as determined by inspection of Giemsa stained preparations. Ranks of activity of the amides on isolated amastigotes were Trp (ED50 = 1.0 mM) > Leu > Phe > Met > Tyr. The amides of Ala, Gly, Val, Ile, His and D-Leu were inactive. This pattern of activity is similar to that of amino acid esters and is compatible with the hypothesis that the same enzymes recognize the two series of compounds. Tryptophanamide was the most interesting compound for studies with infected macrophages, with an ED50 of 2.3 mM and an ED95 of 3.0 mM. Maximal activity required 18 h incubation, contrasting with the far more rapid parasite killing by Leu-OMe and Trp-OMe.

Intracellular amastigotes derived from promastigotes are less sensitive to Leu-OMe

In the course of studies in which macrophages were infected with promastigotes (PM), Liège Quintào found that, for at least 5 days after infection, amastigotes derived from culture PM were less sensitive to Leu-OMe than lesion-derived amastigotes (Quintao and Rabinovitch, in preparation). In a typical experiment, only 60% of macrophages infected with PM were cured by 4.0 mM Leu-Ome, while those infected with lesion amastigotes, were nearly fully cured by 1 mM of the ester. Sensitivity to tryptophanamide was similar in both cases. This observation suggests that sensitivity to amino acid esters may be a useful parameter in the study of amastigote maturation.

Involvement of an Acidified Compartment

In agreement with the work on lysosomes discussed in the previous section, agents which raise the pH within lysosomes (NH4Cl, methylamine or monensin), reduced the killing of isolated amastigotes by Leu-OMe (Rabinovitch et al., 1987). The increase in ED50 was, however, smaller than expected on the basis of work with other cells (e.g., from 0.6 mM in controls to 1.0 mM in parasites treated with 20 mM NH4Cl). Clearly, information is needed on the cytosolic and "lysosomal" pH in amastigotes.

Toxicity of Leu-OMe for Intracellular and Isolated Amastigotes is reduced by certain Esters

A series of amino acid esters, some of which were leishmanicidal by themselves, protected amastigotes against challenge with 1 mM Leu-OMe (Alfieri et al., 1987). Significant protection was obtained with 0.5 mM or less of Tyr-OMe, Gly-OBzl, Ile-OMe or Met-OMe. Other esters were only weakly protective (e.g. Ala-OMe, Gly-OMe, D-Leu-OMe) or inactive (His-OMe, Phe-OMe, Trp-OMe) at several fold higher concentrations. In other experiments it was found that neither Ile-OMe nor several other esters assayed protected amastigotes against killing by Trp-OMe. The findings that

Trp-OMe did not inhibit the killing by Leu-OMe, suggest that Trp-OMe and Leu-OMe are hydrolysed by different enzymes or within different parasite compartments.

We postulated that the protective activities were mediated by inhibition of the enzyme(s) which hydrolyse Leu-OMe. However, we have not excluded the possibility that at higher concentrations, protective esters, similar to ammonia, may raise the pH in the relevant parasite compartments. Experiments involving incubation of amastigotes with tritiated Leu-OMe, to be discussed below, give additional support for the enzyme inhibition theory. In these experiments, as little as 0.1 mM Ile-OMe inhibited the accumulation of 3H-Leu in the amastigotes (Ramazeilles and Rabinovitch, in preparation).

Antipain and Chymostatin Protect Amastigotes form Leu-OMe Toxicity

We have found that the protease inhibitors antipain and chymostatin can protect both intracellular and isolated amastigotes from destruction by Leu-OMe and several other esters (Alfieri et al., 1987; Alfieri, Ramazeilles, Zilberfarb and Rabinovitch, in preparation). Protection of intracellular parasites required at least six hours incubation of infected macrophages with the inhibitors (20-100 μg/ml), suggesting that the peptides have to be pinocytized by the macrophages before thay can reach the parasites. In contrast, protection of isolated amastigotes, required shorter incubation periods. Indeed, as little as 0.2 μg/ml of chymostatin could confer 80% protection.

Studies with Tritiated Esters

Among the factors involved in the leishmanicidal activity of the esters, two, ester uptake and hydrolysis, can be measured with intact parasites incubated with tritiated esters. Hydrolysis is reflected by accumulation of labeled amino acid, conveniently determined by trapping the parasites on glass fiber filters. Direct estimation of ester content by the same procedure is possibly vitiated by preferential loss of the ester species upon washing of the parasites. An oil cushion procedure was developed by Claude Ramazeilles to eliminate the need to wash the parasites. The results suggest that a mechanism similar to that involved in lysosomal disruption operates in the killing of parasites. Indeed, leishmanicidal esters such as Leu-OMe, Trp-OMe or Met-OMe were hydrolysed at much higher rates that non-leishmanicidal compounds such as Ile-OMe or Ala-OMe. Furthermore, hydrolysis of the ester and accumulation of tritiated amino acid were inhibited in amastigotes preincubated with methylamine or ammonium chloride, with Ile-OMe and some other esters, or with antipain (Ramazeilles and Rabinovitch, in preparation).

QUESTIONS AND PROSPECTS

1) **Parasite targets involved in the toxic effects of the esters**

a) **Target organelles.** By analogy with the effects of the compounds on lysosomes and mammalian cells, it is probable that amino acid esters accumulate in "lysosome-like" acidified parasite organelles. The nature of these organelles needs to be clarified. Leishmania mexicana amastigotes contain high activity of several lysosomal enzyme markers. It has been proposed that these enzymes are concentrated in bodies termed "megasomes", previously, defined ultrastructurally by Alexander and Vickerman in 1975 (Pupkis et al., 1986; Coombs et al., 1986). The function of these organelles is as yet unknown. Their rather uniform structure and their lack of accumulation of horseradish peroxidase given to the amastigotes (Jean Claude Antoine, personal communication), suggest that megasomes in lesion amastigotes do not primarily participate in autophagy or in degradation of exogenous macromolecules. It is thus possible that the biological properties of megasomes may differ from those of conventional secondary lysosomes. It should be noted that there is no information on cytosolic pH in amastigotes, which, themselves lodge in acidified phagolysosomes. Were the cytosolic pH in the acid range, the possibility that ester hydrolysis and amino acid accumulation take place in the cytosol cannot be excluded. Ultimately, identification of the primary cellular target(s) within amastigotes will have to rely on combined ultrastuctural, cell fractionation, and biochemical approaches.

b) **Target enzymes.** A second question has to do with the nature of the enzymes which hydrolyse leishmanicidal amino acid derivatives. The term "target" is here loosely employed, leishmanicidal activity may not depend on inhibition or inactivation of parasite enzymes. The report by Jadot et al. (1984) that glycyl-L-phenylalanine 2-naphthylamide, a cathepsin C substrate, disrupts isolated liver lysosomes, suggests that the involvement of the cathepsin in the destruction of Leishmania should be considered. While it is probable that peptide hydrolases are involved in the effects of the esters, it has been shown that purified liver carboxyl esterases can also hydrolyze amino acid esters (Kirsch, 1963; Levy and Ocken, 1969). It is expected that the protection conferred by certain esters, and by the protease inhibitors antipain and chymostatin, against damage of amastigotes by Leu-OMe, may provide "fingerprints" useful in the characterization and isolation of the relevant enzymes. The task ahead is made difficult by the lack of cell fractionation procedures applicable to Leishmania amastigotes. It would be of obvious importance to obtain cytosolic and granular or vacuolar amastigote fractions. Indeed, it is probable, that the enzyme(s) involved in parasite killing by the esters, may represent a minor fraction of the enzyme(s) present in total amastigote extracts.

c) <u>Structure-activity correlations and mechanisms involved in parasite killing</u>. Structure-activity studies may not only lead to more active compounds, but may help understand the mechanisms which underlie toxicity to the parasites. It has been assumed that lysosome disruption reflects osmotic lysis. The fact, however, that damage to lysosomes, NK cells and <u>Leishmania</u> is best induced by esters of hydrophobic amino acids (e.g. Leu, Trp, Met, Phe), indicates that additional mechanisms are involved in the toxicity of the compounds. Dr. Raymond Firestone suggested to us that hydrophobic amino acids and peptides could have a detergent like activity on lysosomal membranes (Miller et al., 1983; Wilson et al., 1987). In addition, as shown by Thiele and Lipsky for NK cells and by us in <u>Leishmania</u>, dipeptide esters are far more active than single amino acid esters. It will be important to examine the hydrolysis of dipeptides in relation to their toxicity. For instance, is hydrolysis of the peptide bond in Leu-Leu-OMe required for toxicity ? Conversely, is Leu-Leu the toxic product ? If the latter is the case, a molecular modification that blocks enzyme hydrolysis (e.g. reduction of the peptide bond), could potentiate the activity.

d) <u>Leishmania species differences</u>. The work discussed here was performed with <u>Leishmania mexicana amazonensis</u>. Preliminary information has shown that <u>Leishmania major</u> amastigotes are slightly less, and <u>Leishmania donovani</u>, much less sensitive to Leu-OMe. However, the sensitivity of <u>L. mexicana</u> and <u>L. donovani</u> to Trp-NH2 was similar.

2) <u>Sensitivity of host cells</u>

There is evidence that amino acid esters accumulate in and are hydrolysed in the lysosomes of several cell types. While it is probable that toxicity of the compounds to mammalian cells is a consequence of lysosomal damage, the involvement of other organelles cannot be excluded. As in the case of <u>Leishmania</u>, there is no information on the nature of the enzymes involved in ester toxicity. Characterization and purification of the enzymes would allow studies of their substrate specificity and detailed cellular distribution. As mentioned, amino acid esters are particularly toxic to certain cell types such as monocytes, NK cells and certain cytotoxic T cells but the reasons for the differences in sensitivity are not apparent.

3) <u>Prospects for chemotherapy</u>

Clarification of the basic mechanisms involved in leishmanicidal activity as well as in the toxicity to host cells, and delineation of structure-activity correlates may permit the design of more selectively parasiticidal molecules. We have assumed that recognition by "specific" parasite enzymes plays a critical role in the leishmanicidal activity. Amastigotes are killed by certain substrates. Will it be possible to find substrates more specific for parasite enzymes (cf Jadot et al. 1984) ? Are there exploitable differences between lysosomes of mammalian cells and those of Leishmania ? A pessimistic view would be that lysosomal enzymes are or should be well conserved in eukaryotic cells. A recent statement, which only applies to a family of extracellular serine proteases, allows us a measure of cautious optimism; "The catalytic domains of the proteases are clearly homologous to each other, as well as to other chymotrypsin-family enzymes, but the substrate specificities of the enzymes are very different and the multiple noncatalytic domains confer different regulatory properties upon these enzymes" (Bond and Butler, 1987).

There is limited information on the toxicity to laboratory animals of amino acid or dipeptide esters injected systemically or locally. That certain esters can reach target organs has been shown in mice injected with glutathione dimethyl or diethyl esters. Liver and kidney glutathione contents in these animals were significantly increased (Puri and Meister, 1983). This is, of course, particularly relevant to systemic administration. It is possible, however, that toxicity of the esters to monocytes and to macrophages would be a desirable feature for local administration of the compounds. Indeed, survival of extracellular parasites is very short, and inhibition of monocyte recruitment leads to the rapid disappearance of viable parasites injected subcutaneously in susceptible mice (Sergio Mendonça, personal communication).

Acknowledgements

This work was supported by INSERM, CNRS, Institut Pasteur, the Rockfeller Foundation, CNPq (Brasil), and the UNDP/World Bank/WHO Special Programme for Research and Training in Tropical Diseases.

The studies reviewed here were performed in collaboration with Silvia C. Alfieri, Jean-Claude Antoine, Claude Ramazeilles, Antoinette Ryter, Liège Galvao Quintao and Vladimir Zilberfarb, all from Institut Pasteur.

REFERENCES

Alfieri, S.C., Zilberfarb, V., and Rabinovitch, M., 1987, Destruction of Leishmania mexicana amazonensis amastigotes by leucine methyl ester: protection by other amino acid esters. Parasitology 95: 31-41.
Alfieri, S.C., Zilberfarb, V., and Rabinovitch, M., 1987, Protease inhibitors protect Leishmania mexicana amastigotes from killing by leucine methyl ester. Abst. Am. Soc. Cell.

Biol., Annual Meeting, November 1987.

Bernar, J., Tietze, F., Kohn, L.D., Bernardini, I., Harper, G.S., Grollman, E.F., and Gahl, W.A., 1986, Characteristics of a lysosomal membrane transport system for tyrosine and other neutral amino acids in rat thyroid cells. J. Biol. Chem. 261: 17107-17112.

Bond, J.S., and Butler, P.E., 1987, Intracellular proteases. Ann. Rev. Physiol. 56: 333-364.

Carmichael, J., Degraff, W.G., Gazdar, A.F., Minna, J.D., and Mitchell, J.B., 1987, Evaluation of a tetrazolium-based semiautomated colorimetric assay: assessment of chemosensitivity testing. Cancer Res. 47: 936-942.

Chance, M.L., Peters, W., and Shchory, L., 1974, Biochemical taxonomy of Leishmania. I: Observations on DNA. Ann. Trop. Med. Parasitol. 68: 307-316.

Charley, M., Thiele, D.L., and Lipsky, P.E., 1986, Prevention of lethal murine graft versus host disease by treatment of donor cells with L-Leucyl-L-Leucine methyl ester. J. Clin. Invest. 78: 1415-1420.

Coombs, G.H., Tetley, L., Moss, V.A., and Vickerman, K., 1986, Three dimensional structure of the Leishmania amastigote as revealed by computer-aided reconstruction from serial sectiuons. Parasitology 92: 13-23.

de Duve, C., de Barsy, T., Poole, B., Trouet, A., Tulkens, P., and Van Hoof, F., 1974, Lysosomotropic agents. Biochem. Pharmacol. 23: 2495-2531.

Gahl, W.A., Tietze, F., Bashan, N., Steinherz, R., and Schulman, J.D., 1982, Defective cystine exodus from isolated lysosome-rich fractions from cystinotic leucocytes. J. Biol. Chem. 257: 9570-9575.

Gahl, W.A., Tietze, F., Bashan, N., Bernardini, I., Raiford, D., and Schulman, J.D., 1983, Characteristics of cystine counter-transport in normal and cystinotic lysosome-rich granular fractions. Biochem. J. 216: 393-400.

Goldman, R., and Kaplan, A., 1973, Rupture of rat liver lysosomes mediated by L-amino acid esters. Biochim. Biophys. Acta 318: 205-216.

Goldman, R., and Naider, F., 1974, Permeation and stereospecificity of hydrolysis of peptide esters within intact lysosomes in vitro. Biochim. Biophys. Acta 338: 224-233.

Jadot, M., Colmant, C., Wattiaux-de Coninck, S., and Wattiaux, R., 1984, Intralysosomal hydrolysis of glycyl-L-phenylalanine 2-naphthylamide. Biochem. J. 219: 965-970.

Jonas, A.J., Smith, M.L., and Schneider, J.A., 1982, ATP-dependent lysosomal cystine efflux is defective in cystinosis. J. Biol. Chem. 257: 13185-13188.

Knight, C.G., 1977, Principles of the design and use of synthetic substrates and inhibitors of tissue proteinases. In Proteinases in mammalian cells and tissues, Ed. A.J., Barrett.

Krisch, K., 1963, Isolierung einer Esterase aus Schweinelebermikrosomen. Biochem. Z. 337: 531545.

Levy, M., and Ocken, P.R., 1969, Purification and properties of pig liver esterase. Arch. Biochem. Biophys. 135: 259-264.

Miller, D.K., Griffiths, E., Lenard, J., and Firestone, R.A., 1983, Cell killing by lysosomotropic detergents. J. Cell. Biol. 97: 1841-1851.

Mosmann, T., 1983, Rapid colorimetric assay for cellular growth and survival: application to proliferation and cytotoxicity assays. J. Immunol. Meth. 65: 55-63.

Pisoni, R.L., Thoene, J.G., and Christensen, H.N., 1985, Detection and characterization of carrrier-mediated cationic amino acid transport in lysosomes of normal and cystinotic human fibroblasts. J. Biol. Chem. 260: 4791-4798.

Pisoni, R.L., Flickinger, K.S., Thoene, J.G., and Christensen, H.N., 1987, Characterization of carrier-mediated transport systems for small neutral amino acids in human fibroblast lysosomes. J. Biol. Chem. 262: 6010-6017.

Pupkis, M.F., Tetley, L., and Coombs, G.H., 1986, Leishmania mexicana: Amastigote hydrolases in unusual lysosomes. Exp. Parasitol. 62: 29-39.

Puri R.N., and Meister, A., 1983, Transport of glutathione, as gamma-glutamylcysteinylglycyl ester, into liver and kidney. Proc. Natl. Acad. Sci. USA 80: 5258-5260.

Rabinovitch, M., 1985, The endocytic system of Leishmania-infected macrophages, in "Mononuclear phagocytes. Characteristics, Physiology and Function". Ralph van Furth, ed. Martinus Nijhoff Publishers, Dordrecht, pp. 611-619.

Rabinovitch, M., Zilberfarb, V., and Ramazeilles, 1986, Destruction of Leishmania mexicana amazonensis amastigotes within macrophages by lysosomotropic amino acid esters. J. Exp. Med. 163: 520-535.

Rabinovitch, M., Zilberfarb, V., and Pouchelet, M., 1987, Leishmania mexicana: Destruction of isolated amastigotes by amino acid esters. Am. J. Trop. med. Hyg. 36: 288-293.

Ransom, J.T., and Reeves, J.P., 1983, Accumulation of amino acids within intracellular lysosomes of rat polymorphonuclear leukocytes incubated with amino acid methyl esters. J. Biol. Chem. 258: 9270-9275.

Reeves, J.P., 1979, Accumulation of amino acids by lysosomes incubated with amino acid methyl esters. J. Biol. Chem. 254: 8914-8921.

Reeves, J.P., Decker, R.S., Crie, J.S., and Wildenthal, K., 1981, Intracellular disruption of rat heart lysosomes by leucine methyl ester: effects on protein degradation. Proc. Natl. Acad. Sci., USA 78: 4426-4429.

Reeves, J.P., and Reames, T., 1981, ATP stimulates amino acid accumulation by lysosomes incubated with amino acid methyl esters. J. Biol. Chem. 256: 6047-6053.

Steinherz, R., Tietze, F., Raiford, D., Gahl, W., and Schulman, J.D., 1982, Patterns of amino acid efflux from isolated normal and cystinotic human leucocyte lysosomes. J. Biol. Chem. 257: 6041-6049.

Thiele, D.L., Kurosaka, M., and Lipsky, P.E., 1983, Phenotype of the accessory cell necessary for mitogen-stimulated T and B cell responses in human peripheral blood: delineation by its sensitivity to the lysosomotropic agent, L-Leucine methyl ester. J. Immunol. 131: 2282-2290.

Thiele, D.L., and Lipsky, P.E., 1985 a, Modulation of human natural killer cell function by L-Leucine methyl ester: monocyte-dependent depletion from human peripheral blood mononuclear cells. J. Immunol. 134: 786-793.

Thiele, D.L., and Lipsky, P.E., 1985 b, Regulation of cellular function by products of lysosomal enzyme activity: elimination of human natural killer cells by a dipeptide methyl ester generated from L-Leucine methyl ester by monocytes or mononuclear leukocytes. Proc. Natl. Acad. Sci. USA 82: 2468-2472.

Thiele, D.L., and Lipsky, P.E., 1986, The immunosuppressive activity of L-Leucyl-L-Leucine methyl ester: selective ablation of cytotoxic lymphocytes and monocytes. J. Immunol. 136: 1038-1048.

Thiele, D.L., Charley, M.R., Calomeni, J.A., and Lipsky, P.E., 1987, Lethal graft-vs-host disease accross major histocompatiblity barriers: requirement for leucyl-leucine methyl ester sensitive cytotoxic cells. J. Immunol. 138: 51-57.

Tietze, F., Rome, L.H., Butler, J.DB., Harper, G.S., and Gahl, W., 1986, Impaired clearance of free cystine from lysosome-enriched granular fractions of I-cell disease fibroblasts. Biochem. J. 237: 9-15.

Wilson, P.D., Firestone, R.A., and Lenard, J., 1987, The role of lysosomal enzymes in killing of mammalian cells by the lysosomotropic detergent N-dodecylimidazole. J. Cell. Biol. 104: 1223-1229.

ANTILEISHMANIAL ACTIVITY OF L-LEUCINE METHYL ESTER AND L-TRYPTOPHANAMIDE

C.A. Hunter, L.M. Macpherson and G.H. Coombs

Department of Zoology
University of Glasgow
Glasgow G12 8QQ, Scotland, U.K.

INTRODUCTION

Rabinovitch and his colleagues have reported that amino acid esters are toxic to Leishmania mexicana amazonensis amastigotes, both when they are residing in macrophages[1] and after isolation[2]. The mechanism underlying this effect is not fully understood, although it is known that the esters are lysosomotropic[3] and it has been suggested that the accumulation in the parasitophorous vacuole or the parasite's lysosomes of free amino acids, resulting from enzymatic hydrolysis of the ester, could lead to osmotic lysis of the cell. The specificity of the compounds towards the parasite, together with the way in which other amino acid esters prevent the killing of amastigotes by L-leucine methyl ester[4], suggest that the activation by hydrolysis of the esters occurs within the amastigote itself. It is likely that this takes place in the unusual lysosome-like organelles present, which have been given the name 'megasomes'[5]. These findings not only provide an interesting lead in the search for new antileishmanial agents but also show that these and related compounds could be useful tools in the study of leishmania parasites and their interaction with the host macrophage.

Our investigations were undertaken in collaboration with Rabinovitch and his colleagues with the aim of extending our knowledge of the antileishmanial action of amino acid esters, the activities of related compounds such as amides which could be activated in a similar manner, and in particular the way in which these amino acid derivatives are metabolised in the leishmania-infected macrophage. It was hoped that the information gained would help us to design compounds with better antiparasite activity. We report here on the comparative activities of one amino acid ester (L-leucine methyl ester, Leu-OMe) and one amino acid amide (L-tryptophanamide) against amastigotes and promastigotes of L. m. mexicana, L. donovani and L. major. The results confirm that L-leucine methyl ester is not equally active against all species and that there is a correlation between the presence of megasomes and susceptibility to the compound.

MATERIALS AND METHODS

Parasites

Promastigotes and amastigotes of L. mexicana mexicana (MNYC/BZ/62/M379), L. major (MHOM/SA/83/RKK2) and L. donovani (MHOM/ET/67/L82) were obtained as described previously[5,6].

Determination of antileishmanial activities of L-leucine methyl ester and L-tryptophanamide

Effects on promastigote growth. Promastigotes were inoculated into HOMEM medium[5], containing 10% (v/v) heat inactivated foetal calf serum, antibacterials and appropriate concentrations of L-leucine methyl ester (Leu-OMe) or L-tryptophanamide HCl, to give an initial parasite density of 5×10^5 ml^{-1}. Incubation was at 25°C under air. Parasite density was determined daily for 8 days, using an improved Neubauer haemocytometer.

Effects on parasite viability, assessed using the tetrazolium salt MTT. The effects of the compounds on the viability of isolated amastigotes and cultured promastigotes were measured using a procedure based upon the metabolism of a tetrazolium salt (MTT) by living cells[7]. Parasites were suspended at approximately 1×10^8 ml^{-1} (amastigotes) or 2×10^7 ml^{-1} (promastigotes) and exposed to the drugs for 1 hour at 37°C (L. donovani amastigotes), 35°C (L. mexicana mexicana amastigotes) or 25°C (promastigotes). The parasites were then washed free from the drug and incubated with MTT at 450 µg ml^{-1} for 3 hours at the appropriate temperature. The formazan product produced by the parasites reducing the MTT was quantified by dissolving it in acid (0.04M HCl) isopropanol and measuring the absorbance at 570 nm. The results are expressed as the reduction of MTT by the treated parasites as a percentage of that by untreated parasites.

Effects on leishmania survival in macrophages. Mouse peritoneal exudate cells (PECs) were obtained from male Balb/c mice and the population pooled. The cells were dispensed into 8-well glass tissue culture slides (Labtek) at a density of 10^5 cells well^{-1} and incubated at 37°C for 24 hours to allow the cells to adhere. Non-adherent cells were then removed and the attached cells exposed for 24 hours to either L. m. mexicana (amastigotes or stationary-phase promastigotes) at 33°C, L. major (amastigotes) at 33°C or L. donovani (amastigotes) at 37°C, using parasite to PECs ratios of between 3/1 and 5/1. Free parasites were then removed by washing and the infected macrophages incubated with drug as indicated in the individual experiments. At the termination of the experiments, cells were fixed with methanol, stained with Giemsa's stain and the number of infected macrophages determined.

Effects on leishmanias in mice. Attempts to detect activity of Leu-OMe against L. donovani in Balb/c mice were made using the methods described previously[8]. This involved administration of drug (1 mg mouse^{-1}) intravenously on days 7 and 8 post-infection and determining the parasite burden in the liver on day 14. Similar experiments were carried out using L. mexicana mexicana, with the drug (2 mg mouse^{-1}) being given subcutaneously on days 7-11 post-infection. Again the parasite burden in the liver was assessed. The susceptibility of L. m. mexicana growing subcutaneously in CBA mice was also determined, the Leu-OMe being given subcutaneously at 5 mg mouse^{-1} on days 7-11 post-infection.

RESULTS

Leu-OMe and L-tryptophanamide both inhibited, at least partially, the growth of promastigotes of all three species. With Leu-OMe the effect was transient, even when the compound was present initially at 10 mM. With L-tryptophanamide at 10 mM, many promastigotes were killed during the first 24 hours and there was no subsequent cell multiplication, although the parasites were not all killed.

Amastigotes and promastigotes of L. m. mexicana and L. donovani were all affected by Leu-OMe, as measured by their reduction of MTT (Figure 1). The amastigotes of L. m. mexicana, however, were apparently the most susceptible to the compound. Exposure of the parasites to L-tryptophanamide also resulted in diminished MTT reduction. With this compound, however, both forms of the two species were affected similarly and significant effects were observed only when concentrations were 5 mM or more.

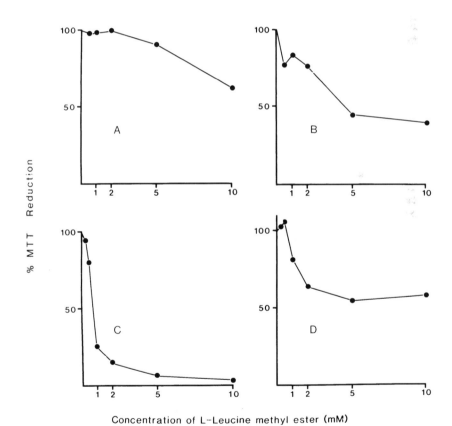

Figure 1. The effect of Leu-OMe on free leishmanias. The viability of the parasites was determined using the method involving the reduction of MTT, as described in the Methods section. Key: A, C, L. mexicana mexicana; B, D, L. donovani; A, B, promastigotes; C, D, amastigotes.

Experiments were performed to determine the sensitivities to Leu-OMe of the three species when residing in macrophages in vitro. PECs were infected by exposure to amastigotes and subsequently treated (24 hours post-infection or later) for 1 hour with 2 mM Leu-OMe. It was found that L. major and L. donovani were unaffected, whereas with L. mexicana mexicana there was a 99% reduction in parasite load whenever the treatment was given. Macrophages infected with L. m. mexicana by exposure to stationary-phase promastigotes responded differently; their susceptibility to 2 mM Leu-OMe increased over the first five days post-infection (Figure 2). Only after this period were they fully susceptible. The effect of Leu-OMe was greater with longer treatments. For instance, exposure of macrophages infected with L. m. mexicana promastigotes to 2 mM Leu-OMe for 1 hour or 24 hours, starting 24 hours post-infection, resulted in reductions in parasite load of 40% and 80%, respectively.

The antileishmanial activity of L-tryptophanamide differed from that of Leu-OMe. Species or stage specificity was not observed, L. donovani and L. m. mexicana being equally susceptible (Figure 3). Again, however, exposure time was important. When L. donovani-infected macrophages were treated with 2 mM L-tryphophanamide for 1, 2 or 24 hours, starting 24 hours post-infection and with the cultures being terminated 48 hours post-infection, there was a reduction in the number of infected macrophages of 0, 33% and 93%, respectively. Similar results were obtained with L. m. mexicana, although this parasite was a little less susceptible.

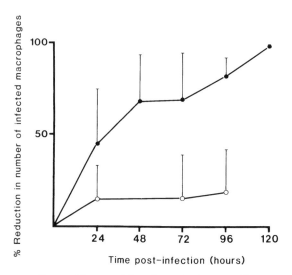

Figure 2. The effect of Leu-OMe on L. mexicana mexicana in PECs. PECs were infected by exposure to stationary-phase promastigotes. Infected PECs were exposed to the ester, at the appropriate concentration, for 1 hour at the times post-infection indicated. Cultures were terminated 6 days post-infection. Key: O, 1 mM; ●, 2 mM.

Both Leu-OMe and L-tryptophanamide exhibited some toxicity towards macrophages. All macrophages were killed by exposure for 24 hours to L-tryptophanamide at 10 mM, whereas some toxicity was observed with drug at 5 mM but none when it was at 2 mM. Leu-OMe at 3 mM caused some adverse effects to macrophages exposed for several days.

Administration of Leu-OMe, using the regimens described, to mice infected with L. donovani or L. m. mexicana had no detectable effect on the course of infection.

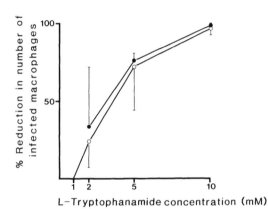

Figure 3. The effects of different concentrations of L-tryptophanamide on intracellular leishmanias. PECs were infected by exposure to L. m. mexicana promastigotes or L. donovani amastigotes and, after removal of free parasites by washing, exposed to the drug at the appropriate concentration for 2 hours. The cultures were terminated 2-3 days post-infection. Key: O, L. m. mexicana; ●, L. donovani.

DISCUSSION

The results presented on the activity of Leu-OMe against L. m. mexicana amastigotes, both free and residing in PECs, are very similar to those of Rabinovitch and his co-workers for L. m. amazonensis[1,2,4]. We modified the viability assay using MTT such that the parasites are incubated with MTT for only three hours; the shorter incubation avoids possible interference from other microorganisms and complications produced by promastigotes dividing. Nevertheless, the results we obtained resemble those of Rabinovitch et al. closely.

The inclusion in these studies of not only promastigotes but also other species has given a deeper insight into how Leu-OMe exerts its antileishmanial effect. We have confirmed that it acts against the parasite directly, but the findings that L. major and L. donovani when residing in PECs are unaffected by Leu-OMe whereas L. mexicana mexicana is highly susceptible, and that this susceptibility appears only slowly after infection of PECs with promastigotes, are perhaps the most crucial. We have reported previously[5] that L. m. mexicana and L. m. amazonensis differ from L. major and L. donovani in that the amastigotes of the former two possess unusual lysosome-like organelles ('megasomes'). These organelles appear to be absent from promastigotes (mid-log stage and metacyclic). Thus there is an apparent correlation between the presence of megasomes and high susceptibility to Leu-OMe. Most intriguingly, we have found that megasomes appear in intracellular parasites, derived from promastigotes of L. mexicana mexicana, only after a few days[9]; similar to the time scale on which susceptibility to Leu-OMe increases. Thus it is proposed that the high susceptibility of L. m. mexicana amastigotes to Leu-OMe is due to the presence of large numbers of megasomes within the amastigote, and that the ester is hydrolysed by an enzyme in this organelle leading to the accumulation of the released amino acid and consequently osmotic lysis of the parasite.

The spectrum of antileishmanial activity of L-tryptophanamide differs markedly from that of Leu-OMe. The results suggest that although the amino acid ester and amino acid amide may exert their antileishmanial activities in a similar manner, involving hydrolysis to the amino acid which causes osmotic stress, they are, as expected, activated by different enzymes. It is probable that the activation process is the key to specificity and likely that compounds activated by enzymes abundant in megasomes of leishmanias will have a reasonable specificity towards this group of parasites. Leu-OMe appears to fall into this category, although neither of the amino acid analogues used in this study seems likely to be a useful antileishmanial drug by itself. It is hoped, however, that further study of how they act, and especially characterisation of the enzymes involved, will provide the information required for the design of more potent and specific antileishmanials. We aim to design compounds that will be activated only by leishmanias; these should be excellent antileishmanial agents. Characterisation of amastigote hydrolases will be an invaluable aid in this approach to providing new antileishmanial drugs.

CONCLUSIONS

Both Leu-OMe and L-tryptophanamide were shown to possess antileishmanial activity against free amastigotes and promastigotes of L. m. mexicana and L. donovani. This was assessed by observing the compounds' effects on promastigote growth and also by measuring parasite viability as determined by their ability to metabolise MTT. There was found to be a direct effect of the compounds on the parasites. L-Tryptophanamide possesses similar activity against both L. m. mexicana and L. donovani, and amastigotes and promastigotes. Relatively high concentrations were required for activity, however, and the chemotherapeutic index was not great. Leu-OMe was found to be especially active against amastigotes of L. m. mexicana, more so than against amastigotes of L. donovani or promastigotes of either species. Amastigotes of L. m. mexicana residing in PECs were as susceptible to the ester as isolated amastigotes, although high susceptibility became apparent only several days after infection if promastigotes were used.

In contrast, neither L. major nor L. donovani in PECs were affected by the ester. The high sensitivity of leishmanias to Leu-OMe appears to correlate with the presence of megasomes within the parasite; it is proposed that the compound is rapidly hydrolysed by an enzyme in these unusual lysosome-like organelles and that the accumulation of the free amino acid in the vacuoles results in osmotic lysis of the parasite. Despite the good activity of Leu-OMe against L. mexicana mexicana in vitro, the compound was found to be inactive against L. m. mexicana and L. donovani in mice.

ACKNOWLEDGEMENTS

This research was supported in part by grants from The Commission of European Communities sub-programme "Medicine, Health and Nutrition in the Tropics" and The Wellcome Trust.

REFERENCES

1. M. Rabinovitch, V. Zilberfarb, and C. Ramazeilles, Destruction of Leishmania mexicana amazonensis within macrophages by lysosomotropic amino acid esters, Journal of Experimental Medicine 163: 520 (1986).
2. M. Rabinovitch, V. Zilberfarb, and M. Pouchelet, Leishmania mexicana: destruction of isolated amastigotes by amino acid esters, American Journal of Tropical Medicine and Hygiene 36: 290 (1987).
3. R. Goldman, and A. Kaplan, Rupture of rat liver lysosomes mediated by L-amino acid esters, Biochimica et Biophysica Acta 318: 205 (1973).
4. S. C. Alfieri, V. Zilberfarb, and M. Rabinovitch, Destruction of Leishmania mexicana amazonensis amastigotes by leucine methyl ester: protection by other amino acid esters, Parasitology 95: 31 (1987).
5. M. Pupkis, L. Tetley, and G.H. Coombs, Leishmania mexicana: amastigote hydrolases in unusual lysosomes, Experimental Parasitology 62: 28 (1986).
6. D. J. Mallinson, and G.H. Coombs, Molecular characterisation of the metacyclic forms of Leishmania, IRCS Medical Science 14: 577 (1986).
7. T. Mossmann, Rapid colorimetric assay for cellular growth and survival: application for proliferation and cytotoxicity assays, Journal of Immunological Methods 65: 55 (1983).
8. A. J. Baillie, G.H. Coombs, T.F. Dolan, C.A. Hunter, T. Laakso, I. Sjoholm, and P. Stjarnkvist, Biodegradable microspheres: Polyarcyl starch microparticles as a delivery system for the antileishmanial drug, sodium stibogluconate, Journal of Pharmacy and Pharmacology 39: in press (1987).
9. L. Tetley, C.A. Hunter, G.H. Coombs, and K. Vickerman, this symposium (1987).

INHIBITION OF LEISHMANIA SPECIES BY α-DIFLUOROMETHYLORNITHINE

Jan S. Keithly and Alan H. Fairlamb[1]

Departments of Medicine and Microbiology
Cornell University Medical College
New York, New York

[1]Department of Medical Protozoology
London School of Hygiene and Tropical Medicine
London, U.K.

INTRODUCTION

DL-α-difluoromethylornithine (DFMO) is a specific, irreversible inhibitor of ornithine decarboxylase (ODC), the rate-limiting enzyme in trypanosome polyamine biosynthesis (reviewed in 1). DFMO cures experimental infections of African trypanosomiasis, and is in phase 1 clinical trials[2]. Although the mechanism of selective toxicity is incompletely known, DFMO has well known effects upon the metabolism and morphology of trypanosomes[1]. Following depletion of the polyamines, putrescine and spermidine, by DFMO, long slender trypomastigotes change into stumpy-like forms which are eliminated by the host. DFMO alters mitochondrial transcripts in these cells[3], and reduces their trypanothione [$T(SH)_2$] levels[4]. As reviewed elsewhere in this volume (Fairlamb, A.H.), $T(SH)_2$ has two important roles in kinetoplastid metabolism: the maintenance of intracellular redox balance and protection against toxic oxygen derivatives and other radicals. The selective toxicity of DFMO for ODC in trypanosomes has also been attributed to this enzyme's slower turnover rate than in mammalian cells[5].

Recently, DFMO was shown to inhibit growth of *Leishmania donovani* promastigotes[6]. Here we report its inhibitory effect upon 3 additional species of *Leishmania*, and extend these data to include suppression of experimental infections in mice.

MATERIALS AND METHODS

Drug Testing in vivo

All experiments were performed in triplicate. P values compare efficacy of treatment with control (untreated, infected) mice. Data were analyzed by the 2-way analysis of variance (Tables 1,2), and by the Neuman-Keuls multiple range and Kruskal-Wallis tests (Tables 3-5). In the latter, significance measures the efficacy of treatment of all dose groups combined, eg. 0.5 through 5.0% DFMO alone, with that of controls.

Visceral Infections. Groups of 5-7 male BALB/cByJ mice were inoculated intracardially with 10 million L. donovani (MHOM/SD/43/WR 130c) infective promastigotes[7] cultivated as previously described[8]. Mice were deprived of water overnight, and the following morning 1 or 3% DFMO was added to the drinking water. Other experimental drugs were given subcutaneously (SC) or intraperitoneally (IP). Dosing began one week prior to, on the day of infection, or 1 week after infection, and was continued for 1 week. Suppression of infection was assessed 8 or 16 days post infection by counting the number of amastigotes in impression smears of liver and spleen, and by culturing as detailed before[9].

Cutaneous Infections. Similar groups of mice were infected intradermally at the shaved base of the tail with 5 million infective promastigotes of either L. braziliensis guyanensis (MHOM/SR/81/CUMC 1) or L. mexicana mexicana (MHOM/BZ/58/WR 183). Mice developed palpable lesions within 5 weeks. At that time, DFMO alone or combined with sodium stibogluconate (Pentostam, Burroughs-Wellcome) was administered. Treatment was continued for 3 weeks, and suppression was assessed 2 weeks after removing drugs (10 weeks after infection). Mice were examined for the presence of parasites in the lesion, blood, and viscera as described previously[9].

Drug Testing in vitro

Primary culture promastigotes[7] of each species were obtained from liquid nitrogen stabilates, and were cultivated in defined medium (RE III to which 1 mg/100 ml hemin had been added[10]). Cells were grown to stationary phase, centrifuged, and the pellet resuspended in 6 duplicate cultures of fresh medium alone, medium containing 5 mM DFMO, or 1 mM putrescine. Samples were removed daily for counting, and extracts (10^9 cells) were prepared by sonication and assayed for trypanothione reductase activity[11]. Thiols were determined by HPLC following derivatization with monobromobimane[4].

RESULTS AND DISCUSSION

Effect of DFMO upon Visceral Infections

Synergism. One percent DFMO combined with Bleomycin (a spermidine-containing, antitumor antibiotic) synergistically suppressed (87%) liver burdens of mice infected with L. donovani (Table 1). DFMO alone suppressed burdens 16%, whereas Bleomycin alone was ineffective. Although the combination did not cure mice of visceral infections, inhibition was as effective as by the antimonial Pentostam, since parasites could still be cultured from spleen homogenates after either treatment (Table 1).

Table 1. Synergistic Effect of DFMO and Bleomycin upon Leishmania donovani Infections in BALB/cByJ Mice

Treatment*	Dose mg/kg/day	Route	Liver Burden Mean + SD	Percent Suppression	Cultures +/Total
Saline alone		SC	308 ± 48	0	3/3
Pentostam alone	140	SC	0	100	2/2
DFMO + Bleomycin	3	IP	41 ± 94	87	2/3
DFMO alone	0		260 ± 238	16	2/2
Bleomycin alone	3	IP	331 ± 148	0	2/2

*DFMO = 1% in drinking water started 24 hours before infection; Bleomycin given at time of infection. Both continued for 7 days.

Additive Effect. Mice infected with L. donovani were also treated with DFMO alone or in combination with a variety of known antikinetoplastid drugs. Without exception, combination of DFMO with Suramin, allopurinol riboside (HPPR), Berenil, or Pentostam improved their ability to suppress experimental infections in mice (Table 2). This was true whether drugs were given before (Table 2) or at time of infection (data not shown). Suramin alone or in combination was also significantly suppressive. As before, none of these treatments cured mice of their infection.

Effect of DFMO upon Cutaneous Infections

We have also extensively tested DFMO alone and in combination with Pentostam against experimental infections of L. b. guyanensis and L. m. mexicana (Tables 3,4), as well as L. donovani (Table 5), to see whether DFMO might lower the Pentostam dose necessary to suppress these infections. In each case, >2% DFMO alone in the drinking water was 20-50% suppressive, and against L. braziliensis guyanensis the effect was striking (p<0.0001; Table 3). This is the first time that an oral, non-toxic alternative to antimony has been identified against mucocutaneous disease.

Table 2. Additive Effect of DFMO and Other Drugs upon Leishmania donovani

Treatment*	Dose mg/kg/day	Liver Burden Mean + SD	Percent Suppressn.	Signif.	Cultures +/Total
Saline alone	---	509 ± 342	0	---	2/2
DFMO alone	---	239 ± 77	53 + 15	---	2/2
Suramin alone	20	151 ± 68	71 + 13	p <0.01	2/2
Suramin + DFMO	20	108 ± 66	79 + 13	p <0.01	2/2
HPPR alone	200	229 ± 214	55 + 44	---	2/2
HPPR + DFMO	200	133 ± 100	74 + 20	p <0.05	2/2
Berenil alone	20	160 ± 70	69 + 14	---	2/2
Berenil + DFMO	20	103 ± 25	80 + 5	p <0.05	2/2
Pentostam alone	20	267 ± 189	48 + 37	---	2/2
Pentostam + DFMO	20	115 ± 105	78 + 21	p <0.01	2/2

*DFMO = 3%; other drugs = SC. All started 7 days before infection.

Table 3. Effect of DFMO and Pentostam upon Lesion Size* of Leishmania braziliensis guyanensis.

DFMO (%)	Pentostam (mg/kg/day)				
	0	6.25	12.5	25	50
0	5.3 ± 3.0	7.8 ± 2.0	6.0 ± 0.9	2.2 ± 2.9	2.1 ± 2.7
0.5	8.3 ± 0.6	8.1 ± 1.8	8.2 ± 1.6	7.7 ± 1.5	8.2 ± 1.4
1.0	0.7 ± 0.6	3.7 ± 5.5	2.9 ± 4.0	3.1 ± 3.6	4.4 ± 3.4
2.0	0.0	7.2 ± 0.3	6.6 ± 0.5	6.2 ± 1.0	0.2 ± 0.3
4.0	3.0 ± 2.0	6.9	9.4 ± 2.6	3.9 ± 2.6	3.8 ± 2.5
5.0	1.0	5.7 ± 1.2	6.4 ± 0.8	6.0 ± 0.4	0.0

Significance: DFMO alone   p <0.0001
              Pentostam alone   p <0.0001
              DFMO + Pentostam   p <0.019

*Diameter in mm

Table 4. Percent Suppression by DFMO and Pentostam of
Leishmania m. mexicana Infections in BALB/cByJ Mice.

DFMO	Pentostam (mg/kg/day)				
(%)	0	40	80	160	320
0	0	14	4	19	20
2	12	18	16	18	38
4	20	6	13	38	39

Significance: DFMO alone $p < 0.046$
Pentostam alone $p < 0.003$
DFMO and Pentostam $p < 0.864$

Table 5. Percent Suppression by DFMO and Pentostam of Leishmania donovani
Infections in BALB/cByJ Mice.

DFMO	Pentostam (mg/kg/day)					
(%)	0	0.1	1.0	10	50	100
0	0	0	0	19	55	98
2	0	43	0	0	48	27
4	51	13	63	17	67	91

Significance: DFMO alone $p < 0.065$
Pentostam alone $p < 0.004$
DFMO and Pentostam $p < 0.040$

Species specific effects. DFMO alone significantly suppressed each experimental infection tested (Tables 3-5), but the effect against L. mexicana infections (Table 4) was less than that for L. b. guyanensis or L. donovani (Tables 3,5). As expected, suppression by Pentostam alone was also highly significant against each of these infections ($p < 0.0001$, 0.003, and 0.004, respectively). When DFMO was combined with Pentostam, however, the effect was additive at best, and in L. mexicana infections suppression was only marginally better than treatment with DFMO or Pentostam alone.

Differences in efficacy upon these infections in vivo may be partly explained by differential drug delivery to tissues, or by a defect in T-cell influx in BALB/c mice infected with L. mexicana[12]. They may also be due to species differences in ODC turnover rates, the enzyme's affinity for DFMO, or the regulation of expression of ODC.

In Vitro Testing

Our in vitro data confirm the difference in efficacy of DFMO against various species of Leishmania (Figs. 1-2). Initial growth of L. donovani and L. b. guyanensis was inhibited >50% by 5 mM DFMO (Fig. 1), whereas growth of L. major and L. m. mexicana was virtually unchanged (data not shown). The reason for this difference is unknown. There was no evidence for differential uptake or concentration of DFMO, nor utilization of alternate enzymatic pathways for polyamine biosynthesis (Keithly and Fairlamb, unpublished data). Others have reported elevated levels of putrescine in late log phase promastigotes of L. mexicana[13]. This could partly explain our observations. Exogenous putrescine (1 mM) reversed growth inhibition of L. donovani and L. b. guyanensis by DFMO (Fig. 2).

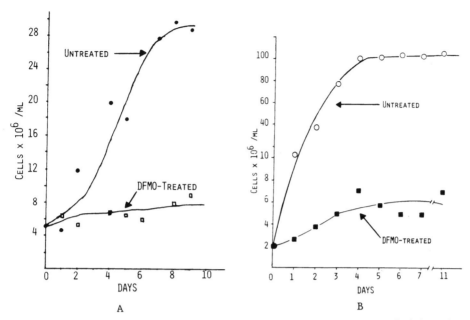

Fig. 1. Effect of 5 mM DFMO upon the growth of L. donovani (A) and L. braziliensis guyanensis (B).

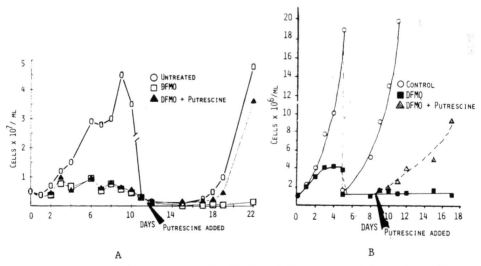

Fig. 2 Inhibition of growth by DFMO and its reversal by putrescine. (A) L. donovani, (B) L. braziliensis guyanensis

Effect of DFMO upon Trypanothione Biosynthesis

Our initial *in vivo* results coincided with the discovery of trypanothione[14], a compound involved in kinetoplastid glutathione metabolism and discussed elsewhere in this volume (Fairlamb, A.H). Trypanothione reductase (TR) is the rate-limiting enzyme for maintaining significant amounts of reduced glutathione (GSH) in trypanosomatids. TR levels in both amastigotes and promastigotes of Leishmania species are high (Table 6). Untreated promastigotes of L. b. guyanensis also contain significant levels of GSH, glutathionyl-spermidine (GSH-SPD), and $T(SH)_2$ (Table 7). Each of these is essential for glutathione metabolism and cell survival. DFMO decreases $T(SH)_2$ and GSH-SPD levels in both log and stationary phase promastigotes to 72% and 61% of controls, respectively, while GSH levels remain unchanged. In addition, significant levels of polyamines are present in untreated promastigotes of three Leishmania species (Table 8). In both log and stationary phase promastigotes, DFMO reduces putrescine to non-detectable levels, and spermidine and spermine to <50% of controls (data not shown).

Table 6. Levels of Trypanothione Reductase in species of Leishmania.

Organisms	Stage	Activity*
L. braziliensis guyanensis	Promastigote	29
L. mexicana amazonensis MHOM/BR/73/M2269	Amastigote	24
L. mexicana amazonensis	Promastigote	27
L. mexicana mexicana	Promastigote	37
L. major MHOM/SN/00/DK 106	Promastigote	31

*$nmol/min/10^9$ cells. Average of 2-3 runs on triplicate samples.

Table 7. Effect of DFMO upon Trypanothione Biosynthesis in Promastigotes of Leishmania braziliensis guyanensis.

Culture Day	Growth Phase	DFMO 5 mM	GSH*	GSH-SPD*	$T(SH)_2$*
3.5	Log	0	1.50	0.61	6.20
		0	2.22	0.63	5.03
3.5	Log	+	1.52	0.36	3.52
		+	1.44	0.39	4.50
8.5	Stationary	0	2.02	0.40	2.64
8.5	Stationary	+	1.08	0.13	1.30

*$nmol/10^8$ cells.

Table 8. Polyamine Levels* in species of Leishmania.

Organisms	Putrescine	Spermidine	Spermine
L. braziliensis guyanensis	7.5	11.2	3.2
L. mexicana amazonensis	8.5	18.5	3.0
L. major	14.0	15.5	3.0

*nmol/10^8 cells

These DFMO-induced changes in metabolite levels are similar to those reported for Trypanosoma b. brucei[4]. The effect of DFMO alone would appear to be cytostatic rather than cytocidal because non-dividing promastigotes can survive in culture for at least 11 days (Fig. 1 A-B). Although the precise mechanism by which DFMO induces cytostasis is unknown, it must be due to a depletion of polyamines and T(SH)$_2$, because its effect can be completely reversed by addition of putrescine (Fig. 2 A-B). These data suggest that it may be necessary to combine DFMO with a cytocidal drug like Bleomycin (Table 1) to effect a complete cure.

CONCLUSIONS

DFMO inhibits in vitro growth and in vivo replication of L. donovani and L. b. guyanensis, but not L. major or L. mexicana. The effect of DFMO alone upon L. braziliensis guyanensis infections is striking. This is the first time an oral, non-toxic, specific alternative to antimonials or Amphotericin B has been identified which is active against experimental mucocutaneous leishmaniasis.

Depending upon the species, DFMO can be synergistic, additive, or have no effect when combined with other drugs. DFMO and the antitumor antibiotic Bleomycin synergistically suppress experimental infections of L. donovani. When used in combination with Suramin, allopurinol riboside, Berenil, or Pentostam, DFMO has an additive effect against experimental visceral leishmaniasis.

Our in vitro data confirm these in vivo effects. DFMO significantly reduces putrescine and trypanothione levels in leishmania. Since leishmania and other trypanosomatids depend upon polyamine and trypanothione metabolism for survival (see Fairlamb, A.H., this volume), we think these should be actively pursued as potential targets for chemotherapy.

ACKOWLEDGMENTS

The authors thank Mr. Simon Paul and Mark Warshofsky for excellent technical assistance, Dr. Peter McCann (Merrell-Dow Research Institute) for supplying DFMO, Dr. Randolph Berens (University of Colorado Medical School) for supplying allopurinol riboside, Dr. Cyrus J. Bacchi (Pace University) for his helpful discussions, and Dr. Miklós Müller (Rockefeller University) for critical reading of the manuscript. This work was supported in part by grants from the Walter Reed Army Institute of Research, Merrell-Dow Institute of Research, the National Institutes of Health (JSK), and UNDP/World Bank/WHO Special Programme for Research and Training in Tropical Diseases (AHF).

REFERENCES

1. Bacchi, C.J. and P.P. McCann. Parasitic protozoa and polyamines, in: Inhibition of polyamine Metabolism. P.P. McCann, A.E. Pegg, and A. Sjoerdsma, eds., Academic Press, San Diego, pages 317-344 (1987).
2. Schechter, P.J., J.L.R. Barlow, and A. Sjoerdsma. Clinical aspects of inhibition of ornithine decarboxylase with emphasis on therapeutic trials of eflornithine (DFMO) in cancer and protozoan diseases, in Inhibition of Polyamine Metabolism, P.P. McCann, A.E. Pegg, and A. Sjoerdsma, eds., Academic Press, San Diego, pages 345-364 (1987).
3. Feagin, J.E., D.P. Jasmer, and K. Stuart. Differential mitochondrial gene expression between slender and stumpy blood forms of Trypanosoma brucei. Mol. Biochem. Parasitol. 20: 207-214 (1986).
4. Fairlamb, A.H., G.B. Henderson, C.J. Bacchi, and A. Cerami. In vivo effects of difluoromethylornithine on trypanothione and polyamine levels in bloodstream forms of Trypanosoma brucei. Mol. Biochem. Parasitol. 24: 185-191 (1987).
5. Phillips, M.A., P. Coffino, and C.C. Wang. Cloning and sequencing of the ornithine decarboxylase gene from Trypanosoma brucei: implications for enzyme turnover and selective difluoromethylornithine inhibition. J. Cell Biol. (in press)
6. Kaur, K., K. Emmett, P.P. McCann, A. Sjoerdsma and Ullman, B. Effects of DL-alpha-difluoromethylornithine on Leishmania donovani promastigotes. J. Protozool., 33: 518-521 (1986).
7. Keithly, J.S. and E.J. Bienen. Infectivity of Leishmania donovani promastigotes for hamsters. Acta Tropica 38: 85-89 (1981).
8. Colomer-Gould, V., L. Galvao-Quintao, J.S. Keithly, and N. Nogueira. A common major surface antigen on amastigotes and promastigotes of Leishmania species. J. Exp. Med. 162: 902-916 (1985).
9. Keithly, J.S. and S.G. Langreth. Inefficacy of metronidazole in experimental infections of Leishmania donovani, L. mexicana, and Trypanosoma brucei brucei. Am. J. Trop. Med. Hyg. 32: 485-495 (1983).
10. Steiger, R.F. and E. Steiger. Cultivation of Leishmania donovani and L. braziliensis in defined media. J. Protozool. 24: 437-441 (1977).
11. Henderson, G.B., A.H. Fairlamb, P. Ulrich and A. Cerami. Substrate specificity of the flavoprotein trypanothione disulphide reductase from Crithidia fasciculata. Biochemistry, 26: 3022-3027 (1987).
12. McElrath, M.J., G. Kaplan, A. Nusrat, and Z.A. Cohn. Cutaneous leishmaniasis. The defect in T-cell influx in BALB/c mice. J. Exp. Med. 165: 546-559 (1987).
13. Coombs, G.H. and B.M. Sanderson. Amine production by Leishmania mexicana. Ann. Trop. Med. Parasitol. 79: 409-415 (1985).
14. Fairlamb, A.H., P. Blackburn, P. Ulrich, B.T. Chait and A. Cerami. Trypanothione: A novel bis(glutathionyl)spermidine cofactor for glutathione reductase in trypanosomatids, Science, 227: 1485-87 (1985).

ANTILEISHMANIAL EFFECT OF SINEFUNGIN AND ITS DERIVATIVES[*]

Malka Robert-Géro, Françoise Lawrence,
Pierre Blanchard, Nérina Dodic,
Philippe Paolantonacci, Halina Malina
and Abdelmalek Mouna

Institut de Chimie des Substances Naturelles
C.N.R.S.
91190 Gif-sur-Yvette   France

INTRODUCTION

Sinefungin 1 is a natural nucleoside isolated from cultures of Streptomyces griseolus at Lilly Research Laboratories in the U.S.[1] and from cultures of S.incarnatus at Rhône-Poulenc Industries in France.[2] This molecule is composed of an adenosine and an orninthine moiety linked together by a carbon-carbon bond at the 5'end of the adenosine part. This structure confers a good chemical and biological stability to this compound.

After its discovery sinefungin was shown to be a potent inhibitor of yeast growth, specially of Candida albicans in vitro and in vivo.[3] Later the inhibitory effect of this antibiotic was demonstrated against various types of viruses such as Rous sarcoma, polyoma, vaccinia and Epstein-Barr viruses in vitro.[4-6] These effects were observed at sinefungin concentrations ranging from 10 to 250 µM. However as it turned out later, the major interest of this antibiotic is its strong antiparasitic activity. In this article we review the results of different laboratories in the world on the antiparasitic activity of sinefungin specially against Leishmania. We will also discuss the problems raised about its use as a chemotherapeutic agent. The mechanism of action of this compound at the cellular and at the molecular level as well as new strategies proposed to overcome the toxic side effects of this molecule are presented in separate chapters in this issue.

---

[*] Dedicated to Professor Edgar Lederer on the occasion of his 80th birthday.

RESULTS AND DISCUSSION

1) Effect of sinefungin in vitro and in vivo

The results concerning the effect of sinefungin on the growth of various parasites in vitro are summarized in Table 1. This antibiotic inhibits different species of Trypanosoma and Leishmania as well as Plasmodium falciparum at concentrations ranging from 10 nM to 7 µM. Much higher concentrations are necessary however for the inhibition of growth of various Amoeba and Giardia intestinalis. Concerning Leishmania, sinefungin affects the growth of promastigotes of all species but its

Table 1. Antiparasitic Effect of Sinefungin in vitro.

Parasite	Dose [µM]	% Inhibition	Reference
Plasmodium falciparum	0.3-1	78-95	7
Leishmania aethiopica pm	3	100	8
Leishmania donovani "	0.13	100	9
Leishmania tropica "	0.26	100	9
Leishmania enrietti "	2.6	100	9
Leishmania mexicana "	0.018	100	L.Nolan "et al." unpublished
Leishmania donovani am	2.4	ED50	10
Trypanosoma cruzi em	1.8-4.8	50	R.A.Neal "et al." unpublished
Trypanosoma cruzi am	7.2	50	10
Trypanosoma gambiense	0.26	30	J. Marr "et al." unpublished
Trypanosoma b. brucei	0.01	100	11
Entamoeba histolytica	20-40	100	12
Naegleria fowleri	65	75	13
Acanthamoeba culbertsoni	525	30	13
Giardia intestinalis	57	50	14

pm : promastigotes.   am : amastigotes.   em : epimastigotes.

effect varies greatly from one species to another. L. mexicana and L. donovani were found to be the most susceptible^9 and L. aethiopica the least. According to our results the growth of promastigotes is arrested within one generation time. Furthermore, when observed under the light microscope, the sinefungin treated promastigotes which were initially elongated, became immobile and spherical. It seems that in both Leishmania and Trypanosoma the amastigote stage is less sensitive to sinefungin than the promastigote or epimastigote forms, but these findings have to be reconfirmed.

The strong in vitro inhibitory effect of the antibiotic prompted several laboratories to undertake the study of its effect in vivo. Data are presented in Table 2. Again the results are quite encouraging. Allison's group showed in 1983 that sinefungin was very efficient against African Trypanosoma, such as T. b. brucei, T. congolense and T. vivax in infected mice. Low doses such as 0.05 to 5 mg/kg given i.p. 3 to 9 times cured the animals.[15] Interestingly sinefungin was not active against T. cruzi in vivo. The effect of sinefungin on L. donovani infected mice was studied by Dr. R.A. Neal who found this nucleoside 73 times more active than sodium stibogluconate. Dr. Neal tested sinefungin also against cutaneous leishmaniasis in mice and demonstrated its activity at relatively low concentration. Quite recently Dr. W.L. Hanson from the University of

Table 2. Antiparasitic Effect of Sinefungin in vivo.

Parasite	Animal	Dose mg/kg	Effect	Reference
Trypanosoma b brucei	mice	5x3 i.p.	cure	15
T. congolense	"	0.05x9 i.p.	"	"
T. vivax	"	5x3 i.p.	"	"
T. cruzi	"	50	slight activity	W. Guttridge unpublished
T. congolense	goat	7.5x8 i.m.	50% cured	16
Leishmania donovani	mice	0.32x5 s.c.	= ED50	17
L. major	"	45 s.c.	44	17
L.b. panamensis	hamster	26 i.m.	84	W.L. Hanson "et al." unpublished
Toxoplasma gondii	mice	2.5x6 i.p.	increase of survival time>28 days	A. Ferrante "et al." unpublished
Plasmodium vinckei petteri	"	1x6 i.p.	No activity	J. Clarck unpublished

Georgia, U.S.A., showed that sinefungin at 26 mg/kg inhibited by 84% the mean lesion area in L. b. panamensis infected hamsters. Furthermore sinefungin seems to inhibit to some extent Toxoplasma gondii in infected mice but was found ineffective against Plasmodium vinckei petteri in vivo. These results show that in mice or hamsters infected with Leishmania and some species of Trypanosoma sinefungin is active and has no toxic side effects. Unfortunately this is not the case when the antibiotic is administered to goats infected with T. congolense.[16] When sinefungin was given at 5 or 7.5 mg/kg twice a day, for 4 consecutive days, 50% of the animals died and the remainder were cured. The authors observed severe nephrotoxic side effects even at subcurative levels and histopathological examinations revealed an acute tubulonephrosis.

2) Toxicity Studies

Toxicity data on sinefungin are rather scarce and unpublished. Most of these studies were performed at Lilly Research Laboratories in the U.S. and at Rhône-Poulenc Industries in France. According to our informations, in single dose (acute toxicity) the compound is well tolerated by mice and rats regardless of the way of administration. Studies on subchronic toxicity gave different results. Low doses ranging from 1 to 4 mg/kg/day for rats and from 0.2 to 0.8 mg/kg/day for dogs during one month provoked nephrosis and bone marrow depression. The latter only in dogs. These effects are probably reversible at least to some extent upon cessation of the treatment. Other observations concerned subchronic toxicity at high doses given orally to rats and to dogs for 5 days and for 3 months. In rats no toxic effects were observed with treatments of 10 mg/kg for 90 days or with 50 mg/kg for 5 days. When increased doses such as 200 mg/kg for 5 days were given, tubular nephrosis was observed in rats but this was generally reversible. Dogs were given either 50 and 200 mg/kg for 5 days or 10 mg/kg for 3 month. In both cases tubular nephrosis was observed and the animals died. Death was associated with haemorrhagic lesions of the intestine.

3) Natural and Synthetic Analogues of Sinefungin

The unpleasant toxic side effects of sinefungin prompted us to undertake a programme to synthesize related molecules with the hope to prepare compounds with good activity and less toxicity. Two parallel ways were chosen to reach this goal : chemical synthesis and microbiological approach. We achieved the total synthesis of sinefungin^{18} and we have now the methodology to introduce modifications into the side chain and to the nucleoside part of the molecule.

The other approach was done by genetic engeneering. We isolated the chromosomal DNA of the producing strain : Streptomyces incarnatus and after appropriate digestion, fragments were introduced into the plasmid vector PIJ61. Protoplasts prepared from S. lividans were transformed by this plasmid vector. Several clones producing sinefungin and other modified nucleosides were isolated. The identification of these compounds is now underway in our laboratory. For this part of our work we collaborate with Dr. J. Davies (Dept. of Genie Microbiologique, Pasteur Institute, Paris).

Fig. 1 shows some structural analogues of sinefungin. The lactam of the antibiotic 2 and the dehydro derivative 3 are natural products isolated respectively from cultures of S. incarnatus and S. griseolus. This latter compound is produced also by a Streptosporangium sp and was isolated at the Schering Corporation in the U.S. This compound has strong antiviral activity but its effect against L. donovani promastigotes is weaker than that of sinefungin. The MLC (minimum leishmanicidal concentration) was higher than 2.6 µM against L. donovani and L. tropica promastigotes and 0.13 µM towards L. enrietti.^{9} According to Dr. Neal's unpublished results the ED50 against macrophages infected with L. donovani amastigotes is 2µM. No toxicity data is available for this compound.

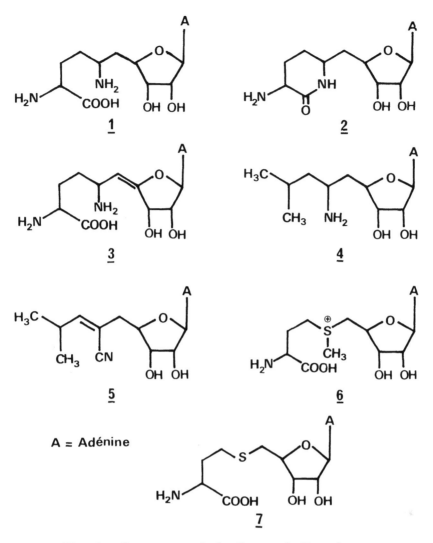

Fig. 1. Structures of the Compounds Tested.

The cyclic derivative of sinefungin, the lactam was more extensively studied. The advantage of this compound is that it can be relatively easily prepared from sinefungin. In all cell systems this molecule was found to be active but at higher concentrations than sinefungin. For example, at concentrations 30 times higher its activity against Candida infected mice is identical to that of sinefungin. With respect of its antileishmanial effect, the MLC against promastigotes of L. donovani is 0.26 µM, against promastigotes of L. donovani and L. enrietti 2.6 µM The ED50 against L. donovani infected macrophages is 0.3 µM. In vivo the ED50 in L. donovani infected mice was achieved with 0.9 mg/kg x 5 (Neal "et al.", unpublished). According to Dr. Hanson's unpublished results 64% inhibition of the mean lesion area was observed on L. b. panamensis infected hamsters with a dose of 26 mg/kg, twice a day for 4 consecutive days. The acute toxicity in mice of this molecule is above 2 g/kg (Rhône-Poulec, France).

Structures 4 and 5 are synthetic analogues prepared in our laboratory several years ago. They have no significant antileishmanial activity. Other side chain analogues are now under biological investigations. S-adenosylmethionine 6 and S-adenosylhomocysteine 7, respectively the substrate and the product of enzymatic transmethylations are presented here to illustrate their structural relationship with sinefungin. They are devoid of antileishmanial activity but 6 antagonises the effect of sinefungin when added together to the cultures at 100 times higher concentration.

It is too early to discuss the structure-activity relationship of these compounds. Nevertheless, the preliminary results indicate that the replacement of the $CH-NH_2$ group by S or by S^+-CH_3 as in 7 or in 6 leads to the loss of the inhibitory activity. The presence of the terminal amino and carboxyl groups are important since the synthetic analogues 4 and 5 lacking these functions are much less active than sinefungin. The cyclization of the side chain preserves but lowers the activity and the presence of a double bond at the 5'end enhances the activity 20 fold against L. enrietti promastigotes in comparison to sinefungin.[9] These preliminary studies suggest that sinefungin and its lactam share commun molecular target(s), at least in L. donovani and L. tropica, sinefungin having a greater affinity. Experiments with additional structural analogues are needed for the clarification of this problem.

MECHANISM OF ACTION

This subject is discussed in detail elsewhere in this issue, yet we would like to summarize in this article the presently available information. Although the exact mechanism of inhibition by sinefungin is not yet completely elucidated, we observed a rapid and severe inhibition of thymidine incorporation into nDNA mainly. This was neither the consequence of reduced uptake of the precursor by treated cells nor of the reduction of the nucleotide triphosphate pool. Thymidine incorporation was also inhibited by the cyclic and by the dehydro derivatives of sinefungin in L. tropica. The lactam but not the dehydro derivative inhibited thymidine incorporation in L. donovani promastigotes while both were inactive in L. enrietti.[10] We observed also inhibition of protein methylases I(arg) and III (lys) in vitro with apparent ki values of 145 µM respectively for sinefungin and of 253 µM for the lactam with respect to the first enzyme, in promastigotes of L. donovani.[9] Sinefungin induced also the rapid overproduction of three main "stress proteins" of approximatively 90, 80 and 70 KDa in L. donovani promastigotes. The cyclic and the dehydro derivatives of sinefungin induced the synthesis of similar proteins, however the intensity of the response varied depending on the protein and on the analogue.[20]

CONCLUSION

According to the results of our and of several other laboratories, sinefungin is a very potent antileishmanial and antitrypanasomal agent in vitro and in vivo. It might become a valuable chemotherapeutic agent. Its serious inconvenience is its toxicity observed in dogs and goats. To overcome this drawback we are actively engaged in the chemical and microbiological synthesis of new analogues. In the meantime we propose to try combined chemotherapy with other drugs or with immunomodulators and also the administration of sinefungin in liposomes or in microcapsules. These approaches will be discussed in a separate chapter in this issue.

ACKNOWLEDGEMENTS

This work was supported by Grants from the World Health Organisation UNDP/World bank/WHO Special Program for Research and Training in Tropical Diseases, from the Fondation pour la Recherche Médicale Française and la Ligue Nationale Française contre le Cancer.

REFERENCES

1. R. Hamill and M. Hoehn, A9145, A New Adenine Containing Antifungal Antibiotic. I. Discovery and Isolation, J. Antibiot., 26:463 (1973).
2. Rhône-Poulenc patent no.7611141, April 1976.
3. R.S. Gordee and T.F. Butler, A9145, A New Adenine Containing Antifungal Antibiotic. II Biological Activity, J. Antibiot., 26:466 (1973).
4. M. Vedel, F. Lawrence, M. Robert-Gero and E. Lederer, The Antifungal Antibiotic Sinefungin as a very Active Inhibitor of Methyltransferases and of the Transformation of Chick Embryo Fibroblasts by Rous sarcoma Virus. Biochem. Biophys. Res. Commun., 85:371 (1978).
5. C.S.G. Pugh, R.T. Borchardt and H.O. Stone, Sinefungin a Potent Inhibitor of virion mRNA (guanine 7) methyltransferase, mRNA (nucleoside 2') methyltransferase and viral Multiplication, J. Biol. Chem., 253:4075 (1978).
6. W.K. Long, G.E. Fronko, R.G. Lindmeyer, R. Wu and E.E. Henderson, Effects of S-adenosylhomocysteine and Analogs on Epstein-Barr Virus-induced Transformation, Expression of the Epstein-Barr virus capsid Antigen, and Methylation of Epstein-Barr Virus DNA, J. Virol., 61:221 (1987).
7. W. Trager, M. Tershakovec, P.K. Chiang and G. Cantoni, Plasmodium falciparum : Antimalarial Activity in Culture of Sinefungin and Other Methylation Inhibitors, Exp. Parasitol., 50:83 (1980).
8. U. Bachrach, L.F. Schnur, J. El-On, C.L. Greenblatt, E. Perlman, M. Robert-Gero and E. Lederer, Inhibitory Activity of Sinefungin and SIBA on the Growth of Promastigotes and Amastigotes of Different Species of Leishmania, FEBS Lett., 121:287 (1980).

9. P. Paolantonacci, F. Lawrence and M. Robert-Gero, Differential Effect of Sinefungin and Its Analogs on the Multiplication of Three Leishmania Species. Antimicrob. Agents Chemother., 28:528 (1985).
10. R.A. Neal and S.L. Croft, An in vitro System for Determining the Activity of Compounds against the Intracellular Amastigote form of Leishmania donovani, J. Antimicrob. Chemother., 14:463 (1984).
11. N.K. Borowy, H. Hirumi, H.K. Waithaka and G. Mkoji, An Assay for Screening Drugs against Animal-infective bloodstream Forms of Trypanosoma brucei brucei in vitro, Drugs Exptl. Clin. Res., 11:155 (1985).
12. A. Ferrante, I. Ljungström, G. Huldt and E. Lederer, Amoebicidal Activity of the Antifungal Antibiotic Sinefungin against Entamoebia histolytica, 78:837 (1984).
13. A. Ferrante, T.J. Abell, B. Robinson and E. Lederer, Effects of Sinefungin and Difluoromethylornithine on Pathogenic Free-living Amoebae in vitro, FEMS Microbiol Letters, 40:67 (1987).
14. P.F.L. Boreham, R.E. Phillips and R.W. Shepherd, A Comparison of the in vitro Activity of Some 5-nitroimidazoles and other Compounds against Giardia intestinalis, J. Antimicrobial Chemother., 16:586 (1985).
15. K.D. Dube, G. Mpimbaza, A.C. Allison, E. Lederer and L. Rovis, Antitrypanosomal Activity of Sinefungin, J. Trop. Med. Hyg., 32:31 (1983).
16. E.D. Zweygarth, D. Schillinger, W. Kaufmann and D. Röttcher, Evaluation of Sinefungin for the Treatment of Trypanosomes (Nannomonas) congolense Infections in Goats, Trop. Med. Parasitol., 37:255 (1986).
17. R.A. Neal, S.L. Croft and D.J. Nelson, Antileishamanial Effect of Allopurinol Ribonucleoside and Related Compounds, Formycin B, Sinefungin and Lepidine WR 6026. Trans. R. Soc., Trop. Med. Hyg., 79:85 (1985).
18. M. Gèze, P. Blanchard, J.-L. Fourrey and M. Robert-Gero, Synthesis of Sinefungin and Its C-6' Epimer, J. Am. Chem. Soc., 105:7638 (1983).
19. P. Paolantonacci, F. Lawrence, L.L. Nolan and M. Robert-Gero, Inhibition of Leishmanial DNA Synthesis by Sinefungin, Biochem. Pharmacol., 36:2813 (1987).
20. F. Lawrence and M. Robert-Gero, Occcurence of Stress Proteins in Leishmania d. donovani upon Sinefungin Treatment, Eur. J. Biochem., Submitted.

EFFECTS OF LANOSTEROL-14α-DEMETHYLATION INHIBITORS ON PROPAGATION AND
STEROL BIOSYNTHESIS OF LEISHMANIA PROMASTIGOTES AND AMASTIGOTES

David H. Beach[1], L. John Goad[2], Jonathan D. Berman[3], and George G. Holz, Jr.[1]

[1]Department of Microbiology and Immunology, S.U.N.Y. Health Science Center at Syracuse, Syracuse, NY 13210 U.S.A.
[2]Department of Biochemistry, University of Liverpool, P.O. Box 147, Liverpool L69 3BX U.K.
3Division of Experimental Therapeutics, Walter Reed Army Institute of Research, Washington, D.C. 20307-5100 U.S.A.

Several membrane lipid classes of Leishmania promastigotes and amastigotes are characteristic of plant cell membranes. Among them are sterols, ω3 and cyclopropane fatty acyl groups of phosphoglycerides and inositolphosphosphingolipids[1]. The enzymatic reactions in the biosynthesis of those lipids are attractive targets for chemotherapeutic drugs, since some reactions are unique to plants and others are more sensitive to drugs than are comparable reactions in vertebrate systems.
The nature of the sterols found in Leishmania[2-4] suggests that they are formed as in fungi; i.e., via the 2,3-epoxidation of squalene, cyclization of the squalene-2,3-epoxide to lanosterol, 4α- and 14α-demethylation of lanosterol, alkylation of the side chain and double bond isomerization, introduction and elimination in the ring system and side chain. This fungal correlation is corroborated by the response of Leishmania to the mycostatic azole drugs; ketoconazole[5], an imidazole, and itraconazole[6] and fluconazole[7], triazoles. The growth and sterol biosynthesis of Leishmania promastigotes in culture[8] and amastigotes in human monocyte derived macrophages[9] and in murine macrophage tumor cells[4] are variously inhibited. As in the case of ketoconazole and its interactions with Candida[10], the inhibitions are influenced by drug dose, duration of drug exposure, numbers exposed, growth phase at exposure, culture medium (composition, pH, osmolarity), temperature and O_2 tension.
An ED_{50} of ~0.01 μg ml^{-1} was noted for L. mexicana mexicana WR227 promastigotes grown in a serum-based medium[4] and the MIC was ~1.0 μg ml^{-1}. Exposure of promastigotes of WHO reference strains of Leishmania to 1 μg ml^{-1} ketoconazole, itraconazole and fluconazole for 5 d from the time of inoculation, and assay of population growth, showed the following hierarchy of inhibitory activity: itraconazole ≥ ketoconazole >>> fluconazole (Table 1; representative strains of each species and subspecies from a total of 50). Of all species tested, the most sensitive to ketoconazole and itraconazole were L. donovani and L. braziliensis.
For amastigotes of L. major WR401 grown in human monocyte derived macrophages[9], the ED_{50} of ketoconazole was 7 μg ml^{-1}, while that of fluconazole was >32 μg ml^{-1}. Itraconazole was as active as ketoconazole but was cytotoxic for the macrophage itself.

Table 1. Effects of azole drugs on population growth of promastigotes of WHO reference and other strains of Leishmania; itraconazole, ketoconazole, fluconazole.

Leishmania	Code	Control[b] (x 10^6 ml^{-1})	Itra[c]	% Control Keto[c]	Fluc[c]
L. aethiopica	MHOM/ET/72/L100	131	34	39	85
L. major	MHOM/SU/73/5-ASKH	104	40	65	77
L. tropica	MHOM/SU/60/LRC-L39	122	4	36	96
L. d. donovani	MHOM/IN/80/DD8	125	8	13	94
L. d. infantum	MHOM/FR/80/LEM200	131	15	14	91
L. d. chagasi	MHOM/BR/00/M2682	163	39	43	86
L. m. amazonensis	IFLA/BR/67/PH8	171	12	35	97
L. m. mexicana	MNYC/BZ/62/M379	181	48	53	92
L. b. braziliensis	MHOM/BR/00/LTB0014	83	3	2	89
L. b. guyanensis	MHOM/SR/79/CUMC1	119	6	6	96
L. b. panamensis	MHOM/PA/71/LS94	77	12	11	94

[a]Modified RE III medium (inactivated fetal bovine serum 10%)[11], Falcon 25 cm^2 flasks, 5 d, 26°C. Initial population 10^6 ml^{-1}.
[b]Averages of triplicate samples, Coulter Counter.
[c]Drug concentration 1 µg ml^{-1}.

As in fungi[12-15], ketoconazole, itraconazole and fluconazole inhibit the cytochrome P-450$_{14DM}$ catalyzed oxidation and removal of the 14α-methyl group of lanosterol in Leishmania sterol biosynthesis[3,4]. This blocks the biosynthesis of episterol, 5-dehydroepisterol and ergosterol, the major sterols of Leishmania promastigotes[2,3,8] and amastigotes[4], and results in their replacement with 14α-methyl sterols (Table 2). The changes in sterol content occur rapidly and progressively through the exposure period (Table 3), and are mirrored precisely in the pattern of incorporation of [2-^{14}C]mevalonic acid into the sterols of promastigotes[3,8] and amastigotes[4] in short term (~1-day) exposures to the drug. There is a rapid and marked shift in the distribution of radioactivity among the 14α-desmethyl and 14α-methyl sterols upon exposure of the parasites to ketoconazole, such that the majority of the radioactivity is sequestered in 4α,14α-dimethylzymosterol. This shift is drug dose dependent and could be detected in the sterols of promastigotes exposed to as little as 0.001 µg ml^{-1} ketoconazole[8].

The reduction in the amount of endogenous 14α-desmethyl sterols to as little as 1% of total free sterols in ketoconazole treated and growth inhibited promastigotes (Table 2), raised the question of whether or not such promastigotes could be subcultured indefinitely. WHO reference strains of Leishmania naturally resistant to ketoconazole (Table 1) were chosen to answer that question and, coincidentally, to find out if their resistance was related to an ability to propagate in the absence of their normal endogenous 14α-desmethyl sterols, or to an ability to continue to form those sterols despite the constant presence of ketoconazole. After 10 subcultures with ketoconazole (1 µg ml^{-1}), their population growth was essentially unchanged and they continued to biosynthesize small amounts of 14α-desmethyl sterols (Table 4).

Table 2. Effects of azoles on the free sterol content of Leishmania mexicana mexicana[a] promastigotes and amastigotes.

Identity by GLC and GC/MS	GLC[b] T_{rr} DB-IN	SPB-5	MS[b] (m/z [M+])	Promastigote Itraconazole 1[d]	Ketoconazole 0	Ketoconazole 1[d]	Fluconazole 10	Amastigote Ketoconazole 0	Ketoconazole 1[e]
Cholest-5-en-3β-ol	1.00	1.00	386	24	27	24	30	40	43
Cholesta-5,24-dien-3β-ol	1.02	1.07	384	1			2	2	1
Cholesta-7,24-dien-3β-ol (& 5,7,24)		1.16			9		9		
Ergosta-5,24(28)-dien-3β-ol	1.055	1.20	398					7	10
Ergosta-5,7,24(28)-trien-3β-ol	1.08	1.31	396	1	61	1	33	7	3
Ergosta-7,24(28)-dien-3β-ol	1.085	1.33	398				4	22	1
Stigmasta-5,7-22-trien-3β-ol	1.12	1.45	410						1
Stigmasta-5,7-dien-3β-ol	1.135	1.55	412					1	2
Stigmasta-5,7,24(28)-trien-3β-ol	1.145	1.57	410					10	12
Stigmasta-7,24(28)-dien-3β-ol	1.165	1.64	412					7	2
14α-Methylcholesta-8,24-dien-3β-ol		1.09				1	6		2
14α-Methylergosta-8,24(28)-dien-3β-ol		1.19				2	4		
4α,14α-Dimethylcholesta-8,24-dien-3β-ol	1.06	1.24	412	36	2	41	10	2	20
4α,14α-Dimethylergosta-8,24(28)-dien-3β-ol	1.09	1.36	426	27		26	1	1	
Lanosta-8,24-dien-3β-ol	1.125	1.49	426	6	1	5	2	1	2

[a]MHOM/PA/80/WR227[16]
[b]Analytical GLC 30 m SPB-5 column; GC/MS 15 m DB-IN column[3,4].
[c]% Total free sterols; µg 10[10] leishmanias, extracted from chloroform/methanol soluble lipids with petroleum ether; promastigotes: control 785, itraconazole 886, ketoconazole 905, fluconazole 768; amastigotes: control 417, ketoconazole 514.
[d]Drug concentration in µg ml^{-1}. Population growth as % of control; ketoconazole 38%, itraconazole 16%, fluconazole 71%. Culture conditions as in footnote a, Table 1, except 200 ml medium in Corning 150 cm^2 flasks.
[e]Exposure to ketoconazole 4 d, amastigotes grown and exposed in J774.A1 cells and isolated by the methods of Chang et al.[17] and Berman et al.[4].

Table 3. Changes in population growth and free sterol content with time of exposure of L. mexicana mexicana[a] promastigotes to ketoconazole.

Sterol identity[b]	Day - 1		Day - 2		Day - 3	
	Free sterols (% total)[c]					
	Control	Keto[d]	Control	Keto	Control	Keto
Exogenous; cholesterol	40	46	38	39	29	25
Endogenous; 14α-desmethyl						
Cholesta-series	6	1	7	2	10	2
Ergosta-series	54	14	55	8	61	3
Endogenous; 14α-methyl						
14α-Monomethyl		7		5		9
4α,14α-Dimethyl		26		38		46
4,4,14α-Trimethyl		6		8		15
Population growth (% control)[e]		87		60		48

[a]MHOM/PA/80/WR227
[b]GLC and GC/MS as described in Table 2.
[c]Obtained and analyzed as described in Table 2.
[d]Ketoconazole 1 μg ml^{-1}.
[e]Promastigotes cultured as described in Table 2.

Table 4. Population growth and free sterol content of Leishmania[a] promastigotes continuously exposed to ketoconazole.

Sterol identity[b]	Free sterols (% total)[c]					
	L. trop. L75		L. aeth. L100		L.m. mex. M379	
	Control	Keto[d]	Control	Keto[d]	Control	Keto[d]
Exogenous; cholesterol	23	38	16	43	15	22
Endogenous; 14α-desmethyl						
Cholesta-series	1		1		2	1
Ergosta-series	67		74	1	79	
Stigmasta-series	5	2	1	1	2	
Endogenous; 14α-methyl						
14α-Monomethyl		16		2		6
4α,14α-Dimethyl	4	40	8	53	2	70
4,4,14α-Trimethyl		4				1
Population growth (% control)[e]		57		45		53

[a]MHOM/IQ/65/L75, MHOM/ET/72/L100, MNYC/BZ/62/M379.
[b]GLC and GC/MS as described in Table 2.
[c]Obtained and analyzed as described in Table 2.
[d]Ketoconazole 1 μg ml^{-1}.
[e]Cultured as described in Tables 1 & 2; subcultured weekly for 9 weeks in 10 ml medium; subculture #10 in 200 ml medium, 5 d; initial population for all cultures 10^6 ml^{-1}. Populations based upon averages of triplicate samples, Coulter Counter.

Ketoconazole[12], itraconazole[13] and fluconazole[15] all display selective toxicity. They are much more active against fungal cytochrome P-450$_{14DM}$ than against the vertebrate enzyme. This would appear to be the case for ketoconazole and the leishmanial enzyme as well. The imidazole impairs the survival of amastigotes in human monocyte derived macrophages[9] and the sterol biosynthesis of amastigotes in murine macrophage tumor cells[4] at concentrations which are not cytotoxic to the host macrophages. Itraconazole, however, was cytotoxic to human monocyte derived macrophages[9] at a concentration as low as 2 µg ml^{-1}. Fluconazole was not cytotoxic at 32 µg ml^{-1}; however, at that concentration it had little effect on amastigote survival[9].

It is generally agreed that the fungistatic action of the azole drugs is caused primarily by their ability to bind to cytochrome P-450$_{14DM}$ and occupy the site normally occupied by lanosterol[12,14]. The formation of ergosterol is blocked thereby, and lanosterol and the 14α-methyl sterol products of its subsequent metabolism accumulate[12,18,19]. Coincidentally, the ergosterol content falls. The cessation of ergosterol biosynthesis has been attributed exclusively to the termination of the formation of the immediate precursors of ergosterol by the inhibition of lanosterol 14α-demethylation. An additional reason may now be considered with the report[20] that inhibition of lanosterol 14α-demethylation in cholesterol biosynthesis, by low concentrations of ketoconazole, is accompanied by the formation of polar sterols that inhibit HMG-CoA reductase, and the presence of HMG-CoA reductase in yeast[21]. Regulatory oxysterols are believed to be generated from the 14α-methyl sterols accumulated as a consequence of the inhibition of cytochrome P-450$_{14DM}$.

The loss of the normal endogenous sterols of leishmanias, the coincident accumulation of 14α-methyl sterols, and the temporal and dose dependent linkage of those events with growth inhibition, suggest a cause and effect relationship. The means by which the radical changes in sterol composition influence growth and reproduction are unknown; however, recent developments in the general study of sterol functions suggest a number of possibilities[22-26]. It is now recognized that sterols have at least two general roles. One, often referred to as the "bulk membrane" function is biophysical in nature and is performed by the cellular free sterols, positioned in the plasma membrane lipid bilayer, with their β-hydroxy groups in the hydrophylic domain and their side chains in the hydrophobic domain. In that site sterols with a wide variety of structures act as spacers between bilayer phospholipids and interact with the phospholipid fatty acyl groups. They buffer against changes in bilayer ordering and help maintain the passive and active barrier properties of the membrane. A second and more recently recognized role, the "metabolic" function, has a more biochemical connotation, though it may not be entirely divorced from the biophysical role, since many enzymes are membrane associated and depend for their activities on the state of ordering of the lipid bilayer. The "metabolic" function is served by smaller amounts of sterols and the sterols must have quite specific structures.

Azole inhibited leishmanias contain large amounts of endogenous 14α-methyl sterols and cholesterol from the culture medium, and small amounts of endogenous C_{28} and C_{29} sterols with ring system and side chain double bonds at positions 5(6), 7(8), 22(23) and 24(28). It would appear from the ability of some leishmanias to continue to reproduce at a rate ~50% of normal in the presence of ketoconazole (1 µg ml^{-1}) for two months, that the 14α-methyl sterols and cholesterol may perform the "bulk membrane" role and the remaining small amount of normal endogenous sterol a "metabolic" role. Sterols with a 14α-methyl group are believed to disorder membrane lipid bilayers as a consequence of the protrusion of the 14α-methyl group from the sterol α-face, compromising sterol interactions with the paraffin chains of the fatty acyl groups of lipid bilayer phospholipids[27]. Consequently, the inhibited growth of azole treated leishmanias is probably a reflection of the imperfect performance of both

leishmanias is probably a reflection of the imperfect performance of both "bulk membrane" and "metabolic" sterol functions.

REFERENCES

1. G. G. Holz, Jr., Lipids of leishmanias, in "Leishmaniasis," K.-P. Chang and R. S. Bray, eds., Elsevier, Amsterdam (1984).
2. L. J. Goad, G. G. Holz, Jr., and D. H. Beach, Sterols of Leishmania species. Implications for biosynthesis, Mol. Biochem. Parasitol. 10:161 (1984).
3. L. J. Goad, G. G. Holz, Jr., and D. H. Beach, Sterols of ketoconazole-inhibited Leishmania mexicana mexicana promastigotes, Mol. Biochem. Parasitol. 15:257 (1985).
4. J. D. Berman, L. J. Goad, D. H. Beach, and G. G. Holz, Jr, Effects of ketoconazole on sterol biosynthesis by Leishmania mexicana mexicana amastigotes in murine macrophage tumor cells, Mol. Biochem. Parasitol. 20:85 (1986).
5. J. Heeres, L. J. J. Backx, J. H. Mostmans, and J. M. Van Cutsem, The synthesis and antifungal activity of ketoconazole, a new potent orally active broad spectrum antifungal agent, J. Med. Chem. 22:1003 (1979).
6. J. Van Cutsem, F. Van Gerven, R. Zaman, J. Heeres, and P. A. J. Janssen, Pharmacological and preclinical results with a new oral and topical broad-spectrum antifungal, R 51 211, in "Proceedings 13th International Congress of Chemotherapy," K. H. Spitzy and K. Karrer, eds., Verlag H. Egermann, Vienna (1983).
7. K. Richardson, K. W. Brammer, M. S. Marriott, and P. F. Troke, Activity of UK-49,858, a bis-triazole derivative, against experimental infections with Candida albicans and Trichophyton mentagrophytes, Antimicrob. Agents Chemother., 27:832 (1985).
8. J. D. Berman, G. G. Holz, Jr., and D. H. Beach, Effects of ketoconazole on growth and sterol biosynthesis of Leishmania promastigotes in culture, Mol. Biochem. Parasitol. 12:1 (1984).
9. J. D. Berman, and J. V. Gallalee, In vitro antileishmanial activity of inhibitors of steroid biosynthesis and combinations of antileishmanial agents, J. Parasitol. 73:671 (1987).
10. C. E. Hughes, R. L. Bennett, and W. H. Beggs, Broth dilution testing of Candida albicans susceptibility to ketoconazole, Antimicrob. Agents Chemother. 31:643 (1987).
11. L. J. Goad, G. G. Holz, Jr., and D. H. Beach, Effect of the allylamine antifungal drug SF 86-327 on the growth and sterol synthesis of Leishmania mexicana mexicana promastigotes, Biochem. Pharmacol. 34:3785 (1985).
12. H. Vanden Bossche, Biochemical targets for antifungal azole derivatives: Hypothesis on the mode of action, in "Current topics in medical mycology," Vol. 1, M. R. McGinnis, ed., Springer-Verlag, Berlin (1985).
13. H. Vanden Bossche, H. Willemsens, P. Marichal, W. Cooks, and W. Lauwers, The molecular basis for the antifungal activities of N-substituted azole derivatives. Focus on R 51 211, in "Mode of action of antifungal agents," J. Ryley and A. P. J. Trinci, eds., Cambridge University Press, Cambridge (1984).
14. Y. Yoshida, and Y. Aoyama, Interaction of azole fungicides with yeast cytochrome P-450 which catalyzes lanosterol 14α-demethylation, in "In vitro and in vivo evaluation of antifungal agents," K. Iwata and H. Vanden Bossche, eds., Elsevier, Amsterdam (1986).

15. M. S. Marriott, G. W. Pye, K. Richardson, and P. F. Troke, The activity of fluconazole (UK-49,858), a novel bis-triazole antifungal and ketoconazole against fungal and mammalian sterol C14 demethylases, in "In vitro and in vivo evaluation of antifungal agents," K. Iwata and H. Vanden Bossche, eds., Elsevier, Amsterdam (1986).
16. E. T. Takafuji, L. D. Hendricks, J. L. Daubek, K. M. McNeil, H. M. Scagliola, and C. L. Diggs, Cutaneous leishmaniasis associated with jungle training, Am. J. Trop. Med. 29:516 (1980).
17. K.-P. Chang, C. A. Nacy, and R. D. Pearson, Intracellular parasitism of macrophages in leishmaniasis: In vitro systems and their applications, Meth. Enzymol. 132:603 (1986).
18. D. Kerridge, Mode of action of clinically important antifungal drugs, Adv. Microb. Physiol. 27:1 (1986).
19. J. D. Weete, Mechanism of fungal growth inhibition by inhibitors of ergosterol biosynthesis, in "Role of lipids in interactions of plants with pests and pathogens," G. Fuller and W. D. Nes, eds., Am. Chem. Soc. Symp. Ser., Washington (1986).
20. A. Gupta, R. C. Sexton, and H. Rudney, Modulation of regulatory oxysterol formation and low density lipoprotein suppression of 3-hydroxy-3-methylglutaryl Coenzyme A (HMG-CoA) reductase activity by ketoconazole. A role for cytochrome p-450 in the regulation of HMG-CoA reductase in rat intestinal epithelial cells, J. Biol. Chem. 261:8343 (1986).
21. P. J. Trocha, and D. B. Sprinson, Location and regulation of early enzymes of sterol biosynthesis in yeast, Arch. Biochem. Biophys. 174:45 (1976).
22. W. J. Pinto, and W. R. Nes, Stereochemical specificity for sterols in Saccharomyces cerevisiae, J. Biol. Chem. 258:4472 (1983).
23. M. Ramgopal, and K. Bloch, Sterol synergism in yeast, J. Biol. Chem. 80:712 (1983).
24. J. S. Dahl, and C. E. Dahl, Coordinate regulation of unsaturated phospholipid, RNA and protein synthesis in Mycoplasma capricolum by cholesterol, Proc. Natl. Acad. Sci. USA 80:692 (1983).
25. R. J. Rodriguez, C. Low, C. D. K. Bottema, and L. W. Parks, Multiple functions for sterols in Saccharomyces cerevisiae, Biochim. Biophys. Acta 837:336 (1985).
26. C. Dahl, H.-P. Biemann, and J. Dahl, A protein kinase antigenically related to pp60^{v-src} possibly involved in yeast cell cycle control: Positive in vivo regulation by sterol, Proc. Natl. Acad. Sci. USA 84:4012 (1987).
27. K. E. Bloch, Sterol structure and membrane function, CRC Crit. Rev. Biochem. 14:47 (1983).

EFFECT OF RIBOSOME-INACTIVATING PROTEINS ON RIBOSOMES
FROM LEISHMANIA AND THEIR POSSIBLE USES IN CHEMOTHERAPY

Pietro Cenini[*] and Fiorenzo Stirpe

Dipartimento di Patologia sperimentale
Università di Bologna
I-40126 Bologna (Italy)

INTRODUCTION

Ribosome-inactivating proteins (RIPs) (1-5) are a group of glycoproteins of plant origin whose biological role is unknown but which possess the peculiarity of inactivating mammalian ribosomes by cleaving the N-glycosidic bond of adenine$_{4324}$ of 28 S rRNA (6,7). RIPs have been found in a great variety of plants and their concentration can vary dramatically between different species (8-10). In some plant families many species contain them in particulary high concentrations and they are purified in large quantities from an ever increasing number of different plants (11).

RIPs can be divided into type 1, which are single-chain proteins, and type 2 (ricin and related toxins) which present an additional galactose-binding chain linked by a disulphide bridge to the ribosome-inactivating one.

Although both types of RIPs are potent inhibitors of ribosome activity in a cell-free system, RIPs type 1 are characterized by a low toxicity to intact cells since, lacking the carbohydrate-binding chain, they have difficulty in binding to the cell membrane and consequently in entering the cytoplasm. However once entered the cell RIPs type 1 are very potent cell killers. As far as toxicity for whole animals is concerned, RIPs type 2 are very toxic while RIPs type 1 generally present a lower in vivo toxicity. The easier preparation in large quantities and absence of problems of contamination with residual intact toxin make RIPs type 1 better candidates for chemotherapic purposes if compared to isolated ribosome-inactivating chains of RIPs type 2.

In the numerous studies carried out in recent years RIPs have been considered for possible uses in chemotherapy (i) as native proteins (without modifications, exploiting differences in toxicity for different cell types) (12), (ii) after some minor modifications (e.g. binding to a carbohydrate, in order to modulate their capacity to enter cells) (13), or (iii) after some major modifications. The latter consist either in their

---

[*]Fellow of the Fondazione Donegani

insertion into liposomes (14), reconstituted Sendai virus envelops (15) or erythrocyte ghosts (16), with consequent enhanced delivery into the cytoplasm and therefore increased toxicity, or in their conjugation to lectins (17), neoglycoproteins (18) or antibodies (19,20), the latter case resulting in the formation of 'immunotoxins' specifically toxic for the cell target of the antibody used.

In the great majority of attempts to use RIPs in chemotherapy the targets of the RIPs were mammalian cells, and the current interest lies mainly in the cure of cancer. The effect of RIPs on mammalian ribosomes is in fact well documented, while little is known as far as ribosomes from other organisms are concerned. However it has been recently shown that ribosomes from organisms phylogenetically very distant from mammals, like fungi and protozoa, can also be inactivated by RIPs (5,21,22).

Amongst protozoa, only two species, namely Acanthamoeba castellanii and Tetrahymena pyriformis, has been so far investigated in this respect. In both cases ribosomes were found to be sensitive to the effect of some although not all of the RIPs used, the intensity of the effect varying greatly from one RIP to the other and, for the same RIP, between the two different species (unpublished data).

These results indicate that most likely some RIPs will be also effective on other protozoan species, hopefully including the ones which are causes of major parasitic diseases. Thus RIPs should be regarded as substances potentially very useful as antiparasitic agents whose possible applications are however still unexplored.

Leishmaniasis represent one of the major parasitic diseases caused by a protozoa for which a definitive drug is still to be found. In addition, Leishmania can be grown, at least at the promastigote stage, in quantities large enough to allow purification of ribosomes for biochemical studies. As a first step in investigating the possibility of using RIPs against a certain protozoa it is in fact necessary to know whether they actually affect its ribosomes and which are the ones most active.

MATERIALS AND METHODS

Parasites

Leishmania infantum promastigotes were obtained from the Istituto Superiore di Sanita' (Rome) and kept in logaritmic growth phase in Evans Modified Tobie's Medium (23) at 24 °C. When a large number of parasites were needed for ribosome purification, promastigotes were passed into 750 ml flasks containing 60 ml of RPMI 1640 supplemented with 30% FCS, and were then harvested at a concentration of 3×10^7 /ml.

RIPs

Viscumin was kindly provided by Dr. P. Ziska, Berlin (DDR). Trichokirin was extracted from seeds of Trichosanthes kirilowii as described by Barbieri et al.(11, and unpublished data). All other RIPs were prepared as in the respective references: momordin (24), gelonin (17), dianthin 30 and dianthin 32 (25), pokeweed antiviral protein from seed (PAP-S) (26), Hordeum vulgare RIP (barley inhibitor) (27), saporin 6 and saporin 9 (28), bryodin (29), ricin (30), abrin (31), modeccin (32) and volkensin (33). Immediately before preforming the protein synthesis assays the sugar binding chains of RIPs type 2 where separated from the ribosome-inactivating chains by incubation for 1 h at 37°C with 1% 2-mercaptoethanol.

Ribosomes

All procedures were carried out at 2-4 °C as quickly as possible. Parasites were harvested by centrifugation at 2,500 g for 15 min, resuspended in 20 ml of buffer solution (20 mM HEPES pH 7.6, 4 mM magnesium acetaacetate, 100 mM KCl, 6 mM 2-mercaptoethanol, 0.25 M RNAse-free sucrose and 1 mg/ml heparin) and disrupted by sonication. The crude sonicate was centrifuged for 10 min at 9,000 g and the supernatant after a further centrifugation at 20,000 g for 20 min was laid on the buffer solution described above in which the concentration of sucrose was increased to 1.8 M while the heparin was omitted. After spinning at 105,000 g for 4 h, ribosomes were resuspended in buffer solution (now without both sucrose and heparin) and their concentration was determined according to Montanaro et al. (34) and adjusted as required. Ribosomes were then immediately used in the in vitro protein synthesis assay. A total of 3×10^{10} promastigotes will yield about 3 mg of ribosomes in a good preparation.

In vitro protein synthesis assay

Ribosome activity was measured by an in vitro polyphenylalanine synthesis assay performed essentially as described by Montanaro et al. (34). Optimal reaction conditions (time, concentrations of ribosomes, magnesium and potassium) were determined by preliminary experiments. The reaction was carried out for 45 min at 24 °C in 100 µl volumes containing 80 mM Tris/HCl buffer pH 7.4, 60 mM KCl, 10 mM magnesium acetate, 2 mM dithiothreitol, 2 mM GTP, 80 µg poly(U), 10 µl of Artemia salina supernatant, $^{14}[C]$-phenylalanyl-tRNA (15,000 d.p.m.), 36 µg of ribosomes and RIPs in scalar concentrations. At the end of the reaction trichloroacetic acid-insoluble radioactivity was measured according to Montanaro et al. (34), and values of zero-time blanks (15-42 d.p.m.) were subtracted. Results are expressed as inhibitor dose 50 (ID_{50}, concentration giving 50% inhibition), which was calculated by linear regression analysis.

Whole protozoa experiments

Promastigotes in logaritmic growth phase were incubated in 24-well plates (250 µl/well; 2.5×10^5 promastigotes/well) for 24 h at 24°C in the absence or presence of the RIPs previously found to be active on isolated ribosomes (1 mg/ml). The culture medium was RPMI 1640 supplemented after the first hour of incubation with 10% FCS. Parasites were radiolabelled at the beginning of the culture by addition to each well of 0.6 µCi of $^{3}[H]$-leucine (specific activity 70 Ci/mM). Triplicate samples were run for each RIP and for controls, and radioactivity at the end of the culture was counted for 10 min in a liquid scintillation spectrometer.

RESULTS

The effects of RIPs on Leishmania infantum ribosomes are shown in Tab.1. While half of the RIPs type 1 tested had little or no effect at the concentration used, saporin 6, saporin 9, dianthin 30, dianthin 32 and PAP-S strongly inhibited in vitro polyphenylalanine synthesis. Amongst RIPs type 2, only the ribosome-inactivating chain of abrin was found to be very active on Leishmania ribosomes. No RIP at the concentration of 1 mg/ml (33.3 µM for type 1 and 17 µM for type 2) was found to hamper the growth of Leishmania promastigotes in culture.

Table 1. Effect of RIPs on in vitro polyphenylalanine synthesis by ribosomes from Leishmania infantum

RIP added	ID_{50} (µM)	RIP added	ID_{50} (µM)
Momordin	>3.330	Saporin 6	0.033
Gelonin	2.590	Saporin 9	0.031
Dianthin 30	0.110		
Dianthin 32	0.027	Ricin	>1.700
PAP-S	0.021	Abrin	0.005
Barley inhibitor	3.330	Modeccin	1.700
Bryodin	>3.330	Viscumin	>1.700
Trichokirin	>3.330	Volkensin	1.700

DISCUSSION

Leishmania infantum ribosomes can be inactivated by RIPs, so indicating that RIPs are potentially useful in the preparation of drugs against Leishmania. The fact that several RIPs type 1 are effective on Leishmania ribosomes is a fortunate circumstance, since these proteins offer several advantages over the ribosome-inactivating chains of toxins. However, the isolated ribosome-inactivating chain of abrin should also be taken into consideration for the preparation of immunotoxins on account of its marked inhibitory effect on leishmanial ribosomes.

The lack of action of RIPs on whole promastigotes indicates that RIPs have difficulty in entering Leishmania cells and that some devise which would facilitate their entrance must be found. However this might not necessarily be the case for extra-macrophagic amastigotes, and studies which would enlighten this point are required. In any case, the use of an immunotoxin made with one of the RIPs here found to be effective on Leishmania ribosome should overcome the problem, as suggested by similar studies on Acanthamoeba castellanii (35).

Comparative studies on ribosomes from Trypanosoma brucei indicate a similarity in the effects of RIPs in the two species of Kinetoplastida (unpublished data). This strongly suggests that the effects of RIPs on ribosomes from different species of the same genus Leishmania are likely to be very similar, and that RIPs should therefore be regarded as potential antiparasitic drugs in the cure of all types of leishmaniasis.

CONCLUSIONS

In this study the possibility of using RIPs against Leishmania was investigated. Ribosomes from Leishmania infantum was purified and the effect of RIPs was tested using a polyphenylalanine polymerization assay. Amongst RIPs type 2 (two chain), only abrin was found to effectively.inhibit the reaction catalized by Leishmania ribosomes, whereas ricin, modeccin, viscumin and volkensin showed no or little effect. Five of the ten RIPs type 1 (single-chain) tested were found to inactivate Leishmania ribosomes (PAP-S, saporin 6, saporin 9, dianthin 32 and, less effectively, dianthin 30) and therefore, together with the ribosome-inactivating chain of abrin, are suitable for the preparation of immunotoxins against Leishmania. Although the results reported here refer to Leishmania infantum, there is indication that RIPs should be also effective in a similar way on ribosomes from the other Leishmania species.

ACKNOWLEDGMENTS

We thank Dr. A. Bolognesi and Prof. L. Barbieri for the preparation of RIPs, Drs. L. Gradoni and M. Gramiccia, Istituto Superiore di Sanita', Rome, for originally providing us with the parasites and with advice on their growth, and Dr. M. Cipone, Istituto di Patologia speciale e Clinica Medica Veterinaria, Bologna, for providing the horse blood. This work was supported by grants from the Ministero della Pubblica Istruzione, Rome, and by a contract from the Commission of the European Communities, Biotechnology Action Programme.

REFERENCES

1. S. Olnes and A. Phil, Toxic lectins and related proteins, in: 'Molecular action of toxins and viruses', P. Cohen and S. van Heyningen, eds., Elsevier, Amsterdam, New York (1982).
2. L. Barbieri and F. Stirpe, Ribosome-inactivating proteins from plant: properties and possible uses, Cancer Surveys 1: 489 (1982).
3. A. Jimenez and D. Vazquez, Plant and fungal protein and glycoprotein toxin inhibiting eukaryote protein synthesis, Ann.Rev.Microbiol. 39: 649 (1985).
4. F. Stirpe and L. Barbieri, Ribosome-inactivating proteins up to date, FEBS Lett. 195: 1 (1986).
5. W.K. Roberts and C.P. Selitrennikoff. Plant proteins that inactivate foreign ribosomes, Biosci.Rep. 6: 19 (1986).
6. Y. Endo, K. Mitsui, M. Motizuki and K. Tsurugi, The mechanism of action of ricin and related toxic lectins on eukaryotic ribosomes, J.Biol.Chem. 262: 5908 (1987).
7. Y. Endo and K. Tsurugi, RNA N-glycosidase activity of ricin A-chain, J.Biol.Chem. 262: 8128 (1987).
8. A. Gasperi-Campani, L. Barbieri, E. Lorenzoni and F. Stirpe, Inhibition of protein synthesis by seed-extracts. A screening study, FEBS Lett. 76: 173 (1977).

9. A. Gasperi-Campani, L. Barbieri, P. Morelli and F. Stirpe, Seed ex-extracts inhibiting protein synthesis in vitro, Biochem. J. 186: 439 (1980).
10. A. Gasperi-Campani, L. Barbieri, M.G. Battelli and F. Stirpe, On the distribution of ribosome-inactivating proteins amongst plants, J. Nat.Prod. 48: 446 (1985).
11. L. Barbieri, C. Stoppa and A. Bolognesi, Large scale chromatographic purification of ribosome-inactivating proteins, J.Chromat. (in the press).
12. F. Spreafico, C. Malfiore, M.L. Moras, L. Marmonti, S. Filippeschi, L. Barbieri, P. Perocco and F. Stirpe, The immunomodulatory activity of the plant proteins Momordica charantia inhibitor and pokeweed antiviral protein, Int.J.Immunopharmac. 5: 335 (1983).
13. J.T. Forbes, R.K. Bretthauer and T.N. Oeltmann, Mannose 6-, fructose 1-and fructose 6-phosphates inhibit human natural cell-mediated cytotoxicity, Proc.Natl. Acad.Sci.USA 78: 5797 (1981).
14. D.P. McIntosh and T.D.Heath, Liposome-mediated delivery of ribosome-inactivating proteins in vitro. Biochem.Biophys. Acta 690: 224 (1982).
15. M. Sangiacomo, L. Barbieri, F. Stirpe and M. Tomasi, Cytotoxicity acquired by ribosome-inactivating proteins carried by reconstituted Sendai virus envelopes, FEBS Lett. 157: 150 (1983).
16. B. Foxwell, J. Long and F. Stirpe, Cytotoxicity of erythrocyte ghosts loaded with ribosome-inactivated proteins following fusion with CHO cells, Biochem.Int. 8: 811 (1984).
17. F. Stirpe, S. Olsnes and A. Pihl, Gelonin, a new inhibitor of protein synthesis, non toxic to intact cells. Isolation, characterization and preparation of cytotoxic conjugates with concavalin A, J.Biol.Chem. 255: 6947 (1980).
18. A.C. Roche, M. Barzilay, S. Midoux, N. Sharon and M. Monsigny, Sugar-specific endocytosis of glycoproteins by Lewis lung carcinoma cells, J.Cell Biochem. 22: 131 (1983).
19. E.S. Vitella and J.W. Uhr, Immunotoxins, Ann.Rev.Immunol. 3: 197 (1985).
20. A.E. Frankel, L.L. Houston, B.F. Issell and G.Fatham, Prospects for immunotoxin therapy in cancer, Ann.Rev.Med. 37:125 (1986).
21. M.D. Howell and C.L. Villemez, Toxicity of ricin, diphteria toxin and alpha-amanitin for Acanthamoeba castellanii, J.Parasitol. 70: 918 (1984).
22. C.L. Villemez, M.A. Russell. L. Barbieri, F. Stirpe, J.D. Irvin and J. D. Robertus, Catalytic toxins for the preparation of protozoan immunotoxins, in: 'Membrane-mediate cytotoxicity', B. Bonavida and R.J. Collier, eds., Alan R. Liss, New York (1987).
23. D.A. Evans, Kinetoplastida, in: 'Methods of cultivating parasites in vitro', A.E.R. Taylor and J.R. Baker, eds., Academic Press, London, New York, San Francisco (1978).
24. L. Barbieri, M. Zamboni, L. Montanaro, S. Sperti and F. Stirpe, Purification and properties of different forms of modeccin, the toxin of Adenia digitata. Separation of subunits with inhibitory and lectin activity, Biochem.J. 185: 203 (1980).

25. F. Stirpe, D.G. Williams, L.J. Onyon, R.F. Legg and W.A. Stevens, Dianthins, ribosome-damaging proteins with antiviral properties from Dianthus caryophyllus L. (carnation), Biochem.J. 195: 339 (1981).
26. L. Barbieri, G.M. Aron, J.D. Irvin and F. Stirpe, Purification and partial characterization of another form of the antiviral protein from the seeds of Phytolacca americana L. (pokeweed), Biochem.J. 203: 55 (1982).
27. K. Asano, B. Svensson and F.M. Poulsen, Isolation and characterization of inhibitors of animal cell-free protein synthesis from barley seeds, Carlsberg Res.Commun. 49: 619 (1984).
28. F. Stirpe, A. Gasperi-Campani, L. Barbieri, A. Falasca, A. Abbondanza and W.A. Stevens, Ribosome-inactivating proteins from the seeds of Saponaria officinalis L. (soapwort), of Agrostemma githago L. (corn cockle) and of Asparagus officinalis L. (asparagus) and from the latex of Hura crepitans L. (sandbox tree), Biochem.J. 216: 617 (1983).
29. F. Stirpe, L. Barbieri, M.G. Battelli, A. Falasca, E. Lorenzoni and W.A. Stevens, Bryodin, a ribosome-inactivating protein from the roots of Bryonia dioica L. (white bryony), Biochem.J. 240: 659 (1986).
30. G.L. Nicolson, J. Blaustein and M. Etzler, Characterization of two plant lectins from Ricinus communis and their quantitative interaction with a murine lymphoma, Biochem. 13: 196 (1974).
31. C.H. Wei, F.C. Hartman, P. Pfuderer and W.-K. Yang, Purification and characterization of two major toxic proteins from seeds of Abrus precatorius, J.Biol.Chem. 249: 3061 (1974).
32. A. Gasperi-Campani, L. Barbieri, E. Lorenzoni, L. Montanaro, S. Sperti, E. Bonetti and F. Stirpe, Modeccin, the toxin of Adenia digitata. Purification toxicity and inhibition of protein synthesis in vitro. Biochem.J. 174: 493 (1978).
33. F. Stirpe, L. Barbieri, A. Abbondanza, A. Falasca, A.N.F. Brown, K. Sandvig, S. Olsnes and A. Pihl, Properties of volkensin, a toxic lectin from Adenia volkensii, J.Biol.Chem. 260: 14589 (1985).
34. L. Montanaro, S. Sperti, M. Zamboni, M. Denaro, G. Testoni, A. Gasperi-Campani and F. Stirpe, Effect of modeccin on the steps of peptide-chain elongation, Biochem.J. 176: 371 (1978).
35. C.L. Villemez and P.L. Carlo, Preparation of an immunotoxin for Acanthamoeba castellanii, Biochem.Biophys.Res.Commun. 125: 25 (1984).

LEISHMANIASIS-AIDS: FAILURE TO RESPOND TO CHEMOTHERAPY

J. Alvar

Centro Nacional de Microbiologia
Virologia & Immunologia Sanitarias
Madrid
Spain

INTRODUCTION
This report is a retrospective analysis of the visceral leishmaniasis cases diagnosed in our laboratory. In the last four years we have diagnosed 62 VL cases from several regions in Spain. Eleven cases (18% of the total) were VL associated with AIDS. The geographical location was closely related to the normal epidemiological distribution of the disease.

RESULTS AND DISCUSSION
According to the serology, we can distinguish two groups: the first one, those (3 cases) with no antibodies against *Leishmania*. These types of response are probably related to both the moment when the individual was infected and the relative impairment of their immune system. No matter when putative infection started, relapses with no apparent response to the normally adequate therapy were common and independent of the drug used. Most of the patients in which the follow up was possible, died some months after the beginning of the symptoms.

To illustrate this point, I would like to describe a clinical history: A thirtyeight year old woman, drug addict, was diagnosed in February 1984 as having hepatitis B and visceral leishmaniasis. She was treated according to standard WHO protocol, with two cycles of Glucantime. Nine months later, in November 1984, she developed fever, splenomegaly, etc. Then, she was treated with Pentamidine, but developed renal failure. Chemotherapy was suspended while she was treated for the kidney complaint. Three months later, in February 1985, the leishmaniasis infection remained unchecked and the strain was isolated in order to monitor its drug sensitivity. The strain showed resistance to Glucantime and a high sensitivity to Ketoconazol and to a lesser degree Amphotericin B. In April 1985 Ketoconazol treatment was started, although its normal use is for cutaneous leishmaniasis. No response was noted and finally treatment with Amphotericine B was started. In August, when the number of parasites had decreased, the patient died of a heroin overdose.

In recent work (Haidaris and Bonventre), T-cell mediated immune responses seem to enhance chemotherapeutic treatment. This could explain the continuous chemotherapeutic failures in HIV positive-patients and their resultant relapses.

LIPOSOMES AND OTHER DRUG DELIVERY SYSTEMS IN THE TREATMENT OF LEISHMANIASIS

S.L. Croft[1], R.A. Neal[2], and L.S. Rao[3]

[1]Department of Biochemical Microbiology, Wellcome Research Laboratories, Beckenham, Kent, U.K.
[2]Department of Medical Protozoology, London School of Hygiene and Tropical Medicine, 395 Hatfield Road St. Albans, Herts, U.K.
[3]Pharmaceutical Development, The Wellcome Foundation Dartford, Kent, U.K.

INTRODUCTION

The identification of a compound showing selective toxicity for a parasite, as determined by biochemical or *in vitro* screening techniques is the first important stage in the development of a new drug. However, the compound must still show that selective anti-parasite activity *in vivo* at a specific site(s) of infection whilst contending with a range of pharmacological factors (e.g. absorption, metabolism, distribution).

To ensure that an effective drug concentration is achieved at the appropriate site of action various delivery systems for (a) sustained drug release and (b) drug targeting have been developed. Most studies with anti-protozoal drugs have concentrated upon specific targeting using carriers to increase the drug concentration at the site of infection, thus improving efficacy whilst reducing the dose and possible adverse effects. Liposomes are perhaps the best known system and have been used widely in the delivery of anti-parasitic drugs (1) but a range of other molecular, particulate, vesicular and cellular carriers have been studied (Table 1). It is in the treatment of visceral leishmaniasis that drug targeting is most likely to produce clinical benefits in the future.

TABLE 1 Targeting of Drugs to Leishmania infections in Experimental Models

Parasite	Drug Delivery System	Drug	Comment	References
Leishmania donovani	liposomes	sodium stibogluconate meglumine antimoniate (MA)	200-700 fold enhanced activity	2,3,4
		amphotericin B + other antifungals	2-4.5 fold enhanced activity	5,6
		WR6026	11.4 fold enhanced activity	7
		other antimicrobials	—	7,8
		muramyl dipeptide + free MA	prophylactic and therapeutic effects	9
		muramyl dipetide	effective	10
	erythrocytes	pentamidine	enhanced activity in vitro and in vivo	11,12
		formycin A	42 fold increase in activity in vitro	13
	niosomes	sodium stibogluconate	—	14
	nanoparticles	dihydroemetine chloride	—	15
	starch microparticles	primaquine	in vitro	16
		sodium stibogluconate	in vivo 100 fold increase in activity	17
	LDL	daunorubicin	in vitro	18
Leishmania major Leishmania mexicana	liposomes	sodium stibogluconate	i.v. route more effective than s.c. route against established lesions	19
Leishmania tropica (= major)	liposomes	amphotericin B	no enhanced activity	20

VISCERAL LEISHMANIASIS

Liposomes and antimonial drugs

A major limitation upon the use of vesicular, cellular and particulate carriers is that following parenteral administration they are normally removed from the blood rapidly and almost exclusively by cells of the reticulo-endothelial system (RES), in particular macrophages of the liver and spleen. Although the distribution can be altered by a number of methods this limitation makes visceral leishmaniasis the ideal disease for passive drug targeting. During 1977-1978 groups in London, Liverpool and Washington showed that antimonials, including sodium stibogluconate ('Pentostam', Wellcome) and meglumine antimoniate ('Glucantime', Rhodia), when encapsulated in liposomes were 200-700 fold more effective than the free drug when comparing single i.v. doses against L.donovani in rodent models (2,3,4). The drugs are entrapped in the aqueous phase of these multi-lamellar phospholipid vesicles. The greatly enhanced efficacy is due, in part, to the direct delivery to the parasitized cells and the lysosomotropic route of the loaded liposomes to the required intracellular site - the parasitophorous vacuole (21,22). Also following liposomal delivery antimony levels in the liver and spleen of mice were 5-20 fold higher than that achieved by free drug and were maintained for up to 14 days (3,23). The slow release of antimony from the liposomes and the long term hepatic and splenic deposition obviously contribute to the improved efficacy. These studies have been reviewed in detail elsewhere (24,25). Liposome-meglumine antimoniate preparations were less effective against virulent L.donovani infections in hamsters in the presence of tissue damage (26).

Wellcome's Liposomal Pentostam

The problems associated with the commercial production of a novel drug delivery system, including liposomal Pentostam, have been reviewed in detail (27,28). Relevant considerations are (a) the feasibility and cost of large scale production (b) characterisation and control of constituent components (c) sterility of production (d) high level of drug encapsulation (e) correct distribution and efficacy of drug-carrier system (f) stability and long shelf-life (h) pharmacology and toxicology to satisfy the requirements of regulatory bodies.

Liposomal Pentostam is prepared by a reverse phase evaporation procedure using synthetic dipalmitoylphosphatidylcholine, cholesterol and dicetyl phosphate in a 9:9:2 molar ratio. Following drug encapsulation the liposomal preparation is dispersed in a 1.8% salt solution (29). The distribution of the liposomes containing ^{125}Sb-sodium stibogluconate was examined in rats following i.v. administration by gamma scintigraphy, indicating a localisation in the liver and spleen (30). Following an injection of the liposomal formulation, 50% of the ^{125}Sb-Pentostam was retained in the body after 40 hours and 40% was still present after 120 hours, whereas 50% of the free drug was removed from the body in 2 hours and 67% in 18 hours. The study also showed that 25% of the free drug was distributed in the liver and spleen whereas following liposomal delivery 40% was in the liver and spleen at 20 hours and 30% at 120 hours after administration.

The efficacy of the Wellcome liposomal Pentostam preparation is comparable with that found in other studies (2,3,4). In the L.donovani-BALB/c mouse model the liposomal formulation was 350 times as active as free drug when comparing single i.v. doses on the basis of ED_{50} values (Table 2). Comparison of five doses on consecutive days showed that liposomal Pentostam was 22-33 fold as active as the free drug. The difference in degree of efficacy when comparing single and multiple doses probably relates to (a) the improved pharmacokinetic profile of free Pentostam following multiple dosing in comparison with an optimum profile achieved by the liposomal preparation after a single delivery and (b) possible detrimental effects of a multi-dose liposome regimen to macrophages including RES blockade and toxicity due to antimonial levels. Previous studies on liposome efficacy have been based upon comparisons of single doses of free and encapsulated drug. To establish whether a second or third dose of liposomal Pentostam gives improved cure over one dose, a series of experiments was carried out in vitro in an amastigote-macrophage model and in vivo in BALB/c mice (Table 3). The results show that on the basis of a comparison of ED_{50} values a second or third dose of liposomal Pentostam does not increase the killing of amastigotes in either in vitro or in vivo models. However, in the in vivo study the ED_{90} value is greatly reduced by a second dose given on either the day immediately after the first dose or four days later. In terms of total mg Sb^V administered the potency of the drug is halved by the second dose when comparing the ED_{50} values but increased 10 fold and 4 fold respectively on the basis of ED_{90} values by second doses given on consecutive days or separated by four days. The implication is that the top dose levels used (2.5 mg Sb^V/kg) were effective following a single administration either in killing the amastigotes directly or in loading the macrophages with sufficient antimony for subsequent killing. At the lower doses (0.1 mg Sb^V/kg and 0.02 mg Sb^V/kg) a second dose still retains efficacy.

TABLE 2 The activity of Wellcome Pentostam liposomes against L.donovani in mice and the effects of storage

Liposome preparations	Dose Regimen	ED_{50} (mg Sb^V/kg) Free	Liposomal
recent	i.v. x 1	61.2	0.17
	i.v. x 5	1.5	0.07
12 months 37°C	i.v. x 1	-	0.10
25°C	i.v. x 1	-	0.10
	s.c. x 5	5.95	-
45 months 4°C	i.v. x 1	-	0.26
	s.c. x 5	17.05	-

A series of studies also examined the stability of the liposomal Pentostam formulation as measured by efficacy in the mouse model. In these experiments a single dose of liposomes administered i.v. was compared with five doses of free Pentostam administered s.c. Preparations kept at 25°C or 37°C for up to 12 months or up to 4 years at 4°C all maintained their efficacy (Table 2). This confirms that the liquid formulation fulfils the stability requirements required for commercial development as assessed biologically.

TABLE 3. Activity of Liposomal Pentostam against L.donovani following multiple dosing

In vitro (macrophage model)

	(mg Sb^V/ml)	
	ED_{50}	ED_{90}
free Pentostam (x 3)	11.25	59.33
liposomal Pentostam (x 1)	0.044	0.406
liposomal Pentostam (x 3)	0.033	0.670

In vivo (mouse model)

	(mg Sb^V/kg)	
	ED_{50}	ED_{90}
free Pentostam (s.c. x 5)	13.78	210.49
liposomal Pentostam (i.v. x 1)	0.12	46.95
liposomal Pentostam (i.v. x 2, consecutive days)	0.14	2.41
liposomal Pentosam (i.v. x 2, 4 days apart)	0.13	5.93

Other drugs in liposomes

A range of other clinically used drugs, experimental compounds and immunomodulators have been tested against L.donovani in rodent models (Table 1). The promising results achieved with amphotericin B liposomes, in which the lipophilic antifungal is incorporated into the lipid envelope, are of particular interest. This drug is occasionally used in the clinical treatment of leishmaniasis despite notable side effects. Recently amphotericin B liposomes have been successfully used in the treatment of systemic mycoses in man (31) and such a formulation is currently under commercial development by Squibb. In studies on visceral leishmaniasis the improved efficacy of encapsulated drug compared with free drug is small (2-4 fold) and the major advantage of the liposome formulation is reduced toxicity (6). In hamster and monkey models Berman et al. (5) have shown that liposomal amphotericin B is respectively 170-750 fold and 60 fold as active as meglumine antimoniate.

Other targeting systems

Although liposomes have so far been the predominant method of drug targeting to visceral leishmaniasis infections other delivery systems have been tried (Table 1). The niosome, a vesicle which has some properties similar to the liposomes, is potentially cheaper than the liposome, being made from a non-ionic surfactant, and is more stable. Niosome encapsulated sodium stibogluconate was more active than free drug against L.donovani in mice, producing a higher and longer antimony concentration in the liver, although the efficacy was not as great as that achieved by liposomal encapsulation in the other studies (14). Erythrocytes have also been studied as carriers of anti-parasitic drugs (Table 1) and may be targeted to macrophages by coating with IgG. In the L.donovani - hamster model a level of 2.5 mg/kg encapsulated pentamidine eliminated nearly all the parasites when the ED_{50} value for the free drug was >50 mg/kg (12). In a further study using erythrocytes Berman et al. (13) incorporated the purine analogue formycin A into IgG coated red blood cells; the drug was retained within the cells, being phosphorylated by erythrocyte enzymes. Tests in an *in vitro* amastigote-macrophage model showed that encapsulated formycin A was 42 fold more active than free drug.

A range of monolithic particulate carriers, prepared from albumin, starch and polymers (e.g. polycyanoacrylate) and termed microspheres or nanoparticles depending on their size, have also been used widely in drug targeting. They are cheap, uniform reproducible systems with a high capacity for drug loading. Sodium stibogluconate covalently coupled to a similar preparation was 100 fold more effective than free drug against *L.donovani* in mice. The microspheres were not toxic (17).

Macromolecular carriers including DNA, albumin, asialofetuin, and low density lipoprotein (LDL) have been used in studies on a range of protozoal infections (Table 1). Soluble macromolecular carriers have the advantage of being able to extravasate and reach cells and sites not accessible to other systems. However, they have a low drug loading capacity and drug attachment must not obscure the targeting moiety of the macromolecule. LDL is the only molecular carrier examined in antileishmanial drug studies, targeting to receptors on the macrophage surface. Daunorubicin attached to LDL was 100-200 fold more active than free drug when tested against intracellular amastigotes in an *in vitro* macrophage model (18).

Sustained Release Systems

One advantage of encapsulating drugs in liposomes is the potential slow release of a drug and increase in plasma half-life. Other drug delivery systems are designed specifically for non-targeted sustained release. Antimony dextran complexes have been used for such a purpose and examined in the treatment of kala-azar and PKDL in man in India (32). Antimony dextran-glycoside (RL-712) was able to confer prophylactic activity in a hamster model (33).

CUTANEOUS LEISHMANIASIS

Liposomes

There have been few studies on drug targeting to cutaneous leishmaniasis. Following parenteral administration liposomes are distributed to the skin (see 24); the problem is in achieving an effective drug concentration particularly in those macrophages at the site of infection. New et al. (19) evaluated a liposome Pentostam preparation against *L.major* and *L.mexicana amazonensis* in TFW mice and observed that the route and time of liposome administration were important in reducing the rate of lesion growth. Drug loaded liposomes administered i.v. were more effective against established lesions in contrast to s.c. administered liposomes which were more effective when given at the time of infection. It has been suggested that the explanation for this particular result lies in the indirect targeting of the antimony via circulating monocytes which take up liposomes and subsequently migrate to the inflammatory lesion (8,19,34). The lack of efficacy of a local injection against an established lesion could be due to either (a) toxicity to macrophages or (b) targeting to macrophages which are not on the migratory route to the inflamed site of infection.

The Wellcome Liposomal Pentostam has also been tested against *L.major* infections in BALB/c mice and administered at the time of infection and against established lesions (5-7 mm diameter). In both cases only i.v. administration produced any reduction in the rate of lesion growth and as in previous studies (19) no cure was observed. When dosing at the time of infection four doses of Liposomal Pentostam (equivalent to 28 mg Sb^V/kg dose) given over a 10 day period delayed the appearance of a lesion by 2 weeks compared with controls; ten daily doses at 100 mg Sb^V/kg of free Pentostam produced the same delay. In tests against established lesions the standard dose of free Pentostam of 400 mg Sb^V/kg for ten days reduced the increase in lesion size during the period of treatment to 13% compared with 33% growth in untreated mice. Treatment of mice with 6 doses and 10 doses of Liposomal Pentostam i.v. over the same period restricted the increase in lesion growth to 19% and 12% respectively. One to two weeks after the termination of treatment the lesions resumed their previous rapid growth. On a simple comparison of levels of Sb^V administered, the Liposomal Pentostam is 10-15 fold more effective than free drug.

Transdermal delivery

A range of delivery systems are under development to aid the percutaneous absorption of drugs. Although most of the simple rate controlling systems are being used for delivery of drugs to the systemic circulation, modifications for the treatment of cutaneous leishmaniasis are not impossible. The skin, particularly the stratum corneum, is by nature of its function a barrier and a number of penetration enhancers, e.g. DMSO, urea, 2-pyrrolidone, have been identified to aid drug diffusion. Although an examination of the history of leishmaniasis chemotherapy reveals that the topical application of drugs, including antimonials and plant products, has been investigated, there is little evidence of the use of penetration enhancers - other than an early example in which sulphuric acid was incorporated into an ointment! However, recently El-On et al. (35) used DMSO to aid the penetration of paromomycin in the successful treatment of L.major lesions in BALB/c mice. Other penetration enhancers, propylene glycol and 'Azone', are known to assist the penetration of the anti-infective drugs metronidazole and 5-fluorouracil across human skin in vitro (36). This approach towards drug delivery should be worthy of further study in the treatment of cutaneous leishmaniasis.

CONCLUSION

Although there are problems in the commercial development of drugs in novel delivery systems, this approach has attracted the interest of the pharmaceutical industry and specialist companies. Several liposome-drug formulations are now in the later stages of development and hopefully those encapsulating Pentostam and amphotericin B will soon be available for clinical trial against visceral leishmaniasis. They offer the obvious advantages of improved efficacy and reduced toxicity but perhaps of equal importance is the chance to reduce a 15-30 day course of treatment down to 1-3 doses. No clinical dosages have been established for liposomal preparations in the treatment of leishmaniasis and there is certainly no guarantee that they will always be effective (26). Obviously a new highly active orally administered anti-leishmanial drug is really required but in its absence and with development costs for a new drug so high, improved delivery systems offer an important less expensive alternative. Apart from liposomes other systems have been tried. Microparticles offer the most pharmaceutically feasible approach (low cost, uniformity, reproducibility) but problems remain regarding their biodegradability, toxicity and the attachment and release of drugs. These systems are unlikely to confer great benefit to the treatment of cutaneous leishmaniasis but the potential of transdermal delivery systems should not be overlooked.

REFERENCES

1. S.L. Croft, Liposomes in the treatment of Parasitic Diseases, Pharm. Int. 7: 229 (1986).

2. C.R. Alving, E.A. Steck, W.L. Chapman Jr, V.B. Waits, L.D. Hendricks, G.M. Swartz Jr, and W.L. Hanson, Therapy of leishmaniasis: Superior efficacies of liposome-encapsulated drugs, Proc. Natl. Acad. Sci. U.S.A. 75: 2959 (1978).

3. C.D.V. Black, G.J. Watson and R.J. Ward, The use of Pentostam liposomes in the chemotherapy of experimental leishmaniasis, Trans. R. Soc. Trop. Med. Hyg. 71: 550 (1977).

4. R.R.C. New, M.L. Chance, S.C. Thomas and W. Peters, Antileishmanial activity of antimonials entrapped in liposomes, Nature. 272: 55 (1978).

5. J.D. Berman, W.L. Hanson, W.L. Chapman, C.R. Alving and G. Lopez-Berestein, Antileishmanial activity of liposome-encapsulated amphotericin B in hamsters and monkeys, Antimicrob. Agents Chemother. 30: 847 (1986).

6. R.R.C. New, M.L. Chance and S. Heath, Antileishmanial activity of amphotericin and other antifungal agents entrapped in liposomes, J. Antimic. Chemoth. 8: 371 (1981).

7. C.R. Alving, E.A. Steck, W.L. Chapman, V.B. Waits, L.D. Hendricks, G.M. Swartz Jr and W.L. Hanson, Liposomes in leishmaniasis: therapeutic effects of antimonial drugs, 8-aminoquinolines and tetracycline, Life Sciences. 26: 2237 (1980).

8. R.R.C. New, M.L. Chance and S. Heath, Liposome Therapy for Experimental Cutaneous and Visceral leishmaniasis, Biol. Cell. 47: 59 (1983).

9. L.E. Adinofli, P.F. Bonventre, M. Vander Pas and D.A. Eppstein, Synergistic effect of glucantime and a liposome-encapsulated muramyl dipeptide analog in therapy of experimental visceral leishmaniasis, Infec. Immun. 48: 409 (1985).

10. M.L. Chance, S. Heath and R.W. Stokes, The effect of liposome entrapped lymphokins and muramyl dipeptide on Leishmania donovani in mice, Trans. R. Soc. Trop. Med. Hyg. 78: 271 (1984)

11. J.D. Berman and M. Aikawa, Activity of immunoglobulin G-coated red cell ghosts containing pentamidine against macrophage-contained Leishmania in vitro, Am. J. Trop. Med. Hyg. 33: 1112 (1984).

12. J.D. Berman, J.C. Gallalee, J.S. Williams and W.D. Hockmeyer, Activity of pentamidine-containing human red cell ghosts against visceral leishmaniasis in the hamster, Am. J. Trop. Med. Hyg. 35: 297 (1986).

13. J.D. Berman and J.V. Gallalee, Antileishmanial activity of Human Red Blood Cells containing Formycin A, J. Infect. Dis. 151: 698 (1985).

14. A. Baille, G.H. Coombs, T.F. Dolan and J. Laurie, Non-ionic surfactant vesicles, niosomes, as a delivery system for the anti-leishmanial drug, sodium stibogluconate, J. Pharm. Pharmacol. 38: 502 (1986).

15. P. Couvreur - personal communication (1985).

16. P. Stjärnkvist, P. Artursson, A. Brunmark, T. Laakso and I. Sjöholm, Biodegradable microspheres VIII: Killing of Leishmania donovani in cultured macrophages by microparticle-bound primaquine, J. Pharm. Sci. (in press) (1987).

17. T.F. Dolan, C.A. Hunter, A.J. Baillie, G.H. Coombs, T. Laasko, I. Sjohölm and P. Stjärnkvist, Biodegradable microspheres IX: Polyacryl starch microparticles as a delivery system for the antileishmanial drug, sodium stibogluconate, J. Pharm. Pharmacol. (in press) (1987).

18. D.T. Hart, Lipoprotein mediated anti-leishmanial chemotherapy, in: 'Host-Parasite Molecular Recognition and Interaction in Protozoal Infections', K-P. Chang, ed. Springer-Verlag. (in press) (1987).

19. R.R.C. New, M.L. Chance and S. Heath, The treatment of experimental cutaneous leishmaniasis with liposome-entrapped Pentostam, Parasitology, 83: 519 (1981).

20. C.B. Panosian, M. Barza, F. Szoka and D.J. Wyler, Treatment of Experimental Cutaneous Leishmaniasis with Liposome-Intercalated Amphotericin B, Antimicrob. Agents Chemother. 25: 655 (1984).

21. S. Heath, M.L. Chance and R.R.C. New, Quantitative and ultrastructural studies on the uptake of drug loaded liposomes by mononuclear phagocytes infected with Leishmania donovani, Molec. Biochem. Parasitol. 12: 49 (1984).

22. J.S. Weldon, J.F. Munnell, W.L. Hanson and C.R. Alving, Liposomal chemotherapy in visceral leishmaniasis: an ultrastructural study of an intracellular pathway, Z. Parasitenkd. 69: 415 (1983).

23. R.J. Ward, C.D.V. Black and G.J. Watson, The determination of free and liposome-entrapped antimony in biological samples and its application to the chemotherapy of experimental leishmaniasis, in: 'Drug Measurement and Drug Effects in Laboratory Health Science', G. Seist and D.S. Young, eds, S. Karger, Basel, (1980).

24. C.R. Alving, Delivery of Liposome - Encapsulated Drugs to macrophages, Pharmacol. Ther. 22: 407 (1983).

25. C.R. Alving, Liposomes as Drug Carriers in Leishmaniasis and Malaria, Parasitol. Today, 2: 101 (1986).

26. C.R. Alving, G.M. Swartz Jr, L.D. Hendricks, W.L. Chapman Jr, V.B. Waits and W.L. Hanson, Liposomes in leishmaniasis: effects of parasite virulence on treatment of experimental leishmaniasis in hamsters, Ann. Trop. Med. Parasit. 78: 279 (1984).

27. G. Poste and R. Kirsh, Site-specific (targeted) drug delivery in cancer therapy, Bio/Technol. 1: 859 (1983).

28. L.S. Rao, Liposomal dosage for development - some practical considerations, J. Parent Sci. Technol. 37: 72 (1983).

29. L.S. Rao, Anti-leishmanial pharmaceutical formulations, U.S. Patent Number: 4, 594, 241 (1986).

30. L.S. Rao, J.G. Hardy and C.G. Wilson, Tissue distribution and fate of free and liposome-encapsulated [^{125}Sb] sodium stibogluconate by gamma scintigraphy, Int. J. Pharmaceut. 17: 283 (1983).

31. G. Lopez-Berestein, V. Fainstein, R. Hopfer, K. Mehta, M.P. Sullivan, M. Keating, M.G. Rosenblum, R. Mehta, M. Luna, E.M. Hersh, J. Reuben, R.L. Juliano and G.P. Bodey, Liposomal Amphotericin B for the treatment of Systemic Fungal Infections in patients with cancer: a preliminary study, J. Infect. Dis. 151: 704 (1985).

32. P.C. Sen Gupta, A. Chatterji and A.M. Mukherjee, Antimony dextran complex in the treatment of leishmaniasis, J. Ind. Med. Assoc. 37: 585 (1961).

33. J.W. Mikhail, N.S. Mansour and M.T. Khayyal, Leishmania donovani: Therapeutic and prophylactic action of antimony dextran glycoside (RL-712) in the golden hamster, Exp. Parasit. 37: 348 (1975).

34. R.R.C. New, M.L. Chance and M. Critchley, The distribution of radiolabelled drug in animals infected with cutaneous leishmaniasis: Comparison of free and liposome-bound sodium stibogluconate, in: 'Radionuclide imaging in drug research', C.G. Wilson, J.G. Hardy, M. Frier and S.S. Davies, eds, Croom Helm London (1981).

35. J. El-On, G.P. Jacobs, E. Witzum and C.L. Greenblatt, Development of topical treatment for cutaneous leishmaniasis caused by Leishmania major in experimental animals, Antimicrob. Agents Chemother. 26: 745 (1984).

36. A. Hoelgaard and B. Møllgaarad, Dermal drug delivery - improvement by choice of vehicle or drug derivative, in: 'Advances in Drug Delivery Systems', J.M. Anderson and S.W. Kim, eds., Elsevier, Amsterdam (1986).

CARRIER MEDIATED THERAPY OF MURINE VISCERAL LEISHMANIASIS

T.F. Dolan[1], C.A. Hunter[2], T. Laakso[3,4] G.H. Coombs[2], A.J. Baillie[1], P. Sjarnkvist[3,4], and I. Sjoholm
[1]Dept. Pharm., Univ. Strathclyde, Glasgow, [2]Dept. Zoology Univ. Glasgow, Glasgow, UK, [3]Dept. Pharmaceutical Biochemistry Univ. Uppsala, Uppsala, [4]Div. Pharmacy, National Board Health and Welfare, Uppsala, Sweden

INTRODUCTION

The response of visceral leishmaniasis to stibogluconate therapy is slow and large quantities of the drug must be administered, usually intramuscularly, to effect a cure. In localities such as Kenya where the disease responds poorly to therapy, continuous 30 day treatments of 10 to 20 mg Sb^V/kg body weight/day have been suggested (Anabwani et al 1983). The dose recommended by the WHO (1984) for general use is 20 mg Sb^V/kg daily. At these high dose levels however toxicity becomes more apparent and it has been suggested (Chulay et al 1985) that in patients receiving 20 mg Sb^V/kg for >20 days, ECG's should be performed regularly to allow early detection of drug induced cardiac arrythmia. Relapse of the disease is common (Chulay et al 1983) and frequently parasites can be obtained from aspirates of spleen (Anabwani et al 1983) and bone marrow (Wickraminghe et al 1987) even after several weeks of daily injections.

Because of the intracellular location of the parasite in the phagocytic cells of the reticuloendothelial system (RES), visceral leishmaniasis is amenable to therapy based on the use of a drug carrier or delivery system. Liposomes of various types have been investigated for this role, and this work was reviewed by Alving (1986). The use of delivery systems such as liposomes in leishmaniasis takes advantage of the avidity of the RES for systemically administered particulates.

As far as stibogluconate is concerned, the potential advantages of carrier-mediated therapy are reduced toxicity, due to a decrease in the total dose of antimony administered, and also perhaps more importantly, a reduction in the number of doses required with practical implications for patient compliance. An ideal formulation of stibogluconate would effect a cure after administration of one dose.

Phospholipids are not unique in their ability to form vesicular molecular aggregates and it is apparent that many surfactants will form liposome-like vesicles under appropriate conditions (Kunitake, 1986). Similarly, liposomes are not unique in their ability to increase the efficacy of entrapped stibogluconate against visceral leishmaniasis and non-ionic surfactant vesicles, niosomes, can be used to achieve similar effects (Baillie et al 1986). Although the development of liposomal drug delivery systems for use in man is well advanced, for example with daunorubicin in cancer chemotherapy and with amphotericin B therapy of systemic mycoses (Lopez-Berestein et al 1985), it has not been established that in visceral leishmaniasis they represent the optimal carrier and indeed in the drug delivery field in general there has been a notable lack of comparison of carrier strategies.

An alternative to vesicular systems such as liposomes and niosomes is the microparticle, which may, by comparison, be regarded as a monolithic structure with drug entrapped within its matrix or bound or adsorbed to the particle surface. Biodegradable polyacryl starch microparticles (Artursson et al 1984) can be used to form a delivery system of this type. It has been shown (Laakso et al 1987) that the low molecular weight, anti-infective drugs primaquine and trimethoprim can be covalently bound to the particles via a peptide spacer. This linkage is stable in serum but can be degraded by lysosomal enzymes to release native drug, thereby conferring a measure of lysosomotropism to drugs administered in this form. This is a pertinent property for a carrier system intended for use against visceral leishmaniasis.

In this paper we report the results of a comparison of the efficacies of free, liposomal, niosomal and microparticulate sodium stibogluconate against visceral leishmaniasis (L. donovani) in a mouse model.

MATERIALS AND METHODS

Materials

Sodium stibogluconate (Pentostam) equivalent to 0.32 mg Sb mg^{-1} was obtained from the Wellcome Foundation, UK., non-ionic surfactants, I, II and III (Fig. 1) from L'Oreal, France and soluble starch (maltodextrin, mol.wt. = 5000) from Stadex B, Sweden. All of these materials were used as received. Synthetic (>99% pure) dipalmitoyl L-α-phosphatidylcholine (DPPC), ash-free cholesterol (CHOL), dicetyl phosphate (DCP, 97% pure by GC) and 1-ethyl-3-(3-dimethylaminopropyl) carbodiimide were obtained from Sigma, UK., N-tert-butyloxycarbonyl-1,6-diaminohexane from Fluka AG, Switzerland and N,N,N',N'-tetramethylene diamine from Merck, Germany. All other reagents were of analytical grade.

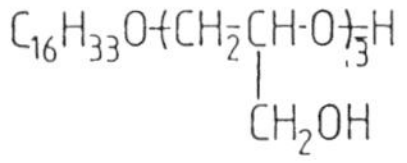

$C_{16}H_{33}O(CH_2CH\text{-}O)_3H$
$\quad\quad\quad\quad\quad |$
$\quad\quad\quad\quad\quad CH_2OH$ 　　　I

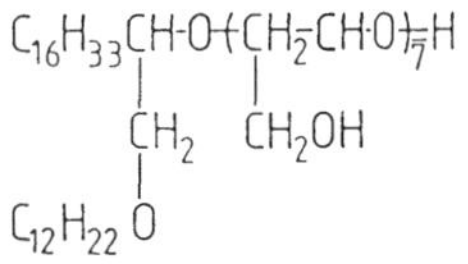

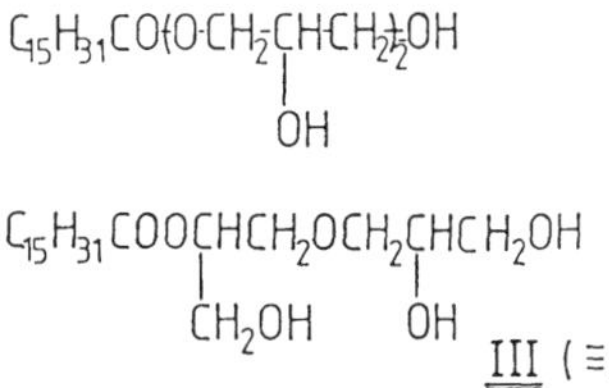

$C_{16}H_{33}CH\text{-}O(CH_2CHO)_7H$
$\quad\quad\quad |\quad\quad\quad\quad |$
$\quad\quad\quad CH_2\quad\quad CH_2OH$
$\quad\quad\quad |$
$C_{12}H_{22}\;O$ 　　　II

$C_{15}H_{31}CO(OCH_2CHCH_2)_2OH$ 　　　A
$\quad\quad\quad\quad\quad\quad\quad |$
$\quad\quad\quad\quad\quad\quad\quad OH$

$C_{15}H_{31}COOCHCH_2OCH_2CHCH_2OH$ 　　　B
$\quad\quad\quad\quad |\quad\quad\quad\quad\quad |$
$\quad\quad\quad CH_2OH\quad\quad\;\; OH$ 　　III ($\equiv$ A:B 92:8)

Figure 1   Three vesicle-forming, non-ionic surfactants synthesised by Vanlerberghe et al (1978). In each case the number of units in the hydrophilic portion is a number average value. Surfactant III contains the isomers in the proportion A:B 92:8.

Methods

Vesicle preparation   Niosomes were prepared by an ether injection method (Baillie et al 1985) in which 450 μmol of surfactant, surfactant-CHOL or surfactant-CHOL-DCP mixture in diethyl ether was injected slowly into 5 ml aqueous stibogluconate solution (300 mg ml^{-1}) at 60°C. Liposomes were prepared by hydrating 114 μmol DPPC-CHOL or DPPC-CHOL-DCP mixtures with 8 ml aqueous stibogluconate solution (300 mg ml^{-1}) at 45-50°C for 2 h under N$_2$, with gentle agitation.

Unentrapped drug was removed by dialysis against 300mM glucose solution. Vesicles were either 'drug-loaded' or 'empty', the latter containing 300mM glucose. Dialysed vesicle suspensions were adjusted to the required drug concentration (Sb content) by dilution with 300 mM glucose solution.

Microparticle preparation   The general procedure followed that of Laakso et al (1986) in which purified acryloylated starch (0.12 acrylic groups/glucose residue) and ADH (synthesised by the method of Stahl, 1978 from the reaction of acrylic acid chloride with N-tert-butyloxy-carbonyl-1,6-diaminohexane) were dissolved in 5 ml 0.2 M, pH 8.5, phosphate buffer containing 10^{-3}M EDTA. After addition of 0.08 M ammonium peroxydisulphate, the aqueous phase was emulsified in 300 ml chloroform:toluene (1:4) with 32 μM Pluronic F68. Polymerisation of monomer in the aqueous phase of the emulsion by the addition of 0.1ml N,N,N',N'-tetramethylene diamine, under N$_2$ formed ADH-polyacryl starch microparticles. To couple drug to particles, 50 mg ADH microparticles and 200 mg sodium stibogluconate were mixed in 10 ml 1M, pH 8, $NaCO_3$ buffer After addition of 5 ml of the same buffer containing 100 mg N-hydroxysuccinimide and 250 mg 1-ethyl-3-(3-dimethylamino-propyl) carbodiimide, the whole suspension was stirred overnight at room temperature. Unreacted drug and coupling reagent were removed by centrifugal washing in normal saline.

<u>Antimony determination</u> Flame atomic absorptiometry (Pye Unicam SP90 atomic absorptiometer) was used to determine antimony contents of microparticles and vesicles. The antimony standard was a solution of $SbCl_3$ in dilute HCl. Method sensitivity was 1 μg Sb ml^{-1}.

<u>Tissue distribution of antimony</u> Mice were sacrificed 24 h after dosing via the tail vein (0.2 ml volumes) with 1 mg sodium stibogluconate, equivalent to 320 mg antimony, in the form of free solution or liposomal or niosomal suspension. The various tissues were removed, weighed into small polythene vials and after freeze drying, reweighed before the vials were sealed by melting the plastic.

The sealed vials were irradiated for a total of 54 h at a nominal flux of 3×10^{12} neutrons cm^{-2} sec^{-2} (Argonaut UTR 300 reactor, Scottish Universities Reactor Centre, East Kilbride). The actual flux was based on the activity of ^{59}Fe (1.099 MeV) in a small piece of pure iron wire attached to the exterior of each vial. Antimony standard, Sb_2O_3 dissolved in HCl, was similarly dried and irradiated in vials.

21 days after irradiation, the vials were counted on a shielded 130 cm^3 Ge-Li detector. Antimony content was based on the activity of ^{124}Sb ($t_{1/2}$ 62.5 days, 1.691 MeV).

<u>Microparticle size determination</u> The size of the microparticles was determined by photon correlation spectroscopy using a Malvern Instruments Type 7027 correlator with 60 channels in conjunction with a He/Cd laser (Linconix) operating at 441.6 nm with a power output of 10mW. The samples were measured in normal saline at 25°C and at an angle of 90° to the incident beam.

<u>Studies of parasite clearance from mice</u> <u>L.donovani</u> (MHOM/ET/67/L82) was maintained by passage through female, Golden Syrian hamsters (<u>Mesocricetus auratus</u>). A suspension of <u>L.donovani</u> (0.4 ml 2×10^8 amastigotes) was administered intraperitoneally to the hamsters which were killed 8-14 weeks after inoculation, the infected spleen being removed and homogenized in PSGEMKA buffer (Hart et al 1981). The released amastigotes were washed and resuspended in PSGEMKA buffer and used to infect further hamsters or to infect mice by tail vein inoculation. Mice were given 0.2 ml parasite suspension containing 2×10^7 <u>L.donovani</u> amastigotes.

Female BALB/c mice (Department of Zoology, University of Glasgow) of about 20g with free access to food and water were used. Treatment with, free drug solution, niosomal, liposomal or microparticulate drug (suspension) or with empty niosomes, liposomes or microparticles was carried out on days 7 and 8 post-infection by tail vein administration of 0.2 ml volumes. The mice were killed on day 14 and multiple liver impression smears prepared and stained using Giemsa's stain. Liver parasite burden, number of parasites per 100 host cell nuclei was assessed by counting ≤2 smears per animal. For all treatment groups there was an untreated control group which had been infected with the same amastigote suspension. The reduction in liver parasite burden achieved in an animal by treatment was calculated relative to the mean parasite burden for the control group (n=5 or 6) and expressed as % parasite suppression. In all cases, the mean parasite suppression for the treatment group is shown.

Parasite suppression in vitro Peritoneal macrophages were obtained after intraperitoneal injection of 5 ml culture medium (RPMI 1640 with 10% foetal calf serum and gentamicin sulphate) into killed male BALB/c mice. The medium, containing cells, was removed via the splenic pocket, pooled from 3 mice and diluted to a cell density of 2.5×10^5 ml^{-1}.

0.4 ml volumes of this suspension were dispensed into the wells of 8-well tissue culture slides (Labtek) which were incubated at 37°C for 24 h, 5% CO_2 in air atmosphere, to allow the cells to adhere. Non-adherent cells were removed by washing with fresh medium and the adherent populations exposed for 24 h, at 37°C, to L.donovani amastigotes, from M.auratus, or at 34°C, to L.mexicana mexicana promastigotes, grown in HOMEM medium (Berens et al 1976). The macrophage:parasite ratio was 1:3 to 1:5. The infected cultures were again washed with fresh medium then exposed at the appropriate temperature to free, liposomal or niosomal stibogluconate. Empty vesicles equivalent to a stibogluconate dose of 50 μg Sb ml^{-1} were also added to infected cultures. Controls comprised untreated cultures.

After 2 h exposure to drug, the cultures were washed and replenished with fresh medium and further incubated until 48 h post-infection. The cells were fixed in methanol and stained with Giemsa's stain. After microscopic examination of the stained slides, the proportion of cells infected after drug treatment was calculated as a % of the proportion infected in the controls.

RESULTS

The activity of free stibogluconate, against L.donovani amastigotes in this mouse model system is shown in Fig. 2. 100% suppression was achieved by a total antimony dose of 1500 to 2000 μg Sb/mouse (ED_{100}) and around 300 μg Sb/mouse was required for 50% suppression (ED_{50}). Although there was some variation in the experimental data due to the nature of the system, the dose response curve for free drug was well established and forms the basis for a comparison of the relative efficacies of the three carrier systems used here.

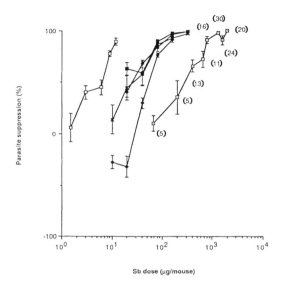

Figure 2 Log_{10} dose-response curves for parasite suppression achieved by administration of four different forms (free, ▣ ; niosomal, surfactant I, ◆ ; surfactant II, ◇ ; surfactant III, ✕ ; liposomal, ■ ; microparticulate, □) of sodium stibogluconate. Vesicles comprised 70 mol % amphiphile (non-ionic surfactant or DPPC) and 30 mol % CHOL. Mice were infected with 2×10^7 L.donovani amastigotes and on days 7 and 8 post-infection, treated by tail-vein injection of 0.2ml volumes of stibogluconate formulation. The total antimony dose, ug/mouse, is shown. Liver parasite burdens, determined on day 14 post-infection, in treated mice were calculated as a proportion (% suppression) of the mean burden for an appropriate control group. Values shown are means ± standard error. The number of observations, (parenthesis for free drug), was ≮4 per datum point.

Fig. 2 shows the data for the suppressive effects of vesicular (liposomes and niosomes, comprising 70 mol % amphiphile and 30 mol % CHOL) and microparticulate forms of the drug. Compared to free drug, liposome and niosome formulations increased apparent efficacy against liver parasites by an order of magnitude and the microparticulate formulation by two orders of magnitude. On the basis of ED_{50} values (ug Sb^V/mouse), free drug = 300, the observed increases in efficacy were :
surfactant I niosomes, ED_{50} = 50, 6x; surfactant II niosomes, ED_{50} = 24, 12.5x; surfactant III niosomes, ED_{50} = 20, 15x; microparticles, ED_{50} = 6, 150x. An ED_{50} was not obtained for liposomes but it can be seen (Fig. 2) that they were equiactive with surfactant III niosomes. ED_{100} values for the carrier formulations were also correspondingly lower than those for free drug.

Manipulation of vesicle composition either in terms of the amphiphile used or admixture of CHOL or DCP appeared to have only a slight effect on the efficacy of the drug-loaded systems especially at the upper end of the dose range,

160-320 μg Sb^V/mouse, used with this type of carrier. At low doses of niosomal drug, it was more apparent that vesicle CHOL content influenced efficacy and vesicles with low CHOL contents had lower antiparasite activity (Fig. 3).

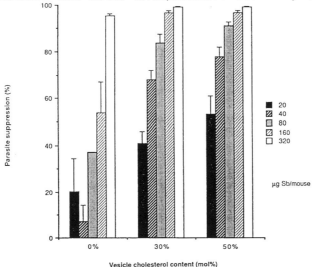

Figure 3 The effect of niosomal CHOL content (0, 30 and 50 mol %) on the antileishmanial activity of stibogluconate loaded surfactant II niosomes. The total antimony dose, ug/mouse is shown. Experimental details as in Fig. 2. Number of observations ⟨5 per datum point.

Drug-loaded surfactant I niosomes (surfactant I + 30 mol % CHOL) at low stibogluconate doses, 10 and 20 ug Sb^V/mouse, gave an apparent negative suppression, i.e. greater liver parasite burdens than untreated controls. This was not found with any other treatment and was not investigated further. A degree of parasite suppression was observed after administration of empty vesicles and in this respect they could be ranked surfactant I niosomes > surfactant II niosomes > surfactant III niosomes = liposomes.

The curve for microparticles (Fig. 2) represents pooled data for high (8.4 ug Sb/mg particles) and low (3.3 ug Sb/mg particles) entrapment efficiency microparticles. The two types were equiactive against liver parasites, the important factor being the total antimony dose/mouse. No evidence was found for an effect on liver parasite burdens of empty, polyacryl starch or ADH-polyacryl starch microparticles, at the dose levels used here.

No acute toxic effects towards mice were observed with stibogluconate loaded vesicles or microparticles.

In vitro, as in vivo against L.donovani, both types of vesicular carrier increased stibogluconate efficacy against L.donovani and L.mex.mexicana infections of macrophages (Fig. 4). This effect was most pronounced against the latter organism, which was unaffected by 2 h exposure to free drug solution at concentrations of up to 1 mg ml^{-1}. The activity of stibogluconate loaded niosomes prepared from surfactants II and III was not significantly different from that of surfactant I niosomes shown in Fig. 4. For the 2 h exposure period used here, empty vesicles had no effect on parasite viability. However at treatment periods of >4h, significant parasite suppression was observed with empty niosomes. At long treatment times and high concentrations of niosomes, toxicity to macrophages and detachment was also observed.

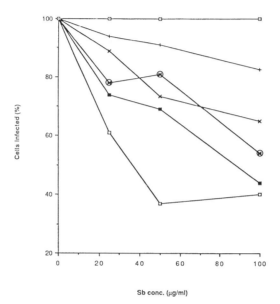

Figure 4   The effect of the tissue culture medium concentration of sodium stibogluconate on the survival of intracellular Leishmania parasites in an in vitro culture of murine peritoneal macrophages. 24 h post-infection, the adherent, infected macrophages were exposed to drug for 2 h then at 48 h post-infection the number of infected macrophages determined after Giemsa's staining. The proportion (%) of infected cells in treated macrophage cultures is shown, where the proportion of cells in untreated cultures was taken as 100%. Macrophages infected with L.mex.mexicana; ☐ , untreated; ■ , liposome treated; ☐ , niosome treated, were incubated at 34°C and macrophages infected with L.donovani; +, untreated; ⊗, liposome treated; ✕, niosome treated, were incubated at 37°C.

The antimony distribution data (Fig. 5), although preliminary, supports earlier findings (Baillie et al, 1986) that compared to free drug, stibogluconate in vesicular form, results in higher levels of antimony in salient tissues such as liver and spleen after i.v. administration. It is reasonable to assume that this finding represents the passive drug delivery to these tissues on which the high antileishmanial activity of the vesicular formulations is based.

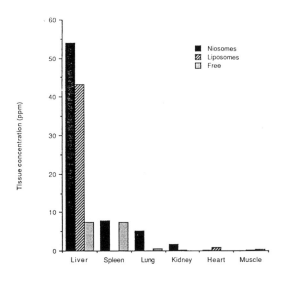

Figure 5 Tissue concentrations (ppm) of antimony determined as ^{124}Sb by neutron activation analysis in the mouse at 24 h after i.v. (tail vein) administration of 1 mg sodium stibogluconate (320ug Sb) as free, liposomal or niosomal drug.

DISCUSSION

The increased efficacy in vivo of the carrier forms of stibogluconate in vivo is in accord with carrier-mediated loading of the infected liver with drug and it would appear that, liposomes, niosomes and microparticles behave similarly in this respect.

The reason for the higher activity of microparticulate stibogluconate is not immediately apparent, although there were marked size differences between this type of carrier, size 1915 nm ±95 (s.d.), niosomes, 333 ± 29 nm and liposomes, 860 ± 42 nm. These mean hydrodynamic diameters, derived from z average diffusion coefficients (Koppel 1972) are weighted towards larger particles. However size differences probably do not contribute significantly to the differences in activity observed between the vesicular and monolithic forms of stibogluconate.

Determination of liver antimony content after administration of niosomal (surfactant I) and liposomal stibogluconate (Baillie et al 1986) showed that, compared to dosing with free drug, a significant antimony content is maintained for a much longer period. Thus the vesicular carriers, in addition to bringing about passive targetting to the liver, appear to counteract the rapid clearance of the drug seen after its administration in free form. The high liver levels achieved after dosing with liposomal and niosomal stibogluconate imply a reduction in Sb excretion rate from this tissue when the drug is given in carrier form. The apparent rates of liver clearance of antimony for vesicular and free drug are shown in Table 1. Compared to free drug, the Sb elimination rate constants (k_{el}) and half-lives ($t_{1/2}$) are some 30x smaller for liposomal and 40x smaller for niosomal drug. The correspondingly greater areas under the tissue concentration-time curves (AUC) for vesicular drug adequately explain the high efficacy of these formulations. Rowland's (1968) data for liver antimony levels after i.p. administration of potassium antimony tartrate give clearance parameters (k_{el} and $t_{1/2}$) for Sb^{III} which are dissimilar to those for Sb^V (Table 1). Ignoring the i.p. route of administration, the data for Sb^{III} reflects the affinity of this form of antimony for liver and its consequent tendency to accumulate in vivo.

In the absence of evidence to the contrary, it would seem reasonable to assume that the microparticles also behave as passive vectors. Indeed it is known that polyacryl starch microparticles are extensively taken up by the liver, mainly by Kupffer cells, after i.v. injection (Laakso et al 1987).

Table 1 Pharmacokinetic parameters for antimony in the liver of the mouse. Based on the data of Baillie et al (1986) for liver Sb^V levels after administration (tail vein) of 1 mg sodium stibogluconate (320 ug Sb^V per mouse) in the form of free, niosomal (surfactant I) or liposomal formulations. The slope of a plot of $\log_{10}$ liver antimony content (µg) against time (h) was used to calculate the apparent elimination rate constant k_{el}(= slopex2.303), half-life $T_{1/2}$(=0.693/k_{el}) and area under the tissue concentration-time curve AUC ($= C_0/k_{el}$). *Based on the data of Rowland (1968) for liver Sb^{III} after i.p. administration of 120µg potassium antimony tartrate.

Formulation	Kel (h^{-1})	T1/2 (h)	AUC (ug liver^{-1} h)
Free	0.509	1.36	15.5
Niosomal	0.013	53.3	723.8
Liposomal	0.018	38.5	473.9
Free*	0.023	30.0	726.1

The pharmacokinetic basis for the increased efficacy of the carrier formulations i.e. tissue loading increased in extent and duration, can be used to explain the observed difference between the vesicular and microparticulate formulations. However to do this the pharmacokinetics at the cellular level are all important since the relevant compartment as far as the antileishmanial activity of stibogluconate is concerned is likely to be the lysosome. The behaviour of the drug loaded carrier in this compartment will influence its performance. Destabilisation of the liposome or niosome bilayer in the hostile lysosomal environment will increase efflux of drug from the vesicles, which, although available for antiparasite activity will also tend to diffuse from the lysosome. This will limit exposure time of parasite to drug and the low activity of drug in niosomes lacking CHOL tends to support this suggestion since CHOL is known to condense liposome and niosome bilayers thereby reducing their permeability to entrapped solute.

By contrast, microparticulate stibogluconate is covalently bound to the carrier and although polyacryl starch is degraded by lysosomal enzymes, some degradation products of mol.wt. >200 (Laakso et al 1986) will remain in the organelle for prolonged periods. Drug attached to these degradation products will have a prolonged lysosomal half-life and duration of action. Thus it is likely that delivery using microparticles prolongs drug-parasite contact.

The _in vitro_ results support those obtained _in vivo_ in that no difference between the carrier functions of liposomes and niosomes could be discerned. The antiparasite activity of carrier formulations _in vitro_ is evidence for endocytic uptake of entrapped drug into the infected phagocyte; the probable route to the parasites for these forms of the drug _in vivo_. The pivotal role of the lysosomal environment in the performance of the stibogluconate carrier is suggested by the difference between the ratio of antileishmanial activities, vesicular form : free form, observed between the _L.donovani_ and _L.mex. mexicana_ systems. Does this reflect differences between conditions in the respective parasitopharous vacoules?

Although microparticulate stibogluconate was not investigated in this _in vitro_ macrophage system, microparticulate primaquine was found, in similar _in vitro_ experiments, to be active although less so than free drug against _L.donovani_ (Stjarnkvist et al 1987). This is further evidence that the efficacy of carrier mediated therapy depends not only on uptake into the infected cell but also on release of drug so that it can affect the parasite. The ideal delivery system for stibogluconate would optimise its uptake by target tissues but would also slowly release it _in situ_, to maintain effective concentrations.

The results presented here suggest that solid particles, such as polyacryl microspheres, may approximate this ideal more closely than vesicular systems. However other factors such as toxicity and ease and cost of manufacture of the putative carrier formulation must also be considered so that although efficacy is of prime importance, the ultimate development of such a dosage form for use in man will acknowledge all of these parameters.

ACKNOWLEDGEMENTS

The donations of Pentostam from the Wellcome Foundation and non-ionic surfactants from L'Oreal, France are gratefully acknowledged. We are indebted to Mr. J. Laurie, Department of Zoology, University of Glasgow for skilled assistance in the animal experiments and to Dr. B.W. East and Mr. I.A. Harris, Scottish Universities Research and Reactor Centre, East Kilbride, Glasgow, for their assistance and advaice in the neutron activation analyses. Support from The

Commission of European Communities sub-Programme "Medicine, Health and Nutrition in the Tropics"; from SERC for T.F.D., and from the Wellcome Foundation from G.H.C. is acknowledged. T.L., I.S. and P.S. were supported by the Swedish Medical Research Council and the Swedish I.F. Foundation.

REFERENCES

Alving, C.R., 1986, Liposomes as drug carriers in leishmaniasis and malaria, Parasitology Today, 2:101.

Anabwani, G.M., Ngira, J.A., Dimiti, G. and Bryceson, A.D.M., 1983, Comparison of two dosage schedules of sodium stibogluconate in the treatment of visceral leishmanisis in Kenya, Lancet, 29 July, 1983, 211.

Artursson, P., Edman, P., Laakso, T. and Sjoholm, I., 1984, Characterization of polyacryl starch microparticles as carriers for proteins and drugs, J.Pharm.Sci., 73:1507.

Baillie, A.J., Florence, A.T., Hume, L.R., Muirhead, G.T. and Rogerson, A., 1985, The preparation and properties of niosomes - non-ionic surfactant vesicles, J.Pharm.Pharmacol., 37:863.

Baillie, A.J., Coombs, G.H., Dolan, T.F. and Laurie, J., 1986, Non-ionic surfactant vesicles, niosomes, as a drug system for the anti-leishmanial drug, sodium stibogluconate, J.Pharm.Pharmacol., 38:502.

Berens, R.L., Brun, R. and Krassner, S.M., 1976, A simple monophasic medium for axenic culture of haemoflagellates, J.Parasit., 62:360.

Chulay, J.D., Bhatt, S.M., Muigal, R., Ho, M., Gochihi, G., Were, J.B., Chunge, C. and Bryceson, A.D.M., 1983, A comparison of three dosage regimens of sodium stibogluconate in the treatment of visceral leishmaniasis in Kenya, J.Infect.Dis., 148:148.

Chulay, J.D., Spencer, H.C. and Mugambi, M., 1985, Electrocardiographic changes during treatment of leishmaniasis with pentavelent antimony (sodium stibogluconate), Am.J.Trop.Med.Hyg., 34:702.

Hart, D.T., Vickerman, K. and Coombs, G.H., 1981, A quick, simple method for purifying leishmania mexicana amastigotes in large numbers, Parasitology, 82:345.

Koppel, D.E., 1972, Analysis of macromolecular polydispersity in intensity correlation spectroscopy - method of cumulants, J.Chem.Phys., 57:4814.

Kunitake, T., 1986, Organisation and functions of synthetic bilayers, Ann.N.Y.Acad.Sci., 471:70.

Laakso, T. Artursson, P. and Sjoholm, T., 1986, Biodegradable microspheres IV : factors affecting the distribution and degradation of polyacryl starch microparticles, J.Pharm.Sci., 75:962.

Laakso, T. Stjarnkvist, P. and Sjoholm, I., 1987, Biodegradable microspheres VI: lysosomal release of covalently bound antiparasitic drugs from starch microparticles, J.Pharm.Sci., 76:134.

Lopez-Berestein, G., Fainstein, V., Hopfer, R., Mehta, K., Sullivan, M.P., Keating, M., Rosenblum, M.G., Mehta, R., Luna, M., Hersh, E.M., Reuben, J., Juliano, R.L. and Bodey, G.P., 1985, Liposomal amphotericin B for the treatment of systemic fungal infections in patients with cancer : a preliminary study, J.Infect.Dis., 151:704.

Rowland, H.A.K., 1968, Stibokinetics III: Trans.Roy.Soc. Trop.Med.Hyg., 62:795

Stahl, G.L., Walter, R. and Smith, C.W., 1978, General procedure for the synthesis of mono-N-acylated 1,6-diaminohexanes, J.Org.Chem., 43: 2285.

Stjarnkvist, P., Artursson, P., Edman, P. and Sjoholm, I. (1987) Biodegradable Microspheres VIII. Killing of Leishmania Donovani in Cultured Macrophages by Microparticle Bound Primaquine.J.Pharm.Sci. (in press).

Vanlerberghe, G., Ribier, A. and Handjani-Vila, R.M., 1978 Les Niosomes, une nouvelle famille de vesicules a base d'amphiphiles non-ioniques. Communication au Colloque du C.N.R.S. sur la Physicochimie des Composes Amphiphiles, Bordeaux

WHO Technical Report Series, No. 701, 1984, "The Leishmaniasis. Report of a WHO Expert Committee" World Health Organisation, Geneva.

Wickraminghe, S.N., Abdalla, S.H. and Kaisili, E.G., 1987, Ultrastructure of bone marrow in patients with visceral leishmaniasis, J.Clin.Path., 40:267.

SITE SPECIFIC ANTILEISHMANIAL DRUG DELIVERY

David Hart and Jayne Lawrence

Drug Delivery Special Interest Group
Departments of Biology and Pharmacy
King's College London (KQC)
Campden Hill Road
London W8 7AH

INTRODUCTION

Over the past decade progress has been made towards the rational development of drug delivery vesicles for the treatment of visceral leishmaniasis. After intravenous (IV) administration, foreign colloidal particles, such as phospholipid vesicles (liposomes) and nanoparticles, are rapidly cleared by the macrophages of the reticuloendothelial system (RES) - particularly those residing in the liver and spleen. While this natural distribution may cause serious limitations for the use of colloidal carriers in the treatment of a number of diseases, including solid tumours or metastases and cutaneous leishmaniasis, it offers considerable advantages in the treatment of visceral leishmaniasis.

To date most effort has centred around the exploitation of liposomes as delivery vesicles for viseral leishmaniasis, however, more recently nonionic surfactant vesicles (niosomes) have also been investigated for their potential as antileishmanial drug carriers (see Croft et al and Dolan et al., in this chapter). Niosomes would seem to be more stable and posses significant cost effective advantages over liposomes, they appear to be, inspite of having a similar biodistribution, somewhat less effective against animal models of the disease.

A major limitation in the use liposomes or niosomes for antileishmanial drug delivery, is the lack of cellular specificity. The ideal antileishmanial drug delivery system should be targeted towards not only the infected organ (or tissue) but should be able to discriminate between the infected and uninfected macrophage populations. Such a delivery system would therefore demonstrate minimal host cytotoxicity and maximal antileishmanial activity.
The chemotherapy of cutaneous leishmaniasis is considerably

more problematic than that of visceral leishmaniasis, presumably because the drug does not reach the subdermal macrophage population in sufficient quantity. Recent studies New et al. (1981, 1983) and Croft, in this chapter) have investigated the properties of liposomally entrapped sodium stibogluconate against a mouse model of cutaneous leishmaniasis. The liposomally encapsulated drug was more effective in all cases when administered IV rather than intralesionaly. This surprising result has been suggested (New et al, 1981) to be due to migration of blood monocytes containing recently endocytosed liposome entrapped drug migrating to the lesion.

Similar disappointing curative effects were also obtained by Panosian et al (1984) investigating the potential of intraperitoneal administration of liposomal entrapped Amphotericin B. Furthermore, there is some evidence to suggest that the cutaneous species of *Leishmania* may have a lower drug susceptibility (eg Neal,in this chapter). The development of a cutaneous targeting system is therefore dependent on either transdermal drug delivery through the skin, that is, topical administration, or lymphotrophic parenteral administration if a mechanism for site specific delivery to only the *Leishmania* infected macrophage populations can be developed.

Macrophages abound with receptor-mediated processes which are used in both the phagocytic antimicrobial activity and endocytic uptake and degradation of macromolecules (see Figure 1). The ligands recognised by macrophage receptors are highly specific and the uptake and degradation processes extremely efficient. Unique or elevated receptor-mediated endocytosis in *Leishmania* infected macrophages could therefore be exploited for the site specific delivery of antileishmanial drugs. Ideally the subcellular topography of the receptor-ligand complex should involve passage through the phagolysosome and result in the release of the prodrug or drug at this subcellular site as is shown in Figure 1. The rational development of site specific antileishmanial drug delivery systems would therefore be facilitated by the identification and characterisation of receptor-mediated processes in *Leishmania* infected macrophages.

We have therefore embarked upon the systematic analysis of the cellular and subcellular biology of *Leishmania* infected macrophages. Thus far several putative receptors have been detected on the surface of infected macrophages, but only the receptors for native and modified low density lipoprotein (LDL) have been characterised and the subcellular topography established. Herein we review current progress in the exploitation of native and modified lipoprotein receptors for site specific delivery of antileishmanial drugs.

MATERIALS AND METHODS

Leishmania
The promastigote stages of *Leishmania donovani* were maintained as described in Hart and Opperdoes (1984). Transformation studies to monitor amastigote viability were carried out as stated in Hart et al (1981).

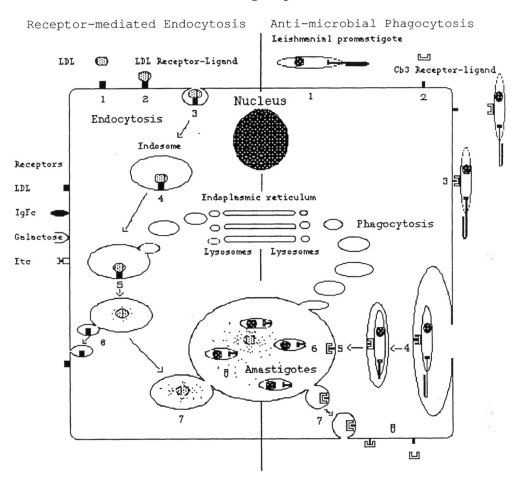

Figure 1 Scheme of Macrophage Receptor-mediated Processes

Receptor-mediated Endocytosis

1 LDL Receptor
2 LDL Receptor-ligand complex
3 Endocytosis
4 Endosome
5 Secondary lysosome
6 Recycling of receptor
7 Fusion with phagolysosome
7 & 8 Degradation of LDL

Antimicrobial Phagocytosis

1 Leishmanial promastigote
2 Cb3 Receptor
3 Cb3 Promastigote complex
4 Phagocytosis
5 Phagosome
6 Amastigote transformation
7 & 8 Recycling of Receptor
8 Cb3 Ligand released

Macrophage-like cell line J774G8

J774G8 were mantained in RPMI 1640 as described by Hart 1987. Late log phase promastigotes (5×10^7/ml) were used to infect the cell line before the cultures had reached confluence (ie $<5 \times 10^6$). Infection ratios of 10:1 were used and drug screening with encapsulated or free Pentostam (100µM) performed 48Hr after infection.

In vivo Studies

Female hamsters were infected by intravenous injection of 10^8 late log phase promastigotes (5×10^7/ml) and drug screening performed 4-6 weeks later by IV injection of Pentostam (10mg/Kg body weight/in saline) in either an unencapsulated or lipoprotein encapsulated formulation. Fractionation of liver cell types was carried out essentially as described by Van Berkel et al (1986) 12 Hr after administration of drug. Liver lobes were spotted on to microscope slides and Giemsa stained. Cytospin centrifuged samples of the fractionated liver cells types were also Giemsa stained and microscopically examined to determine the % infection.

Lipoproteins

Low-density lipoprotein preparations and modifications, including the colloidal gold labeling, were as described in Hart (1987), except for the preparation of triantennary galactose modified lipoproteins which was as stated in Van Berkel et al (1986). Pentostam was encapsulated in freshly prepared native and modified LDL in the aqueous phase and unentrapped drug removed during the dialysis step. The uptake of antimony was measured by atomic absorption spectroscopy of disrupted LDL vesicles.

Niosome and liposome preparation

Nonadecaoxyethyleneglycol mono (1,4,7,10,13 pentaethyl 3,6,9,12,15,18, hexaoxaeicosyl) ether was used to prepare niosomes. Equimolar amounts of distearoyl phosphatidyl chloline and dimyristoyl phosphatidyl choline were used in the preparation of liposomes. Pentostam incorporation was done in the aqueous phase and unentrapped drug removed by dialysis. The antimony content was determined by atomic absorption spectroscopy after disruption of vesicles. Liposomes with the apoprotein moeity from acetylated-LDL incorporated were prepared as above except that the apoprotein was added after the extraction of organic solvents. The vesicles were then characterised by negative staining and examination by electron microscopy. Vesicles were also sized using a Malvern Autosizer.

RESULTS

The occurrence of a native and modified LDL receptor-mediated uptake process in the macrophage cell line J774G8 infected with *Leishmania donovani* is demonstrated in Figure 2. Acetylated LDL was more actively taken up than either native or methylated LDL and clearly demonstrated saturation kinetics. Native and modified LDL receptors have also been demonstrated in *Leishmania mexicana* infected macrophages Hart (1987).

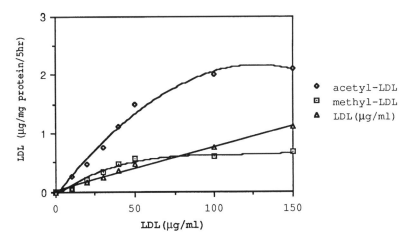

Figure 2 The uptake of native LDL, methlyated LDL and acetylated LDL by J774G8 macrophage infected with Leishmania donovani.

The exploitation of the acetylated LDL receptor-mediated pathway using the conventional carrier systems of liposomes and niosomes was investigated. Liposomes and niosomes containing the antileishmanial drug Pentostam were prepared and characterised for phisicochemical and morphometric properties (eg see Plate 1a, b & c). No significant differences could be detected in morphology and size distribution (data not shown) between the control liposomes and those with the acetyl-LDL apoprotein incorporated, both in the presence and absence of drug. The efficacy of drug action, after the addition of uncapsulated and liposome encapsulated Pentostam, was monitored by amastigote transformation (Figure 3a,b & c).

The ability of amastigotes, freshly isolated from untreated macrophages, to transform to promastigotes is shown in Figure 3a, the reduction in amastigote numbers and the concomitant increase in promastigotes has proved to be a very sensitive assay of amastigote viability. Transformation of amastigotes treated with empty liposomes or acetyl-LDL-liposomes were not significantly different to the untreated controls (data not shown). The addition of Pentostam as an unencapsulated drug (free drug (FD)), resulted in only moderate antileishmanial action after 4 hours exposure to the drug (Figure 3b), while addition of the same drug concentration encapsulated in liposomes (lipo) demonstrated considerable antileishmanial activity (Figure 3b). The antileishmanial activity of Pentostam encapsulated in acetyl-LDL-liposomes (Figure 3c) was even more effective as judged by the extremely low viability of the amastigotes.

The usefulness of low-density lipoproteins as delivery vesicles for the treatment of visceral Leishmaniasis *in vivo* was also investigated. The major site of *Leishmania donovani* infection in our experimental hamster model was found to be the liver with 47+5% of the cells infected,

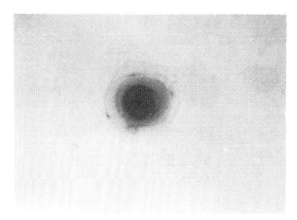

Plate 1a   A typical multilamellar niosome negatively stained and visualised by electron microscopy. (Mag.43,000)

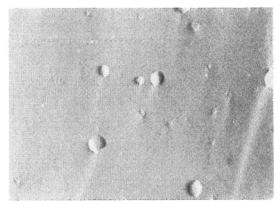

Plate 1b   Typical multilamellar niosomes visualised by freeze fracture replication and electron microscpy. (Mag.98,000)

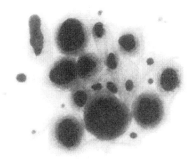

Plate 1c   A typical cluster of multilamellar liposomes negatively stained and visualised by electron microscopy (Mag.43,000)

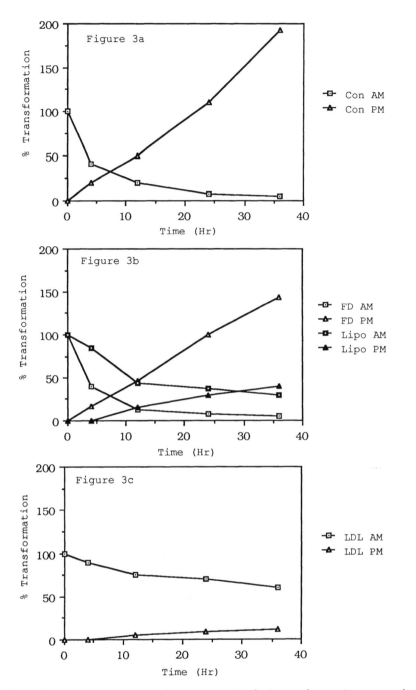

Figure 3 The transformation of *Leishmania donovani* amastigotes (AM) to promastigotes (PM). Fig. 3a untreated controls (Con). Fig. 3b treated with unencapsulated (free drug(FD)) and liposome encapsulated (Lipo) Pentostam (100µg/ml). Fig. 3c acetylated LDL apoprotein incorporated liposome encapsulation (acetyl-LDL-liposomes (LDL)).

while the spleen was found to have a more variable and lower level of infection (21+11%). Fractionation of the liver cells demonstrated that the kupffer cells were the most heavily infected cells (58%) and the parenchymal cell least infected (20%). The antileishmanial activity of Pentostam, encapsulated in either native or modified lipoproteins as the drug delivery vehicles, was determined and is shown in Figure 4.

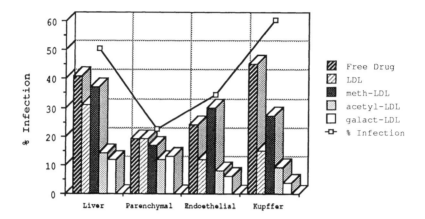

Figure 4 Antileishmanial activity of Pentostam unencapsulated (Free Drug) and encapsulated in native LDL (LDL), methylated LDL (meth-LDL), acetylated LDL (acetyl-LDL), and tris galactose LDL (galact-LDL) as compared to the untreated control (% Infection) of a liver lobe (Liver) and three liver cell types (Parenchymal, Endothelial and Kupffer cells) infected with Leishmania donovani.

Figure 4 shows the % infection with Leishmania donovani amastigotes of a hamster liver lobe and in the fractionated liver cell populations comprising of primarily parenchymal, endothelial and kupffer cells. The efficacy of Pentostam administration in native LDL and modified LDL is higher than with the unencapsulated drug. The efficacy of antileishmanial activity is clearly very much improved via the use of acetyl-LDL or triantennary galactose containing LDL delivery vesicles. Interestingly native and methyl-LDL demonstrated only minor improvements in drug efficacy in the liver, despite the fact that native LDL vehicles demonstrated useful clearance of amastigotes from fractionated kupffer and endothelial cells.

Some differences can be seen in the efficacy of the delivery formulation of Pentostam between the liver lobe and the fractionated liver cell types. This is due to the fact that results are expressed as a % infection of the total cells and should therefore only be compared to the untreated control values. It is strikingly clear from the results that galactose containing and acetylated LDL are highly effective drug delivery vehicles and can demonstrate extremely high clearance of amastigotes from the liver lobe, as well as, all the three liver cell types examined

DISCUSSION

We have shown that lipoprotein receptors abound on *Leishmania* infected macrophages and that the endocytosis of native or modified LDL can be exploited successfully in drug delivery. The LDL receptor-mediated processes would seem to be an excellent target for cell specific delivery due to its elevation in *Leishmania* infected macrophages Hart (1987). In addition our results suggest that the receptor-mediated processes in *Leishmania* infected liver cells may be exploited by the selective modification of the lipoprotein moiety of the delivery vehicle to achieve cell type specific delivery.

Studies on our experimental hamster model suggest that lipoprotein vesicles may be modified to target the encapsulated drug to specific liver cell types. Our observations with *Leishmania donovani* infected liver cells are not dissimilar to those described for normal mammalian liver cells (Van Berkel et al 1986). Therefore the chemotherapeutic potential of exploiting modified lipoproteines and the receptor mediated processes of mammalian macrophages, spleen and liver cells as site specific delivery systems would seem to be considerable.

In addition to the use of lipoprotein delivery vehicles we can demonstrate improved *in vitro* targeting of antileishmanial drugs using the apoprotein moiety from acetylated low-density lipoprotein incorporated into liposomes (and niosomes, data not shown). Furthermore studies in progress suggest that the uptake of acetyl-LDL-liposomes demonstrate classical receptor-mediated characteristics, including saturation kinetics and competition with acetyl-LDL or the isolated apoprotein moiety.

This is the first description of the rational exploitation of a macrophage receptor-mediated process to target and deliver antileishmanial chemotherapy either in a natural delivery vehicle, such as LDL, or a synthetic delivery vesicle, such as liposomes. We are currently investigating several other delivery vesicles including the novel vesicle structure of unsaturated fatty acids (Ufasomes) and extending our search for the most efficient targeting ligand.

Ufasomes are similar to other vesicle structures in that they consist of a series of closed concentric spherules of bilayers formed by the unsaturated fatty acids, separated by aqueous interspaces. Pilot studies have indicated that these vesicles may offer considerable advantages for specific antileishmanial drug delivery. Nonesterified fatty acids would seem to be actively taken up by both leishmanial amastigotes Hart *et al* (1982) and infected macrophages. Prodrugs which are the fatty acid derivatives of antileishmanial drugs have been used effectively for incorporation into delivery vesicles and presumably for the uptake into leishmanial amastigotes Hart (1987).

Topical administration of delivery vesicles could facilitate direct drug delivery for the treatment of cutaneous leishmaniasis. Uptake by absorption transcellularly, or transfollicularly, into the lymphatic system would be an excellent route for the lipophilic ufasomes. This route however may account for about only 1% of the total percutaneous transport and the total amount of drug transdermaly absorbed is generally low, and may be as little as a few milligrams daily.

Topical delivery, however, can be improved by the amount of drug absorbed transcellaularly by the use of penetration enhancers. i.e. compounds such as DMSO, DMF, the surfactant azacycloalkane-2-ones that act by manipulating the barrier properties of the skin at a molecular level thus enabling passage of the drug through the stratum corneum. Recent work by El-On et al. (1984) examined the effect of DMSO on the antileishmanial properties of topically applied paramycin. While treatment was in part successful, the rapid healing achieved may have been due to the presence of the the surfactant methylbenzathonium chloride which exerts its own antileishmanial activity, rather than any increased penetration of paramycin due to DMSO. Further evidence of an improvement of the antileishmanial activity of Ketoconazole due to the presence of DMSO has been published recently (Dutz et al, 1987).

CONCLUSIONS

Many different types of delivery vehicles and routes of administration are therefore at various stages of development. Information on the receptor-mediated processes of *Leishmania* infected macrophages should facilitate the identification and development of site specific ligands which upon incorporation into the delivery vesicle of choice will confer specificity. The apoprotein moiety of modified low-density lipoproteins would seem to be an excellent target for site specific delivery of antileishmanial drugs. Indeed the elevated level of modified lipoprotein metabolism in infected macrophages presumably results in the preferential uptake by these macrophage populations.

Indeed, preliminary results in our laboratories suggest that a novel modification of low-density lipoprotein is specifically recognised by *Leishmania* infected macrophages. The receptors for this modified lipoprotein are absent (or below detection) in normal macrophages and can only be detected on infected or inflamed macrophages. Therefore the rational and expedient development of site specific antileishmanial and anti-inflammatory drug delivery may well be realised via exploitation of the receptor for this novel lipoprotein.

ACKNOWLEDGEMENTS

We thank Sushil Chauhan, Nancy Khammo and Helen Lysandrides for their invaluable assistance to the Antileishmanial Drug Delivery Project.

REFERENCES

Dutz, W., Agarval, N., Bashardost, M.Z., Bently, G. & Kindmark, C.O., (1987)
Topical Therapy of Cutaneous Leishmaniasis with 2% Ketokonazole Oitment and DMSO
Int. J. Dermatology 26, 199

El-On, J., Jacobs, G.J., Witztum, E, and Greenblatt, C.L (1984)
Development of Topical Treatment for Cutaneous Leishmaniasis Caused by *Leishmania major* in Experimental Animals.
Antimicrobial Agents and Chemotherapy 26, 745-751

Hart, D.T., Vickerman, K & Coombs, G.H. (1981)
The in vitro transformation of *Leishmania mexicana mexicana* amastigotes to promastigotes: Nutritional requirements and effect of drugs.
Parasitology 83, 529-541.

Hart, D.T. & Coombs, G.H. (1982)
Leishmania mexicana : Energy metabolism of amastigotes and promastigotes.
Exptl. Parasitol. 54, 397-409.

Hart, D.T. & Opperdoes, F.R. (1984)
The occurrence of glycosomes (microbodies) in the promastigote stage of four major *Leishmania* species.
Mol. Biochem. Parasitol. 13, 159-172.

Hart, D.T. (1987)
Leishmania host-parasite interactions : The development of chemotherapeutic targets and specific drug delivery systems. I. Lipoprotein-mediated antileishmanial chemotherapy. In: Host-Parasite Cellular and Molecular Interactions in Protozoal Infections, eds K-P. Chang & D. Snary, Springer-Verlag, Berlin.

New, R.R.C., Chance, M.L. & Heath, S. (1981)
The Treatment of Experimental Cutaneous Leishmaniasis with Liposome-entrapped Pentostam
Parasitology 83, 519-527

New, R.R.C., Chance, M.L. and Heath, S. (1983)
Liposome Therapy For Experimental Cutaneous and Visceral Leishmaniasis
Biol. Cell 47, 59-64

Panosain, C.B., Barza, M., Szoka, F. & Wyler, D.J. (1984)
Treatment of Experimental Cutaneous Leishmaniasis with Liposome-intercelated Amphotericin B
Antimicrobial Agents and Chemotherapy 25, 655-656

Van Berkel T.J.C., Kruijt J.K., Harkes L., Nagelkerke J.F.,Spanjer H.& Kempen H-J. (1986)
In: Site-specific Drug Delivery. Eds Tomlinson and Davis. John Wiley & Sons Ltd. London.

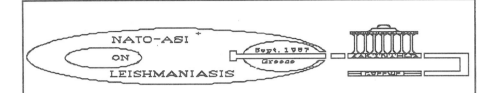

CHAPTER 6
NEW STRATEGIES FOR CONTROL FORUM I
VECTOR CONTROL

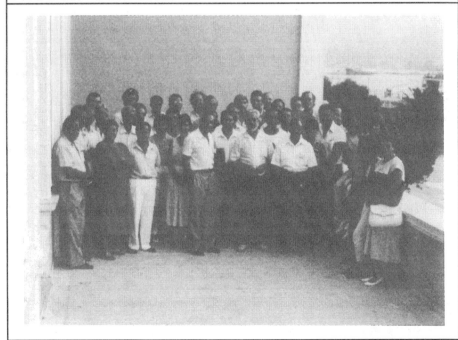

NEW STRATEGIES FOR CONTROL FORUM : VECTOR CONTROL

R. Killick-Kendrick

MRC External Scientific Staff
Department of Pure and Applied Biology
Imperial College at Silwood Park
Ascot
Berks SL5 7DE

Some forms of the leishmaniases were suppressed during house-spraying with insecticides against malaria vectors, only to reappear when spraying was stopped. Thus it appears as if the transmission of leishmaniasis by an endophilic sandfly vector can, in some circumstances, be controlled to the point of no longer being of public health importance. The decision to bear the longterm costs of such intervention depends, among other things, on the numbers of cases and the form of leishmaniasis, with epidemic visceral leishmaniasis as the most dangerous. Since reports of resistance of *Phlebotomus papatasi* (Scopoli) to DDT in India, the assumption that sandflies can never acquire an important degree of resistance to insecticide is no longer tenable and, in any campaign with insecticides, monitoring of resistance is now essential.

The most efficient means of control is the exploitation of the habitat concomittantly rendering it inhospitable to the sandfly. The most notable success of this intervention comes from campaigns in the southern republics of the USSR where the destruction of the gerbil reservoir of zoonotic cutaneous leishmaniasis and their burrows where the vector breeds is followed by agricultural exploitation. In some places, such as parts of the Amazon Basin, there may, however, be a danger of creating conditions for the establishment of a new cycle of transmission of a different form of the disease from that which disappears.

Control aimed at the vector is largely restricted to forms of the leishmaniases with peridomestic transmission. Currently there are trials to reduce risk by means of insecticides / repellents on screens or curtains. Such methods have the advantage that, firstly, they are cheap and, secondly, the control can be achieved by the inhabitants of the focus themselves. Success depends, however, on a basic understanding of the biology of the vector and the customs of the people. If the vector is exophagic and the people sleep outside without mosquito nets during hot weather, this form of control is unlikely to be effective.

Control of the leishmaniases of the Neotropical forests presents special difficulties particularly in foci where the vector or vectors are still unknown or only suspected. It is generally not feasible to use insecticides and, with the present knowledge, methods of so-called biological control cannot be implemented. Almost nothing is known of predators and pathogenic parasites of sandflies and, because of the lack of information on natural larval breeding sites, it is rarely possible to consider attacking preimaginal stages of the vector. BTI toxin has, however, been shown to be lethal to larvae of sandflies of both the genus *Lutzomyia* and the genus *Phlebotomus*.

Truly new strategies for control suitable for use over wide areas are unlikely to be formulated without new knowledge requiring imaginative investigations with no certainty of success. Such research on the leishmaniases is currently difficult to fund in countries where the diseases are of little or no medical importance and cannot be adequately supported by Governments of poor countries of the Third World, in many of which the leishmaniases are a serious public health problem. Progress depends on the support of international funding organisations who must be persuaded to risk more funds than at present on original research with no guarantee of finding a solution. For example, there is a need to find our more about the mechanisms controlling variations in the ability of sandflies to support the development of different species of *Leishmania*. A reasonable working hypothesis is that they are genetically controlled, yet nothing is known of the genetics of susceptibility of sandflies to *Leishmania*, a subject which appears to be outside the current priorities of the Leishmaniasis Component of the UNDP/World Bank/WHO Special Programme for Research and Training in Tropical Diseases. One strategy in the not too distant future may be the introduction of genes of resistance into natural populations of vectors, so diminishing their ability to support the development of the parasite that the infection will disappear with the need to contaminate or destroy the environment. In our present ignorance, this may seem like a dream. But the idea of preventing disease by vaccination was a dream in Jenner's day; it is now commonplace.

In conclusion, current methods of interrupting the transmission of the leishmaniases by attacking the vector are inadequate and, without new imaginative work, are likely to remain so. If there are to be new strategies, more financial support from interested international funding bodies is urgently needed, especially for projects which break new ground.

SQUASH BLOTTING PHLEBOTOMUS PAPATASI TO ESTIMATE RATES OF INFECTION

BY LEISHMANIA MAJOR

P.D. Ready, D.F. Smith*, R. Killick-Kendrick and R. Ben-Ismail**

Dept. Pure & Applied Biology & *Dept. Biochemistry
Imperial College, London SW7 2AZ
** Faculté de Médecine, Tunis, Tunisia

INTRODUCTION

Any attempt to control sandfly vectors of leishmaniasis should include the monitoring of infection rates before, during and after the control programme. Few have tried to measure temporal changes in infection rates during control programmes (Le Pont & Pajot, 1981; Ready et al., 1985). The screening process is slow: each female sandfly examined must be dissected in order to look microscopically for intestinal infections and diagnostic morphological characters. Then, usually, infecting Leishmania must be identified by isoenzyme characterization (Maazoun et al., 1981) or by analysis of extracted kinetoplast (k) DNA (Barker et al., 1986), but this requires at least 10^9 cells that can be difficult to grow either in laboratory rodents or in axenic culture media.

The potential of DNA probes or monoclonal antibodies for identifying infections of Leishmania from sandflies has recently been reported (Barker et al., 1986; Shaw et al., 1987), but the aims have been to identify parasites after dissection and identification of the sandfly.

NEW STRATEGIES

The construction of DNA probes for vectors, however, should provide the means to identify both vector and infecting parasites by sequential hybridization of diagnostic probes to vector and parasite DNA released in one step, achieved simply by squashing the vector on to (nylon) hybridization filters.

We have succeeded in using the squash-blotting technique to identify experimental infections of Leishmania major in laboratory-reared Phlebotomus papatasi, the principal (or sole) vector of L. major over an extensive range, including much of arid north Africa (Ready et al., in press). This summer, we have been testing the method in the field, in active foci of zoonotic cutaneous leishmaniasis in Tunisia. Infected guts, dissected out by conventional methods, were successfully blotted and identified when parasites were abundant in abdominal and/or thoracic midguts. Infection rates given by "blind" squash-blotting were comparable to those shown by conventional dissections, but only if the light infections (<100 parasites) seen microscopically were excluded.

The probes for north African Leishmania have been constructed by cloning diagnostic fragments of highly-repetitive mini-circle "species" of kDNA (Smith et al., in press). For our vector-specific probe we have cloned an intergenic fragment of a ribosomal (r) RNA gene repeat of P. papatasi, which recognises in squash blots only P. papatasi of all the Tunisian species tested (Ready et al., in press).

DISCUSSION

Most females of Phlebotomus species cannot be identified by reference to external characters alone, and so the construction of vector-diagnostic DNA probes permits squash-blot methods to be used not only for screening for infections of Leishmania, but also for identifying sandflies in large scale field studies on vector abundance and behaviour.

The squash blotting technique used for P. papatasi is highly practical. Many flies can be squashed at the same time under sheets of clean plastic, and the solutions required in the preliminary steps are inexpensive and stable in hot climates. The stability of DNA on dry nylon hybridization filters means that samples could be sent by air mail to regional laboratories equipped for using radiolabelled DNA probes.

REFERENCES

Barker, D. C., Gibson, L. J., Kennedy, W. P. K., Nasser, A. A. & Williams, R. H., 1986, The potential of using recombinant DNA species-specific probes for the identification of tropical Leishmania, Parasitology, 91: 139.

Le Pont, F. & Pajot, F. X., 1981, La leishmaniose en Guyane Française. 2. Modalites de la transmission dans un vilage forestier: Cacao, Cah. ORSTOM, sér. Ent. méd. Parasitol., 19: 223.

Maazoun, R., Lanotte, G., Pasteur, N., Rioux, J. A., Kennou, M. F. & Pratlong, F., 1981, Écologie des leishmanioses dans le sud de la France. Ann. Parasitol. Hum. Comp., 56: 131.

Ready, P. D., Arias, J. R. & Freitas, R. A., 1985, A pilot study to control Lutzomyia umbratilis (Diptera: Psychodidae), the major vector of Leishmania braziliensis guyanensis, in a peri-urban rainforest of Manaus, Amazonas State, Brazil, Mems Inst. Oswaldo Cruz, 80: 27.

Ready, P. D., Smith, D. F. & Killick-Kendrick, R., in press, DNA hybridizations on squash-blotted sandflies to identify both insect vector and infecting Leishmania, Med. Vet. Entomol., 1:

Shaw, J. J., Lainson, R., Ryan, L., Braga, R. R., McMahon-Pratt, D. & David, J. R., 1987, Leishmaniasis in Brazil: XXIII. The identification of Leishmania braziliensis braziliensis in wild-caught neotropical sandflies using monoclonal antibodies, Trans. R. Soc. trop. Med. Hyg., 81: 69.

Smith, D. F., Ready, P. D., Searle, S. & Gramiccia, M., in press, Kinetoplast DNA probes diagnostic for Leishmania species, NATO ASI on Leishmaniasis (ed. D. T. Hart), Plenum Publishing Corp, NY.

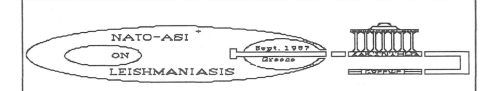

CHAPTER 7
NEW STRATEGIES FOR CONTROL FORUM II
RESERVOIR CONTROL

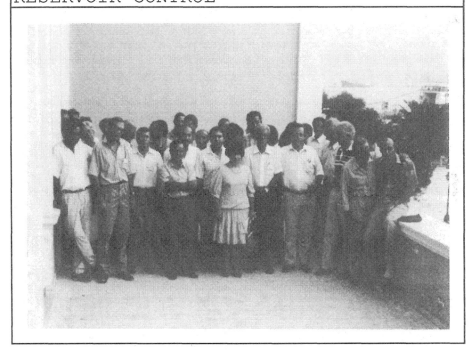

NEW STRATEGIES FOR CONTROL FORUM: RESERVOIR CONTROL

R. W. Ashford

Department of Parasitology
Liverpool School of Tropical Medicine
Pembroke Place, Liverpool, UK

A reservoir of leishmaniasis is a system including sandflies and mammals required for the long term persistence of the parasites. The system contains one or more sandfly species - the vectors, and one or more mammals - the reservoir host. Other mammals may become infected but if they are not required for the long term survival of the parasite, they are incidental hosts. Incidental hosts may well be important as liaison hosts, bring the parasite into contact with man.

In practice it is usually difficult to determine whether a sandfly-mammal-Leishmania system is autonomous (capable of long term persistence) or dependent (requiring repeated introduction of parasites from an autonomous system). This requires quantitative study which has rarely been achieved.

A strategy for control of leishmaniasis is likely to include vector control and case treatment in addition to reservoir or liaison host control. Thus, this Forum is dealing with tactics and techniques of mammal control and may discuss the role of these in an integrated strategy.

There are rather few examples where reservoir host control has been used either alone or in conjunction with other methods so there is limited past experience. Each leishmaniasis situation must be seen individually and assessed according to the structure of the focus, the techniques available, the opinions and requirements of the people, and the funds available.

The discussion in this Forum is organised broadly into the following framework:

TABLE 1. Framework for the discussion of reservoir hosts and _Leishmania_ species to which discussion is applicable

Section	Techs available requiring evaluation & application	Techs requiring development	New techs required or new information on focal structure
1) Sylvatic reservoir hosts excluding rodents		_L. aethiopica_	_L. b. panamensis_, _L. b. guyanensis_ _L. donovani_? _L. tropica_? _L. b. braziliensis_?
2) Synanthropic and wild rodents	_L. major_	_L. major_	_L. mexicana_ sspp
3) Humans as reservoir hosts	_L. d. donovani_ _L. tropica_		_L. tropica_ _L. d. donovani_ _L. major_?
4) Reservoirs maintained by domestic animals, esp. dogs and horses	_L. d. infantum_	_L.b.braziliensis_ _L. d. infantum_	_L.b.braziliensis_ _L. d. infantum_

Section 3 was omitted owing to lack of time and the different concepts involved. The integration of reservoir host control with other control methods, and the evaluation of the effects of control on the incidence of human disease were mentioned only in passing.

1) Sylvatic reservoir hosts excluding rodents

Reduction of number of hyrax in the vicinity of villages has been suggested for the reduction of _L. aethiopica_ transmission (Bray). This could readily be achieved by shooting, but in some counties, e.g. Kenya, these animals are protected by legislation. In South and Central America, sloths of the genus _Bradypus_ could be eliminated by the felling of their favourite food tree, _Cecropia_ spp. _Choloepus_ spp. are less specific in their requirements, but can readily be found and shot (Walton). Oppossums _Didelphis_ spp. are thought to be liaison hosts for _L. b. guyanensis_ and trapping methods are available. No information exists on the numbers to which hosts require to be reduced, nor on the rate of recolonisation of treated areas.

Sylvatic reservoir hosts have been postulated for _L. b. braziliensis_ and for _L. tropica_ in certain localities, but the identity of the animals concerned remains unknown. Imaginative approaches are required for both of these intractable problems.

Wild canids, foxes, jackals and wolves have been postulated as reservoir hosts for _L. d. infantum_ but only in South America has it been demonstrated that these are more than incidental hosts. In southern Europe the red fox _Vulpes vulpes_ has been incriminated but it is generally considered that fox based systems are dependent and would die out if the infection was controlled in domestic dogs. Foxes are becoming synanthropic in their behaviour and dogs are becoming less so; packs of feral dogs roam many areas of southern Europe. The epidemiological implications of these behavioural changes have yet to be assessed.

2) Sylvatic and peridomestic rodents

Successful control of Rhombomys opimus in the USSR was achieved by poisoning with zinc posphide or anticoagulants or by deep ploughing. Reinvasion of control areas was prevented by the construction of water barriers as part of an irrigation scheme. These measures are applicable in part in other countries where R. opimus maintains L. major and to a lesser extent, where other rodents are concerned. Ben Ismail described experimental control measures against Meriones shawi by the systematic application of zinc phosphide to burrow entrances. This treatment eliminated the rodent for a period of four years.

Control of Psammomys obesus is more difficult owing to its reluctance to eat grain. Ben Ismail described measures for the control of P. obesus: zinc phosphide in grain is ineffective, but anticoagulant pellets or wax blocks (Klerat) were placed inside the burrows without blocking them and killed 81% of Psammomys but the rodents recolonised the area in three months. Phostoxin pellets and powdered Phosdrin, two organophosphates were unsuccessful.

A programme is being started in Saudi Arabia (Killick Kendrick) where vegetation will be cleared for an area of 1 km surrounding a village, in the hope of starving P. obesus and achieving leishmaniasis control. Numbers of rodents will be monitored by a standardised system of observation. Jacobson described similar control measures employed by settlers in Israel.

Distribution maps for Psammomys are incomplete owing to the unwillingness of this rodent to enter traps. The distinctive burrows can however indicate the presence of the rodent.

Control of rats Rattus rattus has not been attempted in connection with leishmaniasis; nor has control of forest rodents, Proechimys, Orzyomys, Ototylomys in South or Central America, or Arvicanthis and other reservoir hosts in Africa.

3) Man as a reservoir host

Man is thought to be the source of infection of L. donovani in the epidemic areas of north and east India and, possibly, Sudan and East Africa. Similarly, L. tropica in the traditional parts of its distribution is thought to be dependent on man for its survival. Until recently L. major was not thought to be transmitted from man to man but this is the easiest explanation of the recent outbreaks in Sudan, especially in Khartoum. The remaining Leishmania systems are thought to be zoonotic though, in certain instances the reservoir hosts are unknown.

The role of individuals at various stages of infection, including post kala azar dermal leishmaniaisis in India and East Africa is currently the subject of research by xenodiagnosis.

Control of the human reservoir depends on case detection, treatment and the prevention of re-infection. These procedures have been applied in India and East Africa for L. donovani and in Soviet Transcaucasia for L. tropica. Improved diagnostic methods for field use and for the detection of sub-clinical infections are sorely needed and are being developed.

4) _Reservoirs maintained by domestic animals_

Special constraints apply in the control of domestic animals which commonly have great value, whether monetary or sentimental. The domestic dog maintains _L. d. infantum_ in the Mediterranean basin as well as South America. Elimination of domestic dogs in China, accompanied by other measures, virtually eliminated the disease in man. Less success was achieved in Ceara State, Brazil where some 50,000 seropositive dogs were eliminated, but the operation was interrupted and has recently been started again.

One problem with dogs is that they cannot be cured by antimony therapy. Gradoni described an experiment on the island of Elba where sick dogs were put down, but those with few symptoms or those which were only seropositive were treated. After only two years, the annual incidence of new cases was reduced from 12.4% to 4.6%

Another experience depending on serodiagnosis of infected dogs was described by Ben Ismail in Algeria. By working in close collaboration with primary health care workers, minimal effort was required to collect serum from all 88 dogs in an area of 3 km surrounding the house of a fatal case of visceral leishmaniasis. The serum was examined during the non-transmission season and ten seropositive dogs were identified. A second short visit to the village allowed the examination of the seropositive dogs and their elimination. Seven of the ten were proven to be infected.

Various workers described contrary experiences where people refused to allow their dogs to be examined or where veterinarians charged exorbitant fees for treatment of infected dogs.

In Brazil, dogs and also horses are commonly infected with _L. b. braziliensis_ and may maintain a peridomestic reservoir (Brazil). Horses clearly cannot readily be put down but fortunately have been found to respond well to antimony treatment. Similar infections have been described in pigs; the role of domestic animals in the maintanence and transmission to man of _L. b. braziliensis_ requires extensive quantitative study.

Domestic animals present special opportunities in the development of new control measures, especially those using therapy or prophylaxis; people are commonly willing to invest heavily in the lives of their animals while the strict constraints attaching to human trials do not apply to animals. Thus, there is some experience in the use of targetted chemotherapy and there are plans for vaccine trials on dogs. The results of these studies are not yet available.

Conclusion

The Forum identified a number of opportunities which are ready for application or almost so, and also a number of areas where active development or research is clearly indicated. Opportunities identified include:

Rodent control has reached a high degree of sophistication; with the predictability of _L. major_ outbreaks in development projects in areas occupied by _P. obesus_ presumptive control measures are justified, if the rodents have been shown to be infected.

Control of _Meriones_ spp. in outbreaks in settled areas, by available methods is probably justified.

Control of infection in dogs is feasible and effective in certain circumstances. There are encouraging developments in treatment and protection of dogs on the horizon.

Constraints and areas requiring development or research included:

Ecological, bionomic and ethological studies on mammals in relation to their role as reservoir hosts of leishmaniasis;

Protocols for integration of control measures with agricultural authorities (Meriones spp.) and rabies control services (dogs);

More qualitative information on the structure of sylvatic L. b. braziliensis and L. tropica foci and/or quantitative studies, integrated with human epidemiology and sandfly bionomics in all foci.

The incorporation of primary health care services in control measures is required, as is respect for the local traditions, customs and laws, including envrionmental and conservation legislation. Each leishmaniasis focus will require modification of whatever control measures are used and it must be recognised that no universal strategy is likely to be practical even for any one Leishmania species.

In most instances long term control will require repeated efforts and will have to be part of recurrent budgets. In all cases effective evaluation and long term surveillance of controlled areas will be required. Protocols for surveillance still need to be developed.

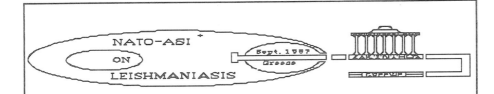

CHAPTER 8
NEW STRATEGIES FOR CONTROL FORUM III
VACCINATION

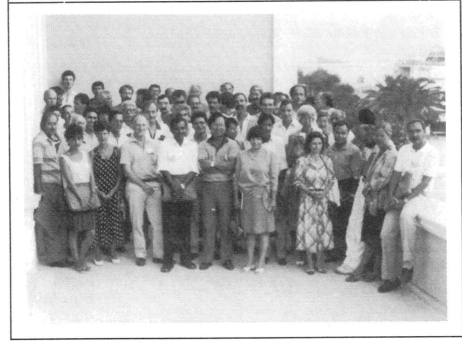

NEW STRATEGY FOR CONTROL FORUM: VACCINATION

F. Y. Liew

Department of Experimental Immunobiology, The Wellcome Research Laboratories, Langley Court, Beckenham, Kent BR3 3BS U.K.

This short article summarises the conclusions reached after a lively discussion in the new strategy for control forum: vaccination. The author acted as the chairman and rapporteur.

FEASIBILITY OF VACCINATION

The fact that life-long protection can be achieved by natural or deliberate infection demonstrates that mass vaccination against leishmaniasis is a strong possibility. This is supported by successful immunisation in the mouse with killed whole culture promastigotes or fractionated antigens against cutaneous leishmaniasis. The recent field trials carried out in Brasil[1,2] with killed L. braziliensis species, although hampered by low incidence rate in the control group, showed that more than 70% of the vaccinees became skin positive and there was no untoward side effect. It should, however, be noted that so far, long-term solid protection has only been achieved with leishmanisation against cutaneous leishmaniasis and that premunition (i.e. persistence of low numbers of parasite) may be needed for such protection. Whether killed vaccine with periodic boosting can achieve similar levels of immunity is at present unknown. In the past, there was a clear relation between leishmanisation and the recrudescence of latent psoriasis or the appearance of new cases[3]. Further, it has been noted that after inoculation against leishmania, the immune response of children receiving their booster to triple vaccine (diphtheria, pertussis and tetanus) is depressed for periods of up to six months[4].

Inspite of these reservations, it is generally felt that the possibility of developing an effective, molecularly defined vaccine against cutaneous leishmaniasis is high.

ANIMAL MODELS

Extensive information on experimental vaccination against cutaneous leishmaniasis is available. It is now routine to obtain substantial protection against L. major and L. mexicana in resistant as well as susceptible strains of mice with killed whole promastigotes or fractionated antigens[5]. Complete protection can also be achieved with more defined antigens such as glycoconjugates on the surface of promatigotes as defined by monoclonal antibody WIC 79.3[6] or a major glycoprotein, gp63 (D. Russell and J. Alexander, submitted). An important point arising from this experimental model is the requirement to administer the antigen via the i.v. or i.p. routes. Immunisation via the s.c. or intramuscular routes is not only ineffective, but frequently exacerbates the disease following challenge infection. Attempts to circumvent this restriction by various adjuvants has only met with partial success. Subcutaneous injection of gp63 incorporated in liposome induced protection against L. mexicana infection in CBA mice but not in the more susceptible BALB/c mice (D. Russell and J. Alexander, submitted). Such a restriction, if extended to molecularly defined antigens in clinical leishmaniasis, will be a formidable obstacle to mass vaccination.

Other experimental models are less well studied. There is an urgent need to extend the investigations into dogs and monkeys. The canine model is of particular interest in view of the increase in prevalence of leishmaniasis in Southern Europe and Central America.

MECHANISM OF ACQUIRED IMMUNITY

The case for cell-mediated immunity playing a causal role in resistance against leishmaniasis is based on an impressive range of clinical and experimental evidence[7]. Protection is mediated by $L3T4^+$ ($CD4^+$) T cells which produce interferon-γ and macrophage activating factor upon leishmania-antigen stimulation. Although antibody has been shown to limit parasite growth in vitro, direct evidence for a corresponding role in vivo is lacking. A secondary protective role for $Lyt-2^+$ T cells remains a possibility.

Evidence is also accumulating that $L3T4^+$ T cells can also be detrimental to the host. Thus, T cells from mice with progressive disease or after s.c. immunisation can exacerbate disease development and inhibit the protective effect of T cells from recovered or i.v. immunised mice. This is demonstrated even more directly with cloned T cell lines. It now appears that the host protective $L3T4^+$ T cells are distinct from the disease enhancing $L3T4^+$ T cells. Understanding of the mechanism of preferential induction of these T cell subsets and their interaction will be the key to rational design of future vaccines.

NEW STRATEGY

In spite of various uncertainties arising from the murine model, there is evidence that these may not be extrapolatable to clinical leishmaniasis. The current practice of leishmanisation in certain high endemic areas offers a unique opportunity in carrying out a limited, well controlled clinical trial for some of the candidate vaccines.

In doing so, the following sequential procedures should be taken:

i.   Preparation of sufficiently large quantities of standard skin test antigen preparation.
ii. Preparation of a standard killed whole promastigote vaccine.
iii. Preparation of various fractionated antigens, e.g. glycoconjugate, gp63 and other soluble cytoplasmic antigens.
iv. Vaccination of monkeys and dogs with these candidate antigens.
v.   Phase I clinical trial:
     (a) Defining acceptable dosage.
     (b) Monitoring cellular and humoral response to different antigens.
vi. Limited phase II clinical trial, using leishmaniasation as challenge.

References

1. Mayrink, W., Da Costa, C. A., et al. (1979) Trans. Roy. Soc. Trop. Med. Hyg. 73:385.
2. Antunes, C. M. et al. (1986) Int. J. Epidemiol. 15:572.
3. Iarmukhamedov, M. A. (1971) Med. Parazitol. (Mosk.) 40:549.
4. Serebryakov, V. A., et al. (1972) Med. Parazitol. (Mosk.) 41:303.
5. Liew, F. Y. (1986) Parasitology Today 2:264.

6. Handman, E. and Mitchell, G. F. (1985) Proc. Natl. Acad. Sci. USA 82:5910.
7. Howard, J. G. (1985) In Leishmaniasis (K-P. Chang and R. S, Bray, Eds.) Elsevier Press, Amsterdam, Pp. 140-162.

VACCINATION AND THE IMMUNOLOGICAL CONTROL OF LEISHMANIASIS

James Alexander

Immunology Division
Strathclyde University
Glasgow

INTRODUCTION

Vaccination against cutaneous leishmaniasis has long been practiced. Accounts in the literature suggest that from as early as the 19th Century children in Baghdad had been vaccinated against "Oriental Sore", by inoculating material from active human lesions into the skin of the arm or thigh (Wenyon, 1911). In this way long-lasting immunity could be induced and the likelihood of developing disfiguring facial scars avoided. To my knowledge there has been only one vaccination study on human visceral leishmaniasis caused by L. donovani. Manson-Bahr (1961) reported that inoculation with a non-visceralising ground squirrel strain of L. donovani protected against challenge with the human parasite. The ground squirrel parasite has, in fact, been identified as L. major using biochemical and serological methods (Chance et al., 1978). However, the use of live material is subject to obvious drawbacks, scarring is inevitable at the site of inoculation and there is always the possibility of a particularly susceptible recipient developing a chronic or severe infection. The problems inherent in the use of virulent vaccines have stimulated trials using attenuated parasites or parasite fractions. Although these have proved disappointing with regard to Old World cutaneous leishmaniasis, recent field trials in South America have produced encouraging results. Using a vaccine consisting of equal parts heat-killed and sonicated promastigotes from five different parasite isolates, Mayrink et al (1985) successfully and significantly protected from infection 70% of the participants that became skin-test positive following vaccination.

Ultimately the development of successful vaccination protocols is dependent on a thorough understanding of the immunological mechanisms determining the growth of leishmania parasites in the host. For obvious reasons it is difficult to study such phenomena in man. This has necessitated the use of laboratory models, particularly inbred mice, for the dissection and investigation of immunological control in leishmaniasis. A wide spectrum of disease profiles develop in mice depending on the genetic background of the host. Although immunity to cutaneous leishmaniasis, L. major, and visceral leishmaniasis, L. donovani, is under the control of different genes, innate susceptibility to both diseases is related to a primary macrophage defect (Gorczynski & MacRae, 1982; Crocker et al., 1984) which in turn gives rise to the generation of T-suppressor cells (Howard et al., 1981; Blackwell & Ulczak, 1984). The overwhelming evidence also indicates that protective immunity is also cell mediated.

Numerous laboratory studies have now shown that immunity can often be induced in normally non-curing leishmaniasis either by selectively depleting T-suppressor cells by prophylactic whole-body irradiation or by promoting the growth of a protective T-cell populations by vaccination (Liew et al., 1985). Most studies have used as vaccines heat-killed, avirulent or radio attenuated promastigotes and protection against cutaneous leishmaniasis could be induced by repeated intravenous or intraperitoneal inoculation. Unfortunately, vaccination via the subcutaneous route was often ineffective or worse exacerbated infections. These reports are troubling with regard to the development of a vaccine for use in humans. Not only are i.v. and i.p. vaccines unacceptable but suitable safe protocols have to be developed which do not risk exacerbating naturally acquired infections.

New Strategies

In order to limit the likelihood of any candidate vaccine enhancing the disease process following infection it is essential that it comprise immunologically characterised purified antigen or its derivatives. Recent studies have shown not only that parasite plasma membrane antigens are capable of inducing protection (Handman and Mitchell, 1985; Russell and Alexander, 1987; Alexander and Russell, 1987), but also soluble non-membrane derived parasite antigens (Scott et al., 1987). However, the antigens responsible for protection in the soluble parasite extract are yet to be identified while protection has been induced by two purified plasma membrane derived antigens, the glycolipid L-GL (formerly EF), and the glycoprotein gp63. Handman and Mitchell (1985) found the L-GL protected mice against L. major if inoculated i.p. with C. parvum. However, lipid free L-GL is a "disease-promoting" antigen (Handman et al., 1987). It was suggested that the crucial role of the lipid moiety was to allow insertion of the polysaccharide complex into cell membranes, resulting in its effective presentation to T cells. By reconstituting L-GL and gp63 in liposomes (phospholipid bilayers) it was anticipated we would further enhance presentation of the antigens to T cells. This has recently been successfully demonstrated in other systems (Hopp, 1984; Watari et al., 1987). In addition, this method of antigen packaging also enabled the isolated membrane components to be inoculated in their native non-denatured configuration anchored in the phospholipid bialyer by their hydrophobic regions. It was reasoned that this method of antigen preparation would direct the immune response to determinants of identical spatial conformation to those occurring on the parasite plasmalemma. Both antigens reconstituted into liposomes were found to be protective even by the subcutaneous route (Russell and Alexander, 1987).

The identification of these 2 candidate antigens for a human vaccine should stimulate experimentation using new technologies in vaccine production (reviewed Liew, 1986; Ada and Jones, 1987; Zanetti et al., 1987). While the Leishmania glycolipid would not easily lend itself to large scale production the polypeptide gp63 would be suitable for experimentation with recombinant or peptide vaccine preparations. This would necessitate the identification of the relevant antigenic determinants as current evidence would suggest that proteins contain not only discrete T and B epitopes but also distinct suppressor determinants. The presence of suppressor determinants in gp63 was suggested by the exacerbated disease produced in mice following vaccination of gp63 together with FCA (Russell and Alexander, 1987).

Distinct determinants responsible for protection and/or suppression following infection with Leishmania have been demonstrated in an elegant study by Gorczynski (1986). Protection rather than suppression was associated with N-linked glycoproteins. The important contribution of sugar residues to the determinants responsible for influencing the disease process may necessitate immunization with parasite glycoprotein expressed by genetically engineered viral vectors. Alternatively, the use of anti-idiotypic vaccines which mimic the molecular configuration of antigenic determinants would circumvent the requirement for carbohydrates.

Although synthetic or sub-unit vaccines may have the specificity of the antigen from which they are derived it is unlikely that they will have the same immunological potency. It is likely they will have to be attached to suitable carriers or presented in association with adjuvants to maximise their immunogenicity. Among those being considered for use in humans are liposomes. These greatly enhance the T cell responses to parasite plasma membrane antigen (Russell and Alexander, 1987). Iscoms (immunostimulating complexes) formed by the interaction of the hydrophobic portion of membrane proteins with a glycoside matrix (Morein et al., 1984) are promising alternatives. Bacterial derivatives are also useful immunopotentiators. Thus the antigenicity of L-GL has been increased through a non-covalent ionic association with poly L-lysine to the adjuvant MDP (Greenblatt et al., 1983). An alternative approach may be to link purified derivative of tuberculin (PPD) to antigen. These preparations greatly enhance immune responses to animals pre-exposed to BCG (Lachmann et al., 1986).

DISCUSSION

Leishmania has the tremendous advantage over many other parasites of being relatively easy to grow in culture. The large quantities of readily available parasite material have allowed tremendous progress in the fields of molecular biology, biochemistry and immunology in recent years. Thus biologically important antigens, particularly those on the parasite surface membrane and involved in interactions with the macrophage host cell have been described. As these antigens are crucial to the parasite's successful entry into macrophages they have been thought the most likely candidates for a vaccine. The two antigens described, L-GL and gp63, are found in related forms in all species of Leishmania examined to date (Etges et al., 1985; Colomer-Gould et al., 1985; Handman et al., 1984) and may ultimately form the basis of a cross-protective vaccine. In the studies reported in this volume and elsewhere (Russell and Alexander, 1987) we have demonstrated the immunizing potential of these antigens when they are suitably packaged for presentation to the immune system. What is more we successfully vaccinated mice by the subcutaneous route.
While these results in mouse models of leishmaniasis are encouraging are they directly applicable to the development of a human vaccine? This is a debatable point and one which has to be examined carefully. For example, bacterial polysaccharide antigens that are immunosuppressive in mice are protective in man (reviewd Handman et al., 1987). Vaccine trials in man will therefore have to be approached with considerable caution. The numerous problems associated with vaccine development, production and administration are superbly reviewed by Liew (1986). Nevertheless the apparent success of a human field trial using crude parasite antigens from several isolates is extremely promising (Mayrink et al., 1985).

REFERENCES

Ada, G.L. and Jones, P.D., 1987, Vaccines for the future - an update, Immunol. Cell Biol., 65:11.

Alexander, J. and Russell, D.G., 1987, A novel method of vaccination using parasite membrane antigens, This volume.

Blackwell, J. and Ulczak, O.M., 1984, Immunoregulation of genetically controlled acquired responses to Leishmania donovani infection in mice: demonstration and characterisation of suppressor T cells in non-cure mice, Infec. Immun., 44:97.

Chance, M.L., Schnur, L.F., Thomas, S.C. and Peters, W., 1978, The biochemical and serological taxonomy of Leishmania from the Aethiopian zoogeographical region of Africa, Ann. Trop. Med. and Parasitol., 72;533.

Colomer-Gould, V., Quintass, L.G., Keithly, J. and Noguiera, N., 1985, A common surface antigen on amastigotes and promastigotes of Leishmania species, J. Exp. Med., 162:902.

Etges, R.J., Bouvier, J., Hoffman, R. and Bordier, L., 1985, Evidence that the major surface proteins of three Leishmania species are structurally related, Mol. Biochem. Parasitol., 14:141.

Crocker, P.R., Blackwell, J.M. and Bradley, D.J., 1984, Expression of the natural resistance gene Lsh in resident tissue macrophages, Infec Immun., 43:1033.

Gorczynski, R.M., 1986, Do sugar residues contribute to the antigenic determinants responsible for protection and/or abolition of protection in Leishmania infected BALB/c mice, J. Immunol., 137:1010.

Gorczynski, R.M. and MacRae, S., 1982, Analysis of subpopulations of glass adherent mouse skin cells controlling resistance/susceptibility to infection with Leishmania tropica and correlation with the development of independent proliferative signals to Lyt-1^+/Lyt-2^+ T lymphocytes, Cell Immunol., 67:74.

Handman, E. and Mitchell, G.F., 1985, Immunization with Leishmania receptor for macrophages protects mice against cutaneous leishmaniasis, Proc. Natl. Acad. Sci. USA., 82:5910.

Handman, E., Greenblatt, C.H. and Goding, J., 1984, An amphipathic sulphated glycoconjugate of Leishmania: characterisation with monoclonal antibodies, EMBO J., 3:1206.

Handman, E., McConville, M.J. and Goding, J.W., 1987, Carbohydrate antigens as possible parasite vaccines, Immunol. Today, 8:181.

Hopp, T.P., 1984, Immunogenicity of a synthetic HBsAg peptide : enhancement by conjugation to a fatty acid carrier, Mol. Immunol., 31:13.

Howard, J.G., Hale, C. and Liew, F.Y., 1981, Immunological regulation of experimental cutaneous leishmaniasis IV Prophylactic effect of sublethal irradiation as a result of abrogation of suppressor T cell generation in mice genetically susceptible to Leishmania tropica, J. Exp. Med., 153:557.

Lachman, P.J., Strangeways, L., Vyakarnam, A. and Evan, G.I., 1986, Raising antibodies by coupling peptides to PPD and immunizing BCG-sensitised animals, Ciba Foundation Symp., 119:25.

Liew, F.Y., 1986, New aspects of vaccine development, Clin. Exp. Immunol., 62:225.

Liew, F.Y., Hale, C. and Howard, J.G., 1985, Prophylactic immunization against experimental leishmaniasis. IV subcutaneous immunization prevents the induction of protective immunity against fatal Leishmania major infection, J. Immunol., 135:2095.

Manson-Bahr, P.E.C., 1961, Immunity in Kala-Azar, Trans. R. Soc. Trop. Med. Hyg., 55:550.

Mayrink, W., Williams, P., Da Costa, C.A., Magalpaes, P.A., Melr, M.N., Dias, M., Oliveira Lima, A., Michaelick, M.S.M., Ferriera Carvahlo,

E., Barros, G.C., Sessa, P.A. and De Alencar, J.T.A., 1985, An experimental vaccine against American dermal leishmaniasis : experience in the State of Espirito Santo, Brazil, Ann. Trop. Med. Parasitol., 79:255.

Morein, B., Sundquist, B., Hoglund, S., Dalsgaard, K. and Osterhaus, A., 1984, Iscom, a novel structure for antigenic presentation of membrane proteins from enveloped viruses, Nature, 308:457.

Russell, D.G. and Alexander, J., 1987, Effective immunization against cutaneous leishmaniasis with defined membrane antigens reconstituted into liposomes, J. Immunol. (submitted).

Scott, P., Pearce, E., Natovitz, P. and Sher, A., 1987, Vaccination against cutaneous leishmaniasis in a murine model 1. Induction of protective immunity with a soluble extract of promastigotes, J. Immunol., 139:221.

Watari, E., Dietzschold, B., Szoham, G. and Heber-Katz, E., 1987, A synthetic peptide induces long-term protection from lethal infection with Herpes simplex virus 2, J. Exp. Med., 165:459.

Wenyon, C.M., 1911, Oriental Sore in Baghdad, together with observations on a gregarine in Stegomyia fasciata the haemogregarine of dogs and flagellates of house flies, Parasit., 4:273.

Zanetti, M., Sercarz, E. and Jonas Salk, 1987, The immunology of new generation vaccines, Immunol. Today, 8:18.

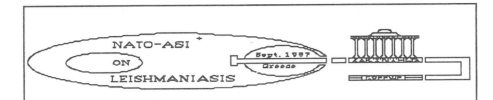

CHAPTER 9
NEW STRATEGIES FOR CONTROL FORUM IV
CHEMOTHERAPY

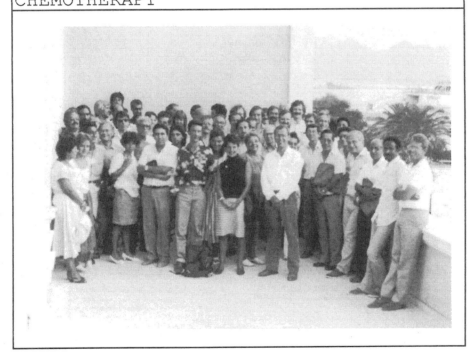

NEW STRATEGIES FOR CONTROL FORUM : CHEMOTHERAPY

Simon L. Croft and Ralph A. Neal

Electron Microscopy Laboratory and Department of Medical
Protozoology, London School of Hygiene and Tropical Medicine
London WC1E 7HT, U.K.

In 1937 sodium antimonyl gluconate ('Solustibosan') was first used in the treatment of leishmaniasis in India and China[1,2]. It is a remarkable condemnation of our progress that fifty years later improved dosing regimens for the pentavalent antimonial derivatives of 'Solubstibosan', sodium stibogluconate ('Pentostam',Wellcome) and meglumine antimoniate ('Glucantime',Rhone-Poulenc), can still create such interest and be considered an advance. Despite the long courses, parenteral administration, difficulties in chemical synthesis and low activities against cutaneous disease, these pentavalent antimonials remain the first line treatment for leishmaniasis[3]. Attempts to identify alternatives have produced a number of new drugs for the disease currently or about to undergo clinical trial. These include the pyrazolopyrimidines allopurinol and allopurinol riboside, the antifungal imidazole ketoconazole and the 4-methyl-8-aminoquinoline WR6026. Clinical evaluation of the compounds is not complete and whether they will replace the antimonials or be added to the 'second line' list along with pentamidine and amphotericin B is uncertain. Allopurinol may have a future in combination with 'Pentostam'[4], but along with it's riboside derivative this drug has the pharmacokinetic problems of rapid excretion and metabolism by host xanthine oxidase. In a clinical trial in which allopurinol riboside was used to treat cutaneous leishmaniasis, one group of patients also received probenicid which reduces the renal tubular clearance of some purine analogues, and elevated plasma levels of the pyrazolopyrimidine were shown along with an improved cure rate[5]. Other purine analogues have also shown promising results , including 9-deazainosine in rodent and monkey models[6]. This group of compounds continue to show potential and further patent applications have been submitted recently for the antileishmanial activity of a variety of inosine and guanosine analogues. Another group of compounds which has shown potential in the treatment of leishmaniasis is the sterol synthesis inhibiting imidazoles. Ketoconazole is under clinical trial in Saudi Arabia[7] and the related compounds miconazole and itraconazole have also been shown to be effective. The determination of a similar sterol synthesis pathway in <u>Leishmania</u> as in fungi[8] has led to the examination of other known inhibitors including the antifungal allylamines (see D.H. Beach et al., this volume).

The last decade has seen an enormous growth in our understanding of the biochemistry of protozoan parasites and accompanying this the identification of possible chemotherapeutic targets. The list of approaches is large and many were outlined in the forum by Dr.G.Coombs and Dr.F.Opperdoes (this volume) in addition to those mentioned above. In the forum further comments were made by Dr.A.Fairlamb on polyamine synthesis as a chemotherapeutic target especially since the relationship of polyamines to oxidative defence mechanisms through trypanothione has been established. Targets in the metabolic pathways associated with the glycosome were summarised by Drs. Opperdoes and Hart. Dr.D.T.Hart described the mechanism of action of some drugs, including Pentostam, on glycosomal pathways as well as emphasising the potential of molecular graphics in drug design. Dr.S.Beverley, whose recent molecular approach to the understanding of methotrexate resistance in promastigotes has helped to revive interest in folate metabolism as a chemotherapeutic target in Leishmania, described recent studies characterising folate and methotrexate uptake by these organisms. The importance of the ATPase proton pump present on the cytoplasmic surface of the plasmamembrane was described by Dr.D.Zilberstein. The enzyme which has critical roles in the nutrition and pH control of parasites can be inhibited by tricyclic antidepressants indicating the basis for another new approach to chemotherapy.

Although one has faith that the rational approach will identify an ideal selectively toxic compound with good pharmacological characteristics, there remains a further obstacle to the development of an antileishmanial drug. The cost of development of a new drug is so high that for most tropical diseases it is not an economic proposition. Development of a specific antileishmanial is only likely to be possible through cooperation between a pharmaceutical company and international organisations. A drug with a wider activity to encompass trypanosomiasis with a profitable veterinary market is more feasible. One alternative to this impasse is the empirical screening of drugs designed and clinically used for other diseases and serendipity. A further alternative is to package current antileishmanial drugs in new delivery systems which improve their efficacy and reduce their toxicity. A new formulation for topical use has been developed for paromomycin with a quaternary ammonium compound which[9] has proved to be successful experimentally and in preliminary clinical trials. The targeting of pentavalent antimonials and amphotericin B in liposomes and other carriers to the infected macrophages of the liver and spleen has been enormously successful in experimental models of visceral leishmaniasis and hopefully soon there will be clinical trials to evaluate this approach (see S.L.Croft et al. and C.A.Hunter et al. this volume).

REFERENCES

1. W.Kikuth and H.Schmidt, Contribution to the progress of antimony therapy of kala-azar, Chinese Med. J., 52:425 (1937)
2. L.E.Napier, R.Chaudhui and M.N.Rai Chaudhui, A stable solution of antimony for the treatment of kala-azar, Indian Med. Gaz., 72:462 (1937)
3. WHO Technical Report Series, 701, The Leishmaniases (1984)
4. C.N.Chunge, G.Gachihi, K.Wasunna, J.R.Rashid, J.D.Chulay, G.Anabwani, C.N.Oster and A.D.M.Bryceson, Visceral leishmaniasis unresponsive to antimonial drugs III. Successful treatment using a combination of sodium stibogluconate plus allopurinol, Trans.R.Soc.Trop.Med.Hyg., 79:715 (1985)
5. R.E.Saenz, H.Paz, C.M.Johnson, J.J.Marr, D.J.Nelson, M.D.Rogers and K.H.Pattishall, Treatment of American cutaneous leishmaniasis with orally-administered allopurinol riboside, submitted for publication (1987)
6. J.D.Berman, W.L.Hanson, J.K.Lovelace, V.B.Waits, J.E.Jackson, W.L.Chapman Jr. and R.S.Klein, Activity of purine analogs against Leishmania donovani in vivo, Antimicrob.Agents Chemoth., 31:111 (1987)
7. R.Kubba, Y.Al-Gindan, A.M.El-Hassan and A.elH.S.Omer, Ketoconazole in cutaneous leishmaniasis : Results of a pilot study, Saudi Med.J., 7:596 (1986)

8. J.D.Berman, L.J.Goad, D.H.Beach and G.G.Holz Jr., Effects of ketoconazole on sterol biosynthesis by Leishmania mexicana mexicana amastigotes in murine macrophage tumor cells, Molec.Biochem.Parasit., 20:85 (1986)
9. J.El-On, R.Livshin, Z.Even-Paz, D.Hamburger and L.Weinrauch, Topical treatment of cutaneous leishmaniasis, J.Invest.Dermatol., 87:284 (1986)

STRATEGIES FOR THE DESIGN OF NEW ANTILEISHMANIAL DRUGS

Graham H. Coombs

Department of Zoology
University of Glasgow
Glasgow G12 8QQ
Scotland, U.K.

INTRODUCTION

The need for new antileishmanial drugs is well known and undisputed. There has been renewed interest in the problem during recent years and several promising new antileishmanial compounds and formulations have emerged as candidate drugs, notably allopurinol riboside, ketoconazole and the use of liposomes as a delivery system for drugs against visceral leishmaniasis. Some of these are still undergoing trials, but as yet none has proved to be the answer to leishmaniasis. Nevertheless, the information gained from these studies, together with that arising from the increased number of investigations of the biochemistry and cell biology of the parasites, go someway towards providing the baseline data that will enable us to identify key differences between the parasite and host that we should be able to exploit with drugs.

This so-called "rational approach to chemotherapy" has been widely advocated, but much criticised as not bearing fruit. Such criticism seems premature and unreasonable. The approach is totally dependent upon a detailed knowledge of the biochemistry of the infective organism and such information takes a long time to accumulate. It is, however, a progressive process which should speed up. Nevertheless, it has to be accepted that we are investing today for the good of tomorrow; not an altogether popular concept in the modern world.

Certainly more studies on the biochemistry of the leishmanias and the leishmaniases are required, and undoubtedly these will increase our understanding, but nevertheless it seems an appropriate time to review the possibilities that have already been revealed for designing drugs to act specifically against the parasite. It is to be hoped that this will help to stimulate new lines of investigation and provide direction for attempts to apply our current knowledge.

STRATEGIES

The blocking of any enzyme-catalysed reaction occurring in a parasite is likely to have severe consequences and so compounds that do this selectively have potential as antiparasitic agents. Thus there have been many investigations aimed at finding parasite-specific features, in particular enzymes with no mammalian equivalent or which differ from their mammalian counterpart in significant ways. The antibacterial activities of the penicillins, sulphonamides and trimethoprim provide fine examples of how successfully such enzymes can be exploited.

Several leishmanial enzymes that appear to fall into this category have been discovered already. Notable amongst them are 3'-nucleotidase, adenase, xanthine phosphoribosyltransferase, nucleoside phosphotransferase, trypanothione-specific enzymes and enzymes involved with sterol biosynthesis; all of these catalyse reactions that apparently do not occur in mammals. In addition, leishmanial dihydrofolate reductase, thymidylate synthetase, dihydroorotate dehydrogenase, orotate phosphoribosyltransferase and orotidine-5'-phosphate decarboxylase have been shown to differ very markedly from the isofunctional mammalian enzymes. Inhibitors of many of these parasite enzymes are known, but none has so far proved to be the answer to leishmaniasis. The usual problem is lack of specificity. Compounds that inhibit enzymes present only in the parasite should possess excellent selective toxicity, but only if they effect no other enzymes; this rarely is so.

In some cases, blocking the enzyme has no apparent effect on the parasite. This suggests that the enzyme is not required, certainly under the conditions of the test. This latter point highlights a major difficulty, many models used for assessing the activity of putative antiparasitic drugs bear rather little resemblance to the natural infection. It may be that key adaptations of a parasite for existence in a host are of no importance when the parasite is growing axenically in vitro. An alternative explanation is that parasites possess functionless, unnecessary enzymes, although I prefer to consider that there are likely to be few, if any; such enzymes are very likely to be lost during the course of evolution. Another possible explanation is that the enzyme in question is present in all stages of the parasite, but necessary in only some - for instance those in the sandfly. There are, however, many examples of proteins that are developmentally regulated during parasite life cycles, suggesting that this is the more cost-effective method of adaptation. Clearly there are many uncertainties, but for the present it seems reasonable to have the working hypothesis that if it's there, it's important.

Perhaps the main reason that we have not so far been very successful at purposefully producing enzyme inhibitors that are good drugs is that we are not yet good enough at designing appropriate inhibitors. This is partly because we do not have sufficient information on the enzymes. It is to be expected, therefore, that the situation will improve with time and should be helped considerably by the advent of techniques such as computer-graphics. The approach itself seems basically right.

So far I have concentrated on the situation were parasite enzymes themselves are unusual. There are, however, other ways in which enzymes can differ from their host equivalent, for instance in their amount and location, and these also provide opportunities for drug design. Perhaps the best studied examples in leishmanias are the enzymes on the surface of the parasite and those associated with the organelles known as glycosomes and 'megasomes'.

The surface location of an enzyme, as is known to be the case for several leishmanial enzymes including acid phosphatase, 3'-nucleotidase, 5'-nucleotidase, phospholipases and a proteinase[1], means that it can be severely affected by compounds that are unable to enter cells. One can envisage how this could be a good means of achieving selectivity against several parasites, although less easily for leishmania as it is itself intracellular. Nevertheless, exogenous material that does not enter into the cytoplasm of macrophages can permeate to the parasitophorous vacuole. Presenting such a formulation to the infected macrophage in vivo, however, would presumably necessitate injection, not the ideal route for an antileishmanial drug.

The glycosomes of leishmanias have been investigated much less extensively than those of trypanosomes, nevertheless it is clear already that there are many similarities between the organelles of the two groups of parasites[2,3]. Those of leishmania possess not only several glycolytic enzymes and associated enzymes such as phosphoenolpyruvate carboxykinase and malate dehydrogenase but also some enzymes involved in purine salvage and pyrimidine biosynthesis[4]. The association of these enzymes with glycosomes is a major difference from their mammalian counterparts and this must be reflected in their structures as well as the occurrence of proteins with related functions, such as transporters into the organelle. It may also be possible to design drugs that are accumulated in the organelles and so disrupt their functioning.

Such an approach has been widely discussed and demonstrated for lysosomes, of which the 'megasomes' of L. mexicana seem to be a class[6]. The main rationale for testing lysosomotropic agents against leishmania was that the amastigote lives in a vacuole apparently equivalent to a secondary lysosome, so a lysosomotropic agent would accumulate in the vacuole and the parasite would be exposed to it at high concentration. Several compounds thought to work in this way were found to be toxic to leishmania amastigotes in macrophages. Some of these may act simply by changing the conditions, for instance pH, within the vacuole in such a way as the parasite is unable to survive. Even modulating the environment to make it less extreme, such as raising the pH, may have adverse effects on the parasite if it is adapted for the natural conditions. This approach does not appear to have been investigated fully. Ammonia apparently aids initial survival of L. mexicana in macrophages[7], but how is subsequent growth affected? How do similar amines affect other leishmanias that may be adapted differently for life in macrophages?

The finding that amastigotes themselves, at least those of the L. mexicana complex, have an extensive and well developed lysosomal network and contain relatively high activities of several lysosomal enzymes[6], notably proteinases, provides further support for the suggestion that lysosomotropic agents could be potent antileishmanials. It may well be, however, that the activity of such compounds would be mediated through their accumulation in parasite lysosomes rather than simply the parasitophorous vacuole. This is thought to be the case for L-leucine methyl ester and related compounds, which are highly toxic to amastigotes of L. m. mexicana and L. m. amazonensis[8,9,10]. Their toxicity is apparently mediated by rapid hydrolysis within the amastigote lysosomes with the release and accumulation of the free amino acid; this results in lysis of the parasite through osmotic stress.

The leishmanial habitat within macrophages offers other opportunities for targetting drugs to the parasite. One potentially exploitable character is the phagocytic ability of the host cell. It has been convincingly proven that an antimonial entrapped in liposomes (phospholipid-containing vesicles) is more efficacious than the free drug against visceral leishmaniasis[11]. This increase in activity appears to be due to the liposome-entrapped drug being taken up to a much greater extent by the liver and spleen. A liposome-Pentostam (sodium stibogluconate) formulation is currently undergoing clinical trials. Similar levels of targetting can be achieved with vesicles known as niosomes, which are made from non-ionic surfactants and cholesterol[12,13]. These latter vesicles, however, may have advantages over liposomes in being potentially more stable in vitro, having a longer half life in vivo and possessing less toxicity towards mammalian systems. There are indications that polyacryl starch microparticles may provide an even better delivery system for antimonials against visceral leishmaniasis[13].

A similar approach to targetting antileishmanials is to make use of the ability of macrophages to take up acetyl-low density lipoprotein (acetyl-LDL), a feature not shared by many other cells[14]. Thus a drug attached to this lipid is likely to be concentrated in macrophages and so leishmanial amastigotes could be exposed to it at high concentrations. It may be that the amastigotes themselves are also able to endocytose exogenous material, as yet we know little about their phagocytic ability. Clearly, however, any compound specifically taken up by both the macrophage and the parasite is likely to have a good degree of specifity. These approaches to targetting appear to have high potential for use in the treatment of visceral leishmaniasis, but current evidence suggests that they may be less effective for the cutaneous leishmaniases. Perhaps more hopeful as a means of targetting drugs against these diseases are the attempts to use topical treatments. Even then, however, some means of increasing the uptake of the drug into the infected macrophage is likely to have a beneficial effect.

Another strategy is to design parasite-activated drugs. In many ways this is one of the most attractive approaches to drug design, as the pro-drug should be non-toxic and if the activation is carried out only by the parasite then the active drug will be produced only in its locality. Perhaps the best known parasite-activated drugs are the 5-nitroimidazoles. These appear to be reductively activated only under anaerobic conditions and so are selective to anaerobes. Can this approach be applied to the leishmanias? The answer is clearly yes. The studies on inosine analogues and other pyrazolopyrimidines confirm this[15]. These compounds are metabolised by parasite enzymes involved in purine salvage to yield rogue nucleotides that are toxic to the cell. Mammalian enzymes have stricter substrate specificities and incorporate the substrate analogues much less well. Unfortunately, the species differences in the ability to use the compounds is not absolute and some of the best antileishmanials have unacceptable toxicity to mammals. Allopurinol riboside, however, is currently undergoing clinical trials.

Table 1 LEISHMANIA: TARGETS FOR CHEMOTHERAPEUTIC ATTACK

1. COMPONENTS PRESENT ONLY IN LEISHMANIAS e.g. glycosomes, kinetoplast, 'megasomes', 3'-nucleotidase, xanthine phosphoribosyltransferase, trypanothione and related enzymes, sterols and biosynthetic enzymes.

2. COMPONENTS THAT DIFFER STRUCTURALLY FROM MAMMALIAN COMPONENTS e.g. dihydrofolate reductase/thymidylate synthetase, dihydroorotate dehydrogenase, orotate phosphoribosyltransferase, orotidine-5'-phosphate decarboxylase, tubulin.

3. ENZYMES WITH DIFFERENT SPECIFICITIES TO MAMMALIAN COUNTERPARTS e.g. purine-metabolising enzymes, nucleoside transporter.

4. ENZYMES THAT DIFFER IN LOCATION FROM MAMMALIAN COUNTERPARTS e.g. surface acid phosphatase, glycosomal enzymes.

6. ENZYMES DIFFERING QUANTITATIVELY FROM ISOFUNCTIONAL MAMMALIAN ENZYME e.g. hydrolases in 'megasomes'.

7. EXISTENCE OF AMASTIGOTE IN A PARASITOPHOROUS VACUOLE IN A MACROPHAGE.

Other possibilities for drug activation can be envisaged. It has been postulated that the high proteinase activity of L. mexicana amastigotes could be used to activate a peptide-blocked drug[16]. It may also be feasible to exploit the surface-located 3'-nucleotidase. Phosphorylated compounds are not taken up well usually and so a toxic nucleoside phosphorylated at the 3'-position is likely to have little effect on mammalian cells. In contrast, the 3'-nucleotidase on the surface of the parasite could release the free nucleoside, which would be transported into and kill the cell. A similar approach could be made to exploiting the surface acid phosphatase. In order to design the best compounds, however, we need more information on the two enzymes, particularly with respect to the substrates they will handle. So we are back to the requirement for more research.

The search for and development of synergistic drug combinations is a strategy that has been pursued with vigour in some areas of parasitology, but to date such an approach has received relatively little attention in the search for new antileishmanials. Whilst it is widely accepted that the use of drugs in combination is a means of slowing down the advent of drug resistance problems, there are financial drawbacks to their production. These considerations, together with worries that combinations synergistic against a parasite will also be synergistic against the host, probably explain the lack of interest shown so far. Nevertheless, there have been a few interesting reports of drugs with synergistic activity against leishmanias[17] and possibilities for other combinations that could show synergy specifically against leishmania have recently become apparent.

Table 2   LEISHMANIA: STRATEGIES FOR RATIONAL DRUG DESIGN

---

1. COMPOUNDS ACTING SPECIFICALLY AGAINST PARASITE FEATURE e.g. enzyme inhibitors.

2. COMPOUNDS CONCENTRATED IN PARASITE OR PARASITOPHOROUS VACUOLE e.g. targetted (using liposomes, niosomes, microparticles, antibodies, or lipoproteins), glycosomotropic or lysosomotropic (parasitophorous vacuole or parasite lysosomes) drugs.

3. PRODRUGS: COMPOUNDS ACTIVATED BY PARASITE FEATURE e.g. through incorporation (purine analogues), reduction (nitroheterocyclic compounds) or hydrolysis (by amastigote proteinases or other hydrolases [e.g. amino acid esters], by surface-located phosphomonoesterases).

4. DRUG COMBINATIONS e.g. toxin and inhibitor of uptake into mammalian cells (tubercidin/nitrobenzylthioinosine).

The finding that the nucleoside transporters of leishmanias differ from the mammalian equivalent in not being inhibited by 4-nitrobenzylthioinosine(NBMPR) or dipyridamole[18] suggests that a combination such as tubercidin and NBMPR may have a good chemotherapeutic index. Similarly, it may well be that the ornithine decarboxylase inhibitor ∝-difluoromethylornithine(DFMO) given in conjunction with other compounds interfering with polyamine metabolism could prove of therapeutic value. The antileishmanial diamidines reported to inhibit S-adenosylmethionine decarboxylase[19] would seem good candidates to be included, as would compounds with specificity towards trypanothione or related enzymes. Similar combinations involving DFMO are known to have interesting antitrypanosomal activity[20].

One of the major disincentives concerning drug combinations, that of cost of development, could be partially avoided if the combination involved established drugs already in clinical use. A complementary aim is to find ways of reducing the dose required of the standard antileishmanial drugs, such that toxicity to the host is reduced whilst the efficacy against the parasite is retained. The use of delivery systems, such as liposomes with Pentostam, is one way of achieving both aims; it may also be possible to design drug combinations that give similar results. One difficulty is that the precise modes of action of the major antileishmanial drugs have not yet been elucidated, which makes rational selection of combinations difficult. Finding out how the antileishmanial antimonials act would be a useful advance, again more basic science is required. The discovery of compounds synergistic with the antimonials against leishmanias would be helpful in this matter, as well as providing a means of using the drugs better in treatment of the disease.

DISCUSSION

Many promising drug targets have been identified already, as described above and summarised in Table 1, and a variety of stategies for their exploitation have been postulated (summarised in Table 2). In most instances, however, the detail available on the parasite features is not sufficient to allow the design of compounds with good specifity towards leishmanias. More biochemical investigations are essential and there should be continuing and closer collaboration between biochemists and chemists in the design and synthesis of putative new antileishmanials.

There is ample to attract and interest scientists, and a real goal for them to aim for, but the problem of funding remains. Leishmaniasis does not affect the right people to attract large-scale research support, indeed it is not even the AIDS of tropical medicine. It should be noted, however, that several of the approaches I have discussed above (such as exploiting the presence of glycosomes, 3'-nucleotidase and trypanothione) could be applied with equal validity to trypanosomes; indeed, some of them are well advanced. It is to be hoped that a concerted antitrypanosomatid programme could be the answer to the suffering of millions.

ACKNOWLEDGEMENTS

I thank The Wellcome Trust for financial support.

REFERENCES

1. D. M. Dwyer, The roles of surface membrane enzymes and transporters in the survival of Leishmania, in: "Host-parasite cellular and molecular interactions in protozoal infections", K-P Chang, and D. Snary, eds, Springer Verlag, Heidleberg.
2. D. T. Hart, and F. R. Opperdoes, The occurrence of glycosomes (microbodies) in the promastigote stage of four major Leishmania species, Mol. Biochem. Parasitol., 13: 159 (1984).
3. J. C. Mottram, and G. H. Coombs, Leishmania mexicana mexicana: Subcellular distribution of enzymes in amastigotes and promastigotes, Exp. Parasitol., 59: 265 (1985).
4. H. F. Hassan, J. C. Mottram, and G.H. Coombs, Subcellular localisation of purine-metabolising enzymes in Leishmania mexicana mexicana, Comp. Biochem. Physiol., 81B: 1037 (1985).
5. H. F. Hassan, and G.H. Coombs, Purine and pyrimidine metabolism in parasitic protozoa, FEMS Microbiol. Rev., in press (1987).
6. M. Pupkis, L. Tetley, and G. H. Coombs, Leishmania mexicana: amastigote hydrolases in unusual lysosomes, Exp. Parasitol., 62: 28 (1986).
7. J. Alexander, Leishmania mexicana: inhibition and stimulation of phagosome-lysosome fusion in infected macrophages, Exp. Parasitol., 52: 261 (1981).
8. M. Rabinovitch, V. Zilberfarb, and C. Ramazeilles, Destruction of Leishmania mexicana amazonensis within macrophages by lysosomotropic amino acid esters, J. Exp. Med., 163: 520 (1986).

9. M. Rabinovitch, V. Zilberfarb, and M. Pouchelet, Leishmania mexicana: destruction of isolated amastigotes by amino acid esters, Amer. J. Trop. Med. Hyg., 36: 290 (1987).
10. C. A. Hunter, L. M. Macpherson, and G. H. Coombs, Antileishmanial activity of L-leucine methyl ester and L-tryptophanamide, This symposium, (1987).
11. C. R. Alving, Liposomes as drug carriers in leishmaniasis and malaria, Parasitol. Today, 2: 101 (1986).
12. A. J. Baillie, G. H. Coombs, T. F. Dolan, and J. Laurie, Nonionic surfactant vesicles, niosomes, as a delivery system for the antileishmanial drug, sodium stibogluconate, J. Pharm. Pharmacol., 38: 502 (1986).
13. C. A. Hunter, T. F. Dolan, T. Laakso, A. J. Baillie, G. H. Coombs, I. Sjoholm, and P. Stjarnkvist, A comparison of delivery systems for sodium stibogluconate in the therapy of experimental murine leishmaniasis, This symposium, (1987).
14. D. T. Hart, Antileishmanial drug design and delivery, J. Royal Army Med. Corps, 132: 149 (1986).
15. D. L. Looker, J. J. Marr, and R. L. Berens, Mechanisms of action of pyrazolopyrimidines in Leishmania donovani, J. Biol. Chem., 261: 9412 (1986).
16. G. H. Coombs, The biochemical approach to the discovery of antileishmanial drugs, J. Royal Army Med. Corps, 132: 147 (1986).
17. J. El-On, Growth inhibition of Leishmania tropica amastigotes in vitro with rifampicin combined with amphotericin B, Ann. Trop. Med. Parasitol., 78: 93 (1984).
18. B. Aronow, K. Kaur, K. McCartan, and B. Ullman, Two high affinity nucleoside transporters in Leishmania donovani, Mol. Biochem. Parasit., 22: 29 (1984).
19. A. J. Bitonti, J. A. Dumont, and P. P. McCann, Characterisation of Trypanosoma brucei brucei S-adenosyl-L-methionine decarboxylase and its inhibition by Berenil, pentamidine and methylglyoxal bis(guanylhydrazone), Biochem. J., 237: 685 (1986).
20. P. P. McCann, C. J. Bacchi, H. C. Nathan, and A. Sjoerdsma, Difluoromethylornithine and the rational development of polyamine antagonists for the cure of protozoan infection, in: "Mechanisms of drug action", T. P. Singer and R. N. Ondarza, eds, Academic Press, New York, p 159 (1983).

THE GLYCOSOME OF LEISHMANIA AS A POSSIBLE TARGET FOR CHEMOTHERAPEUTIC ATTACK

Fred R. Opperdoes

Research Unit for Tropical Diseases
International Institute of Cellular and Molecular Pathology
1200 Brussels, Belgium

INTRODUCTION

Basic studies over the last ten years have revealed that all Trypanosomatidae harbour a number of biochemical features unique in Nature. Several of these peculiarities, as found in the genus Trypanosoma, have been the subject of a recent review (1). One of them, a peculiar microbody-like organelle, called glycosome (2), has since been studied extensively, mainly in Trypanosoma brucei. This paper gives a short review of what is known about the glycosome, with special reference to the organelle of the genus Leishmania.

THE GLYCOSOME

Glycosomes are microbody-like organelles with no mammalian counterpart. They were described for the first time in 1977 in the bloodstream form of Trypanosoma brucei (2). Subsequently, organelles with similar functional properties have been reported for other trypanosome species and related genera such as Crithidia and Leishmania. (Table 1). Together they constitute the major representatives of the Trypanosomatid family. It is now generally accepted that glycosomes are present in all Trypanosomatidae and it is even likely that they are a general property of all the Kinetoplastida.

The name "glycosome" was coined because of the fact that although these organelles resembled peroxisomes in morphology, they lacked such typical peroxisomal enzymes as catalase and hydrogen-peroxide producing oxidases. Instead they contained nine enzymes involved in the conversion of glucose and glycerol to phosphoglycerate. In the vertebrate stage of T. brucei these organelles are highly specialized in glycolysis. Ninety percent or more of their entire protein content is involved in this pathway (8). The insect stage of this parasite is capable of oxidizing amino acids in addition to glucose, owing to a derepression of mitochondrial respiratory chain and Krebs' cycle activities. Despite of the fact that glycolysis plays a role of lesser importance in this stage of the life cycle, glycosomes are present in these cells (9). Several additional enzymes and pathways have been

TABLE 1

Trypanosomatid species for which glycosomes have been reported

Species	Reference
Trypanosoma brucei	2
Crithidia luciliae	3
Crithidia fasciculata	4
Trypanosoma cruzi	4
Trypanosoma cruzi	5
Leishmania mexicana	6,7
Leishmania major	7
Leishmania donovani	7
Leishmania braziliensis	7

identified in such insect-stage glycosomes, and are summarized in Table 2.

From a comparison of the enzymes and pathways associated with glycosomes of various representatives of the Trypanosomatid family the following picture emerges. Only the glycosomes of the vertebrate stage of the African trypanosomes are highly specialized in glycolysis, while those of the insect stage of the same organism and those of the other genera are much less specialized and have additional functions (Table 2). Such other functions are carbon-dioxide fixation, pyrimidine biosynthesis, purine salvage, beta-oxidation of fatty acids and the biosynthesis of ether lipids. The glycosomes of Crithidia spp. are, until now, the only ones within the entire family that have been shown biochemically to contain catalase.

Limited information is available on the number of glycosomes within the various cells. In T. brucei bloodstream forms it has been estimated that some 240 glycosomes are present per cell (13). This represented approximately 4% of the total cell volume or 9% of the protein, while in the insect stage a similar contribution to the total protein has been reported (9).

THE GLYCOSOME OF LEISHMANIA

In Leishmania major promastigotes 50 to 100 glycosomes were estimated per cell (7), while serial sections of L. mexicana amastigotes revealed only 10 glycosomes (14). Although this seems a small number compared to the promastigote stage or to the various stages of T. brucei, this still represents 1% of the total cell volume, when one takes into account the relatively small size of this intracellular stage.

Subcellular fractionation experiments carried out on promastigote forms of the various representatives of the genus Leishmania have shown that the glycosomes of the different species resemble each other in function (7). They all contained the early enzymes of the glycolytic pathway and glycerol kinase and glycerol-3-phosphate dehydrogenase; an enzyme involved in CO2 fixation: phosphoenolpyruvate kinase and possibly malate dehydrogenase. Several enzymes of the beta-oxidation of

TABLE 2

Enzymes biochemically localized in glycosomes of the Trypanosomatidae

Pathway	Enzyme	Organism*
Glycolysis	Hexokinase	Tb, Tc, L, Cl
	Phosphoglucose isomerase	Tb, L, Cl
	Phosphofructokinase	Tb, L, Cl
	Aldolase	Tb, L, Cl
	Triosephosphate isomerase	Tb, L, Cl
	Glyceraldehyde-phosphate dehydrogenase	Tb, L, Cl
	Phosphoglycerate kinase	Tb, L, Cl
Glycerol Metabolism	Glycerol-3-phosphate dehydrogenase	Tb, L, Cl
	Glycerol kinase	Tb, L,
CO_2 fixation	Phosphoenolpyruvate carboxykinase	Tb, Tc, L, Cl
	Malate dehydrogenase	Tb
Pyrimidine Synthesis	Orotate phosphoribosyltransferase	Tb, Tc, L, Cf
	Orotidine-5'-phosphate decarboxylase	Tb, Tc, L, Cf
Purine Salvage	Hypoxanthine guanine phosphoribosyl transferase	Tb, Tc, L
Etherlipid Synthesis	DHAP acyltransferase	Tb, L
	Acyl/alkyl DHAP reductase	Tb
	Acyl CoA reductase	Tb
Oxidation of Fatty acids	Palmitoyl CoA synthetase	L
	Beta-OH-butyrateCoA dehydrogenase	L
Others	Adenylate kinase	Tb, L
	Catalase	Cl
	Phosphomannose isomerase	Tb

* Tb, *T. brucei*; Tc, *T. cruzi*; L, *Leishmania* spp; Cl, *C. luciliae*; Cf, *C. fasciculata*.

fatty acids were partly associated with glycosomes and partly with the mitochondrial fraction. In addition it has been demonstrated that dihydroxyacetone-phosphate acyltransferase (7), orotate decarboxylase and orotidine phosphoribosyltransferase (15) are associated with these organelles. Together this suggests that the biochemical pathways associated with the glycosomes of Leishmania are similar to those described for the African trypanosomes.

Nothing is known about the biochemical composition of the glycosomes of the amastigote stage of Leishmania. This is mainly due to the the great difficulty of breaking the amastigotes prior to cell fractionation. It is likely, however, that the enzyme content of amastigote glycosomes will only differ in quantitative aspects from those of promastigotes. It is generally accepted that the metabolism of these two life-cycle stages is not too different from each other. Some quantitative differences have been observed by Hart et al (6) that suggest that the intracellular stages are more dependent on the oxidation of fatty acids than on that of carbohydrates. The rate of fatty-acid oxidation in amastigotes of L. mexicana was 10-fold higher than in promastigotes stages of the same strain. It would be of interest to know whether that part of the beta-oxidation that is associated with the glycosomes, and not that of the mitochondria, would be responsible for this increased activity. A similar situation has been described for clofibrate-induced peroxisomes of mammals.

THE GLYCOSOME AS DRUG TARGET

In Leishmania spp. the glycosome fulfils an essential role in both energy metabolism and biosynthetic processes. Therefore any disturbance of glycosomal functions may interfere directly with the growth of the parasite. In this respect it is of interest to note that Pentostam, the pentavalent arsenical that is used for the treatment of leishmaniasis, inhibits glycolysis and fatty acid oxidation (Berman, J.D., in this book; Hart and Opperdoes, unpublished observations), pathways that are both associated with the glycosomes of Leishmania. It is not yet known whether Pentostam interferes with the activity of individual enzymes of these pathways or with glycosomal function in general.

The uniqueness of the glycosome and its important function in several essential catabolic and anabolic pathways renders it an excellent target for the development of new antileishmanial drugs. An additional advantage is that glycosomes are also found in other representatives of the Trypanosomatidae responsible for major diseases of mankind, such as sleeping sickness in Africa and Chagas' disease in South America. Any such drug, effective in the treatment of leishmaniasis, therefore, may have at least some effect on the course of these other diseases.

ACKNOWLEDGEMENT

Part of the work carried out in the author's laboratory received the financial support from the UNDP/World Bank/WHO Special Programme for Research and Training in Tropical Diseases.

REFERENCES

1. Opperdoes, F.R. (1985) Brit. Med. Bull. 41, 130-136.
2. Opperdoes, F.R. and Borst, P. (1977) FEBS Lett. 80, 360-364.
3. Opperdoes, F.R., Borst, P., Bakker, S. and Leene, W. (1977) Eur. J. Biochem. 76, 29-39.
4. Taylor, M.B., Berghausen, H., Heyworth, P., Messenger, N., Rees, L.J. and Gutteridge, W.E. (1979) J. Biochem. 11, 117-120.
5. Cannata, J.J.B., Valle, E., Docampo, R. and Cazullo, J.J. (1982) Mol. Biochem. Parasitol. 6, 151-160.
6. **Hart, D.T., Vickerman, K. and Coombs, G.H. (1986) Mol. Biochem. Parasitol. 13, 159-172.**
7. Hart, D.T. and Opperdoes, F.R. (1984) Mol. Biochem. Parasitol. 13, 159-172.

8. Opperdoes, F.R. (1987) Ann. Rev. Microbiol. 41, 127-151.
9. Hart, D.T., Misset, O., Edwards, S. and Opperdoes, F.R. (1984) Mol. Biochem. Parasitol. 12, 25-35.
10. Opperdoes, F.R., Markos, A., Steiger, R.F. (1981) Mol. Biochem. Parasitol. 4, 291-309.
11. Opperdoes, F.R. and Cottem, D. (1982) FEBS Lett. 143, 60-64.
12. Opperdoes, F.R. (1984) FEBS Lett. 169, 35-39.
13. Opperdoes, F.R., Baudhuin, P., Coppens, I., DeRoe, C., Edwards, S.W., Weijers, P.J. and Misset, O. (1984) J. Cell Biol. 98, 1178-1184.
14. Tetley, L. and Coombs, G.H. (1983) Parasitol. 87, XXXVI.
15. Hammond, D.J., Gutteridge, W.E. and Opperdoes, F.R. (1981) FEBS Lett. 128, 27-29.

MOLECULAR STRATEGIES FOR ANTILEISHMANIAL DRUG DESIGN

David Hart, Andrew Langridge, David Barlow
and Brian Sutton

Drug Design Special Interest Group
Departments of Biology, Biophysics
Pharmacology and Pharmacy
King's College London (KQC)
Campden Hill Road
London W8 7AH U.K.

INTRODUCTION

Leishmaniasis is the cause of considerable morbidity and mortality in current world health. The chemotherapy of Leishmaniasis is heavily dependent upon the antimonial drugs Pentostam (sodium stibogluconate) and Glucantime (meglumine antimoniate). Despite the considerable clinical importance of these antimonials their mechanism(s) of action are not known. Similarly, the antileishmanial mode of action of the second line drugs Pentamidine and Amphotericin B await elucidation.

The antimonials have been in use for more than 50 years (see Croft and Neal, this chapter) and administration is via intravenous or intramuscular injection at a adult dose regime of 10mg/kg/day. Recent studies have shown that peak serum levels are approximately 10mg of antimony/l, and that more than 90% of the antimony is excreted within 6hr. It is important to monitor ECG, as well as liver and kidney function following antimonial administration as the side effects observed include arrhymthmia and acute renal failure. In addition to adverse host cytotoxicity reports drug resistance strains of *Leishmania* have been observed

Clearly, there is an urgent need to develop new and effective antileishmanial chemotherapy. We have therefore embarked upon a nonempirical programme for antileishmanial drug design. The programme has two parallel molecular approaches. Firstly, the mechanisms of action of the aforementioned drugs are being elucidated to facilitate the rational design of more potent derivatives. Secondly, unique and essential aspects of the parasites' metabolism, which are at variance with the metabolism of the host, are being identified and exploited to design putative new drugs.

RESULTS AND DISCUSSION

Antileishmanial Drug Mechanisms of Action

The antimonial drugs are actively taken up by both promastigotes and amastigote with the latter being considerably more sensitive. Indeed, promastigotes and amastigotes we found in our experimental system to have accumulated an intracellular concentrations of antimony more than 10 and 30 fold higher than the extracellular medium. These data are in good agreement with previous values (Croft et al 1981 Berman et al 1987) and suggest that the higher accumulation of drug in the amastigote may explain the higher sensitivity of this stage. The site of action and mode of action of antimony was investigated and a summary of the effects of several antileishmanial drugs on the intermediary and energy metabolism of Leishmania mexicana promastigotes is shown in Table 1.

Table 1 The effects of Pentostam, Triostam, Pentamidine and Amphotericin B on *Leishmania mexicana* promastigote intermediary and energy metabolism.*

% Inhibition (100µM)

	Pentostam	Triostam	Pentamidine	Amphotericin B
Glycolytic Pathway	35%	75%	22%	9%
Pentose Phosphate Pathway	3%	10%	6%	7%
ß-oxidation of NEFA [+]	39%	59%	19%	7%
Amino Acid Catabolism[#]	5%	7%	10%	5%
Fixation of CO_2 [≠]	25%	52%	9%	3%

* Radiosubstrate assay and expressed as the percentage inhibition of control rate of CO_2 produced from each respective substrate.
+ With palmitate as substrate.
\# With proline as substrate
≠ Assayed as Hart and Opperdoes (1984)

The antimonial drugs Pentostam and Triostam can be seen in Table 1 to perturb the three primarily glycosomal pathways of glycolysis, ß-oxidation of fatty acids and CO_2 fixation. In contrast antimony had little effect on the cytosolic, pentose phosphate pathway, and the primarily mitochondrial, catabolism of amino acids. An even more dramatic perturbation profile was found with *Leishmania mexicana* amastigote intermediary and energy metabolism (data not shown).

The subcellular distribution of antimony in *Leishmania mexicana* promastigotes was investigated (Figure 1a & b) by following the distribution of Pentostam.

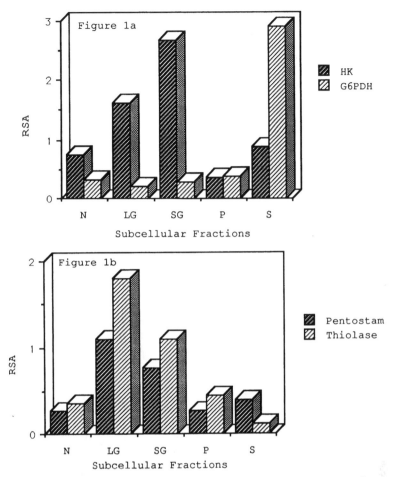

Figure 1a & b The subcellular distribution of marker enzymes and Pentostam. **Fig. 1a.** The glycosomal marker enzyme hexokinase (HK) and the cytosolic marker glucose-6-phosphate dehydrogenase(G6PDH) **Fig 1b.** The mitochondrial and glycosomal enzyme thiolase and the drug Pentostam. The abbreviations used are N, nuclear fraction. LG, Large granular or mitochondrial fraction. SG, Small granular fraction or glycosomal fraction. P, Particulate fraction and S, Soluble or cytosolic fraction.

The distribution of Pentostam was compared to the marker enzymes and found to be primarily glycosomal and mitochondrial in distribution (Hart, Hammond and Mayer, manuscript in preparation). The subcellular distribution of

Pentostam was strikingly similar to the ß-oxidation enzyme thiolase (Figure 1b), and other glycosomal and mitochondrial enzymes (data not shown).

Interestingly these antimonal drugs were not found to inhibit individual glycosomal enzymes in cell free homogenates (data not shown). At comparable drug concentrations to those which inhibit glycosomal flux in whole cell Opperdoesnon no significant inhibition of any of the major glycolytic, ß-oxidation or CO_2 fixation enzymes were observed (Hammond and Hart, unpublished data). These results are supported by previous results with the leishmanial glycosomal enzymes hexokinase, phosphofructokinase and phosphenolpyruvate carboxykinase (Mottram and Coombs 1985). These results suggest that antimony action may be dependent upon the viability of subcellular organelles or that the concentration of antimony found within the organelles is higher than those tested.

The accumulation of Pentostam in mitochondrial and glycosomal compartments therefore suggests that antimony may be at extremely high levels in these organelles. Morphometric analysis of leishmanial promastigotes suggests that the glycosome represents approximately 1% of the total cell volume and yet more than 30% of the cellular drug concentration could be accumulated in these essential organelles. The high concentration of Pentostam in the glycosome and mitochondria could therefore be involved in the drugs mechanism of action.

The difference in sensitivity between the amastigote and promastigote stage could therefore be due to the higher overall subcelluar accumulation of antimony within amastigote organelles. Subcellular accumulation could for example be due to binding of antimony to target proteins and differences in glycosomal and mitochondrial polypeptide composition between the two stages. Differences in the composition of glycosomal polypeptides have been demonstrated between the bloodstream and culture forms of *Trypanosoma brucei* (Hart et al 1984) and preliminary comparisons suggest that a simmilar situation occurs in leishmanial glycosomes (Hart et al, unpublished data).

Antiglycosomal Drug Design Strategies

The glycosome is an excellent target for rational drug design (see Opperdoes, this chapter) due to the essential nature of the intermediary and energy pathways located within the organelle and the absence of a mammalian counterpart. Therefore unique molecular properties of glycosomal enzymes could be used as a basis for nonempirical drug design. In our laboratories the genes for several glycosomal enzymes have been cloned and selected from cDNA and genomic libraries using heterologous probes. The respective nucleotide sequences are being determined so that the amino acid sequences can be derived.

From these sequence data, and based upon homology with enzymes of known tertiary structure, atomic models will be constructed using molecular graphics techniques. Differences in the tertiary structure of glycosomal enzymes their mammalian homolog will then be exploited in the design of highly specific drugs. The atomic models of the antileishmanial drugs which we are constructing will be modelled with the glycosomal enzymes to investigate their mode of action. Target enzyme and drug models will finally be used to design highly specific derivatives with improved antileishmanial activity.

Molecular Modelling Strategies

We have constructed molecular models of Pentostam using a combination of conformational energy calculations and sub-structure searches in the Cambridge Crystallographic Database. In addition we have recently embarked upon the construction of models of the related antimonials Triostam and Glucantime. The preliminary models obtained for Pentostam are shown in Figures 2a, b and c. Of the three putative structures shown the polymeric form illustrated in Figure 2c complies best with the available physicochemical data. Similar modelling exercises have been performed on the second and third line antileishmanial drugs Pentamidine and Amphotericin B (Figures 2d and e respectively). The antitrypanosomal drug Suramin is also shown in Figure 2f.

Molecular models of the glycosomal enzymes, including phosphoglycerate kinase (see Figure 2g), for which homologous structures are available, are being constructed using an Evans & Sutherland PS390 graphics system and the software packages Frodo, Insight and Discover. These programmes include facilities for sub-structure searches within the Brookhaven Protein Databank, and energy calculation and minimisation. Experience with the sequences of glycosomal enzymes from *Trypanosoma brucei* (Osinga et al 1985) unequivocally demonstrate that the degree of homology will be sufficient to allow confident modelling of the structures. Most of the insertions and deletions should therefore be confined to surface loops which can be modelled by analogy (cf Del la Paz et al 1985, Blundell & Barlow 1986 and Thornton et al 1988).

To construct molecular models of glycosomal enzymes where no homologous structures are available crystallographic studies will be performed to obtain the molecular coodinates. We are currently developing enzyme purification procedures based on hydrophobic interaction chromatography and hope to crystalize purified glycosomal enzymes for analysis by X-ray diffraction. Furthermore, crystals of the glycosomal enzymes complexed with, for example, Pentostam and Triostam will be used to study molecular interactions and elucidate the mechanism of antimony action.

Drug Design Strategies

The modelled and experimentally determined structures of the glycosomal enzymes will open many routes to the design of drugs specifically targeted at the glycosome. The possible binding sites, and therefore the potential mode of action, of antimony will be investigated using the atomic models of both

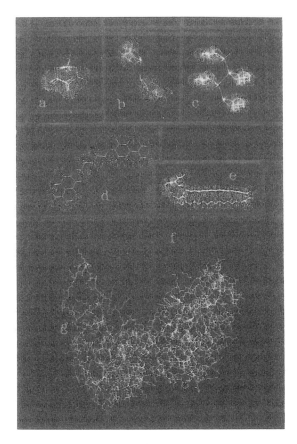

Figure 2 Molecular Models of Pentostam (a,b&c), Pemtamidine(d), Amphotericin B(e), Suramin(f) & Trypanosomal PGK(g).

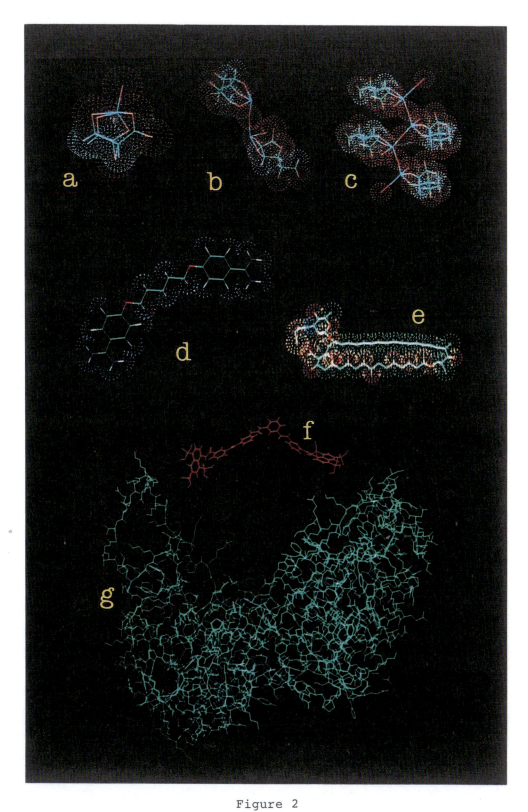

Figure 2

target enzymes and drugs. The physicochemical and kinetic data together with the atomic models will be used to design highly specific analogues which mimic the antiglycosomal enzyme interactions but which are devoid of interaction with mammalian counterparts.

Common features in the atomic structures of the glycosomal polypeptides which, for example, constitute the topogenic signal for translocation during glycosomal biogenesis (Hart et al, 1987), will be exploited to design highly specific and novel antiglycosomal drugs. The glycosomal enzymes from *Trypanosoma brucei* appear to possess two distinctive regions of positively charged residues on their surface (Wierenga et al, 1987). These positively charged regions are 40Å apart, with a characteristic 7Å separation between the charges within each cluster, and could be involved in the translocation mechanism. Work in progress (Hart et al, unpublished data) indicates that the topogenic signal(s) on leishmanial glycosomal proteins is unlikely to involve two such large positive charge clusters.

Preliminary modelling of glycosomal PGK from *Trypanosoma brucei* and the antitrypanosomal drug Suramin suggest a striking complementarity in the disposition of the positively charged amino acids on the surface of the enzyme and the negatively charged suphonic groups on the drug which are approximately 40Å apart with a further 7Å separation between two of the negative charges at each end of drug. It is tentatively proposed therefore that Suramin could exert its mechanism of action via bridging the two domains of glycosomal PGK, as schematically shown in Figure 1f+g, and thus perturb glycosomal enzyme function or translocation. Thus, after several decades of use the molecular mechanism of action of Suramin is, at least in part, being elucidated via the use of molecular modelling techniques.

CONCLUSIONS

The recent discovery (Hart and Opperdoes, 1984) that all the clinically important species of *Leishmania* possess glycosomes offers considerable hope for the exploitation of this unique and essential aspect of leishmanial metabolism in rational drug design. Subsequently we have shown that the accumulation of antimony and perturbation of glycosomal function could be involved in the mode of action of Pentostam. It is therefore hoped that the construction of molecular models of the glycosomal proteins from *Leishmania* and the antimony drugs will facilitate the elucidation of the molecular mechanism of action of antimony. In addition, differences between the molecular structure of the glycosomal enzymes and their mammalian counterparts will be used as rational targets for the design of new and highly effective antileishmanial drugs.

ACKNOWLEDGEMENTS

We wish to thank Mark Hammond and Nishi Mayer for their invaluable assistance to the Antileishmanial Drug Design Project.

REFERENCES

Berman J.D., Gallalee J.V. & Hansen B.D. 1987
    Exptl. Parasitol. 64, 127-131.

Blundell T. & Barlow D.J. 1986
    Phil.Trans.Roy.Soc.Lond.A317. 333-334.

Croft S.L., Neame K.D. & Homewod C.A. 1981
    Comp.Biochem. Physiol. 68, 95-98.

De la Paz, Sutton B.J., Darley & Rees A. 1985
    EMBO J. 5, 415-425

Hart, D.T., Misset, O., Edwards, S.W. and Opperdoes, F.R.(1984)
    Mol. and Biochem. Parasitol. 12, 25-35

Hart, D.T. & Opperdoes, F.R.1984
    Mol. Biochem. Parasitol. 13, 159-172.

Hart, D.T., Baudhuin, P., Opperdoes, F.R. & de Duve, C.1987
    EMBO J. 6, 1403-1411.

Mottram J.C. & Coombs G.H. 1985
    Exptl. Parasitol. 59,151-160.

Osinga K A, Swinkles B.W., Gibson W.C., Borst P, Veeneman G.H, Van Boom J H, Michaels P.A.M. & Opperdoes F.R.1985
    EMBO J 4, 3811-3817

Wierenga R.C. Swinkles B. Michaels P.A.M. Osinga K. Misset O. Van Beeumen J. Gibson W. C. Postma J.P.M. Borst P. Opperdoes F.R. & Hols W.G.J. 1987
    EMBO J 6, 215-221

Thornton J.M., Sibanda B.L., Edwards M.S. & Barlow D.J. 1988
    BioEssays 8, 63-70.

UNSTABLE AND STABLE GENE AMPLIFICATION IN METHOTREXATE-RESISTANT LEISHMANIA MAJOR AND NATURAL ISOLATES OF LEISHMANIA TARENTOLAE

Stephen M. Beverley[1], Thomas E. Ellenberger[1] and Maria Petrillo-Peixoto[1,2]

[1]Department of Biological Chemistry and Molecular Pharmacology, Harvard Medical School, Boston, MA 02115 USA and [2]Departamento de Microbiologia, ICB, CP 2486, Universidade Federal de Minas Gerais, 30.000, Belo Horizonte, Brasil

One mechanism that cells and organisms can employ to increase the level of gene expression is that of specific gene amplification. This process has been most intensively studied in tumor cells exhibiting amplification of cellular oncogenes and cultured mammalian cells selected for resistance to drugs (1,2), though it also occurs in a developmentally-regulated manner in Xenopus (3) and Drosophila (4). In the laboratory gene amplification has been shown to occur in human parasites, including drug-resistant lines of three species of Leishmania (5-8) and in Plasmodium falciparum (9).

Leishmania major selected for resistance to the folate analog methotrexate frequently exhibit amplification of two regions of DNA (7,10,11). One of these, the R region, includes the gene encoding the novel bifunctional dihydrofolate reductase-thymidylate synthase (DHFR-TS; 12,13), the DHFR domain being the presumed cellular target of MTX. The R region amplification has also been found in cells selected with an inhibitor of thymidylate synthase (14). In the MTX-resistant Leishmania the R amplification frequently exists initially as a 30 kb extra-chromosomal circular DNA, formed by recombination between repetitive sequences flanking the DHFR-TS gene (11,15).

The second amplified region, the H region, encodes a MTX resistance determinant distinct from the DHFR-TS (6,12). Amplification of this region of DNA has also been found in certain isolates of the lizard parasite Leishmania tarentolae (5), showing that amplification occurs and is likely to be significant in parasites outside the laboratory. Current data indicate that the H region may encode a form of multi-drug resistance, as it is also amplified in lines of Leishmania selected with two structurally and mechanistically unrelated drugs. The biochemical mechanism of resistance provided by H-amplification is unknown, although it does not mediate decreased drug accumulation (16) and is therefore distinct from that encoded by the amplification-associated multi-drug resistance of cultured mammalian cells (17,18). The H amplified DNA is found as an 85 kb extra-chromosomal circular inverted repeat (6,10).

The amplified R and H DNAs present in the MTX-resistant R1000-3 line of L. major are initially unstable in the absence of drug pressure, though after lengthy propagation in MTX (yielding the R1000-11 line) they show greatly increased stability (10). Our early experiments, employing density gradient centrifugation in CsCl/ethidium bromide, suggested that the unstable amplified DNA was extra-chromosomal and circular, whereas the stably-amplified DNA associated with the chromosomal DNA (10). Though several models were consistent with these data, by analogy with the results obtained with cultured mammalian cells (1,2) we proposed that the stably-amplified DNA had integrated into the chromosome, thereby acquiring the segregational stability provided by centromeres and presumably lacking in the circular amplified DNA.

Recently, powerful new methods for the separation of large DNAs have been developed, such as pulsed-field gradient electrophoresis (PFGE;19) and orthogonal field alternating gel electrophoresis (OFAGE;20). These methods allow the resolution of chromosome-sized DNAs of yeast and Leishmania (19-25). Application of OFAGE to the study of stabilization of amplified DNAs has called into question the integration model presented in the preceding paragraph (26). We have employed PFGE and the related technique of CHEF electrophoresis (27) to study this question (15), the results of which are summarized below.

First, employing non-amplified probes specific for the wild-type R and H chromosomes, closely flanking the amplified region but not themselves amplified, we find that the wild-type chromosomes do not increase in size in the stably-amplified R1000-11 line. In combination with previous results (10) these data show that integration of the amplified DNA into chromosomal DNA has not occurred.

Secondly, we (15) and others (26) find that the R region exists as an extra-chromosomal circular DNA in the stably-amplified R1000-11 line. However, we find that the stable R amplification consists of a series of oligomeric circular molecules bearing up to 8 copies of the basic monomeric 30 kb circular amplification found in the unstably amplified R1000-3 line. As chromosomal size has been found to be an important determinant of stability in artificial yeast chromosomes (28-30), it is possible that increased size is one factor contributing to stabilization of this amplified region.

Thirdly, we find that the H region has the same structure in both the unstably and stably-amplified lines, indicating that at least for this region size cannot be the sole determinant of chromosomal stability in Leishmania. That multimeric inverted amplifications can occur is shown by the structure of the H amplification in Leishmania tarentolae, which consists of a tetrameric inverted repeat, which is stable during laboratory culture (5).

Fourthly, the R or H amplifications have identical restriction maps in unstable and stably-amplified lines, as revealed by extensive blot hybridization analysis using 10 6-base restriction endonucleases and probes encompassing the entire amplifications. This suggests that the stable DNAs have not acquired any new genetic information, such as new sequences which could provide centromeric function.

How are we then to explain the stabilization process at the molecular level? Presumably the processes involved in normal chromosomal segregation must be responsible in some manner. One model would be that small genetic alterations conferring centromeric function have occurred in the stably-amplified DNAs, but in a manner undetectable by our blot hybridization experiments, such as point mutations or insertions of less than about 100 bp. We have not yet tested this model by fine structure restriction mapping or large-scale DNA sequencing, nor could any alterations detected be tested for function with methods currently available in Leishmania. Another model proposes that the molecular mechanisms which determine chromosome stability operate in a different manner in Leishmania and the Trypanosomatidae than in species possessing a single, localized centromere on each chromosome. There is ample precedent for this model, as many species of insects (Heteroptera and Homoptera) and nematodes possess chromosomes in which centromeric function is non-localized and distributed over much of the chromosome (31). As in many other areas of trypanosomatid biology, it is possible that the Leishmania have employed novel and surprising mechanisms.

Clearly, our ability to address the problem of stability of amplified DNAs is dependent upon knowledge of the genetic and cytological properties of centromeres of the chromosomes. Current knowledge of centomere location and function in the Trypanosomatidae is limited, although there are reports of kinetochore-like structures revealed by electron microscopy in Trypanosoma cruzi (32). Interestingly, the number of "kinetochores" per nucleus appears to be significantly less than the number of chromosomes revealed by PFGE analysis (33).

Small DNAs such as the amplified extra-chromosomal circular DNAs present in Leishmania major (10,14), L. tarentolae (5), and L. mexicana (8), or the small DNAs found within certain isolates of L. donovani (34,35), L. braziliensis (34,35) and Endotrypanum (36) constitute true mini-chromosomes, as they contain expressed genes and all elements necessary for chromosome replication (origins, telomeres) and (in some cases) segregation. Analysis of each of these elemental genetic functions in the Leishmania would be greatly aided by the ability to perform DNA-mediated transformation, and these small DNAs may potentially offer excellent systems for the realization of this goal.

Acknowledgements We thank G.M. Kapler for reading this manuscript. Supported by a grant from the US-NIH (SMB) and fellowships from Brazil MEC-Capes (MPP) and the Pharmaceutical Manufacturer's Association (TEE). SMB is a Burroughs-Wellcome Scholar in Molecular Parasitology.

REFERENCES

1. Schimke, R.T., "Gene amplification in cultured animal cells", Cell 37: 705-713 (1984).
2. Stark, G.R. and G.M. Wahl, "Gene Amplification", Ann. Rev. Bioch. 53: 447-91 (1984).
3. Brown, D.D. and I.B. Dawid, "Specific gene amplification in oocytes", Science 198: 739-742 (1968).
4. Spradling, A.C. and A.P. Mahowald, "Amplification of genes for chorion proteins during oogenesis in Drosophila melanogaster", Proc. Natl. Acad. Sci. USA 77: 1096-2002 (1980).
5. Peixoto, M. P. and S.M. Beverley, manuscript submitted.
6. Ellenberger, T.E. and S.M. Beverley, in preparation.
7. Coderre, J.A., S.M. Beverley, R.T. Schimke and D.V. Santi, "Overproduction of a bifunctional thymidylate synthetase-dihydrofolate reductase and DNA amplification in methotrexate-resistant Leishmania", Proc. Natl. Acad. Sci. USA 80: 2132-6 (1983).
8. Kink, J.A. and K-P. Chang, "Tunicamycin-resistant Leishmania mexicana amazonensis: expression of virulence associated with an increased activity of N-acetylglucoasminyltransferase and amplification of its presumptive gene", Proc. Natl. Acad. Sci. USA 84: 1253-1257 (1987).
9. Inselburg, J., D.J. Bzik and T. Horii, "Pyrimethamine-resistant Plasmodium falciparum: overproduction of DHFR by a gene duplication", Molec. Bioch. Parasit., in press.
10. Beverley, S.M., J.A. Coderre, D.V. Santi and R.T. Schimke, "Unstable DNA amplifications in methotrexate-resistant Leishmania consist of extra-chromosomal circles which relocalize during stabilization", Cell 38: 431-439 (1984).
11. Beverley, S.M, T.E. Ellenberger, D.M. Iovannisci, G.M. Kapler, M.P. Peixoto, and B.J. Sina, "Gene amplification in Leishmania", in Englund, P.T. and Sher, A. (eds.), Biology of Parasitism, MBL Lectures in Biology, in press (1988).
12. Beverley, S.M., T.E. Ellenberger, and J.S. Cordingley, "Primary structure of the gene encoding the bifunctional dihydrofolate reductase-thymidylate synthase of Leishmania major", Proc. Natl. Acad. Sci. USA 83: 2584-2588 (1986).

13. Grumont, R, W.L. Washtien, D. Caput and D.V. Santi, "Bifunctional thymidylate synthase-dihydrofolate reductase from Leishmania: sequence homology with the corresponding monofunctional proteins", Proc. Natl Acad. Sci USA 83: 5387-5391 (1986).
14. Garvey, E.P., J.A. Coderre and D.V. Santi, "Selection and properties of Leishmania resistant to 10-propargyl-5,8-dideazafolate, an inhibitor of thymidylate synthetase", Molec. Bioch. Parasitology 17: 79-91 (1985).
15. Beverley, S.M., in preparation.
16. Ellenberger, T.E. and S.M. Beverley, "Reductions in Methotrexate and folate influx in methotrexate-resistant lines of Leishmania major are independent of R or H region amplification", J. Biol. Chem. 262: 13501-13506 (1987).
17. Fojo, A., A. Shin-ichi, M.M. Gottesman and I. Pastan, "Reduced drug accumualtion in multiply drug-resistant human KB carcinoma cell lines", Cancer Res. 45, 3002-3007 (1985).
18. Riordan, J.R. and V. Ling, "Genetic and biochemical characterization of multidrug resistance", Pharmac. Ther. 28, 51-75 (1985).
19. Schwartz, D.C. and C.R. Cantor, "Separation of yeast chromosome-sized DNAs by pulsed field gradient gel electrophoresis", Cell 37: 67-75 (1984).
20. Carle, G.F. and M.V. Olson, "Separation of chromosomal DNA molecules from yeast by orthogonal-field-alternation gel electrophoresis", Nucleic Acids Research 12: 5647-5664 (1984).
21. Scholler, J.K., S.G. Reed and K. Stuart, "Molecular karyotype of species and subspecies of Leishmania", Molec. Bioch. Parasitol. 20: 279-293 (1986).
22. Comeau, A.M., S.I. Miller and D.F. Wirth, "The chromosome location of four genes in Leishmania, Molec. Bioch. Parasitol. 21: 161-169 (1986).
23. Beverley, S.M., manuscript submitted.
24. Spithill, T.W. and N. Samaras, " The molecular karyotype of Leishmania major and mapping of alpha and beta-tubulin gene families to multiple unlinked chromosomal loci", Nucleic Acids. Research 13: 4155-4169 (1985).
25. Giannini, S.H., M. Schittini, J.S. Keithly, P.W. Warburton, C.R. Cantor and L.H.T. Van der Ploeg, "Karyotype analysis of Leishmania species and its use in classification and clinical diagnosis", Science 232: 762-765 (1986).
26. Garvey, E.P. and D.V. Santi, "Stable amplified DNA in drug-resistant Leishmania exists as extra-chromosomal circles. Science 233: 535-540 (1986).
27. Chu, G., Vollrath, D. and R.W. Davis, "Separation of large DNA molecules by contour-clamped homogeneous electric fields", Science 234: 1582-1585 (1986).
28. Hieter, P., C. Mann, M. Snyder and R.W. Davis, "Mitotic stability of yeast chromosomes: a colony color assay that measures nondisjunction and chromosome loss". Cell 40: 381-392 (1985).
29. Murray A.W., N.P Schultes and J.W. Szostak, "Chromosome length controls mitotic chromosome segreation in yeast", Cell 45: 529-536 (1986).
30. Zakian, V.A., H.M. Blanton, L. Wetzel and G. Dani, "Size threshold for Saccharomyces cerevisiae chromosomes: generation of telocentric chromosomes from an unstable minichromosome", Molec. Cell. Biol. 6: 925-932 (1986).
31. White, M.J.D., Animal Cytology and Evolution, Cambridge University Press, London (1973).
32. Solari, A.J., "The 3-dimensional fine structure of the mitotic spindle in Trypanosoma cruzi, Chromosoma 78: 239-255 (1980).
33. Gibson, W.C. and M.A. Miles, "The karyotype and ploidy of Trypanosoma cruzi, EMBO J. 5: 1299-1305 (1986).

34. Stuart, K., S. Karp, R. Aline Jr., B. Smiley, J. Scholler and J. Keithly, "Small nucleic acids in <u>Leishmania</u>, in <u>Leishmaniasis: the first centenary 1885-1985, New Strategies for Control</u>, D.T. Hart, ed., Plenum Press, N.Y., in press.
35. Hamers, R., N. Gajendran, J-C. Dujardin, K. Stuart, "Circular and linear forms of small nucleic acids in <u>Leishmania</u>", in <u>Leishmaniasis: the first centenary 1885-1985, New Strategies for Control</u>, D.T. Hart, ed., Plenum Press, N.Y., in press.
36. Lopes, A., D.M. Iovannisci, D. McMahon-Pratt and S.M. Beverley, in preparation.

POTENTIAL CLINICAL USE OF SINEFUNGIN : REDUCTION OF TOXICITY

AND ENHANCEMENT OF ACTIVITY

        Malka Robert-Gero, Françoise Lawrence
        and Edgar Lederer

        Institut de Chimie des Substances Naturelles
        C.N.R.S.
        91190 Gif-sur-Yvette, France

INTRODUCTION

    Sinefungin was shown to be a potent antiparasitic agent in vitro and in vivo.[1] The severe toxic side effects observed in dogs and goats hampers its clinical use. Yet this antibiotic has great advantages: it can be produced in large quantities by fermentation with relatively low cost, it is highly water-soluble and can be orally administered. These properties justify an effort to find a way to lower the toxicity and enhance the therapeutic value of this antibiotic. The development of new therapeutic agents is also highly desirable because of the emergence of drug resistant parasite strains. To achieve this goal, we propose to consider two strategies : combined chemotherapy with other drugs or with immunomodulators and the administration of sinefungin in drug carriers such as liposomes and microcapsules.

1) Combined Chemotherapy

    Ideally enzymes specific for the parasite should be selected as targets for chemotherapy. Alternatively drugs which have higher affinities for parasite than host enzymes should be selected. If this is not feasible combined therapy should be attempted.
    It was recently reported that the combination of two ornithine-decarboxylase (ODC) inhibitors difluoromethylornithine (DFMO) or monomethyldehydroornithine methyl ester with suramin acted synergistically and cured Trypanosoma b. brucei infected mice.[2] Suramin was shown to inhibit enzymes involved in NADH oxidation.[3] A synergistic effect was reported also with DFMO and bleomycin in a mouse model of central nervous system (CNS) African trypanosomiasis.[4] According to Dr. Bacchi's preliminary results, sinefungin also acts synergistically with DFMO in this same system. These results suggest that the effect of sinefungin might be potentiated against African trypanosomiasis by combining it to one of the above mentioned compounds, DFMO or its analogues, suramin or bleomycin.

Although the exact mechanism of action of sinefungin in Leishmania is not yet completely understood, its main inhibitory effect was shown to be on DNA synthesis.[5] Thus, it is highly probable that the combination of this antibiotic with molecules affecting enzymes of purine metabolism of this parasite such as allopurinol riboside, formycin B and thiopurinol riboside[6] will enhance its inhibitory effect, and might decrease its toxicity. With respect to Leishmania b. panamensis infections, experiments are now underway in Dr. Hanson's laboratory to combine sinefungin and its cyclic derivative with DFMO and its analogues to treat infected hamsters. As paromomycin an aminoglycoside antibiotic was also shown to affect polyamine levels in mouse skin infected with L. tropica it would be worthwhile to test for a synergistic effect with sinefungin. Furthermore the combination of sinefungin with antimonial drugs should also be attempted in order to lower the undesirable side effects of the former.

2. Combined Chemo and Immunotherapy

The probability that immunostimulation resulting in macrophage activation combined with chemotherapy will provide superior results than either one alone was predicted by one of us several years ago[8]. The validity of this hypothesis can now be illustrated with several examples. In the case of visceral leishmaniasis L. donovani infected mice were treated either with Corynebacterium parvum, sodium stibogluconate (Pentostam),[9] or a combination of immunostimulant and drug. According to the authors immunostimulation reduced by about 50% the amount of antimonial required to reduce the amastigote burden in the liver. Combined therapy resulted in an approximate 100-fold reduction in the severity of infection when compared to untreated animals. In contrast the efficiency of amphotericin B could not be enhanced by immunostimulation. Furthermore immunostimulation could not enhance the effect of Glucantime in treatment of cutaneous leishmaniasis of mice.[10] This is probably due to the restricted localisation of the lesions distant from the activated macrophage system. Thus, it seems that visceral leishmaniasis will be more amenable to the combined therapy since infection involves primarly those organs where the activated macrophage system is expressed. The choice of the immunomodulator to use in the combined therapy is not predictable. Good results were obtained with whole bacterial cells or crude extracts, but the use of chemically defined natural or synthetic compounds which were shown to strongly stimulate non specific immunity are certainly preferable. The immunomodulation by muramyl peptides and trehalose diesters and their use in parasitic infections was recently reviewed extensively.[11,12] It is highly probable that the toxicity of sinefungin can be reduced by combination with a well choosen immunomodulator.

3) Drug Carriers

In the past several years, phospholipid vesicles (liposomes) have attracted considerable interest for the selective delivery of drugs and immunomodulators to macrophages.[13] Liposomes are synthetic lipid spheres that can encapsulate either the drug or the immunopotentiating compound.

They are nontoxic and nonimmunogenic. These attractive properties prompted several laboratories to evaluate their efficiency in cancer, and bacterial, fungal or parasitic infections.[13] In the case of leishmaniasis several groups reported that liposome containing antimonial compounds had increased efficiencies in the treatment of animals infected with <u>L. donovani</u>. After encapsulation in liposomes less than 0.15% of the normal therapeutic dose produced the same effect in hamsters[16] and dogs.[15] In addition to pentavalent antimonials such as Glucantime and Pentostam other drugs have been successfully entrapped within liposomes for treatment of experimental leishmaniasis. These are trivalent antimonials, 8-aminoquinoline derivatives, amphotericin B, 5-fluorocytosine, griseofulvin and pentamidine.[17] It was recently shown that liposome encapsulated amphotericin B has very low toxicity and could be used in humans.[18] In contrast, free amphotericin B is extremely toxic and has very low therapeutic index. Another example of reduced drug toxicity upon liposome incorporation was reported with valinomycin.[19] The encapsulation of this antibiotic into liposomes composed of dimyristoyl phosphatidyl choline : cholesterol : phosphatidyl serine resulted in a profound reduction in toxicity with maintainance or enhancement of its antitumor activity against P388 leukemia in mice. These results suggest that liposome encapsulated sinefungin should be prepared and tested.

As it was mentioned above, immunomodulators can also be encapsulated into liposomes. It was reported that a lipophilic analogue of muramyl dipeptide (MDP) combined with Glucantime was more effective against <u>L. donovani</u> infection than was either of the two treatments applied individually. This was demonstrated <u>in vitro</u> and <u>in vivo</u> in mice and hamsters.[20]

Other drug carriers are microcapsules, which are biodegradable polymers, for example, poly(DL lactide-co-glycolide).[21] Drugs can be distributed within this polymeric matrix at known concentrations. Upon injection to animals the microcapsule will slowly release the active compound. The therapeutic efficacy of these long-acting microcapsule preparations in rats with prostate cancer was recently demonstrated.[22] Such microcapsules were prepared with sinefungin in Debiopharm Lausanne, Switzerland, and kindly supplied by Dr. R. Deghengi. These sinefungin microcapsules will now be tested in animal models.

We hope that one of the strategies discussed in this article will permit the clinical application of sinefungin as an antiparasitic agent in humans.

REFERENCES

1. P. Blanchard, N. Dodic, J.-L. Fourrey, M. Gèze, F. Lawrence, H. Malina, P. Paolantonacci, M. Vedel, C. Tempête, M. Robert-Gero and E. Lederer, Sinefungin and Derivatives : Synthesis, Biosynthesis and Molecular Target Studies in <u>Leishmania</u>, in: Biological Methylation and Drug Design, R.T. Borchardt, C.R. Creveling and P.M. Ueland Ed., Humana Press Clifton, New Jersey (1986).

2. C.J. Bacchi, H.C. Nathan, A.B. Clarkson, Jr, E.J. Bienen, A.J. Bitonti, P.P. McCann and A. Sjoerdsma, Effects of the Ornithine Decarboxylase Inhibitors DL-α-difluoromethylornithine and α-monofluoromethyldehydroornithine Methyl Ester alone and Combination with Suramin against Trypanosoma brucei brucei Central Nervous System Models, Am. J. Trop. Med. Hyg., 36:46 (1987).
3. A.H. Fairlamb, I.B.R. Bowman, Trypanosoma brucei: Suramin and Other Trypanocidal Compound's Effect on sn Glycerol-3-phosphate oxidase, Exp. Parasitol., 43:353 (1977).
4. A.B. Clarkson, C.J. Bacchi, G.H. Mellow, H.C. Nathan, P.P. McCann and A. Sjoerdsma, Efficacy of DFMO + Bleomycin in a Mouse Model of Central Nervous System African Trypanosomiasis, Proc. Natl. Acad. Sci, USA, 80:5729 (1983).
5. P. Paolantonacci, F. Lawrence, L.L. Nolan and M. Robert-Gero, Inhibition of Leishmanial DNA Synthesis by Sinefungin, Biochem. Pharmacol., 36:2813 (1987).
6. D.J. Nelson, C.J.L. Buggé, G.B. Elion, R.L. Berens and J.J. Marr, Metabolism of Pyrazolo(3,4-d)pyrimidines in Leishmania braziliensis and Leishmania donovani, J. Biol. Chem., 254:3959 (1979).
7. U. Bachrach, L. Abu-Elheiga and L.F. Schnur, Leishmania tropica major : Effect of Paromomycin and Pentamidine on Polyamine Levels in the Skin of Normal and Infected Mice, Exp. Parasitol., 55:280 (1983).
8. E. Lederer, Natural and Synthetic Immunostimulants and Transmethylase Inhibitors as Antiparasitic Agents in Animal Models, in "The Biochemistry of Parasites", G.M. Slutzky Ed., Pergamon Press, Oxford and New York (1981).
9. C.G. Haidaris and P.F. Bonventre, Efficacy of Combined Immunostimulation and Chemotherapy in Experimental Visceral Leishmaniasis, Am. J. Trop. Med. Hyg., 32:286 (1983).
10. J.L. Avila, F. Biondo, H. Monzon and J. Convit, Cutaneous Leishmaniasis in Mice : Resistance to Glucan Immunotherapy, Either Alone or Combined with Chemotherapy, Am. J. Trop. Med. Hyg., 31:53 (1982).
11. E. Lederer, Immunomodulation of Muramyl Peptides and Trehalose Diesters in Experimental Parasitology, Int. J. Immunotherapy, 2:267 (1986).
12. P. Lefrancier and E. Lederer, Muramyl-peptides, Pure & Appl. Chem., 53:449 (1987).
13. H.K. Kimelberg and E. Mayhew, Properties and Biological Effects of Liposomes and Their Use in Pharmacology and Toxicology, Int. Rev. Toxicol., 6:25 (1978).
14. C.R. Alving, E.A. Steck, W.L. Hanson, P.S. Loizeaux, W.L. Chapman Jr. and W.B. Waits, Improved Therapy of Experimental Leishmaniasis by Use of a Liposome-encapsulated antimonial drug, Life Sci., 22:1021 (1978).
15. W.L. Chapman Jr., W.L. Hanson, C.R. Alving and L.D. Hendricks, Antileishmanial Activity of Liposome Encapsulated Meglumine Antimonate in the Dog, Am. J. Vet. Res., 45:1028 (1984).
16. W.L. Chapman Jr., V.B. Waits and W.L. Hanson, Liposomes in Leishmaniasis Effects of Parasite Virulence on Treatment of Experimental Leishmaniasis in Hamsters, Ann. Trop. Med. Parasitol., 78:279 (1984).
17. C.R. Alving, Liposomes as Drug Carriers in Leishmaniasis and Malaria, Parasitology Today, 2:101 (1986).

18. G. Lopez-Berestein, V. Fainstein, R. Hopfer, K. Mehta, M.P. Sullivan, M. Keating, M.G. Rosenblum, R. Mehta, M. Luna, E.M. Hersh, J. Reuben, R.L. Juliano and G.P. Bodey, Liposomal Amphotericin B for the treatment of Systemic Fungal Infections in Patients with Cancer : a Preliminary Study, J. Infect. Dis., 151:704 (1985).
19. S.S. Daoud and R.L. Juliano, Reduced Toxicity and Enhanced Antitumor Effects in Mice of the Ionophoric Drug Valinomycin When Incorporated in Liposomes, Cancer Res., 46:5518 (1986).
20. L.E. Adinolfi, P.F. Bonventre, M. Vander Pas, D.A. Eppstein, Synergistic Effect of Glucantime and a Liposome-encapsulated Muramyl Dipeptide Analog in Therapy of Experimental Visceral Leishmaniasis, Infect. Immun., 48:409 (1985).
21. T.W. Redding, A.V. Schally, T.R. Tice and W.E. Meyers, Long-acting Delivery Systems for Peptides : Inhibition of Rat Prostate Tumors by Controlled Release of [D-Trp^6]-luteinizing Hormone-releasing Hormone from Injectable Microcapsules, Proc. Natl. Acad. Sci., USA, 81:5845 (1984).
22. A.V. Schally, A.I. Kook, E. Monje, T.W. Redding and J.I. Paz-Bouza, Combination of a Long-acting Delivery System for Luteinizing Hormone-releasing Hormone agonist with Novantrone Chemotherapy : Increased Efficacy in the Rat Prostate Cancer Model, Proc. Natl. Acad. Sci., USA, 83:8764 (1986).

EFFECTS OF A SQUALENE-2,3-EPOXIDASE INHIBITOR ON PROPAGATION AND STEROL BIOSYNTHESIS OF LEISHMANIA PROMASTIGOTES AND AMASTIGOTES

David H. Beach[1], L. John Goad[2], Jonathan D. Berman[3], Thomas E. Ellenberger[4], Steven M. Beverley[4], and George G. Holz, Jr.[1]

[1]Department of Microbiology and Immunology, S.U.N.Y. Health Science Center at Syracuse, Syracuse, NY 13210 U.S.A.
[2]Department of Biochemistry, University of Liverpool, P.O. Box 147, Liverpool L69 3BX U.K.
[3]Division of Experimental Therapeutics, Walter Reed Army Institute of Research, Washington, D.C. 20307-5100 U.S.A.
[4]Department of Biological Chemistry and Molecular Pharmacology Harvard Medical School, 250 Longwood Ave., Boston, MA 02115 U.S.A.

A new class of antimycotic agents, the allylamines, are fungistatic or fungicidal for many different pathogenic dermatophytes and yeasts. Their primary mode of action is the inhibition of microsomal squalene-2,3-epoxidase, with accumulation of squalene and loss of cellular ergosterol accompanied by inhibition of growth and reproduction[1]. Cessation of cell growth and loss of viability coincide with the accumulation of squalene in some species (e.g. Candida parapsilosis), while in others (Candida albicans) complete growth inhibition requires the total cessation of ergosterol synthesis and minimum cellular ergosterol content[1]. The allylamines also demonstrate selective toxicity. Terbinafine SF 86-327, which is being developed for oral administration against systemic fungal infections, has a negligible effect on the squalene-2,3-epoxidase of vertebrate cholesterol biosynthesis at concentrations greater than the maximal serum concentrations that have been recorded in vitro[1].

Terbinafine is also active against growth and sterol biosynthesis in Leishmania species; the promastigote stage in culture[2] and the amastigote stage in cultured human monocyte derived macrophages[3] and in murine macrophage tumor cells[4]. For promastigotes of L. mexicana mexicana WR227, the ED_{50} for growth inhibition was ~3 µg ml^{-1} and the MIC ~10 µg ml^{-1}, while for survival of L. major WR401 amastigotes[3] in human monocyte-derived macrophages the ED_{50} was ~9 µg ml^{-1}. Among promastigotes of WHO reference and other strains (Table 1) the sensitivity to terbinafine varied widely. Until a larger sample of strains has been examined, the association between terbinafine sensitivity and different species of Leishmania remains open.

Accompanying terbinafine inhibition of the growth of Leishmania promastigotes is an accumulation of squalene and a loss of the characteristic endogenous sterols of promastigotes[2] (Table 2). In the presence of a concentration of terbinafine inhibiting population growth by 52% at 5 d, L. mexicana mexicana WR227 promastigotes contained six times as much squalene as control promastigotes. All the endogenous free sterols, and the cholesterol incorporated from the culture medium, were present in smaller amounts in the terbinafine inhibited promastigotes than in the controls.

Table 1. Effects of terbinafine on population growth of promastigotes of WHO reference and other strains of Leishmania

Leishmania	Code	Population growth[a] Control[b] (x 10^6 ml^{-1})	Terbinafine[c] (% Control)
L. aethiopica	MHOM/ET/72/L100	155	10
L. major	MHOM/IL/67/JerichoII	97	48
L. major	MHOM/SU/73/5-ASKH	172	10
L. tropica	MHOM/SU/60/LRC-L39	176	7
L. tropica	MHOM/IQ/65/L75	158	8
L. d. donovani	MHOM/IN/80/DD8	133	61
L. d. infantum	MHOM/FR/80/LEM200	106	15
L. d. chagasi	MHOM/BR/00/M2682	149	10
L. m. amazonensis	IFLA/BR/67/PH8	241	26
L. m. mexicana	MNYC/BZ/62/M379	148	74
L. b. braziliensis	MHOM/BR/00/LTB0014	88	28
L. b. guyanensis	MHOM/BR/75/M4147	137	51
L. b. panamensis	MHOM/PA/71/LS94	108	59

[a] Modified RE III medium (inactivated fetal bovine serum 10%)[2], 10 ml in Falcon 25 cm^2 flasks, 6 d, 26°C. Initial population 10^6 ml^{-1}.
[b] Averages of triplicate samples, Coulter counter.
[c] Terbinafine 8 µg ml^{-1}. Drug was a gift of Dr. Neil Ryder, Sandozforschungsinstitut.

The same phenomena were observed when murine macrophage tumor cells (J774.A1) infected with L. mexicana mexicana amastigotes were exposed to terbinafine for a shorter time interval (2 d). Amastigotes freed from the macrophage-like cells after drug exposure were found to contain three times as much squalene as control amastigotes and less free sterol. Control and terbinafine-exposed amastigotes were notably richer in squalene than promastigotes. The effects of terbinafine on cellular squalene and free sterol content have also been examined at the metabolic level[2]. Coincident exposure of logarithmic growth phase L. mexicana mexicana WR227 promastigotes to terbinafine and [2-^{14}C]mevalonic acid for 20 h resulted in a greater incorporation of radioactivity into squalene and a lesser incorporation into free sterols than was the case for control promastigotes.

It is inferred from the results of the effects of terbinafine on Leishmania squalene and sterol metabolism that, as in fungi, the allylamine inhibits the leishmanial microsomal squalene-2,3-epoxidase. Instructive in this regard are the observations that terbinafine was inactive in an assay[8] for inhibition of growth of the bloodstream stage of Trypanosoma brucei (N. Borowy, personal communication), but inhibited the growth and sterol biosynthesis of the epimastigote stage of T. cruzi (D. H. Beach, L. J. Goad and G. G. Holz, Jr.; unpublished observation). African salivarian trypanosome bloodstream trypomastigotes do not biosynthesize sterols[9], while T. cruzi epimastigotes form a variety of fungal-type sterols[10].

Generally speaking, the development of resistance to antimycotic drugs by pathogenic fungi has not been a serious clinical problem[11] though instances of resistance to ketoconazole have been reported[12].

Table 2. Effects of terbinafine on the squalene and free sterol content of Leishmania mexicana mexicana[a] promastigotes and amastigotes and macrophage tumor cells

Identity by GLC and GC/MS	GLC[b] T_{rr} DB-IN	GLC[b] T_{rr} SPB-5	MS[b] (m/z [M+])	Promastigotes Terbinafine 0	Promastigotes Terbinafine 3[d]	Amastigotes Terbinafine 0	Amastigotes Terbinafine 2[e]	Macrophages Terbinafine 0	Macrophages Terbinafine 2[e]
Terbinafine[f]	—	0.37	—	—	+	—	tr	—	tr
Squalene	0.94	0.63	410	20	117	72	192	43	71
Cholest-5-en-3β-ol	1.00	1.00	386	278	218	202	153	221	180
Cholesta-5,24-dien-3β-ol	1.02	1.07	384	—	—	5	3	14	13
Cholesta-7,24-dien-3β-ol (& Δ5,7,24)		1.16		90	66				
Ergosta-5,24(28)-dien-3β-ol	1.06	1.20	398	24	18	13	9		
4α,14α-Dimethylcholesta-8,24-dien-3β-ol	1.07	1.24	412	314	175	3	3		
Ergosta-5,7,24(28)-trien-3β-ol	1.08	1.31	396	86	43	33	26		
Ergosta-7,24(28)-dien-3β-ol	1.09	1.33	398	18	6	132	84		
Lanosta-8,24-dien-3β-ol	1.13	1.49	426	11	9	50	41		
Stigmasta-5,7,24(28)-trien-3β-ol	1.15	1.57	410	14	8	66	19		
Stigmasta-7,24(28)-dien-β-ol	1.16	1.64	412						
Total free sterols				835	543	504	338	239	193
Endogenous sterols/squalene				28	4	4	1		

[a]MHOM/PA/80/WR227[5].
[b]Analytical GLC, 30 m SPB-5 column; GC/MS, 15 m DB-IN column[4,6].
[c]Quantified by analytical GLC (SPB-5) with an internal standard (5α-cholestane); μg 10^{10} leishmanias^{-1} or mg 10^{10} macrophages^{-1}; extracted from chloroform-methanol soluble lipids with petroleum ether.
[d]Growth 48% of control at 5 d, conditions in footnote a, Table 1, except 200 ml medium in Corning 150 cm^2 flasks.
[e]Exposure to terbinafine 2 d, amastigotes grown and exposed in J774.Al cells and isolated by the methods of Chang et al.[7] and Berman et al.[4].
[f]Identified provisionally by analytical GLC with a terbinafine standard, not quantified.

Table 3. The squalene and free sterol content of Leishmania major[a], wild type and terbinafine-resistant promastigotes.

	GLC[b] T_{rr}		MS[b] (m/z [M$^+$])	Lipids[c] (μg 10^{10} pro^{-1})	
Identity by GLC and GC/MS	BP-5	SPB-5		Wild type[d]	Terb. resist.[e]
Terbinafine[f]		0.37		0	457
Squalene	0.91	0.63	410	9	130
Cholest-5-en-3β-ol	1.00	1.00	386	34	40
Ergosta-5,7,22-trien-3β-ol	1.03	1.18	396	143	94
4α,14α-Dimethylzymosterol	1.04	1.24	412 }	8	
Ergosta-7,22-dien-3β-ol	1.04	1.24	398		25
Ergosta 5,7,24(28)-trien-3β-ol	1.06	1.31	396 }	182	61
Ergosta-5,7-dien-3β-ol	1.06	1.31	398		
Stigmasta-5,7,22-trien-3β-ol	1.07	1.45	410	6	17
Lanosta-8,24-dien-3β-ol	1.08		426		
Stigmasta-5,7-dien-3β-ol	1.10	1.54	412	8	4
Stigmasta-5,7,24(28)-trien-3β-ol	1.10	1.57	410	20	14
Stigmasta-7,24(28)-dien-3β-ol	1.11	1.64	412	19	20
Total free sterols				420	275
Endogenous sterols/squalene				43	2

[a] MHOM/IR/83/LT252[13].
[b] Analytical GLC, 30 m SPB-5 column, GC/MS, 12 m BP-5 column[4,6].
[c] Footnote c, Table 2.
[d] Grown in modified Medium 199, fetal bovine serum (20%)[14], 200 ml Corning 150 cm^2 flasks, 7 d, 26°C.
[e] Grown as for wild type except terbinafine added, 30 μg ml^{-1}; population at harvest 47% that of control.
[f] Identified provisionally by analytical GLC with a terbinafine standard.

To initiate experimental studies of the ability of Leishmania to become resistant to terbinafine, cells were selected in a stepwise manner, following a protocol similar to that described for the selection of methotrexate-resistance in L. major[14] (note that this strain was originally termed L. tropica). Promastigotes of the LT252 line of L. major were exposed continuously to 4 μg ml^{-1} of terbinafine, a dose which caused substantial growth inhibition. Cells which eventually grew out at this concentration were repassaged in the presence of drug, and this process was repeated until rapid initial growth suggestive of the development of resistance was attained (about 10 passages). The selection was then repeated at higher drug concentrations, using 10, 20 and 30 μg ml^{-1} terbinafine, ultimately yielding the SF-R30 line. At 30 μg ml^{-1}, a concentration lethal to the wild-type cells, the SF-R30 line achieves a density of about 47% that of the wild-type cells grown in the absence of the drug. Preliminary results indicate that in the presence of 30 μg ml^{-1} terbinafine the SF-R30 cells suffer an accumulation of squalene and a loss of endogenous sterols, of the same nature and magnitude observed for promastigotes of L. mexicana mexicana WR227 exposed for the first time to terbinafine (3 μg ml^{-1}; Table 2). At face value these experiments suggest that 10-fold higher concentrations of terbinafine are required for the

SF-R30 line to evidence the metabolic alterations characteristic of terbinafine action. Further experiments, examining the squalene and free sterol content of the wild-type LT252 line in the presence of terbinafine and the SF-R30 line in the absence of drug and in the presence of low concentrations of drug, are required in order to firmly establish the mechanism(s) of resistance. For example, it is possible that the resistant line has somehow adapted to the alterations in the membrane sterol composition induced by terbinafine. Other possibilities include metabolism of terbinafine to an inactive form, or decreased drug accumulation or decreased accessibility to squalene-2,3-epoxidase. The genetic basis of terbinafine resistance, including the possible involvement of gene amplification as a resistance mechanism, is also under investigation.

In the course of experiments on the metabolism of [2-^{14}C]mevalonate by terbinafine-inhibited promastigotes of L. mexicana mexicana WR227[2] it was observed that terbinafine itself was taken up by the promastigotes and could be demonstrated by TLC in a steryl ester containing fraction from the alumina column chromatography of a petroleum ether extract of promastigote lipids (L. J. Goad, unpublished observation). Substantial amounts of terbinafine were also recognized by GLC of petroleum ether extracts of promastigote lipids (Tables 2 & 3). The cellular localization of the terbinafine is unknown, but given its strongly lipophilic character it may be assumed to be concentrated in the plasma and organellar membranes. Of interest was the failure to observe notable amounts of terbinafine associated with L. mexicana mexicana WR227 amastigotes that had suffered squalene accumulation as a consequence of exposure of their macrophage host cells to terbinafine (Table 2). Terbinafine treated uninfected macrophages also contained little terbinafine.

The cytotoxic action of terbinafine on the fungal cell is thought to have a dual causality, the accumulation of squalene and the loss of free sterol[1]. Squalene can become intercalated among the hydrocarbon chains in the hydrophobic region of a lipid bilayer and be oriented perpendicular to the surface of the bilayer[15]. Among the consequences leading therefrom would be alteration of the ordering of the bilayer and coincident changes in passive and active barrier properties of the membrane. Support for this view is found in the report that naftifine, another allylamine antimycotic, increases the fragility of the Candida parapsilosis plasma membrane[16]. The loss of membrane sterols from terbinafine treated cells also would be expected to disrupt cellular membrane structure and function since sterols act to buffer against extreme changes in the ordering of the lipid bilayer[17]. The loss may also be linked to requirements for small amounts of sterols with quite specific structural characteristics necessary for important metabolic processes and physiological functions[18-25].

REFERENCES

1. N. S. Ryder, Biochemical mode of action of the allylamine antimycotic agents naftifine and SF 86-237, in "In vitro and in vivo evaluation of antifungal agents," K. Iwata and H. Vanden Bossche, eds., Elsevier, Amsterdam (1986).
2. L. J. Goad, G. G. Holz, Jr., and D. H. Beach, Effect of the allylamine antifungal drug SF 86-327 on the growth and sterol synthesis of Leishmania mexicana mexicana promastigotes, Biochem. Pharmacol. 34:3785 (1985).
3. J. D. Berman, and J. V. Gallalee, In vitro antileishmanial activity of inhibitors of steroid biosynthesis and combinations of antileishmanial agents, J. Parasitol. 73:671 (1987).
4. J. D. Berman, L. J. Goad, D. H. Beach, and G. G. Holz, Jr, Effects of ketoconazole on sterol biosynthesis by Leishmania mexicana mexicana amastigotes in murine macrophage tumor cells, Mol. Biochem. Parasitol. 20:85 (1986).

5. E. T. Takafuji, L. D. Hendricks, J. L. Daubek, K. M. McNeil, H. M. Scagliola, and C. L. Diggs, Cutaneous leishmaniasis associated with jungle training, Am. J. Trop. Med. 29:516 (1980).
6. L. J. Goad, G. G. Holz, Jr., and D. H. Beach, Sterols of ketoconazole-inhibited Leishmania mexicana mexicana promastigotes, Mol. Biochem. Parasitol. 15:257 (1985).
7. K. P. Chang, C. A. Nacy, and R. D. Pearson, Intracellular parasitism of macrophages in leishmaniasis: In vitro systems and their applications, Meth. Enzymol. 132:603 (1986).
8. N. K. Borowy, E. Fink, and H. Hirumi, Trypanosoma brucei: Five commonly used trypanosides assayed in vitro with a mammalian feeder layer system for the the cultivation of bloodstream forms, Exp. Parasitol. 60:323 (1985).
9. H. Dixon, C. D. Ginger, and J. Williamson, Trypanosome sterols and their metabolic origins, Comp. Biochem. Physiol. 41B:1 (1972).
10. D. H. Beach, L. J. Goad, and G. G. Holz, Jr., Effects of ketoconazole on sterol biosynthesis of Trypanosoma cruzi epimastigotes, Biochem. Biophys. Res. Commun 136:851 (1986).
11. K. Iwata, Drug resistance in human pathogenic fungi, in "In vitro and in vivo evaluation of antifungal agents," K. Iwata and H. Vanden Bossche, eds., Elsevier, Amsterdam (1986).
12. J. F. Ryley, R. G Wilson, and K. J. Barrett-Bee, Azole resistance in Candida albicans, Sabouraudia 22:53 (1984).
13. A. Ebrahimzadeh, and T. C. Jones, A comparative study of different Leishmania tropica isolates from Iran: Correlation between infectivity and cytochemical properties, Am J. Trop. Med. Hyg. 32:694 (1983).
14. J. A. Coderre, S. M. Beverley, R. T. Schimke, and D. V. Santi, Overproduction of a bifunctional thymidylate-synthetase-dihydrofolate reductase and DNA amplification in methotrexate-resistant Leishmania tropica, Proc. Natl. Acad. Sci. USA 80:2132 (1983).
15. J. K. Lanyi, W. Z. Plachy, and M. Kates, Lipid interactions in membranes of extremely halophilic bacteria. II. Modification of the bilayer structure by squalene, Biochemistry 13:4914 (1974).
16. G. Daum, Lipids of mitochondria, Biochim. Biophys. Acta 822:1 (1985).
17. P. L. Yeagle, Cholesterol and the cell membrane. Biochim. Biophys. Acta 822:267 (1985).
18. G. G. Holz, Jr., J. A. Erwin, B. Wagner, and N. Rosenbaum, The nutrition of Tetrahymena setifera HZ-1, J. Protozool. 9:359 (1962).
19. W. J. Pinto, and W. R. Nes, Stereochemical specificity for sterols in Saccaromyces cerevisiae, J. Biol. Chem. 258:4472 (1983).
20. M. Ramgopal, and K. Bloch, Sterol synergism in yeast, J. Biol. Chem. 80:712 (1983).
21. J. S. Dahl, and C. E. Dahl, Coordinate regulation of unsaturated phospholipid, RNA and protein synthesis in Mycoplasma capricolum by cholesterol, Proc. Natl. Acad. Sci. USA 80:692 (1983).
22. R. J. Rodriguez, C. Low, C. D. K. Bottema, and L. W. Parks, Multiple functions for sterols in Saccharomyces cerevisiae, Biochim. Biophys. Acta 837:336 (1985).
23. W. D. Nes, and R. C. Heupel, Physiological requirements for biosynthesis of multiple 24β-methyl sterols in Gibberella fujikuroi, Arch. Biochem. Biophys. 244:211 (1986).
24. C. Dahl, H.-P. Biemann, and J. Dahl, A protein kinase antigenically related to pp60^{v-src} possibly involved in yeast cell cycle control: Positive in vivo regulation by sterol, Proc. Natl. Acad. Sci. USA 84:4012 (1987).
25. P. A. Haughan, J. R. Lenton, and L. J. Goad, Paclobutrazol inhibition of sterol biosynthesis in a cell suspension culture and evidence of an essential role for 24-ethylsterol in plant cell division, Biochem. Biophys. Res. Commun. 146:510 (1987).

RIBOSOME-INACTIVATING PROTEINS AND LEISHMANIA:

NEW STRATEGIES FOR FUTURE RESEARCH

Pietro Cenini* and Fiorenzo Stirpe
Dipartimento di Patologia sperimentale
Università di Bologna
I-40126 Bologna Italy

INTRODUCTION

Few drugs are under investigation for the cure of leishmaniasis and none has so far proved to be totally satisfactory. Researchers are therefore still looking for new substances which could be employed as antileishmanial agents. We now draw attention to a group of proteins extracted from plants and known as ribosome-inactivating proteins (RIPs) which have recently given great interest for their wide potential uses in chemotherapy (1-5).

RIPs are known to catalytically inactivate eukaryotic ribosomes and act by cleaving the N-glycosidic bond of adenine$_{4324}$ of 28 S rRNA (6,7). They are widely distributed in plants (9-10) where they exist either as single-chain or as A-chains linked to galactose-binding B-chains in concentrations sometimes high enough to allow purification in large quantities (11). While two-chain RIPs are highly toxic, single-chain ones present a relatively low toxicity to intact cells due to the absence of the binding chain. Macrophages represent an exception, possibly because of their high phagocytic activity. A-chains or single-chain RIPs have proved to be very useful in the preparation of immunotoxins since they can be conjugated to antibodies with consequent aquisition of a selective toxicity for the target cells (12,13).

Due to their general characteristics and to recent results on fungi and protozoa (5,14-16, and unpublished data) we think that RIPs may be considered as potentially useful antiparasitic agents and that the appli-application in the struggle against <u>Leishmania</u> is worth investigating.

NEW STRATEGIES

It was first necessary to know whether leishmanial ribosomes are sensitive to their effects. We found that the two-chain RIP abrin and five

---
*Fellow of the Fondazione Donegani

out of ten single-chain RIPs tested (pokeweed antiviral protein from seeds, saporin 6, saporin 9, dianthin 30 and dianthin 32) inhibited activity of ribosomes from Leishmania infantum in an in vitro polyphenylalanine synthesis assay (see 'Effect of ribosome-inactivating proteins on ribosomes from Leishmania and their possible uses in chemotherapy' in the volume). We are now investigating whether these RIPs can act on whole amastigotes and reduce the infectivity, using an in vitro macrophage model. One way of specifically delivering these effective RIPs inside the leishmanial cells could be the use of immunotoxins formed by conjugation with monoclonal antibodies.

A totally different approach to the chemotherapy of leishmaniasis could be the use of macrophages as target cells for the RIPs, and in this case the RIPs uneffective on Leishmania ribosomes could also be used. In our laboratory experiments are now in progress to investigate whether there is a difference in sensitivity to RIPs by infected versus uninfected macrophages; if so, then it might be possible to obtain a reduction of infection with doses of RIPs non toxic for other cell types. The employment of liposomes might become useful in this approach since they are easily taken up by macrophages (17) and have been succesfully used in the past for encapsulating RIPs and achieving cytotoxicity with otherwise non-toxic doses (18,19).

DISCUSSION

RIPs may be considered as potential antileishmanial agents.

Experiments on Leishmania promastigotes suggest that RIPs would have difficulty in entering amastigotes. As indicated by similar studies on Acanthamoeba castellanii (20), the use of an immunotoxin would probably allow specific entrance of the RIP into the extra-microphage Leishmania cells and therefore possibly affect the infectivity to other macrophages; the degree of unspecific toxicity of the immunotoxin itself would largely depend on the type of RIP used.

The employment of RIPs against infected macrophages depends on the possibility of delivering them into the cytoplasm and on the fate of amastigotes once the host cell has been killed. The possibility of using liposomes is supported by the fact that they have been succesfully used for delivering RIPs into the cytoplasm (18,19). On the other hand, the enhanced efficiency of classic antileishmanial drugs after encapsulation into liposomes is well documented (21).

The possible utilization of RIPs or their derivatives as topical drugs in localised lesions should be considered, in view (i) of the great need for such drugs in cutaneous leishmaniasis and (ii) of the probably low general toxicity of RIPs administrated in this way.

REFERENCES

1. S. Olnes and A. Phil, Toxic lectins and related proteins, in: 'Molecular action of toxins and viruses', P. Cohen and S. van Heyningen, eds., Elsevier, Amsterdam, New York (1982).

2. L. Barbieri and F. Stirpe, Ribosome-inactivating proteins from plants: properties and possible uses, Cancer Surveys 1: 489 (1982).
3. A. Jimenez and D. Vazquez, Plant and fungal protein and glycoprotein toxin inhibiting eukaryote protein synthesis, Ann.Rev.Microbiol. 39: 649 (1985).
4. F. Stirpe and L. Barbieri, Ribosome-inactivating proteins up to date, FEBS Lett. 195: 1 (1986).
5. W.K. Roberts and C.P. Selitrennikoff. Plant proteins that inactivate foreign ribosomes, Biosci.Rep. 6: 19 (1986).
6. Y. Endo, K. Mitsui, M. Motizuki, and K. Tsurugi, The mechanism of action of ricin and related toxic lectins on eukaryotic ribosomes, J.Biol.Chem. 262: 5908 (1987).
7. Y. Endo and K. Tsurugi, RNA N-glycosidase activity of ricin A-chain, J.Biol.Chem. 262: 8128 (1987).
8. A. Gasperi-Campani, L. Barbieri, E. Lorenzoni and F. Stirpe, Inhibition of protein synthesis by seed-extracts. A screening study, FEBS Lett. 76: 173 (1977).
9. A. Gasperi-Campani, L. Barbieri, P. Morelli and F. Stirpe, Seed extracts inhibiting protein synthesis in vitro, Biochem. J. 186: 439 (1980).
10. A. Gasperi-Campani, L. Barbieri, M.G. Battelli and F. Stirpe, On the distribution of ribosome-inactivating proteins amongst plants, J. Nat.Prod. 48:446 (1985).
11. L. Barbieri, C. Stoppa and A. Bolognesi, Large scale chromatographic purification of ribosome-inactivating proteins,J. Chromat.(in the press).
12. E.S. Vitella and J.W. Uhr, Immunotoxins, Ann.Rev.Immunol.3: 197 (1985).
13. A.E. Frankel, L.L. Houston, B.F. Issell and G. Fatham, Prospects for immunotoxin therapy in cancer, Ann.Rev.Med. 37: 125 (1986).
14. W.K. Roberts and C.P. Selitrennikoff, Isolation and partial characterization of two antifungal proteins from barley, Biochem.Biophys. Acta 880: 161 (1986).
15. M.D. Howell and C.L. Villemez, Toxicity of ricin, diptheria toxin and alpha-amanitin for Acanthamoeba castellanii, J.Parasitol. 70: 918 (1984).
16. C.L. Villemez, M.A. Russell. L. Barbieri, F. Stirpe, J.D. Irvin and J.D. Robertus, Catalytic toxins for the preparation of protozoan immunotoxins, in: 'Membrane-mediated cytotoxicity', B. Bonavida and R.J. Collier, eds., Alan R. Liss, New York (1987).
17. T. De Barsy, P. Devos and F. van Hoof, A morphological and biochemical study on the fate of antibody-bearing liposomes, Lab.Invest. 34: 273 (1976).
18. G.L. Nicolson and G. Poste, Mechanism of resistance to ricin toxin in selected mouse lymphoma cell lines, J.Supramolec.Struc. 8: 235 (1978).
19. D.P. McIntosh and T.D.Heath, Liposome-mediated delivery of ribosome-inactivating proteins in vitro. Biochem.Biophys. Acta 690: 224 (1982).
20. C.L. Villemez and P.L. Carlo, Preparation of an immunotoxin for Acanthamoeba castellanii, Biochem.Biophys.Res.Commun. 125: 25 (1984).
21. C.R. Alving, E.A. Steck, W.L. Chapman Jr., V.B. Waits, L.D. Hendricks, G.M. Swartz Jr. and W.L. Hanson, Therapy of leishmaniasis: superior efficiencies of liposome-encapsulated drugs, Proc.Natl.Aca. Sci.USA 75: 2959 (1978).

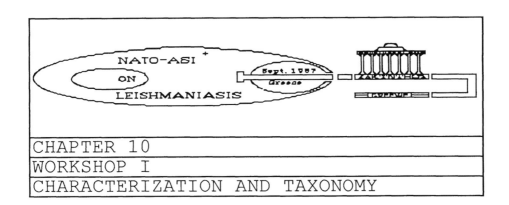

CHAPTER 10
WORKSHOP I
CHARACTERIZATION AND TAXONOMY

WORKSHOP I: CHARACTERISATION AND TAXONOMY OF LEISHMANIA

David A. Evans

Department of Medical Protozoology
London School of Hygiene and Tropical Medicine
Keppel Street, London WC1E 7HT, U.K.

The main aims of this workshop were to define the areas where characterization and taxonomy of leishmanial organisms had important roles to play, and to examine the methods currently available for use in leishmanial taxonomy. The following is an overview of the main points of discussion which came up during the ninety minutes allotted to this workshop. Technical details of some of the methods described at the workshop, such as those of Barker and Anthony, are given in the main body of papers issuing from the A.S.I.

The first subject tackled was an attempt to define a Leishmania species, and not surprisingly no one was prepared do this. The concensus was that, at present, there is no better definition than that a leishmanial species is what a competent taxonomist says it is! An opinion was expressed that species do not exist in Leishmania, and that we should just refer to them as taxa, but retain the present binomial system of 'labelling' the organisms. It was further stated that there was no formal definition of what comprised a leishmanial species, and that their present day names were based on non-biological criteria such as clinical picture and geographical distribution but, as we have the names, we really need to keep them. It was thought that giving the organisms code numbers rather than names was not reasonable as: (a) names are easier to remember than numbers; (b) we are really obliged to use binomial nomenclature as we are referring to organisms in the animal kingdom and are so bound by the International Rules of Zoological Nomenclature. The question was then asked as to what were the requirements when someone wished to name a new 'species' of Leishmania, how different does it have to be before it is justified as being named a new 'species'. This was thought to be an impossible question to answer, and no definite rules could or should be laid down - go ahead and describe it and time would tell whether or not other experts would accept it, was the advice given.

Since at this stage it was apparent that many of the participants were confusing taxonomy with systematics, identification with classification etc., definitions of terminology were given:

Taxonomy is the overall process of dealing with organisms and covers everything from their collection to the publication of descriptions.

Systematics is the scientific interpretation of the study of diverse kinds of organisms, including their distinction, grouping into taxa and their evolution.

Classification is the placing of organisms into groups, or taxa, using common relationships between organisms, following an examination of their various features and peculiarities.

Thus classification provides a series of predictions; identification indicates which of these apply to a given organism/isolate. Leishmania classification was thought best achieved at present by using isoenzymes together with numerical or cladistic analysis of a large series of results. None of the new methods has so far superseded isoenzymes for the purpose of classification. Identification is dependent on a valid classification and may use other methods such as a single enzyme, monoclonal antibodies, DNA probes etc.

The genuine taxonomists in the audience stated how amazed they were that leishmaniacs in general seemed to have ignored the concept of 'types', and in so doing were making life very much more difficult for themselves. It was suggested that we should sit down, use the International Rules of Zoological Nomencalture, and designate some type material for Leishmania. It was hoped that the decisions taken at the Montpellier meeting held in July 1984 on reference strains of Leishmania would be endorsed, and thought given to designating these strains as Neotypes, the Holotypes having been lost in antiquity. The need for good Leishmania reference centres with banks of well documented characterized strains was thought to be of paramount importance. The importance of referring to stocks and strains of Leishmania by their international codes and up to date taxonomic name was stressed, this being especially important when publishing information, as failure to do this in the past has led to the great amount of confusion which exists in the literature. Editors of scientific journals should be requested to ensure this is done in all future publications on Leishmania.

The remainder of the meeting was taken up with with more specific topics. Leishmania chagasi and its relationship to L.infantum and L.donovani of the Old World. No evidence was presented that was suggestive of L.chagasi being other than an import from the Old World. Isoenzyme, kinetoplast and nuclear DNA studies all pointed to an extremely close relationship between L.chagasi and L.infantum, although preliminary work from one laboratory using a very limited number of strains appeared to show a somewhat greater similarity of L.chagasi to L.donovani than to L.infantum. It was reported that more than 100 isolates of L.chagasi had been examined using isoenzyme techniques, and that no polymorphisms were seen between L.infantum and L.chagasi in the 18 loci examined. It was also pointed out that one year after Carlos Chagas first described L.chagasi as a new species, he withdrew this, as he was convinced that the organism was synonomous with L.infantum. There was then some discussion on cutaneous leishmaniasis (CL) caused by L.infantum. In Italy it was found that all the recent cases of human autochthonous CL isolated by workers in one laboratory were caused by L.infantum belonging to three different zymodemes. The most frequently occuring zymodeme was MON24, which was also found in isolates made from CL cases in the northern regions of Algeria and Tunisia. At the present time in Italy the annual number of CL cases is about twice that of VL, although it is not known how many of the CL cases are caused by L.infantum. The strains of L.infantum isolated from CL patients behaved quite differently from those from VL patients. The strains isolated from cutaneous lesions failed to grow in conventional biphasic culture medium and grew only in all liquid medium.

The question was also raised of L.tropica causing VL in man. Over the past few years there have been odd reports of L.tropica being isolated from the bone marrow or spleen of kala-azar patients. The precise histories of these strains was always in doubt, but, at this meeting, the history was given of an Israeli soldier with acute VL and the isolation from his spleen and bone marrow of a definite L.tropica.

The remainder of the workshop was taken up with brief descriptions of some of the latest techniques which may speed up identification of leishmanial organisms - e.g. a technique using photobiotinylated kDNA probes for rapid (12 hour) identification of Leishmania by in situ hybridization on microscope slides; the use of flow cytometry to monitor surface antigen expression by Leishmania; the use of molecular karyotyping for identifying Leishmania; the development of new highly specific monoclonal antibodies for identification of L.tropica. It was the opinion of those attending the workshop that DNA probes and monoclonal antibodies developed for identification purposes be made available to anyone wishing to use them.

CHARACTERISATION BY LIGHT MICROSCOPE "IN SITU" HYBRIDISATION WITHIN 12 HOURS OF LIVE LEISHMANIA OBSERVATION

Douglas C Barker

MRC Outstation of NIMR, Molteno Laboratory
Department of Pathology, University of Cambridge
Cambridge, CB2 3EE

INTRODUCTION

We have previously reported [1] that, in a double blind trial carried out in Brazil in 1985, we non-ambiguously identified 10 strains of cultured promastigotes, 5 strains of promastigotes in dissected guts of Lutzomyia flaviscutellata and Lu. furcata and 5 strains of amastigotes taken from hamster lesions using recombinant DNA probes and Biotin-16-dUTP nick translated probes. We now have to report that Biotin-16-dUTP has a limited shelf life and recommend the use of the commercially available (BRL) Biotin-11-dUTP nucleotide or photobiotin (BRESA). Computer generated data sheets of our hybridisation results on several hundred isolates we have tested will be available in mid 1988.

The kinetoplast of Leishmania proved to be an ideal target for 'in situ' hybridisation. It is eminently visible microscopically, using an X40, or even better an X100 oil immersion objective, as a 1-2 μm diameter disc or rod at the base of the flagellum. It also can be seen in amastigotes, usually as a dense, discrete rod quite separate from the nucleus. The kinetoplast contains a network of 10,000 minicircles each of some 700 base pairs (bp) so there are at least 7×10^6 bp of mitochondrial DNA available as a hybridisation target [1-6].

It is important to remember that most 'in situ' hybridisation seen in scientific papers is concerned with localising material in large embryonic fields of cells, where each cell is about 25 μm and each field may contain up to 100 cells. The resolution demanded (10 to 100 um) is, therefore, one or two orders of magnitude less than we need to localise 'in situ' hybridisation in an object as small as 1-2 μm.

kDNA has other unique features which make it suitable for DNA probes. There are a small number of sequence classes in Leishmania, between 3 and 10, and 80% of these minicircles are usually of one or two major classes [2, 3, 4, 5]. There is rapid sequence divergence between minicircle DNA sequences in fairly closely related Leishmania [1, 5, 6, 7]. The utilisation of these features has made it possible to detect kDNA sequences in the kinetoplast of a morphologically recognisable organism complementary to kDNA sequences labelled with biotin from WHO reference stocks, which are acknowledged internationally as causal agent of a particular form of leishmaniasis.

Recently 'in situ' hybridisation was discussed by Wirth et al. [5] as an alternative method for leishmaniasis diagnosis since it could be a way of limiting the number of false positive reactions in dot blot analysis. These false positives may indeed not be false but could be due to the fact that DNA probes are more sensitive indicators than other methods. The possibility exists for binding labelled DNA non-specifically to tissue or blood stuck to the nitrocellulose during dot blotting. The 'in situ' hybridisation method as previously published [1, 8, 9], appeared to be both time consuming and requiring expertise [5]. In this communication we attempt to answer these criticisms. We show that the method need not be time consuming and can be adapted to a large number of samples. In our laboratory it is not yet possible to complete the entire procedure between 09.00 and 17.00 hours but it can be done between 08.00 and 20.00 hours in a single day. Indeed Van Eys et al. [10], using a streptavidin-biotinylated horseradish peroxidase complex detection system, have claimed that the assay can be done in 4-6 hours using total DNA probes.

MATERIALS AND METHODS

General methods for making radioactive and standard non-radioactive DNA probes and the preparation of organisms for hybridisation, are all given in full in a laboratory manual of simplified methods for the characterisation of leishmania [4], available at the NATO-ASI and free of charge from the Director, WHO/TDR Programme 1211 Geneva 27, Switzerland. Only new methods or substantial alterations to methods are given below.

Photobiotinylation of DNA Probes

"Photobiotin" was obtained from BRESA, Adelaide, Australia and the following protocol developed from the excellent comprehensive manufacturer's instructions. Under very subdued light or any darkroom red safe light conditions (Kodak, ISo 906), the dry Photobiotin acetate was dissolved in glass distilled water (1 mg/ml) and aliquots of 100 ul (containing 100 ug) transferred to eppendorf tubes. The Photobiotin solutions were kept in light-tight boxes (Agar Scientific) at $-20\,°C$ except for the one in current use which was kept at $4\,°C$ in a light-tight 35 mm film cassette holder. Because of the extreme reactivity of the nitrine group during photoactivation, the DNA to be photobiotinylated must be as free as possible of all other organic compounds such as RNA, proteins, lipids, carbohydrates and organic buffers. DNA at a concentration of approximately 0.5 $\mu g/\mu l$ was mixed with an equal volume of the photobiotin solution in an open plastic eppendorf tube in subdued light. Once mixed, the photobiotinylation starts immediately under normal day light or room illumination. To achieve maximum labelling the tube was placed, surrounded by ice to absorb heat from the lamps, under direct illumination from an ultraviolet/visible light source. The manufacturer recommends suitable lamps and we have achieved excellent results from a 50 year old plus sun lamp (HOMESUN, HANOVIA) and the mercury bulb in a light source, (LEITZ, LAMPENHAUS 250), from a fluorescence microscope. The light, from a distance of about 10 cm, shone directly onto the solution in the bottom of the tube for 10 minutes. The solution in our laboratory turned from orange to light brown when good photobiotinylation of the DNA had been achieved. The solution was made up to 5 times its volume with 100 mM TRIS and unused photobiotin removed by 2 sequential extractions with equal volumes of sec Butan -2-ol. This procedure reduced the volume to approximately half the original and the labelled DNA was precipitated at $-20\,°C$ with two and a half volumes of ethanol and 300 mM sodium acetate. The labelled DNA was resuspended at a concentration of 0.5 $\mu g/\mu l$ in 0.1 mM EDTA. This DNA can then be used as probe DNA for hybridisation using identical methods to those given in our manual of methods [17] for nick translated Biotin labelled DNA probes.

Expanded Protocol for "12 hour" Identification

Fixation. 1 - Smear promastigotes from culture or in a dissected sandfly gut, or amastigotes from infected tissue, on to a microscope slide as for blood smears or Geimsa staining. 2 - Fix for 15 minutes by total immersion in 3 parts ethanol, 1 part acetic acid and then dry. It is convenient to take the slides in batches of 25 through the rest of the protocol.

Pretreatment. 3 - Wash the slides for 5 minutes in 2 x SSC (SSC = 0.15 M NaCl, 0.015 M Na citrate pH 7). 4 - Predenature the DNA within the organism with 0.07 N NaOH for exactly 5 minutes. 5 - Dehydrate in 70% ethanol for 5 minutes followed by 96% ethanol for 5 minutes and dry. Check that organisms are still on the slides by Geimsa staining one replicate slide of each isolate.

Hybridisation. 6 - Micropipette 50 µl of biotin-11-dUTP or photobiotin labelled DNA probe in hybridisation buffer (5 x SSC, Denhardts, 10% Dextran sulphate, phosphate buffer, calf thymes DNA and 50% formamide [4]) on to the area of the slide containing the organisms, cover with a coverslip and seal with rubber cement or waterproof tape.
7 - Place 8 to 10 slides at a time on a wire mesh support 2 cm above the water level of a 90-95°C covered water bath for 10 minutes to simultaneously denature the probe DNA and DNA in the organisms. The slides will be at approximately 85°C in a steam atmosphere. 8 - Place the slides on glass rod supports above wet filter paper in square petri dishes and hybridise for a minimum of one and a half hours at 42°C.

Stringency washes. 9 - Ease off the rubber cement or tape, never lift the coverslip but allow it to float off in 2 x SSC, and wash in 2 x SSC for 5 minutes. 10 - Stringency wash the slides in 2 x SSC at 65°C for 15 minutes and rinse in 2 x SSC to get rid of non-hybridised probe DNA. 11 - Wash in 2 x SSC for 5 minutes. 12 - Wash the slides for 5 minutes in ice cold TCA (Trichloroacetic acid) kept below 5°C in an ice bucket to reduce later background staining. 13 - Wash the slide in 2 x SSC for 5 minutes to get rid of cold TCA soluble material.

Detection. Essentially as in the BRL detection kit instructions but with time modification. 14 - Soak the slides in 3% bovine serum albumin in AP.7.5 buffer (100 mM Tris, 100 mM NaCl, 2 mM $MgCl_2$ pH 7.5) for 5 minutes. 15 - Return the slides to the glass supports in the moist chambers, flood the slide with 200 µl of streptavidin (2 µg/µl), cover with parafilm cut to the size of a coverslip and incubate for 10 minutes at 42°C. 16 - Remove the parafilm by flotation, and wash the slides three times, 5 minutes each, in excess AP7.5 buffer containing 0.05% Triton-X-100 (eg 25 slides/250 mls). 17 - Return the slides to the glass supports in the moist chambers and flood the slide with 200 µl of biotinylated polymerised alkaline phosphatase. Cover with fresh parafilm and incubate for 10 minutes at 42°C. 18 - Remove the parafilm coverslip and wash twice, 5 minutes each, with AP7.5/0.05% Triton buffer and once with AP9.5 (100 mM Tris, 100 mM NaCl 50 mM $MgCl_2$, pH 9.5). 19 - Return the slides to the glass supports and flood with the freshly made up enzyme substrate (to 7.5 ml of AP9.5 buffer add 33 µl of 75 mg/ml solution of nitroblue tetrazolium (NBT) and 25 µl of a 50 mg/ml solution of 5-bromo-4-chloro-3-indolyl phosphate (BCIP). Cover with a fresh parafilm coverslip and incubate at 42°C or leave at room temperature for 2 hours or until colour develops. 20 - Rinse the slides in distilled water, add one drop of liquid parafin and cover with a glass coverslip.

Microscopy

It is much easier to find the organisms first using phase contrast microscopy before visualising positive hybridisation by observing the stained kinetoplast under bright field illumination. NOTE Bacteria contain alkaline phosphatase and will stain, therefore, it is very necessary to keep solutions as sterile as possible.

RESULTS

Test of Photobiotinylation of DNA Probes

One advantage of photobiotinylation of DNA probes is that, because the DNA is not subjected to the enzyme DNase treatment during the labelling process, the probe DNA is intact. The photobiotin labelled probe DNA can, therefore, be digested with endonuclease and an aliquot electrophoresed on the same gel as the experimental samples. After Southern transfer of the fragments to a nitrocellulose filter the photobiotinylated fragments act as an internal standard. If all fragments are labelled then the detection system will show stain on every fragment. This also tests the efficiency of the detection system. By comparing the intensity of colour in the probe DNA track with the intensity of colour in the fragments which have been hybridised some subjective measure of the efficiency of hybridisation can also be gained. It must be remembered, however, that in the probe photobiotinylated fragments both strands of the DNA helix are labelled whereas after hybridisation only one strand of the DNA is labelled. The colour intensity on hybridised fragments is, therefore, always one half that on probe DNA.

Figure 1 illustrates these points. In this experiment the first seven tracks contained aliquots of endonuclease Hae III digested PM2 DNA which were loaded onto a 2% agarose gel in decreasing quantities (1. 1000 ng, 2. 500 ng, 3. 100 ng, 4. 50 ng, 5. 10 ng, 6. 5 ng, 7. 1 ng). Track 8 was loaded with 1000 ng of photobiotinylated PM2, Hae III digested DNA. The photograph (Figure 1a), taken in ultraviolet light of the gel after electrophoretic separation and ethidium bromide staining of the DNA, showed clearly the fragments in the first four tracks, ie the Hae III digested fragments from 50 ng of PM2 DNA could be visualised. Tracks 1, 2 and 8 showed very similar staining intensity with ethidium bromide. Figure 1b is a photograph of the fragments from the gel Southern transferred and hybridised, with a 1000 ng aliquot of the same photobiotinylated PM2 DNA in track 8, and subjected to the normal streptavidin, alkaline phosphatase, chromogenic substrate detection system. There was intense staining of all eight major fragments in the probe DNA and the detection system had detected at least four other partial digestion fragments not seen in the ethidium stained gel. The tear drop artifact between bands 2 and 3 in track one was due to a bubble appearing between the gel and the nitrocellulose paper during Southern transfer. All eight major fragments were well stained in tracks one and two and the bands were progressively less stained in tracks 3-7. However, this indicates that photobiotinylated probe DNA can, by hybridisation and non-radioactive detection, detect a band containing a fraction of a nanogram of DNA.

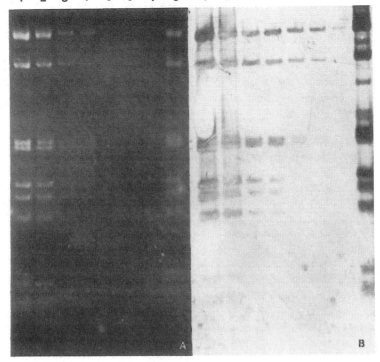

Fig. 1. (a) Photograph taken under ultraviolet light of ethidium bromide stained fragments of bacteriophage PM2 - DNA previously digested with the endonuclease Hae III and electrophoresed in a 2% agarose gel. Track 8 contains PM2 probe DNA photobiotinylated before digestion. The other tracks contain serial dilutions of PM2 DNA endonuclease fragments as indicated in the text. (b) After Southern transfer the nitrocellulose filter was hybridised with the same photobiotinylated PM2 DNA as in track 8. These results indicate that homologous DNA can be detected at the level of fractions of a nanogram by this method.

'In situ' Hybridisation Identification In A Day

Biotin-11-dUTP probes. Figure 2 illustrates the excellent discrimination which can be obtained using the 12 hour protocol given in the methods. Promastigotes of four internationally recognised reference strains, L. b. braziliensis MHOM/BR/75/M2903 and L. b. guyanensis MHOM/BR/75/M4147 representing the braziliensis complex, L. m. mexicana NYC/BZ/62/M379 and L. m. amazonensis IFLA/BR/67/PH8 clone 5, were smeared on microscope slides. Replicate sets of slides of all four isolates were hybridised with either Biotin-11-dUTP labelled kDNA of L. m. mexicana or L. b. guyanensis. The L. m. mexicana Bio-11 probe hybridised to the kinetoplasts of the homologous organism (Figure 2a) giving an intense coloration of the kinetoplast after using the streptavidin/alkaline phosphatase/chromogenic substrate detection. The same probe gave coloration of the kinetoplast of the other mexicana complex strain L. m. amazonensis (Figure 2b). No colour could be detected in either of the braziliensis complex strains L. b. braziliensis (Figure 2c) or L. b. guyanensis (not illustrated). The L. b. guyanensis Bio-11 probe hybridised strongly to the homologous kinetoplasts (not illustrated) and

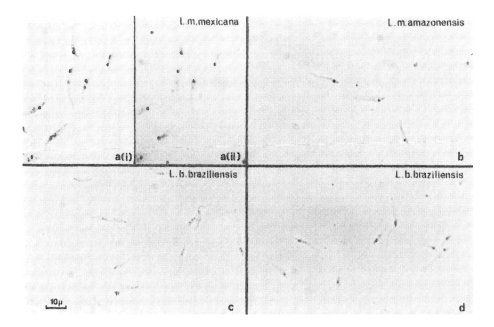

Fig. 2. Promastigotes of a - L. m. mexicana M379, b - L. m. amazonensis PH8, c - L. b. braziliensis M2903 hybridised with biotin-11-dUTP labelled kDNA from L. m. mexicana M379 and d - L. b. braziliensis M2903 hybridised with biotin-11-dUTP labelled kDNA from L. b. guyanensis M4147. After application of the detection system intense colouration of the kinetoplast can be seen whereever hybridisation has taken place ie in a, b and d. a (i) is a phase image and a (ii) the bright field image as are b, c and d.

to the kinetoplasts of L. b. braziliensis (Figure 2d) giving an equally intense staining after the detection system had been applied. No colour was detected in the kinetoplasts of either of the mexicana complex strains (not illustrated).

Photobiotinylated kDNA probes. Promastigotes of the same four reference strains as those used above were smeared on microscope slides. Replicate sets of slides were hybridised with photobiotinylated kDNA probes from L. b. guyanensis and L. m. mexicana. Figure 3 illustrates the equally excellent results which can be obtained using the 12 hour protocol given in the methods. The L. b. guyanensis probe DNA hybridised to the kinetoplast in the cells of both L. b. guyanensis (Figure 3a) and L. b. braziliensis (Figure 3b) giving intense coloured organelles

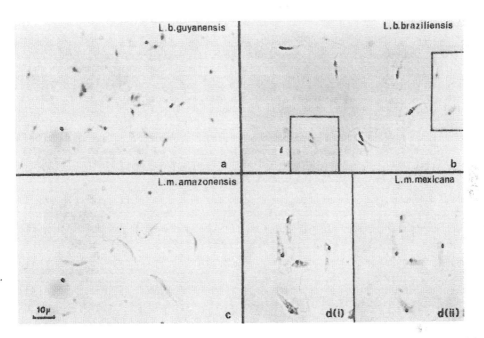

Fig. 3. Promastigotes of reference strains of Leishmania: a - L. b. guyanensis M4147, b - L. b. braziliensis M2903, c - L. m. amazonensis PH8 hybridised with photobiotinylated kDNA of L. b. guyanensis M4147 and d - L. m. mexicana M379 hybridised with photobiotinylated DNA from L. m. mexicana M379. After application of the detection system intense colouration of the kinetoplast can be seen wherever hybridisation has taken place ie in a, b and d. d (i) is the phase image and d (ii) the bright field image as are a and c. B is phase image with corresponding bright field inserts

after the detection system had been used. No colour was seen on the kinetoplast of L. m. amazonensis (Figure 3c) nor on the kinetoplast of L. m. mexicana (not illustrated). The L. m. mexicana probe hybridised with the kinetoplast in the homologous promastigotes giving intense coloration of the organelle after use of the detection system (Figure 3d). Colour on the kinetoplast was also seen in L. m. amazonensis kinetoplasts but not in either of the braziliensis strains kinetoplasts (not illustrated).

DISCUSSION

The evidence given in this paper seeks to establish that light microscope 'in situ' hybridisation has now become a relatively simple and rapid means of identifying Leishmania. The use of photobiotinylated kDNA or recombinant DNA probes and non-radioactive detection systems has reduced the time necessary for this assay to under 12 hours. Provided that Leishmania amastigotes or promastigotes can be seen in microscope smears, this technique can show the presence or absence of DNA sequences within a single kinetoplast, which are homologous to appropriate probe DNA sequences. The specificity of the technique is now entirely dependent on the production of complex, species, subspecies or isolate specific DNA sequences according to the needs of the clinician or the epidemiologist.

CONCLUSIONS

The diagnostic use of Biotin-11-dUTP or Photobiotin labelled kDNA probes with a streptavidin/alkaline phosphatase/chromogenic substrate system is now feasible. The technque can detect a fraction of a nanogram of homologous minicircle sequence in endonuclease fragments by filter hybridisation. Homologous minicircle sequences within a single kinetoplast in an individual leishmania can also be detected. The entire assay from live Leishmania to 'in situ' hybridisation identification by microscopy can be completed in less than 12 hours.

Future research in the molecular field should concentrate on the production for distribtion of cheap recombinant DNA photobiotinylated probes with defined sequence specificities.

REFERENCES

1. Barker, D.C., Gibson, L.J., Kennedy, W.P.K, Nasser, A.A.A. and Williams, R.H. (1986) The potential of using recombiantnt DNA species-specific probes for the identification of tropical Leishmania. Parasitology 91:S139-S174
2. Barker, D.C. and Butcher, J. (1983) The use of DNA probes in the identification of leishmaniasis: discrimination between isolates of the Leishmania mexicana and L. braziliensis complexes. Trans. R. Soc. Trop. Med. Hyg. 77:285-297
3. Spithill, T.W. and Grumont, R.J. (1984) Identification of species, strains and clones of Leishmania by characterization of kinetoplast DNA mini-circles. Mol. Biochem. Parasitol. 12:217-236
4. Lopes, U.G. and Wirth, D.F. (1986) Identification of visceral Leishmania species with cloned sequences of kinetoplast DNA. Mol. Biochem. Parasitol. 20:77-84
5. Wirth, D.F., Rogers, W.O., Barker, R., Dourado, H., Suesbang, L. and Albuquerque, B. (1986) Leishmaniasis and Malaria: New tools for epidemiological analysis. Science 234:975-979
6. Wirth, D.F. and Rogers, W.O. (1985) "Rapid identification of infectious agents" Kingsburg, D.T. and Falbow, S., eds 127-137, Academic Press, New York
7. Barker, D.C. (1987) DNA diagnosis of human leishmaniasis. Parasitology Today. 3:177-184
8. Kennedy, W.P.K. (1984) Novel identification of differences in the kinetoplast DNA of Leishmania isolated by recombinant DNA techniques and 'in situ' hybridisation. Mol. Biochem. Parasitol. 12:313-325
9. Barker, D.C. (1986) in: "Characterisation of Leishmania sp. by DNA

hybridisation probes" pp 57, WHO, Geneva

10 van Eys, G.J.J.M., Schoone, G.J., Lighart, G.S., Laarman, J.J. and Terpstra, W.J. (1987) Detection of Leishmania parasites by DNA in situ hybridization with non-radioactive probes. Parasitol. Res. 73:199-202

ACKNOWLEDGEMENTS

I am grateful that the investigations received the financial support of the Medical Research Council (UK) and the UNDP/WORLD BANK/WHO/TRD programme ID 840412. I would like to thank Lorna Gibson and Roger Williams for their active participation in this work and for their sometimes sceptical and always critical evaluation of our results. My thanks is also due to Miss Tracy Askin for typing this manuscript.

ENZYME ELECTROPHORETIC EVIDENCE FOR THE IMPORTATION OF

L.infantum INTO THE NEW WORLD

Hooman Momen and Gabriel Grimaldi Jr

Instituto Oswaldo Cruz, (FIOCRUZ)
Av. Brasil, 4365, Cx. Postal 926
21040 Rio de Janeiro, RJ, Brazil

INTRODUCTION

There exists a controversy as to whether the aetiological agent of American Visceral Leishmaniasis (AVL) was recently introduced to the New World or has an ancient origin (Reviewed by Lainson, 1983; Deane & Grimaldi, 1985). If it arrived at the time of the European colonization the parasite would have diverged from L.infantum less than 500 years ago. If the parasite arrived at the time of the introduction of canids into S.America then it would have diverged from the Mediterranean parasite several million years ago. Molecular evolution studies have shown that when populations are geographically separated their genomes begin to diverge. This divergence is dependent on time and therefore by measuring the genetic distance between the two populations the time of their divergence can be estimated (Sarich, 1977).

Here we present the results of a mutilocus enzyme electrophoresis study to determine the genetic similarity between isolates from cases of AVL and associated animals refered to here as L.chagasi and the WHO recommended reference strains of L.infantum and L.chagasi. The analysis was made on over 100 isolates of L.chagasi for which data on at least 11 and up to 16 enzyme loci were available. The isolates came from the major endemic areas of AVL in Brazil and were isolated from both humans and animals.

MATERIALS AND METHODS

Leishmania stocks

Over 100 isolates of "L.chagasi" from humans, dogs and opossums were analysed. The strains came from the major endemic areas of Brazil as well as from Honduras. Full clinical and epidemiological details on the isolates have been published previously (Grimaldi et al., 1987). W.H.O. recommended reference strains for L.chagasi MHOM/BR/74/PP75 and L.infantum MHOM/TN/80/IPTI were also included.

Isolation of parasites

The primary isolation was made by *in vitro* culture of samples from the visceral and cutaneous lesions. In the case of visceral infections, the sample was obtained by aspiration of bone marrow and inoculated directly into the medium. In the case of the cutaneous lesions the material was washed several times in a balanced salt solution containing relatively high amounts of antibiotics: penicillin (1.000 Units/ml) and streptomycin (1.000 µg/ml). The tissue was then cut into small pieces and the epidermis removed. The pieces were then rewashed in the same solution and finally introduced aseptically into tubes containing the culture medium.

In vitro cultivation

Stocks were initially cultivated in brain heart infusion agar (Difco), 5.2% to which 15% rabbit blood was added. An overlay of modified liquid LIT medium (Jaffe et al., 1984) containing 10% heat-inactivated fetal bovine serum (FBS) was used. Samples of overlay were examined at regular intervals to check both the parasite growth and the presence of contaminants. Promastigotes were cultured repeatedly and when an optimal rate of growth was achieved the parasites were transferred to an enriched liquid, the Schneider's drosophila medium (Gibco) (Hendricks et al., 1978), supplemented with 20% FBS, and incubated at $24°C$.

Preparation of samples

When the promastigotes were in the log phase of growth in Schneider's medium, they were harvested by centrifugation (1500g for 10 minutes at 4 C) and washed twice in phosphate buffered saline (PBS), pH 7.3. The final pellet was resuspended in lysis buffer containing 0.04M NaCl, 0.01M sodium ethylene diamine tetra-acetate (EDTA) and 0.1M Tris pH 8.0 for enzyme electrophoresis.

Enzyme electrophoresis

Electrophoresis was carried out in agarose gels according to the procedure described by Momen et al. (1985). Sixteen enzymes were found to produce clear distinct bands useful for parasite identification (see Table I). The buffers and stains used for the enzymes were as described in Salles et al. (1986) except for nucleoside hydrolase and the peptidases where the procedures used by Miles et al. (1979) were followed. The leishmanial extracts were run in many separate experiments and the order of the extracts was interchanged to allow side-by-side comparisons for all variants. All variants having mobilities similar enough to preclude consistent separation were conservatively scored as the same enzyme band. All isolates were studied with at least eleven of the enzymes given in Table I.

TABLE I
Enzymes used in the identification of Leishmania parasites

Name	Abreviation	Enzyme Comission (E.C.) Number
Malate dehydrogenase	MDH	1.1.1.37.
Malic enzyme	ME	1.1.1.39.
Isocitrate dehydrogenase	IDH	1.1.1.40.
6-phosphogluconate dehydrogenase	6PGDH	1.1.1.44.
Glucose-6-phosphate dehydrogenase	G6PDH	1.1.1.49.
Phosphoglucomutase	PGM	2.7.5.1.
Carboxyl esterase	EST	3.1.1.1.
Nucleoside hydrolase (Two loci)	NH1 & NH2	3.2.2.2.
Proline dipeptidase	PEP D	3.4.13.9.
Peptidase (as substrate:		3.4.11.
leucyl-leucyl-leucine	PEP 1	or 13.
leucyl-leucyl-alanine	PEP 2	
leucyl-alanine)	PEP 3	
Aconitate hydratase	ACON	4.2.1.3.
Mannose phosphate isomerase	MPI	5.3.1.8.
Glucose phosphate isomerase	GPI	5.3.1.9.

RESULTS

All isolates were examined for at least 11 loci and selected isolates for up to 17 loci. No evidence for polymorphism was found at any of the loci examined. All isolates had the same enzyme profile as the WHO reference strains for L.chagasi and L.infantum.

DISCUSSION

Molecular techniques of parasite characterization allow an objective method to determine similarities between parasites and can be applied to determine the identity of L.chagasi and its relationship to L.infantum. The exact rate of genomic evolution is not known in Leishmania however if L.chagasi has an ancient origin one would expect isolates of L.chagasi to possess a) genetic diversity reflected in polymorphic alleles and b) genomic divergence from L.infantum.

The best measurement of this would be by direct analysis of the DNA however such studies have yielded conflicting results. This is probably due to the fact that a) Mitochondrial (kinetoplast) DNA and nuclear DNA evolve at different rates. Kinetoplast DNA evolves much faster and often shows interpopulation heterogeneity; b)Too few isolates of each species were analysed. Unless a representative sample of each species is analyzed to determine intraspecific heterogeneity the significance of interspecific differences can not be determined. For example Beverley et al. (1987) compared nuclear DNA restriction fragment patterns and suggested that L.infantum and L.chagasi may be as closely related to each other as two random individuals from the same population; c) Because of the quantity of parasites usually required, studies are often carried out with strains that have been laboratory adapted over many years to grow well in culture media. These strains because of selection, adaption or contamination may not be truly representative of field isolates.

The only studies using large numbers of field isolates of L.chagasi are those involving serodeme analysis with monoclonal antibodies and enzyme electrophoresis. Grimaldi et al. (1987) using a panel of 16 L.donovani (s.l.) species-specific monoclonal antibodies examined 110 isolates of L.chagasi as well as the reference strain of L.infantum. They did not find any significant difference in the reactivity pattern to the monoclonals. As enzyme electrophoretic studies measure amino acid variation which is a direct expression of the genome, they can be used to indirectly measure genetic diversity and distance among Leishmania species. Besides the results presented here we can add those of previously published studies in particular those of Kreutzer et al. (1987, 20 isolates & 20 loci), Desjeux et al. (1984, 7 isolates & 13 loci) and Braga et al. (1986, 11 isolates & 6 loci). Except for one loci in the report by Kreutzer et al. (1987) no other evidence for polymorphism in L.chagasi was found. These results show the homogeniety of L.chagasi isolates from the New World and their identity with the WHO reference strains for L.chagasi and/or L.infantum.

The above studies taken together have examined about 150 different isolates originating from a wide variety of hosts and geographical areas namely, humans, dogs, opossums, foxes and sandflies as well as from Honduras, Panama, Colombia, Bolivia and all the major endemic areas of Brazil. A total of 27 enzymatic loci were also studied representing most of the loci that can be resolved electrophoretically in Leishmania with current techniques as well as 5 out of the 6 classes of enzymes. If we consider the isolates as representative of L.chagasi and the loci examined as representative of the genome then we can infer that there has been practically no genomic divergence between L.chagasi and the reference strain of L.infantum.

These results would support the theory of the recent origin of AVL in the New World due to the importation of L.infantum The apparent homogeneity of the isolates of AVL so far studied is further support for this theory. It is already known that L.infantum can infect and develop in Lu. longipalpis (Killick-Kendrick et al.,1980). There have also been reports of the importation of canine visceral leishmaniasis from the Mediterranean region into the New World including the apparent transmission of the parasite within a dog kennel in the U.S.A. (Anderson et al.,1980; Zeledon, 1985). This suggests that AVL may have a multiple origin having been introduced on several occassions during the European colonization. L.infantum is known to be polymorphic in the Old World (Bellazoug et al., 1985). We may therefore expect to find in the future polymorphic loci in the New World which should correspond to alleles already described in the Old World.

There may well exist among the diversity of leishmanial parasites of S.America an indigenous species capable of causing visceral leishmaniasis in man as suggested by Lainson (1983). Such a parasite however remains to be isolated and identified. The view that the causative agent of AVL was indigenous to the New World was first proposed by Cunha & Chagas (1937). However the following year Cunha (1938a,b) retracted this point of view. In these papers ,having managed to establish the infection experimentally in dogs, which he had previously failed to do, he was able to show that the diseaese followed the same pattern as that described for L.infantum in dogs. He also managed to obtain a recent isolate of L.infantum and was able to show that the previous antigenic differences reported between the Mediterranean and New World parasites were in fact due to the age of the respective culture and that fresh isolates of both parasites behaved identically.

We may therefore finish by citing from the English abstract of Cunha's 1938a paper: "Thus, we feel authorized to conclude that the agent of visceral american leishmaniasis is identical with L.infantum."

Acknowledgements

This work received financial support from CNPq, and FINEP (Brazil) and the UNDP/WORLD BANK/WHO Special Programme for Research and Training in Tropical Diseases. We are grateful to Prof. Leonidas M. Deane for drawing our attention to the early Brazilian literature and to Andiaria R. da Silva and Maria G.R. de Miranda for technical assistance.

REFERENCES

Anderson, D. C., Buckner, R. G., Glenn, B. L. and MacVean, D. W., 1980, Endemic Canine Leishmaniasis, Vet. Path. 17:94-96

Bellazzoug, S., Lanotte, G., Maazoun, R., Pratlong, F. and Rioux, J.A., 1985, A new enzymatic variant of Leishmania infantum (Nicole, 1908) causative organism of cutaneous leishmaniasis, Ann. Parasit. hum. comp. 60:1-3.

Beverley, S. M., Ismach, R. D. and McMahon-Pratt, D., 1987, Evolution of the genus Leishmania as revealed by comparisons of nuclear DNA restriction fragment patterns, Proc. Natl. Acad. Sci. 84:484-488.

Braga, R. R., Lainson, R., Shaw, J. J., Ryan L. and Silveira, F. T., 1986, Leishmaniasis in Brazil XXII: Characterization of Leishmania from Man, dogs and the sandfly Lutzomia longipalpis (Lutz & Neiva, 1912) isolated during an out break of visceral Leishmaniasis in Santarem, Para State, Trans. R. Soc. Trop. Med. Hyg. 80:143-145.

Cunha, A. M., 1938a, Infecções experimentais na Leishmaniose visceral americana, Mem. Inst. Oswaldo Cruz 33:581-616.

Cunha, A. M., 1938b, A aglutinação e o diagnostico diferencial das leishmanias, Brasil-Médico 52:849-855.

Cunha, A. M. and Chagas, E. 1937, Nova especie de protozoario do genero Leishmania pathogenico para o homen. Leishmania chagasi n.sp. Nota Previa. O Hospital. Rio de Janeiro 11, 3-9.

Deane, L. M. and Grimaldi, Jr. G., 1985, Leishmaniasis in Brazil, in: "Leishmaniasis" Chang, K. P. and Bray, R. S. Eds, Elsevier Science Publishers, Amsterdam.

Desjeux, P., Le Pont , F., Mollinedo, S. and Tibayrenc,

M., 1984, Las Leishmania da Bolivia II. *Annuario 1983-84. Instituto Boliviano de Biologia de la Altura*. 163-170.

Grimaldi, Jr. G., David, J. R. and McMahon-Pratt, D., 1987, Identification and distribution of New World *Leishmania* species characterized by serodeme analysis using monoclonal antibodies, *Am. J. Trop. Med. Hyg.*, 36:270-287.

Hendricks, L. D., Wood, D. E. and Hadjuk, M.E., 1978, Haemoflagellates commercially available liquid media for rapid cultivation, *Parasitology*, 76:309-316.

Jaffe, C. L., Grimaldi, Jr. G. and McMahon-Pratt, D., 1984, The cultivation and cloning of *Leishmania*, in: "Genes and Antigens of parasites. A Laboratory Manual", Morel, C. M., ed., Fundacao Oswaldo Cruz, Rio de Janeiro.

Killick-Kendrick, R., Molyneux, D. H., Rioux, J. A. and Lanotte, G., 1980, Possible origins of *Leishmania chagasi*, *Ann. Trop. Med. Parasit.*, 74:563-564.

Kreutzer, R. D., Souraty, N. and Semko, M. E., 1987, Biochemical identities and differences amongst *Leishmania* species and subspecies, *Am. J. Trop. Med.Hyg.*, 36:22-32.

Lainson, R., 1983, The American Leishmaniases: some observations on their ecology and epidemiology *Trans. R. Soc. Trop. Med. Hyg.*, 77:569-596.

Miles, M. A., Lanham, S. M., de Souza, A. A. and Povoa, M., 1980, Further enzymic characters of *Trypanosoma cruzi* and their evaluation for strain identification, *Trans. R. Soc. Trop. Med. Hyg.*, 74:221-237

Momen, H., Grimaldi, Jr. G., Pacheco, R. S., Jaffe, C. L., McMahon-Pratt, D. and Marzochi, M. C. A., 1985, Brazilian *Leishmania* stocks phenotypically similar to *Leishmania major*. *Am. J. Trop. Med. Hyg.*, 34:1076-1084.

Salles, C. A., da Silva, A. R. and Momen, H., 1986, Enzyme typing and phenetic relationships in *Vibbrio cholerae*. *Rev. Bras. Genet.*, 9:407-419.

Sarich, V. M., 1977, Rates, sample sizes and the neutrality hypothesis for electrophoresis in evolutionary studies. *Nature*, 265:24-28.

Zeledon, R., 1985, Leishmaniasis in North America, Central America and the Caribbean Islands, in: "Leishmaniasis" Chang, K. P. and Bray, R. S., Eds, Elsevier Science Publishers, Amsterdam.

CHROMOSOME SIZE HOMOLOGIES IN LEISHMANIA MAJOR DETERMINED BY MOLECULAR KARYOTYPING

Suzanne Holmes Giannini

Department of Medicine
University of Maryland School of Medicine
 and Center for Vaccine Development
Baltimore MD 21201

INTRODUCTION

Each isolate of Leishmania species has a distinctive and unique molecular karyotype [1-6]. Chromosome size polymorphisms occur in Leishmania such that each stock may differ from even closely related isolates, by one or more bands. Indeed, even clones of the same stock may have slightly different karyotypes [2]. The molecular karyotypes of closely related stocks, however, are clearly similar, enough so that unidentified isolates of Leishmania have been successfully typed by pulsed field gradient gel (PFG) analysis [1,6]. This finding suggests that karyotypes among members of the same Leishmania species are similar but not identical. (Throughout the paper Leishmania species will be those proposed by Lainson and Shaw [7], equivalent to subspecies in the 1964 nomenclature approved by the Society of Protozoologists [8] and recommended by the World Health Organization [9]).

I propose that there might be species-specific molecular karyotypes, that is, chromosome bands that are conserved in size among all isolates of a given species. I decided to test this hypothesis by comparing L. major isolates, which have relatively few variations in biochemical, excretion factor and isoenzyme markers compared with other Leishmania species. Because phenotype reflects the underlying genotype, the hypothesis predicts that isolates of this relatively homogeneous species should display a high degree of chromosome size concordance.

MATERIALS AND METHODS

Reference stocks. L. major Neal (Strain MRHO/SU/59/P) and LRC-L137 (Strain MHOM/IL/67/Jericho II) [10] were received as cloned stocks. The L. major stocks D-1 [11], WR300 [12] and Bokkara [13] were cloned by limiting dilution. Stocks were cryopreserved in liquid nitrogen. Reference stocks have been previously characterized by kDNA hybridization, isoenzyme typing, EF (excretion factor) analysis, and/or monoclonal antibodies. To prepare samples for pulsed field gradient gel electrophoresis (PFG), promastigotes were cultivated at $24^o \pm 2^oC$ in Schneider's medium, supplemented with 1% of a 100x antibiotic-antimycotic solution (both from GIBCO, Grand Island NY) and 20% fetal bovine serum (Hyclone, Sterile Systems, Logan UT), and harvested from late log phase. PFG karyotypes of promastigotes from culture, and of amastigotes from culture and from skin lesions, are the same [1].

Molecular weight standards. Annealed multimers of bacteriophage lambda DNA ("lambda ladders") were included as standards for each PFG gel [14]. The DNA of our phage lambda is ~50kb in size, so that the multimeric "rungs" of the lambda ladders subdivide the length of the gel into intervals of ~50 kb. Lambda ladders of 18 to 22 multimers are obtained, permitting sizing of chromosomes up to about 1100 kb. The WR300 isolate was also included as an internal standard on all gels.

Karyotyping. Complete details for sample preparation and PFG karyotyping have been published elsewhere [15, 16]. Samples were electrophoresed horizontally at 15ºC in 1% agarose gels of 20 cm x 20 cm size. Electrophoresis was at 12 volts/cm in a double inhomogeneous electrode box. The pulse frequency was 45 sec, which optimally separates chromosomes between 50 and 1000 kb, for which we have accurate size standards.
At the end of each run, gels were ethidium stained and photographed using 665 film (Polaroid Corporation, Cambridge MA).

Computing chromosome size distribution. Photographs of PFG gels were printed to actual size. Using the multimers of the lambda ladders as size standards, each sample lane was first divided into 18 to 22 intervals depending on the upper limit for annealed multimers. Because all the DNA in a single leishmanial chromosome band migrated within an interval spanning <25 kb, each 50 kb size interval was further subdivided in half, making a total of 36 to 44 size intervals of ~25 kb. Photographs of a typical PFG gel before and after its subdivision into appropriate size intervals are shown in Fig. 1. Each interval in the sample lane was then scored as 0 (no chromosome present, 1 (one chromosome present) or 2 (non-stoichiometrically stained chromosome, indicating more than one chromosome present).

RESULTS

Reliability and validity of chromosome size estimation by PFG. Reproducibility of DNA band size distribution from replicate samples and for gels run at different pulse frequencies was good, with individual DNA bands being measured with <5% coefficient of variation. Although the electrophoretic mobilities of chromosomes separated by PFG were reproducible, absolute sizing of chromosomes by PFG analysis might not be possible. Along with size, apparently also the nucleotide structure of DNA affects its migration. For example, chromosome 12 in yeast migrates abnormally slowly, probably due to its large tandem ribosomal DNA (rDNA) cluster [15]. A similar phenomenon occurs in Trypanosoma brucei, where an rDNA-containing chromosome migrates abnormally [16]. The high molecular weight chromosomes >2000 kb may be subject to shear, with loss of DNA. These chromosomes stain non-stoichiometrically with ethidium bromide. However, the size determinations of leishmanial chromosomes, and those of other species, although not to be taken as precise measurements of their molecular weights, are not affected by these artefacts when restricted to the smaller DNA molecules between 50 and 1500 kb.
Regardless of their absolute molecular weights, homologous chromosomes would be expected to share both size and nucleotide structure, and to migrate similarily.

Size distributions for chromosomes of stocks of L. major. From inspection of the smaller DNA molecules between 50 and 1100 kb, which can be accurately sized, a remarkable pattern emerged (Table I).

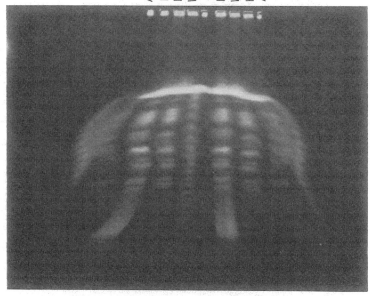

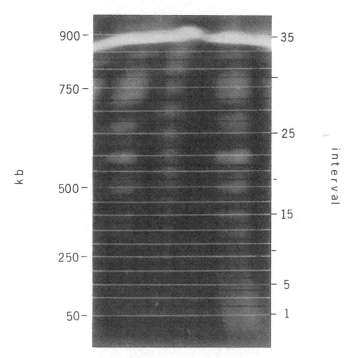

FIGURE 1. PFG sizing of chromosomes from two L. major stocks (D-1 and WR300) and one L. donovani stock (Khartoum) by comparing their relative mobilities with those of lambda ladders (λ).
  Upper panel: ethidium bromide stained PFG, 45 second pulse frequency.
  Lower panel: center three lanes of PFG, subdivided into intervals by comparison with mobilities of lambda ladders. Results are in Table I.

TABLE I. COMPARISON OF CHROMOSOME SIZES AND STAINING INTENSITIES IN SIX STOCKS OF LEISHMANIA

	Size interval	Apparent size	Lambda multimer	Leishmania major					L.d.+ Khar	#
				D-1	WR300	Neal	Bokk	L137		
	36	900 kb	18	n.r.	n.r.	n.r.	n.r.	n.r.	1	
	35			0	n.r.	0	1	0	0	
*	34	850 kb	17	1	1	1	1	0	0	
o	33			0	0	0	0	0	1	
	32	800 kb	16	0	0	0	0	1	1	
	31			1	1	1	1	0	0	
*	30	750 kb	15	1	1	2	1	1	1	_P.f.
*	29			1	1	1	1	1	0	
	28	700 kb	14	0	0	0	1	1	1	
*	27			2	1	1	1	1	0	
o	26	650 kb	13	0	0	0	0	0	1	
	25			0	1	1	0	0	1	
**	24	600 kb	12	2	2	2	2	2	0	
	23			0	0	1	0	0	0	
*	22	550 kb	11	1	1	1	1	1	1	
o	21			0	0	0	0	0	1	
*	20	500 kb	10	1	1	1	2	1	1	
o	19			0	0	0	0	0	0	
o	18	450 kb	9	0	0	0	0	0	0	
o	17			0	0	0	0	0	2	
*	16	400 kb	8	1	1	1	2	1	0	
	15			0	1	0	0	1	1	
*	14	350 kb	7	1	1	1	1	1	0	_L.ma.
	13			0	0	0	0	0	0	
	12	300 kb	6	0	0	0	0	0	0	_L.br.
	11			0	0	0	0	0	0	
	10	250 kb	5	0	0	0	0	0	0	-L.me.
	9			0	0	0	0	0	0	
	8	200 kb	4	0	0	0	0	0	0	
	7			0	0	0	0	0	0	
	6	150 kb	3	0	0	0	0	0	0	
	5			0	0	0	0	0	0	
	4	100 kb	2	0	0	0	0	0	0	
	3			0	0	0	0	0	0	
	2	50 kb	1	0	0	0	0	0	0	_T.b.
	1	<50 kb		0	0	0	0	0	0	

+ L.d., L. donovani Khartoum strain [17]
* chromosome band present in this interval in all stocks of L. major
o no chromosomes present in this interval in any stock of L. major
lower size limit reported for DNA bands of Plasmodium falciparum (P.f.) [22], L. major (L.ma.), L. braziliensis (L.br.) [1], L. mexicana (L.me.) [19], and Trypanosoma brucei minichromosomes (T.b.) [16]

A high proportion of resolved chromosome bands (8 of 14) were found to be size-homologous in all 5 stocks of L. major, indicated by asterisks in Table I. For example, a chromosome of ~350 kb is found in size interval 14 in all 5 L. major stocks.

The remainder of the chromosome bands were variable, being found in some but not all isolates. For example, a chromosome of ~375 kb occurs in size interval 15 in the WR300 and L357 stocks, but not in the D-1, Neal or Bokkara stocks (Table I).

Species-specificity of the L. major karyotype. The molecular karyotype of L. donovani Khartoum strain [17] was compared with those of the L. major isolates. Only 3 of its chromosomes fell in the size ranges for the conserved chromosomes of L. major, in size intervals 20, 22 and 30 (Table I).

DISCUSSION

Our data suggest that the majority of the chromosomes of L. major may be highly conserved in size among all isolates, thereby permitting identification of a species-specific karyotype. Of course many more stocks need to be karyotyped to confirm the hypothesis of a conserved karyotype for Leishmania species. Using the accurate estimates of apparent size distribution of chromosomes, our analysis revealed significant karyotype concordances among different stocks of L. major. Such a high level of size concordance is even more striking when we consider that the marker strains were isolated over a 25 year period, and originated in widely separated geographic areas over ranges of 80° of longitude and 25° of latitude (Senegal, Egypt, Israel and Turkestan). Such evidence argues strongly for a species-specific "consensus" karyotype in Leishmania.

Similarities in the karyotypes of members of the same species are great enough that members and non-members can be distinguished readily by molecular karyotyping. Indeed, PFG analysis has been used to type unidentified clinical isolates by comparison with known marker stocks [1,6].

The hypothesis of a species-specific "consensus" karyotype predicts that chromosomes that are highly conserved in size, will also have homologous DNA sequences. It is clear for L. major that chromosomes of the same size have high levels of DNA sequence homology because DNA eluted from a conserved chromosome band on PFG gels hybridizes preferentially with the corresponding sized chromosomes in other stocks of L. major [Giannini, unpublished observations]. Furthermore, the genes for α, β tubulin, for Hsp 70 (coding sequences for the 70 kD heat shock protein) and Pr8 (ribosomal RNA gene), all occur on the same size chromosomes of different stocks when these are closely related [1].

It is also clear that a high degree of plasticity exists in the genome of L. major [Table I; 1, 2], and also in the genomes of L. donovani [4, 5, 18], L. braziliensis and L. mexicana [1,3,6,19]. For each of these species, individual stocks have unique karyotypes, even though having a large proportion of size-homologous chromosomes.

Interestingly, when chromosome specific DNA is purified from hypervariable chromosome bands, it can hybridize to chromosomes of other sizes as well as to the size-homologous chromosome band in the stock from which the DNA was derived (e.g., Fig. 2 in [2]). Hypervariable chromosome DNA also hybridizes in other stocks to chromosomes that are not size-homologous [2].

Another indication of the plasticity of the L. major genome is the occurrence of stock- and clone-specific karyotypes [Table I; 2]. A comparison of the stocks identified as Neal and Bokkara in Table I reveal a number of differences in chromosome presence or copy number (intervals 16,20,23,25, 28 and 30). These stocks are both of strain MRHO/SU/59/-NealP, and were received from different laboratories, one in the USA, the other in Belgium. These two lines of strain MRHO/SU/59/NealP seem to have diverged considerably since being isolated by Professor Neal in 1959. Thus changes in the hypervariable chromosomes seem to occur readily in

Leishmania populations from discrete geographic locales, and/or under laboratory conditions.

Several non-sexual mechanisms have been identified that can lead to diversity in size and number of chromosomes in Leishmania. Integration into chromosomes of amplified dihydrofolate reductase-thymidylate synthase genes in methotrexate-resistant L. major can lead to an increase in apparent size of chromosomes, while extrachromosomal multimers of amplified genes can appear as a new chromosome band [20]. Chromosomal translocation can lead to alterations in apparent size of chromosomes [2,5]. Independently replicating DNAs (possibly of episomal or viral origin) occur as circular DNA, appearing as a band in the molecular karyotype of some Leishmania stocks. In other stocks, the independently replicating DNA may be integrated into the DNA of one of several different chromosomes [18,19,21].

CONCLUSIONS

We have hypothesized that the karyotype of each Leishmania species consists of a basic set of highly conserved chromosomes, augmented by an idiosyncratic set of hypervariable chromosomes unique to each isolate. Data on five stocks of L. major support this model. If the model proves to be correct, we shall need to identify the relationships between these two sets of genetic information, and the mechanisms for maintaining them. Then we can better define what is a Leishmania species, and design and interpret experiments to evaluate ploidy and genetic recombination.

ACKNOWLEDGEMENTS

This work was supported by USPHS Grant AI23956, by a grant from the Charles and Catherine MacArthur Foundation, and an award from the University of Maryland Biotechnology Center. We thank Drs. David Hart, now at King's College, London; Tosson A. Morsy, Ain Shams University, Cairo; Jan S. Keithly, Cornell University Medical College, New York; Phillip Scott, National Institutes of Health, Bethesda; Lionel Schnur and Charles Greenblatt, Hebrew University, Jerusalem, for supplying stocks of L. major. Drs. Mary G.S. Lee and David Glass of Columbia University College of Physicians & Surgeons, New York, provided much helpful advice. The expert technical assistance of Ms. Susie A. Mathews is gratefully acknowledged. A special word of thanks is due to Dr. Lex H.T. Van der Ploeg of Columbia University College of Physicians & Surgeons for a critical review of the manuscript, as well as for many inspiring discussions and generous loans of PFG boxes.

REFERENCES

1. Giannini, S.H., Schittini, M., Keithly, J.S., Warburton, P.W., Cantor, C.R., and Van der Ploeg, L.H.T. 1986. Science 232: 761-765.
2. Spithill, T.W., and Samaras, N. 1987. UCLA Symp. Mol. Cell. Biol. 42: 269-278.
3. Scholler, J.K., Reed, S.G., and Stuart, K. 1986. Mol. Biochem. Parasitol. 20: 279-283.
4. Bishop, R.P., and Miles, M.A. 1987. Mol. Biochem. Parasitol. (in press)
5. Bishop, R.P. 1987. In D.T. Hart [ed.]. Leishmaniasis: The First Centenary (1885-1985) New Strategies for Control. NATO ASI Series A: Life Sciences. London: Plenum Publishing Co. Ltd. (in press).
6. Dujardin, J.C., Gajendran, N., Matthijsen, G., Hamers, R., Urjel, R., Recacoechea, M., Villaroel, G., Desjeux, P., Bermudez, H., Le Ray, D.

1987. In D.T. Hart [ed.]. Leishmaniasis: The First Centenary (1885-1985) New Strategies for Control. NATO ASI Series A: Life Sciences. London: Plenum Publishing Co. Ltd. (in press).

7. Lainson, R., and Shaw, J.J. 1987. In W. Peters and R. Killick-Kendrick [eds.] Leishmaniasis in Biology and Medicine, Vol. 1, Biology and Epidemiology. New York: Academic Press (in press).
8. Honigberg, B.M. and Committee. 1964. A revised classification of the phylum Protozoa. J. Protozool. 11: 7-20.
9. World Health Organization. 1984. The Leishmaniases. WHO Tech. Rep. Ser. 701.
10. World Health Organization. 1985. Report of the Sixth Meeting of the Scientific Working Group on the Leishmaniases (Reference Strains of Leishmania). Cyclostyled document TDR/LEISH/STRAINS/SWG(6)/84.3. Geneva.
11. Schnur, L.F., Morsy, T.A., Feinsod, F.M., and El Missiri, A.G. 1985. Trans. R. Soc. Trop. Med. Hyg. 79: 134-135.
12. Strobel, M., Ndiaye, B., Renaud-Steens, C., Dedet, J.P. and Marchand, J.P. 1978. Medecine Maladies Infectieuses 8: 98.
13. Hart, D.T., and Opperdoes, F.R. 1984. Mol. Biochem. Parasitol. 13: 159-172.
14. Smith, C.L., Warburton, P.E., Gaal, A., and Cantor, C.R. 1986. In J.K. Setlow and A. Hollaender [eds.] Genetic Engineering: Principles and Methods, Vol. 8. New York: Plenum Press, pp. 45-70.
15. Schwartz, D.C., and Cantor, C.R. 1984. Cell 37: 67-75.
16. Van der Ploeg, L.H.T., Cornelissen, A.W.C.A., Barry, J.D. and Borst, P. 1984. EMBO Journal 13: 3109-3115.
17. Stauber, L.A. 1966. Exp. Parasitol. 18: 1-11.
18. Gajendran, N., Dujardin, J.P., Le Ray, D., Matthyssens, G., and Hamers, R. 1987. In D.T. Hart [ed.]. Leishmaniasis: The First Centenary (1885-1985) New Strategies for Control. NATO ASI Series A: Life Sciences. London: Plenum Publishing Co. Ltd. (in press).
19. Stuart, K. 1987. In D.T. Hart [ed.]. Leishmaniasis: The First Centenary(1885-1985) New Strategies for Control. NATO ASI Series A: Life Sciences. London: Plenum Publishing Co. Ltd. (in press).
20. Beverley, S.M. 1987. In D.T. Hart [ed.]. Leishmaniasis: The First Centenary(1885-1985) New Strategies for Control. NATO ASI Series A: Life Sciences. London: Plenum Publishing Co. Ltd. (in press).
21. Hamers, R. 1987. Discussion of Workshop 3: Molecular Genetics of Leishmania Development. NATO ASI on Leishmaniasis, Zakinthos, Greece.
22. Van der Ploeg, L.H.T., Smits, M., Ponnudurae, T., Vermeulen, A., Meuwissen, J.H.E.T. and Langsley, G. 1985. Science 229: 658-661.

IDENTIFICATION OF LEISHMANIA TROPICA BY SPECIES SPECIFIC MONOCLONAL ANTIBODIES

Rive Sarfstein and Charles L. Jaffe

Department of Biophysics and MacArthur Center
for Molecular Biology of Tropical Diseases
Weizmann Institute of Science, Rehovot 76100
Israel

INTRODUCTION

Leishmanial species can be typed by several methods[1] including isoenzymes,[2,3] nuclear or kinetoplast DNA hybridization,[4,5] excreted factor serotypes[6] and monoclonal antibodies.[7,8] Identification of parasite species is important in epidemiological studies and clinical treatment or follow up. Monoclonal antibodies now exist to several Old and New World species and subspecies of Leishmania. Using these antibodies, parasite typing can be carried out on small numbers of organisms by routine laboratory procedures. Species specific monoclonal antibodies to L. tropica are described which will complement existing L. donovani[9] and L. major[10] antibodies for the identification of Old World parasites.

MATERIAL AND METHODS

Parasites. Promastigotes of Leishmania were obtained primarily from Dr. Lionel Schnur at the WHO Leishmania Reference Center, Hadassah Medical School, Jerusalem, Israel and are summarized in Tables I and II. Parasites were cultured in Schneider's Drosophila medium at 26°C supplemented with 10% fetal calf serum and antibiotics.

Monoclonal Antibodies. Antibodies were produced to the membranes of various leishmanial species as previously described.[9-11] Hybridoma culture supernatants were used in all studies.

Preparation of Antigen. Lysates of whole promastigotes were prepared by washing $2-10 \times 10^8$ organisms twice with phosphate buffered saline, pH 7.2 (PBS) and resuspending in 1-2ml lysis buffer.[9] The cells were snap frozen in liquid N_2 and stored at either -70 or -190°C until use. Prior to coating of the microtiter plates the aliqouts to be tested were thawed, sonicated briefly to disrupt the parasites using an E/MC sonicator bath and the protein concentration determined.[12] Antigen was then diluted to a final protein concentration of 0.05 to 0.08mg/ml with PBS-azide.

Assays for Monoclonal Antibody Binding. Indirect radioimmune assays and enzyme-linked immunosorbent assays (ELSIA) were both carried out as described elsewhere.[10,11] Briefly, microtiter plates (96 well U-bottomed polyvinyl chloride) were coated with antigen overnight at 4°C. The plates were washed twice with 0.1% Tween-20 in PBS (PBS-Tween) and blocked with 2% fetal calf serum in PBS-azide. After rinsing with PBS-Tween, monoclonal antibody (50νl diluted 1:2) was incubated with the antigen either 2h or overnight. Excess monoclonal antibody was removed and the radioactive or enzyme-conjugated second antibody added for 1h. The plates were washed with PBS-Tween and in the case of the enzyme-conjugate a substrate, ABTS, was added.

RESULTS AND DISCUSSION

Four monoclonal antibodies to membranes of L.tropica LRC-L36 were produced (T11, T13 to T15).[11] These antibodies only react with parasites of the species L. tropica and do not react with lysates obtained from other Leishmania species (Table I, II). Ratios less than 3.0 are considered negative. Antibody T11 was tested on the largest number of isolates (45), including 16 L. tropica. All of the L.tropica examined reacted strongly with this antibody with binding ratios from 11.2 (LRC-L493I) to 124.3 (LRC-L159). No correlation was observed between the intensity of reaction and the clinical history, zymodeme or geographical origin of the parasite. Similar results were obtained using the remaining three L. tropica species-specific monoclonal antibodies. Antibody T15 consistently reacted weaker than T11, T13 and T14 with the exception of one isolate, Ben-Ami, recently isolated from the spleen of a patient with kala-azar. This isolate was also characterized as a L. tropica by isoenzymes and excreted factor serotyping (L.Schnur, personal communication). All four antibodies appear to recognized a similar membrane glycoconjugate[11] which is also present on excreted factor.[13]

The availability of L. tropica specific monoclonal antibodies will facilitate the identification of Old World Leishmania. Monoclonal antibodies specific for L. donovani[9] and L. major[10,14,15] exist which react with isolates obtained from diverse geographic origins. However L. major specific antibodies may crossreact on selected isolates of L. tropica.[10,14] In fact monoclonal antibodies specific to L. major show a spectrum of reactivities with L. tropica (see T1, Table I). **This demonstrates the necessity of combinding** several species-specific monoclonal antibodies into a panel when screening new isolates for reactivity.

Interestingly L. tropica shows a high level of complexity, not found by monoclonal antibodies, when zymodeme analysis is carried out. Le Blancq and Peters[16] have identified 18 different zymodemes in 27 stocks of L. tropica and several zymodemes may be present in one restricted region. This finding suggests that monoclonal antibodies may be

Table I. Specificity of Monoclonal Antibody Binding to Leishmania tropica stocks

Species Reference No. Local;WHO	T1	Binding Ratio* T11	T13	T14	T15	Notes[+]
L. tropica						
LRC-L5;MCAN/IQ/30/Lourie-11	n.d.	26.8	53.0	35.5	15.2	—
LRC-L7;MHOM/IN/3?/India-23	1.4	30.1	n.d.	n.d.	n.d.	CL
LRC-L8;MHOM/AF/??/Afghan-31	4.7	30.2	n.d.	n.d.	n.d.	CL
LRC-L18;MHOM/IL/52/Yonah-141	7.9	90.1	n.d.	n.d.	n.d.	CL
LRC-L32;MHOM/IQ/65/A. Sinai I	22.9	29.1	59.6	40.1	7.0	LR
LRC-L36;MHOM/IL/67/Jericho I	4.0	77.0	34.0	28.2	14.1	CL
LRC-L39;MHOM/SU/60/LRC-L39	6.9	56.9	40.0	20.1	10.1	CL
LRC-L43;MHOM/IL/49/Abu Ghosh-123	14.2	47.0	76.1	63.7	18.9	KA
LRC-L156;MHOM/IN/69/Ali	1.4	58.3	n.d.	n.d.	n.d.	KA
LRC-L159;MHOM/IN/67/Samanta	6.3	124.3	59.0	45.6	20.1	PKDL
LRC-L286;MHOM/IL/79/A. Sinai IV	22.9	40.5	n.d.	n.d.	n.d.	LR
LRC-L435;MHOM/GR/84/LA170	n.d.	40.3	70.2	46.1	10.0	CL
LRC-L440;MHOM/GR/84/LA180	n.d.	39.0	82.5	52.2	11.3	CL
LRC-L493;MHOM/IL/85/Katzav-I	n.d.	11.2	19.3	9.0	0.9	LR
LRC-L529;MHOM/IL/86/Ben Ami	n.d.	11.3	7.5	6.5	17.1	KA
Ackerman;MHOM/AF/??/NIH-AC	n.d.	73.0	n.d.	n.d.	n.d.	CL

* Binding Ratio - Positive monoclonal antibody (cpm or $Abs_{405-490}$)/ Negative monoclonal antibody (cpm or $Abs_{405-490}$).

[+] CL, cutaneous leishmaniasis; LR, leishmaniasis recidivans; KA, Kala-azar; PKDL, post kala-azar dermal leishmaniasis.

n.d. not determined; parasites were obtained from Dr. L. Schnur, WHO Ref. Center, Israel.

Table II. Specificity of Monoclonal Antibody binding to other *Leishmania* species

Species Reference No. Local; WHO	T11	Binding Ratio[+] T13	T14	T15	Source[+]
L. major					
LRC-L38;MRHO/SU/59/Neal P	0.7	–	–	–	a
LRC-L137;MHOM/IL/67/Jericho II	1.4	–	–	–	a
LRC-L207;MHOM/IL/77/LRC-L207	1.1	–	–	–	a
LRC-L223;MHOM/IL/78/Friedman	1.7	–	–	–	a
LRC-L241 MMAS/SN/77/DK110	1.4	–	–	–	a
LRC-L304;MHOM/IL/80/Meirson	1.1	–	–	–	a
LRC-L329;MHOM/SD/??/3S	1.0	–	–	–	a
LRC-L352;MHOM/SA/??/??	0.6	–	–	–	a
LRC-L505;MHOM/EG/84/Roa	1.2	2.1	2.1	1.0	a
IOC-L134;MHOM/SN/??/??	1.2	3.0	1.3	0.9	b
WR260B;MHOM/IL/67/Jericho II	0.6	0.9	1.0	1.5	c
WR309;MHOM/IL/79/Perlstein	1.5	1.1	1.3	1.6	c
L. aethiopia					
LRC-L134;MHOM/ET/??/TWG	1.8	1.0	0.9	1.5	a
LRC-L147;MHOM/ET/71/L100	1.8	–	–	–	a
LRC-L494;MHOM/ET/85/Avata	1.0	0.9	1.1	1.0	a
LRC-L495;MHOM/ET/85/Vasa	0.9	0.8	1.0	1.3	a
Gede; MHOM/ET/??/Gede	1.1	1.1	0.9	1.1	d
Kassaye;MHOM/ET/??/Kassaye	1.0	1.3	1.3	1.2	d
L. donovani					
LRC-L47;MHOM/FR/62/SXI	1.6	–	–	–	a
LRC-L52;MHOM/IN/54/Sc23	1.4	–	–	–	a
LRC-L133;MHOM/ET/67/HU3	1.3	–	–	–	a
Edmael;MHOM/BR/??/Edmael	2.0	1.0	1.5	1.1	g
WR168c;MHOM/SN/??/WR168	1.5	–	–	–	c
WR352;MHOM/IN/??/WHO Strain	1.1	1.2	1.3	0.9	c
Khartoum;MHOM/SD/??/Khartoum	2.1	1.3	1.7	2.7	h
LRC-L307;MHOM/GR/80/L24	1.0	–	–	–	a
LV9 MHOM/ET/67/HU3	1.6	1.3	1.0	1.7	e
NLB 125;MHOM/KE/??/NLB125	1.6	–	–	–	f

* Binding Ration - See Table I

[+] Source. (a) Dr. L. Schnur, WHO *Leishmania* Ref. Center, Israel. (b) Dr. L. Hendricks, WRAIR, Washington, D.C. (c) Dr. G.Grimaldi, Fundacao Oswaldo Cruz, Brazil, (d) Dr. F. Neva, LPD, NIH, Maryland. (e) Dr. M. Hommel, Liverpool School Tropical Medicine, England. (f) Dr. D. Koech, Clinical Research Center, Kenya. (g) Dr. S. Reed, Seattle Biomedical Res. Inst. Washington. (h) Dr. J. Kiethly, Cornell Medical School, New York.

especially convenient for the typing of L. tropica by any of the immunochemical techniques currently available.

Acknowledgements. This work was supported in part by the John and Catherine T. MacArthur Foundation, the Minerva Foundation and the US-Israel Binational Science Foundation. The authors would like to thank Lee Schnur for helping with the WHO nomenclature.

REFERENCES

1. M.L.Chance and B.C.Walton, eds.(1982) "Biochemical Identification of Leishmania," UNDP/WORLD BANK/WHO, Geneva, Switzerland.
2. R.D.Kreutzer, N.Souraty and M.E.Semko (1987) Am.J.Trop. Med.Hyg. 36: 22-32.
3. S.M.Le Blancq and W.Peters (1986) Trans.Roy.Soc.Trop.Med. Hyg. 80: 113-119.
4. D.C.Barker, L.J.Gibson, W.P.K.Kennedy, A.A.A.Nasser and R.H.Williams (1986) Parasitology 91: 8139-8174.
5. D.F.Wirth, W.O.Rogers, R.Barker, H.Dourado, K.Susubang and B.Albuquerque (1986) Science 234: 975-979.
6. L.Schnur "The Immunological identification and characterization oof leishmaniala stocks and strains, with special reference to excreted factor serotyping," In: Biochemcial Characterization of Leishmania, M.L.Chance and B.C.Walton, eds.(1982) UNDP/WORLD BANK/WHO, Geneva.
7. D.McMahon-Pratt and J.R.David (1981) Nature 291: 581-583.
8. D.McMahon-Pratt, Grimaldi
9. C.L.Jaffe, E.Bennett, Gabriel Grimaldi and D.Mcmahon-Pratt (1984) J.Immunol. 133: 440-447.
10. C.L.Jaffe and D.Mcmahon-Pratt (1983) J.Immunol. 131: 1987-1993.
11. C.L.Jaffe and R.Sarfstein (1987) J.Immunol. 138: 1310-1319.
12. M.Bradford (1976) Anal.Biochem. 72: 248-254.
13. L.Schnur, R.Sarfstein and C.L.Jaffe (1986) Isr.J.Med.Sci. 22: 849
14. E.Handman and R.E.Hocking (1982) Inf.Imm. 37: 28-33.
15. A.A.L.de Ibarra, J.G.Howard and D.Snary (1982) Parasitology 65: 523-531.

FLOW CYTOMETRIC ANALYSIS OF LEISHMANIA SURFACE MEMBRANE ANTIGEN

EXPRESSION

>Ronald. L. Anthony and John B. Sacci Jr.

>Department of Pathology
>University of Maryland School of Medicine
>Baltimore, Maryland 21201 USA

INTRODUCTION

The advent of cell fusion technology for the construction of hybridomas synthesizing monoclonal antibodies (Kohler and Milstein, 1975) has provided the immunoparasitologist with the means to detect subtle antigenic differences on the surface membrane of the leishmania parasites which cause human disease. Use of these antibodies in radioimmune binding assays (McMahon-Pratt and David, 1981; Jaffe and McMahon-Pratt 1983; Jaffe et al., 1984; Pan et al., 1984; McMahon-Pratt et al., 1985; Grimaldi et al., 1987), immunofluorescent antibody assays (Handman and Hocking, 1982; de Ibarra et al., 1982; Lemesre et al., 1985) and enzyme linked immunosorbant assays (Fong and Chang, 1982; Anthony et al., 1985) has now culminated in the identification of a sizeable composite of species-specific, subspecies-specific and stage-specific epitopes. Most importantly, the ability to demonstrate such epitopes on parasites taken directly from the patient's lesion (Lynch et al., 1986; Anthony et al., 1987) permits a prompt diagnosis of the infection. Such diagnoses are critical when attempting to decide regimens of treatment, management of the patient and prognosis.

In most of those earlier studies, specificity of the monoclonal antibodies was assessed on the basis of their reactivity with either isolated membranes or gluteraldehyde-fixed intact parasites. While the methods were semi-quantitative, the number of parasites within any given specimen or culture which were actually recognized by the antibody, and thereby contributed to positivity, could not be determined. Similarly, we had to assume that all parasites within the culture were binding equal amounts of the monoclonal antibody. Demonstration of quantitative differences in intensity of surface membrane reactivity among the promastigotes within a particular culture would have necessitated analysis of individual, living cells.

We have now developed a dual parameter immunofluorescent flow cytometric procedure for quantitating the binding of monoclonal antibodies to the surface membrane of living leishmania promastigotes. This procedure distinguishes between viable and non-viable cells and the intensity of the fluorescent signal emitted by each parasite, which is a function of the number of epitopes displayed, is quantitated. We have now begun to apply this technology for the speciation of leishmania isolates and for monitoring the kinetics of antigen expression throughout parasite differentiation.

METHODS

Fifty microliters from a culture of promastigotes, maintained at 26 C in medium 199 containing 10 mM Hepes with 20% fetal calf serum and antibiotics, are centrifuged at 800 g for 5 min at room temperature. After washing three times in 1 ml phosphate buffered saline (PBS), pH 7.2, the pellet of parasites is resuspended in 500 ul of the monoclonal antibody (media supporting the cloned hybridoma). The reaction is allowed to proceed for 30 min at room temperature and the washing cycle is repeated. The promastigotes are then covered with 100 ul of a goat anti-mouse immunoglobulin serum labeled with fluorescein isothiocyanate (FITC) diluted in PBS containing ethidium bromide (10 ug/ml). Incubation continues for another 30 min at room temperature and following one wash in PBS, the parasites are fixed, for ten seconds, in 250 ul paraformaldehyde. After two final washes, the pellet is resuspended in 500 ul PBS and analysed in the Epics Profile Flow Cytometer (Coulter Laboratories, Hialeah, Florida.).

RESULTS AND DISCUSSION

Each point in Histogram A of Figure 1 represents a promastigote of a specific size (FS = forward angle light scatter) and density (SS = 90 degree angle side scatter). The bit-map in the lower left corner (circle 1) encloses the homogeneous population which has been selected (gated) for analysis of fluorescent signals. This particular culture was comprised of stationary phase promastigotes of L. mexicana amazonensis (WRAIR isolate 303).

Each of the 3,062 points in Histogram B represents a promastigote which fell within the gated bit-map of Histogram A. This time, however, the promastigotes are separated upon the basis of their red fluorescence (LFL1), which is an indicator of ethidium bromide incorporation or cell death, and green fluorescence (LFL2) which is a measure of the amount of the FITC conjugate bound to the monoclonal antibody-surface antigen complex. The U9B3 monoclonal antibody, which recognizes the gp63 surface glycoprotein (Bouvier et al., 1985), was used in this analysis. The viable cells (86.8%) are limited to quadrants 3 and 4 (lack of red fluorescence) whereas antigen bearing cells (47.6%) fall within quadrants 2 and 4 (green fluorescence). Quadrant 1 includes 34 dead promastigotes (1.1%) which were negative for antibody reactivity. Of the 1,426 antigen positive promastigotes, 369 (26%) were dead and 1,057 (74%) were viable. The data headings "min" and "max" represent the channel numbers, on both the X and Y axis, assigned to each of the four quadrants. The "mean" channel number for promastigotes falling within a given quadrant and the standard deviation (SD) are calculated also. The percent half-peak coefficient of variaton (% HPCV) is the coefficient of variation in the channel number through which promastigotes, one-half way across the delimiter, are falling .

The separation of viable promastigotes from dead promastigotes is clearly evident in the two peaks of Histogram C. The delimiter (├──────┤) re-calculates the percentage of cells emitting the red signal; in this case 12.9%. The slightly higher percentage of dead parasites calculated in Histogram B (13.2%) is due to the lack of precision used in the manual positioning of the horizontal delimiter which separates quadrants 2 and 4.

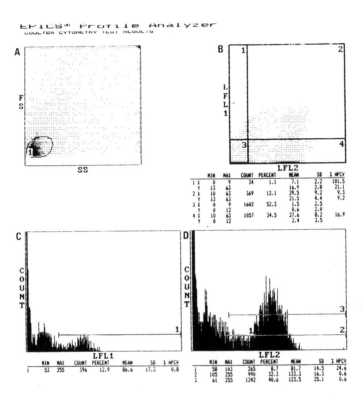

Fig. 1. Flow cytometric analysis of gp63 expression on surface membranes of stationary phase promastigotes of L. mexicana amazonensis.

In Histrogram D, delimiter #3 was positioned above all of the promastigotes (40.6%) which were emitting a green signal and therefore were displaying the epitope reactive with the monoclonal antibody. However, the wide range of channels (61-255) into which the antibody-positive cells were sorted establishes that the 1,242 promastigotes analysed were quite heterogeneous with respect to the quantity of the epitope they were expressing. Delimiter #2 marks the 32.3% of the promastigotes displaying the highest density of the epitope; e.g. highest channels for green fluorescence. The weak fluorescent signal emitted by the 265 promastigotes marked by delimiter #1 confirms that the epitope is present but sparse.

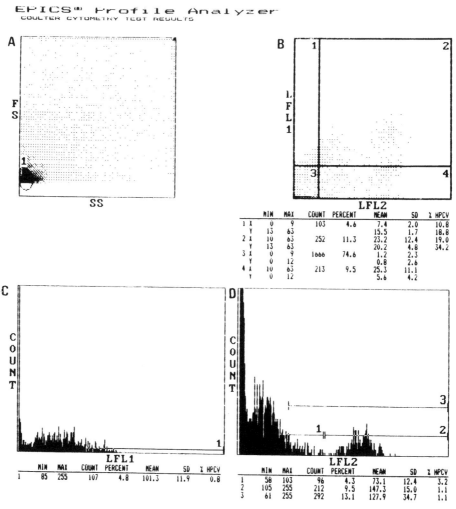

Fig. 2. Flow cytometric analysis of gp63 expression on surface membranes of logarithmic phase promastigotes of L. mexicana amazonensis.

These quantitative differences in antigen expression are further exemplified by analysis of histograms for the corresponding log phase culture of WRAIR 303 (Figure 2). In contrast to 40.6% of the stationary phase organisms, only 13.1% of the log-stage parasites were reactive with the monoclonal antibody. Although such comparative analysis in not affected by the number of parasites counted, it is essential that the channel numbers defining the 3 delimiters remained unchanged. Nine and one-half percent of the cells were strongly reactive with the U9B3; 4.3% were weakly reactive. Note that only 5% of the parasites in the log phase culture were non-viable (delimiter 1 of Histogram C). Again, the inability to precisely position the delimiters in Histogram B creates some discrepancy when comparing the data analysis with that of Histograms C and D.

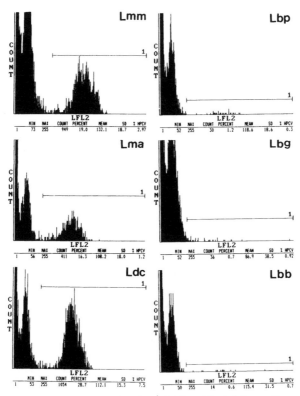

Fig. 3. Flow cytometric analysis of the 10-15kd surface antigen expression on stationary phase promastigotes of New World Leishmania.

Figure 3 is a composite of histograms depicting the reactivity of monoclonal antibody U7D5 (Williams, 1986), generated against an enriched pellicular membrane preparation of L. mexicana mexicana promastigotes (WRAIR 222), with living promastigotes of L. mexicana mexicana (WRAIR 222), L. mexicana amazonensis (WRAIR 303), L. donovani chagasi (WRAIR 685 -WHO reference strain), L. braziliensis panamensis (WRAIR 676 -WHO reference strain), L. braziliensis braziliensis (WRAIR 608 - WHO reference strain) and L. braziliensis guyanensis (WRAIR -677 - WHO reference strain). The reactive epitope, as confirmed by Western blot, is displayed on the immuodominant 10-15kd glycoconjugate (Turco et al., 1984). Although the reactivity of L. donovani and L. mexicana parasites is clearly evident, a significant percentage of promastigotes from these cultures did fail to bind the monoclonal antibody. Inhibition of capping by incubation at 4C did not have a significant effect. Since these non-reactive parasites would not be detected in the radioimmune binding assays or enzyme linked immunosorbent assays, we are forced to conclude that prior reports of species-specificity of monoclonal antibodies were based on reactivity of only some of the parasites representative of the culture. On the other hand, cultures appearing to be negative for reactivity with a specific antibody invariably contain a few promastigotes, < 3%, which clearly express the epitope (e.g. L. b. panamensis in Figure 3). Again, these parasites would never be detected in antibody assays wherein isolated membranes or parasite extracts were used as the antigen substrate. On the other hand, visualization of an occasional reactive promastigote (air-dried) on an otherwise negative IFA slide is not uncommon.

CONCLUSIONS

It would seem that speciation of leishmania parasites on the basis of their reactivity with murine monoclonal antibodies might be best accomplished by analysis of living promastigotes in flow cytometric assays. In contrast to methods utilizing isolated membranes or fixed parasites, this technology permits selection of a homogeneous population of parasites, the number of cells examined can be pre-set, dead cells can be excluded from analysis, and quantitative variations in antigen expression among promastigotes representative of a single specimen or culture can be detected. We suspect that such variations in the epitopic phenotype are common among promastigotes representative of a single isolate and that they have a significant influence on infectivity and pathogenesis of human disease.

REFERENCES

Anthony, R.L., Williams, K.M. Sacci, J.B., and Rubin, D.C., 1985, Subcellular and taxonomic specificity of monoclonal antibodies to New World Leishmania, Am. J. Trop. Med. Hyg., 34:1085.

Anthony, R.L., Grogl, M., Sacci, J.B., and Ballou,R.W., 1987, Rapid detection of Leishmania amastigotes in fluid aspirates and biopsies of human tisues, Am. J. Trop. Med. Hyg., 37:271.

Bouvier, J., Etges, R.J., and Bordier, C., 1985, Identification and purification of membrane and soluble forms of the major surface protein of Leishmania promastigotes, J. Biol. Chem., 260:15504.

de Ibarra, A.A.L., Howard, J.G., and Snary, D., 1982, Monoclonal antibodies to Leishmania tropica major. Specificities and antigen location, Parasitol., 85:523.

Fong, D., and Chang, K.P., 1982, Surface antigen change during differentiation of a parasitic protozoan, Leishmania mexicana: Identification by monoclonal antibodies, Proc. Natl. Acad. Sci., 79:7366.

Grimaldi, G., David, J.D., and McMahon-Pratt, D., 1987, Identification and distribution of New World Leishmania species characterized by serodeme analysis using monoclonal antibodies, Am. J. Trop. Med. Hyg., 36:270.

Handman, E., and Hocking, R.E., 1982, Stage-specific, strain-specific and cross-reactive antigens of Leishmania species identified by monoclonal antibodies, Infect. Immun., 37:28.

Jaffe, C.L., and McMahon-Pratt, D., 1983, Monoclonal antibodies specific for Leishmania tropica. I. Characterization of antigens associated with stage- and species-specific determinants, J. Immunol., 131:1987.

Jaffe, C.L., Bennett, E., Grimaldi, G., and McMahon-Pratt, D., 1984, Production and characterization of species-specific monoclonal antibodies against Leishmania donovani for immunodiagnosis, J. Immunol., 133:440.

Kohler, G., and Milstein, C., 1975, Derivation of specific antibody producing tissue culture and tumor lines by cell fusion, Europ. J. Immunol., 6:511.

Lemesre, J.L., Rizvi, F.S., Afchain, D., Sadigurski, M., Capron, A., and Santoro, F., 1985, Subspecies-specific surface antigens of promastigotes of the Leishmania donovani complex, Infect. Immun., 50:136.

Lynch, N.R., Malave, C., Ifante, R.B., Modlin, R.L., and Convit, J., 1986, In situ detection of amastigotes in American cutaneous leishmaniasis using monoclonal antibodies, Trans. Roy. Soc. Trop. Med., 80:6.

McMahon-Pratt, D., and David, J.R., 1981, Monoclonal antibodies that distinguish between New World species of Leishmania, Nature, 291:581.

McMahon-Pratt, D., Bennett, E., Grimaldi, G., and Jaffe, C.L., 1985, Subspecies- and species-specific antigens of Leishmania mexicana characterized by monoclonal antibodies, J. Immunol., 134:1935.

Pan, A.A., McMahon-Pratt, D., and Hornigberg, B.M., 1984, Leishmania mexicana pifanoi: Antigenic characterization of promastigote and amastigote stages by solid phase radioimmunoassay, J. Parasitol., 70:834.

Turco, S.J., Wilkerson, M.A., and Clawson, D.R., 1984, Expression of an unusual acidic glycoconjugate in Leishmania donovani, J. Biol. Chem., 259: 3883.

Williams, K.M., Sacci, J.B., and Anthony, R.L., 1986, Characterization and quantitation of membrane antigens of New World Leishmania species by using monoclonal antibodies in Western blot and flow microfluorometric assays, J. Protozool., 33:490.

ON THE CLINICAL MANIFESTATIONS AND PARASITES OF OLD WORLD LEISHMANIASES
AND LEISHMANIA TROPICA CAUSING VISCERAL LEISHMANIASIS

L.F.Schnur

Department of Parasitology, The Kuvin Centre
Hebrew University-Hadassah Medical School
Jerusalem, Israel

Leishmanial parasites were first discovered in the Old World by Cunningham (1885) and with this the first defined cases of leishmaniasis began to be described. By the turn of the century, two distinct leishmaniases were recognized: cutaneous leishmaniasis (CL)(Borovsky,1898, cited and translated by Hoare, 1938; Wright, 1903) and visceral leishmaniasis (VL) (Leishman, 1903; Donovan,1903). This was before the generic name Leishmania was ever applied to the parasites causing them (Ross,1903). Since the clinical manifestations of these two leishmaniases were so distinct, their parasites were named as separate species: L.tropica for those causing CL; L.donovani for those causing VL, despite their similar morphology. So distinct were these in the minds of practitioners that the two species names became synonymous with the two diseases. Even today they are often applied to uncharacterized organisms solely according to clinical condition and the organs in which the parasites are found.

Yakimoff and Schokhor (1914) described two types of leishmanial parasite from skin lesions: one with small amastigotes, maximal size 3.9 x 3.1 μm; the other with large amastigotes, maximal size 5.5 x 3.9 μm. These they named respectively L.tropica var. minor and L.tropica var. major on account of amastigotic size. Kojevnikov (1941, reviewed Hoare,1944) noted that two basic types of lesion existed: dry nodular ones and wet ulcerating ones. Later, he and his co-workers (Kojevnikov et al.,1947; Kojevnikov, 1963) linked the morphological types to the lesional differences seen in Russian foci, although Adler and Katzenellenbogen (1952) could not substantiate this by observations made in Israel. However, differences in the epidemiology and ecology of the two varieties were also seen to exist (Latyshev and Kriukova, 1941). Lesions caused by the small amastigotic variety tended to originate in urban environments and those by the large amastigotic variety in rural environments, where wild rodents were also infected and served as a reservoir of human infection. On account of these differences, Bray et al. (1973a) separated the two varieties into two species: L.tropica and L.major, respectively. This greater separation was endorsed and shown to be justified by serological and biochemical characterisation that exposed intrinsic differences between the two species. In man, L.major has only ever been known to cause simple CL. L.tropica has also been isolated from cases of leishmaniasis recidivans(LR)a non-self-healing, recurrent leishmaniasis first described by Dostrovsky (1934,1936). In fact, only L.tropica has ever been known to cause LR, just as only L.aethiopica has ever been found to cause Old World diffuse cutaneous leishmaniasis (DCL) (Balzer et al.,1960; Bryceson,1969; Bray et al., 1973a). In most cases L.aethiopica causes simple CL like that caused by L.tropica and L.major. Human simple CL has also been recorded in Namibia (Grove, 1970). Its parasite is quite distinct from the other species associated with Old World CL, LR and DCL (Chance et al., 1978) and probably constitutes a further species of Leishmania.

Leishmania donovani sensu lato is the parasite of VL throughout the world, but has also been shown to be associated with particular cutaneous leishmaniases. Abdulla (1982) showed the parasite of Sudanese naso-oral, also called mucosal, leishmaniasis (Christopherson, 1914; Milošev et al., 1969) to be L.donovani. The dermal condition post-kala-azar dermal leishmaniasis (PKDL) that appears as a sequela in some treated, cured cases of VL, first described by Bramachari (1922), is another. Cahill (1964) even showed that L.d.donovani from Sudan can cause simple CL, without concomitant signs of VL. This has now also been established for L.d.infantum in France (Rioux et al., 1980) and Italy (Gramiccia et al., 1987). That L.donovani s.l. can be cutaneous as well as visceralize in man was established long ago but forgotten. Benhamou et al.(1935) and Benhamou and Fourès (1935) showed that stained smears of tissue taken from normal, healthy skin of infants with VL contained amastigotes and helped to confirm diagnosis.

With all the Old World species of Leishmania known to cause leishmaniasis in man having been mentioned, it would seem that this brief perspective is finished. However, just as L.donovani visceralizes but tends towards dermatotropism, so L.tropica is dermatotropic with a tendency to visceralize. Evidence for this comes from four sources. Bray et al. (1973b) studied eight Bengali strains, four from VL cases and four from cases of PKDL. Using an indirect haemagglutination test to type them, they showed all eight to be essentially similar, but different from an Ethiopian L.donovani strain (i.e. MHOM/ET/67/HU3 = L82 = LV9 = LRC-L133) that serves as an international reference strain of this species. When typed by excreted factor (EF) serotyping (Schnur et al., 1972; Schnur, 1982) and enzyme analysis (Schnur et al., 1981), they proved to be L.tropica, producing sub-serotype A_2 EF. This is characteristic of all L.tropica strains, including those from LR cases (Schnur et al., 1973; Zuckerman, 1975). Four Israeli strains from infantile cases of VL were identified as L.tropica by EF serotyping, showing that they, too, produced sub-serotype A_2 EF (Schnur et al., 1973, 1981) and enzyme analysis (Schnur et al., 1981). Two Iraqi strains from children with VL were shown to be L.tropica by enzyme analysis (Algeboori and Evans, 1980a, 1980b). On receiving and typing these two strains serologically, I found they, too, produced sub-serotype A_2 EF. Lastly, Balazzoug (1982, cited Al-Hussayni et al., 1987), working on Algerian strains, has also reported that L.tropica can visceralize.

There is some doubt concerning the authenticity of these visceralizing strains of L.tropica, as they have either been in strain collections for many years or have been sent to different institutions and passaged many times, allowing for errors during handling. This is compounded by traditional thinking, in which it is accepted that L.donovani causes VL and L.tropica CL. However, the following case supplies definitive proof of L.tropica being able to visceralize and adds credence to the cases cited above.

On 5th February, 1987, I was given two biopsy samples from a 20-year old Israeli male patient, who had been hospitalized some weeks before with signs of VL, including splenomegaly. One was a piece of lymph gland, the other a piece of spleen. Previously, smears and cultures of bone marrow aspirates had proved negative for leishmanial parasites. I made smears and cultures of the lymph gland and spleen samples. The smears of both organs were negative, as was the lymph gland culture. However, the culture of splenic tissue grew promastigotes after seven days. On testing the used culture medium overlay from this isolation culture for the presence of leishmanial EF and its type, it proved to contain sub-serotype A_2 EF, the type specific for L.tropica. Since the material tested came directly from the primary culture, mishandling could be excluded. That the strain was L.tropica was corroborated by enzyme analysis, although the strain had some enzymic differences compared with the reference strain used. This patient could only have acquired his infection in Israel.

Recently, Barral et al. (1986) described the isolation of L.mexicana amazonensis, a species causing CL and DCL in the New World, from the bone marrow of a VL case.

While the cases cited might be extraordinary, care must be taken in concluding leishmanial types by clinical manifestations only and strain typing is imperative.

ACKNOWLEDGEMENT

The diagnosis of leishmaniasis and typing of leishmanial strains done in Jerusalem was supported by:the WHO, contract TRY L3/181/2; the leishmaniases component of the UNDP/World Bank/WHO Special Programme TDR;and research contract NOI AI-22668-NIH-NIAID on the Epidemiology and Control of Arthropod Borne Diseases.

REFERENCES

Adler, S., and Katzenellenbogen, I., 1952, The problem of the association between particular strains of Leishmania tropica and clinical manifestations produced by them, Ann. Trop. Med. Parasit.,46:25.

Algeboori, T.I., and Evans, D.A., 1980a, Leishmania spp. in Iraq. Electrophoretic isoenzyme patterns. I. Visceral leishmaniasis. Trans. R. Soc. Trop. Med. Hyg.,74:169.

Algeboori, T.I., and Evans, D.A., 1980b, Leishmania spp. in Iraq. Electrophoretic isoenzyme patterns. II. Cutaneous leishmaniasis, Trans. R. Soc. Trop. Med. Hyg., 74:178.

Al-Hussayni, N.K., Rassam, M.B., Jawdat, S.Z., and Wahid F.N., 1987, Numerical taxonomy of some Old World Leishmania spp., Trans. R. Soc. Trop. Med. Hyg., 81:581.

Balzer, R.J., Destombes, P., Schaller, K.F. and Série, C., 1960. Leishmaniose cutanée pseudolepromateuse en Ethiopie, Bull. Soc. Path. Exot., 53:293.

Barral, A., Badaro, R., Barrel-Netto, M., Grimaldi Jr, G., Momen, H., and Carvalho, E.M., 1986, Isolation of Leishmania mexicana amazonensis from the bone marrow in a case of American visceral leishmaniasis, Am. J. Trop. Med. Hyg., 34:732.

Benhamou, E., Faugère, R., and Choussat, F., 1935, Le diagnostic du kala-azar par les frottis dermiques, Bull. et Mem. Soc. Méd. Hôpit. de Paris, 3eme series, No 25:1326.

Benhamou, E., and Fourès, R., 1935, A propos d'un nouveau cas de kala-azar vérifié par les frottis dermiques. L'ascite leishmanienne, Bull. Soc. Path. Exot., 28:706.

Brahmachari, U.N., 1922, A new form of cutaneous leishmaniasis-dermal leishmanoid, Indian Med. Gaz., 57:125.

Bray, R.S., Ashford, R.W. and Bray, M.A., 1973a, The parasite causing cutaneous leishmaniasis in Ethiopia, Trans. R. Soc. Trop. Med. Hyg., 67:345.

Bray, R.S., Ashford, R.W., Mukherjee, A.M., and Sen Gupta, P.C., 1973b, Studies on the immunology and serology of leishmaniasis IX. Serological investigation of the parasites of Indian kala-azar and Indian post-kala-azar dermal leishmaniasis. Trans.R.Soc.Trop.Med.Hyg.,67:125.

Bryceson, A.D.M., 1969, Diffuse cutaneous leishmaniasis in Ethiopia. I. The clinical and histopathological features of the disease, Trans. R. Soc. Trop. Med. Hyg., 63:708.

Cahill, K.M., 1964, Leishmaniasis in the Sudan Republic. XXI. Infection in American personnel, Am. J. Trop. Med. Hyg., 13:794.

Chance, M.L., Schnur, L.F., Thomas, S.C., and Peters, W., 1978, The biochemical and serological taxonomy of Leishmania from the Aethiopian zoogeographical region of Africa, Ann. Trop. Med. Parasit., 72:533.

Christopherson,J.B.,1914,On a case of naso-oral leishmaniasis (corresponding to the description of espundia);and a case of Oriental sore both originating in the Anglo-Egyptian Sudan, Ann. Trop. Med. Parasit., 8:458.

Cunningham, D.D., 1885, On the presence of peculiar parasitic organisms in the tissue of a specimen of Dehli boil, Scient. Mem. Med. Offrs Army India, 1:21.

Donovan, C., 1903, On the possibility of the occurrence of trypanosomiasis in India, Br. Med. J.,ii:79.

Dostrovsky, A., 1934, Leishmania recidiva of the skin, Harefuah, 8:118. In Hebrew, English summary, p.1.

Dostrovsky, A., 1936, Relapses in cutaneous leishmaniasis, Ann. Trop. Med. Parasit., 30:267.

Gramiccia, M., Gradoni, L., and Pozio, E, 1987, Leishmania infantum sensu lato as an agent of cutaneous leishmaniasis in Abruzzi region (Italy), Trans. R. Soc. Trop. Med. Hyg., 81:235.

Grové, S.S. 1970, Cutaneous leishmaniasis in South West Africa, S. Afr. Med. J., 44:206.

Hoare, C.A., 1938, Early discoveries regarding the parasite of Oriental sore (with an English translation of the memoir by P.F.Borovsky: "On Sart sore." 1898) Trans. R. Soc. Trop. Med. Hyg.,32:67.

Hoare, C.A., 1944, Cutaneous leishmaniasis (critical review of recent Russian work), Trop. Dis. Bull., 41:331.

Kojevnikov, P.V., 1963, Two nosological forms of cutaneous leishmaniasis, Am. J. Trop. Med. Hyg.,12:719.

Kojevnikov, P.V., Dobrotvorkaya, N.V., and Latyshev, N.I., 1947, "Cutaneous Leishmaniasis: a Treatise for Physicians and Biologists," State Publishers of Medical Literature, Moscow. In Russian, abstracted in Trop. Dis. Bull. 44:940.

Latyshev, N.I., and Kriukova, A.P., 1941, On the epidemiology of cutaneous leishmaniasis: cutaneous leishmaniasis as a zoonotic disease of wild rodents in Turkmenia, Trav. Acad. Milit. Méd. Armée Rouge U.R.S.S., 25:229. In Russian, abstracted in Trop. Dis. Bull., 40:24.

Leishman, W.B., 1903, On the possibility of the occurrence of trypanosomiasis in India, Br. Med. J.,i:1252.

Milošev, B., Daoud, E.H., El Hadi, A., El Hassan, A.M., and Sati, M.H., 1969, Mucosal leishmaniasis in the Sudan, Ann. Trop. Med. Parasit., 63:123.

Rioux, J.-A., Lanotte, G., Maazoun, R., Perello, R., and Pratlong, F.,1980, Leishmania infantum Nicolle, 1908, agent du bouton d'Orient autochthone. A propos de l'identification biochemique de deux souches isolées dans les Pyrenées-Orientales, C.R.Acad. Sci. Paris,291:701.

Ross, R., 1903, Further notes on Leishman's bodies, Br. Med. J.,ii:1401.

Schnur, L.F.,Chance, M.L., Thomas, S.C., and Peters, W., 1981., The biochemical and serological taxonomy of visceralizing Leishmania, Ann. Trop. Med. Parasit., 75:131.

Schnur, L.F., Zuckerman, A., and Greenblatt, C.L., 1972, Leishmanial serotypes as distinguished by the gel diffusion of factors excreted in vitro and in vivo. Israel J. Med. Sci., 8:932.

Schnur, L.F., Zuckerman, A., and Greenblatt, C.L., 1973, The relationship between the clinical types and serotypes of Leishmania, J.Protozool. (Suppl.), 20:534.

Wright, J.H., 1903, Protozoa in a case of tropical ulcer ("Dehli Sore"), J. Med. Res., 10:472.

Yakimoff, W.L., and Schokhor, N.I., 1914, Récherches sur les maladies tropicales humaines et animales au Turkestan – II. La leishmaniose cutanée (bouton d'Orient) spontanée du chien au Turkestan, Bull. Soc. Path. Exot., 7:186.

Zuckerman, A., 1975, Current status of the immunology of blood and tissue protozoa. I. Leishmania, Expl. Parasit., 38:370.

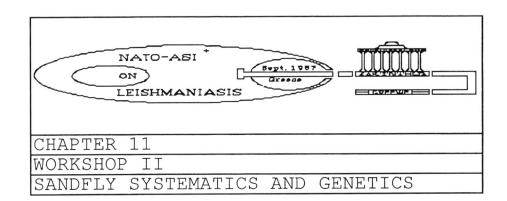

CHAPTER 11
WORKSHOP II
SANDFLY SYSTEMATICS AND GENETICS

WORKSHOP II : SANDFLY SYSTEMATICS AND GENETICS

Richard D. Ward

Department of Medical Entomology
Liverpool School of Tropical Medicine
Liverpool L3 5QA, U.K.

Since 1786 when Scopoli first described <u>Bibio</u> (=<u>Phlebotomus</u>) <u>papatasi</u>, sandfly systematics have passed through three main phases. Initially taxa were distinguished by reference to external morphology, either qualitative and/or quantitative. Further distinguishing characteristics became available in the mid-1920's when Adler and Theodor (1926) showed the value of internal structures of sandflies. In the mid-1970's a third phase bagan as a response to the need for methods to distinguish between individuals in species groups and complexes. As a result, the application of crossing experiments, cytogenetics, electrophoresis, gas chromatography, multivariate statistics and molecular techniques have been investigated with varying degrees of success.

The invited participants to the workshop reflected this recent change in emphasis in their presentations and the current interest in new methods was evident in the discussions that followed. Dr. Richard Lane, who introduced the subject, presented a synthesis of our current knowledge from the theoretical and practical standpoint and concluded with his views on future needs.

The main impetus for interest in sandfly systematics is clearly the relationship to disease transmission. This has led for example to significantly greater interest in the phlebotomines when compared to the rest of the Family Psychodidae. It was emphasised that sandfly systematics, if they are to be of practical use, should be predictive at the generic, sub-generic and species levels. Thus we generally expect the genus <u>Phlebotomus</u> to be potential vectors of <u>Leishmania</u> and at the sub-generic level Adlerius is mainly associated with parasites causing visceral leishmaniasis. At the species level we may often extrapolate that a known vector in one geographic zone may reasonably be suspected as responsible for transmission of a similar parasite elsewhere. When such predictions are confirmed as correct then we have an indication that systematics are establishing a useful and practical framework. Definition of species in the sub-family has until recently been mainly upon morphological criteria. With the establishment of thriving colonies greater interest is now being shown in biological definition of species using crossing experiments (Ward et al.,1986; Ready et al., 1986). However, it was emphasised that the current status of sandfly systematics is probably comparable to the stage reached by mosquito systematists in the early 1940's. For example, there have been few biogeographic studies of single species and there is as yet little understanding of phylogenetic relationships.

Attempts to apply new techniques to sandflies have nonetheless begun to yield results and there was optimism about the potential for future progress. For example, although early studies of larval salivary gland chromosomes produced poor results, recent observations on adults are showing polytenes of improved clarity (Lane unpublished observations). Electrophoretic techniques have been applied mainly to differentiate members of species groups and have been successful in distinguishing female Lu. carrerai from Lu. yucumensis in Bolivia (Caillard et al., 1986). When applied to populations of P. perfiliewi and Lu. longipalpis from different parts of Italy and Colombia respectively, signiiicant allele frequency differences have been demonstrated (Ward et al., 1981; Ward in press). The relevance, if any, of such results is however unknown. The application of gas chromatography to identify cuticular hydrocarbons has been successful in distinguishing between members of the squamiventris group in Brazil (Ryan et al., 1986) and has indicated differences between domestic and silvatic populations of P. ariasi in France (Kamhawi et al., 1987). This technique in conjunction with mass spectroscopy has also been applied to show the existence of two pheromone types in the Lu. longipalpis complex (Phillips et al., 1986). The use of multivariate statistics has been applied to phlebotomines with disappointing results so far and numerical taxonomy remains to be tested. At the species group level, individual egg batch rearing is now more widely applied and has often resulted in the correct association of previously undefined pairs. Sandfly systematists have also begun to pay renewed attention to fine structures at the light microscope level revealing new spermathecal duct structures (Leger et al., 1983) and significant ascoid length differences between P. papatasi and the closely related P. bergeroti (Lane and Fritz, 1986). Scanning electron microscopy has been applied to the chorionic sculpturing of eggs (Ward & Ready, 1975; Zimmerman et al., 1977; Irungu et al., 1986) and to the caudal setae of some sandfly larvae (Killick-Kendrick unpublished observations. Such studies on immature stages have not yet reached the point where they can be incorporated into and correlated with the systematics of adults. With the exception of Chaika (1975) and Boufana & Ward (unpublished observations) who studied antennal morphology and Lane & Ward (1984) who examined male Lu. longipalpis tergites the SEM has not been widely applied to adults. Amongst the newest methods to be applied to the sub-family is the use of DNA probes for identification and this subject was well represented in presentations by Dr. P. Ready and Dr. J.M. Crampton.

Dr. Lane concluded his introduction by emphasising the need to consolidate faunistic studies and to rewrite the major monographs on the different geographic zones. On the basis that it is a source of confusion to those studying leishmaniasis he made a plea that workers should be conservative with the raising of new genera, which is currently also a point of some dispute amongst those who study blackflies. Finally, it was noted that our current fascination with infra-specific variation should not be allowed to over-ride the need to define its significance in relation to the leishmanial epidemiologies that we study.

Dr. Leger, who ably chaired the session, then described the significance of her new spermathecal duct characters which are proving of value in the differentiation of members of the subgenus Larrousius. Dr. Killick-Kendrick, who is also interested in this group, again emphasised the importance of individual egg batch rearing, which has recently revealed morphological differences between immature stages of this group.

Dr. Paul Ready described the results of his work with Dr. D. Smith on rDNA sequence polymoprhism as population markers for P. papatasi from Tunisia, Saudi Arabia and Iraq. In addition their work has identified a diagnostic non-transcribed spacer fragment of the rDNA of P. papatasi which distinguishes it from closely related species in an endemic zone for leishmaniasis in Tunisia. The alternative 'shot gun' approach to the development of DNA probes was then described by Dr. Crampton who together with Ms T. Knapp and Dr. R. Ward has begun to apply this technique to Lu. longipalpis populations. This involves the comparison of repetitive genomic DNA sequences to distinguish species specific characters, regardless of whether the sequences are functional or not. The relative merits of the two different approaches are discussed in both papers. The speakers emphasised that DNA probes should not be regarded as magic bullets that will solve all systematists problems overnight, but rather should be used wisely as a powerful new tool in conjunction with existing techniques for species identification. Professor D. Molyneux echoed this sentiment in a short presentation that followed on the application of cuticular hydrocarbons to vector identification.

In his concluding comments Professor J.A. Rioux drew attention to the need for systematists to consider the co-evolution and in consequence co-adaptation of sandflies with the Leishmania that they transmit; this theme having been the subject of a recent review by Dr. Killick-Kendrick (1985). The session ended therefore with the contributors focusing on the need for systematics within the sub-family to reflect and predict associations with Leishmania and mirror correlations between similar epidemiologies. The advent and the application of new technologies to sandfly systematics will initially produce an abundance of new data. However, relating this information to similarly new developments in the identification of parasites will be a long and interesting task for "Leishmaniacs" - retired, functioning and lying unaware in their cradles.

REFERENCES

Adler, S. and Theodor, O., 1926, On the minutus group of the genus Phlebotomus in Palestine, Bull.Entomol.Res., 16: 399-405.

Caillard, T., Tibayrenc, M., Le Pont, F., Dujardin, J.P., Deseux, P. and Ayala, F.J., 1986, Diagnosis by isozyme methods of two cryptic species, Psychodopygus carrerai and P. yucumensis (Diptera: Psychodidae), J.Med.Entomol., 23: 489-492.

Chaika, S.Y., 1975, Electron microscopic investigation of the olfactory sensilla of the sandfly (Diptera: Phlebotomidae) (in Russian), Insect Chemoreception No.2. (Proc. 2nd All-Union Symp. on Insect Chemoreception., Vilnius., pp 69-75.

Irungu, L.W., Mutinga, M.J. and Kokwaro, E.D., 1986, Chorionic sculpturing of eggs of some Kenyan Phlebotomine sandflies, Insect Sci.Applic., 1: 45-48.

Kamhawi, S., Molyneux, D.H., Killick-Kendrick, R., Milligan, P.J.M., Phillips, A., Wilkes, T.J. and Killick-Kendrick, M., 1987, Two populations of Phlebotomus ariasi in the Cevennes focus of leishmaniasis in the south of France revealed by analysis of cuticular hydrocarbons, Med.Vet.Entomol., 1: 97-102.

Killick-Kendrick, R., 1985, Some epidemiological consequences of the evolutionary fit between leishmaniae and their phlebotomine vectors, Bull.Soc.Path.exot., 78: 747-755.

Lane, R.P. and Fritz, G.N., 1986, The differentiation of the leishmaniasis vector P. papatasi from the suspected vector P. bergeroti (Diptera: Phlebotominae), Systematic Entomol., 11: 439-445.

Lane, R.P. and Ward, R.D., 1984, The morphology and possible function of abdominal patches in males of two forms of the leishmaniasis vector Lutzomyia longipalpis (Diptera: Phlebotominae), Cah. O.R.S.T.O.M. ser.Ent.med et Parasitol., 22: 245-249.

Leger, N., Pesson, B., Madulo-Leblond, G. and Abonnenc, E., 1983, Sur la differenciation des femelles du sous-genre Larroussius Nitzulescu, 1931 (Diptera-Phlebotomidae) de la region mediterraneenne, Ann. Parasitol.Hum.Comp., 58: 611-623.

Ready, P.D., Killick-Kendrick, R., Smith, D.F. and Bailly, M. 1986, rDNA structural polymorphisms as diagnostic markers for populations of Phlebotomus papatasi from areas endemic and non-endemic for zoonotic cutaneous leishmaniasis, Trans.R.Soc.trop.Med.Hyg., 80: 341-342.

Ryan, L., Phillips, A., Milligan, P., Lainson, R., Molyneux, D.H. and Shaw, J.J., 1986, Separation of female Psychodopygus wellcomei and P. complexus by cuticular hydrocarbon analysis, Acta Tropica, 43: 85-89.

Scopoli, J.D., 1786, Delicae faunae et florae insubricae 1: 85 pp.

Ward, R.D., 1986, Mate recognition in a sandfly (Diptera: Psychodidae), J. R. Army Cps., 132: 132-134.

Ward, R.D. (in press), Genetic diversity in phlebotomine sandflies (Diptera: Psychodidae), Ann.Parasitol.Hum.Comp.

Ward, R.D., Bettini, S., Maroli, M., McGarry, J.W. and Draper, A., 1981, Phosphoglucomutase polymorphism in Phlebotomus perfiliewi perfiliewi Parrot (Diptera: Psychodidae) from central and northern Italy, Ann.Trop.Med.Parasit., 75: 653-661.

Ward, R.D. and Ready, P.A., 1975, Chorionic sculpturing in some sandfly eggs (Diptera: Psychodidae), J.Ent. (A), 50: 127-134.

Zimmerman, J.H., Newson, H.D., Hooper, G.R. and Christensen, H.A., 1977, A comparison of the egg surface structure of six anthropophilic phlebotomine sandflies (Lutzomyia) with the scanning electron microscope (Diptera: Psychodidae), J.Med.Entomol., 13: 574-579.

SANDFLY SYSTEMATICS: EPIDEMIOLOGICAL REQUIREMENTS AND CURRENT DEVELOPMENTS

R.P. Lane

Department of Entomology
London School of Hygiene & Tropical Medicine
London WC1
U.K.

The raison d'etre of sandfly studies is the role of phlebotomines as vectors of parasites, both *Leishmania* and viruses. Without this impetus their small size, retiring behaviour and difficult identification would surely have relegated sandflies to taxonomic obscurity, as are the other members of the family Psychodidae. The interest shown in sandflies by many different disciplines brings considerable responsibility and difficultires to phlebotomine systematists to produce a useable and predictive classification.

A classification has two fundamental objectives: Firstly, it should be a clear and effective means of communication, and therefore easy to use by non-specialists, and secondly, like any theory, it should be predictive and testable. Often these two aspects conflict, a workable classification is often a compromise.

The predictive qualities of a classification is important in relation to epidemiological studies at several levels:

The genus level: The genera *Phlebotomus* and *Lutzomyia* both contain species which transmit *Leishmania* capable of infecting man. Species of *Sergentomyia, Brumptomyia* and *Warilya* are not known to transmit such *Leishmania* even though a few species will bite man. Hence, species of the latter three genera may be omitted from epidemiological investigations (at least initially).

The subgenus level: At this level the predictive ability is maintained, e.g. species of the sub genus *Lutzomyia (Nyssomyia)* are found in lowland neotropical forests and are often vectors of the *Leishmania mexicana* group and *Leishmania (Viannia)* species. In the Old World, the taxonomic distribution of vectors is greater, wioth species from most of the sub-genera of *Phlebotomus* incriminated (see Lewis & Ward, 1987; Killick-Kendrick, 1985). Nevertheless some clear predictions can be made e.g. species of the subgenus *Phlebotomus* (s.s) are only known to transmit *L. major* and are most likely to transmit *L. donovani*.

The species level: The predictive requirements here are of two types: between species and within species. The taxonomic affinity of a species with a proven vector aids compilation of a shortlist of "potential" vectors in a disease focus. If a species is a proven vector in one area it is likely to be a vector in another ecologically similar area also, assuming homogeneity of the species and access to the appropriate reservoir. These two predictions rely heavily on the assumption that taxonomists have recognised what is in fact a species and secondly, that the affinity of species is correctly determined.

How are sandfly species defined?

At present sandfly species are defined morphologically, there are no 'non-morphological' species based on isoenzyme or chrosomal criteria as for example, there are in the Simulidae of Culicidae. The steady increase in the number of described species based on morphology alone since the beginning of the century shows no sign of abating (Figure 1.) and the introduction of the new techniques summarised below will no doubt hasten the increase. At present there is little understanding of the biological basis of species differences in sandflies but this is changing; detailed work is now being carried out on some species involving cross mating and behavioural studies (Ward et al., in press). The potentially misleading emphasis on morphology is well recognised. For example the effect of environmental factors on morphology has been examined both observationally (Artemiev, 1972; Rioux et al., 1975) and, to a limited extent, experimentally (Lane, in press).

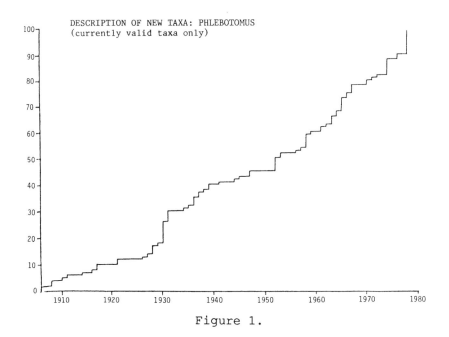

Figure 1.

The rank of some taxa (either species or genera) is a contentious matter in several instances, although there is often little disagreement over composition of the taxa (e.g. *Psychodopygus*, Lewis et al., 1977; Ready et al., 1980). The higher classification of sandflies is poorly studied as are biogeography or faunal relationships, or of sandfly phylogony. There are numerous examples in sandflies of difficulties in differentiating species in both sexes, males are often separable but females are not. This is a major problem for workers in the field investigating the epidemiology of leishmaniasis. However, this is a problem of identification, not of classification, which can often be resolved by detailed morphological studies or by the application of new, more refined, techniques.

Recently Applied Techniques in Phlebotomine Systematics

Recently, several new techniques have been applied in sandfly systematics. Initially the introduction of such techniques was slow, certainly in comparison with work on the Simulidae and Culicidae, but their use is now increasing.

Cytology: White and Killick-Kendrick (1975) reported polytene chromosomes in fourth instar larvae of *Lutzomyai longipalpis* but did not make comparisons with other species of sandflies.

Electrophoresis: This technique has been adopted in several studies to examine variation in isoenzymes both within and between species. Miles and Ward (1978) introduced the technique to sandfly systematics which has subsequently been used in studies in Tunisia, Italy, Congo, French Guiana, Bolivia and Panama. The principal enzymes varying both within and between species most clearly are PGM, PGI, MDH, HK and ME (refs in Lane, 1986). Caillard et al. (1986) have demonstrated the specific status of two sympatric species, one of which is a presumed vector of *Le. braziliensis*, originally recognised as colour morphs of *Lutzomyia (Psychodopygus) carrerai*.

Electron microscopy: This is essentially an extension of light microscopy of slide mounted specimens to examine fine detail morphology. Chaika (1975) used both SEM and TEM on the sensilla of adult sandflies but did not make interspecific comparisons. Although Lane and Ward (1985) demonstrated differences in the surface detail of two populations of *L. longipalpis* by SEM which ultimately led to the discovery of pheromones in this recently discovered 'complex', Ward et al. (in press) later showed morphology to be irrelevant in distinguishing the reproductively isolated populations.

Morphometrics: Phlebotometry, the practice of using biometric data to differentiate sandfly species during the first half of this century, considered characters ub a univariate manner. Lane and Ready (1985) introduced multivariate methods to distinguish females of *Lutzomyia complexus* and *wwllcomei* reared from iso-female broods. Traditional phenetic numerical taxonomic methods have not been applied.

Laboratory rearing and colonisation: Improved methods of rearing iso-female broods has allowed conspecific males and females to be correctly associated. This has also produced unambiguously identified specimens of species in which the females are indistinguishable for subsequent analysis by more powerful techniques such as enzyme electrophoresis or multivariate statistical analysis. These improvements have also produced some thorough studies of immature stages. Ward and Ready (1975) and Zimmerman (1977) have examined eggs under the SEM and several groups have made excellent studies of larvae e.g. Trouillet (1979); Ward (1976). When the present descriptive phase has passed, information on immature stages should be of considerable use in substantiating supra-specific taxa (sub-genera etc.). Cross mating studies of different populations have only been feasible since the introduction of efficient methods for laboratory colonisation of sandflies (Ward et al., in press).

Gas chromatography: Following the pioneering work of Carlson and associates working on *Glossina* and Culicidae, the use of gas chromatography of cuticular hydrocarbons has been used to differentiate several species or populations in which one or both sexes are morphologically indistinguishable (Ryan et al., 1987; Kamhawi, 1987).

The use of DNA hybridisation techniques are only just beginning to be applied to sandlfies.

Outstanding problems in sandfly systematics

There are several outstanding problems in phlebotomine systematics. Well revised and clearly illustrated faunal studies are required for many regions of the world to update existing works and to incorporate the considerable quantity of recent information on the variation and distribution of species. The higher classification of the Phlebotominae is an undeveloped topic requiring the application of both new techniques and a re-evaluation of data from existing techniques.
The stability of nomenclature, especially the conservation of genera will need to be addressed, perhaps as a consequence of more profound studies of higher classification, to ensure that a functional and yet scientifically acceptable classification is produced.
One of the most exciting future challenges to sandfly systematics will be the discovery and definition of species complexes of vector species and the associated biological information using the new techniques at our disposal.

References

Artemiev, M.M. 1972. Spiracular index and size in *Phlebotomus papatasi* (Diptera: Psychodidae) in villages and in the wild. Medskaya Parazit., 41 : 300-303.

Calliard, T., Tibayrenc, M., Le Pont, F., Dujardin, J.P., Desjeux, P. & Ayala, F.J. 1986. Diagnosis by isoenzyme methods of two cryptic species *Psychodopygus carrerai* and *P. yucamensis* (Diptera: Psychodidae). J. med. Ent., 23 : 489-492.

Chaika, S.Y. 1975. Electron microscpic investigation of the olfactory sensilla of the sandflies (Diptera: Phlebotomidae). In: Proceedings of the 2nd All-Union Symposium on insect chemoreception, Vilinius, pp. 69-75.

Kamhawi, S., Molyneux, D.H., Killick-Kendtick, R., Milligan, P.J.M., Phillips, A., Wilkes, T.J. & Killick-Kendrick, M. 1987. Two populations of *Phlebotomus ariasi* in the Cevennes focus of leishmaniasis in the south of France revealed by analysis of cuticular hydrocarbons. Med. Vet. Ent., 1 : 97-102.

Killick-Kendrick, R. 1985. Some epidemiological consequences of the evolutionary fit between leishmaniae and their phlebotomine vectors. Bull. Path. exot., 78 : 747-755.

Lane, R.P. 1986. Recent advances in the systematics of phlebotomine sandflies. Insect Sci.Applic., 7 : 225-230.

Lane, R.P. in press. Geographic variation in Old World phlebotomine sandlfies. In: "Biosystematics of heamatophagous arthropods". M. Service ed., Oxford University Press.

Lane, R.P. & Ready, R.D. 1985. Multivariate discrimination between *Lutzomyia wellcomei*, a vector of mucocutaneous leishmaniasis, and *Lu. complexus* (Diptera: Phlebotominae). Ann. trop. Med. Parasit., 79 : 469-472.

Lane, R.P. & Ward, R.D. 1984. The morphology and possible function of abdominal patches in males of two forms of the leishmaniasis vector *Lutzomyia longipalpis* (Diptera: Phlebotominae). Cah. O.R.S.T.O.M. ser..Ent. med. Parasit., 22 : 245-249.

Lewis, D.J. & Ward, R.D. 1987. Transmission and vectors. pp. 235-262. In: "The leishmaniases in biology and medicine". W. Peters & R. Killick-Kendrick eds. Academic Press, London.

Lewis, D.J., Young, D.G., Fairchild, G.B. & Minter, D.M. 1977. Proposals for a stable classification of phlebotomine sandlfies (Diptera: Psychodidae). Syst. Ent., 2 : 319-332.

Miles, M. & Ward, R.D. 1978. Preliminary isoenzyme studies on phlebotomine sandflies (Diptera: Psychodidae). Ann. trop. Med. Parasit., 72 : 398-399.

Ready, P.D., Fraiha, H., Lainson, R. & Shaw, J.J. 1980. *Psychodopygus* as a genus: reasons for a flexible classification of the phlebotomine sandflies (Diptera: Psychodidae). J. med. Ent., 17 : 75-88.

Rioux, J.A., Croset, H., Leger, N. & Maistre, M. 1975. Remarques sur la taxonomie infraspecifique de *Sergentomyia minuta, Sergentomyia africana* et *Sergentomyia antennata*. Ann. parasit. hum. comp., 50 : 635-641.

Ryan, L., Phillips, A., Milligan, P., Lainson, R., Molyneux, D. & Shaw, J.J. 1987. Separation of female *Psychodopygus wellcomei* and *P. complexus* (Diptera: Psychodidae) by cuticular hydrocarbons. Acta trop. 43 : 85-89.

Trouillet, J. 1979. *Sergentomyia (Rondanomyia) ingrami* Newstead, *Sergentomyia (Rondanomyia) dureni* Parrot et *Sergentomyia hamoni* Abonnenc (Diptera: Phlebotomidae). Etude morphologique des stades pre-imaginaux et notes bioecologiques. Annls Parasit., 54 : 353-373.

Ward, R.D. 1976. A revised numerical chaetotaxy for Neotropical phlebotomine sandfly larvae (Diptera: Psychodidae). Syst. Ent., 50 : 127-134.

Ward, R.D., Philips, A., Burnet, B. & Brisola, C.M. in press. The *Lutzomyia longipalpis* complex: reproduction and distribution. In: "Biosystematics of haematophagous arthropods". M. Service ed., Oxford University Press.

Ward, R.D. & Ready, P.A. 1975. Chorionic sculpturing in some sandfly eggs (Diptera: Psychodidae). J. Ent., 50 : 127-134.

White, G.B. & Killick-Kendrick, R. 1975. Polytene chromosomes of the sandfly *Lutzomyia longipalpis* and the cytogenetics of Psychodidae in relation to other Diptera. J. Ent., 50 : 187-196.

Zimmerman, J.H., Newson, H.D., Hooper, G.R. & Christensen, H.A. 1977. A comparison of the surface structure of six anthropophilic phlebotomine sandflies (*Lutzomyia*) with the scanning electron microscope (Diptera: Psychodidae). J. med. Ent. PS., 13 : 574-579.

DNA PROBES FOR VECTOR TAXONOMY

Julian Crampton, Teresa Knapp and Richard Ward

Wolfson Unit of Molecular Genetics
Department of Medical Entomology
Liverpool School of Tropical Medicine, LIVERPOOL, L3 5QA

INTRODUCTION

The use of DNA probes is now becoming established as one means for the identification of insect vectors of disease particularly where more traditional methods are not available[1,2,3]. Currently, their use involves the application of either a portion of the fly specimen or purified DNA from the specimen onto nitrocellulose. The DNA in the sample is then denatured with alkali and immobilised by baking at 80°C for 2 hours. Subsequently, a radioactive DNA probe is hybridised to the nitrocellulose and identification results from inspection of the autoradiographic signal obtained.

There are essentially two methods for the preparation of such DNA probes. The first involves the prior identification of DNA sequences whose variation may be expected to be of use for identification purposes. One example of this is the use of the non-transcribed spacer region of the ribosomal gene repeat which can vary both within populations and between species[4]. Such variation, whether in repeat number or base sequence may form the basis of a species-specific probe and the work of Ready et al (this volume) amply illustrates the power of this technique when applied to the identification of <u>Phlebotomous paptasi</u>. The advantage of this strategy is that it is very simple to clone and analyse this gene sequence so that probe development is not time consuming or particularly expensive. Another advantage is that the probe developed is based on the detection of a repeated sequence (the ribosomal genes are, for example, repeated 450 times in mosquitoes) which means that the probe is sensitive and may be used to identify the vector species using a portion of the specimen. The importance of this is that the remainder of the specimen can be used in other tests to support the DNA identification of the vector species, in conjunction with the use of DNA probes to detect and identify parasites in the infected insect (see Ready et al, this volume). The problem is that this approach has not always proved successful particularly in closely related species and between sibling species, for example in the <u>Simulium damnosum</u> complex and the <u>Anopheles gambiae</u> species complex[1,2,5]. This problem has necessitated the development of an alternative approach to the development of diagnostic DNA probes.

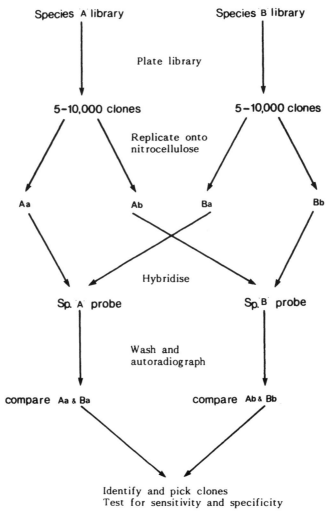

Figure 1   Scheme for the identification of random DNA sequences of diagnostic potential.

The second method for developing species-specific probes may be called a 'shot gun' approach. It is based on the notion of comparing the repetitive sequences present in the two, or more, species which need to be distinguished. Using this method any DNA sequence which exhibits species specificity, no matter whether it has a function or not, can be identified and used as the basis of a test system. This approach is illustrated in Figure 1 and in practice involves the preparation of DNA clone banks from DNA derived from each of the species of interest e.g. A and B. Each library is then screened in duplicate with radioactive probes prepared from total DNA from species A and B. Following autoradiography the screens are compared and clones identified which hybridise to the radioactive DNA from one species and not the other. The importance of this type of screening is that only repetitive sequences are detected and the intensity of the signal is indicative of the copy number of the repetitive sequence in the genome of the insect. The higher the copy number of the sequence which is used as a probe the more sensitive the final probe will be i.e. the quicker a test can be performed or the smaller the portion of the sample required for the test. Once clones have been identified which contain species-specific DNA sequences, these can then be isolated, grown in quantity and their true usefulness assessed. DNA probes which exhibit the required levels of specificity and sensitivity may then be used in a dot blot or squash blot assay to determine the species of specimens collected in the field. Eventually the probe may be further refined. This can involve sequencing the probe, identifying the repetitive sequence of interest and then constructing a synthetic oligo-nucleotide probe based on the sequence data. Such oligo probes have a number of advantages in use and these are discussed below.

The shot gun approach to probe development is clearly more time consumming but has been applied successfully not only to develop probes for vector taxonomy but also for parasite identification and diagnosis. DNA probes have now been developed in this way for the identifcation of species within the Anopheles gambiae complex of species[5], the Anopheles darus complex[3], and the Simulium damnosum backfly complex in West Africa[1,6]. These studies have indicated that the probes which have been developed using this method may have a number of advantages over probes based on the ribosomal gene sequences.

Perhaps the major advantage is that the repetitive sequences which have shown potential as species-specific probes in general seem to be present at very high copy number. For example, the Anopheles arabiensis specific sequence, pAnal, described by Gale and Crampton[2] is present in over 200,000 copies per haploid genome compared with 450 copies for the ribosomal genes[7]. This means that such probes are very sensitive, to such an extent that very small portions of a fly specimen need be used in determining the insect vector species using this probe. Indeed, the pAnal probe is so sensitive that the species of the female can be inferred from identifying the species of male sperm DNA present in the spermathecae[8]. Therefore, in this example only the terminal segment of the abdomen need be used for identification with the DNA probe, the remainder can be used for hydrocarbon analysis, dissection, blood meal determination, cytogenetic studies etc. The other implication of very high copy number probes is that autoradiographic exposure times can be kept very short so as to speed up species determination. Where biotinylated[9], rather than radioactive probes, are used only very short incubation times are needed.

The second advantage of shot-gun probes is that the species-specific, repetitive sequences appear to be short, often between 30 and 200 bases in length. Again, using the Anopheles arabiensis specific probe as an example, the repetitive sequence present in this probe is only 46 bases in length, of which 21 bases are invariant between different members of the repeat family[10]. The advantage of such short sequences as probes lies in the fact that they lend themselves to the preparation of synthetic oligo-nucleotides derived from the sequence data. Such oligo-probes are cheap to prepare, better defined, may be labelled during synthesis and can be used with very short hybridisation times (as little as 30 minutes) at relatively low temperatures.

We are interested in the studying the Lutzomyia longipalpis complex of sandfly populations in South America, in particular in developing ways

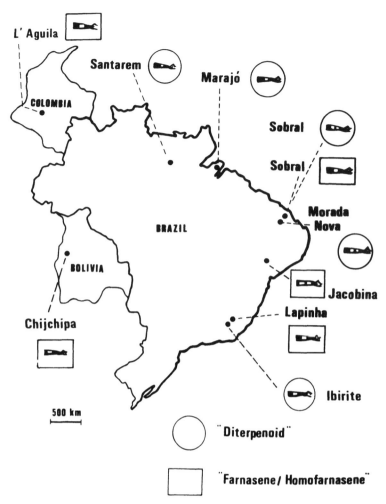

Figure 2   Summary map of the Lutzomya longipalpis populations studied in South America[11] with respect to their 'spot number' or number of light tergal patches (shown in the boxes) and their pheromone type (shown by the shape of the boxes).

of identifying the females of the different populations and in determining which are the major vectors of leishmaniasis. Populations of Lu. longipalpis from a number of different locations in Brazil, Bolivia and Colombia have already been studied and described in some detail with respect to their mating characteristics, male abdominal tergal spot patterns found in each population as well as the identity of some of the pheromones employed by the males[11]. We have begun a study aimed at the development of DNA probes which may be used to distinguish the females of each species and which, when used in conjunction with Leishmania specific DNA probes, may elucidate the vectorial significance of each population.

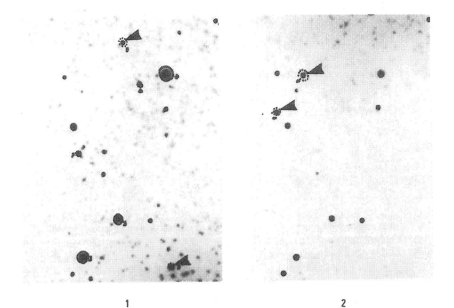

Figure 3   Duplicate, high density screening of the Morada Nova gene bank with DNA probes derived from Morada Nova sandfly total DNA (1) and Chijchipa sandfly total DNA (2). The arrow heads indicate clones of interest.

MATERIALS AND METHODS

Sandflies

Laboratory stocks of Lu. longipalpis raised from wild caught individuals were maintained as previously described[11]. Stocks derived from Chijchipa, Morada Nova, Sobral, Marajo, Lapinha Jacobina (see Fig.2) were used in this study.

DNA preparations

DNA from laboratory stocks was prepared from 20-50 pooled adults by the method of Bingham et al[12]. DNA from 1-5 individuals was prepared by the method of Ish-Horowicz[13].

Construction of Sandfly genomic libraries

Genomic DNA prepared from each of the sandfly populations was sheared by sonication to an average length of 1Kb, blunt-ended using the Klenow-fragment of DNA polymerase I and ligated to EcoRI linkers using standard methods. Cohesive sites were generated by excess EcoRI digestion and the resulting molecules ligated into the EcoRI site of the insertional lambda vector, NM1149. The recombinant DNA was packaged in vitro and plated on standard host cells. Recombinant phage were screened at high density using the method of Benton and Davis[14], washed and autoradiographed at -70°C with an intensifying screen.

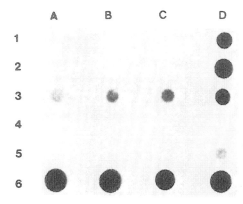

Figure 4   Dot blots of sandfly DNAs from (A) Morada Nova, (B) Sobral, (C) Lapinha and (D) Chijchipa probed with cloned DNAs (1) MN7A, (2) MN7B, (3) MN11, (4) MN12, (5) MN16 and (6) the spacer region from a Morada Nova ribosomal gene, MN17.

Radiolabelling and hybridisation of DNA probes

Double-stranded DNA was radiolabelled by the procedure of nick-translation[15]. The probes were boiled before use and hybridisations were performed overnight in 5 x SSC, 50% formamide, 1mM EDTA and 100ug/ml denatured, sonicated herring sperm DNA at 43°C in a heat sealed bag.

Dot blots

Total sandfly DNA was denatured for 10 minutes in 0.5M NaOH, 5 x SSC at room temperature. The solution was neutralised and dotted onto nitrocellulose using a dot blot manifold connected to a suction pump. The nitrocellulose was rinsed briefly in 6 x SSC and baked at 80°C for 2 hours.

RESULTS

Replicate copies of 50,000 recombinant clones derived from Morada Nova DNA were screened at high density with radioactive, total genomic DNA probes from the six sandfly populations listed in Materials and Methods. An example of the type of results obtained is shown in Figure 3. This shows a small section of an autoradiograph obtained after hybridising replicate copies of a number of clones with total DNA probes derived from Morada Nova and Chijchipa sandfly populations. The arrows in the figure indicate clones which hybridise strongly with one of the probes but not the other in each case. Clones such as these were picked, plaque purified and phage DNA prepared. The clones were further analysed by dotting the clone DNA onto nitrocellulose and hybridising each of these to the same genomic probes used above. In this way, clones showing potential as species-specific probes were identified.

Subsequently, sandfly DNA derived from each of the populations being studied were dot blotted onto nitrocellulose and hybridised with radioactive DNA prepared from the clones described above. An example of the results obtained is shown in Figure 4 and shows clearly that, for example, probe MN7B hybridises specifically to the Chijchipa sandfly DNA and does not hybridise to any of the DNAs from the other populations. Also included in this Figure is the result obtained when the same sandfly DNAs are hybridised with a probe derived from the spacer region of the ribosomal gene present in Morada Nova sandflies. This probe hybridises equally to the DNAs from all the different populations.

DISCUSSION

This study is in it's early stages but it is clear that this type of approach may prove useful in developing DNA probes for distinguishing the different populations of Lu. longipalpis in South America. Such probes, used in conjunction with Leishmania probes, should help to elucidate the nature and importance of these populations as vectors of leishmaniasis in this area. Further probes are currently under development and existing probes are being refined so that they may eventually be of use in a field situation.

REFERENCES

1. R.J. Post, DNA probes for vector identification, Parasitology Today 1:89 (1985)
2. K.R. Gale and J.M. Crampton, DNA probes for species identification of mosquitoes in the Anopheles gambiae complex, Med. and Vet. Entomol. 1:127 (1987)
3. S. Panyim, S. Yasothornsrikul and V Baimai, DNA probes for species identification in the Anopheles dirus complex, "Biosystematics of haematophagous insects" Oxford University Press, (In Press)
4. E.S. Coen, T. Strachan and G.A. Dover, The dynamics of concerted evolution in the ribosomal and histone gene families in the Drosophila melanogaster species subgroup, J. Mol. Biol. 158:17 (1982)
5. K.R. Gale and J.M. Crampton, A DNA probe to distinguish the species Anopheles quadriannulatus from other species of the Anopheles gambiae complex, Trans. R. Soc. Trop. Med. Hyg. 3: (1987) In Press
6. R.J. Post and J.M. Crampton, The taxonomic use of variation in repetitive DNA sequences in the Simulium damnosum complex, "Biosystematics of Haematophgous Insects" Oxford University Press, (In Press)
7. K.R. Gale and J.M. Crampton, The ribosomal genes in some species of mosquito, (Submitted for publication)
8. K.R. Gale and J.M. Crampton, Use of a male-specific DNA probe to distinguish female mosquiotes of the Anopheles gambiae species complex, Med. Vet. Entomol., 2: (1988) In press.
9. M. Renz and C. Kurz, A colorimetric method for DNA hybridisation, Nucleic Acids Res. 12:3435 (1984)
10. J.M. Crampton, T.F. Knapp and K.R.Gale, A male-specific repetitive sequence family in the genome of Anopheles arabiensis, (In preparation)
11. R.D. Ward, A. Phillips, B. Burnet and C.B. Marcondes, The Lutzomyia longipalpis complex: reproduction and distribution, "Biosystematics of Haematophagous Insects", Oxford University Press, (In Press)

12. P.M. Bingham, R. Lewis and G.M. Rubin, Cloning of DNA sequences from the white locus of Drosophila melanogaster by a novel and general method, Cell 25:693 (1981)
13. D. Ish-Horowicz, Personal communication in: Rate turnover of structural variants in the rDNA gene family of Drosophila melanogaster, Nature 295:564 (1982)
14. W.D. Benton and R.W. Davis, Screening lambda gt recombinant clones by hybridisation to single plaques in situ, Science 196:180 (1977)
15. P.W.J. Rigby, M. Deckmann, C. Rhodes and P. Berg, Labelling DNA to high specific activity in vitro by nick-translation with DNA polymerase I, J. Mol. Biol. 113:1237 (1977)

DNA SEQUENCE POLYMORPHISMS AS GENOTYPIC MARKERS FOR PHLEBOTOMINE
VECTORS OF LEISHMANIA

P.D. Ready and D.F. Smith*

Dept. Pure & Applied Biology & *Dept. Biochemistry
Imperial College of Science & Technology
London SW7 2AZ, UK

INTRODUCTION

Phlebetomine sandflies cannot be high on the list of candidates for pure research on genetics: they are not known to have any unique genetic mechanisms and their generation times are long. DNA technology is expensive, solutions to the public health problems posed by leishmaniasis should be pressing and, consequently, it is important not to waste resources by using new technology blindly. This paper seeks to explain some limitations of using DNA sequence polymorphisms as practical taxonomic characters.

Sandflies are morphologically conservative, their polytene chromosomes are relatively fragile and indistinctly banded (White & Killick-Kendrick, 1976) and only limited isoenzyme variation has been demonstrated (see Ready & da Silva, 1984). It is natural, therefore, to turn to DNA, with its wealth of sequence variation, in order to find polmorphisms diagnostic for species, or intra-specific populations, with medically-important traits. Measurement of biochemical variation is often thought to be "objective", because the biochemist's results can be more reproducible than the biologist's, and "intrinsic" characters are loosely equated with genomic characters. However, given the independent segregation of many genes, it is often no easy task to demonstrate even a non-causal linkage between a genotypic character and a trait that has epidemiological importance. DNA complicates matters further: much of it is not even inherited in a Mendelian fashion, and so the discovery of unique DNA sequences, spread throughout a population, does not automatically signify a biological identity.

TABLE 1. Common DNA techniques and their uses (References in Maniatis et al., 1982 and Ready et al., in press)

TECHNIQUE	PRELIMINARY PROCESS-ING OF DNA	VARIATION IDENTIFIED	TAXONOMIC USES
1. Southern hybridization	extraction, purification, digestion of DNA from single flies	absence/presence and location of restriction sites	restriction fragment length analysis for systematics, pop. genetics, identification
2. Dot blotting	extraction and purification of DNA from single flies	nucleotide sequence abundance/absence	identification; systematics - distribution/abundance of specific sequences
3. Squash blotting	DNA released from single flies by squashing	ditto	ditto
4. Construction of homologous gene probes using:			
a) differential screen of genomic libraries	extraction, purification, digestion, cloning of DNA from 20-400 flies (followed by restriction mapping, sequencing)	population specific sequences; shared sequences	diagnostic, or specific, gene probes for 1,2,3 above; systematics - comparative sequence analysis
b) heterologous gene probe to find homologous gene in genomic library	ditto	ditto, but for DNA of known function	ditto

MATERIALS AND METHODS

The variations normally measured are in the primary structure of DNA in the sequence of nucleotide bases along the molecule. The common techniques and their uses are outlined in Table 1. Watson et al. (1982) and Lewin (1987) are primers for those with a non-molecular vocabulary, and Maniatis et al. (1982) provide the basic techniques.

Pieces of cloned DNA can be sequenced and compared directly. This approach is expensive and lengthy. More often, sequence variations are measured indirectly by comparing the strength of hybridization (the degree of homology) between pairs of denatured, single-stranded DNA molecules, and by comparing the distribution of endonuclease restriction sites between regions that share some sequence homology. Populations can show diagnostic restriction fragment length polymorphisms (RFLPs), which can be demonstrated by restriction digestion, electrophoretic separation and Southern hybridization.

RESULTS AND DISCUSSION

Types of DNA studied and significance of sequence variation

The rapid techniques of diagnostic hybridization (using dot blot or squash blot procedures) demand the use of sequences that are multicopy in the genome, otherwise no appreciable hybridization signal can be obtained. Sequence diversity in mitichondrial DNA can be useful for population genetics (DeSalle et al., 1986), but this DNA has the limitation of being maternally inherited. Many multicopy nuclear sequences are transcribed (e.g. genes for ribosomal RNA and histones) but even more have no known function (the so-called "junk" DNA that does not code for proteins). Multicopy sequences are often fast evolving, with many polymorphisms occurring in the sequences that flank coding regions (e.g. Coen et al., 1982).

Non-coding, multicopy DNA falls into two broad classes. Highly repetitive sequences are often found in heterochromatin blocks, in just a few chromosomal locations, and can be isolated as satellite DNAs in caesium chloride gradients. The nucleotide sequences of the highly-repeated elements can vary slightly between species and, therefore, direct sequence comparisons could be useful in deciding taxonomic relationships, but overall homology means that these elements are unlikely to be diagnostic in dot/squash blots for (sibling) species within a complex or group (Lewin, 1987; Strachan et al., 1982). The second class of non-coding, multicopy sequence is that of middle repetitive DNA, which is usually more dispersed in the genome than the highly-repetitive DNA. Middle repetitive sequences will often be isolated when genomic libraries of two related species are differentially screened for diagnostic sequences using radiolabelled total DNA of each as probes.

It is important to be aware that multicopy sequences are the ones most likely to be inherited in a non-Mendelian fashion: a variety of mechanisms of non-reciprocal DNA transfer, within and between chromosomes, can permit mutations to spread "selfishly" and "ignorantly" through a family of genes (= homogenization) and through a population (= fixation), a process termed molecular drive; the resulting molecular coevolution can be independent of natural selection and genetic drift, it is thought (Dover, 1986) (Fig. 1).

Some useful DNA polymorphisms in sandflies

In many insects studied, hundreds of genes for ribosomal (r) RNA occur in the nucleolus organisers of the sex chromosomes as tandem repeats (e.g.

MOLECULAR DRIVE   applies mainly to   FAMILIES OF REPETITIVE SEQUENCES

Process by which mutations spread through a family of genes (homogenization) and through a population (fixation)

Consist of multigene families and 'junk' DNA

Mechanism Non-reciprocal DNA transfer by gene conversion, unequal crossing-over, transposition, slippage replication, RNA-mediated exchange

Origins Duplicative transposition ('selfish' genes), rolling circle amplification, RNA reverse transcription, telomeric growth of simple sequences ('ignorant')

Features Multilineage process, with coevolution of molecules dependent neither on Natural Selection nor on Genetic Drift

Features Non-Mendelian segregation of genes resulting from non-reciprocal DNA transfer both within and between chromosomes

(Review by Dover, 1986)

Fig. 1. Molecular Drive and its effect on repetitive DNA sequences

Coen et al., 1982). Each gene repeat is separated by an intergenic "non-transcribed spacer" (NTS) containing multiple promoters/enhancers and species-specific sequences; and, in several groups of species, there exists a molecular incompatibility between the rDNA of one species and the transcription factors of another (see Dover, 1986). The NTS region of rDNA, then, is a candidate for population-specific probes.

We have cloned a rDNA gene repeat of *Phlebotomus* (*Phlebotomus*) *papatasi*, the sandfly vector of *Leishmania major* over a wide geographical range. A fragment of the NTS region is diagnostic for *P. papatasi*, there being no homologous sequences detectable in the closely-related *P.* (*P.*) *duboscqi* or in 8 other species of sandflies (of 4 subgenera) which predominate in Tunisian foci of zoonotic cutaneous leishmaniasis due to *L. major* (Ready et al., in press).

As in *Drosophila* species (Coen & Dover, 1983), the NTS region of *P. papatasi* shows much variation in (restriction fragment) length and copy number, both within and between individuals of the same population (Fig. 2). However, there are RFLPs diagnostic for populations (Fig. 3). These are potentially useful for identifying hybridization between adjacent populations. In this way, following the end of a sandfly control programme, RFLP analysis of rDNA could be used to show whether the reappearance of *P. papatasi* had resulted from recovery of the local population or from immigration from adjacent areas.

Phylogenies

It is widely believed that DNA sequences not under much selection pressure (including silent sites in three-base codons) will passively accumulate mutations in a clock-like manner (Lewin, 1987). The theory of molecular drive predicts that each gene family is different in its rates of change (Dover, 1986). If this is so, easy solutions to phylogenetic controversies are unlikely to be found by analysing sequence polymorphisms in and around one or a few genes.

CONCLUSIONS

There must be a temptation to believe that the analysis of DNA polymorphisms should provide instant solutions to taxonomic problems. By differentially screening genomic libraries it will often be possible to find (middle) repetitive DNA sequences that are unique to each of the populations being compared. However, there is a good chance that the cloned sequences will be diagnostic only quantitatively, or only for some populations of a species, or for one sex alone (Post, 1985; Gale & Crampton, 1987). The non-coding nature of much DNA and the ubiquity of non-reciprocal DNA transfer together signify that we cannot assume that repetitive DNA sequences are allelic and occur in frequencies that approach Hardy-Weinberg equilibria. Deviations from Mendelian ratios will not in themselves suggest barriers to gene flow or taxonomic identity.

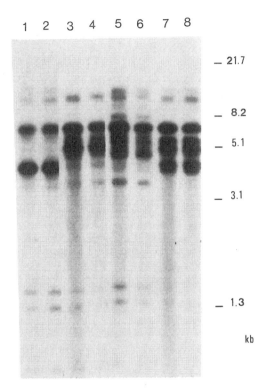

Fig. 2. RFLPs of rDNA of individual females of P. papatasi, after digestion with Xho I, electrophoretic separation on a 0.6% agarose gel, blotting and hybridization with a cloned homologous rDNA probe (PpλC) at 42°C in 50% formamide (see Ready et al., in press), washing in 0.2xSSC/65°C and autoradiographic exposure overnight (Tracks: 3-8, pairs of sisters bred from 3 mothers caught in Tunisia; 1&2, two females from laboratory colony started with flies caught in Saudi Arabia). DNA was radiolabelled with ^{32}P by nick-translation.

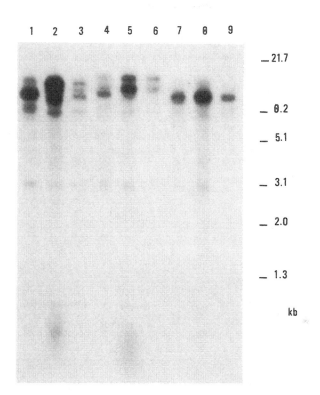

Fig. 3. RFPLs of rDNA of laboratory-bred P. papatasi. Techniques as in Fig. 2, except that digests were with Pst I/Eco RI and the probe was pDm238, a rDNA gene repeat of D. melanogaster. (Tracks: 1-3, Saudi colony; 4-6, Indian colony; 7-9, Iraq colony. 1 female in tracks 3,6,9; 3 females in tracks 2,5,8; 3 males in tracks 1,4,7)

REFERENCES

Coen, E. S. and Dover, G. A., 1983, Unequal exchanges and the coevolution of X and Y rDNA arrays in Drosophila melanogaster, Cell, 33: 849.

Coen, E. S., Strachan, T. and Dover, G. A., 1982, The dynamics of concerted evolution in the ribosomal and histone gene families in the Drosophila melanogaster species subgroup, J. Mol. Biol., 158: 17.

DeSalle, R., Giddings, L. and Templeton, A. R., 1986, Mitochondrial DNA variability in natural populations of Hawaiian Drosophila. 1., Heredity, 56: 75.

Dover, G. A., 1986, Molecular drive in multigene families: how biological novelties arise, spread and are assimilated, Trends in Genetics, 2: 159.

Gale, K. R. and Crampton, J. M., 1987, DNA probes for species identifica of mosquitoes in the Anopheles gambiae complex, Med. Vet. Entomol., 1: 127.

Lewin, B., 1987,"Genes III," John Wiley & Sons, New York.

Maniatis, T., Fritsch, E. F. and Sambrook, J., 1982, "Molecular cloning. A laboratory manual," Cold Spring Harbor Laboratory.

Post, R. J., 1985, DNA probes for vector identification, Parasitology Today, 1: 89.

Ready, P. D. and da Silva, R. M. R., 1984, An alloenzymic comparison of Psychodopygus wellcomei - an incriminated vector of Leishmania braziliensis in Para State, Brazil - and the sympatric morphospecies Ps. complexus (Diptera, Psychodidae), Cahiers ORSTOM, ser. Ent. med. Parasit., 22: 1.

Ready, P. D., Smith, D. F. and Killick-Kendrick, R., in press, DNA hybridizations on squash-blotted sandflies to identify both insect vector and infecting Leishmania, Med. Vet. Entomol., 1:

Strachan, T., Coen, E. S., Webb, D. and Dover, G. A., 1982, Modes and rates of change of complex DNA families of Drosophila, J. Mol. Biol., 158: 37.

Watson, J. D., Tooze, J. and Kurtz, D. T., 1983, "Recombinant DNA. A short course," W. H. Freeman and Company, New York.

White, G. B. and Killick-Kendrick, R., 1976, Polytene chromosomes of the sandfly Lutzomyia longipalpis and the cytogenetics of Psychodidae in relation to other Diptera, J. Entomol. A, 50: 187.

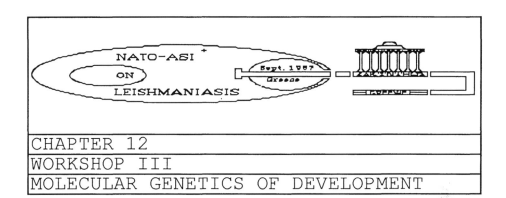

CHAPTER 12
WORKSHOP III
MOLECULAR GENETICS OF DEVELOPMENT

WORKSHOP III: MOLECULAR GENETICS OF LEISHMANIA DEVELOPMENT

Deborah Smith and Paul D. Ready

Departments of Biochemistry, Pure and Applied Biology
Imperial College of Science and Technology
London SW7 2AZ

In order to understand how Leishmania genes and their products may vary during the parasite life cycle, the techniques of molecular genetics are being widely applied in an attempt to answer questions relating to the structure, expression and regulation of parasite genes. That this is by no means a simple task has been shown in work on Trypanosoma brucei, which not only exhibits a sophisticated genetic mechanism with which to vary its surface antigenic coat, but also displays the unusual (in eukaryotes) property of discontinuous transcription.

In the Leishmania species, the fundamental mechanisms controlling gene expression and replication are at present poorly understood. This "state of the art" was reflected at this workshop by the relative paucity of speakers on some topics e.g. discontinuous transcription, regulatory sequences, in vitro transcription systems. Within these limitations, a lively and informed discussion took place.

The first presentation (Stuart, Seattle) concerned post-transcriptional modification in Leishmania (manuscript included). The addition of uridines to the mRNAs encoding cytochrome b may be important in controlling the expression of this gene and, by analogy to T. brucei, could be developmentally regulated. Uridine addition to the cytochrome oxidase mRNA was also reported (Opperdoes, Brussels). Stuart has no evidence as yet that this mechanism also modifies nuclear gene transcripts.

Modification at the 3' end of transcripts, by polyadenylation, was also discussed. Stuart reported some evidence for developmentally-regulated polyadenylation in T. brucei: relatively few mitochondrial transcripts from bloodstream forms are polyadenylated whereas many procyclic mitochondrial transcripts are. Smith (London) described mRNAs in Leishmania major which appear to be present as both polyadenylated and non-polyadenylated molecules.

It is known that most if not all Leishmania mRNAs so far characterised have an independently coded 'mini-exon' at their 5' ends. This short 35 bp sequence could prove a useful target for hybridisation with an anti-sense RNA, which would presumably inhibit the discontinuous transcriptional process, as shown in T. brucei. It was reported, from the UCLA parasitology conference (1987), that an oligonucleotide complementary to the mini-exon sequence in Leishmania does alter transcription and that this has a chemotherapeutic effect.

The next presentation described the identification and molecular cloning of a developmentally-regulated antigen from L. donovani (Kelly, London). Sera from patients with visceral leishmaniasis were used to screen lambda gt11 expression libraries (as described by Kelly, Blaxter and Miles, this volume). One of the cDNA clones thus selected encoded a promastigote-specific, peripheral membrane antigen of 67/68 Kd. This protein is translated from a 3.6 Kb polyadenylated transcript, which is encoded by a tandemly-repeated gene in L. donovani. Hybridisation studies demonstrate the existence of a similar gene in Crithidia fasciculata, T. cruzi and T. brucei, each being found at a single chromosomal location, as shown by pulsed-field gradient electrophoresis.

Discussion then turned to the search for a method for the genetic transformation of Leishmania. In order to test and understand the function of parasite DNA sequences in vivo, it will be essential to be able to reintroduce in vitro manipulated molecules back into the Leishmania cell. Many workers have attempted such experiments, using a variety of techniques to introduce DNA into the cells and a range of selectable markers. However, success has so far been fairly limited.

Stuart (Seattle) and Hamers (Brussels) caused some excitement in this workshop with their independent observations on the identification and occurrence of small nucleic acids in Leishmania (manuscript included). These molecules, which have been found in isolates of the L. donovani/L. infantum complex and in L. braziliensis braziliensis, can exist as circles as well as being integrated into linear chromosomal DNA and may, therefore, be derived from either plasmids or viruses. Evidence in support of the presence of a virus in Leishmania cells comes from the detailed study of a single-stranded RNA by Stuart et al. (this volume). This molecule shows all the characteristics expected of the nucleic acid component of a single-stranded RNA virus and has an open reading frame for protein synthesis which shares homology with the L-protein of vesicular stomatitis virus (VSV).

Stuart quoted some results from the laboratory of R. Tesh (Department of Epidemiology, Yale), which described the identification of VSV in many different human serum samples, 40% of which were taken from patients suffering from leishmaniasis. Could the sandfly be a vector for VSV or a VSV-like virus? Keithly (Cornell) reported some experiments involving the experimental infection of sandflies with isolates of L. b. guyanensis containing the small nucleic acids described above. After cloning individual parasites from these infected flies, it was found that one clone had lost the putative genetic element following passage through the insect vector, but others had not. It was suggested that Warburg and Schlein (Hadassah Madical School, Jerusalem) might have observed viral particles in Phlebotomus papatasi infected with L. major. Molyneux (Salford) reminded the audience of the reported finding of similar particles in L. hertigi.

In conclusion, there now appears to be good evidence in favour of the existence of one or more naturally-occuring, transmissable agents in Leishmania. The prospects for the rapid development of a useful molecular cloning vector appear much more promising as a result of this work. It should be remembered, however, that until we know more about gene expression and replication in Leishmania, even the most sophisticated methods of molecular biology will not aid us in our understanding of the factors controlling the differentiation of this parasite, in both its insect vector and the host macrophage.

TRANSCRIPT ALTERATION IN LEISHMANIA

K. Stuart, and J.E. Feagin

Seattle Biomedical Research Institute
4 Nickerson St.
Seattle, WA 98109-1651 USA

INTRODUCTION

Recent studies of mitochondrial transcripts, initially in African trypanosomes, have revealed that nucleotides (uridines) not encoded in the genes are added to their transcripts. This transcript alteration is developmentally regulated for some genes, such as the apocytochrome b and cytochrome oxidase II genes, but not others such as MURF2 (Feagin et al., 1987 and 1988; Feagin and Stuart, 1988). In addition, this uridine addition does not occur for all genes. These studies indicate the existence of a genetic regulatory process in Kinetoplastidae unlike any previously described. It has been suggested that the transcript alteration creates initiation codons, corrects frameshifts, and alters the 3' untranslated regions of transcripts (Benne et al., 1986; Feagin et al., 1987; Feagin and Stuart, 1988). These processes could thus affect the transcript translatability, the nature of the protein product or the stability of the transcripts. In African trypanosomes, where developmental regulation of the production of the mitochondrial respiratory system is apparent (Vickerman, 1985), the transcript alteration process probably plays a role in this regulation. However, little is known about possible developmental regulation of the production of the mitochondrial respiratory system in Leishmania, including those that infect humans (see Blum et al., 1987). We extended our studies to Crithidia fasciculata and Leishmania tarentolae to further examine the hypothesis that the initiation codons are created in the cytochrome b transcripts by uridine addition and found that this occurred in each case (Feagin et al., 1988). We have now examined the cytochrome b transcripts of L. mexicana amazonenesis, L. tropica, and L. major and find that uridines are added within the 5' coding sequence of cytochrome b transcripts of these species, creating initiation codons.

MATERIALS AND METHODS

L. tarentolae (U.C. strain) was grown in Brain Heart Infusion with 10 ug/ml hemin. L. mexicana amazonensis MHOM/BR/78/Josefa C11, L. major MHOM/IL/67/Jericho II, and L. tropica MHOM/SU/60/LRC-L39 were grown in medium 199 supplemented with 20% fetal calf serum. Cells were harvested by centrifugation and stored at -80°C until used. Total RNA was prepared, hybridized to synthetic oligonucleotide primers, and sequenced, using M-MLV reverse transcriptase (Bethesda Research Laboratories), by the dideoxy chain termination method in the presence of [^{32}P]dATP, as described in Feagin et al., 1987.

RESULTS

The cytochrome b transcript sequences of L.tarentolae, L.mexicana amazonensis, L. major, and L. tropica were determined using an

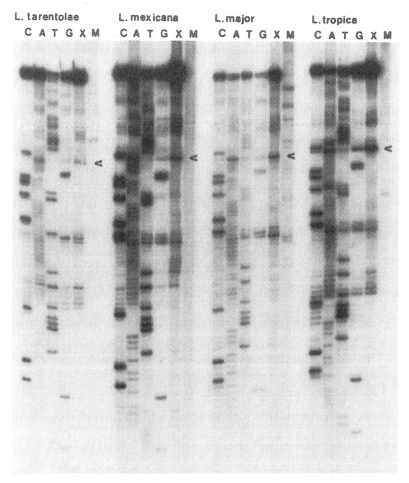

Figure 1. Sequence of cytochrome b transcripts from four Leishmania species. The sequencing was performed using 30 micrograms of total RNA and 50 nanograms of LtCYb-CS primer (see Feagin et al. 1987 for details). Didexoynucleotides were omitted in lanes X and primer was omitted in lanes M. The location of the extension product corresponding to transcripts without additional uridines is indicated with an arrowhead for each sequence set.

oligonucleotide primer, LtCYb-CS (Feagin et al., 1988), which is complementary to the L. tarentolae cytochrome b transcript near its 5' end (Fig. 1). The L. tarentolae RNA contains 39 uridines, represented by many of the bands in the A lane, that are not present in the gene. The cytochrome b transcripts from the other species have a sequence that is very similar to that of L. tarentolae. The genomic sequence has not been determined for the cytochrome b genes of these species. However, since the genomic sequences are highly conserved among T. brucei, C. fasciculata and

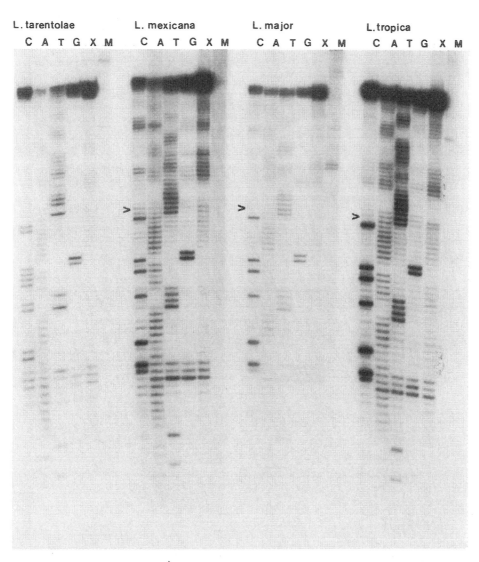

Figure 2. Sequence of (U)$^+$ cytochrome b transcripts from four Leishmania species. Sequencing was performed as described in the legend to figure 1 except the LtCYb-R primer was used. The arrowheads indicate the location of the AUG created by uridine addition in L. tarentolae and the corresponding position in the other species.

Leishmania tarentolae

```
ATAAATTTAATTTAAATTTTAAATAATTATAAA A G        CG G AGA     G A      A A  AGAAA    A G  G C TTTAAC  DNA
NNNNAUUUAAUUUAAAUUUAAAUUAUAAUuGuuuuuuCGuGuuAGAuuuuuGuuAuuuuuuuuAuuAuuuAGAAuuuAuGuuGuCuUUUAAC       RNA
```

Leishmania mexicana amazonensis

```
                                                    *                             *
       ......NNNNNAAAAAAWGUUUUUUCSUGUUARAAUUUUGUUGNUUUUUUAUUAUUUAGAAUUUAUGUUGUCUUUUAAC  RNA
```

Leishmania major

```
                                                 *                             *
       ......NNNNNNNAAAAAWGUUUUUUCSUGUUARAAUUUUGUUGNUUUUUUAUUAUUUAGAAUUUAUGUUGUCUUUUAAC  RNA
```

Leishmania tropica

```
                                                 *                             *
       ......NNNNNNAAAAAWGUUUUUUCSUGUUWRAAUUUUGUUGNUUUUUUAUUAUUUNGAAUUUAUGUUGUCUUUUAAC  RNA
```

N = A,C,G,U
W = A or U
S = C or G
R = G or A

Figure 3. Comparison of cytochrome b sequences from four species of Leishmania. The RNA and 7uDNA sequences of L. tarentolae are aligned with gaps left in the DNA sequence where uridines are added. The added uridines are shown in lower case in the RNA sequence and the created AUG is underlined. The RNA sequences of the other four species are aligned below that of L. tarentolae. Most of the uridines are probably added but are not shown as lower case since the DNA sequences are not known. The two nucleotide positions that differ from L. tarentolae are marked with asterisks.

L. tarentolae, these transcripts also almost certainly contain uridines that are not present in the gene.

The RNA from all species contains a minor component (arrow) that is about 40 nts shorter than the 5' end of the major transcript. This product corresponds to the transcript without additional uridines since it is not seen using a primer (LtCYb-R; see Feagin et al., 1988) that hybridizes only to the RNA with additional uridines (Fig. 2). Thus, all the Leishmania contain two classes of cytochrome b transcripts; those with and without additional uridines. This suggests that uridines are added to all but a small fraction of cytochrome b transcripts in these species.

Sequencing with the LtCYb-R primer reveals great similarity among the cytochrome b transcripts of the Leishmania species (Fig. 2). This similarity deteriorates within the 5' 40 nucleotides. There is considerable sequence ambiguity which probably reflects sequence diversity resulting from the uridine addition process and/or reverse transcriptase pausing during the sequencing. The ambiguity is particularly pronounced in the 5' end of the sequence but it is evident that there is considerable sequence divergence among the species in this region. In addition, the mini exon or spliced leader sequence (Parsons, et al., 1984) is not found at the 5' terminus of the mRNA.

The sequences for all four species that were compiled from data obtained using both primers are shown in Fig. 3. The uridine additions to the L. tarentolae cytochrome b transcript create an AUG codon near the 5' end (arrow, Fig. 2). This is probably the functional initiation codon since the gene lacks such a codon and AUG codons are created at about the same position in C. fasciculata and T. brucei (Feagin et al., 1988). The uridine additions appear to create AUGs in the three human infective Leishmania but the sequences are ambiguous in this area, probably reflecting transcript diversity or reverse transcriptase pausing.

DISCUSSION

The evolutionary conservation among the Kinetoplastidae of uridine addition that creates an in frame AUG strongly suggests that human Leishmania also employ this process to create functional transcripts. The uridine additions to cytochrome b transcripts of L. tarentolae, T. brucei, and C. fasciculata create AUG codons in the same region of the transcripts of genes lacking such codons and the sequence is conserved among species 3' but not 5' to this AUG (Feagin et al., 1988). The ambiguities in the created AUG region in human Leishmania transcript sequences probably reflect greater transcript diversity than in the other species since the great sequence similarity would appear to preclude differential reverse transcriptase pausing among species. The significance of such diversity is not clear. Uridine addition may occur co- or posttranscriptionally but the existence of transcripts lacking added uridines implies that it is posttranscriptional.

The cytochrome b transcript sequences from the four Leishmania species examined here are quite similar. All of the ambiguous positions in the human Leishmania sequences have as one possible interpretation a sequence which is the same as that of L. tarentolae. All the human Leishmania have the same sequence 3' of the possible AUG and differ at only two nucleotides from the L. tarentolae sequence; one is an A/G transition and the other an A/U transversion, where the U is an added nucleotide. At both of these sites, the sequence is unambiguous. This suggests, as expected, that the human Leishmania are more similar to each other than to L. tarentolae and also demonstrates that positions where uridines are added in one species may have nucleotides encoded in other species, as has been previously shown for L. tarentolae, T. brucei, and C. fasciculata cytochrome b transcripts (Feagin et al., 1988).

Uridine addition into cytochrome b transcripts is developmentally regulated in T. brucei where the mitochondrial respiratory system is produced only in some stages of the life cycle (Feagin et al., 1987). The respiratory changes during the life cycle of Leishmania have not been completely elucidated (see Blum et al., 1987) but the similarity in uridine additions between Leishmania and T. brucei suggest that the possibility of developmental regulation of uridine addition should be examined in Leishmania. If such developmental regulation exists, it implies there may also be stage-regulated production of the respiratory system in Leishmania.

Mitochondrial transcript alteration by uridine addition has now been found in African trypanosomes, Crithidia, and Leishmania (Benne et al., 1986; Feagin et al., 1987 and 1988; Feagin and Stuart, 1988) indicating that this process is widespread among the Kinetoplastidae. It is not yet known if it occurs in all parasitic protozoa (with mitochondria), in free living protozoa or in any metazoans. However, a possibly analogous process has been described for the apolipoprotein-B48 transcript in the intestine of mammals (Powell et al., 1987). There are two general although not mutually exclusive alternatives. The presence of this process may reflect an evolutionary lineage characterized by the presence of this genetic regulatory process. Alternatively, it may reflect a physiological process associated with control of the respiratory system that is common to many parasitic protozoa and possibly other organisms.

CONCLUSION

Human Leishmania and other parasitic kinetoplastids create potential initiation codons in the cytochrome b transcripts by addition of uridines that are not encoded in the gene. This process is developmentally regulated in T. brucei and the possibility of similar developmental regulation needs to be examined in Leishmania. The uridine addition activity appears vital to the parasite and, if it does not occur in human mitochondria, may be a target for intervention.

ACKNOWLEDGEMENTS

We thank Dr. S. Reed for the human Leishmania. This work was supported by NIH grant AI14102. KS is a recipient of a Special Fellowship from the Burroughs Wellcome Fund.

REFERENCES

Benne, R., Van den Burg, J., Brakenhoff, J.B.J., Sloof, P., Van Boom, J.H., Tromp, M.C., 1986, Major transcript of the frameshifted coxII gene from trypanosome mitochondria contains four nucleotides that are not encoded in the DNA, Cell, 46: 819.

Blum, J.J., Davis, D.G., Darling, T.N., and London R.E., 1987, Interrrelationships between glucose and alanine catabolism, ammonia production, and the D-lactate pathway in Leishmania braziliensis, in Leishmaniasis: The first centenary (1885-1985) new strategies for control, Plenum Press, London.

Feagin, J.E., Jasmer, D.P., and Stuart,K., 1987, Developmentally regulated addition of nucleotides within apocytochrome b transcripts in Trypanosoma brucei, Cell, 49: 337.

Feagin, J.E., Shaw, J.M., Simpson, L. and Stuart, K. 1988, Creation of AUG initiation codons by addition of uridines within cytochrome b transcripts of kinetoplastids, Proc. Natl. Acad. Sci. USA (in press).

Feagin, J.E. and Stuart, K., 1988, Developmental aspects of uridine addition within mitochondrial transcripts of Trypanosoma brucei, Mol. Cell. Biol. (submitted).

Parsons, M., Nelson, R.G., Watkins, K.P., and Agabian, N., 1984, Trypanosome mRNAs share a common 5' spliced leader sequence, Cell 38: 309.

Powell, L.M., Wallis, S.C., Pease, R.J., Edwards, Y.,H., Knott, T.J., and Scott, J., 1987, A novel form of tissue-specifiec RNA processing produces apolipoprotein-B48 in intestine, Cell, 50: 831.

Vickerman, K., 1985, Developmental cycles and biology of pathogenic trypanosomes, Brit. Med. Bull., 41:105.

CIRCULAR AND LINEAR FORMS OF SMALL NUCLEIC ACIDS IN

LEISHMANIA

R. Hamers, N. Gajendran, +J.C. Dujardin, and

*K. Stuart

Vrije Universiteit Brussel, Instituut voor
Moleculaire Biologie Paardenstraat 65
1640 Sint-Genesius-Rode BELGIUM
* Seattle Biomedical Research Institute
4 Nickerson Street Seattle, WA 98109-1651 USA
+ Institute of Tropical Medecine
Nationalestraat 155, 2000 Antwerpen, Belgium

INTRODUCTION

We wish to elucidate the process that control the expression of parasite genes since these processes may differ from those of the host and thus be targets for intervention. Several laboratories have attempted DNA transformation of parasitic protozoa with limited success. Recombinant plasmid DNA has been transformed into Leishmania tarentolae whereupon it became altered (Hughes and Simpson, 1986) and minichromosome DNA, which is not convenient for manipulation, was transformed into Trypanosoma brucei (Gibson et al, 1987). These difficulties as well as the early stage of understanding of genetic exchange that may naturally occur in parasites (Jenni et al., 1987) makes the alternative approach of searching for naturally occuring transmissible agents such as viruses or plasmids more attractive especially since virus like particles have been observed in a number of parasitic protozoa (Molyneux, 1974, Diamond and Mattern, 1976). Such agents are not only potentially useful tools for molecular studies but also may be relevant to the biological and clinical aspects of Leishmanias. In this paper we report the discovery of a potentially transmissible DNA that occurs in several Leishmania isolates either in a circular form or integrated into chromosomal DNA.

MATERIALS AND METHODS

The parasites used in this study are described in Gajendran et al. (1987 this volume) and Scholler et al. (1986). They were grown as promastigotes at 26 C in GLSH medium (Le Ray, 1975) or in Schneider's medium supplemented with 10% fetal calf serum. The parasites were harvested at late log phase, prepared for and examined by pulsed field gel electrophoresis as described in Scholler et al. (1986). The CD1 from L. donovani ITMAP 263 is described in Gajendran et al. (1987). It was radiolabelled by nick translation and used as a probe on blots of the pulse field gels.

RESULTS

As reported in more detail elsewhere (Gajendran et al. 1987 and Stuart et al. 1987) two classes of stock specific nucleic acids have been detected by pulse field gel electrophoresis. One class appears to be circular DNA based on its mobility which results in it being offset from the track followed by the linear chromosomal DNAs. We call this CD1 (circular DNA 1) and find it in 6 isolates of the L.donovani/L.infantum-complex (K 42; 1-S; LRC-L51; VP74, LRC-61; Tunis; ITMAP 263). The other class of DNA is linear and is detected by hybridization with the labelled DNA of CD1 from ITMAP 263. Hybridization to linear DNAs is found in the other seven isolates of L. donovani (MOM/IN/80/DD8; L13; LRC-L133/ITMAP 1899; CRC L64; Khartoum LV711; L28; MHOM/BR/74/PP75) that were examined. None of 14 isolates of five other Leishmania species contained CD1. However, one isolated of L.b. braziliensis (MHOM/BR/75/M 2903) contained a linear DNA that hybridized to the CD1 probe while the other twelve did not. The size of the linear chromosome that hybridized to CD1 was quite variable among stocks. In addition, the chromosome to which CD1 hybridized was present in comparable amounts compared to the other chromosomal DNAs except in L.b. braziliensis MHOM/BR/75/M 2903. In the latter case the linear DNA to which the CD1 probe hybridizes (fig.1B) is multicopy as previously noted (Scholler et al., 1986) and has been referred to as LD1 (Leishmania DNA 1 - Stuart et al. 1987).

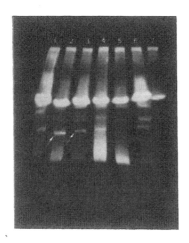

Fig.1A. An OFAGE gel with:
Lane1 : L.b.b. 704
Lane2 : L.b.b. M2903
Lane3 : L.b.b. 17/L.chagasi
Lane4 : L.b.guanensis M4147
Lane5 : L.b.pan. M4037
Lane6 : L.sp. ITMAP 2063
Lane7 : S.cerevisiae

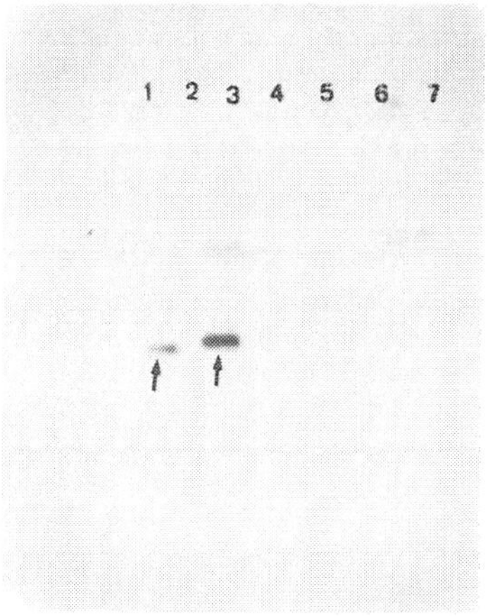

Fig.1B. Southern hybridization with the labelled CD1 Arrows point to linear DNA in M2903 and in the mixed population with L.d.chagasi/L.b.b.

DISCUSSION

The hybridization of CD1 probes with circular and linear DNAs from some but not all stocks and species of Leishmania indicates that the elements designated CD1 and LD1 are related. Since these related sequences are not widespread but were only found in the L. donovani/L.infantum-complex and a strain of L.b.braziliensis suggest that they are acquired rather than endogenous sequences. The existence of these sequences in either circular or linear DNA but not both is highly reminiscent of plasmid and viral DNAs that have the ability to independently replicate or to integrate into chromosomes.

The presence of the integrated sequences in chromosomes of different sizes suggests that the integrated form does not occur at a unique site or chromosome. However, we cannot at this time exclude the possibility that the DNA is integrated at a unique site with a variety of subsequent events leading to differences in the sizes of the resulting chromosomes. It is intriguing that LD1 is the smallest linear DNA containing CD1 sequences and is also multicopy. This may indicate that replication of this chromosome is under the control of the CD1 rather than the chromosomal sequences. This notion is plausible since CD1 also appears multicopy based on its staining intensity with ethidium bromide compared to its size which is greater than 20 kb but probably less than 50 kb as deduced from restriction enzyme digests.

CONCLUSIONS

Some stocks of the L.donovani/L.infantum-complex contain a circular DNA which is integrated into linear chromosomal DNA in the other L. donovani stocks examined and in one strain of L.b.braziliensis but not in 14 other Leishmania isolates. These DNA sequences are integrated into a 250 kb linear DNA a L.b. braziliensis perhaps leading to the multicopy nature of this DNA. These data strongly suggest that the DNA is an acquired genetic element such as a plasmid or virus that can exist in either a circular DNA or be integrated into chromosomal DNA.

ACKNOWLEDGEMENTS

KS wishes to thank R.A.Sutherland for excellent technical assistance, NIH AI24771 and the Rockefeller Foundation for support, and a Special Fellowship from the Burroughs Wellcome Trust. The Belgian group acknowledges financial support from EEC programme TSD M 002-B and FGWO contracts 3.0082.85 and 3.0027.85.

REFERENCES

Diamond, L., and Mattern, C., 1976.: Protozan Viruses. Advances in virus research, 20 (87).

Gajendran, N., Dujardin, J.C., Le Ray, D., Matthyssens, G., and Hamers, R., 1987, Abnormally migrating chromosomes identify Leishmania donovani strains, in : "LEISHMANIASIS : THE FIRST CENTENARY (1885-1985) NEW STRATEGIES FOR CONTROL", Plenum Press, New York.

Gibson, W.C., White, T.C., Laird, P.W., and Borst, P., 1987 Stable introduction of exogenous DNA in <u>Trypanosoma brucei</u>, EMBO J. 6:2457.

Hughes, D.E. and Simpson, L., 1986, Introduction of plasmid DNA into the trypanosomatid protozoan <u>Crithidia fasciculata</u>, Proc.Natl.Acad.Sci.USA, 83:6058.

Jenni, L., Marti, S., Schweizer, J., Bretschart, B., Le Page, R.W.F., Wells, J.M., Tait, A., Paindavoine, P., Pays, E., Steinert, M., 1986, Hybrid formation between African Trypanosomes during cyclic transmission. Nature 322 : 173.

Le Ray, D., 1975, Structures antigeniques de <u>Trypanosoma brucei</u> (Protozoa, Kinetoplastida). Analyse immunoelectrophoretique et etude comparative, Ann. Soc. Belge Med. Trop., 55, 158-160.

Molyneux, D.H., 1974, Virus-like particles in Leishmania parasites, Nature, 249:588.

Scholler, J.K., Reed, S.G., and Stuart, K., 1986, Molecular karyotype of species and subspecies of Leishmania, Molec. Biochem. Parasitol., 20:279.

Stuart, K., Tarr, P., Aline, R., Smiley, B., and Scholler, J.K., 1987, Small nucleic acids in Leishmania, in : "LEISHMANIAS : THE FIRST CENTENARY (1885-1985) NEW STRATEGIES FOR CONTROL", "Plenum Press, New York.

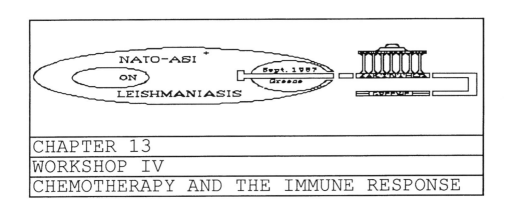

CHAPTER 13
WORKSHOP IV
CHEMOTHERAPY AND THE IMMUNE RESPONSE

WORKSHOP IV : CHEMOTHERAPY AND THE IMMUNE RESPONSE

J.Alexander[1] and S.L.Croft[2]

[1] Immunology Division, University of Strathclyde
Glasgow G4 ONR, Scotland
[2] London School of Hygiene and Tropical Medicine, Keppel Street, London WC1E 7HT, England

The success of any chemotherapeutic regime is often dependent on the potential or latent immunological response of the patient. Thus successful treatment of visceral leishmaniasis is associated with the acquisition of a positve skin-test response and a drop in antibody levels (1). If the patient cannot develop a protective immune response, as in the case with AIDS victims, drug therapy may be completely ineffective (2). Successful therapy in man, however, results in the generation of antigen specific T cells (3) while liver macrophages (Kupffer cells) are activated in BALB/c mice following sodium stibogluconate treatment (4). This close association between chemotherapy and cell mediated immunity has indicated that a dual approach to therapy could be advantageous. Adinolfi et al.(5) have shown the synergistic activity of meglumine antimoniate and the immunopotentiator muramyl dipeptide encapsulated in liposomes in experimental visceral leishmaniasis. Another derivative of the mycobacterial cell wall, trehalose-6, 6'-dimycolate, was used together with BCG to restore delayed-type hypersensitivity in a DCL case prior to chemotherapy (6). Other immunomodulators including levamisole, Corynebacterium parvum, lipoidal amine CP-46,665-1, and cyclosporin A have also been tried either alone or in combination with chemotherapeutic agents in studies on leishmaniasis with varying success. However, the list of enhancing agents with defined activity on the immunological pathways is long (7) and many are suitable candidates for dual therapy in the treatment of leishmaniasis.

Chemotherapy has been greatly enhanced in recent years by encapsulating drugs in liposomes (8). The implication being that liposomes are rapidly sequestered by macrophages and thus the drugs are targetted directly to the parasites in the phagolysosomes. However, liposomes have also been shown to have adjuvant activity and this has stimulated their use as carriers for candidate vaccines (9). These carrier systems are therefore currently providing an area of overlapping interest for those workers studying either immunological or chemical prophylaxis and therapy. As leishmanias parasitise macrophages and therefore cells which play a pivotal role in the immune response, it is more than likely that these two aspects of therapy are interdependent. Professor Peters rightly emphasised that this is an area requiring, but yet to achieve, thorough interdisciplinary investigation.

REFERENCES

1. P.E.C.Manson-Bahr, East African kala-azar with special reference to the pathology, prophylaxis and treatment, Trans.R.Soc.Trop.Med.Hyg., 53:123 (1959).
2. J.Alvar, Leishmaniasis-AIDS association: new epidemiological perspectives (this volume).
3. D.L.Sacks,S.L.Lal, S.N.Shrivastava, J.Blackwell and F.Neva, An analysis of T cell responsiveness in Indian Kala-azar, J.Immunol., 138:908 (1987)
4. K.C.Carter, A.J.Baillie, J.Alexander and T.F.Dolan, Clearance of L.donovani from the liver of BALB/c mice results in local resistance to re-infection, (this volume).
5. L.E.Adinolfi, P.F.Bonventre, M.Vander Pas and D.A.Eppstein, Synergistic effect of Glucantime and Liposome-Encapsulated Muramyl Dipeptide analog in the therapy of Experimental Visceral Leishmaniasis, Infec.Immun., 48:409 (1985).
6. H.A.Cohen, Induction of delayed-type sensitivity to Leishmania parasite in a case of Leishmaniasis Cutanea Diffusa with BCG and Cord-Factor (trehalose-6,6'-dimycolate), Acta Dermatovener., 59:547 (1979).
7. M.A.Chirigos and J.E.Talmadge, Immunotherapeutic Agents: Their role in cellular immunity and their therapeutic potential, Springer Semin. Immunopathol., 8:327 (1985).
8. C.R.Alving, Delivery of liposome-encapsulated drugs to macrophages, Trends Pharm.Sci., 22:407 (1983).
9. J.Alexander and D.J.Russell, A novel method of vaccination using parasite membrane antigens, (this volume).

CLEARANCE OF L. DONOVANI FROM THE LIVER OF BALB/c MICE RESULTS IN
LOCAL RESISTANCE TO RE-INFECTION

K.C. Carter [1,2], A.J. Baillie [1], J. Alexander [2] and T.F. Dolan [1]

[1]Pharmacy Department and [2]Immunology Division
Strathclyde University
Glasgow

INTRODUCTION

Relapse occurs in 5-30% of cases of visceral leishmaniasis (Chulay et al., 1983; Sanyal and Arora, 1979). This could be caused either by treatment failure, or because patients become re-infected after successful chemotherapy. As the majority of individuals who acquire Leishmania donovani infections live in endemic areas, it is highly likely that they would be exposed to the parasite again, but what effect chemotheraphy has on the immunity of the host and resistance to re-infection has received little attention. However, it is well known that many of the immunological responses depressed during active infection are increased following chemotherapy. Thus after treatment patients develop positive responses in delayed hypersensitivity skin tests (Manson-Bahr, 1959) and their lymphocytes respond to in vitro stimulation with specific antigen (Sacks et al., 1987).

In this study we investigated what effect sodium stibogluconate treatment would have on subsequent immunity to re-infection in L. donovani susceptible BALB/c mice.

MATERIALS AND METHODS
Materials

Sodium stibogluconate (Pentostam) equivalent to 0.32 mg Sb mg^{-1} was obtained from the Wellcome Foundation, U.K. ^{125}I-labelled horseradish peroxidase immune complex (HRP immune complex) was kindly provided by Professor W.H. Stimson, Immunology Department, University of Strathclyde. These materials were used as received. All other reagents were of analytical grade.

Animals

Eight to ten week-old female inhouse bred BALB/c mice were used throughout experiments. Golden syrian hamsters (Mesocricetus auratus) obtained from the Anatomy Department, Glasgow University were used to maintain the parasite.

Parasite

Leishmania donovani (MHOM/ET/67/L82 = LV9) obtained from Dr. G. Coombs, Glasgow University was harvested and maintained as described by Carter et al. (1987). Mice were injected into the tail vein (without anaesthetic) with $1-2 \times 10^7$ amastigotes in 0.2ml.

Parasite distribution

The method of determining parasite burdens (numbers/1000 host cell nuclei) in liver, spleen and bone marrow has been described by Carter et al., 1987. The number of Leishman-Donovan units (LDU) was calculated per organ for the liver and spleen using the formuala: LDU = number of amastigotes per 1000 host cell nuclei x the organ weight gm. (Bradley and Kirkley, 1977).

Experimental design

Parasite suppression

In a typical experiment mice were injected into the tail vein (without anaesthetic) on days 7 and 8 post-infection with 0.2ml of either distilled water (controls) or sodium stibogluconate solution (equivalent to 5mg antimony ml^{-1}). On day 14 post-infection, two groups (control and drug treated) were killed to determine the efficacy of drug treatment.

Also on day 14 post infection, a second group of drug treated animals was re-infected with $1-2 \times 10^7$ L. donovani amastigotes. This is described as the challenge infection. In addition, an age and sex-matched uninfected group was infected as a control for the challenge group. Parasite burdens in these groups (challenge and controls) were assessed twenty-three days later.

In vivo phagocytic activity of macrophages

Mice infected with 2×10^7 L. donovani were treated (0.2ml via tail vein) on days 30 and 31 post-infection, along with age and sex-matched uninfected controls, with either drug solution (5mg antimony ml^{-1}) or distilled water. On day 6 post-treatment, drug treated and control mice were injected into the tail vein (without anaesthetic) with 25μl of labelled HRP immune complex (8.01×10^5 cpm/mouse). The mice were killed two hours later, the liver, spleen, and both femurs removed, and placed in vials. The amount of label present (as cpm/organ) was obtained using a gamma counter (Packard BPGD 00217). The concentration of label (cpm/gm) in spleen and liver was calculated to allow for the hepatosplenomegaly caused by L. donovani.

Presentation and statistical analysis of data

Parasite burden of the spleen and liver is expressed as mean LDU/organ $\pm$ standard error, whereas the bone marrow counts are expressed as mean number of parasites/1000 host cells $\pm$ standard error. Both parasite data and radioactive counts were analysed using an independent 't' test or a one way analysis of variance on the $\log_{10}$ transformed data.

RESULTS

The results obtained on day 14 post-infection showed that treatment with free sodium stibogluconate (2mg antimony/mouse) caused a

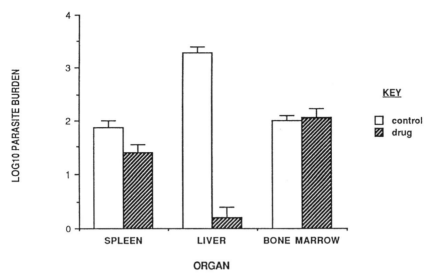

Fig. 1 The effect of treatment of L. donovani infected BALB/c mice with free sodium stiogluconate on parasite burden on day 14 post-infection. Mice, infected with 2×10^7 L. donovani, were treated on days 7 and 8 post-infection with either water (controls) or sodium stibogluconate solution (equivalent to a total antimony dose of 2mg/mouse). Parasite numbers were determined on day 14 post-infection. The data is expressed as the mean $\log_{10}$ LDU/organ + standard error for the liver, and as the mean $\log_{10}$ number of amastigotes/1000 host cell nuclei + standard error for the bone marrow.

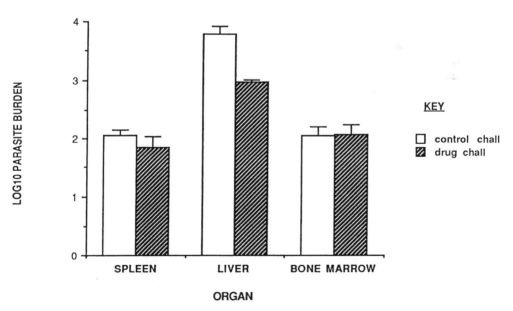

Fig. 2 The effect of sodium stibogluconate chemotherapy of L. donovani infected BALB/c mice on immunity to subsequent challenge infection. Infected mice drug treated as described in Fig. 1 were re-infected, along with corresponding uninfected controls, with 1.2×10^7 L.donovani. 23 days later parasite numbers were determined as described in Fig. 1.

significant reduction in the liver parasite number compared with primary controls (p<0.001, Fig. 1) but had little effect on spleen and bone marrow parasite burdens (p>0.05).

When sodium stibogluconate treated mice were rechallenged with 2×10^7 L. donovani amastigotes, assessment of parasite numbers twenty-three days later showed that significantly fewer parasites were found in the liver of these animals compared with controls given their first infection (p<0.001, Fig. 2). There was however no significant difference in spleen and bone marrow parasite burdens of challenged animals and controls (not shown) which suggested that parasites from the challenge infection were unable to add to the parasite populations still present in these sites following drug treatment.

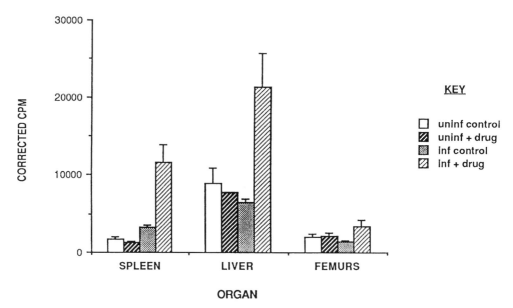

Fig. 2 The effect of sodium stibogluconate therapy on the in vivo phagocytic activity of macrophages of L. donovani infected BALB/c mice. Uninfected (unin) and infected mice (inf, infected with 2×10^7 L. donovani amastigotes 30 days previously), were treated with either water (controls) or free sodium stibogluconate (+ drug, equivalent to a total antimony dose of 2mg/mouse); on days 1 and 2. Six days later the mice were injected with ^{125}I-labelled horseradish peroxidase immune complex (equivalent to 8.01×10^5 cpm). Two hours afterwards the mice were killed and the amount of radioactivity present in each organ determined and corrected for background (226 +10 cpm). Results are expressed as the mean corrected counts per minute/organ (cpm) + standard error.

Drug treatment itself seemed to have no effect on macrophage activity in vivo as measured by phagocytosis since a similar amount of labelled HRP immune complex was taken up by the organs of both groups (drug treated and untreated) of uninfected mice (p>0.10, Fig. 3).

However, macrophage function as measured by phagocytosis was markedly altered in drug treated infected animals. Results obtained for the spleen showed that infected animals took up significantly more of the complex than uninfected controls (p<0.001) and this function was enhanced even further in drug treated infected animals (p<0.01). Drug treated infected animals also had significantly higher liver phagocytosis indices compared with the other groups (p<0.05). Calculation of spleen and liver uptake in terms of cpm/gm did not significantly alter the results. No differences were recorded in the uptake of immune complex in the femur bone marrow of any experimental groups (p>0.10).

DISCUSSION

The therapeutic effect of sodium stiboglucoante in BALB/c mice infected with L. donovani is organ dependent. A dose of 2mg antimony/mouse over two days suppressed parasite numbers in the liver but had little effect on parasites residing in spleen and bone marrow.

Following re-infection signifantly fewer parasites were recovered from the liver of drug treated animals compared with controls given their first infection. This suggested that some factor(s) induced by chemotherapy increased the liver's resistance to re-infection. It is unlikely that residual drug could have killed the challenge parasites in re-infected animals as sodium stibogluconate is rapidly cleared from the tissue (95% of the drug is excreted in the urine within 6 hours of an intravenous injection, D'Arcy and Harron, 1983). Resistance to re-infection as demonstrated in the liver may also have occurred in spleen and bone marrow. Re-infection of drug treated animals did not increase parasite numbers in these organs above that of controls. There may however simply be an upper limit to the number of parasites which can infect macrophages in these tissues at any time. Following chemotherapy there was an increase in macrophage activity in spleen and liver, though not bone marrow, as measured by the in vivo uptake of ^{125}I-labelled horseradish peroxidase immune complex. However, if the spleen was activated following drug treatment why were parasites not cleared from this organ to a similar extent as from the liver? Perhaps this reflects heterogeneity in the macrophage populations of these organs. It has been demonstrated for example that Leishmania parasite survival and growth in vitro is dependent on the tissue origin of the macrophage population (Alexander, 1981). In addition, macrophage activation as measured by one parameter, does not necessarily indicate that all functions associated with macrophage activation are in operation. Thus while increased tumoricidal activity corresponded with the ability to kill L. major in vitro (Pappas et al., 1983), similarly activated macrophages were unable to kill L. donovani (Haidaris and Bonventre, 1981). Further the ability to kill existing intra-cellular parasites and the ability to withstand re-infection may be regarded as two different phenomena. These are not mutually exclusive but they can operate independently and it has been suggested from work using L. major that these two functions are controlled by different lymphokines (Nacy et al., 1984). This may explain the apparent dissociation between drug induced levels of resistance to re-infection and parasite clearance in the spleen and livers of BALB/c mice. The close relationship between drug therapy and macrophage activation has been demonstrated by Adinolfi et al. (1985) since treatment with the drug, glucantime and the macrophage stimulator, muramyl dipeptide, had a synergistic therapeutic effect in experimental visceral leishmaniasis.

CONCLUSIONS

The response of L. donovani infected BALB/c mice, treated with sodium stibogluconate, to re-infection was investigated. The efficacy of drug treatment of infected mice on days 7 and 8 was established by determination of liver, spleen and bone marrow parasite burdens on day 14 post-infection. A dose of 2mg antimony/mouse reduced parasite numbers in the liver, but had little effect on those residing in spleen and bone marrow. Significantly fewer liver parasites were found in re-infected animals, which had previously been drug treated, compared with controls given their first infection. An in vivo assay showed that the sodium stibogluconate treatment of infected animals caused a significant increase in the uptake of HRP-immune complex by liver and spleen. It is proposed that drug treatment not only has a direct leishmanicidal effect but also indirectly promotes macrophage activation.

ACKNOWLEDGEMENTS

This study was supported by the Medical Research Council. J. Alexander holds a Wellcome Trust Lectureship and T.F. Dolan is supported by SERC. The donations of Pentostam and HRP immune complex are gratefully acknowledged.

REFERENCES

Adinolfi, L.E., Bonventre, P.F., Vander Pas, M., and Epstein, D. (1985) Syngergistic effect of glucantime and liposome-encapsulated muramyl dipeptide analog in the therapy of visceral leishmaniasis. Immun., 48, 409.

Alexander, J. (1981) Interaction of Leishmania mexicana mexicana with mouse macrophages in vitro. In Heterogeneity of mononuclear phagocytes, Editor Forster, D. and Landy, M. Academic Press p447.

Bradley, D.J. and Kirkley, J. (1977) Regulation of Leishmania populations within the host. 1. The variable course of Leishmania donovani infections in mice. Clin. Exp. Immunol., 30, 119.

Carter, K.C., Baillie, A.J., Alexander, J. and Dolan, T.F. (1987) The therapeutic effect of sodium stibogluconate in BALB/c mice infected with L. donovani. Submitted J. Pharm. Pharmacol.

Chulay, J.D., Bhatt, S.M., Muigai, R., HO, M., Gochihi, G., Were, J.B., Chunge, C. and Bryceson, A.D. (1983) A comparison of three dosage regimens of sodium stibogluconate in the treatment of visceral leishmaniasis in Kenya. J. Inf. Dis., 148, 148.

D'Arcy, P.F. and Harron, D.W.G. (1983) Leishmaniasis. Pharm. Int., 4, 238.

Haidaris, C.G. and Bonventre, P.F. (1981) Elimination of Leishmania donovani amastigotes by activated macrophages. Infect. Immunity, 33, 918.

Manson-Bahr, P.E.E. (1959) East African Kala-azar with special reference to the pathology, prophylaxis and treatment. Trans. Roy. Soc. Trop. Med. Hyg., 53, 123.

Nacy, C.A., Meltzer, m.S. and Fortier, A.H. (1984) Macrophage activation to kill Leishmania tropica: characterisation of P/J mouse macrophage defects for lymphokine-induced antimicrobial activities against Leishmania tropica amastigotes. J. Immunol., 133, 3344.

Pappas, M.G., Oster, C.N. and Nacy, C.A. (1983) Intra-cellular destruction of Leishmania tropica by macrophages activated in vivo

with Mycobacterium bovis strain BCG. Adv. Exp. Biol. 162, 425.
Sacks, D.L., Lal, S.L., Shrivastava, S.N., Blackwell, J. and Neva, F.A. (1987). An analysis of T cell responsiveness in Indian Kala-azar. J. Immunol., 138, 908.
Sanyal, R.K. and Arora, R.R. (1979) Assessment of drug therapy of Kala-azar in current epidemic in Bihar. J. Commun. Dis., 11, 198.

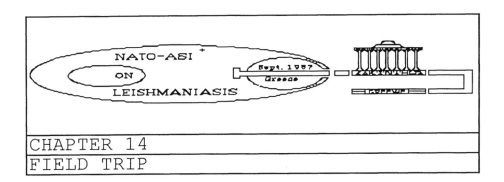

CHAPTER 14
FIELD TRIP

I - THE FIELD TRIP

Nicole Leger , rapporteur

Laboratoire de Parasitologie
U.E.R. de Pharmacie de Reims
51096 Reims Cedex France

Four short speeches introduced the field trip .
Two of the speakers presented the techniques in use for trapping sandflies
(Pr. N. Leger) and for taking samples from dogs (Pr. R. Houin) .
Then Dr. Garifallou and Dr. Schnur presented the leishmanian focus of Zakinthos and the results of their investigations

I - HOW TO CATCH SANDFLIES IN THE MEDITERRANEAN AREA by N. Leger .

The various techniques employed have been briefly reviewed by means of diapositives :
- the oily traps (castor oil traps) :
    - how to make them ,
1   - the strategy of the trapping along a transect itinerary,
    -how to set traps in the resting places : in walls " barbacanes",
between disjointed stones , in houses and ruins ,
    - the collection of the traps,
2   - how to gather the sandflies on the oily papers and to pack them
- the manual capture :
    - presentation of the equipment,
3   - how to catch sandflies at day time in the resting places,
    - how to catch them at night time on the walls or on a human bait,
- the light trapping :
    - presentation of the CDC trap,
4   - how to put it in a well , in a henhouse , under a tree ,
    - the lighted oily paper chain .

- People in charge of the organization of the field trip :
        Dr. Garifallou and Dr. Hatziandoniou (itinerary, local contacts,
choice of places for demonstrations)
        Pr. Houin (demonstrations on dogs)
        Pr. Leger , Pr. Killick-Kendrick et M. Killick-Kendrick (demonstrations on sandflies) .

- Itinerary :
The map n°I gives the route of the trip with the stations where demonstrations took place

- Programme of practical demonstrations :
Demonstrations on the field consisted of two parts : the sampling of sandflies and the canine enquiry .

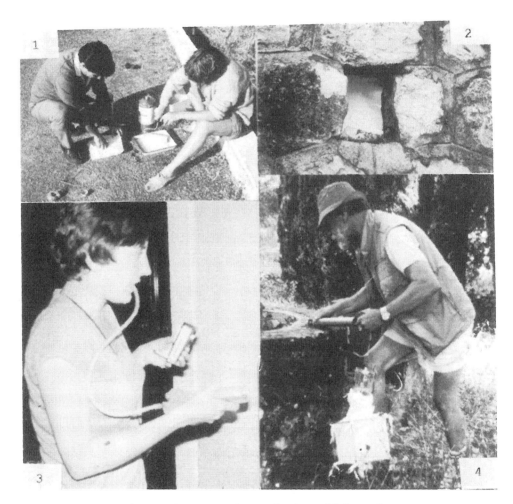

Figure 1   Examples of the slides shown.

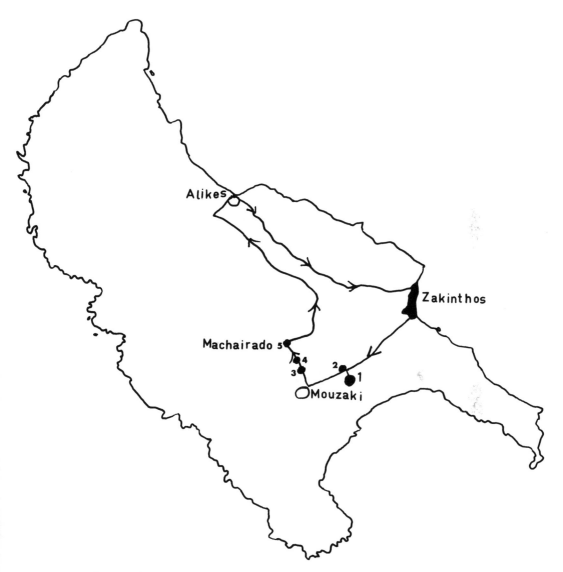

Figure 2 Map of the route used for the Field Trip

I- Sampling of sandflies :
　　　　A- by the technique of the oily traps :
Sheets of paper coated with castor oil had been put in place two days before the trip in five stations (see numbers of the stations on the map) : I in a ruin situated near the farm where the gathering of the dogs was planed , 2 in the "barbacanes" of a wall near station I , 3 between the disjoined stones of an enclosure lining the road , 4 in the "barbacanes" of a roughcast wall under a house , 5 around the church of Machairado .
These oily papers have been taken along the trip and the sandflies have been collected on them the next day .
It has been shown that the best place to collect sandflies by this mean is the "barbacanes" .
　　　　B- by the technique of light traps :
Four light traps have been placed in wells situated in the location I . They worked during three days and have been inspected every day .
Some of the trapped sandflies served for demonstrations of dissections set up for people who have asked for it .
271 of the sandflies have been identified in order to have an idea of the faunistic distribution at this time of the year . We identified : Phlebotomus major neglectus , the suspected vector (1,5%) , P.perfiliewi (4%) , P.tobbi (57,5%) , Sergentomyia minuta (36,5%) and S.dentata (0,5%) .

　　　　2- Canine enquiry :
The demonstration took place in a farm situated near Mouzaki (I on the map) where Dr. Garifallou had organized the gathering of some dogs , one of them suffering of leishmaniasis .
Pr. Houin carried out the bleeding of the dogs and the preparation of the sera .
Pr. Rioux performed a ponction of a lymph node on the ill dog with a subsequent culture .

The practical demonstrations (collection of the sandflies and sampling on the dogs) were followed by a trip across the most active part of the leishmanian focus of the island .

II - FERAL RESERVOIRS OF LEISHMANIASIS ON THE ISLAND OF ZAKINTHOS

L.F. Schnur[1], C. Stamatopoulos[2], A. Garifallou[3],
M. Patrikoussis[3] and R.L. Jacobson[1]

1. Kuvin Centre, Hebrew University-Hadassah Medical School
   Jerusalem, Israel
2. Department of Zoology, University of Patras
   Patras, Greece
3. Institute Pasteur Hellenique
   Athens, Greece

Cutaneous leishmaniasis (CL) caused by Leishmania tropica (Garifallou et al., 1984) and visceral leishmaniasis (VL) caused by L.donovani (Tzamouranis et al., 1984) both occur in Greece generally, including the Ionian Island of Zakinthos. Dogs infected with L.d.infantum serve as a domestic reservoir of human VL. Since dogs show no resistance to infection, succumbing readily, it is doubtful that they are the primary reservoir of L.d.infantum. Foxes and jackals have been found infected in other parts of the world and carnivores like these are probably the primary source of VL, which is transmitted to dogs and then to man (see Abranches, this publication). L.tropica is said to be anthroponotic, but the paucity of human cases in many places suggests that it, too, is a zoonosis and has a wild reservoir. The search for possible feral hosts of leishmanial parasites in a small island like Zakinthos is simplified, since relatively few possibilities exist. Only 12 wild mammalian species have been recorded on Zakinthos, two of which are carnivores and five are rodents (Table 1). Besides man, carnivores and rodents are the only mammalian orders known to be infected with leishmanial parasites in the Old World.

None of 80 wild mammals caught on Zakinthos between 1983 and 1986 proved to be infected (Table 2). The rodents were Apodemus sp., Mus sp., Rattus rattus and R.norvegicus. The only carnivore was a stone marten, Martes foina (Figure 1). Two hedgehogs, Erinaceus concolor, insectivores, were also examined. Though shown to be parasitologically negative by the examination of stained smears and blood-agar cultures of tissue from the skin, spleen, liver and bone marrow, the stone marten displayed a positive titre of anti-leishmaial antibody, measured by a radioimmunoassay (Fig. 2). If a feral reservoir of L.d.infantum exists on Zakinthos, the stone marten is a promising candidate.

ACKNOWLEDGEMENT

Supported by the EEC R&D programme for Science and Technology Development and the leishmaniases component of the UNDP/World Bank/WHO Special Programme for Research and Training in Tropical Diseases.

Table 1. Wild mammals known to exist on Zakinthos Island, Greece

Order Carnivora:
  Family Mustelidae
    <u>Mustela nivalis</u>
    <u>Martes foina</u>
Order Rodentia:
  Family Muridae
    <u>Mus musculus domesticus</u>
    <u>Apodemus sylvaticus</u>
    <u>A. flavicolis</u>
    <u>A. mystacinus</u>
    <u>Rattus norvegicus</u>
    <u>Rattus rattus</u>

Order Lagomorpha:
  Family Leporidae
    <u>Lepus carpensis</u>
Order Chiroptera
  Family Vespertilionidae
    <u>Miniopterus schreibersii</u>
    <u>Pipistrellus kuhli kuhli</u>
Order Insectivora:
  Family Erinaceidae
    <u>Erinaceus concolor</u>

Table 2. Wild animals trapped and examined for <u>Leishmania</u> parasites on Zakinthos Island, Greece

	Jun.1983	Sep.1983	Sep.1985	Oct.1986	Total
<u>Apodemus</u> sp.	9	14	3	0	26
<u>Mus</u> sp.	8	8	1	0	17
<u>Rattus rattus</u>	2	0	7	0	9
<u>Rattus norvegicus</u>	1	13	2	9	25
<u>Erinaceus concolor</u>	0	0	0	2	2
<u>Martes foina</u>	0	0	0	1	1
				Grand Total	80

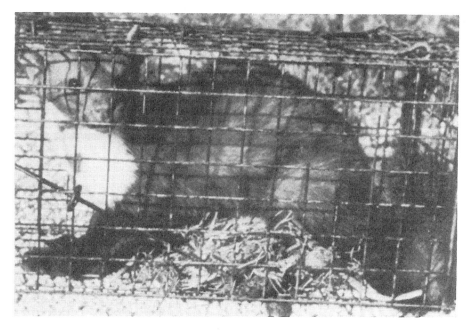

Figure 1. <u>Martes foina</u> (Stone marten) from Meso Gerakari, a focus of canine and human leishmaniasis.

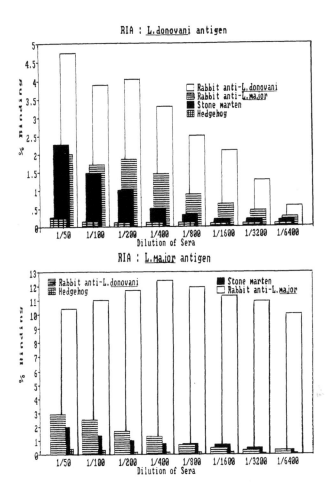

Fig. 2. A solid phase radioimmunoassay (El-On et al., 1983) was used. The antigen, leishmanial excreted factor (EF), was coated onto microplate wells (solid phase); test antibodies were added; after incubation wells were washed 3X with PBS-Tween; ^{125}I Protein A added; after further incubation washed 3X and adhering radioactivity measured. Anti-L.donovani and anti-L.major sera raised in rabbits served as positive controls. Normal rabbit (not shown) was used as negative controls; hedgehog sera included for comparison.

REFERENCES

El-On, J., Zehavi, U., Avraham, H., and Greenblatt, C.L., 1983, Leishmania tropica and L.donovani: Solid phase radioimmunoassay using leishmanial excreted factor, Expl Parasit., 55: 270.

Garifallou, A., Schnur, L.F., Stratigos, J.D., Hadziandoniou, M., Savigos, M., Stavrianeas, M., and Série, C., 1984, Leishmaniasis in Greece II. Isolation and identification of the parasite causing cutaneous leishmaniasis in man, Ann. Trop. Med. Parasit., 78:369.

Tzamouranis, N., Schnur, L.F., Garifallou, A., Pateraki, E., and Série, C., Leishmaniasis in Greece I. Isolation and identification of the parasite causing human and canine leishmaniasis, Ann. Trop. Med. Parasit.,78:363.

III - EPIDEMIOLOGY OF HUMAN AND CANINE LEISHMANIASIS ON THE ISLAND OF ZAKINTHOS

A. Garifallou[1], M. Hadziandoniou[1], L.F. Schnur[2], B. Yuval[2],
A. Warburg[2], R.L. Jacobson[2], E. Pateraki[1], M. Patrikoussis[1],
Y. Schlein[2] and C. Sérié[1]

1. Institut Pasteur Hellenique, Athens, Greece
2. Kuvin Centre, Hebrew University, Jerusalem, Israel

INTRODUCTION

Canine, human visceral (VL) and human cutaneous (CL) leishmaniases all occur widely on the mainland of Greece and many of the Greek islands. Their quite extensive history has been reviewed briefly by Tzamouranis et al. (1984) and Garifallou et al. (1984). Human cases are usually infants and young children. More dogs have been found infected than people and they are the main source of human infection (Papantonakis, 1935; Adler, 1936,1964).

We began our epidemiological survey of leishmaniasis on the Island of Zakinthos after a case of human CL reminiscent of leishmaniasis recidivans (LR) was discovered on the island at Mousaki that was shown to be caused by Leishmania tropica (Garifallou et al.,1984) and on hearing reports of human VL. Studies were initiated in autumn 1982 on a very brief visit to the island, during which a second case of CL, also shown to be caused by L.tropica (unpublished data), was seen by us. This was a rather 'atypical' lesion on the eyelid of an old woman living in the town of Zakinthos, the Island's capital. We also examined a very sick dog and isolated a strain from its popliteal lymph node that proved to be L.donovani infantum (unpublished data). Serum taken from this dog showed a high antileishmanial antibody titre in immunofluorescent antibody (IFA) and ELISA tests.

Our main studies were carried out during 1983 to 1986 and covered four main sapects: a survey of the human population in selected areas of the Island; a simultaneous survey of the dogs, which are many and all domesticated and cared for; a search for the sandfly vectors of both L.donovani infantum and L.tropica on the Island; and a search for possible feral reservoirs of these two leishmanial species on the Island. The fourth aspect is covered in a brief report by Schnur et al. (this publication) and will not be reconsidered here. No leishmanial parasites were isolated from the 80 wild animals caught on the Island so far.

THE ISLAND OF ZAKINTHOS AND STUDY AREAS

The Island of Zakinthos is the southernmost island of the seven Ionian Islands, lying just off the north-western coast of the Peloponnesus. Our studies were concentrated in three areas chosen for their different geographical settings (Fig. 1). Area 1 included the villages of Mousaki and Pantokrator, where 311 people and 111 dogs were examined; Area 2, the villages of Vanato, Kalipado, Mesogerakari and Tragaki, where 280 people and 85 dogs were examined; Area 3, the village of Pigadakia, where 68 people and 19 dogs were examined. All the dogs examined were owned and were kept on leads and chains in farmyards close to the homes of their owners. Every homestead had a well for its water supply. Sand flies were caught in abundance in these wells, which seemed to be a favoured resting site and, possibly, the main breeding site. Catches were much less abundant in the fields and orchards.

SURVEYING THE HUMAN AND DOG POPULATIONS

A total of 665 people and 215 dogs were examined. This was done in households, with a complete record of each family and its dogs being made, including medical histories. People and dogs were examined and bled. The families were visited every year over the four year period and the people and dogs were bled on each occasion if possible. Thus, up to four samples of sera were tested and anywhere between none to all four samples could be positive. Sera were tested for antileishmanial antibodies using immunofluorescence (IFA), where a positive result was measured as a dilution greater than or equal to 1/100, and ELISA tests, where a positive result was greater than or equal to an optical density (OD) of 250 for a given serum dilution, and were tested against L.d.infantum and L.tropica promastigote antigens.

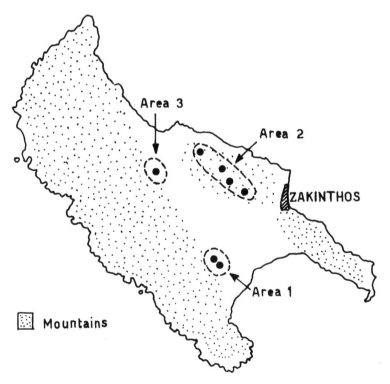

Fig. 1. The Island of Zakinthos showing the three study areas. One case of CL caused by L.tropica was seen in the town of Zakinthos; 25 people having shown indications of VL, 4 infected dogs and 1 human case of LR caused by L.tropica came from Area 1; 8 people having shown indications of VL, 2 infected dogs and 1 infected sand fly (Phlebotomus major) came from Area 2; 4 people having shown indications of VL and 2 infected dogs came from Area 3.

Table 1. Human Serology

No. of times serum was positive out of 4	Immunofluorescence (IFA)				ELISA			
	L.d.infantum antigen		L.tropica antigen		L.d.infantum antigen		L.tropica antigen	
	No.	%	No.	%	No.	%	No.	%
0 Positives	425	72	335	57	261	45	360	62
1 Positive	126	21	196	33	265	45	181	31
2 Positives	27	4	46	7	49	8	35	6
3 Positives	5	0.8	5	0.8	3	0.5	2	0.3
4 Positives	0	0	1	0.2	1	0.2	0	0
TOTAL	583	100	583	100	579	100	578	100

Many of the adults screened were also skin tested with leishmanin to check for delayed hypersensitivity to leishmanial antigens, comparing this with serum antibody levels. Subjects received two types of leishmanin: one made with L.d.infantum promastigotes; the other with L.tropica promastigotes, both at 10^6 per ml, made up in 0.5% phenol-saline, which was also given separately as a phenol-saline control. Some subjects were also skin tested on subsequent occasions.

Dogs showing signs of disease were checked parasitologically by making and checking stained smears and blood-agar cultures of popliteal lymph node aspirates.

SEROLOGICAL TESTING

Table 1 presents all the data on human serum antileishmanial positivity and negativity under both test systems and with both types of antigen. The results, while being difficult to interpret, do indicate a high degree of positivity with both test systems. The IFA system gave more positives when the L.d.infantum antigen was used and the ELISA system when the L.tropica antigen was used. Even so, very few subjects showed a consistant antibody level over the four times sera were collected. Some showed an increase with time, some a deminution and some constancy. One would have to analyse these fluctuations of antibody level in order to begin to understand the significance of the serology. We are currently working on a complete analysis of this information in terms of geographical distribution, familial groupings, age, sex, relationship with canine serum positivity and the presence of proven human cases and sick dogs.

SKIN TESTING

The results of skin testing have also proved difficult to interpret and are also being analysed in relation to all the factors mentioned above, owing to the large number of subjects showing some reactivity, i.e., granuloma formation, persistent erythema or both. Of the 594 subjects skin tested, approximately 25% showed reactivity to L.d.infantum leishmanin and approximately 20% showed reactivity to L.tropica leishmanin, with many showing reactivity to both. Some reactions were massive, with granulomatous plaques over 20mm in diameter and surrounding persistent erythema being 40mm or more in diameter.

INDICATIONS OF VISCERAL LEISHMANIASIS IN MAN

The absolute proof of leishmaniasis in people is parasitological diagnosis demonstrating the presence of leishmanial parasites. By culturing

Table 2. Canine Serology

No. of times serum was positive out of 4	IFA No.	%	ELISA No.	%
0 Positives	194	90.0	147	68.7
1 Positive	12	5.6	49	22.9
2 Positives	8	3.7	10	4.7
3 Positives	0	0	6	2.8
4 Positives	0	0	2	1.0
TOTAL	214	100	214	100

infected tissues, strains are made available for typing and the causative agent can be identified and named to complete diagnosis. Often this does not happen and cases are diagnosed on clinical evidence alone. The cases considered here were not diagnosed by us and parasites were not available for typing. We recorded 37 (6.7%) 'cases' amongst the 562 subjects whose medical records we were able to consider. No records were available for 103 people. Of the 254 from Area 1, 25 (10%) had shown indications of VL. Of the 240 from Area 2, eight had shown indications, one being a seven-year old girl just recovered after treatment. Of the 68 from Area 3, 4 (6%) had shown indications, one being an eight-year old boy just recovered after treatment. It is interesting to note that of eight infected dogs examined by us and from which strains were isolated, four came from Area 1, two came from Area 2 and two from Area 3. Also, the one infected sandfly caught by us during the whole survey came from Area 2.

CANINE LEISHMANIASIS

Of the 215 dogs examined, eight were found to be infected. Sick dogs were found in all three areas, as mentioned above. The amount of anti-leishmanial sero-positivity among 214 of the dogs is given in Table 2. Little to no difference was seen between using L.donovani infantum and and L.tropica antigen and only the overall testing is indicated. The IFA test revealed 20 positive dogs, while the ELISA discerned 67. A complete evaluation of this has yet to be done with regard to the increase, stability and reduction of antileishmanial antibodies over the four times dogs were bled.

Culture of lymph node aspirates from two of the eight infected dogs yielded two stocks. Biochemical and serological typing by cellulose acetate enzyme electrophoresis and excreted factor (EF) serotyping showed these isolated flagellate stocks to be identical to one another and very similar, but not identical, to two international reference strains, an Ethiopian L.d.donovani strain (MHOM/ET/67/HU3) and a Tunisian L.d.infantum strain (MHOM/TN/80/IPT1). In fact, the strains from the dogs lie enzymically between these two reference strains in type and probably constitute a new zymodeme.

THE SEARCH FOR VECTORS OF L.DONOVANI AND L.TROPICA

Before the onset of the Zakinthos project, no proven vectors of leishmaniases in Greece were known. However, Phlebotomus sergenti females were suspected of being the vectors of L.tropica, the cause of cutaneous leishmaniasis in Greece, and P.major females were suspected of being the vectors of L.donovani, the cause of visceral leishmaniasis in Greece. Experimental infection of each type of suspected vector with its corresponding Leishmania sp. was achieved during the 1930's.

A survey of phlebotomine species on Zakinthos undertaken in June 1983, showed the presence of four species of Phlebotomus. A total of 1286 males and 392 females were found, giving a male:female ratio of 3.28:1. Of these, 50.9% were P.tobbi, 46.4% were P.perfiliewi, 2.0% were P.major and 0.46% were P.sergenti. 302 Sergentomyia spp. sand flies were caught, but these are not known or considered to be vectors of leishmanial parasites. This survey was taxonomic only and none of the sand flies were dissected in search of leishmanial infections.

In September 1983, over 5000 sand flies were caught, mostly in CDC light traps. Oiled papers were also used. The species composition was 59% P.tobbi, 28% P.perfiliewi, 5% P.major and 8% Sergentomyia spp. No P.sergenti were caught. Some 300 females were dissected, none of which harboured flagellate infections.

In September 1985, 994 male and 360 female Phlebotomus were caught giving a ratio of 2.76 males to each female. Dissection of the females exposed one infected P.major. Biochemical and serological typing by cellulose acetate enzyme electrophoresis and excreted factor serotyping showed this isolated flagellate stock to be absolutely identical to the two strains isolated from the dogs described above. This is the first time ever that a naturally infected P.major has been definitely incriminated as a vector of L.donovani sensu lato. The infected sand fly was caught in a CDC light trap set up in a disused house on the outskirts of the village of Mesogerakari in Area 2. This was the only female P.major caught there. Twenty seven males were caught there, as were 1 female and 17 male P.tobbi, and 1 male P.perfiliewi. Some Sergentomyia spp. sand flies were also caught.

In October 1986, trapping was done in the same general location where the infected P.major female was caught in 1985. Two hundred and sixty-four male and 92 female phlebotomine sand flies were caught, giving a ratio of 2.86 males to each female. All the females were dissected, none of which harboured flagellate infections. Two of the eight infected dogs were found in this location in 1986.

ACKNOWLEDGEMENT

Supported by the EEC R&D Programme for Science and Technology Development and the leishmaniases component of the UNDP/World Bank/WHO Special Programme for Research and Training in Tropical Diseases.

REFERENCES

Adler, S., 1936, Canine visceral leishmaniasis with special reference to its relationship to human visceral leishmaniasis, Proc. Third Intl Congr. Comp. Path., p.3, The Eleftheroudakis Company, Athens.
Adler, S. 1964, Leishmania, Adv. Parasit., 2:35.
Garifallou, A., Schnur, L.F., Stratigos, J.D., Hadziandoniou, M., Savigos,M., Stavrianeas, N., and Série, C., 1984, Leishmaniasis in Greece II. Isolation and identification of the parasite causing cutaneous leishmaniasis in man, Ann. Trop. Med. Parasit., 78:369.
Papantonakis, E., 1935, Observation on leishmaniasis in the district of Canea (Crete), Ann. Trop. Med. Parasit., 29:191.
Tzamouranis, N., Schnur, L.F., Garifallou, A., Pateraki, E., and Série, C., Leishmaniasis in Greece I. Isolation and identification of the parasite causing human and canine visceral leishmaniasis, Ann. Trop. Med. Parasit., 78:363.

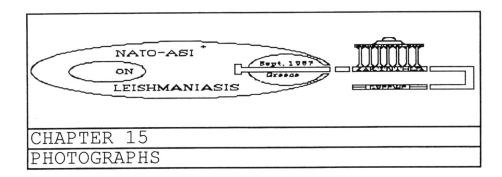

CHAPTER 15
PHOTOGRAPHS

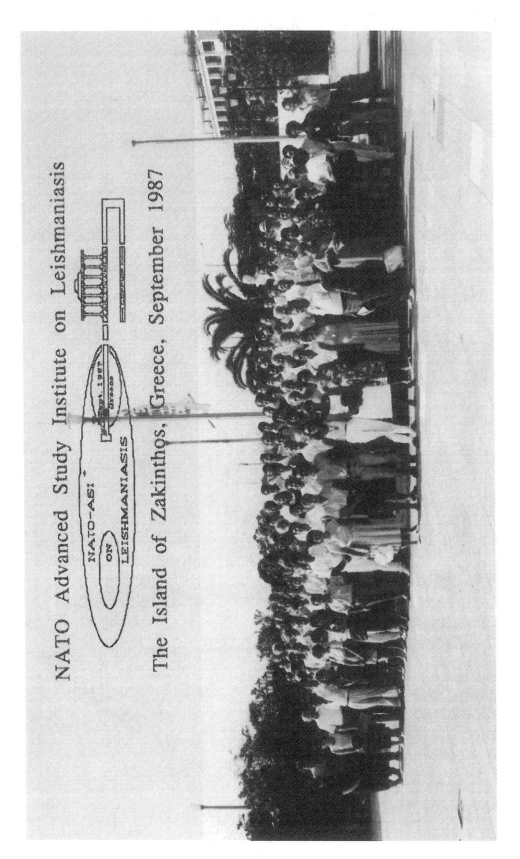

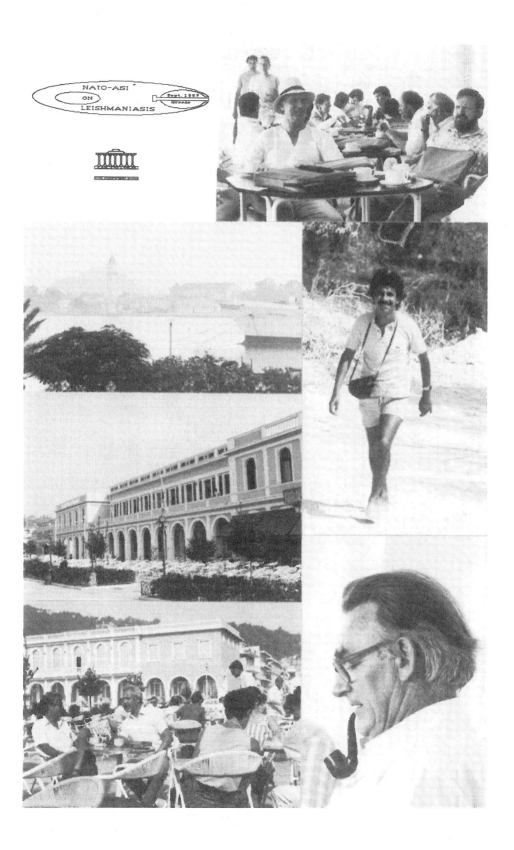

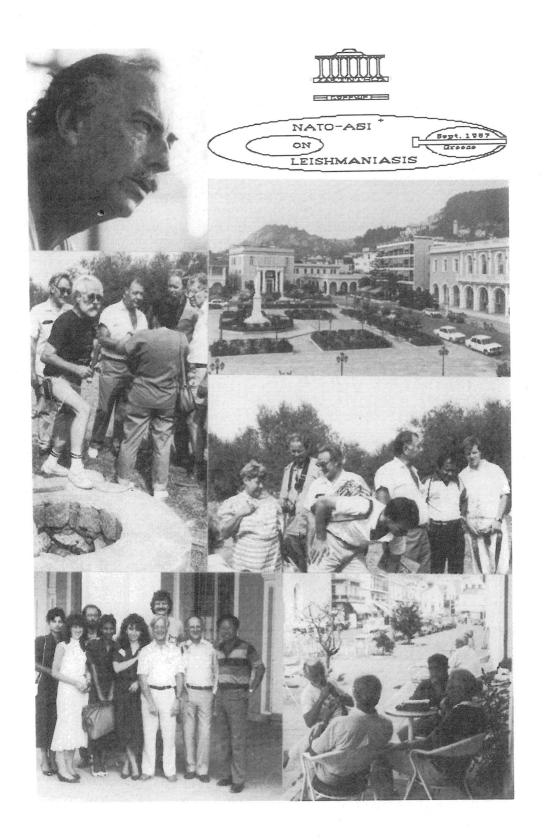

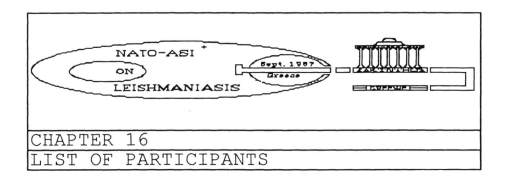

CHAPTER 16
LIST OF PARTICIPANTS

PARTICIPANTS

Professor P. Abranches
Disciplina de Protozoologia
Inst. de Higiene e Med. Trop.
96, Rua da Junqueira
1300 Lisboa
PORTUGAL

Dr S.S. Ahmed
School of Parasitology
Department of Zoology
Univeristy of Sind
Jamshoro
Pakistan

Dr M.L.C. de Almeida
Escola Paulista de Medicina
R. Botucatu, 862 8º andar
04023 - Sao Paulo
BRAZIL

Dr J. Alvar
Department of Parasitology
National Center of Microbiology
28220 Majadahonda
Madrid
SPAIN

Dr R.L. Anthony
Univ. of Maryland
Department of Biology
10 South Pine Street
Baltimore, MD 21201
U.S.A.

Dr R.W. Ashford
Liverpool School of Trop. Med.
Pembroke Place
Liverpool L3 5QA
U.K.

Dr P.A. Bates
Laboratory of Parasitic Diseases
N.I.A.I.D.
Building 5, Room 114
N.I.H.
Bethesda, MD 20892
U.S.A.

Dr J.D. Berman
Walter Reed Army Inst. of Research
Division of Expertl. Therapeutics
Washington, DC 20307-5100
U.S.A.

Dr A.G.H. Ahmed
P.O. Box 5198
Khartoum
SOUTH SUDAN

Dr J. Alexander
Immunology Division
Todd Centre
University of Strathclyde
Glasgow G4 0NR
U.K.

Dr J.M. Alunda
Dpto. Sandidad Animal
Fac. Veterinaria
Univ. Complutense
28040 Madrid
SPAIN

Dr A.J.O. de Andrade
Servico de Anatomia
Hospital Militar Principal
Largo da Estrela
1200 Lisboa
PORTUGAL

Dr J.L. Arevalo
Instituto de Medicina Tropical
"Alexander von Humboldt"
Universidad Peruana Cayetano Heredia
P.O. Box 5045
Lima 100
PERU

Dr D.C. Barker
MRC, Nat. Inst. Medical Research
Molteno Laboratory Outstation
Department of Pathology
University of Cambridge
Cambridge CB2 3EE
U.K.

Dr S. Belazzoug
Parasitology Department
Institut Pasteur
Rue du Dr Laveran
Alger
ALGERIA

Dr H. Bermudez
Entomology Department
CENETROP
Casilla 2974
Santa Cruz
BOLOVIA

Professor S. Bettini
Istituto Superiore di Sanita
Viale Regina Elena, 299
00161 Rome
ITALY

Dr S.M. Beverley
Department of Pharmacology
Harvard Medical School
250 Longwood Ave.
Boston, MA 02115
U.S.A.

Dr R. Bishop
Wolfson Unit.
London Sch. of Hygiene & Trop. Med
Keppel Street
London WC1E 7HT
U.K.

Mr M.L. Blaxter
Wolfson Unit.
London Sch. of Hygiene & Trop. Med
Keppel Street
London WC1E 7HT
U.K.

Dr C. Bordier
Institut de Biochimie
Universite de Lausanne
CH-1066 Epalinges
SWITZERLAND

Professor D.J. Bradley
London Sch. of Hygiene & Trop. Med
Keppel Street
London WC1E 7HT
U.K.

Dr R.S. Bray
150 Kew Rd.
Richmond
Surrey TW9 2AU
U.K.

Dr L.L. Button
Department of Medical Genetics
226 Wasbrook Building
6174 University Boulevard
University of British Columbia
Vancouver, BC
CANADA V6T 1W5

Professor L. Ceci
Inst. di Clinica Medica Veterinaria
Facolta di Medicina Veterinaria
via Caduti di Tutte le Guerre 1
70126 Bari
ITALY

Miss E. Beveridge
6 Moira Court
Balham High Road
London SW17 7AH
U.K.

Dr G.H. Bigaignon
ICP-TROP UNIT
Avenue Hippocrate 74.39
B-1200 Brussels
BELGIUM

Dr J.M. Blackwell
Department of Tropical Hygiene
London Sch. of Hygiene & Trop. Med
Keppel Street
London WC1E 7HT
U.K.

Dr J.J. Blum
Department of Physiology
Duke University Medical Center
Durham, NC 27710
U.S.A.

Dr B.S. Boufana
Liverpool School of Trop. Med.
Pembroke Place
Liverpool L3 5QA
U.K.

Dr O. Brandonisio
Parassitologia Medica
Universita di Bari
Medical School
Policlinico
70124 Bari
ITALY

Dr R.P. Brazil
Department Parasitologia - ICB-CCS
University Rederal do Rio de Janeiro
Rio de Janeiro 21941
BRAZIL

Dr K.C. Carter
Immunology Division
Todd Centre
University of Strathclyde
Glasgow G4 0NR
U.K.

Dr P. Cenini
Dipart. di Patologia Sperimentale
Universita di Bologna
via S. Giacomo, 14
I-40126 Bologna
ITALY

Dr K.-P. Chang
Department of Microbio-Immunology
UHS/Chicago Medical School
3333, Green Bay Road
North Chicago, IL 60064
U.S.A.

Dr C. Chapman
Department of Medical Protozoology
London Sch. of Hygiene & Trop. Med
Keppel Street
London WC1E 7HT
U.K.

Dr J.M. Conlon
US Naval EPMU-7 Box 41
Via E. Scarfoglio
80125 Agnano-Napoli
ITALY

Ms A. Cooper
Department of Tropical Hygiene
London Sch. of Hygiene & Trop. Med
Keppel Street
London WC1E 7HT
U.K.

Dr J.M. Crampton
Wolfson Molecular Genetics Unit
Liverpool School of Trop. Med.
Pembroke Place
Liverpool L3 5QA
U.K.

Dr A. Llanos-Cuentas
Instituto de Medicina Tropical
"Alexander von Humboldt"
Uni. Peruana Cayetano Heredia
P.O. Box 5045
Lima 100
PERU

Dr P. Desjeux
Inst. o Boliviano de Biol. de Altura
c/o Embajada de Francia
Casilla 824
La Paz
BOLIVIA

Dr J-C. Dujardin
Laboratory of Protozoology
Institute of Tropical Medicine
155, Nationalestraat
2000 Antwerpen
BELGIUM

Dr M.L. Chance
Department of Parasitology
Liverpool School of Trop. Medicine
Pembroke Place
Liverpool L3 5QA
U.K.

Dr G. Colella
Ist. i Malattie Inf. e Parassitarie
degli Animali Domestici
Facolta di Medicina Veterinaria
Via Casamassima Km 3
70010 Valenzano
ITALY

Dr G.H. Coombs
Department of Zoology
University of Glasgow
Glasgow G12 8QQ
U.K.

Professor F.E.G. Cox
Department of Biophysics
King's College London
26 Drury Lane
London WC2B 5RL
U.K.

Dr S. Croft
Department of Biochem. Microbiology
Wellcome Research Laboratories
Beckenham
Kent BR3 3BS
U.K.

Dr N. Daldal
Department of Parasitology
Faculty of Medicine
Ege University
Bornova
Izmir
TURKEY

Dr C.M. Dye
London Sch. of Hygiene & Trop. Med
Keppel Street
London WC1E 7HT
U.K.

Dr D.A. Evans
Department of Medical Protozoology
London Sch. of Hygiene & Trop. Med
Keppel Street
London WC1E 7HT
U.K.

Dr R. Etges
Institut de Biochimie
Universite de Lausanne
CH-1066 Epalinges
SWITZERLAND

Dr G.J.J.M. van Eys
Laboratory of Tropical Hygiene
Royal Tropical Institute
Meibergdreef, 39
1105 AZ Amsterdam
HOLLAND

Dr J. Farrell
Department of Pathology
University of Pennsylvania
3800 Spruce Street
Philadelphia, PA 19104
U.S.A.

Dr N. Gajendran
Vrije Universiteit Brussel
Instituut voor Moleculaire Biologie
Paardenstraat 65
1640 st-Genesius-Rode
BELGIUM

Dr M. Robert-Gero
Inst. de Chimie des Sub. Naturelles
C.N.R.S.
91190 Gif-sur-Yvette
FRANCE

Dr S.H. Giannini
Center for Vaccine Development
Univ.of Maryland School of Medicine
10 South Pine Street
Baltimore, MD 21201
U.S.A.

Dr L.J. Goad
Department of Biochemistry
University of Liverpool
P.O. Box 147
Liverpool L69 3BX
U.K.

Dr G.M. Santos Gomes
Disciplina de Protozoologia
Inst. de Higiene e Medicina Tropical
96, Rua da Junqueira
1300 Lisboa
PORTUGAL

Dr A. Fairlamb
Department of Medical Protozoology
London Sch. of Hygiene & Trop. Med
Keppel Street
London WC1E 7HT
U.K.

Dr T.E. Fehniger
Armauer Hansen Research Institute
P.O. Box 1005
Addis Ababa
ETHIOPA

Dr A. Garifallou
Hellenic Pasteur Institute
127, Av. Vassilissis Sofias
Athens 11521
GREECE

Dr A. Giangaspero
Ist. i Malattie Inf. e Parassitarie
degli Animali Domestici
Facolta di Medicina Veterinaria
Via Casamassima Km 3
70010 Valenzano
ITALY

Dr Y. Al-Gindan
King Abdulaziz City for Science & Tech
King Faisal University
SAUDI ARABIA

Dr E. Minter-Goedbloed
49 Spooners Drive
Park Street
St Alband
Herts AL2 2HX
U.K.

Dr L.G. Goodwin
Shepperlands Farm
Park Lane
Finchampstead
Berks RG11 4QF
U.K.

Dr M. Gramiccia
Laboratorio di Parassitologia
Istituto Superiore di Sanita
Viale Regina Elena 299
00161 Rome
ITALY

Dr L. Gradoni
Laboratorio di Parassitologia
Istituto Superiore di Sanita
Viale Regina Elena 299
00161 Rome
ITALY

Dr F. Grimm
Swiss Tropical Institute
Socinstr. 57
Ch-4051 Basel
SWITZERLAND

Dr J.P. Haldar
Schie Eye Institute
University of Pennsylvania
51 N. 39th Street
Philadelphia, PA 19104
U.S.A.

Dr M. Hatziandoniou
Hellenic Pasteur Institute
127, Av. Vassilissis Sofias
Athens 11521
GREECE

Dr G.G. Holz
Dept Microbiology and Immunology
SUNY Health Center at Syracuse
Syracuse, NY 13210
U.S.A.

Mr M.K. Howard
Department of Medical Protozoology
London Sch. of Hygiene & Trop. Med
Keppel Street
London WC1E 7HT
U.K.

Dr I.C. Irfanoglu
YeniFoca sok. No=3/9
Gaziosmanpasa
Ankara
TURKEY

Dr R.L. Jacobson
Department of Parasitology
The Kuvin Centre
Hadassah Medical School
Jerusalem
ISRAEL

Dr P.A. Kager
NH Swellengrebel Lab.Trop.Hyg.
Meibergdreef 39
1105 AZ Amsterdam
HOLLAND

Mr M. Guy
Department of Tropical Hygiene
London Sch. of Hygiene & Trop. Med
Keppel Street
London WC1E 7HT
U.K.

Dr R. Hamers
Vrije Universiteit Brussel
Instituut voor Moleculaire Biologie
Paardenstraat 65
1640 st-Genesius-Rode
BELGIUM

Dr I. Bonsch - Heermes
Inst. f. Med. Parasitrologie
Universitat Bonn
Simmund Freud Str 25
D 5300 Bonn 1
W.G.R.

Professor R. Houin
Labo. de Parasitol. et de Mycologie
Centre Hospitalier et Uni. de Cerete
6, Rue Du General Sarrail
94010 Creteil
CEDEX
FRANCE

Mr C.A. Hunter
Department of Zoology
University of Glasgow
Glasgow G12 8QQ
U.K.

Dr R. Ben-Ismail
Department de Parasitologie
Faculte de Medecine
9, Rue Z. Essafi
Tunis
TUNISIA

Dr C.l. Jaffe
Department of Biophysics
Weizmann Institute of Science
Rehovot 76100
ISRAEL

Dr L.P. Kahl
Dept. of Experimental Immunobiology
Wellcome Research Laboratories
Langley Court
Beckenham
Kent BR3 3BS
U.K.

Ms Kamhawi
Department of Biological Sciences
University of Salford
Salford M5 4WT
U.K.

Dr P. Kaye
Department of Tropical Hygiene
London School of Hygiene & Trop. Med
Keppel Street
London WC1E 7HT
U.K.

Dr R. Killick-Kendrick
Imperial College at Silwood Park
Ashurst Lodge
Ascot
Berks SL5 7PY
U.K.

Dr A.F. Kiderlen
Fraunhofer Institut fur Toxikologie
Nikolai-Fuchs-Str. 1
D-3000 Hannover 61
F.R.G.

Dr A. Kharazmi
Department of Clinical Microbiology
Rigshopitalet, Afsnit 7806
Tagensvej 20, DK 2200
Copenhagen N
DENMARK

Dr R.P. Lane
Entomology Department
London Sch. of Hygiene & Trop. Med
Keppel Street
London WC1E 7HT
U.K.

Dr F. Lawrence
Inst.de Chimie des Sub.Naturelles
C.N.R.S.
91190 Gif-sur-Yvette
FRANCE

Professor N. Leger
Faculty de Pharmacie de Reims
63, Avenue Pierre Semard
94210 La Varenne St-Hilaire
FRANCE

Professor M.V. Londner
Department of Parasitology
Kuvin Centre, Hebrew University
Hadassah Medical School
Jerusalem 91010
ISRAEL

Dr J.S. Keithly
Cornell University Medical College
Division of International Med.
1300 York Avenue
New York City 10021
U.S.A.

Dr J.M. Kelly
Department of Medical Protozoology
London Sch. of Hygiene & Trop. Med
Keppel Street
London WC1E 7HT
U.K.

Ms N. Khammo
Department of Biology
King's College London (KQC)
Campden Hill Road
London W8 7AH
U.K.

Dr V.I. Kontos
Department of Clinical Studies
Aristotelian Uni. of Thessaloniki
11 S. Voutyra str. 546 27
Thessaloniki
GREECE

Mr A. Langridge
Department of Biology
King's College London
Campden Hill Road
London W8 7AH
U.K.

Dr M.J. Lawrence
Department of Pharmacy
King's College London
Manresa Road
London SW3 6LX
U.K.

Dr F.Y. Liew
Dept. of Experimental Immunobiology
Wellcome Research Laboratories
Langley Court
Beckenham
Kent BR3 3BS U.K.

Dr J. Louis
WHO Immunol. Res. & Training Centre
Institute of Biochemistry
Chemin des Boveresses
CH-1066 Epalinges
SWITZERLAND

Dr U. Lucatelli
Ist. i Malattie Inf. e Parassitarie
degli Animali Domestici
Facolta di Medicina Veterinaria
Via Casamassima Km 3
70010 Valenzano
ITALY

Professor P.D. Marsden
Nuclao de Med. Trop. e Nutricao
Universidade de Brasilia
C.P. 153121
70.910 Brasilia-DF
BRAZIL

Dr F. Marsilio
Facolta di Medicina Veterinaria
Via Casamassima Km 3
70010 Valenzano
ITALY

Dr M.J. McElrath
Lab. of Cellular Physiol.& Immunol.
Box 280
Rockefeller University
New York, NY 10021
U.S.A.

Dr D.M. Minter
Department of Entomology
London School of Hygiene & Trop. Med
Keppel Street
London WC1E 7HT
U.K.

Professor D.H. Molyneux
Department of Biological Sciences
University of Salford
Salford M5 4WT
U.K.

Dr A.J. Mukkada
Department of Biological Sciences
University of Cincinnati
Cincinnati
Ohio 45221
U.S.A.

Dr R.A. Neal
Department of Medical Protozoology
London School of Hygiene & Trop. Med
Winches Farm Laboratories
395 Hatfield Road
St. Albans
Herts AL4 0XQ U.K.

Dr F. Martin-Luengo
Department of Microbiology
Faculty of Medicine
University of Murcia
Murcia
SPAIN

Dr M. Maroli
Istituto Superiore di Sanita
Laboratorio di Parassitologia
Viale Regina Elena 299
00161 Roma
ITALY

Ms N. Mayer
Department of Biology
King's College London
London W8 7AH
U.K.

Dr M.A. Miles
Wolfson Unit
London School of Hygiene & Trop. Med
Keppel Street
London WC1E 7HT
U.K.

Dr F. Modabber
T.D.R.
World Health Organization
1211 Geneva
27- Switzerland

Dr H. Momen
Department of Biochem & Mol. Biol.
Fundacao Oswaldo Cruz
Cx Postal 926
21040 Rio de Janeiro
BRAZIL

Dr M.A. Munir
Entomologist
Public Health Division
National Institute of Health
Islamabad
PAKISTAN

Dr M. Nitti
Ist. i Malattie Inf. e Parassitarie
degli Animali Domestici
Facolta di Medicina Veterinaria
Via Casamassima Km 3
70010 Valenzano
ITALY

Dr T. Nolan
Department of Parasitology
School of Veterinary Medicine
University of Pennsylvania
3800 Spruce Street
Philadelphia, PA 19104
U.S.A.

Dr R.W. Olafson
Department of Biochem & Microbiol.
University of Victoria
Victoria
British Columbia V8W 2Y2
CANADA

Dr A. Nonroy-Ostria
Departamento de Immunologia
Escuela Nacional de Ciencias Biol.
Col. Nueva Santa Maria
Mexico D.F. 02800 Apdo.
MEXICO

Dr A. Nurdan Ozer
Hacettepe University
Parasitology Department
Beytepe-Ankara
TURKEY

Professor J. Papavassiliou
Department of Microbiology
University of Athens
P.O. Box 8540
10010 Athens
GREECE

Dr E. Pateraki
Hellenic Pasteur Institute
127, Av. Vassilissis Sofias
Athens 11521
GREECE

Professor W. Peters
Department of Medical Protozoology
London Sch. of Hygiene & Trop. Med
Keppel Street
London WC1E 7HT
U.K.

Dr P. Pirson
UCL Unite BEPC 75.43
75, Ave Hippocrate
B-1200 Bruxelles
BELGIUM

Dr M.J. North
Department of Biological Science
University of Stirling
Stirling FK9 4LA
U.K.

Dr F.R. Opperdoes
ICP-TROP
Ave Hippocrate 74.39
B-1200 Brussels
BELGIUM

Dr Y. Ozbel
Department of Parasitology
Medical Faculty of Ege University
Bornova-Izmir
TURKEY

Dr C. Papadopoulou
Department of Microbiology
Medical School
University of Ioannina
Ioannina
GREECE

Dr K.B. Pastakia
National Institute of Health
Bldg.5, Rm 203
9000, Rockville Pike
Bethesda, Maryland 20892
U.S.A.

Dr M.C.D. Silva Pereira
Instituto de Higiene e Med. Trop.
96, Rua da Junqueira
1300 Lisboa
PORTUGAL

Dr A. Phillips
Department of Biological Sciences
University of Salford
Salford M5 4WT
U.K.

Dr D. McMahon-Pratt
Dept.of Epidemiol.& Public Health
School of Medicine
60 College St
P.O. Box 3333
New Haven
Connecticut 06510
U.S.A.

Dr V. Puccini
Ist. i Malattie Inf. e Parassitarie
degli Animali Domestici
Facolta di Medicina Veterinaria
Via Casamassima Km 3
70010 Valenzano
ITALY

Dr D. Le Ray
Laboratory of Protozoology
Institute of Tropical Medicine
155, Nationalestraat
2000 Antwerpen
BELGIUM

Dr P.D. Ready
c/o Department of Biochemistry
Imperial College of Science & Tech.
Prince Consort Rd
London SW7 2AZ
U.K.

Dr L. Rivas
Yale School of Medicine
Dept Epidemiology & Public Health
Yale Arbovirus Research Unit
60 College Street
New Haven, CT 06510
U.S.A.

Dr T. Roach
Department of Tropical Hygiene
London Sch. of Hygiene & Trop. Med
Keppel Street
London WC1E 7HT
U.K.

Dr A. Sabarti
Hellenic Pasteur Institute
127, Av. Vassilissis Sofias
Athens 11521
GREECE

Dr G. Sarti
Ist. i Malattie Inf. e Parassitarie
degli Animali Domestici
Facolta di Medicina Veterinaria
Via Casamassima Km 3
70010 Valenzano

Dr L.F. Schnur
The Kuvin Centre
Hadassah Medical School
P.O. Box 1172
Jerusalem
ISRAEL

Dr M. Rabinovitch
Unite de Immunophysiologie Cellulaire
25 rue du Docteur Roux
75724 Paris Cedex
FRANCE

Dr M.S. Ben Rachid
Departement de Parasitologie
Faculte de Medicine
9, rue Z. Essafi
Tunis
TUNISIA

Dr J-A. Rioux
Faculte de Medicine de Montpellier
Laboratoire de Parasitologie
Institut de Botanique
163, Rue Auguste Broussonet
34000 Montpellier
FRANCE

Dr D. Rivier
Institut de Biochimie
Universite de Lausanne
CH-1066 Epalinges
SWITZERLAND

Ms M. Roberts
Department of Tropical Hygiene
London Sch. of Hygiene & Trop. Med
Keppel Street
London WC1E 7HT
U.K.

Dr D.L. Sacks
Laboratory of Parasitic Diseases
Nat. Inst.of Allergy & Infect. Diseaes
National Institute of Health
Bethesda, MD 20892
U.S.A.

Dr Y. Schlein
Department of Parasitology
Hadassah Medical School
P.O. Box 1172
Jerusalem
ISRAEL

Professor C. Serie
Hellenic Pasteur Institute
127, Av. Vassilissis Sofias
Athens 11521
GREECE

Dr M. Shapira
Department of Chemical Immunology
Weizmann Institute of Science
Rehovot, 76100
ISRAEL

Dr D.F. Smith
Department of Biochemistry
Imperial College of Science & Tech.
Prince Consort Road
London SW7 2AZ
U.K.

Professor A.G. Spais
Emeritus Prof. of Veterinary Med.
St. Voutira 11 546 27
Thessaloniki
GREECE

Dr P. Tassi
Ist. i Malattie Inf. e Parassitarie
degli Animali Domestici
Facolta di Medicina Veterinaria
Via Casamassima Km 3
70010 Valenzano
ITALY

Dr S. Turco
Department of Biochemistry
Uni. of Kentucky Med. Center
Lexington, Kentucky 40536
U.S.A.

Dr B. Ullman
Department of Biochemistry
School of Medicine
Oregon Health Sciences University
3181 S.W. Sam Jackson Park Road
Portland, Oregon 97201
U.S.A.

Dr B.C. Walton
771 Barlow Drive
Lake Heritage
Gettysburg, PA 17325
U.S.A.

Ms S. Wirth
WHO Immunol. Res.& Training Centre
Institute of Biochemistry
Chemin des Boveresses
CH-1066 Epalinges
SWITZERLAND

Prof S. Yasarol
Department of Parasitology
Faculty of Medicine
Ege University
Bornova, Izmir
TURKEY

Dr F.M. Conceicao Silva
Instituto de Higiene e Med. Tropical
96, Rua da Junqueira
1300 Lisboa
PORTUGAL

Dr K.Ph. Soteriadou
Hellenic Pasteur Institute
127, Av. Vassilissis Sofias
Athens 11521
GREECE

Dr K. Stuart
Seattle Biomedical Research Institute
4 Nickerson Street
Seattle, Washington 98109-1651
U.S.A.

Dr L. Tavares
Department of Infectious Diseases
Hospital Santa Maria
Ave Prof Egas Moniz
1600 Lisboa
PORTUGAL

Dr A.K. Tzinia
Hellenic Pasteur Institute
127, Av. Vassilissis Sofias
Athens 11521
GREECE

Dr J.G. Wallace
US Naval EPMU-7 Box 41
Via E. Scarfoglio
80125 Agnano-Napoli
ITALY

Dr R.D. Ward
Department of Medical Entomology
Liverpool Sch. of Tropical Medicine
Pembroke Place
Liverpool L3 5QA
U.K.

Professor K. Vickerman
Department of Zoology
University of Glasgow
Glasgow G12 8QQ
U.K.

Dr D. Zilberstein
Department of Biology
Technion-Israel Institute of Tech.
Haifa 3200
ISRAEL

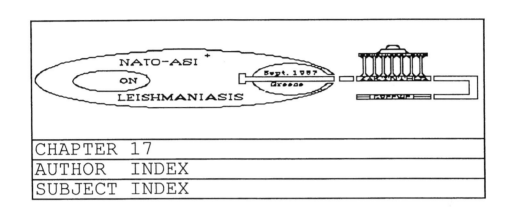

CHAPTER 17
AUTHOR INDEX
SUBJECT INDEX

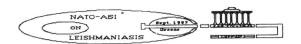

AUTHOR INDEX

Abranches	61	De Doncker	109,137
Aguilar	131	De Fabo.	677
Alexander	359,721,839,991,993	De Memezes.	159
Aline	555	De Oliveira	159
Allen	711	Desjeux	131,137
Altamura	395	Didisheim	423
Alvar	781	Dodic	757
Anderson	667	Dolan	721,793,993,
Angelici	21	Dujardin	95,131,137,539,985,
Anthony	281,931	Dwek	619
Antonaci	395	Dwyer	651
Arevalo	525	Dye	245
Argov	295	Eitrem	207
Ashford.	827	Ellenberger	873,885
Baillie	721,793,993	Ellis	589
Balderrama.	103,109,131	Etges	423,627
Barker	503,901	Evans	549,685,897
Barlow	864	Fairlamb	487,749
Beach	495,765,885	Farrell	345
Ben Ismail	39,823	Feagin	977
Ben Rachid	39	Fehniger	581
Ben Said	39	Ferguson.	619
Berman	473,495,699,765,885	Frankenburg	367
Bermudez	95,117,121,129,131,137	Gajendran	137,539,985
Bettini	179	Garifallou	1007,1011
Beverley	873,885	Gessesse	581
Bishop	533	Ghafoor	47
Blackwell	259, 271,335	Ghose.	387
Blanchard	757	Giannini	677,917
Blaxter	597	Githure1	89
Blum	659	Glaser	667
Bordier	423, 627	Goad	495,885,765
Bouvier	627	Goodwin	693
Bradley	3	Gouvea	159
Brandonisio	395	Gradoni	21,71
Bray	57	Gramiccia	21,71
Brazil	159	Greenblatt	367,401
Burney	47	Grimaldi	911
Button	611	Grogl.	473
Campos	563	Guevara	353
Carrasco	131	Hadziandoniou	603
Carter	721,993	Hadziandoniou	1011
Carvalho	705	Haldar	387
Ceci	395	Hamers,	137,539,985
Cenini	773,891	Haral-abidis	83
Chance	409	Harith	89
Chang	417,619	Hart	807,864
Chapman	549	Heath	409
Claure	117,123,129	Holz	495,765,885
Cohn.	325	Hommel	409
Coombs	449,469,635,741,793,851	Houin	165
Cooper	271	Howard	267
Coulson	563	Hunter	449,741,793
Cox	255,309	Iha	89
Crampton	409,589,957	Iqbal	47
Croft	783,847,991	Jacobson	401,1007
Croop	345	Jacquet	109
Darling	659	Jaffe	295,575,925
Davis	659	Jirillo	395
De Almeida	159	Kager	89

Kahl	417	Nolan	345
Kamhawi	225	North	635
Kaye	259,335	Olafson	611,619
Keithly.	495,555,749	Opperdoes	859
Kellet	597	Paolantonacci	757
Kelly	597	Pastakia	651
Kennedy	549	Pateraki	1011
Khan	47	Patrikoussis	1007,1011
Kharazmi	441	Paz	353
Kiderlen	457	Pedrazzini	329
Killick-Kendrick	175,685,821,823	Perkins 1	89
Kindler	329	Peters	9,685
Kirkpatrick.	345	Petrillo-Peixoto	873
Kiugu	89	Phillips	225
Knapp	957	Pieri	71
Koech	89	Rab	47
Kontos	77	Rabinovitch.	729
Kontos	83	Rachamim	295
Koptopoulos	83	Rademacher	619
Krup	295	Rao	783
Laakso	793	Ready	563,823,965,975
Lancaster	235	Recacoechea	95,103,109,117,131,137
Lane	217,951	Rivero	123,129
Langridge	864	Rivier	423
Lawrence (F)	479,757,879	Roach	271,335
Lawrence(MJ)	807	Robert-Gero	479,757,879
Lawyer	189	Roberts	259
LE Ray.	95,109,131,137,539	Rocha	117,123
Lederer.	879	Rosen	367
Leeuwenburg	89,189	Russell	359
Leger	1003	Sacci	281,931
Liew.	315,417,835	Saha	387
Ligthart	515	Sarfstein	911
Llanos-Cuentas	525	Sayers	267
Llanos	353	Schalken	515
Lockwood	635	Schlein	1011
Lohmann-Matthes	457	Schnur	379,401,939,1007,1011
Londner	367	Scholler	555
London	659	Schoone	515
Lopez	525	Searle	563
Louis.	329	Serie.	1011
Macpherson	741	Sevlever	367
Malina	757	Shapira	575
Mallinson	635	Shoenfeld	295
Mancianti	71	Sjoholm	793
Marchal	329	Smiley	555
Mariam	581	Smith (DF)	563,685,823,965,975
Maroli	217	Smith (P)	235
Matthijsen	137	Sorensen	441
Matthyssens	539	Soteriadou	603
Mauel	423	Spais	77,83
McElrath	325	Stamatopoulos	1007
McEwen	575	Stirpe	773,891
McMaster	611	Stjarnkvist	793
Mebrahtu	189	Stuart	555,977,985
Mengistu	581	Sutton.	864
Miles	267,533,597	Swift.	235
Milligan	225	Tarr	555
Milon	259,329	Tavares	705
Minter	207	Terpstra.	515
Molyneux	225	Tetley	449
Momen	911	Turco	643
Monroy-Ostria	431,335	Tzartos	603
Montalban	117,123,129	Tzinia	603
Monteiro	705	Urjel	95,109,129,131,137
Montoya	525	Van Eys	515
Morton	235	Vassalli	329
Mouna	757	Velasco1	49
Mugai	89	Velez-Castro	431
Muigail	89	Vickerman	449
Mukkada	667	Villarroel	95,103,109,131,137
Munir	47	Walton	149
Murray	325	Warburg	1011
Muyldermans	539	Ward	35,947,957
Mwaniki	89	Wells	667
Neal	685,783,847,711	Williams.	281
Negesse	581	Wozencraft	271
Nielsen	441	Yuval	1011
Nieto	353	Zalis	295

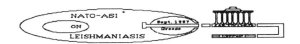

SUBJECT INDEX

Acidic adaptations	667	Dermotropic	28
Adoptive transfer	360	Diagnosis	502, 515, 549, 823, 901
Aids (HIV)	781		
Alanine catabolism	659	Diffuse cutaneous	149
Allopurinol	695, 699, 847	Difluoromethylornithine	491, 696, 749, 879
Allylamines	847	Direct Agglutination Test	89
Amino acid esters	721	DNA electrophoresis	551
Aminoquinoline	696, 847	DNA fingerprinting	593
Ammonia production	659	DNA In situ hybridization	503, 526, 901
Amphotericin B	781, 865	Domestic sandfly	159
Anthroponotic (CL)	9, 41, 51	Dot blot hybridization	503
Antibodies	353	Drug delivery	783, 793, 807
Antigens	295, 359, 388, 409, 423, 432, 581, 603, 611, 931	Drug design	851, 859, 865
		Drug screening	713, 721, 741, 749, 795
Antigen presentation	262	DTT spraying	48
Antigen purification	297	Electron microscopy	450
Antigen specific T cells	264	ELISA	84, 296, 336, 353, 369, 388
Antimonial	473, 695, 699, 711, 721, 785, 793, 847, 867	Excreted factor	368, 401
		Field trip	1003
B10 D2 mouse model	722	Flow cytometric analysis	288, 402, 931
BALB/c mouse model	268, 272, 317, 325, 348, 361, 432, 722	Fluconazole	765
		Flupentixol	443
Biotinylated kDNA	502, 525, 907	GLC	225
Bleomycin	879	Gel chromatography	474, 604
C57 BL-6 mouse model	259, 325, 335, 432	Gene amplification	873
Candida albicans	397, 757	Gene expression	563, 576, 581, 597
Canine leishmaniasis	71, 395	Genome	589
control measures	71	Glucantine	694, 699, 705, 781, 785, 847, 865, 880
epizootiological study	77		
Italy	71	Glucose catabolism	659
Northern Greece	77	Glycoconjugates	401
serology	73	Glycosome	471, 853, 859, 867
CBA-Ca mouse model	361	GP63	417, 423, 611, 619, 627, 835, 840, 932
Chemotherapy	441, 473, 479, 495, 693, 699, 705, 711, 721, 729, 741, 757, 765, 773, 781, 783, 793, 847	Heat shock protein (HSP 70)	570, 576
		HPLC	619
		Histopathology	431
		Hybrids	685
Chemotherapy & Immunity	991, 993	IgG, IgM	353, 388
Chloroquine	443	Imidazole	495
Chlorpromazine	443	Immunity	
Chlorprothixene	443	H-11 susceptibility	259
Chromosomes	539	cell-mediated	315
Clinical manifestations	937	non specific	395
Cloning	551, 564, 590, 612, 868	protective	316, 834
		Immunocytochemistry	261
Clopenthixol	443	Immunodominant epitopes	281
Colony stim. factor assay	346	Immunoelectron microscopy	284
Complement receptor (CR3)	271	Immunofluorescence assay	80
Complement-mediated lysis	268	Immunoidentification	925
Counter-immunoelectrophor.	401	Immunoprecipitation	654
Cutaneous	39, 47, 549	Infective promastigotes	267, 272, 563
Cutaneous anthroponotic	41, 51	Interferon-Gamma	312, 315, 327, 351, 457
Cutaneous sporadic	41		
Cutaneous zoonotic	41	Intracellular pH	671
D-lactate metabolism	659	Isoenzymes	9, 21, 132, 687, 911
Delayed type hypersensitivity	309, 315, 319, 330, 370, 388, 437		

Itraconazole	765, 847	Lysosomes	729
Karyotypes	140, 533, 539, 917	Macrophage activation	261
kDNA analysis	21, 502, 549	Malaria	309
Ketoconazole	495, 695, 699, 765, 781, 847	Megasomes (lysozomes)	449, 853
		Membranes	441, 611, 619
L-leucine methyl esters	696, 741	Methotrexate	873
L-tryptophanamide	741	Microparticles	795
Leishmania		Molecular genetics	975
L. aethiopica	22, 189, 581	Molecular graphics	869
L. arabica	10, 550, 685	Niosome	724, 793, 807, 854
L. b. guyanensis	17, 496, 505, 556, 749	NMR analysis	474, 659
		Northern blotting	564, 590, 598
L. b. panamensis	154, 659, 711	Nucleic acids	555, 985
L. braziliensis	14, 97, 317, 353, 525, 529, 556, 699, 711	Nucleotidase	651, 853
		Olfactometer	235
		Oligonucleotide synthesis	590
L. chagasi	14, 911	Oxidative damage	488
L. donovani	22, 189, 259, 267, 271, 296, 327, 337, 359, 387, 409, 461, 479, 533, 539, 581, 589, 597, 635, 643, 651, 667, 699, 741, 757, 839	*Phlebotomus*	
		P. adlerius longiductus	54
		P. alexandri	14, 54
		P. andrejevi	14
		P. ariasi	27
		P. caucasicus	14
		P. grimmi	14
L. enriettii	438, 757	P. larrousius	14, 54
L. gerbilli	10	P. longicuspis	42
L. infantum	10, 21, 42, 396, 603, 774	P. mongolensis	14
		P. papatasi	12, 42, 54
L. m. pifanoi	153	P. perniciosus	24, 67, 72
L. major	10, 22, 42, 189, 271, 296, 317, 328, 345, 359, 367, 380, 417, 423, 442, 459, 550, 563, 581, 611, 685, 711, 741, 839, 873, 917	P. perphiliewi	27, 42, 67
		P. sergenti africana	55
		P. s. clydei	55
		P. s dentata	55
		P. s. squamipleuris	55
		P. salehi	55
		P. sergenti sp	14, 42
L. mexicana	97, 153, 317, 359, 380, 431, 449, 476, 496, 505, 529, 635, 699, 741	P. tobbi	29
		P388D cell line	268
		Pentamidine	847, 865
		Pentostam	473, 694, 699, 705, 785, 793, 847, 865, 880
L. mexicana amazonensis	100, 153, 296, 325, 417, 576, 729		
L. peruviana	14, 154	Peridomestic sandflys	159
L. sp. USSR	10	Permethrin	217
L. tarentolae	873	*Plasmodium* sp.	309
L. tropica	10, 42, 189, 380, 550, 581, 699, 925	PNA lectin	272, 563
		Polymorphism	534
Lambda gt 11 expression vector	597	Post Kala-Azar	387
Lanosterol	765	Premunition	379
Leishmaniasis		Pro-drug	854
Bolivia	95, 103, 109, 117, 129, 131, 137	Proline transport	670
		Promastigote uptake	441
Brazil	159	Prostaglandins (PGE2)	345
Central America	149, 353	Protein labelling	369, 566, 577, 604
Central Italy	217	Protein sequencing	612
Cyprus	207	Proteinase assay	636
India	387	Proteinases	635, 853
Kenya	189	Proton gradients	669
Mediterranean	21, 705	*Psammomys obesus*	12
Middle East	9	Pulse Field Gradient Electroph.	132, 137, 540, 555, 598, 918
Pakistan	47		
USSR	9	Recombinant DNA probes	515
Tunisia	39	Repetitive DNA	589
Zakinthos	1011	Reservoir	
Lectin agglutination	268	Apodemus sp.	1007
Lipophosphoglycan (LPG)	643	Canidae	62, 165
Liposomes	359, 417, 695, 724, 783, 793, 807, 854, 880	Citellus citellus	83
		Dog	13
		Fan-tailed sand rat	12
Low density lipoprotein (LDL)	788, 807, 854	Fox	27
Lutzomyia sp.	100, 117, 123, 161, 175, 182, 225, 235	Gerbil	12
		Ground squirrel	83
Lutzomyia sp. identification	117, 525	Meriones sp.	15, 53, 829
Lymphoblast transformation	370	M. libycus	42, 53
Lymphocyte proliferation	260, 285, 339, 388, 426	M. shawi	42
		Matres foina	1007
Lymphokines	315, 331, 335	Mus musculus	53, 1007
Lymphotoxin	312	Rat	13, 24, 53, 1007

Rattus rattus	13, 24, 53, 829, 1007
Rhombomys opimus	12, 53, 828
Tatera indica	53
Vulpes vulpes	27, 828
Reservoirs	
control	827
Feral	1007
USSR	12
Zakinthos	1007
man	62
others	63
rodents	63
Restriction enzymes	23, 550, 564
Ribosome-inactivating protein	773, 891
RNA extraction	563
Sandfly	
breeding sites	179
cuticular hydrocarbon analysis	225
DNA probes	957, 965
genetics	947
genotypic markers	965
key (Cyprus)	215
pheromones	235
systematics	947, 951
taxonomy	897 957
vectorial capacity	245
Schizodeme	29
SDS-PAGE	281, 297, 369, 425, 582, 604, 612, 653
Serology	84, 89, 295, 354
Sinefungin	479, 695, 757, 879
Site specific drug delivery	807
Skin test	432
Southern blot hybridization	503, 541, 551, 598
Squalene epoxidase	885
Sterols	495, 765, 885
Suramin	870, 879
Surface membrane	281
Surface proteases	627
Sylvatic cycle	100
Systematics	897
T-Lymphocytes	312, 315, 325, 329, 335
Thin layer chromatography	369
Total DNA probes	515
Transcription	977
Transdermal drug delivery	789
Triostam	695
Trypanothione (reductase)	470, 487
UV irradiation	677
V8 protease digestion	604
Vaccination	16, 359, 379, 835, 839
Vector control	821
Vectors	12, 13
Visceral Leishmaniasis	39, 47, 89, 409
infantile	42
reservoirs	61
African	90
Viscerotropic	24
Western blotting	284, 369, 577, 582, 598, 604
Zoonoses	57
Zoonotic Cut. Leishmaniasis	9
Zymodeme	29